Mosby's

2006 Medical Drug Reference

Allan J. Ellsworth, Pharm.D., PA-C

Professor of Pharmacy and Family Medicine
University of Washington Schools of Pharmacy and Medicine
Seattle, Washington

Daniel M. Witt, Pharm.D., FCCP

Clinical Pharmacy Services Manager
Kaiser Permanente of Colorado
Aurora, Colorado

David C. Dugdale, M.D.

Associate Professor of Medicine
University of Washington School of Medicine
Seattle, Washington

Lynn M. Oliver, M.D.

Associate Professor of Family Medicine
University of Washington School of Medicine
Seattle, Washington

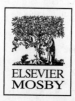

ELSEVIER
MOSBY

ELSEVIER
MOSBY

1600 John F. Kennedy Blvd.
Suite 1800
Philadelphia, PA 19103-2899

MOSBY'S 2006 MEDICAL DRUG REFERENCE   ISBN 0-323-02222-7
Copyright 2006 by Mosby, Inc.

NOTICE

Knowledge and best practice in this field are constantly changing. As new
research and experience broaden our knowledge, changes in practice,
treatment, and drug therapy may become necessary or appropriate. Readers
are advised to check the most current information provided (i) on procedures featured or (ii) by the manufacturer of each product to be administered, to verify the recommended dose or formula, the method and
duration of administration, and contraindications. It is the responsibility of
the practitioner, relying on their own experience and knowledge of the
patient, to make diagnoses, to determine dosages and the best treatment for
each individual patient, and to take all appropriate safety precautions. To
the fullest extent of the law, neither the Publisher nor the Editors assumes
any liability for any injury and/or damage to persons or property arising
out of or related to any use of the material contained in this book.

Some material was previously published.

International Standard Book Number: 0-323-02222-7

Senior Acquisitions Editor: Rolla Couchman
Developmental Editor: Amy Cannon
Publishing Services Manager: Julie Eddy
Project Manager: Joy Moore
Senior Designer: Julia Dummitt
Multimedia Producer: Adrienne Simon

Printed in the United States of America

Last digit is the print number: 9 8 7 6 5 4 3 2 1

Instructions for Use

Mosby's Medical Drug Reference was conceived in the primary care environment in response to the demands of physicians and other healthcare providers who require an up-to-date, authoritative, comprehensive, portable drug prescribing reference for use at the point of care. This compact, easily accessible manual has been created in part from the renowned and objective drug database, *Mosby's Drug Consult,* which is updated quarterly to provide timely drug information for accurate and efficient prescribing. As a standard reference, *Mosby's Drug Consult* is indispensable in its print and PDA formats; for those situations when the demands of patient care require a more portable drug prescribing guide, we proudly present *Mosby's 2006 Medical Drug Reference.*

Mosby's 2006 Medical Drug Reference is organized into several highly functional parts. The body of the book is an alphabetical listing, by generic name, of over 850 drugs in common clinical use, representing over 2800 products. An appendix of the book contains tables of comparative drug data and other information useful for choosing drug therapy. The comprehensive index provides rapid reference by listing all generic and trade names; index searches are further aided by the colored index paper. The inside front and back covers contain formulas for calculating drug dosages and useful conversion information. The comprehensive Therapeutic Index allows prescribers to locate drugs appropriate for a broad range of clinical indications.

Drug monographs in *Mosby's 2006 Medical Drug Reference* are organized uniformly as follows (when there is no information in a category applicable to a given drug, the category is deleted entirely):

Drug Name (generic)
Pronunciation (phonetic)
Trade Names
Chemical Class
Therapeutic Class
DEA Schedule (if applicable, see p. ix)
Clinical Pharmacology (including information about the mechanism of action and pharmacokinetics of the drug)
Indications and Dosages (non–FDA-approved uses marked with * if applicable)
Available Forms and Cost of Therapy (the range of average wholesale prices [AWPs] of generic brands are given)

Contraindications (if the only contraindication is hypersensitivity, this category has been deleted; hypersensitivity to the drug is always a contraindication)

Precautions

Pregnancy and Lactation (see p. ix)

Side Effects/Adverse Reactions (listed by organ system; anaphylaxis and hypersensitivity reactions are potentially possible for all drugs and have not been included routinely)

Drug Interactions, if applicable. The clinical significance of each drug interaction is derived from data presented in Hansten PD, Horn JR: Drug interactions analysis and management. Interactions are classified by potential severity as: ▲—Avoid combination, risk always outweighs benefit; ❷—Usually avoid combination, use combination only under special circumstances; or ❸—Minimize risk, take action as necessary to reduce risk of adverse outcome as a result of drug interaction. Interactions of lesser significance, either because they are minor or poorly documented, are not included. If no drug interactions are known, or if the interactions are of minimal risk, this category has been deleted.

Special Considerations (if applicable) such as patient education or monitoring or information about the place of the drug in therapy.

Every possible effort has been made to ensure the accuracy and currency of the information contained within *Mosby's 2006 Medical Drug Reference*. However, drug information is constantly changing and is subject to interpretation. The authors, editors, or publishers cannot be responsible for information that has either changed or been erroneously published or for the consequences of such errors. Decisions regarding drug therapy for a specific patient must be based on the independent judgment of the clinician.

Allan J. Ellsworth
Daniel M. Witt
David C. Dugdale
Lynn M. Oliver

ACKNOWLEDGMENTS

We are grateful for the support, stimulus, and suggestions of our colleagues in the Departments of Family Medicine, Medicine, and Pharmacy, University of Washington, Seattle, Washington, and the Medical and Pharmacy Staff of Kaiser Permanente of Colorado, Denver, Colorado. As usual, we also thank our families and friends for their continued support, patience, love, and understanding for time spent on *Mosby's 2006 Medical Drug Reference*.

Abbreviations

ABG	arterial blood gas	**CPK**	creatine phosphokinase
ac	before meals	**CrCl**	creatinine clearance
ACE	angiotensin-converting enzyme	**cre**	cream
		CRP	c-reactive protein
ACTH	adrenocorticotropic hormone	**Creat**	creatinine
AD	right ear	**CSF**	cerebrospinal fluid
ADH	antidiuretic hormone	**CV**	cardiovascular
aer	aerosol	**CVA**	cerebrovascular accident
AIDS	acquired immunodeficiency syndrome	**CVP**	central venous pressure
		CXR	chest x-ray
ALT	alanine aminotransferase, serum	**D5W**	5% dextrose in water
		DIC	disseminated intravascular coagulation
ANA	antinuclear antibody		
aPTT	activated partial thromboplastin time	**dL**	deciliter
		D_LCO	diffusing capacity of carbon monoxide
ARB	angiotensin receptor blocker		
AS	left ear	**DMARDs**	disease-modifying antirheumatic drugs
AST	aspartate aminotransferase, serum		
		DNA	deoxyribonucleic acid
AT II	angiotensin II	**DUB**	dysfunctional uterine bleeding
AU	each ear		
AUC	area under curve	**ECG**	electrocardiogram
AV	atrioventricular	**EDTA**	ethylenediaminetetraacetic acid
bid	twice a day		
BP	blood pressure	**EEG**	electroencephalogram
BUN	blood urea nitrogen	**EENT**	eye, ear, nose, throat
c-AMP	cyclic adenosine monophosphate	**elix**	elixir
		ESR	erythrocyte sedimentation rate
cap	capsule		
°C	degrees Celsius (centigrade)	**ET**	via endotracheal tube
Ca	calcium	**EXT REL**	extended release
CAD	coronary artery disease	**°F**	degrees Fahrenheit
cath	catheterize	FEV_1	forced expiratory volume in 1 second
cc	cubic centimeter		
CBC	complete blood count	**FSH**	follicle stimulating hormone
chew tab	tablet, chewable		
CHF	congestive heart failure	**g**	gram
Cl	chloride	**G6PD**	glucose-6-phosphate dehydrogenase
cm	centimeter		
CMV	cytomegalovirus	**GGTP**	gamma glutamyl transpeptidase
CNS	central nervous system		
CO_2	carbon dioxide	**GI**	gastrointestinal
COPD	chronic obstructive pulmonary disease	**gtt**	drop
		GU	genitourinary
CPAP	continuous positive airway pressure	H_2	histamine$_2$
		Hct	hematocrit

HCG	human chorionic gonadotropin	**MS**	musculoskeletal
HEME	hematologic	**Na**	sodium
Hgb	hemoglobin	**neb**	nebulizer
5-HIAA	5-hydroxyindoleacetic acid	**NPO**	nothing by mouth
HIV	human immunodeficiency virus	**NS**	normal saline
H₂O	water	**NSAID**	nonsteroidal antiinflammatory drug
HMG CoA	3-hydroxy-3-methylglutaryl coenzyme A	**O₂**	oxygen
HPA	hypothalamic-pituitary-adrenal	**OD**	right eye
hr	hour	**oint**	ointment
hs	at bedtime	**OS**	left eye
HSV	herpes simplex virus	**OTC**	over the counter
IgG	immunoglobulin G	**OU**	each eye
IL-1	interleukin-1	**oz**	ounce
IM	intramuscular	**PaCO₂**	arterial partial pressure of carbon dioxide
in	inch	**PaO₂**	arterial partial pressure of oxygen
INF	infusion	**pc**	after meals
INH	inhalation	**PCWP**	pulmonary capillary wedge pressure
inj	injection	**Pᵢ**	inorganic phosphorus
INR	international normalized ratio	**po**	by mouth
IO	intraosseous	**PO₄**	phosphate
IPPB	intermittent positive pressure breathing	**pr**	per rectum
IU	international units	**prn**	as needed
IV	intravenous	**PT**	prothrombin time
K	potassium	**PTH**	parathyroid hormone
kg	kilogram	**PTT**	partial thromboplastin time
L	liter	**PVC**	premature ventricular contraction
LA	long acting	**q**	every
lb	pound	**qAM**	every morning
LDH	lactate dehydrogenase	**qday**	every day
LDL	low density lipoprotein	**qh**	every hour
LFTs	liver function tests	**qid**	four times a day
LH	luteinizing hormone	**qod**	every other day
liq	liquid	**qPM**	every night
LMP	last menstrual period	**q2h**	every 2 hours
loz	lozenge	**q3h**	every 3 hours
lyphl	lyophilized	**q4h**	every 4 hours
m	meter	**q6h**	every 6 hours
m²	square meter	**q8h**	every 8 hours
MAOI	monoamine oxidase inhibitor	**q12h**	every 12 hours
mcg	microgram	**RAIU**	radioactive iodine uptake
MDI	metered dose inhaler	**RBC**	red blood cell count
mEq	milliequivalent	**RESP**	respiratory
mg	milligram	**RNA**	ribonucleic acid
Mg	magnesium	**sc**	subcutaneous
MI	myocardial infarction	**sl**	sublingual
min	minute	**sol**	solution
ml (mL)	milliliter	**SO₄**	sulfate
mm	millimeter	**ss**	one half
mmol	millimole	**SSRI**	selective serotonin reuptake inhibitor
mo	month	**supp**	suppository

sus rel	sustained release	**U**	unit
susp	suspension	**UA**	urinalysis
sust	sustained	**URI**	upper respiratory infection
syr	syrup	**UTI**	urinary tract infection
T₃	triiodothyronine	**UV**	ultraviolet
T₄	thyroxine	**vag**	vaginal
tab	tablet	**VMA**	vanillylmandelic acid
TCA	tricyclic antidepressant	**vol**	volume
tid	three times a day	**VS**	vital signs
tinc	tincture	**WBC**	white blood cell count
top	topical	**wk**	week
trans	transdermal	**-XL, -XR**	extended release preparations
TSH	thyroid stimulating hormone	**yr**	year
TT	thrombin time		

Federal Controlled Substances Act
Drug Enforcement Administration (DEA), U.S. Department of Justice
Schedules

SCHEDULE I: No accepted medical use in the United States and a high abuse potential. Examples include heroin, marijuana, LSD, peyote, mescaline, psilocybin, and methaqualone.

SCHEDULE II: High abuse potential with severe dependence liability, but currently accepted medical use. Examples include opium, morphine, codeine, fentanyl, hydromorphone, methadone, meperidine, oxycodone, oxymorphone, cocaine, amphetamine, methamphetamine, phenmetrazine, methylphenidate, phencyclidine, amobarbital, pentobarbital, and secobarbital.

SCHEDULE III: Lesser abuse potential with moderate dependence liability, but currently accepted medical use. Examples include compounds containing limited quantities of certain opiates and other sedative-hypnotic drugs. Examples include codeine and hydrocodone with aspirin or acetaminophen, barbiturates, glutethimide, methyprylon, nalorphine, benzphetamine, chlorphentermine, clortermine, phendimetrazine, and paregoric; suppository dosage form containing amobarbital, secobarbital, or pentobarbital. Anabolic steroids are also included here.

SCHEDULE IV: Low abuse potential. Examples include barbital, phenobarbital, mephobarbital, chloral hydrate, ethchlorvynol, ethinamate, meprobamate, paraldehyde, methohexital, fenfluramine, diethylpropion, phentermine, chlordiazepoxide, diazepam, oxazepam, clorazepate, flurazepam, clonazepam, prazepam, lorazepam, alprazolam, halazepam, temazepam, triazolam, propoxyphene, pentazocine, zaleplon, and zolpidem.

SCHEDULE V: Low abuse potential. These products contain limited quantities of certain opiate drugs generally for antitussive or antidiarrheal purposes. The over-the-counter cough medicines with codeine are classified schedule V.

FDA Pregnancy Categories

A: Adequate studies in pregnant women have not demonstrated a risk to the fetus in the first trimester of pregnancy, and there is no evidence of risk in later trimesters.

B: Animal studies have not demonstrated a risk to the fetus, but there are no adequate studies in pregnant women; **OR** animal studies have shown an adverse effect, but adequate studies in pregnant women have not demonstrated a risk to the fetus during the first trimester of pregnancy, and there is no evidence of risk in later trimesters.

C: Animal studies have shown an adverse effect on the fetus, but there are no adequate studies in humans; **OR** there are no animal reproduction studies and no adequate studies in humans.

D: There is evidence of human fetal risk, but the potential benefits from the use of the drug in pregnant women may be acceptable despite its potential risks.

X: Studies in animals or humans demonstrate fetal abnormalities or adverse reaction; reports indicate evidence of fetal risk. The risk of use in a pregnant woman clearly outweighs any possible benefit.

Contents

abacavir
(ah-bah'cah-veer)
Rx: Ziagen
Combinations
Rx: with lamivudine (Epzicom); with zidovudine and lamivudine (Trizivir)
Chemical Class: Nucleoside analog
Therapeutic Class: Antiretroviral

CLINICAL PHARMACOLOGY
Mechanism of Action: An antiretroviral that inhibits the activity of HIV-1 reverse transcriptase by competing with the natural substrate deoxyguanosine-5'-triphosphate (dGTP) and by its incorporation into viral DNA. *Therapeutic Effect:* Inhibits viral DNA growth.

Pharmacokinetics
Rapidly and extensively absorbed after PO administration. Protein binding: 50%. Widely distributed, including to CSF and erythrocytes. Metabolized in the liver to inactive metabolites. Primarily excreted in urine. Unknown if removed by hemodialysis. **Half-life:** 1.5 hrs.

INDICATIONS AND DOSAGES
HIV Infection (in combination with other antiretrovirals)
PO
Adults. 300 mg twice a day.
Children (3 mo-16 yr) 8 mg/kg twice a day. Maximum: 300 mg twice a day.

Dosage in liver impairment
Mild dysfunction: 200 mg 2 times/day.
Moderate to severe dysfunction: Not recommended.

S **AVAILABLE FORMS/COST**
• Liq—Oral: 20 mg/ml, 240 ml: **$111.64**
• Tab—Oral: 300 mg, 60's: **$424.69**

CONTRAINDICATIONS: Hypersensitivity to abacavir or its components

PREGNANCY AND LACTATION: Pregnancy category C; breast-feeding not recommended due to drug secretion and potential for HIV transmission

SIDE EFFECTS
Adult
Frequent
Nausea (47%), nausea with vomiting (16%), diarrhea (12%), decreased appetite (11%)
Occasional
Insomnia (7%)
Children
Frequent
Nausea with vomiting (39%), fever (19%), headache, diarrhea (16%), rash (11%)
Occasional
Decreased appetite (9%)

SERIOUS REACTIONS
• A hypersensitivity reaction may be life-threatening. Signs and symptoms include fever, rash, fatigue, intractable nausea and vomiting, severe diarrhea, abdominal pain, cough, pharyngitis, and dyspnea.
• Life-threatening hypotension may occur.
• Lactic acidosis and severe hepatomegaly may occur.

INTERACTIONS
Drugs
3 *Amprenavir:* Mild increase in amprenavir plasma level with co-administration

SPECIAL CONSIDERATIONS
PATIENT/FAMILY EDUCATION
• May administer without regard for food
• If you miss a dose: take the missed dose as soon as you remember, then go back to your normal dosing schedule; skip the missed dose if it is time for your next dose; do not take 2 doses at the same time

MONITORING PARAMETERS
• CBC, metabolic panel, CD4 lymphocyte count, HIV RNA level

---

abciximab
(ab-six'ih-mab)
Rx: ReoPro
Chemical Class: Glycoprotein (GP) IIb/IIIa inhibitor
Therapeutic Class: Antiplatelet agent

CLINICAL PHARMACOLOGY
Mechanism of Action: A glycoprotein IIb/IIIa receptor inhibitor that rapidly inhibs platelet aggregation by preventing the binding of fibrinogen to GP IIb/IIIa receptor sites on platelets. *Therapeutic Effect:* Prevents closure of treated coronary arteries. Prevents acute cardiac ischemic complications.

Pharmacokinetics
Rapidly cleared from plasma. Initial-phase half-life is less than 10 min; second-phase half-life is 30 min. Platelet function generally returns within 48 hr.

INDICATIONS AND DOSAGES
Percutaneous coronary intervention (PCI)
IV bolus
Adults. 0.25 mg/kg 10–60 min before angioplasty or atherectomy, then 12-hr IV infusion of 0.125 mcg/kg/min. Maximum: 10 mcg/min.

PCI (unstable angina)
IV bolus
Adults. 0.25 mg/kg, followed by 18- to 24-hr infusion of 10 mcg/min, ending 1 hr after procedure.

S AVAILABLE FORMS/COST
• Sol, Inj-IV: 2 mg/ml, 5 ml: **$579.38**
CONTRAINDICATIONS: Active internal bleeding, arteriovenous malformation or aneurysm, cerebrovascular accident (CVA) with residual neurologic defect, history of CVA (within the past 2 years) or oral anticoagulant use within the past 7 days unless PT is less than $1.2 \times$ control, history of vasculitis, intracranial neoplasm, prior IV dextran use before or during PTCA, recent surgery or trauma (within the past 6 weeks), recent (within the past 6 weeks or less) GI or GU bleeding, thrombocytopenia (less than 100,000 cells/mcl), and severe uncontrolled hypertension

PREGNANCY AND LACTATION: Pregnancy category C; excretion into breast milk unknown, use caution in nursing mothers

SIDE EFFECTS
Frequent
Nausea (16%), hypotension (12%)
Occasional (9%)
Vomiting
Rare (3%)
Bradycardia, confusion, dizziness, pain, peripheral edema, urinary tract infection

SERIOUS REACTIONS
• Major bleeding complications may occur. If complications occur, stop the infusion immediately.
• Hypersensitivity reaction may occur.
• Atrial fibrillation or flutter, pulmonary edema, and complete atrioventricular block occur occasionally.

INTERACTIONS
Drugs
3 *Antithrombotics (aspirin, heparin, warfarin, ticlopidine, clopidogrel):* Increased risk of bleeding

SPECIAL CONSIDERATIONS
• Fab fragment of the chimeric human-murine monoclonal antibody 7E3
• Intended to be used with aspirin and heparin

- Discontinue if bleeding occurs that is not controlled by compression
- Discontinue if PTCA fails
- Eptifibitide, tirofiban, and abciximab can all decrease the incidence of cardiac events associated with acute coronary syndromes; direct comparisons are needed to establish which, if any, is superior; for angioplasty, until more data become available, abciximab appears to be the drug of choice

MONITORING PARAMETERS
- Baseline platelet count, prothrombin time, aPTT; during INF closely monitor platelet count and aPTT (heparin therapy)

---

acamprosate
(ah-cam′pro-sate)
Rx: Campral
Chemical Class: Amino acid derivative
Therapeutic Class: Alcohol deterrent

CLINICAL PHARMACOLOGY
Mechanism of Action: An alcohol abuse deterrent that appears to interact with glutamate and gamma-aminobutyric acid neurotransmitter systems centrally, restoring their balance. *Therapeutic Effect:* Reduces alcohol dependence.
Pharmacokinetics
Slowly absorbed from the GI tract. Steady-state plasma concentrations are reached within 5 days. Does not undergo metabolism. Excreted in urine. **Half-life:** 20-33 hr.

INDICATIONS AND DOSAGES
Maintenance of alcohol abstinence in alcohol-dependent patients who are abstinent at initiation of treatment.
PO
Adults, Elderly: Two tablets 3 times a day.

Dosage in renal impairment
For patients with creatinine clearance of 30-49 ml/min, dosage is decreased to one tablet 3 times a day.

CONTRAINDICATIONS: Severe renal impairment (creatinine clearance of 30 ml/min or less)

PREGNANCY AND LACTATION: Pregnancy category C; teratogenicity has been demonstrated in animals; excreted in the milk of lactating rats; excretion into human milk is unknown; use caution in nursing mothers

SIDE EFFECTS
Frequent (17%)
Diarrhea
Occasional (6%-4%)
Insomnia, asthenia, fatigue, anxiety, flatulence, nausea, depression, pruritus
Rare (3%-1%)
Dizziness, anorexia, paresthesia, diaphoresis, dry mouth

SERIOUS REACTIONS
- None known.

SPECIAL CONSIDERATIONS
- Does not cause disulfiram-like reaction with ingestion of alcohol
- Higher doses appear to be more effective for maintaining abstinence
- The optimal time to initiate therapy has not been identified

PATIENT/FAMILY EDUCATION
- Use caution operating hazardous machinery, including automobiles, until there is reasonable certainty that acamprosate will not affect ability to engage in such activities
- Continue use even in the event of a relapse and discuss any renewed drinking with prescriber
- To be used as part of a treatment program that includes psychosocial support

MONITORING PARAMETERS
- Maintenance of alcohol abstinence

acarbose

(a-car′bose)

Rx: Precose

Chemical Class: α-amylase inhibitor; α-glucosidase inhibitor

Therapeutic Class: Antidiabetic; hypoglycemic

CLINICAL PHARMACOLOGY

Mechanism of Action: An alpha glucosidase inhibitor that delays glucose absorption and digestion of carbohydrates, resulting in a smaller rise in blood glucose concentration after meals. *Therapeutic Effect:* Lowers postprandial hyperglycemia.

INDICATIONS AND DOSAGES

Diabetes mellitus

PO

Adults, Elderly. Initially, 25 mg 3 times a day with first bite of each main meal. Increase at 4- to 8-wk intervals. Maximum: For patients weighing more than 60 kg, 100 mg 3 times a day; for patients weighing 60 kg or less, 50 mg 3 times a day.

[$] **AVAILABLE FORMS/COST**

• Tab—Oral: 25 mg, 100's: **$67.35**; 50 mg, 100's: **$72.54**; 100 mg, 100's: **$86.86**

CONTRAINDICATIONS: Chronic intestinal diseases associated with marked disorders of digestion or absorption, cirrhosis, colonic ulceration, conditions that may deteriorate as a result of increased gas formation in the intestine, diabetic ketoacidosis, hypersensitivity to acarbose, inflammatory bowel disease, partial intestinal obstruction or predisposition to intestinal obstruction, significant renal dysfunction (serum creatinine level greater than 2 mg/dl)

PREGNANCY AND LACTATION: Pregnancy category B; excreted into breast milk in rats; no human data available

SIDE EFFECTS

Side effects diminish in frequency and intensity over time.

Frequent

Transient GI disturbances: flatulence (77%), diarrhea (33%), abdominal pain (21%)

SERIOUS REACTIONS

• None known.

INTERACTIONS

Drugs

[3] *Charcoal, digestive enzyme preparations:* Reduced effects of acarbose

[3] *Cholestyramine:* Enhanced side effects of acarbose

[3] *Neomycin:* Enhanced reduction of postprandial blood glucose and exacerbation of adverse effects

[3] *Metformin:* Decreased metformin peak serum and AUC concentrations

SPECIAL CONSIDERATIONS

• Does not cause hypoglycemia

• Reduces HbAlc 0.5-1%

MONITORING PARAMETERS

• Blood glucose; HbAlc 3-6 mo

• Consider ALT/AST during first yr

PATIENT/FAMILY EDUCATION

• Take glucose rather than complex carbohydrates to abort hypoglycemic episodes

• Decrease adverse GI effects by reducing dietary starch content

acebutolol
(a-se-byoo'toe-lole)
Rx: Sectral
Chemical Class: β₁-adrenergic blocker, cardioselective
Therapeutic Class: Antianginal; antihypertensive

CLINICAL PHARMACOLOGY
Mechanism of Action: A beta₁-adrenergic blocker that competitively blocks beta₁-adrenergic receptors in cardiac tissue Reduces the rate of spontaneous firing of the sinus pacemaker and delays AV conduction. *Therapeutic Effect:* Slows heart rate, decreases cardiac output, decreases BP, and exhibits antiarrhythmic activity.

Pharmacokinetics

Route	Onset	Peak	Duration
PO (hypotensive)	1–1.5 hr	2–8 hr	24 hr
PO (antiarrhythmic)	1 hr	4–6 hr	10 hr

Well absorbed from the GI tract. Protein binding: 26%. Undergoes extensive first-pass liver metabolism to active metabolite. Eliminated via bile, secreted into GI tract via intestine, and excreted in urine. Removed by hemodialysis. **Half-life:** 3–4 hr; metabolite, 8–13 hr.

INDICATIONS AND DOSAGES
Mild to moderate hypertension
PO
• *Adults* . Initially, 400 mg/day in 12 divided doses. Range: Up to 1,200 mg/day in 2 divided doses. Maintenance: 400–800 mg/day.
Ventricular arrhythmias
PO
Adults. Initially, 200 mg q12h. Increase gradually to 600–1,200 mg/day in 2 divided doses.

Elderly. Initially, 200–400 mg/day. Maximum: 800 mg/day.
Dosage in renal impairment
Dosage is modified based on creatinine clearance.

Creatinine Clearance	% of Usual Dosage
less than 50 ml/min	50
less than 25 ml/min	25

AVAILABLE FORMS/COST
• Cap, Gel—Oral: 200 mg, 100's: **$29.73-$252.38**; 400 mg, 100's: **$44.29-$279.63**

UNLABELED USES: Treatment of anxiety, chronic angina pectoris, hypertrophic cardiomyopathy, MI, pheochromocytoma, syndrome of mitral valve prolapse, thyrotoxicosis, tremors

CONTRAINDICATIONS: Cardiogenic shock, heart block greater than first degree, overt heart failure, severe bradycardia

PREGNANCY AND LACTATION: Pregnancy category D; frequently used in the third trimester for treatment of hypertension; long-term use associated with intrauterine growth retardation; excreted into breast milk

SIDE EFFECTS
Frequent
Hypotension manifested as dizziness, nausea, diaphoresis, headache, cold extremities, fatigue, constipation, or diarrhea
Occasional
Insomnia, urinary frequency, impotence or decreased libido
Rare
Rash, arthralgia, myalgia, confusion (especially in the elderly), altered taste

SERIOUS REACTIONS
• Overdose may produce profound bradycardia and hypotension.

- Abrupt withdrawal may result in diaphoresis, palpitations, headache, and tremors.
- Acebutolol administration may precipitate CHF or MI in patients with heart disease; thyroid storm in those with thyrotoxicosis; or peripheral ischemia in those with existing peripheral vascular disease.
- Hypoglycemia may occur in patients with previously controlled diabetes.
- Signs of thrombocytopenia, such as unusual bleeding or bruising, occur rarely.

INTERACTIONS

Drugs

■ *α₁-adrenergic blockers:* Potential enhanced first dose response (marked initial drop in blood pressure, particularly on standing [especially prazosin])

■ *Amiodarone:* Bradycardia/ventricular dysrhythmia

■ *Anesthetics, local:* Enhanced sympathomimetic effects, hypertension due to unopposed α-receptor stimulation

■ *Antacids:* May reduce β-blocker absorption

■ *Antidiabetics:* Delayed recovery from hypoglycemia, hyperglycemia, attenuated tachycardia during hypoglycemia, hypertension during hypoglycemia

■ *Clonidine:* Rebound hypertension; discontinue β-blocker prior to clonidine withdrawl

■ *Digoxin:* Additive prolongation of atrioventricular (AV) conduction time

■ *Dihydropyridine calcium channel blockers:* Severe hypotension or impaired cardiac performance; most prevalent with impaired left ventricular function, cardiac arrhythmias, or aortic stenosis

■ *Dipyridamole:* Bradycardia

■ *Disopyramide:* Additive decreases in cardiac output

■ *Epinephrine:* Enhanced pressor response resulting in hypertension

■ *Neostigmine:* Bradycardia

■ *Neuroleptics:* Increased serum levels of both resulting in accentuated pharmacologic response to both drugs

■ *NSAIDs:* Reduced hypotensive effects

■ *Phenylephrine:* Acute hypertensive episodes

■ *Tacrine:* Additive bradycardia

❷ *Theophylline:* Antagonist pharmacodynamics

SPECIAL CONSIDERATIONS

- Fewer CNS and bronchospastic effects than other β-blockers

MONITORING PARAMETERS

- Heart rate, blood pressure

PATIENT/FAMILY EDUCATION

- Do not discontinue abruptly; may require taper; rapid withdrawal may produce rebound hypertension or angina

acetaminophen
(ah-seet'ah-min-oh-fen)

OTC: Acephen, Apacet, Arthritis Pain Formula, Aspirin Free Pain Relief, Feverall, Genapap, Liquiprin, Neopap, Panadol, Tapanol Tempra, Tylenol
Combinations

Rx: with butalbital (Phrenilin); with butalbital and caffeine (Fioricet, Esgic, Isocet); with butalbital, caffeine and codeine (Amaphen, Fioricet w/codeine); with codeine (Tylenol, Phenaphen No. 2,3,4); with dichloralphenazone and isometheptene (Midrin, Midchlor); with hydrocodone (Vicodin, Lorcet, Lortab); with oxycodone (Percocet, Roxicet, Tylox); with pentazocine (Talacen); with propoxyphene (Wygesic, Darvocet-N)

OTC: with pamabrom + pyrilamine (Midol PMS, Pamprin); with antihistamine and decongestant (Actifed Plus, Drixoral Cold & Flu, Benadryl Sinus, Sine-Off, Sinarest); with decongestant, antihistamine, dextromethorphan (Nyquil)

Chemical Class: Para-aminophenol derivative
Therapeutic Class: Antipyretic; nonnarcotic analgesic

CLINICAL PHARMACOLOGY
Mechanism of Action: A central analgesic whose exact mechanism is unknown, but appears to inhibit prostaglandin synthesis in the central nervous system (CNS) and, to a lesser extent, block pain impulses through peripheral action. Acetaminophen acts centrally on hypothalamic heat-regulating center, producing peripheral vasodilation (heat loss, skin erythema, sweating). *Therapeutic Effect:* Results in antipyresis. Produces analgesic effect. Results in antipyresis.

Pharmacokinetics

Route	Onset	Peak	Duration
PO	15-30 mins	1-1.5 hrs	4-6 hrs

Rapidly, completely absorbed from gastrointestinal (GI) tract; rectal absorption variable. Protein binding: 20%-50%. Widely distributed to most body tissues. Metabolized in liver; excreted in urine. Removed by hemodialysis. **Half-life:** 1-4 hrs (half-life is increased in those with liver disease, elderly, neonates; decreased in children).

INDICATIONS AND DOSAGES
Analgesia and antipyresis
PO
Adults, Elderly. 325-650 mg q4-6h or 1 g 3-4 times/day. Maximum: 4 g/day.
Children. 10-15 mg/kg/dose q4-6h as needed. Maximum: 5 doses/24 hrs.
Neonates. 10-15 mg/kg/dose q6-8h as needed.
Rectal
Adults. 650 mg q4-6h. Maximum: 6 doses/24 hrs.
Children. 10-20 mg/kg/dose q4-6h as needed.
Neonates. 10-15 mg/kg/dose q6-8h as needed.

Dosage in renal impairment

Creatinine Clearance	Frequency
10-50 ml/min	q6h
less than 10 ml/min	q8h

$ AVAILABLE FORMS/COST

• Cap—Oral: 500 mg, 100's: **$2.80-$6.99**

• Drops—Oral: 80 mg/0.8 ml, 15 ml: **$1.25-$5.99**

• Elixir—Oral: 160 mg/5 ml, 120 ml: **$1.21-$11.29**; 500 mg/15 ml, 240 ml: **$3.24-$12.77**

• Supp—Rect: 80 mg, 6's: **$4.81-$5.25**; 120 mg, 12's: **$3.36-$10.54**; 325 mg, 12's: **$3.80-$9.48**; 650 mg, 12's: **$3.41-$11.60**

• Tab—Oral: 325 mg, 100's: **$0.70-$10.88**; 500 mg, 100's: **$1.13-$26.47**

• Tab, Sus Action-Oral: 650 mg, 100's: **$9.58**

• Tab, Chewable—Oral: 80 mg, 30's: **$0.84-$3.69**; 160 mg, 24's: **$2.64-$4.28**

CONTRAINDICATIONS: Active alcoholism, liver disease, or viral hepatitis, all of which increase the risk of hepatotoxicity

PREGNANCY AND LACTATION: Pregnancy category B; low concentrations in breast milk (1%-2% of maternal dose); compatible with breast-feeding

SIDE EFFECTS

Rare

Hypersensitivity reaction

SERIOUS REACTIONS

• Acetaminophen toxicity is the primary serious reaction.

• Early signs and symptoms of acetaminophen toxicity include anorexia, nausea, diaphoresis, and generalized weakness within the first 12 to 24 hrs.

• Later signs of acetaminophen toxicity include vomiting, right upper quadrant tenderness, and elevated liver function tests within 48 to 72 hrs after ingestion.

• The antidote to acetaminophen toxicity is acetylcysteine.

INTERACTIONS

Drugs

3 *Anticoagulants:* Enhanced hypoprothrombinemic response

3 *Anticonvulsants, Barbiturates, Rifabutin, Rifampin:* Enhanced hepatoxic potential in overdose

3 *Cholestyramine/Colestipol:* Reduced acetaminophen levels and response

3 *Ethanol:* Increased hepatotoxicity in chronic, excessive alcohol ingestion

3 *Isoniazid:* Increased acetaminophen levels & hepatotoxicity

Labs

• *False decrease:* Amylase

• *False increase:* Urine 5-HIAA

• *Interference:* Cannot assay ticarillin levels

SPECIAL CONSIDERATIONS

PATIENT/FAMILY EDUCATION

• Many OTC drugs contain acetaminophen; additive dosage may exceed 4 g/day maximum and increase risk of hepatotoxicity

---

acetazolamide

(ah-seat-ah-zole-ah-myd)

Rx: AK-Zol, Diamox, Storzolamide

Chemical Class: Carbonic anhydrase inhibitor; sulfonamide derivative

Therapeutic Class: Anticonvulsant; antiglaucoma agent; diuretic

CLINICAL PHARMACOLOGY

Mechanism of Action: A carbonic anhydrase inhibitor that reduces formation of hydrogen and bicarbonate ions from carbon dioxide and water by inhibiting, in proximal renal tubule, the enzyme carbonic anhydrase, thereby promoting renal excretion of sodium, potassium, bicarbonate, water. Ocular: Reduces rate of aqueous humor formation, lowers intraocular pressure. *Therapeutic Effect:* Produces anticonvulsant activity.

Pharmacokinetics

Rapidly absorbed. Protein binding: 95%. Widely distributed throughout body tisses including erythrocytes, kidneys, and blood brain barrier. Not metabolized. Excreted in unchanged in urine. Removed by hemodialysis. **Half-life:** 2.4-5.8 hrs.

INDICATIONS AND DOSAGES

Glaucoma

PO

Adults. 250 mg 1-4 times/day. Extended-Release: 500 mg 1-2 times/day usually given in morning and evening.

Secondary glaucoma, preop treatment of acute congestive glaucoma

PO/IV

Adults. 250 mg q4h, 250 mg q12h; or 500 mg, then 125-250 mg q4h.

PO

Children. 10-15 mg/kg/day in divided doses.

IV

Children. 5-10 mg/kg q6h.

Edema

IV

Adults. 25-375 mg once daily.

Children. 5 mg/kg or 150 mg/m2 once daily.

Epilepsy

Oral

Adults, Children. 375-1,000 mg/day in 1-4 divided doses.

Acute mountain sickness

PO

Adults. 500-1,000 mg/day in divided doses. If possible, begin 24-48 hrs before ascent; continue at least 48 hrs at high altitude.

Usual elderly dosage

PO

Initially, 250 mg 2 times/day; use lowest effective dose.

Dosage in renal impairment

Creatinine Clearance	Dosage Interval
10- 50 ml/min	q12h
less than 10 ml/min	avoid use

$ AVAILABLE FORMS/COST

• Cap, Gel, Sus Action—Oral: 500 mg, 100's: **$161.23**
• Powder, Inj-IV: 500 mg, 1 vial: **$22.50**
• Tab-Oral: 125 mg, 100's: **$12.50-$21.10**; 250 mg, 100's: **$4.00-$43.60**

UNLABELED USES: Urine alkalinization, respiratory stimulant in COPD

CONTRAINDICATIONS: Severe renal disease, adrenal insufficiency, hypochloremic acidosis, hypersensitivity to acetazolamide, to any component of the formulation, or to sulfonamides.

PREGNANCY AND LACTATION: Pregnancy category C; premature delivery and congenital anomalies in humans; teratogenic (defects of the limbs) in mice, rats, hamsters, and rabbits; not recommended for nursing mothers

SIDE EFFECTS

Frequent

Unusually tired/weak, diarrhea, increased urination/frequency, decreased appetite/weight, altered taste (metallic), nausea, vomiting, numbness in extremities, lips, mouth

Occasional

Depression, drowsiness

Rare

Headache, photosensitivity, confusion, tinnitus, severe muscle weakness, loss of taste

SERIOUS REACTIONS

• Long-term therapy may result in acidotic state.

• Nephrotoxicity/hepatotoxicity occurs occasionally, manifested as dark urine/stools, pain in lower back, jaundice, dysuria, crystalluria, renal colic/calculi.

• Bone marrow depression may be manifested as aplastic anemia, thrombocytopenia, thrombocytopenic purpura, leukopenia, agranulocytosis, hemolytic anemia.

INTERACTIONS
Drugs
⬛ *Cyclosporine:* Increased trough cyclosporine levels with potential for neurotoxicity and nephropathy

⬛ *Flecainide, quinidine:* Alkalinization of urine increases quinidine serum levels

⬛ *Methenamine compounds:* Alkalinization of urine decreases antibacterial effects

⬛ *Phenytoin:* Increased risk of osteomalacia

⬛ *Primidone:* Decreased primidone levels

② *Salicylates:* Increased serum levels of acetazolamide—CNS toxicity

Labs
• *False increase:* 17 hydroxysteroid

SPECIAL CONSIDERATIONS
PATIENT/FAMILY EDUCATION
• Carbonated beverages taste flat
• If GI symptoms occur, take with food

MONITORING PARAMETERS
• Serum electrolytes, creatinine

---

acetic acid
(a-cee′-tik as′-id)

Rx: Acetasol, Burow's Otic, VoSol
Combinations
  Rx: with hydrocortisone (VoSol HC Otic, AA HC Otic, Acetasol HC) with oxyquinolone (Aci-Jel)
Chemical Class: Organic acid
Therapeutic Class: Antibacterial; antifungal

CLINICAL PHARMACOLOGY
Mechanism of Action: The mechanism by which acetic acid exerts it antibacterial and antifungal actions is unknown. *Therapeutic effect:* Antibacterial and antifungal.

Pharmacokinetics
Unknown.

INDICATIONS AND DOSAGES
Superficial infections of the external auditory canal
Topical

Adults, Elderly, Children. Carefully remove all cerumen and debris to allow acetic acid to contact infected surfaces directly. To promote continuous contact, insert a wick saturated with acetic acid into the ear canal; the wick may also be saturated after insertion. Instruct the patient to keep the wick in for at least 24 hours and to keep it moist by adding 3-5 drops of acetic acid every 4-6 hours. The wick may be removed after 24 hours but the patient should continue to instill 5 drops of acetic acid 3 or 4 times daily thereafter, for as long as indicated. Dosing should be tapered gradually after apparent response to avoid relapse.

Ⓢ **AVAILABLE FORMS/COST**
• Gel—Vaginal: 0.92%, 85 g: **$25.02-$34.90**

A

• Otic drops: 2%, 15 ml: **$1.73-$31.00**
• Sol, Bladder Irrigation: 0.25%, 1000 ml: **$2.51-$3.09**
CONTRAINDICATIONS: Hypersensitivity to acetic acid or any of the ingredients. Perforated tympanic membrane is frequently considered a contraindication to the use of any medication in the external ear canal.
PREGNANCY AND LACTATION: Pregnancy category C when combined with oxyquinoline
SIDE EFFECTS
Occasional
Stinging or burning
Rare
Local irritation, superinfection
SERIOUS REACTIONS
• Super infection with prolonged use
Alert
Discontinue promptly it sensitization or irritation occurs.

---

acetylcysteine
(a-see-til-sis'tay-een)
Rx: Acetadote, Mucomyst, Mucosil
Chemical Class: Amino acid, L-cysteine
Therapeutic Class: Antidote, acetaminophen; mucolytic

CLINICAL PHARMACOLOGY
Mechanism of Action: An intratracheal respiratory inhalant that splits the linkage of mucoproteins, reducing the viscosity of pulmonary secretions. *Therapeutic Effect:* Facilitates the removal of pulmonary secretions by coughing, postural drainage, mechanical means. Protects against acetaminophen overdose–induced hepatotoxicity.

INDICATIONS AND DOSAGES
Adjunctive treatment of viscid mucus secretions from chronic bronchopulmonary disease and for pulmonary complications of cystic fibrosis
Nebulization
Adults, Elderly, Children. 3–5 ml (20% solution) 3–4 times a day or 6–10 ml (10% solution) 3–4 times a day. Range: 1–10 ml (20% solution) q2–6h or 2–20 ml (10% solution) q2–6h.
Infants. 1–2 ml (20%) or 2–4 ml (10%) 3–4 times a day.
Treatment of viscid mucus secretions in patients with a tracheostomy
Intratracheal
Adults, Children. 1–2 ml of 10% or 20% solution instilled into tracheostomy q1–4h.
Acetaminophen overdose
PO (Oral solution 5%)
Adults, Elderly, Children. Loading dose of 140 mg/kg, followed in 4 hr by maintenance dose of 70 mg/kg q4h for 17 additional doses (unless acetaminophen assay reveals nontoxic level).
IV
Adults, Elderly, Children. 150 mg/kg infused over 15 minutes, then 50 mg/kg infused over 4 hr, then 100 mg/kg infused over 16 hr. See administration and handling. Repeat dose if emesis occurs within 1 hr of administration. Continue until all doses are given, even if acetaminophen plasma level drops below toxic range.
Prevention of renal damage from dyes used during certain diagnostic tests
PO (Oral solution 5%)
Adults, Elderly. 600 mg twice a day for 4 doses starting the day before the procedure.

§ **AVAILABLE FORMS/COST**
• Sol, INH—Oral: 10%, 4 ml, 10 ml, 30 ml: **$9.12-$35.00**/30 ml
• Sol, INH—Oral: 20%, 4 ml, 10 ml, 30 ml: **$7.81-$42.81**/30 ml
UNLABELED USES: Prevention of renal damage from dyes given during certain diagnostic tests (such as CT scans)
CONTRAINDICATIONS: None known.
PREGNANCY AND LACTATION: Pregnancy category B
SIDE EFFECTS
Frequent
Inhalation: Stickiness on face, transient unpleasant odor
Occasional
Inhalation: Increased bronchial secretions, throat irritation, nausea, vomiting, rhinorrhea
Rare
Inhalation: Rash
Oral: Facial edema, bronchospasm, wheezing
SERIOUS REACTIONS
• Large doses may produce severe nausea and vomiting.
INTERACTIONS
• Avoid contact with iron, copper, rubber
SPECIAL CONSIDERATIONS
• Disagreeable odor may be noted
• Solution in opened bottle may change color; of no significance

---

acitretin
(a-si-tre'tin)
Rx: Soriatane
Chemical Class: Retinoid anolog
Therapeutic Class: Antipsoriatic

CLINICAL PHARMACOLOGY
Mechanism of Action: A second-generation retinoid that adjusts factors influencing epidermal proliferation, RNA/DNA synthesis, controls glycoprotein, and governs immune response. *Therapeutic Effect:* Regulates keratinocyte growth and differentiation.
Pharmacokinetics
Well absorbed from the gastrointestinal (GI) tract. Food increases rate of absorption. Protein binding: greater than 99%. Metabolized in liver. Excreted in bile and urine. Not removed by hemodialysis. **Half-life:** 49 hrs.
INDICATIONS AND DOSAGES
Psoriasis
PO
Adults, Elderly. 25-50 mg/day as a single dose with main meal. May increase to 75 mg/day if necessary and dose tolerated. Maintenance: 25-50 mg/day after the initial response is noted. Continue until lesions have resolved.
§ **AVAILABLE FORMS/COST**
• Cap—Oral: 10 mg, 30's: **$354.16**; 25 mg, 30's: **$465.93**
UNLABELED USES: Treatment of Darier's disease, palmoplantar pustulosis, lichen planus; children with lameliar ichthyosis, nonbullous and bullous ichthyosiform erythroderma, Sjogren-Larsson syndrome
CONTRAINDICATIONS: Pregnancy or those who intend to become pregnant within 3 years fol-

lowing discontinuation of therapy, severely impaired liver or kidney function, chronic abnormal elevated lipid levels, concomitant use of methotrexate or tetracyclines, ingestion of alcohol (in females of reproductive potential), hypersensitivity to acitretin, etretinate or other retinoids, sensitivity to parabenz (used as preservative in gelatin capsule)

PREGNANCY AND LACTATION:
Pregnancy category X; breast milk excretion unknown

SIDE EFFECTS

Frequent

Lip inflammation, alopecia, skin peeling, shakiness, dry eyes, rash, hyperesthesia, paresthesia, sticky skin, dry mouth, epistaxis, dryness/thickening of conjunctiva

Occasional

Eye irritation, brow and lash loss, sweating, chills, sensation of cold, flushing, edema, blurred vision, diarrhea, nausea, thirst

SERIOUS REACTIONS

• Benign intracranial hypertension (pseudotumor cerebri) occurs rarely.

INTERACTIONS

Drugs

❷ *Methotrexate:* Increased potential for hepatotoxicity

❷ *Ethanol:* Drastically increases the $t_{1/2}$ of acitretin metabolite, etretinate

❷ *Progestin only contraceptives:* Decreased contraceptive effects

SPECIAL CONSIDERATIONS

PATIENT/FAMILY EDUCATION

• Avoid progestin only contraceptives

MONITORING PARAMETERS

• Transaminase levels monthly for first 6 mo then every 3 mo
• Lipid levels monthly for first 4 mo then every 2-3 mo

• Yearly radiographs to monitor for drug-induced vertebral abnormalities
• In children, measure PO_4, Ca levels in blood and urine and vitamin D and PTH levels every 6 mo

---

acyclovir

(ay-sye′kloe-ver)

Rx: Zovirax
Chemical Class: Acyclic purine nucleoside analog
Therapeutic Class: Antiviral

CLINICAL PHARMACOLOGY

Mechanism of Action: A synthetic nucleoside that converts to acyclovir triphosphate, becoming part of the DNA chain. *Therapeutic Effect:* Interferes with DNA synthesis and viral replication. Virustatic.

Pharmacokinetics

Poorly absorbed from the GI tract; minimal absorption following topical application. Protein binding: 9%-36%. Widely distributed. Partially metabolized in liver. Excreted primarily in urine. Removed by hemodialysis. **Half-life:** 2.5 hr (increased in impaired renal function).

INDICATIONS AND DOSAGES

Genital herpes (initial episode)

IV

Adults, Elderly, Children 12 yr and older. 5 mg/kg q8h for 5 days.

PO

Adults, Elderly, Children 12 yr and older. 200 mg q4h 5 times a day.

Genital herpes (recurrent)

Less than 6 episodes per year:

PO

Adults, Elderly, Children 12 yr and older. 200 mg q4h 5 times a day for 5 days.

6 episodes or more per year:

PO

Adults, Elderly, Children 12 yr and older. 400 mg 2 times a day or 200 mg 3-5 times a day for up to 12 months.

Herpes simplex mucocutaneous
IV
Adults, Elderly, Children 12 yr and older. 5 mg/kg/dose q8h for 7 days.
Children younger than 12 yr. 10 mg/kg q8h for 7 days.

Herpes simplex neonatal
IV
Children younger than 4 mo. 10 mg/kg q8h for 10 days.

Herpes simplex encephalitis
IV
Adults, Elderly, Children 12 yr and older. 10 mg/kg q8h for 10 days.
Children 3 mos - younger than 12 yr. 20 mg/kg q8h for 10 days.

Herpes zoster (caused by varicella)
IV
Adults, Elderly, Children 12 yr and older. 10 mg/kg q8h for 7 days.
Children younger than 12 yr. 20 mg/kg q8h for 7 days.

Herpes zoster (shingles)
PO
Adults, Elderly, Children 12 yr and older. 800 mg q4h 5 times a day for 7-10 days.
Topical
Adults, Elderly. Apply to affected area 3-6 times a day for 7 days.

Varicella (chickenpox)
PO
Adults, Elderly, Children older than 12 yr or children 2-12 yr, weighing 40 kg or more. 800 mg 4 times a day for 5 days.
Children 2-12 yr, weighing less than 40 kg. 20 mg/kg 4 times a day for 5 days. Maximum: 800 mg/dose.
Children younger than 2 yr. 80 mg/kg/day.

Dosage in renal impairment
Dosage and frequency are modified based on severity of infection and degree of renal impairment.

PO
For creatinine clearance of 10 ml/min or less, dosage is 200 mg q12h.
IV

Creatinine Clearance	Dosage Percent	Dosage Interval
greater than 50 ml/min	100	8 hr
25-50 ml/min	100	12 hr
10-25 ml/min	100	24 hr
less than 10 ml/min	50	24 hr

$ AVAILABLE FORMS/COST
• Cap, Gel—Oral: 200 mg, 100's: **$97.20-$260.00**
• Cream-Top: 5%, 2 g, 5 g: **$35.28**/2 g
• Powder, Inj-IV: 500 mg: **$10.00-$70.42**; 1000 mg: **$20.00-$120.21**
• Oint—Top: 5%, 3 g, 15 g: **$26.51-$27.57**/3 g
• Susp—Oral: 200 mg/5 ml, 473 ml: **$118.55-$138.49**
• Tab-Oral: 400 mg, 100's: **$36.88-$308.90**; 800 mg, 100's: **$72.50-$600.65**

UNLABELED USES: Treatment of herpes simplex ocular infections, infectious mononucleosis

CONTRAINDICATIONS: Use in neonates when acyclovir is reconstituted with bacteriostatic water containing benzyl alcohol.

PREGNANCY AND LACTATION: Pregnancy category B; excreted into breast milk; compatible with breast-feeding

SIDE EFFECTS
Frequent
Parenteral (9%-7%): Phlebitis or inflammation at IV site, nausea, vomiting
Topical (28%): Burning, stinging
Occasional
Parenteral (3%): Pruritus, rash, urticaria

Oral (12%-6%): Malaise, nausea

Topical (4%): Pruritus

Rare

Oral (3%-1%): Vomiting, rash, diarrhea, headache

Parenteral (2%-1%): Confusion, hallucinations, seizures, tremors

Topical (less than 1%): Rash

SERIOUS REACTIONS

• Rapid parenteral administration, excessively high doses, or fluid and electrolyte imbalance may produce renal failure exhibited by such signs and symptoms as abdominal pain, decreased urination, decreased appetite, increased thirst, nausea, and vomiting.

• Toxicity has not been reported with oral or topical use.

SPECIAL CONSIDERATIONS

• In recurrent herpes genitalis and herpes labialis in non-immunocompromised patients, no evidence of clinical benefit from topical acyclovir

---

adalimumab

Rx: Humira

Chemical Class: Monoclonal antibody

Therapeutic Class: Disease-modifying antirheumatic drug (DMARD); immunomodulatory agent

---

CLINICAL PHARMACOLOGY

Mechanism of Action: A monoclonal antibody that binds specifically to tumor necrosis factor (TNF) alpha, blocking its interaction with cell surface TNF receptors. *Therapeutic Effect:* Reduces inflammation, tenderness, and swelling of joints; slows or prevents progressive destruction of joints in rheumatoid arthritis.

Pharmacokinetics

Half-life: 10–20 days.

INDICATIONS AND DOSAGES

Rheumatoid arthritis

Subcutaneous

Adults, Elderly. 40 mg every other week. Dose may be increased to 40 mg/wk in those not taking methotrexate.

AVAILABLE FORMS/COST

• Sol, Inj-SC: 40 mg/0.8 ml: **$657.90**

CONTRAINDICATIONS: Active infections

PREGNANCY AND LACTATION: Pregnancy category B; breast milk excretion unknown

SIDE EFFECTS

Frequent (20%)

Injection site, erythema, pruritus, pain, and swelling

Occasional (12%–9%)

Headache, rash, sinusitis, nausea

Rare (7%–5%)

Abdominal or back pain, hypertension

SERIOUS REACTIONS

• Rare reactions include hypersensitivity reactions, malignancies, respiratory tract infections, bronchitis, UTIs, and more serious infections (such as pneumonia, tuberculosis, cellulitis, pyelonephritis, and septic arthritis).

INTERACTIONS

Drugs

Methotrexate: Reduced apparent clearance after single and multiple dosing by 29% and 44% respectively

SPECIAL CONSIDERATIONS

• Evaluate for latent tuberculosis infection with a tuberculin skin test before initiation of therapy

• Adalimumab does not contain preservatives — unused portions of drug should be discarded

PATIENT/FAMILY EDUCATION
• Injection sites should be rotated and injections should never be given into areas where the skin is tender, bruised, red or hard
• Intended for use under the guidance and supervision of clinician; patients may self-inject if appropriate and with medical follow-up, after proper training in injection technique, including proper syringe and needle disposal

MONITORING PARAMETERS
• *Therapeutic:* Rheumatoid arthritis signs and symptoms (joint stiffness, pain, swollen/tender joints), mobility, quality of life, radiographs of affected joints, ESR, CRP
• *Toxicity:* Temperature, blood pressure periodically, signs and symptoms of respiratory infection, including tuberculosis, hypersensitivity, anti-adalimumab antibodies (ELISA) at least once during therapy, anti-dsDNA antibody determinations in patients presenting with lupus-like symptoms (*e.g.,* tiredness, rash, bone pain), CBC, routine blood chemistry periodically during long-term therapy

---

adapalene
(a-dap′pa-leen)
Rx: Differin
Chemical Class: Naphthoic acid derivative (retinoid-like)
Therapeutic Class: Antiacne agent

CLINICAL PHARMACOLOGY
Mechanism of Action: Binds to retinoic acid receptors in cell nuclei modulating cell differentiation, keratinization. Possesses anti-inflammatory properties. *Therapeutic effect:* Normalizes differentiation of follicular epithelial cells.

Pharmacokinetics
Absorption through the skin is low. Trace amount found in plasma following topical application. Excreted primarily by biliary route.

INDICATIONS AND DOSAGES
Acne vulgaris
Topical
Adults, elderly, children > 12 years. Apply to affected area once daily at bedtime after washing.

$ AVAILABLE FORMS/COST
• Cre—Top: 0.1%, 15, 45 g: **$342.19**/15 g
• Gel—Top: 0.1%, 15, 45 g: **$27.31-$42.19**/15 g
• Sol—Top: 0.1%, 30 ml: **$86.19**

CONTRAINDICATIONS: Hypersensitivity to adapalene, vitamin A or any one of its componenets.

PREGNANCY AND LACTATION: Pregnancy category C; excretion in breast milk unknown

SIDE EFFECTS
Frequent
Erythema, scaling, dryness, pruritis, burning (likely to occur first 2-4 weeks, lessens with continued use)
Occasional
Skin irritation, stinging, sunburn, acne flares, erythema, photosensitivity, pruritis, xerosis

SERIOUS REACTIONS
• Concurrent use of other potential irritating topical products (soaps, cleansers, aftershave, cosmetics may produce severe topical irritation.

SPECIAL CONSIDERATIONS
• Avoid excessive exposure to sunlight
• Do not apply to lips or mucous membranes, or to cut, abraded, or sunburned skin
• May aggravate acne early in course of therapy
• Therapeutic results noticed in 8-12 wks

adefovir
(ah-deh'foh-veer)
Rx: Hepsera
Chemical Class: Nucleotide analog
Therapeutic Class: Antiviral

CLINICAL PHARMACOLOGY
Mechanism of Action: An antiviral that inhibits the enzyme DNA polymerase, causing DNA chain termination after its incorporation into viral DNA. *Therapeutic Effect:* Prevents cell replication of viral DNA.
Pharmacokinetics
Binds to proteins after PO administration. Excreted in urine. **Half-life:** 7 hr (increased in impaired renal function).

INDICATIONS AND DOSAGES
Chronic hepatitis B in patients with normal renal function
PO
Adults, Elderly. 10 mg once a day.
Chronic hepatitis B in patients with impaired renal function
Adults, Elderly with creatinine clearance 20-49 ml/min. 10 mg q48h.
Adults, Elderly with creatinine clearance 10-19 ml/min. 10 mg q72h.
Adults, Elderly on hemodialysis. 10 mg every 7 days following dialysis.
S AVAILABLE FORMS/COST
• Tab-Oral: 10 mg, 30's: **$555.23**
CONTRAINDICATIONS: None known.
PREGNANCY AND LACTATION: Pregnancy category C; breast milk excretion unknown but breast-feeding not recommended
SIDE EFFECTS
Frequent (13%)
Asthenia
Occasional (9%-4%)
Headache, abdominal pain, nausea, flatulence
Rare (3%)
Diarrhea, dyspepsia
SERIOUS REACTIONS
• Nephrotoxicity (characterized by increased serum creatinine and decreased serum phosphorus levels) is a treatment-limiting toxicity of adefovir therapy.
• Lactic acidosis and severe hepatomegaly occur rarely, particularly in female patients.
INTERACTIONS
Drugs
3 *Ibuprofen:* Ibuprofen increases adefovir exposure by 23%
SPECIAL CONSIDERATIONS
• Offer HIV testing before treatment
• Effective in patients with HBV resistant to lamivudine
• Histologic improvement seen in 60% of treated patients, but long-term effect unknown
PATIENT/FAMILY EDUCATION
• Avoid behavior that may cause exposure to HIV
MONITORING PARAMETERS
• ALT, AST, bilirubin, HBV DNA level, INR, renal function

adenosine
(ah-den'oh-seen)
Rx: Adenocard
Chemical Class: Endogenous nucleoside
Therapeutic Class: Antiarrhythmic

CLINICAL PHARMACOLOGY
Mechanism of Action: A cardiac agent that slows impulse formation in the SA node and conduction time through the AV node. Adenosine also acts as a diagnostic aid in myocardial perfusion imaging or stress echocardiography. *Therapeutic Ef-*

fect: Depresses left ventricular function and restores normal sinus rhythm.

INDICATIONS AND DOSAGES
Paroxysmal supraventricular tachycardia (PSVT)
Rapid IV bolus
Adults, Elderly. Initially, 6 mg given over 1–2 sec. If first dose does not convert within 1–2 min, give 12 mg; may repeat 12-mg dose in 1–2 min if no response has occurred.
Children. Initially 0.1 mg/kg (maximum: 6 mg). If ineffective, may give 0.2 mg/kg (maximum: 12 mg).
Diagnostic testing
IV infusion
Adults. 140 mcg/kg/min for 6 min.

$ AVAILABLE FORMS/COST
• Sol, Inj-IM: 25 mg/ml, 10 ml: **$4.98-$15.95**
• Sol, Inj-IV: 3 mg/ml, 2 ml: **$26.97-$40.94**

CONTRAINDICATIONS: Atrial fibrillation or flutter, second- or third-degree AV block or sick sinus syndrome (with functioning pacemaker), ventricular tachycardia

PREGNANCY AND LACTATION: Pregnancy category C; fetal effects unlikely

SIDE EFFECTS
Frequent (18%–12%)
Facial flushing, dyspnea
Occasional (7%–2%)
Headache, nausea, light-headedness, chest pressure
Rare (less than or equal to 1%)
Numbness or tingling in arms; dizziness; diaphoresis; hypotension; palpitations; chest, jaw, or neck pain

SERIOUS REACTIONS
• May produce short-lasting heart block.

INTERACTIONS
Drugs
▣ β-*blockers:* Bradycardia

▣ *Dipyridamole:* Increased serum adenosine levels, potentiates pharmacologic effects of adenosine
▣ *Nicotine:* Greater hemodynamic response to adenosine (hypotension, chest pain)
▣ *Theophylline/caffeine:* Inhibits hemodynamic effects of adenosine

---

albendazole
(all-ben′-dah-zole)
Rx: Albenza
Chemical Class: Benzimidazole derivative
Therapeutic Class: Antihelmintic

CLINICAL PHARMACOLOGY
Mechanism of Action: A benzimidazole carbamate anthelmintic that degrades parasite cytoplasmic microtubules, irreversibly blocks cholinesterase secretion, glucose uptake in helminth and larvae (depletes glycogen, decreases ATP production, depletes energy). Vermicidal. *Therapeutic Effect:* Immobilizes and kills worms.
Pharmacokinetics
Poorly and variable absorbed gastrointestinal (GI) tract. Widely distributed, cyst fluid and including cerebrospinal fluid (CSF). Protein binding: 70%. Extensively metabolized in liver. Primarily excreted in urine and bile. Not removed by hemodialysis. **Half-life:** 8-12 hrs.

INDICATIONS AND DOSAGES
Neurocysticercosis
PO
Adults, Elderly more than 60 kg. 400 mg 2 times/day. Continue for 28 days, rest 14 days, repeat cycle 3 times.
Adults, Elderly less than 60 kg. 15 mg/kg/day. Continue for 28 days, rest 14 days, repeat cycle 3 times.

Cystic hydatid
PO

Adults, Elderly more than 60 kg. 400 mg 2 times/day. Continue for 8-30 days.

Adults, Elderly less than 60 kg. 15 mg/kg/day. Continue for 8-30 days.

AVAILABLE FORMS/COST
• Tab-Oral: 200 mg, 112's: **$167.16**

UNLABELED USES: Angiostrongyliasis, cysticercosis, gnathostomiasis, liver flukes, trichuriasis

CONTRAINDICATIONS: Hypersensitivity to albendazole or any component of the formulation, pregnancy

PREGNANCY AND LACTATION: Pregnancy category C, excreted in breast milk

SIDE EFFECTS
Frequent

Neurocysticerosis: Nausea, vomiting, headache

Hydatid: Abnormal liver function tests, abdominal pain, nausea, vomiting

Occasional

Neurocysticerosis: Increased intracranial pressure, meningeal signs

Hydatid: Headache, dizziness, alopecia, fever

SERIOUS REACTIONS
• Pancytopenia occurs rarely.
• In presence of cysticerosis, drug may produce retinal damage in presence of retinal lesions.

INTERACTIONS
Drugs

▣ *Dexamethasone:* 56% increase in serum level of albendazole

▣ *Praziquantel:* 50% increase in serum level of albendazole

SPECIAL CONSIDERATIONS
• For appropriate infections, retest stool 3 wk after treatment to detect residual ova
• Patients treated for neurocystircercosis should receive steroid and anticonvulsant therapy

---

albuterol

(al-byoo'ter-ole)

Rx: Airet, Proventil, Proventil-HFA, Proventil Repetabs, Respirol, Ventolin, Ventolin Rotacaps, Volmax Combinations

  Rx: with ipratropium (Combivent)

Chemical Class: Sympathomimetic amine; β_2-adrenergic agonist

Therapeutic Class: Antiasthmatic; bronchodilator

CLINICAL PHARMACOLOGY
Mechanism of Action: A sympathomimetic that stimulates beta$_2$-adrenergic receptors in the lungs, resulting in relaxation of bronchial smooth muscle. *Therapeutic Effect:* Relieves bronchospasm and reduces airway resistance.

Pharmacokinetics

Route	Onset	Peak	Duration
PO	15–30 min	2–3 hr	4–6 hr
PO (extended-release)	30 min	2–4 hr	12 hr
Inhalation	5–15 min	0.5–2 hr	2–5 hr

Rapidly, well absorbed from the GI tract; gradually absorbed from the bronchi after inhalation. Metabolized in the liver. Primarily excreted in urine. **Half-life:** 2.7–5 hr (PO); 3.8 hr (inhalation).

INDICATIONS AND DOSAGES
Bronchospasm
PO

Adults, Children older than 12 yr. 2–4 mg 3–4 times a day. Maximum: 8 mg 4 times/day.

Elderly. 2 mg 3–4 times a day. Maximum: 8 mg 4 times a day.

Children 6–12 yr. 2 mg 3–4 times a day. Maximum: 24 mg/day.

PO (Extended-Release)

Adults, Children older than 12 yr. 4-8 mg q12h.

Inhalation

Adults, Elderly, Children older than 12 yr. 1-2 puffs by metered dose inhaler q4-6h as needed.

Children 4-12 yr. 1–2 puffs 4 times a day.

Nebulization

Adults, Elderly, Children older than 12 yr. 2.5 mg 3-4 times a day.

Children 2-12 yr. 0.63-1.25 mg 3-4 times a day.

Exercise-induced bronchospasm

Inhalation

Adults, Elderly, Children 4 yr and older. 2 puffs 15-30 min before exercise.

Ⓢ AVAILABLE FORMS/COST

• Cap, Gel—INH: 0.2 mg/puff, 100's: **$37.92**
• MDI—INH: 0.09 mg/puff, 17 g (200 puffs): **$8.19-$39.90**
• MDI-INH (albuterol sulfate HFA): 0.108 mg/puff (equivalent to 0.09 mg of the base, 18 g (200 puffs): **$8.19-$39.90**
• MDI—INH (with ipratropium): 103 mcg-18 mcg/puff, 14.7 g (200 puffs): **$51.38-$59.91**
• Sol—INH: 0.021%, 0.042%, both 3 ml: **$1.60**; 0.083%, 3 ml: **$0.36-$2.25**; 0.5%, 20 ml: **$7.24-$23.58**
• Syr—Oral: 2 mg/5 ml, 480 ml: **$7.37-$40.15**
• Tab, Coated, Sus Action—Oral: 4 mg, 100's: **$91.45-$109.21**; 8 mg, 100's: **$188.05-$218.42**
• Tab-Oral: 2 mg, 100's: **$4.37-$48.92**; 4 mg, 100's: **$5.63-$86.77**

CONTRAINDICATIONS: History of hypersensitivity to sympathomimetics

PREGNANCY AND LACTATION: Pregnancy category C; excretion into breast milk unknown

SIDE EFFECTS

Frequent

Headache (27%); nausea (15%); restlessness, nervousness, tremors (20%); dizziness (less than 7%); throat dryness and irritation, pharyngitis (less than 6%); BP changes, including hypertension (5%–3%); heartburn, transient wheezing (less than 5%)

Occasional (3%–2%)

Insomnia, asthenia, altered taste
Inhalation: Dry, irritated mouth or throat; cough; bronchial irritation

Rare

Somnolence, diarrhea, dry mouth, flushing, diaphoresis, anorexia

SERIOUS REACTIONS

• Excessive sympathomimetic stimulation may produce palpitations, extrasystole, tachycardia, chest pain, a slight increase in BP followed by a substantial decrease, chills, diaphoresis, and blanching of skin.

• Too-frequent or excessive use may lead to decreased bronchodilating effectiveness and severe, paradoxical bronchoconstriction.

INTERACTIONS

Drugs

❸ *β-blockers:* Decreased action of albuterol, cardioselective β-blockers preferable if concurrent use necessary

❸ *Furosemide:* Potential for additive hypokalemia

❸ *MAOIs:* Action of albuterol on the vascular system may be potentiated, caution if administered concomitantly or within 2 weeks of discontinuation of MAOIs

❸ *Tricyclic antidepressants:* Action of albuterol on the vascular system may be potentiated, caution if administered concomitantly or within 2 weeks of discontinuation of Tricyclics

SPECIAL CONSIDERATIONS
• Inhalation technique critical
• Consider spacer devices

PATIENT/FAMILY EDUCATION
• See clinician if using ≥4 inhalations/day on regular basis or >1 canister (200 inhalations) in 8 wks

alclometasone
(al-kloe-met'a-sone)
Rx: Aclovate
Chemical Class: Corticosteroid, synthetic
Therapeutic Class: Corticosteroid, topical

CLINICAL PHARMACOLOGY
Mechanism of Action: Topical corticosteroids exhibit anti-inflammatory, antipruritic, and vasoconstrictive properties. Clinically, these actions correspond to decreased edema, erythema, pruritus, plaque formation and scaling of the affected skin.
Pharmacokinetics
Approximately 3% is absorbed during an 8 hours period. Metabolized in the liver. Excreted in the urine.

INDICATIONS AND DOSAGES
Atopic dermatitis, contact dermatitis, dermatitis, discoid lupus erythematosus, eczema, exfoliative dermatitis, granuloma annulare, lichen planus, lichen simplex, polymorphous light eruption, pruritis, psoriasis, Rhus dermatitis, seborrheic dermatitis, xerosis
Topical
Adults, adolescents, children 1 year and older. Apply a thin film to the affected area 2-3 times a day.

[$] **AVAILABLE FORMS/COST**
• Cre/Oint—Top: 0.05%, 15, 45, 60 g: **$18.79-$19.70**/15 g

CONTRAINDICATIONS: Hypersensitivity to alclometasone, other corticosteroids, or any of its components.

PREGNANCY AND LACTATION: Pregnancy category C; unknown whether topical application could result in sufficient systemic absorption to produce detectable amounts in breast milk (systemic corticosteroids are secreted into breast milk in quantities not likely to have detrimental effects on infant)

SIDE EFFECTS
Frequent
Burning, erythema, maculopapular rash, pruritis, skin irritation, xerosis
Occasional
Acneiform rash, contact dermatitis, folliculitis, glycosuria, growth inhibition, headache, hyperglycemia, infection, miliaria, papilledema, skin atrophy, skin hypopigmentation, skin ulcer, striae, telangiectasia
Rare
Adrenalcortical insufficiency, increased intracranial pressure, pseudotumor cerebri, impaired wound healing, Cushing's syndrome, HPA suppression, skin ulcers, tolerance, withdrawal, visual impairment, ocular hypertension, cataracts

SPECIAL CONSIDERATIONS

PATIENT/FAMILY EDUCATION
• Apply sparingly only to affected area
• Avoid contact with the eyes
• Do not put bandages or dressings over treated area unless directed by clinician
• Discontinue drug, notify clinician if local irritation or fever develops
• Do not use on weeping, denuded, or infected areas

alefacept

Rx: Amevive
Chemical Class: Dimeric fusion protein
Therapeutic Class: Antipsoriatic; immunomodulatory agent

CLINICAL PHARMACOLOGY

Mechanism of Action: An immunologic agent that interferes with the activation of T lymphocytes by binding to the lymphocyte antigen, thus reducing the number of circulating T lymphocytes. *Therapeutic Effect:* Prevents T cells from becoming overactive, which may help reduce symptoms of chronic plaque psoriasis.

Pharmacokinetics
Half-life: 270 hr.

INDICATIONS AND DOSAGES

Plaque psoriasis
IV
Adults, Elderly. 7.5 mg once weekly for 12 wk.
IM
Adults, Elderly. 15 mg once weekly for 12 wk.

$ **AVAILABLE FORMS/COST**

• Powder, Inj-IM: 7.5 mg/vial: **$1,072.50** Powder, Inj-IM: 15 mg/vial: **$1,038.75**

CONTRAINDICATIONS: History of systemic malignancy, concurrent use of immunosuppressive agents or phototherapy

PREGNANCY AND LACTATION: Pregnancy category B; effect on pregnancy and fetal development unknown (Biogen Pregnancy Registry available: 1-866-263-8483)

SIDE EFFECTS

Frequent (16%)
Injection site pain and inflammation (with IM administration)
Occasional (5%)
Chills

Rare (2% or less)
Pharyngitis, dizziness, cough, nausea, myalgia

SERIOUS REACTIONS

• Rare reactions include hypersensitivity reactions, lymphopenia, malignancies, and serious infections requiring hospitalization (such as abscess, pneumonia, and postoperative wound infection).

• Coronary artery disease and MI occur in fewer than 1% of patients.

INTERACTIONS

Drugs

▣ *Immunosuppressive agents (steroids, chemotherapy, radiation):* potential excessive immunosuppression

▣ *Phototherapy; photochemotherapy (light or laser):* potential excessive immunosuppression

▣ *Vaccines, live or live-attenuated:* potential risk of disease

SPECIAL CONSIDERATIONS

PATIENT/FAMILY EDUCATION

• Inform patients of the need for monitoring of lymphocyte counts during therapy; increased risk of infection or a malignancy

MONITORING PARAMETERS

• *Efficacy:* Psoriasis Area and Severity Index (PASI) - extent of area affected and severity of erythema, scaling, and thickness of plaques

• *Toxicity:* CD4+ lymphocyte counts weekly during 12 week course; withhold therapy if counts below 250 cells/μl

alendronate
(a-len′dro-nate)
Rx: Fosamax
Chemical Class: Pyrophosphate analog
Therapeutic Class: Antiosteoporotic; bisphosphonate; bone resorption inhibitor

CLINICAL PHARMACOLOGY
Mechanism of Action: A bisphosphonate that inhibits normal and abnormal bone resorption, without retarding mineralization. *Therapeutic Effect:* Leads to significantly increased bone mineral density; reverses the progression of osteoporosis.

Pharmacokinetics
Poorly absorbed after oral administration. Protein binding: 78%. After oral administration, rapidly taken into bone, with uptake greatest at sites of active bone turnover. Excreted in urine. **Terminal half-life:** Greater than 10 yr (reflects release from skeleton as bone is resorbed).

INDICATIONS AND DOSAGES
Osteoporosis (in men)
PO
Adults, Elderly. 10 mg once a day in the morning.
Glucocorticoid-induced osteoporosis
PO
Adults, Elderly. 5 mg once a day in the morning.
Post-menopausal women not receiving estrogen. 10 mg once a day in the morning.
Post menopausal osteoporosis
PO (treatment)
Adults, Elderly. 10 mg once a day in the morning or 70 mg weekly.
PO (prevention)
Adults, Elderly. 5 mg once a day in the morning or 35 mg weekly.

Paget's disease
PO
Adults, Elderly. 40 mg once a day in the morning.

Ⓢ **AVAILABLE FORMS/COST**
• Tab—Oral: 5 mg, 100's: **$251.32**; 10 mg, 100's: **$251.32**; 35 mg, 20's: **$366.56**; 40 mg, 30's: **$169.97**; 70 mg, 20's: **$366.56**

UNLABELED USES: Treatment of breast cancer

CONTRAINDICATIONS: GI disease, including dysphagia, frequent heartburn, gastrointestinal reflux disease, hiatal hernia, and ulcers, inability to stand or sit upright for at least 30 minutes; renal impairment; sensitivity to alendronate

PREGNANCY AND LACTATION: Pregnancy category C; contraindicated in nursing mothers

SIDE EFFECTS
Frequent (8%–7%)
Back pain, abdominal pain
Occasional (3%–2%)
Nausea, abdominal distention, constipation, diarrhea, flatulence
Rare (Less than 2%)
Rash

SERIOUS REACTIONS
• Overdose causes hypocalcemia, hypophosphatemia, and significant GI disturbances.
• Esophageal irritation occurs if alendronate is not given with 6–8 ounces of plain water or if the patient lies down within 30 minutes of drug administration.

INTERACTIONS
Drugs
▣ *Antacids:* Calcium, magnesium and aluminum bind alendronate and reduce absorption
▣ *Food (including coffee and orange juice):* Decreases bioavailability of alendronate by 40%-60%
▣ *Aspirin:* Increased risk of upper GI adverse effects

SPECIAL CONSIDERATIONS
PATIENT/FAMILY EDUCATION
• Patients should receive supplemental calcium and vitamin D if dietary intake is inadequate
• Administer 30 min before the first food/beverage/medication of the day with 6-8 oz plain water; avoid lying down for at least 30 min
• Weekly administration may be an advantage
• Some expert recommend cessation of therapy after 5 yrs due to theoretical concerns of poor quality bone formation with prolonged therapy

---

alfuzosin

Rx: Uroxatral
Chemical Class: Quinazoline
Therapeutic Class: α_1-adrenergic blocker

CLINICAL PHARMACOLOGY
Mechanism of Action: An alpha$_1$ antagonist that targets receptors around bladder neck and prostate capsule. *Therapeutic Effect:* Relaxes smooth muscle and improves urinary flow and symptoms of prostatic hyperplasia.

Pharmacokinetics
Rapidly absorbed and widely distributed. Protein binding: 90%. Extensively metabolized in the liver. Primarily excreted in urine. **Half-life:** 3–9 hr.

INDICATIONS AND DOSAGES
Benign prostatic hyperplasia
PO
Adults. 10 mg once a day, approximately 30 min after same meal each day.

ⓢ AVAILABLE FORMS/COST
• Tab, Sus Action-Oral: 10 mg, 100's: **$186.25**

CONTRAINDICATIONS: History of hypersensitivity to alfuzosin
PREGNANCY AND LACTATION:
Pregnancy category B, but not indicated for use in women
SIDE EFFECTS
Frequent (7%–6%)
Dizziness, headache, malaise
Occasional (4%)
Dry mouth
Rare (3%–2%)
Nausea, dyspepsia (such as heartburn, and epigastric discomfort), diarrhea, orthostatic hypotension, tachycardia, drowsiness
SERIOUS REACTIONS
• Ischemia-related chest pain may occur rarely.
INTERACTIONS
Drugs
🔳 *Atenolol:* Atenolol increases peak plasma alfuzosin level by 25%; alfuzosin increases plasma atenolol levels by 25%
🔳 *Cimetidine:* Cimetidine increases peak plasma alfuzosin level by 20%
❷ *Diltiazem:* Diltiazem increases peak plasma alfuzosin level by 50%; alfuzosin increases plasma diltiazem level by 50%
⚠ *Itraconazole:* Itraconazole markedly increases plasma alfuzosin level
⚠ *Ketoconazole:* Ketoconazole markedly increases plasma alfuzosin level
⚠ *Ritonavir:* Ritonavir markedly increases plasma alfuzosin level
SPECIAL CONSIDERATIONS
• In clinical trials, peak flow rates increase from a baseline of 10 ml/sec to 12 ml/sec; American Urological Association (AUA) scores decreased by 4-7 points from a baseline of 18
PATIENT/FAMILY EDUCATION
• Take immediately after the same meal each day

• Hypotension or postural hypotension may occur with first doses
MONITORING PARAMETERS
• Liver function

---

allopurinol
(al-oh-pure′i-nole)
Rx: Aloprim, Lopurin, Zurinol, Zyloprim
Chemical Class: Hypoxanthine isomer; xanthine oxidase inhibitor
Therapeutic Class: Antigout agent

CLINICAL PHARMACOLOGY
Mechanism of Action: A xanthine oxidase inhibitor that decreases uric acid production by inhibiting xanthine oxidase, an enzyme. *Therapeutic Effect:* Reduces uric acid concentrations in both serum and urine.
Pharmacokinetics

Route	Onset	Peak	Duration
PO/IV	2–3 days	1–3 wk	1–2 wk

Well absorbed from the GI tract. Widely distributed. Metabolized in the liver to active metabolite. Excreted primarily in urine. Removed by hemodialysis. **Half-life:** 1–3 hr; metabolite, 12–30 hr.
INDICATIONS AND DOSAGES
Chronic gouty arthritis
PO
Adults, Children older than 10 yr. Initially, 100 mg/day; may increase by 100 mg/day at weekly intervals. Maximum: 800 mg/day. Maintenance: 100–200 mg 2–3 times a day or 300 mg/day.
To prevent uric acid nephropathy during chemotherapy
PO
Adults: Initially, 600–800 mg/day starting 2–3 days before initiation of chemotherapy or radiation therapy.

Children 6–10 yr. 100 mg 3 times a day or 300 mg once a day.
Children less than 6 yr. 50 mg 3 times a day.
IV
Adults. 200–400 mg/m^2/day beginning 24–48 hr befo initiation of chemotherapy.
Children. 200 mg/m^2/day. Maximum: 600 mg/day.
Prevention of uric acid calculi
PO
Adults. 100–200 mg 1–4 times a day or 300 mg once a day.
Recurrent calcium oxalate calculi
PO
Adults. 200–300 mg/day.
Elderly. Initially, 100 mg/day, gradually increased until optimal uric acid level is reached.
Dosage in renal impairment
Dosage is modified based on creatinine clearance.

Creatinine Clearance	Dosage Adjustment
10-20 ml/min	200 mg/day
3-9 ml/min	100 mg/day
Less than 3 ml/min	100 mg at extended intervals

S **AVAILABLE FORMS/COST**
• Powder, Inj-IV: 500 mg/vial: **$500.00**
• Tab-Oral: 100 mg, 100's: **$4.26-$60.50**; 300 mg, 100's: **$8.05-$108.45**
UNLABELED USES: In mouthwash following fluorouracil therapy to prevent stomatitis
CONTRAINDICATIONS: Asymptomatic hyperuricemia
PREGNANCY AND LACTATION: Pregnancy category C; allopurinol and oxypurinol have been found in the milk of a mother who was receiving allopurinol
SIDE EFFECTS
Occasional
Oral: Somnolence, unusual hair loss

IV: Rash, nausea, vomiting
Rare
Diarrhea, headache
SERIOUS REACTIONS
• Pruritic maculopapular rash possibly accompanied by malaise, fever, chills, joint pain, nausea, and vomiting should be considered a toxic reaction.
• Severe hypersensitivity may follow appearance of rash.
• Bone marrow depression, hepatic toxicity, peripheral neuritis, and acute renal failure occur rarely.
INTERACTIONS
Drugs
❷ *Angiotensin-converting enzyme inhibitors:* Predisposed to hypersensitivity reactions including Stevens-Johnson syndrome, skin eruptions, fever, and arthralgias
❸ *Antacids:* Aluminum hydroxide inhibits the response to allopurinol
❷ *Azathioprine:* Increased toxicity of azathioprine; requires dose adjustment
❸ *Cyclophosphamide:* May increase cyclophosphamide toxicity
❸ *Cyclosporine/tacrolimus:* Increased toxicity of immunosuppressive drug
❷ *Mercaptopurine:* Increased effect of mercaptopurine with increased risk of toxicity
❸ *Oral anticoagulants:* Enhanced hypoprothrombinemic response
❸ *Theophylline:* Large doses may increase serum theophylline levels
SPECIAL CONSIDERATIONS
• Increased acute attacks of gout during early stages of allopurinol administration—cover with colchicine
• Maintenance doses of colchicine (0.6 mg qday-bid) should be given prophylactically along with starting with low doses of allopurinol

• To reduce risk of flare, begin with 100 mg qday and increase by 100 mg qwk until serum uric acid ≤6mg/dl
• Parenteral formulation available as orphan drug and in Canada
MONITORING PARAMETERS
• Serum uric acid; can usually be achieved in 1-3 wks

---

almotriptan
(al-moe-trip′tan)
Rx: Axert
Chemical Class: Serotonin derivative
Therapeutic Class: Antimigraine agent

CLINICAL PHARMACOLOGY
Mechanism of Action: A serotonin receptor agonist that binds selectively to vascular receptors, producing a vasoconstrictive effect on cranial blood vessels. *Therapeutic Effect:* Produces relief of migraine headache.
Pharmacokinetics
Well absorbed after PO administration. Metabolized by the liver, excreted in urine. **Half-life:** 3-4 hr.
INDICATIONS AND DOSAGES
Migraine headache
PO
Adults, Elderly. 6.25–12.5 mg. If headache improves but then returns, dose may be repeated after 2 hr. Maximum: 2 doses/24 hr.
Dosage in renal impairment
For adult and elderly patients, recommended initial dose is 6.25 mg and maximum daily dose is 12.5 mg.
Ⓢ **AVAILABLE FORMS/COST**
• Tab—Oral: 12.5 mg, 6's: **$110.63**
CONTRAINDICATIONS: Arrhythmias associated with conduction disorders, hemiplegic or basilar migraine, ischemic heart disease (including angina pectoris, history of

MI, silent ischemia, and Prinzmetal's angina), uncontrolled hypertension, use within 24 hours of ergotamine-containing preparation or another serotonin receptor antagonist, use within 14 days of MAOIs, Wolff-Parkinson-White syndrome

PREGNANCY AND LACTATION: Pregnancy category C; excretion in human breast milk unknown (but excreted into milk in lactating rats), use caution in nursing mothers

SIDE EFFECTS

Frequent

Nausea, dry mouth, paresthesia, flushing

Occasional

Changes in temperature sensation, asthenia, dizziness

SERIOUS REACTIONS

• Excessive dosage may produce tremor, red extremities, reduced respirations, cyanosis, seizures, and chest pain.

• Serious arrhythmias occur rarely, particularly in patients with hypertension or diabetes, obese patients, smokers, and those with a strong family history of coronary artery disease.

INTERACTIONS

Drugs

⚠ *Egotomine-containing drugs:* Increased vasoconstriction

⚠ *Other 5-HT$_1$-agonists:* Increased vasoconstriction

▣ *MAO inhibitors:* Decreased almotriptan clearance

▣ *Ketoconazole, itraconazole, ritonavir, erythromycin:* Increased plasma concentrations of almotriptan

❷ *Sibutramine:* Theoretical increase in the risk of serotonin syndrome

SPECIAL CONSIDERATIONS

• Safety of treating, on average, more than 4 headaches in a 30-day period has not been established

• Controlled trials have not adequately established the effectiveness of a second dose if the initial dose is ineffective

• Superiority over other triptan migraine headache agents has not been demonstrated

PATIENT/FAMILY EDUCATION

• Use only to treat migraine headache, not for prevention

---

alprazolam

(al-pray'zoe-lam)

Rx: Xanax

Chemical Class: Benzodiazepine

Therapeutic Class: Anxiolytic

DEA Class: Schedule IV

CLINICAL PHARMACOLOGY

Mechanism of Action: A benzodiazepine that enhances the action of the inhibitory neurotransmitter gamma-aminobutyric acid in the brain. *Therapeutic Effect*: Produces anxiolytic effect from its CNS depressant action.

Pharmacokinetics

Well absorbed from GI tract. Protein binding: 80%. Metabolized in the liver. Primarily excreted in urine. Minimal removal by hemodialysis. **Half-life:** 11–16 hr.

INDICATIONS AND DOSAGES

Anxiety disorders

PO

Adults (immediate release). Initially, 0.25–0.5 mg 3 times a day. May titrate q3-4 days. Maximum: 4 mg/day in divided doses.

Elderly, Debilitated patients, Patients with hepatic disease or low serum albumin. Initially, 0.25 mg 2–3 times a day. Gradually increase to optimum therapeutic response.

Panic disorder

PO, immediate release

Adults. Initially, 0.5 mg 3 times a day. May increase at 3- to 4-day intervals. Range: 5-6 mg/day. Maximum: 10 mg/day.

PO, extended release

Adults. Initially, 0.5-1 mg once a day. May titrate at 3- to 4-day intervals. Range: 3-6 mg/day. Maximum: 10 mg/day.

Elderly. Initially, 0.125–0.25 mg 2 times a day; may increase in 0.125-mg increments until desired effect attained.

Premenstrual syndrome
PO

Adults. 0.25 mg 3 times a day.

§ AVAILABLE FORMS/COST

• Sol—Oral: 0.5 mg/5ml, 500 ml: **$51.75**
• Sol, Concentrate-Oral: 1 mg/ml w/dropper, 30 ml: **$65.08**
• Tab, Plain Coated—Oral: 0.25 mg, 100's: **$6.42-$106.95**; 0.5 mg, 100's: **$6.58-$133.24**; 1 mg, 100's: **$25.75-$177.78**; 2 mg, 100's: **$136.28-$302.26**

UNLABELED USES: Management of premenstrual syndrome symptoms (mood disturbances, insomnia, and cramps), irritable bowel syndrome

CONTRAINDICATIONS: Acute alcohol intoxication with depressed vital signs, acute angle-closure glaucoma, concurrent use of itraconazole or ketoconazole, myasthenia gravis, severe COPD

PREGNANCY AND LACTATION: Pregnancy category D; children born of a mother receiving benzodiazepines may be at risk for withdrawal symptoms; neonatal flaccidity and respiratory problems have been reported; chronic administration of diazepam to nursing mothers has been reported to cause infants to become lethargic and lose weight

SIDE EFFECTS

Frequent

Ataxia); lightheadedness; transient, mild somnolence; slurred speech (particularly in elderly or debilitated patients)

Occasional

Confusion, depression, blurred vision, constipation, diarrhea, dry mouth, headache, nausea

Rare

Behavioral problems such as anger, impaired memory, paradoxical reactions such as insomnia, nervousness, or irritability

SERIOUS REACTIONS

• Abrupt or too rapid withdrawal may result in pronounced restlessness, irritability, insomnia, hand tremors, abdominal and muscle cramps, diaphoresis, vomiting, and seizures.

• Overdose results in somnolence, confusion, diminished reflexes, and coma.

• Blood dyscrasias have been reported rarely.

INTERACTIONS

Drugs

⬛ *Cimetidine:* Cimetidine inhibits metabolism, increases plasma levels

⬛ *Digoxin:* Inconsistently raises digoxin levels

⬛ *Erythromycin, clarithromycin, troleandomycin:* Possible increased sedation

⬛ *Ethanol:* Enhanced adverse psychomotor effects; difficulty performing tasks that require alertness

⬛ *Fluoxetine, fluvoxamine, ketoconazole, itraconazole, nefazadone (see contraindications):* Increases alprazolam plasma concentrations; increases in psychomotor impairment

⬛ *Grapefruit juice:* Increased alprazolam levels due to inhibition of presystemic (intestinal) enzyme CYP34A

[3] *Phenytoin, carbamazepine:* Decreased benzodiazepine effect

SPECIAL CONSIDERATIONS

PATIENT/FAMILY EDUCATION

• Not for "everyday" stress or longer than 3 mo; avoid driving, activities that require alertness

• Caution when medication discontinued abruptly after long-term (>4 wks) use—may precipitate withdrawal syndrome

alprostadil

(al-pros'ta-dil)

Rx: Caverject, Edex, MUSE, Prostin VR Pediatric

Chemical Class: Prostaglandin E_1

Therapeutic Class: Anti-impotence agent; patent ductus arteriosus

CLINICAL PHARMACOLOGY

Mechanism of Action: A prostaglandin that directly affects vascular and ductus arteriosus smooth muscle and relaxes trabecular smooth muscle. *Therapeutic Effect:* Causes vasodilation; dilates cavernosal arteries, allowing blood flow to and entrapment in the lacunar spaces of the penis.

INDICATIONS AND DOSAGES

Maintain patency of ductus arteriosus

IV infusion

Neonates. Initially, 0.05–0.1 mcg/kg/min. Maintenance: 0.01 - 0.4 mcg/kg/min. Maximum: 0.4 mcg/kg/min.

Impotence

Pellet, Intracavernosal

Adults. Dosage is individualized.

[$] **AVAILABLE FORMS/COST**

• Sol, Inj-IV: 0.5 mg/ml, 1 ml: **$225.00**

• Inj, Kit—Intracavernosal: 5 mcg/ml: **$12.44**; 10 mcg/ml: **$18.10-$42.18**; 20 mcg/ml: **$24.24-$56.99**; 40 mcg/ml: **$36.17-$39.36**

• Pellet, Intraurethral: 125 mcg, 6's: **$128.25**; 250 mcg, 6's: **$124.13**; 500 mcg, 6's: **$143.63**; 1000 mcg, 6's: **$154.88**

UNLABELED USES: Treatment of atherosclerosis, gangrene, pain due to severe peripheral arterial occlusive disease

CONTRAINDICATIONS: Conditions predisposing to anatomic deformation of penis, hyaline membrane disease, penile implants, priapism, respiratory distress syndrome

SIDE EFFECTS

Frequent

Intracavernosal (4%–1%): Penile pain (37%), prolonged erection, hypertension, localized pain, penile fibrosis, injection site hematoma or ecchymosis, headache, respiratory infection, flu-like symptoms

Intraurethral (3%): Penile pain (36%), urethral pain or burning, testicular pain, urethral bleeding, headache, dizziness, respiratory infection, flu-like symptoms

Systemic (greater than 1%): Fever, seizures, flushing, bradycardia, hypotension, tachycardia, apnea, diarrhea, sepsis

Occasional

Intracavernosal (less than 1%): Hypotension, pelvic pain, back pain, dizziness, cough, nasal congestion

Intraurethral (less than 3%): Fainting, sinusitis, back and pelvic pain

Systemic (less than 1%): Anxiety, lethargy, myalgia, arrhythmias, respiratory depression, anemia, bleeding, thrombocytopenia, hematuria

SERIOUS REACTIONS

• Overdose is manifested as apnea, flushing of the face and arms, and bradycardia.

• Cardiac arrest and sepsis occur rarely.

SPECIAL CONSIDERATIONS

• For intracavernosal use administer 1st dose under medical supervision. Use ½-inch 27-30 gauge needle along dorso-lateral aspect of proximal third of penis. Alternate sides
• Urinate prior to intraurethral use to disperse pellet
• Use lowest dose allowing satisfactory erection lasting ≥1 h

MONITORING PARAMETERS

• Infant ABG's, arterial pH, arterial pressure, continuous ECG

---

alteplase

(al-teep′lase)

Rx: Activase
Chemical Class: Tissue plasminogen activator (tPA)
Therapeutic Class: Thrombolytic

CLINICAL PHARMACOLOGY
Mechanism of Action: A tissue plasminogen activator that acts as a thrombolytic by binding to the fibrin in a thrombus and converting entrapped plasminogen to plasmin. This process initiates fibrinolysis. *Therapeutic Effect:* Degrades fibrin clots, fibrinogen, and other plasma proteins.

Pharmacokinetics
Rapidly metabolized in the liver. Primarily excreted in urine. **Half-life:** 35 min.

INDICATIONS AND DOSAGES
Acute MI
IV infusion
Adults weighing greater than 67 kg. 100 mg over 90 min, starting with 15-mg bolus over 1–2 min, then 50 mg over 30 min, then 35 mg over 60 min. Or a 3-hour infusion, giving 60 mg over first hr (6-10 mg as bolus over 1-2 min), 20 mg over second hr, and 20 mg over third hr.
Adults weighing 67 kg or less: 100 mg over 90 min, starting with 15-mg bolus, then 0.75 mg/kg over 30 min (maximum: 50 mg), then 0.5 mg/kg over 60 min (maximum: 35 mg). Or 3-hour infusion of 1.25 mg/kg giving 60% of dose over first hr (6%–10% as 1- to 2-min bolus), 20% over second hr, and 20% over third hr.

Acute pulmonary emboli
IV infusion
Adults. 100 mg over 2 hr. Institute or reinstitute heparin near end or immediately after infusion when aPTT or thrombin time (TT) returns to twice normal or less.

Acute ischemic stroke
IV infusion
Adults. 0.9 mg/kg over 60 min (10% total dose as initial IV bolus over 1 min).

Central venous catheter clearance
IV
Adults, Elderly. 2 mg; may repeat after 2 hr.

 AVAILABLE FORMS/COST
• Powder, Inj-IV: 1 mg/ml, 50 mg: **$1,487.06**; 1 mg/ml, 100 mg: **$2,974.13**

UNLABELED USES: Coronary thrombolysis, to decrease ischemic events in unstable angina

CONTRAINDICATIONS: Active internal bleeding, AV malformation or aneurysm, bleeding diathesis, intracranial neoplasm, intracranial or intraspinal surgery or trauma, recent (within past 2 months) cerebrovascular accident, severe uncontrolled hypertension

PREGNANCY AND LACTATION: Pregnancy category C; unknown if excreted in breast milk

SIDE EFFECTS
Frequent
Superficial bleeding at puncture sites, decreased BP
Occasional
Allergic reaction, such as rash or wheezing; bruising
SERIOUS REACTIONS
• Severe internal hemorrhage may occur.
• Lysis of coronary thrombi may produce atrial or ventricular arrhythmias or stroke.
INTERACTIONS
Drugs
▣ *Heparin, oral anticoagulants, drugs that alter platelet function (i.e., aspirin, dipyridamole, abciximab, eptifibitide, tirofiban):* May increase the risk of bleeding
Labs
• *Decrease:* Fibrinogen (mitigated by collecting blood in presence of aprotinin)
SPECIAL CONSIDERATIONS
• Heparin (in doses sufficient to prolong the aPTT to 1.5-2 times control value) is usually administered in conjunction with thrombolytic therapy; aspirin may also be administered to inhibit platelet aggregation during and/or following post-thrombolytic therapy
• Compress arterial puncture sites at least 30 min
MONITORING PARAMETERS
• Prior to initiation of therapy: coagulation tests, hematocrit, platelet count

aluminum chloride hexahydrate
Rx: Drysol (20%), Xerac AC (6.25%)
Chemical Class: Trivalent cation
Therapeutic Class: Antihidrotic

CLINICAL PHARMACOLOGY
Mechanism of Action: Aluminum salts cause an obstruction of the distal sweat gland. This obstruction causes metal ions to precipitate with mucopolysaccharides, damaging epithelial cells along the lumen of the duct, and forming a plug to block sweat output. *Therapeutic Effect:* Results in decreased secretion of the sweat glands.
Pharmacokinetics
Not known.
INDICATIONS AND DOSAGES
Antiperspirant
Topical
Adults, Elderly, Children 12 yrs and older. Apply to each underarm once a day, at bedtime.
Hyperhidrosis
Topical
Adults, Elderly, Children 12 yrs and older. Apply to affected areas once a day, at bedtime.
Ⓢ AVAILABLE FORMS/COST
• Sol—Top: 6.25%, 35, 60 ml: **$6.28**/35 ml; 20%, 35, 60 ml: **$6.44**/35 ml
CONTRAINDICATIONS: Hypersensitivity to aluminum chloride or any one of its components.
SIDE EFFECTS
Frequent
Itching, burning, tingling sensation
Occasional
Rash
SERIOUS REACTIONS
• Hypersensitivity reaction, such as rash may occur.

SPECIAL CONSIDERATIONS
PATIENT/FAMILY EDUCATION
• Do not apply to broken or irritated skin
• For maximum effect, cover treated area with saran wrap held in place by snug-fitting shirt, mitten or sock (never hold saran wrap in place with tape)
• Avoid contact with eyes

---

aluminum salts
OTC: *Aluminum hydroxide:* AlternaGEL, Alu-Cap, Alu-Tab, Amphojel
OTC: *Aluminum carbonate:* Basaljel
Combinations
  OTC: with magnesium hydroxide (Maalox, Rulox, Mylanta, Gelusil, Aludrox)
Chemical Class: Trivalent cation
Therapeutic Class: Antacid; phosphate adsorbent

CLINICAL PHARMACOLOGY
Mechanism of Action: An antacid that reduces gastric acid by binding with phosphate in the intestine, and then is excreted as aluminum carbonate in feces. Aluminum carbonate may increase the absorption of calcium due to decreased serum phosphate levels. The drug also has astringent and adsorbent properties. *Therapeutic Effect:* Neutralizes or increases gastric pH; reduces phosphates in urine, preventing formation of phosphate urinary stones; reduces serum phosphate levels; decreases fluidity of stools.
Pharmacokinetics
Varies in each formulation.

INDICATIONS AND DOSAGES
Aluminum hydroxide
Peptic ulcer disease: PO: *Adults, Elderly. Children.* 5- 15 ml as above.: 15- 45 ml q3-6h or 1 and 3 hrs after meals and at bedtime.
Antacid: PO: *Adults, Elderly.* 30 ml 1 and 3 hrs after meals and at bedtime.
Gastrointestinal (GI) bleeding prevention: PO: *Adults, Elderly.* 30- 60 ml/hr.: *Children.* 5- 15 ml. q1-2h.
Hyperphosphatemia: PO: *Adults, Elderly.* 500-1 800 mg 1 and 3 hrs after meals and at bedtime.: Children. 50-150 mg/kg/ 24 hrs q4-6h.
Aluminum acetate & acetic acid
Superficial infections of the external auditory canal
Otic
Adults, Elderly. Instill 4-6 drops in ear(s) q2-3h.
Aluminum hydroxide & magnesium carbonate
Antacid: PO: *Adults, Elderly.* 15-30 ml 4 times/day of the liquid; chew 2-4 tablets 4 times/day.
Aluminum hydroxide & magnesium hydroxide
Antacid: PO: *Adults, Elderly.* 5-10 ml 4-6 times/day.
Aluminum hydroxide & magnesium trisillicate
Antacid: PO: *Adults, Elderly.* Chew 2-4 tablets 4 times/day or as directed.
Aluminum hydroxide, magnesium hydroxide, and simethicone
Antacid (with flatulence): PO: *Adults, Elderly.* 10-20 ml or 2-4 tablets 4-6 times/day.
Aluminum sulfate & calcium acetate
Inflammtory skin conditions with weeping that occurs in dermatitis
Topical
Adults, Elderly. Soak affected area in solution 2-4 times/day for 15-30 min or apply wet dressing soaked in solution 2-4 times/day for 30 min

treatment periods. Domeboro: Saturate dressing and apply to affected area and saturate every 15-30 minutes; or soak for 15-30 min 3 times/day.

$ AVAILABLE FORMS/COST
Aluminum Acetate
• Sol-Top: 480 ml: **$2.45-$9.80**
Aluminum Carbonate Gel
• Cap—Oral: 500 mg, 100's: **$20.66**
• Tab—Oral: 500 mg, 100's: **$20.44**
Aluminum Hydroxide
• Cap-Oral: 400 mg, 100's: **$19.62**; 500 mg, 100's: **$17.22**
• Susp—Oral: 320 mg/5 ml, 480 ml: **$5.09-$9.80**; 400 mg/5 ml, 480 ml: **$4.51**; 600 mg/5 ml, 480 ml: **$8.00**
• Tab—Oral: 300 mg, 100's: **$4.29**
CONTRAINDICATIONS: Children age 6 yrs or younger, intestinal obstruction, hypersensitivity to aluminum or any component of the formulation
PREGNANCY AND LACTATION: Pregnancy category C
SIDE EFFECTS
Frequent
PO: Chalky taste, mild constipation, stomach cramps
Topical: Burning, itching
Occasional
PO: Nausea, vomiting, speckling or whitish discoloration of stools
Otic: Burning or stinging in ear
Topical: New or continued redness, skin dryness
Rare
Otic: Skin rash, redness, swelling or pain in ear
SERIOUS REACTIONS
• Prolonged constipation may result in intestinal obstruction.
• Excessive or chronic use may produce hypophosphatemia manifested as anorexia, malaise, muscle weakness or bone pain and resulting in osteomalacia and osteoporosis.
• Prolonged use may produce urinary calculi.

INTERACTIONS
Drugs
▣ *Allopurinol, atenolol, ketoconazole, itraconazole (not fluconazole):* Aluminum hydroxide inhibits GI absorption
▣ *Cefpodoxime, cefuroxime:* Reduced antibiotic bioavailability and serum concentration
▣ *Cyclosporine:* Reduced cyclosporine blood concentrations possible
▣ *Glipizide, glyburide:* Enhanced absorption of hypoglycemic agent
▣ *Iron:* Reduced GI absorption of iron; separate doses by 1-2 hr
▣ *Isoniazid:* Some antacids reduce plasma concentration of isoniazid
▣ *Penicillamine:* Reduced penicillamine bioavailability
▣ *Quinolones:* Reduced serum concentration of antibiotics
▣ *Salicylates:* Decreased serum salicylate concentrations
▣ *Sodium polystyrene sulfonate resin:* Combined use may result in systemic alkalosis
▣ *Tetracycline:* Reduced serum concentration and efficacy of tetracycline
▣ *Vitamin C:* Increases aluminum absorption
SPECIAL CONSIDERATIONS
PATIENT/FAMILY EDUCATION
• Thoroughly chew chewable tablets before swallowing, follow with a glass of water
• May impair absorption of many drugs; do not take other drugs within 1-4 hr of aluminum hydroxide administration
• Stools may appear white or speckled
MONITORING PARAMETERS
• Consider monitoring for hypophosphatemia

amantadine

(a-man'ta-deen)

Rx: Symmetrel
Chemical Class: Adamantane derivative; tricyclic amine
Therapeutic Class: Anti-Parkinson's agent; antiviral

CLINICAL PHARMACOLOGY

Mechanism of Action: A dopaminergic agonist that blocks the uncoating of influenza A virus, preventing penetration into the host and inhibiting M2 protein in the assembly of progeny virions. Amantadine also blocks the reuptake of dopamine into presynaptic neurons and causes direct stimulation of postsynaptic receptors. *Therapeutic Effect:* Antiviral and antiparkinsonian activity.

Pharmacokinetics

Rapidly and completely absorbed from the GI tract. Protein binding: 67%. Widely distributed. Primarily excreted in urine. Minimally removed by hemodialysis. **Half-life:** 11-15 hr (increased in the elderly, decreased in impaired renal function).

INDICATIONS AND DOSAGES

Prevention and symptomatic treatment of respiratory illness due to influenza A virus

PO

Adults older than 64 yr. 100 mg/day.
Adults 13-64 yr. 200 mg/day.
Children 10-12 yr and older. 5 mg/kg/day up to 200 mg/day.
Children 1-9 yr. 5 mg/kg/day (up to 150 mg/day).

Parkinson's disease, extrapyramidal symptoms

PO

Adults, Elderly. 100 mg twice a day. May increase up to 300 mg/day in divided doses.

Dosage in renal impairment

Dose and frequency are modified based on creatinine clearance.

Creatinine Clearance	Dosage
30-50 ml/min	200 mg first day; 100 mg/day thereafter
15-29 ml/min	200 mg first day; 100 mg on alternate days
less than 15 ml/min	200 mg every 7 days

S AVAILABLE FORMS/COST

• Cap—Oral: 100 mg, 100's: **$29.00-$84.72**
• Syr—Oral: 50 mg/5 ml, 480 ml: **$22.44-$125.75**

UNLABELED USES: Treatment of ADHD. Fatigue associated with multiple sclerosis

CONTRAINDICATIONS: None known.

PREGNANCY AND LACTATION: Pregnancy category C; excreted in human milk; exercise caution when administering to nursing mothers because of potential for urinary retention, vomiting, and skin rash

SIDE EFFECTS

Frequent (10%-5%)

Nausea, dizziness, poor concentration, insomnia, nervousness

Occasional (5%-1%)

Orthostatic hypotension, anorexia, headache, livedo reticularis (reddish blue, netlike blotching of skin), blurred vision, urine retention, dry mouth or nose

Rare

Vomiting, depression, irritation or swelling of eyes, rash

SERIOUS REACTIONS

• CHF, leukopenia, and neutropenia occur rarely.
• Hyperexcitability, seizures, and ventricular arrhythmias may occur.

INTERACTIONS

Drugs

3 *Benztropine:* Potentiation of amantadine's CNS side effects

[3] *Triamterene:* Increased amantadine toxicity

[3] *Trihexyphenidyl:* Potentiation of amantadine's CNS side effects

SPECIAL CONSIDERATIONS

PATIENT/FAMILY EDUCATION
• Administer at least 4 hr before bedtime to prevent insomnia
• Take with meals for better absorption and to decrease GI symptoms
• Arise slowly from a reclining position; avoid hazardous activities if dizziness or blurred vision occurs
• Do not discontinue abruptly in Parkinson's disease

---

ambenonium
(am-be-noe′-nee-um)
Rx: Mytelase
Chemical Class: Cholinesterase inhibitor; quaternary ammonium compound
Therapeutic Class: Cholinergic

CLINICAL PHARMACOLOGY
Mechanism of Action: A cholinesterase inhibitor that enhances and prolongs cholinergic function by increasing the concentration of acetylcholine through inhibition of the hydrolysis of acetylcholine. *Therapeutic Effect:* Increases muscle strength in myasthenia gravis.

Pharmacokinetics
Poorly absorbed after PO administration.

INDICATIONS AND DOSAGES
Myasthenia gravis
PO
Adults. 5-25 mg 3 or 4 times a day. If well tolerated, after 1 or 2 days, may increase to 50-75 mg 3 times a day. Range: 5-200 mg/day in divided doses.

[$] **AVAILABLE FORMS/COST**
• Tab, Scored—Oral: 10 mg, 100's: **$128.06**

CONTRAINDICATIONS: Not recommended in patients receiving routine administration of atropine or other belladonna derivatives. Not recommended in patients receiving mecamylamine.

PREGNANCY AND LACTATION: Pregnancy category C; would not be expected to cross placenta or be excreted into breast milk because it is ionized at physiologic pH; although apparently safe for the fetus, may cause transient muscle weakness in the newborn

SIDE EFFECTS
Frequent
Abdominal pain, diarrhea, increased salivation, miosis, sweating, and vomiting
Occasional
Anxiety, blurred vision, and urinary urgency
Rare
Trembling, difficulty moving or controlling movement of the tongue, neck, or arms

SERIOUS REACTIONS
• Overdosage may result in cholinergic crisis, characterized by severe nausea, vomiting, diarrhea, increased salivation, diaphoresis, bradycardia, hypotension, flushed skin, stomach pain, respiratory depression, seizures, and paralysis of muscles.
• Increasing muscle weakness of myasthenia gravis may occur. Antidote: 0.5-1mg IV atropine sulfate with other supportive treatment.

INTERACTIONS
Drugs
[3] *Tacrine:* Increased cholinergic effects

SPECIAL CONSIDERATIONS
PATIENT/FAMILY EDUCATION
• Notify clinician of nausea, vomiting, diarrhea, sweating, increased salivation, irregular heartbeat, muscle weakness, severe abdominal pain or difficulty in breathing
• Administer on an empty stomach

MONITORING PARAMETERS
• Narrow margin between 1st appearance of side effects and serious toxicity
• Symptoms of increasing muscle weakness may be due to cholinergic crisis (overdosage) or myasthenic crisis (increased disease severity); if crisis is myasthenia, patient will improve after 1-2 mg edrophonium; if cholinergic, withdraw ambenonium and administer atropine

---

amcinonide
(am-sin′oh-nide)
Chemical Class: Corticosteroid, synthetic
Therapeutic Class: Corticosteroid, topical

CLINICAL PHARMACOLOGY
Mechanism of Action: Topical corticosteroids have anti-inflammatory, antipruritic, and vasoconstrictive properties. The exact mechanism of the anti-inflammatory process is unclear. *Therapeutic Effect:* Reduces or prevents tissue response to inflammatory process.

Pharmacokinetics
Well absorbed systemically. Large variation in absorption among sites: forearm 1%; scalp 4%; forehead 7%; scrotum 36%. Greatest penetration occurs at groin, axillae, and face. Protein binding in varying degrees. Metabolized in liver. Primarily excreted in urine.

INDICATIONS AND DOSAGES
Dermatoses
Topical
Adults, Elderly. Apply sparingly 2-3 times/day.

Ⓢ AVAILABLE FORMS/COST
• Cre-Top: 0.1%, 15, 30 and 60 g: **$18.42-$20.57**/15 g
• Lotion-Top: 0.1%, 20 and 60ml: **$23.83**/20 ml
• Oint-Top: 0.1%, 15, 30 and 60 g: **$19.60**/15 g

CONTRAINDICATIONS: History of hypersensitivity to amcinonide or other corticosteroids.

PREGNANCY AND LACTATION: Pregnancy category C; unknown whether topical application could result in sufficient systemic absorption to produce detectable amounts in breast milk (systemic corticosteroids are secreted into breast milk in quantities unlikely to have detrimental effects on breast-feeding infant)

SIDE EFFECTS
Frequent
Itching, redness, irritation, burning
Occasional
Dryness, folliculitis, hypertrichosis, acneiform eruptions, hypopigmentation, perioral dermatitis
Rare
Allergic contact dermatitis, maceration of the skin, secondary infection, skin atrophy.
Systemic: Absorption more likely with occlusive dressings or extensive application in young children.

SERIOUS REACTIONS
• The serious reactions of long-term therapy and the addition of occlusive dressings are reversible hypothalamic-pituitary-adrenal (HPA) axis suppression, manifestations of Cushing's syndrome, hyperglycemia and glucosuria.

• Abruptly withdrawing the drug after long-term therapy may require supplemental systemic corticosteroids.

SPECIAL CONSIDERATIONS
PATIENT/FAMILY EDUCATION

• Apply sparingly only to affected area
• Avoid contact with eyes
• Do not put bandages or dressings over treated area unless directed by clinician
• Do not use on weeping, denuded, or infected areas

---

amikacin
(am-i-kay'sin)
Rx: Amikin
Chemical Class: Aminoglycoside
Therapeutic Class: Antibiotic

CLINICAL PHARMACOLOGY
Mechanism of Action: An aminoglycoside antibiotic that irreversibly binds to protein on bacterial ribosomes. *Therapeutic Effect:* Interferes with protein synthesis of susceptible microorganisms.
Pharmacokinetics
Rapid, complete absorption after IM administration. Protein binding: 0%-10%. Widely distributed (doesn't cross blood-brain barrier, low concentrations in CSF). Excreted unchanged in urine. Removed by hemodialysis. **Half-life:** 2-4 hr (increased in impaired renal function and neonates; decreased in cystic fibrosis and burn or febrile patients).
INDICATIONS AND DOSAGES
UTIs
IV, IM
Adults, Elderly. 250 mg q12h.

Moderate to severe infections
IV, IM
Adults, Elderly. 15 mg/kg/day in divided doses q8-12h. Maximum 1.5 g/day.
Children,   Infants: 15-22.5 mg/kg/day in divided doses q8h.
Neonates   7.5-10   mg/kg/dose q8-24h.
Dosage in Renal Impairment
Dosage and frequency are modified based on the degree of renal impairment and serum drug concentration. After a loading dose of 5-7.5 mg/kg, the maintenance dose and frequency are based on serum creatinine levels and creatinine clearance.
$ AVAILABLE FORMS/COST
• Sol, Inj-IM, IV: 50 mg/ml, 2 ml: **$8.75-$33.04**; 250 mg/ml, 2 ml: **$6.00-$34.26**
CONTRAINDICATIONS: Hypersensitivity to amikacin, or other aminoglycosides (cross-sensitivity), or their components.
PREGNANCY AND LACTATION: Pregnancy category C; although fetal ototoxicity has occurred after *in utero* exposure to other aminoglycosides, 8th cranial nerve toxicity has not been reported with amikacin; excreted into breast milk in low concentrations; poor oral bioavailability reduces potential for ototoxicity for the infant
SIDE EFFECTS
Frequent
IM: Pain, induration
IV: Phlebitis, thrombophlebitis
Occasional
Hypersensitivity reactions (rash, fever, urticaria, pruritus)
Rare
Neuromuscular blockade (difficulty breathing, drowsiness, weakness)
SERIOUS REACTIONS
• Serious reactions may include nephrotoxicity (as evidenced by increased thirst, decreased appetite,

nausea, vomiting, increased BUN and serum creatinine levels, and decreased creatinine clearance); neurotoxicity (manifested as muscle twitching, visual disturbances, seizures, and tingling); and ototoxicity (as evidenced by tinnitus, dizziness, and loss of hearing).

INTERACTIONS

Drugs

▣ *Amphotericin B:* Synergistic nephrotoxicity

② *Atracurium:* Amikacin potentiates respiratory depression by atracurium

▣ *Carbenicillin:* Potential for inactivation of amikacin in patients with renal failure

▣ *Carboplatin, Cisplatin:* Additive nephrotoxicity or ototoxicity

▣ *Cephalosporins:* Increased potential for nephrotoxicity in patients with preexisting renal disease

▣ *Cyclosporine:* Additive nephrotoxicity

② *Ethacrynic acid:* Additive ototoxicity

▣ *Indomethacin:* Reduced renal clearance of amikacin in premature infants

▣ *Methoxyflurane:* Additive nephrotoxicity

▣ *Neuromuscular blocking agents:* Amikacin potentiates respiratory depression by neuromuscular blocking agents

▣ *NSAIDs:* May reduce renal clearance of amikacin

▣ *Penicillins (extended spectrum):* Potential for inactivation of amikacin in patients with renal failure

▣ *Piperacillin:* Potential for inactivation of amikacin in patients with renal failure

② *Succinylcholine:* Amikacin potentiates respiratory depression by succinylcholine

▣ *Ticarcillin:* Potential for inactivation of amikacin in patients with renal failure

▣ *Vancomycin:* Additive nephrotoxicity or ototoxicity

② *Vecuronium:* Amikacin potentiates respiratory depression by vecuronium

Labs

• *False increase:* Urine amino acids
• *False decrease:* Bilirubin, cholesterol, serum creatine kinase, serum glucose, LDH, BUN
• *False positive:* Urine oligosaccharides
• *Interference:* Serum tobramycin, kanamycin

SPECIAL CONSIDERATIONS

MONITORING PARAMETERS

• Urine output, serum creat
• Serum peak, drawn 30-60 min after IV INF or 60 min after IM inj; trough level drawn just before next dose; adjust dosage per levels (usual therapeutic plasma levels; peak 20-35 mg/L, trough ≤10 mg/L)

---

amiloride
(a-mill'oh-ride)
Rx: Midamor
Combinations
   Rx: with hydrochlorothiazide (Moduretic)
Chemical Class: Pyrazine
Therapeutic Class: Antihypertensive; diuretic, potassium-sparing

CLINICAL PHARMACOLOGY

Mechanism of Action: A guanidine derivative that acts as a potassium-sparing diuretic, antihypertensive, and antihypokalemic by directly interfering with sodium reabsorption in the distal tubule. *Therapeutic Ef-*

fect: Increases sodium and water excretion and decreases potassium excretion.

Pharmacokinetics

Route	Onset	Peak	Duration
PO	2 hrs	6–10 hrs	24 hrs

Incompletely absorbed from gastrointestinal (GI) tract. Protein binding: Minimal. Primarily excreted in urine; partially eliminated in feces.
Half-life: 6–9 hrs.

INDICATIONS AND DOSAGES

To counteract potassium loss induced by other diuretics
PO

Adults, Children weighing more than 20 kg. 5–10 mg/day up to 20 mg.
Elderly. Initially, 5 mg/day or every other day.
Children weighing 6–20 kg. 0.625 mg/kg/day. Maximum: 10 mg/day.

Dosage in renal impairment

Creatinine Clearance	Dosage
10–50 ml/min	50% of normal
less than 10 ml/min	avoid use

$ AVAILABLE FORMS/COST
• Tab-Oral: 5 mg, 100's: **$28.00–$57.65**
UNLABELED USES: Treatment of edema associated with congestive heart failure (CHF), liver cirrhosis, and nephrotic syndrome; treatment of hypertension, reduces lithium-induced polyuria, slows pulmonary function reduction in cystic fibrosis
CONTRAINDICATIONS: Acute or chronic renal insufficiency, anuria, diabetic nephropathy, patients on other potassium-sparing diuretics, serum potassium greater than 5.5 mEq/L
PREGNANCY AND LACTATION: Pregnancy category B; therapy for preexisting hypertension can be continued throughout pregnancy with minimal risk; initiating for simple edema not recommended; few unequivocal indications for diuretic therapy in pregnancy except for pulmonary edema or congestive heart failure; excretion into breast milk unknown; use caution in nursing mothers

SIDE EFFECTS
Frequent (8%–3%)
Headache, nausea, diarrhea, vomiting, decreased appetite
Occasional (3%–1%)
Dizziness, constipation, abdominal pain, weakness, fatigue, cough, impotence
Rare (less than 1%)
Tremors, vertigo, confusion, nervousness, insomnia, thirst, dry mouth, heartburn, shortness of breath, increased urination, hypotension, rash

SERIOUS REACTIONS
• Severe hyperkalemia may produce irritability, anxiety, a feeling of heaviness in the legs, paresthesia of hands, face, and lips, hypotension, bradycardia, tented T waves, widening of QRS, and ST depression.

INTERACTIONS
Drugs
☒ *ACE inhibitors:* Hyperkalemia in predisposed patients
☒ *Angiotensin II receptor antagonists:* Increased risk of hyperkalemia
❷ *Potassium preparations:* Hyperkalemia in predisposed patients
☒ *Quinidine:* Increased ventricular arrhythmias

SPECIAL CONSIDERATIONS
PATIENT/FAMILY EDUCATION
• Notify clinician of muscle weakness, fatigue, flaccid paralysis
• Take with food or milk for GI symptoms
• Take early in day to prevent nocturia

• Avoid large quantities of potassium-rich foods: oranges, bananas, salt substitutes

MONITORING PARAMETERS
• Electrolytes

---

aminocaproic acid
(a-mee-noe-ka-proe'ik)
Rx: Amicar
Chemical Class: Monoaminocarboxylic acid, synthetic
Therapeutic Class: Hemostatic

CLINICAL PHARMACOLOGY
Mechanism of Action: A systemic hemostatic that acts as an antifibrinolytic and antihemorrhagic by inhibiting the activation of plasminogen activator substances. *Therapeutic Effect:* Prevents formation of fibrin clots.

INDICATIONS AND DOSAGES
Acute bleeding
PO, IV infusion
Adults, Elderly. 4–5 g over first hr; then 1–1.25 g/hr. Continue for 8 hr or until bleeding is controlled. Maximum: 30 g/24 hr.
Children. 3 g/m^2 over first hr; then 1 g/m^2/hr. Maximum: 18 g/m^2/24 hr.
Dosage in renal impairment
Decrease dose to 25% of normal.

S AVAILABLE FORMS/COST
• Sol, Inj-IV: 250 mg/ml, 20 ml: **$17.70**
• Syr—Oral: 1.25 g/5 ml, 480 ml: **$371.89**
• Tab-Oral: 500 mg, 100's: **$153.79**
UNLABELED USES: Prevention of recurrence of subarachnoid hemorrhage, prevention of hemorrhage in hemophiliacs following dental surgery
CONTRAINDICATIONS: Evidence of active intravascular clotting process, disseminated intravascular coagulation without concurrent heparin therapy, hematuria of upper urinary tract origin (unless benefit outweighs risk); newborns (parenteral form).

PREGNANCY AND LACTATION: Pregnancy category C; excretion in milk unknown; use caution in nursing mothers

SIDE EFFECTS
Occasional
Nausea, diarrhea, cramps, decreased urination, decreased BP, dizziness, headache, muscle fatigue and weakness, myopathy, bloodshot eyes

SERIOUS REACTIONS
• Too rapid IV administration produces tinnitus, rash, arrhythmias, unusual fatigue, and weakness.
• Rarely, a grand mal seizure occurs, generally preceded by weakness, dizziness, and headache.

INTERACTIONS
Labs
• *False increase:* Urine amino acids
SPECIAL CONSIDERATIONS
PATIENT/FAMILY EDUCATION
• Report any signs of bleeding or myopathy
• Change position slowly to decrease orthostatic hypotension
• No need to adjust INR in warfarin anticoagulated patients with topical hemostatic mouthwash use
MONITORING PARAMETERS
• Do **not** administer without a definite diagnosis and laboratory findings indicative of hyperfibrinolysis
• Blood studies including coagulation factors, platelets, fibrinolysin; CPK, urinalysis

aminophylline
(am-in-off'i-lin)
Rx: Truphylline
Chemical Class: Ethylenedi-
amine derivative
Therapeutic Class: COPD
agent; antiasthmatic; bronchodilator

CLINICAL PHARMACOLOGY

Mechanism of Action: A xanthine
derivative that acts as a bronchodilator by directly relaxing smooth muscle of the bronchial airways and pulmonary blood vessels. *Therapeutic
Effect:* Relieves bronchospasm and
increases vital capacity.

INDICATIONS AND DOSAGES

Chronic bronchospasm

PO

Adults, Elderly, Children. 16 mg/kg
or 400 mg/day (whichever is less) in
3–4 divided doses (8-hr intervals);
may increase by 25% every 2–3
days. Maximum: 13 mg/kg/day
(children 13-16 yr); 18 mg/kg/day
(children 9-12 yr); 20 mg/kg/day
(children 1-8 yr). Maximum dosages are based on serum theophylline concentrations, clinical condition, and presence of toxicity.

*Acute bronchospasm in patients
not currently taking theophylline*

PO

Adults, children older than 1 yr. Initially, loading dose of 5 mg/kg (theophylline); then maintenance dosage
of theophylline based on patient
group (shown below).

Patient Group	Maintenance Theo-phylline Dosage
Healthy, nonsmok-ing adults	3 mg/kg q8h
Elderly patients, patients with cor pulmonale	2 mg/kg q8h
Patients with CHF or hepatic disease	1–2 mg/kg q12h
Children 9–16 yr, young adult smokers	3 mg/kg q6h
Children 1–8 yr	4 mg/kg q6h

IV

Adults, Children older than 1 yr. Initially, loading dose of 6 mg/kg (aminophylline); maintenance dosage of
aminophylline based on patient
group (shown below).

Patient Group	Maintenance Ami-nophylline Dosage
Healthy, nonsmok-ing adults	0.7 mg/kg/hr
Elderly patients, patients with cor pulmonale, CHF, or hepatic impairment	0.25 mg/kg/hr
Children 13–16 yr	0.7 mg/kg/hr
Children 9–12 yr, young adult smokers	0.9 mg/kg/hr
Children 1–8 yr	1–1.2 mg/kg/hr
Children 6 mo–1 yr	0.6–0.7 mg/kg/hr
Children 6 wk–6 mo	0.5 mg/kg/hr
Neonates	5 mg/kg q12h

*Acute bronchospasm in patients
currently taking theophylline*

PO, IV

Adults, children older than 1 yr. Obtain serum theophylline level. If not
possible and patient is in respiratory
distress and not experiencing toxic
effects, may give 2.5 mg/kg dose.
Maintenance: Dosage based on peak
serum theophylline concentration,
clinical condition, and presence of
toxicity.

S **AVAILABLE FORMS/COST**

• Sol, Inj-IV: 25 mg/ml, 10 ml:
$0.79-$1.68

• Sol-Oral: 105 mg/5 ml, 240 ml:
$10.05

• Supp-Rect: 250 mg, 10's: **$13.12-
$14.34**

• Tab-Oral: 100 mg, 100's:
$4.20-$6.05; 200 mg, 100's: **$3.31-
$6.79**

UNLABELED USES: Treatment of apnea in neonates

CONTRAINDICATIONS: History of hypersensitivity to caffeine or xanthine

PREGNANCY AND LACTATION: Pregnancy category C; pharmacokinetics of theophylline may be altered during pregnancy, monitor serum concentrations carefully; excreted into breast milk; may cause irritability in the nursing infant, otherwise compatible with breast-feeding

SIDE EFFECTS

Frequent

Altered smell (during IV administration), restlessness, tachycardia, tremor

Occasional

Heartburn, vomiting, headache, mild diuresis, insomnia, nausea

SERIOUS REACTIONS

• Too-rapid IV administration may produce marked hypotension with accompanying faintness, light-headedness, palpitations, tachycardia, hyperventilation, nausea, vomiting, angina-like pain, seizures, ventricular fibrillation, and cardiac standstill.

INTERACTIONS

Drugs

🔳 *Adenosine:* Decreased hemodynamic effects of adenosine

🔳 *Allopurinol, Amiodarone, Cimetidine, Ciprofloxacin, Disulfiram, Erythromycin, Interferon alfa, Isoniazid, Methimazole, Metoprolol, Norfloxacin, Pefloxacin, Pentoxifylline, Propafenone, Propylthiouracil, Radioactive iodine, Tacrine, Thiabendazole, Ticlopidine, Verapamil:* Increased theophylline concentrations

🔳 *Aminoglutethamide, Barbiturates, Carbamazepine, Moricizine, Phenytoin, Rifampin, Ritonavir,*

Thyroid hormone: Reduced theophylline concentrations; decreased serum phenytoin levels

🔳 *β-blockers:* Reduced bronchodilating response to theophylline

② *Enoxacin, Fluvoxamine, Mexiletine, Propranolol, Troleandomycin:* Markedly increased theophylline concentrations

🔳 *Imipenem:* Some patients on theophylline have developed seizures following addition of imipenem

🔳 *Lithium:* Reduced lithium concentrations

🔳 *Smoking:* Increased aminophylline dosing requirements

SPECIAL CONSIDERATIONS

PATIENT/FAMILY EDUCATION

• Avoid large amounts of caffeine-containing products

• If GI upset occurs, take with 8 oz water

• Notify clinician if nausea, vomiting, insomnia, jitteriness, headache, rash, palpitations occur

MONITORING PARAMETERS

• Serum theophylline concentrations every 6-12 mo or with status changes (therapeutic level is 10-20 mcg/ml); toxicity may occur with small increase above 20 mcg/ml, especially in the elderly

• Serious side effects (ventricular dysrhythmias, seizures, death) may occur without preceding signs of less serious toxicity (nausea, restlessness)

aminosalicylic acid

(a-mee-noe-sal-i-sil-ik as-id)

Rx: Aminosalicylic Acid, Paser D/R

Chemical Class: Salicylate derivative

Therapeutic Class: Antituberculosis agent

CLINICAL PHARMACOLOGY

Mechanism of Action: An antitubercular agent active against M. tuberculosis. Thought to exhibit competitive antagonism of folic acid synthesis. *Therapeutic Effect:* Bacteriostatic activity in susceptible microorganisms.

Pharmacokinetics

Readily absorbed from the gastrointestinal (GI) tract. Protein binding: 50-60%. Widely distributed (including cerebrospinal fluid [CSF]). Metabolized in liver. Primarily excreted in urine. Removed by hemodialysis. **Half-life:** 1.1-1.62 hrs.

INDICATIONS AND DOSAGES

Tuberculosis

PO

Adults, Elderly. 4 g in divided doses 3 times/day.

Children. 150 mg/kg/day in divided doses 3 times/day. Maximum: 12 g/day.

$ **AVAILABLE FORMS/COST**

• Granules, Sus Action-Oral: 4 g/packet, 30's: **$112.13**

UNLABELED USES: Crohn's disease, hyperlipidemia, ulcerative colitis

CONTRAINDICATIONS: End-stage renal disease, hypersensitivity to aminosalicylic acid products

PREGNANCY AND LACTATION: Pregnancy category C; excreted into breast milk; use caution in nursing mothers

SIDE EFFECTS

Occasional

Abdominal pain, diarrhea, nausea, vomiting

Rare

Hypersensitivity reactions, hepatotoxicity, thrombocytopenia

SERIOUS REACTIONS

• Liver toxicity and hepatitis, blood dyscrasias occur rarely.

• Agranulocytosis, methemoglobinemia, thrombocytopenia have been reported.

INTERACTIONS

Drugs

[2] *Vitamin B_{12}:* Vitamin B_{12} absorption reduced by 55%; Vitamin B_{12} maintenance should be considered for therapy of more than 1 month

[3] *Digoxin:* Reduced digoxin levels

Labs

• Aminosalicylic acid has been reported to interfere technically with the serum determinations of albumin by dye-binding, SGOT by the azoene dye method and with qualitative urine test for ketones, bilirubin, urobilinogen or porphobilinogen

SPECIAL CONSIDERATIONS

• If recognized promptly drug-induced hepatitis resolves quickly; 21% mortality if the reaction is unrecognized

• Desensitization has been accomplished with 10 mg aminosalicylic acid given as a single dose; double the dose q2 days until total of 1 gram then follow the regular schedule of administration; if a mild temperature rise or skin reaction develops, drop back one level or hold the progression for one cycle; reactions are rare after a total dosage of 1.5 g

PATIENT/FAMILY EDUCATION
• Sprinkle granules on apple sauce or yogurt or add to acidic juice such as orange, tomato, grape, apple, grapefruit, or cranberry; swirl well, granules sink
• Protect from moisture, light, and extremes of temperature; do not use if packets are swollen or if granules turn dark brown or purple
• Notify clinician if fever, sore throat, unusual bleeding, bruising, or skin rashes occur
• The skeleton of the granules may be seen in the stool

MONITORING PARAMETERS
• Monitor carefully in first 3 mo of therapy for signs of intolerance/drug-induced hepatitis (rash, fever, jaundice, hepatomegaly)

amiodarone
(a-mee'oh-da-rone)
Rx: Amiodarone Hydrochloride, Cordarone, Pacerone
Chemical Class: Iodinated benzofuran derivative
Therapeutic Class: Antiarrhythmic, class III

CLINICAL PHARMACOLOGY
Mechanism of Action: A cardiac agent that prolongs duration of myocardial cell action potential and refractory period by acting directly on all cardiac tissue. Decreases AV and sinus node function. *Therapeutic Effect:* Suppresses arrhythmias.
Pharmacokinetics

Route	*Onset*	*Peak*	*Duration*
PO	3 days–3 wk	1 wk–5 mo	7–50 days after discontinuation

Slowly, variably absorbed from GI tract. Protein binding: 96%. Extensively metabolized in the liver to active metabolite. Excreted via bile; not removed by hemodialysis. **Half-life:** 26–107 days; metabolite, 61 days.

INDICATIONS AND DOSAGES
Life-threatening recurrent ventricular fibrillation or hemodynamically unstable ventricular tachycardia
PO
Adults, Elderly. Initially, 800–1,600 mg/day in 2–4 divided doses for 1–3 wk. After arrhythmia is controlled or side effects occur, reduce to 600–800 mg/day for about 4 wk. Maintenance: 200–600 mg/day.
Children. Initially, 10–15 mg/kg/day for 4–14 days, then 5 mg/kg/day for several wk. Maintenance: 2.5 mg/kg or lowest effective maintenance dose for 5 of 7 days/wk.
IV infusion
Adults. Initially, 1,050 mg over 24 hr; 150 mg over 10 min, then 360 mg over 6 hr; then 540 mg over 18 hr. May continue at 0.5 mg/min for up to 2–3 wk regardless of age or renal or left ventricular function.

[$] AVAILABLE FORMS/COST
• Sol, Inj-IV: 50 mg/ml, 3 ml: **$8.38-$105.71**
• Tab-Oral: 200 mg, 100's: **$200.66-$405.00**; 400 mg, 30's: **$211.85**

UNLABELED USES: Treatment and prevention of supraventricular arrhythmias and symptomatic atrial flutter refractory to conventional treatment

CONTRAINDICATIONS: Bradycardia-induced syncope (except in the presence of a pacemaker), second- and third-degree AV block, severe hepatic disease, severe sinus-node dysfunction

PREGNANCY AND LACTATION: Pregnancy category D; due to a very long $t_{1/2}$, amiodarone should be discontinued several months prior to conception to avoid early gestational exposure, reserve for refractory dysrhythmias; newborns exposed to amiodarone should have TFTs; excreted into breast milk; contains high proportions of iodine; breast-feeding not recommended

SIDE EFFECTS

Expected

Corneal microdeposits are noted in almost all patients treated for more than 6 months (can lead to blurry vision).

Frequent (greater than 3%)

Parenteral: Hypotension, nausea, fever, bradycardia.

Oral: Constipation, headache, decreased appetite, nausea, vomiting, paresthesias, photosensitivity, muscular incoordination.

Occasional (less than 3%)

Oral: Bitter or metallic taste; decreased libido; dizziness; facial flushing; blue-gray coloring of skin (face, arms, and neck); blurred vision; bradycardia; asymptomatic corneal deposits.

Rare (less than 1%)

Oral: Rash, vision loss, blindness.

SERIOUS REACTIONS

• Serious, potentially fatal pulmonary toxicity (alveolitis, pulmonary fibrosis, pneumonitis, acute respiratory distress syndrome) may begin with progressive dyspnea and cough with crackles, decreased breath sounds, pleurisy, CHF or hepatotoxicity.

• Amiodarone may worsen existing arrhythmias or produce new arrhythmias (called proarrhythmias).

INTERACTIONS

Drugs

▣ *Aprinidine:* Increased aprinidine concentrations

▣ *β-adrenergic blockers:* Bradycardia, cardiac arrest, or ventricular arrhythmia shortly after initiation of β-adrenergic blockers that undergo extensive hepatic metabolism (propranolol, sotalol, metoprolol)

▣ *Calcium channel blockers:* Cardiotoxicity with bradycardia and decreased cardiac output with diltiazem and, potentially, verapamil

▣ *Cholestyramine, Colestipol:* Decreased amiodarone plasma concentrations

▣ *Cimetidine:* Increased amiodarone plasma concentrations (other H_2 blockers likely have no effect)

▣ *Cyclosporine, Tacrolimus:* Increased cyclosporine, tacrolimus concentrations

▣ *Digitalis glycosides:* Accumulation of digoxin

▣ *Fentanyl:* In combination with amiodarone may cause hypotension, bradycardia, and decreased cardiac output

▣ *Flecainide, Ecainide:* Increased flecainide, ecainide serum concentrations

▣ *Methotrexate:* Impaired methotrexate metabolism with >2 weeks oral amiodarone administration

▣ *Oral anticoagulants:* Enhanced hypoprothrombinemic response to warfarin (prothrombin time increased 100%), reduce warfarin dose 1/3-1/2

▣ *Phenytoin:* Increased serum phenytoin concentrations, decreased amiodarone concentrations

▣ *Procainamide:* Increased procainamide concentrations

▣ *Protease inhibitors (Indinavir):* Inceased amiodarone plasma concentrations

3 *Quinidine:* Increased quinidine plasma concentrations, reduce quinidine dose by ⅓

3 *Rifampin:* Decreased amiodarone plasma concentrations

3 *St. John's Wort (Hypericum perforatum):* Potential for decreased amiodarone plasma concentrations

3 *Theophylline:* Increased theophylline levels

3 *Volatile anesthetic agents:* Increased sensitivity to myocardial depressant and conduction effects of halogenated inhalational anesthetics

Labs
• *Increase:* Serum T4 and serum reverse T3
• *Decrease:* Serum T3

SPECIAL CONSIDERATIONS
• **Should be administered only by clinicians experienced in treatment of life-threatening dysrhythmias who are thoroughly familiar with the risks and benefits of amiodarone therapy**
• IV amiodarone contains the preservative benzyl alcohol which has been associated with fatal gasping syndrome in neonates

PATIENT/FAMILY EDUCATION
• Take with food and/or divide doses if GI intolerance occurs, do not take oral form with grapefruit juice
• Use sunscreen or stay out of sun to prevent burns
• Report side effects immediately
• Skin discoloration is usually reversible

MONITORING PARAMETERS
• Chest x-ray, ophth referral, and PFTs (baseline and q3 mo)
• Electrolytes
• LFTs
• ECG; QT interval prolongation of 10%-15% suggests therapeutic effect
• TFTs
• CNS symptoms

amitriptyline
(a-mee-trip'ti-leen)

Rx: Elavil
Combinations
  Rx: with chlordiazepoxide (Limbitrol); with perphenazine (Triavil)
Chemical Class: Dibenzocycloheptene derivative; tertiary amine
Therapeutic Class: Antidepressant, tricyclic; antineurolgic; anxiolytic

CLINICAL PHARMACOLOGY
Mechanism of Action: A tricyclic antidepressant that blocks the reuptake of neurotransmitters, including norepinephrine and serotonin, at presynaptic membranes, thus increasing their availability at postsynaptic receptor sites. Also has strong anticholinergic activity. *Therapeutic Effect:* Relieves depression.

Pharmacokinetics
Rapidly and well absorbed from the GI tract. Protein binding: 90%. Undergoes first-pass metabolism in the liver. Primarily excreted in urine. Minimal removal by hemodialysis. **Half-life:** 10–26 hr.

INDICATIONS AND DOSAGES
Depression
PO
Adults. 30–100 mg/day as a single dose at bedtime or in divided doses. May gradually increase up to 300 mg/day. Titrate to lowest effective dosage.
Elderly. Initially, 10–25 mg at bedtime. May increase by 10–25 mg at weekly intervals. Range: 25–150 mg/day.
Children 6–12 yr. 1–5 mg/kg/day in 2 divided doses.

IM
Adults. 20–30 mg 4 times a day.
Pain management
PO
Adults, Elderly. 25–100 mg at bedtime.

$ AVAILABLE FORMS/COST
• Sol, Inj-IM: 10 mg/ml, 10 ml: **$4.50**
• Tab, Coated-Oral: 10 mg, 100's: **$2.25-$27.51**; 25 mg, 100's: **$1.96-$69.95**; 50 mg, 100's: **$3.25-$116.45**; 75 mg, 100's: **$3.75-$134.43**; 100 mg, 100's: **$6.00-$133.50**; 150 mg, 100's: **$7.75-$206.67**

UNLABELED USES: Relief of neuropathic pain, such as that experienced by patients with diabetic neuropathy or postherpetic neuralgia; treatment of bulimia nervosa

CONTRAINDICATIONS: Acute recovery period after MI, use within 14 days of MAOIs

PREGNANCY AND LACTATION: Pregnancy category D; excreted into breast milk; effect on nursing infant unknown but may be of concern

SIDE EFFECTS
Frequent
Dizziness, somnolence, dry mouth, orthostatic hypotension, headache, increased appetite, weight gain, nausea, unusual fatigue, unpleasant taste
Occasional
Blurred vision, confusion, constipation, hallucinations, delayed micturition, eye pain, arrhythmias, fine muscle tremors, parkinsonian syndrome, anxiety, diarrhea, diaphoresis, heartburn, insomnia
Rare
Hypersensitivity, alopecia, tinnitus, breast enlargement, photosensitivity

SERIOUS REACTIONS
• Overdose may produce confusion, seizures, severe somnolence, arrhythmias, fever, hallucinations, agitation, dyspnea, vomiting, and unusual fatigue or weakness.
• Abrupt discontinuation after prolonged therapy may produce headache, malaise, nausea, vomiting, and vivid dreams.
• Blood dyscrasias and cholestatic jaundice occur rarely.

INTERACTIONS
Drugs
③ *Altretamine:* Orthostatic hypotension
③ *Amphetamines:* Theoretical increase in effect of amphetamines, clinical evidence lacking
③ *Anticholinergics:* Excessive anticholinergic effects
③ *Barbiturates:* Reduced serum concentrations of cyclic antidepressants
② *Bethanidine:* Reduced antihypertensive effect of bethanidine
③ *Carbamazepine:* Reduced antidepressant serum concentrations
③ *Cimetidine (other H_2 blockers less likely to have effect):* Inhibition of TCA metabolism
② *Clonidine:* Reduced antihypertensive response to clonidine; enhanced hypertensive response with abrupt clonidine withdrawal
② *Epinephrine, norepinephrine:* Enhanced pressor response
③ *Ethanol:* Additive impairment of motor skills; abstinent alcoholics may eliminate cyclic antidepressants more rapidly than non-alcoholics
③ *Fluoxetine, paroxetine:* Marked increases in cyclic antidepressant plasma concentrations
③ *Guanabenz, guanfacine, debrisoquin:* Inhibition of antihypertensive effect

❷ *Guanethidine, guanadrel:* Inhibited antihypertensive response to guanethidine

❸ *Hypoglycemics:* Enhanced hypoglemic effects

❸ *Isoproterenol:* Increased cardiac arrhythmias

❸ *Lithium:* Increased risk of neurotoxicity

❷ *MAOIs:* Excessive sympathetic response, mania, or hyperpyrexia possible

❷ *Moclobemide:* Potential association with fatal or non-fatal serotonin syndrome

❸ *Neuroleptics:* Increased therapeutic and toxic effects of both drugs

❷ *Norepinephrine:* Markedly enhanced pressor response to norepinephrine

❸ *Phenylephrine:* Enhanced pressor response

❸ *Propoxyphene:* Enhanced effect of cyclic antidepressants

❸ *Quinidine:* Increased cyclic antidepressant serum concentrations

❸ *Rifampin:* Possible decreased TCA levels

❸ *Ritonavir, indinavir:* Increased TCA levels

Labs

• *False increase:* Carbamazepine levels

SPECIAL CONSIDERATIONS

PATIENT/FAMILY EDUCATION

• Therapeutic effects may take 2-3 wk

• Use caution in driving or other activities requiring alertness

• Avoid rising quickly from sitting to standing, especially elderly

• Avoid alcohol ingestion, other CNS depressants

• Do not discontinue abruptly after long-term use

• Wear sunscreen or large hat to prevent photosensitivity

• Increase fluids, bulk in diet if constipation occurs

• Gum, hard sugarless candy, or frequent sips of water for dry mouth

MONITORING PARAMETERS

• Mental status: mood, sensorium, affect, suicidal tendencies

• Determination of amitriptyline plasma concentrations is not routinely recommended but may be useful in identifying toxicity, drug interactions, or noncompliance (adjustments in dosage should be made according to clinical response not plasma concentrations)

• Therapeutic plasma levels 125-250 mcg/L (including active metabolites)

---

amlexanox

(am-lecks-ah-knocks)

Rx: Aphthasol

Chemical Class: Benzopyrano-bipyridine carboxylic acid derivative

Therapeutic Class: Antiinflammatory

CLINICAL PHARMACOLOGY

Mechanism of Action: A mouth agent that has anti-allergic and antiinflammatory properties. Appears to inhibit formation and/or release of inflammatory mediators (e.g., histamine) from mast cells, neutrophils, mononuclear cells. *Therapeutic Effect:* Alleviates signs and symptoms of aphthous ulcers.

Pharmacokinetics

After topical application, most systemic absorption occurs from the gastrointestinal (GI) tract. Metabolized to inactive metabolite. Excreted in urine. **Half-life:** 3.5 hrs.

INDICATIONS AND DOSAGES

Aphthous ulcers

Topical

Adults, Elderly. Administer ¼ inch directly to ulcers 4 times/day (after meals and at bedtime) following oral hygiene.

[$] **AVAILABLE FORMS/COST**

• Paste-Top: 5%, 5g: **$20.88**

CONTRAINDICATIONS: Hypersensitivity to amlexanox or any component of the formulation

SIDE EFFECTS

Rare

Stinging, burning at administration site, transient pain, rash

SERIOUS REACTIONS

• Ingestion of a full tube would result in nausea, vomiting, and diarrhea.

amlodipine

(am-low′di-peen)

Rx: Norvasc

Combinations

Rx: with atorvastatin (Caduet); with benazepril (Lotrel)

Chemical Class: Dihydropyridine

Therapeutic Class: Antianginal; antihypertensive; calcium channel blocker

CLINICAL PHARMACOLOGY

Mechanism of Action: A calcium channel blocker that inhibits calcium movement across cardiac and vascular smooth-muscle cell membranes. *Therapeutic Effect:* Relieves angina by dilating coronary arteries, peripheral arteries, and arterioles. Decreases total peripheral vascular resistance and BP by vasodilation.

Pharmacokinetics

Route	Onset	Peak	Duration
PO	0.5–1 hr	6–12 hr	24 hr

Slowly absorbed from the GI tract. Protein binding: 93%. Undergoes first-pass metabolism in the liver. Excreted primarily in urine. Not removed by hemodialysis. **Half-life:** 30–50 hr (increased in the elderly and those with liver cirrhosis).

INDICATIONS AND DOSAGES

Hypertension

PO

Adults. Initially, 5 mg/day as a single dose. Maximum: 10 mg/day.

Small-Frame, Fragile, Elderly. Initially, 2.5 mg/day as a single dose.

Angina (chronic stable or vasospastic)

PO

Adults. 5–10 mg/day as a single dose.

Elderly, Patients with hepatic insufficiency: 5 mg/day as a single dose.

Dosage in renal impairment

For adults and elderly patients, give 2.5 mg/day.

[$] **AVAILABLE FORMS/COST**

• Tab-Oral: 2.5 mg, 90's: **$142.60**; 5 mg, 100's: **$145.11-$154.73**; 10 mg, 90's: **$195.70**

CONTRAINDICATIONS: Severe hypotension

PREGNANCY AND LACTATION: Pregnancy category C; unknown if excreted into milk; use caution in nursing mothers

SIDE EFFECTS

Frequent (greater than 5%)

Peripheral edema, headache, flushing

Occasional (less than 5%)

Dizziness, palpitations, nausea, unusual fatigue or weakness (asthenia)

Rare (less than 1%)

Chest pain, bradycardia, orthostatic hypotension

SERIOUS REACTIONS

• Overdose may produce excessive peripheral vasodilation and marked hypotension with reflex tachycardia.

INTERACTIONS

Drugs

▣ *Barbiturates:* Reduced plasma concentrations of amlodipine

▣ *Diltiazem:* Reduced clearance of amlodipine

▣ *Erythromycin:* Reduced clearance of amlodipine

▣ *Fentanyl:* Severe hypotension or increased fluid volume requirements

▣ *Grapefruit juice:* Reduced clearance of amlodipine

▣ *H₂ blockers:* Increased plasma concentration of amlodipine possible

▣ *Proton pump inhibitors:* Increased plasma concentration of amlodipine possible

▣ *Quinidine:* Increased plasma concentration of amlodipine; reduced plasma quinidine level

▣ *Rifampin:* Reduced plasma concentration of amlodipine

▣ *Vincristine:* Reduced vincristine clearance

SPECIAL CONSIDERATIONS
PATIENT/FAMILY EDUCATION

• Notify clinician of irregular heart beat, shortness of breath, swelling of feet and hands, pronounced dizziness, hypotension

ammonium lactate
Rx: Lac-Hydrin
Chemical Class: α-hydroxy acid
Therapeutic Class: Emollient

CLINICAL PHARMACOLOGY

Mechanism of Action: Lactic acid is an alpha-hydroxy acid that influences hydration, decreases corneocyte cohesion, reduces excessive epidermal keratinization in hyperkeratotic conditions, and induces synthesis of mucopolysaccharides and collagen in photodamaged skin. The exact mechanism is not known. *Therapeutic Effect:* Increases hydration of the skin.

Pharmacokinetics

Not known.

INDICATIONS AND DOSAGES

Treatment of ichthyosis vulgaris and xerosis

PO

Adults, Elderly. Apply sparingly and rub into area thoroughly q12h.

🅢 **AVAILABLE FORMS/COST**

• Cre-Top: 12%, 140, 280, 385 g: **$58.06**/385 g

• Lotion-Top: 12%, 225, 400 ml: **$10.84-$46.39**/225 ml; 5%, 120, 226 ml: **$5.81**/120 ml

• Sol: 500, 2500 ml: **$27.85**/500 ml

CONTRAINDICATIONS: Hypersensitivity to ammonium lactate.

PREGNANCY AND LACTATION: Pregnancy category C; unknown if excreted in breast milk; lactic acid is a normal constituent of blood and tissues

SIDE EFFECTS

Occasional (15%-2%)

Burning, stinging, rash, dry skin

SPECIAL CONSIDERATIONS
• Side effects greater in fair-skinned individuals, if applied to abraded or inflamed areas, and in ichthyosis (where incidence of burning, stinging, and erythema is 10%)

---

amobarbital
(am-oh-bar'bi-tal)
Rx: Amytal
Combinations
  Rx: with secobarbital (Tuinal)
Chemical Class: Barbituric acid derivative
Therapeutic Class: Sedative/hypnotic
DEA Class: Schedule II

CLINICAL PHARMACOLOGY
Mechanism of Action: A barbiturate that depresses the sensory cortex, decreases motor activity, and alters cerebellar function. *Therapeutic Effect:* Produces drowsiness, sedation, and hypnosis.
Pharmacokinetics
Readily absorbed from the gastrointestinal (GI) tract and distributed. Protein binding: 60%. Metabolized in liver primarily by the hepatic microsomal enzyme system. Primarily excreted in urine. **Half-life:** 16-40 hrs.

INDICATIONS AND DOSAGES
Hypnotic
IM/IV
Adults, Children older than 6 yrs. 65 to 200 mg at bedtime.
IM: Administer deeply into a large muscle. Do not use more than 5 ml at any single site (may cause tissue damage). Maximum: 500 mg.
IV: Use only when IM administration is not feasible. Administer by slow IV injection. Maximum: 50 mg/min in adults.

Children younger than 6 yrs. 2 to 3 mg/kg/dose.
Preanesthetic
IM/IV
Adults, Children older than 6 yrs. 65 to 500 mg at bedtime.
Sedative
IV
Adults. 30 to 50 mg given 2 or 3 times/day.

$ AVAILABLE FORMS/COST
• Powder, Inj-IM, IV: 0.5 g/vial: **$11.00**

UNLABELED USES: Anticonvulsant

CONTRAINDICATIONS: History of manifest or latent porphyria, marked liver dysfunction, marked respiratory disease in which dyspnea or obstruction is evident, and hypersensitivity to amobarbital products.

PREGNANCY AND LACTATION: Pregnancy category D; small amount excreted in breast milk, use caution in nursing mothers

SIDE EFFECTS
Frequent
Somnolence, headache, confusion, dizziness
Occasional
Nausea, vomiting, visual abnormalities, such as spots before eyes, difficulty focusing, blurred vision, dry mouth or pharynx, tongue irritation, water retention, increased sweating, constipation, or diarrhea

SERIOUS REACTIONS
• Overdosage results in severe respiratory depression, skeletal muscle flaccidity, bronchospasm, cardiovascular disturbances, such as congestive heart failure (CHF), hypotension or hypertension, arrhythmias, cold and clammy skin, cyanosis, and coma.
• Tolerance may occur with repeated use.

INTERACTIONS
Drugs

▪ *Acetaminophen:* Enhanced hepatotoxic potential of acetaminophen overdoses

▪ *Antidepressants:* Reduced serum concentration of cyclic antidepressants

▪ *β-adrenergic blockers:* Reduced serum concentrations of β-blockers which are extensively metabolized

▪ *Calcium channel blockers:* Reduced serum concentrations of verapamil and dihydropyridines

▪ *Chloramphenicol:* Increased barbiturate concentrations; reduced serum chloramphenicol concentrations

▪ *Corticosteroids:* Reduced serum concentrations of corticosteroids; may impair therapeutic effect

▪ *Cyclosporine:* Reduced serum concentration of cyclosporine

▪ *Digitoxin:* Reduced serum concentration of digitoxin

▪ *Disopyramide:* Reduced serum concentrations of disopyramide

▪ *Doxycycline:* Reduced serum doxycycline concentrations

▪ *Estrogen:* Reduced serum concentration of estrogen

▪ *Ethanol:* Excessive CNS depression

▪ *Griseofulvin:* Reduced griseofulvin absorption

▪ *Methoxyflurane:* Enhanced nephrotoxic effect

▪ *MAOIs:* Prolonged effect of barbiturates

▪ *Narcotic analgesics:* Increased toxicity of meperidine; reduced effect of methadone; additive CNS depression

▪ *Neuroleptics:* Reduced effect of either drug

❷ *Oral anticoagulants:* Decreased hypoprothrombinemic response to oral anticoagulants

▪ *Oral contraceptives:* Reduced efficacy of oral contraceptives

▪ *Phenytoin:* Unpredictable effect on serum phenytoin levels

▪ *Propafenone:* Reduced serum concentration of propafenone

▪ *Quinidine:* Reduced quinidine plasma concentrations

▪ *Tacrolimus:* Reduced serum concentration of tacrolimus

▪ *Theophylline:* Reduced serum theophylline concentrations

▪ *Valproic acid:* Increased serum concentration of amobarbital

❷ *Warfarin:* See oral anticoagulants

SPECIAL CONSIDERATIONS

PATIENT/FAMILY EDUCATION

• Indicated only for short-term treatment of insomnia; probably ineffective after 2 wk; physical dependency may result when used for extended time (45-90 days depending on dose)

• Avoid driving or other activities requiring alertness

• Avoid alcohol ingestion or CNS depressants

• Do not discontinue medication abruptly after long-term use

MONITORING PARAMETERS

• Serum folate, vitamin D (if on long-term therapy)

• PT in patients receiving anticoagulants

amoxapine
(a-moks-a-peen)
Rx: Asendin
Chemical Class: Dibenzocycloheptene derivative; secondary
amine
Therapeutic Class: Antidepressant, tricyclic

CLINICAL PHARMACOLOGY
Mechanism of Action: A tricyclic
antidepressant that blocks the reuptake of neurotransmitters, such as
norepinephrine and serotonin, at
central nervous system (CNS) presynaptic membranes, increasing
their availability at postsynaptic receptor sites. The metabolite, 7-OH-
amoxapine has significant dopamine receptor blocking activity similar to haloperidol. *Therapeutic Effect:* Produces antidepressant effects.

Pharmacokinetics
Rapidly, well absorbed from the
gastrointestinal (GI) tract. Protein
binding: 90%. Metabolized in liver.
Excreted in urine and feces. **Half-
life:** 8 hrs.

INDICATIONS AND DOSAGES
Depression
PO
Adults. 25 mg 2-3 times/day. May
icrease to 100 mg 2-3 times/day.
Adolescents. Initially, 25-50 mg/day
as single or divided doses. May increase to 100 mg/day.
Elderly. Initially, 25 mg at bedtime.
May increase by 25 mg/day q3-7
days. Maximum: 400 mg/day (outpatient), 600 mg/day (inpatient).
Ⓢ AVAILABLE FORMS/COST
• Tab-Oral: 25 mg, 100's: **$49.20-
$61.51**; 50 mg, 100's: **$84.20-
$99.95**; 100 mg, 100's: **$134.80-
$166.95**; 150 mg, 30's: **$62.95-
$78.99**

UNLABELED USES: Panic disorder
CONTRAINDICATIONS: Acute recovery period following myocardial
infarction (MI), within 14 days of
MAOI ingestion, hypersensitivity to
dibenzoxazepine compounds
PREGNANCY AND LACTATION:
Pregnancy category C; excreted into
breast milk; effect on nursing infant
unknown but may be of concern
SIDE EFFECTS
Frequent
Drowsiness, fatigue, xerostomia,
constipation, weight gain
Occasional
Nausea, dizziness, headache, confusion, nervousness, restlessness, insomnia, edema, tremor, blurred vision, aggressiveness, muscle weakness
Rare
Paradoxical reactions (agitation,
restlessness, nightmares, insomnia,
extrapyramidal symptoms, particularly fine hand tremor), laryngitis,
seizures
SERIOUS REACTIONS
• High dosage may produce cardiovascular effects, including severe
postural hypotension, dizziness,
tachycardia, palpitations, and arrhythmias, and seizures. High dosage may also result in altered temperature regulation, such as hyperpyrexia or hypothermia.
• Abrupt withdrawal from prolonged therapy may produce headache, malaise, nausea, vomiting,
and vivid dreams.
INTERACTIONS
Drugs
③ *Barbiturates:* Reduced serum
concentrations of cyclic antidepressants
② *Bethanidine:* Reduced antihypertensive effect of bethanidine
③ *Carbamazepine:* Reduced serum
concentrations of cyclic antidepressants

3 *Cimetidine:* Increased serum concentrations of cyclic antidepressants

3 *Clonidine:* Reduced antihypertensive effect of clonidine; enhanced hypertensive response with abrupt clonidine withdrawal

3 *Debrisoquin:* Reduced antihypertensive effect of debrisoquin

3 *Dilitiazem:* Increased serum concentrations of cyclic antidepressants

2 *Epinephrine:* Markedly enhanced pressor response to IV epinephrine

3 *Ethanol:* Additive impairment of motor skills; abstinent alcoholics may eliminate cyclic antidepressants more rapidly than non-alcoholics

3 *Fluoxetine:* Marked increases in serum concentrations of cyclic antidepressants

3 *Fluvoxamine:* Marked increases in serum concentrations of cyclic antidepressants

3 *Guanabenz, guanadrel, guanethidine, guanfacine:* Reduced antihypertensive effect

3 *Lithium:* Increased risk of neurotoxicity

2 *Moclobemide:* Potential association with fatal or non-fatal serotonin syndrome

⚠ *MAOIs:* Excessive sympathetic response, mania, or hyperpyrexia possible

3 *Neuroleptics:* Increased therapeutic and toxic effects of both drugs

2 *Norepinephrine:* Markedly enhanced pressor response to IV norepinephrine

3 *Paroxetine:* Marked increases in serum concentrations of cyclic antidepressants

3 *Propoxyphene:* Increased serum concentrations of cyclic antidepressants

3 *Quinidine:* Increased serum concentrations of cyclic antidepressants

3 *Rifampin:* Reduced serum concentrations of cyclic antidepressants

3 *Ritonavir:* Marked increases in serum concentrations of cyclic antidepressants

3 *Sulfonylureas:* Cyclic antidepressants may increase hypoglycemic effect

SPECIAL CONSIDERATIONS

PATIENT/FAMILY EDUCATION

• Therapeutic effects may take 2-3 wk

• Use caution in driving or other activities requiring alertness

• Avoid rising quickly from sitting to standing, especially elderly

• Avoid alcohol ingestion, other CNS depressants

• Do not discontinue abruptly after long-term use

• Wear sunscreen or large hat to prevent photosensitivity

• Increase fluids, bulk in diet if constipation occurs

• Use gum, hard sugarless candy, or frequent sips of water for dry mouth

• Potential for tardive dyskinesia

---

amoxicillin

(a-mox'i-sill-in)

Rx: Amoxil, Moxilin, Senox, Trimox, Wymox

Chemical Class: Penicillin derivative, aminopenicillin

Therapeutic Class: Antibiotic

CLINICAL PHARMACOLOGY

Mechanism of Action: A penicillin that inhibits bacterial cell wall synthesis. *Therapeutic Effect:* Bactericidal in susceptible microorganisms.

[A]

Pharmacokinetics

Well absorbed from the GI tract. Protein binding: 20%. Partially metabolized in the liver. Primarily excreted in urine. Removed by hemodialysis. **Half-life:** 1-1.3 hr (increased in impaired renal function).

INDICATIONS AND DOSAGES

Ear, nose, throat, GU, skin, and skin-structure infections

PO

Adults, Elderly, Children weighing more than 20 kg. 250-500 mg q8h or 500-875 mg (tablets) twice a day

Children weighing less than 20 kg. 20-40 mg/kg/day in divided doses q8-12h.

Lower respiratory tract infections

PO

Adults, Elderly, Children weighing more than 20 kg. 500 mg q8h or 875 mg (tablets) twice a day.

Children weighing less than 20 kg. 40 mg/kg/day in divided doses q8-12h.

Acute, uncomplicated gonorrhea

PO

Adults. 3 g one time with 1 g probenecid. Follow with tetracycline or erythromycin therapy.

Children 2 yr and older. 50 mg/kg plus probenecid 25 mg/kg as a single dose.

Acute otitis media

PO

Children. 80-90 mg/kg/day in divided doses q12h.

Helicobacter pylori infection

PO

Adults, Elderly. 1 g twice a day for 10 days (in combination with other antibiotics).

Prevention of endocarditis

PO

Adults, Elderly. 2 g 1 hr before procedure.

Children. 50 mg/kg 1 hr before procedure.

Usual pediatric dosage

Children younger than 3 mo, Neonates. 20-30 mg/kg/day in divided doses q12h.

Dosage in renal impairment

Dosage interval is modified based on creatinine clearance.

Creatinine clearance 10-30 ml/min. Usual dose q12h.

Creatinine clearance less than 10 ml/min. Usual dose q24h.

$ **AVAILABLE FORMS/COST**

- Cap, Gel—Oral: 250 mg, 100's: **$5.82-$33.25**; 500 mg, 100's: **$8.65-$58.75**; 875 mg, 100's: **$87.21-$96.90**
- Powder, Reconst—Oral: 50 mg/ml, 15, 30 ml: **$1.80-$2.65**/15 ml; 125 mg/5 ml, 80, 100, 150 ml: **$2.49-$9.55**/150 ml; 200 mg/5 ml, 50, 75, 100 ml: **$9.14-$10.15**/100 ml; 250 mg/5 ml, 80, 100, 150, 200 ml: **$2.81-$10.43**/150 ml; 400 mg/5 ml; 50, 75, 100 ml: **$9.81-$10.90**/100 ml
- Tab-Oral: 500 mg, 100's: **$49.81-$55.35**; 875 mg, 100's: **$87.21-$96.90**
- Tab, Chewable—Oral: 125 mg, 100's: **$11.00-$24.65**; 200 mg, 100's: **$50.75**; 250 mg, 100's: **$22.82-$45.00**; 400 mg, 100's: **$62.00**

UNLABELED USES: Treatment of Lyme disease and typhoid fever

CONTRAINDICATIONS: Hypersensitivity to any penicillin, infectious mononucleosis

PREGNANCY AND LACTATION: Pregnancy category B; excreted into breast milk in low concentrations; no adverse effects have been observed, but potential exists for modification of bowel flora and allergy/sensitization in nursing infant

SIDE EFFECTS

Frequent

GI disturbances (mild diarrhea, nausea, or vomiting), headache, oral or vaginal candidiasis

Occasional

Generalized rash, urticaria

SERIOUS REACTIONS

• Antibiotic-associated colitis and other superinfections may result from altered bacterial balance.

• Severe hypersensitivity reactions, including anaphylaxis and acute interstitial nephritis occur rarely.

INTERACTIONS

Drugs

▣ *Atenolol:* Reduced serum concentration of atenolol

▣ *Chloramphenicol:* Inhibited antibacterial activity of amoxicillin; administer amoxicillin 3 hours before chloramphenicol

▣ *Macrolide antibiotics:* Inhibited antibacterial activity of amoxicillin; administer amoxicillin 3 hours before macrolides

▣ *Methotrexate:* Increased serum methotrexate concentrations

▣ *Oral contraceptives:* Occasional impairment of oral contraceptive efficacy; consider use of supplementary contraception during cycles in which amoxicillin is used

▣ *Tetracyclines:* Inhibited antibacterial activity of amoxicillin; administer amoxicillin 3 hours before tetracycline

SPECIAL CONSIDERATIONS

PATIENT/FAMILY EDUCATION

• May administer on a full or empty stomach

• Administer at even intervals

• Shake oral suspensions well before administering; discard after 14 days

• High rates of rash in patients on allopurinol, with mononucleosis, lymphocytic leukemia

amoxicillin/ clavulanate

(a-mox'i-sill-in clav-u-lan'ate)

Rx: Augmentin, Augmentin XR, Augmentin ES-600

Chemical Class: Penicillin derivative, aminopenicillin; β-lactamase inhibitor (clavulanate)

Therapeutic Class: Antibiotic

CLINICAL PHARMACOLOGY

Mechanism of Action: Amoxicillin inhibits bacterial cell wall synthesis, while clavulanate inhibits bacterial beta-lactamase. *Therapeutic Effect:* Amoxicillin is bactericidal in susceptible microorganisms. Clavulanate protects amoxicillin from enzymatic degradation.

Pharmacokinetics

Well absorbed from the GI tract. Protein binding: 20%. Partially metabolized in the liver. Primarily excreted in urine. Removed by hemodialysis. **Half-life:** 1–1.3 hr (increased in impaired renal function).

INDICATIONS AND DOSAGES

Mild to moderate infections

PO

Adults, Elderly, Children weighing more than 40 kg. 250 mg q8h or 500 mg q12h.

Children weighing less than 40 kg. 20 mg/kg/day in divided doses q8h.

Respiratory tract and other severe infections

PO

Adults, Elderly, Children weighing more than 40 kg. 500 mg q8h or 875 mg q12h.

Children weighing less than 40 kg. 40 mg/kg/day in divided doses q8h.

Otitis media

PO

Children. 90 mg/kg/day in divided doses q12h for 10 days.

Sinusitis, lower respiratory tract infections
PO
Children. 40 mg/kg/day in divided doses q8h or 45 mg/kg/day in divided doses q12h.
Usual neonate dosage
PO
Neonates, Children younger than 3 mos. 30 mg/kg/day in divided doses q12h.
Dosage in renal impairment
Dosage and frequency are modified based on creatinine clearance.
Creatinine clearance 10–30 ml/min: 250–500 mg q12h.
Creatinine clearance less than 10 ml/min: 250–500 mg q24h.

§ AVAILABLE FORMS/COST
• Powder, Reconst—Oral: 125 mg-31.25 mg/5 ml, 75, 100, 150 ml: **$32.24-$43.20**/150 ml; 200 mg-28.5 mg/5 ml, 50, 75, 100 ml: **$36.17-$41.80**/100 ml; 250 mg-62.5 mg/5 ml, 75, 100, 150 ml: **$61.98-$87.24**/150 ml; 400 mg-57 mg/5 ml, 50, 75, 100 ml: **$56.15-$85.77**/100 ml; 600 mg-42.9 mg/5 ml, 75, 125, 200 ml: **$65.04**/125 ml
• Tab, Chewable—Oral: 125 mg-31.25 mg, 30's: **$30.20-$41.54**; 200 mg-28.5 mg, 20's: **$41.80**; 250 mg-62.5 mg, 30's: **$52.51-$92.27**; 400 mg-57 mg, 20's: **$79.65**
• Tab-Oral: 250 mg-125 mg, 100's: **$255.48**; 500 mg-125 mg, 100's: **$332.32**; 875 mg-125 mg, 20's: **$101.03-$119.13**
• Tab, Sus Action—Oral: 1000 mg-62.5 mg, 28's: **$78.46**
NOTE: Due to clavulanate strength, 2×250 mg tabs do not equal a 500 mg tab
UNLABELED USES: Treatment of bronchitis and chancroid
CONTRAINDICATIONS: Hypersensitivity to any penicillins, infectious mononucleosis

PREGNANCY AND LACTATION: Pregnancy category B; excreted into breast milk in low concentrations; no adverse effects have been observed
SIDE EFFECTS
Frequent
GI disturbances (mild diarrhea, nausea, vomiting), headache, oral or vaginal candidiasis
Occasional
Generalized rash, urticaria
SERIOUS REACTIONS
• Antibiotic-associated colitis and other superinfections may result from altered bacterial balance.
• Severe hypersensitivity reactions, including anaphylaxis and acute interstitial nephritis occur rarely.
INTERACTIONS
Drugs
▣ *Atenolol:* Reduced serum concentration of atenolol
▣ *Chloramphenicol:* Inhibited antibacterial activity of amoxicillin; administer amoxicillin 3 hours before chloramphenicol
▣ *Macrolide antibiotics:* Inhibited antibacterial activity of amoxicillin; administer amoxicillin 3 hours before macrolides
▣ *Methotrexate:* Increased serum methotrexate concentrations
▣ *Oral contraceptives:* Occasional impairment of oral contraceptive efficacy; consider use of supplementary contraception during cycles in which amoxicillin is used
▣ *Tetracyclines:* Inhibited antibacterial activity of amoxicillin; administer amoxicillin 3 hours before tetracycline
SPECIAL CONSIDERATIONS
• Augmentin XR indicated for treatment of community acquired pneumonia or bacterial sinusitis due to β-lactamase-producing strains with reduced penicillin susceptibility

• Augmentin ES indicated for otitis media (AOM) in pediatric patients with antibiotic treatment for AOM in previous 3 mos and either ≤age 2 or attending daycare

PATIENT/FAMILY EDUCATION

• Administer with food to decrease GI side effects
• Administer at even intervals
• Shake oral suspensions well before administering; discard after 14 days; must be refrigerated

---

amphetamine

(am-fet'ah-meen)
Combinations

Rx: with dextroamphetamine: (Adderall, Adderall XR)
Chemical Class: β-phenyliso-propylamine (racemic)
Therapeutic Class: Central nervous system stimulant
DEA Class: Schedule II

CLINICAL PHARMACOLOGY
Mechanism of Action: A sympatho-mimetic amine that produces central nervous system (CNS) and respiratory stimulation, mydriasis, bronchodilation, a pressor response, and contraction of the urinary sphincter. Directly effects alpha and beta receptor sites in peripheral system. Enhances release of norepinephrine by blocking reuptake, inhibiting monoamine oxidase. *Therapeutic Effect:* Increases motor activity, mental alertness; decreases drowsiness, fatigue.

Pharmacokinetics

Well absorbed from the gastrointestinal (GI) tract. Protein binding: 20%. Widely distributed (including CSF). Metabolized in liver. Excreted in urine. Unknown if removed by hemodialysis. **Half-life:** 7-31 hrs.

INDICATIONS AND DOSAGES
Attention-deficit hyperactivity disorder (ADHD)
PO
Adults. 5-20 mg 1-3 times/day.
Adults, Children older than 12 yrs. Initially, 5 mg twice a day. Increase by 10 mg at weekly intervals until therapeutic response achieved.
Children 6-12 yrs. Initially, 2.5 mg twice a day. Increase by 5 mg/day at weekly intervals until therapeutic response achieved.
Children 3-6 yrs. Initially, 2.5 mg twice a day. Increase by 2.5 mg/day at weekly intervals until therapeutic response achieved.

Narcolepsy
PO
Adults. 5-20 mg 1-3 times/day.
Adults, Children older than 12 yrs. Initially, 5 mg twice a day. Increase by 10 mg at weekly intervals until therapeutic response achieved.
Children 6-12 yrs. Initially, 2.5 mg twice a day. Increase by 5 mg/day at weekly intervals until therapeutic response achieved.

S AVAILABLE FORMS/COST
• Tab, with dextroamphetamine— Oral: 5-1.25 mg, 7.5-1.875 mg, 10-2.5 mg, 12.5-3.125 mg, 15-3.75 mg, 20-5 mg, 30-7.5 mg, 100's; all: **$181.74**
• Tab, with dextroamphetamine— Sus Action: 5-1.25 mg, 10-2.5 mg, 15-3.75 mg, 20-5 mg, 25-6.25 mg, 30-7.5 mg, 100's; all: **$298.61**

UNLABELED USES: Depression, obsessive-compulsive disorder

CONTRAINDICATIONS: Advanced arteriosclerosis, agitated states, glaucoma, history of drug abuse, history of hypersensitivity to sympathomimetic amines, hyperthyroidism, moderate to severe hypertension, symptomatic cardiovascular disease, within 14 days following discontinuation of an MAOI

PREGNANCY AND LACTATION:
Pregnancy category C; use of amphetamine for medical indications not a significant risk to the fetus for congenital anomalies, mild withdrawal symptoms may be observed in the newborn; illicit maternal use presents significant risks to the fetus and newborn, including intrauterine growth retardation, premature delivery, and the potential for increased maternal, fetal, and neonatal morbidity; concentrated in breast milk; contraindicated during breastfeeding

SIDE EFFECTS

Frequent

Irregular pulse, increased motor activity, talkativeness, nervousness, mild euphoria, insomnia

Occasional

Headache, chills, dry mouth, gastrointestinal (GI) distress, worsening depression in patients who are clinically depressed, tachycardia, palpitations, chest pain

SERIOUS REACTIONS

• Overdose may produce skin pallor or flushing, arrhythmias, and psychosis.

• Abrupt withdrawal following prolonged administration of high dosage may produce lethargy (may last for weeks).

• Prolonged administration to children with ADHD may produce a temporary suppression of normal weight and height patterns.

INTERACTIONS

Drugs

3 *Antacids:* May inhibit amphetamine excretion

3 *Ethosuximide:* Intestinal absorption of ethosuximide may be delayed

3 *Furazolidone:* Hypertensive reactions

3 *Guanadrel:* Inhibits antihypertensive response to guanadrel

3 *Guanethidine:* Inhibits antihypertensive response to guanethidine

3 *Lithium:* May inhibit effects of amphetamines

⚠ *MAOIs:* Severe hypertensive reactions possible

3 *Methenamine:* Urinary excretion of amphetamine is increased by acidifying agents

2 *Norepinephrine:* Adrenergic effect of norepinephrine enhanced

3 *Phenobarbital:* Intestinal absorption of phenobarbital may be delayed; synergistic anticonvulsant effect possible

3 *Phenytoin:* Intestinal absorption of phenytoin may be delayed; synergistic anticonvulsant effect possible

⚠ *Propoxyphene:* In cases of propoxyphene overdosage, amphetamine CNS stimulation is potentiated, fatal convulsions can occur

2 *Selegiline:* Severe hypertensive reactions possible

3 *Sodium bicarbonate:* May inhibit amphetamine excretion

2 *Tricyclic antidepressants:* May enhance activity of tricyclics; increased amphetamine levels in the brain; CV effects potentiated

Labs

• *False positive:* Urine amino acids

• May interfere with urinary steroid determinations

SPECIAL CONSIDERATIONS

PATIENT/FAMILY EDUCATION

• Take early in the day

• Do not discontinue abruptly

• Avoid hazardous activities until stabilized on medication

amphotericin B / amphotericin B cholesteryl / amphotericin B lipid complex / liposomal amphotericin B

Rx: Abelcet (ABLC);
AmBisome, Amphotec,
Fungizone (IV and topical)
Chemical Class: Amphoteric
polyene lipid complex (ABLC)
Therapeutic Class: Antifungal

CLINICAL PHARMACOLOGY

Mechanism of Action: The amphotericin B group is antifungal and antiprotozoal and generally fungistatic but may become fungicidal with high dosages or very susceptible microorganisms. This drug binds to sterols in the fungal cell membrane. *Therapeutic Effect:* Increases fungal cell-membrane permeability, allowing loss of potassium, and other cellular components.

Pharmacokinetics

Protein binding: 90%. Widely distributed. Metabolic fate unknown. Cleared by nonrenal pathways. Minimal removal by hemodialysis. Amphotec and Abelcet are not dialyzable. **Half-life:** 24 hrs (half-life increased in neonates, children). Amphotec **half-life:** 26-28 hrs. Abelcet **half-life:** 7.2 days. AmBisome **half-life:** 100-153 hrs.

INDICATIONS AND DOSAGES

Invasive fungal infections unresponsive or intolerant to Fungizone (Abelcet)
IV Infusion
Adults, Children. 5 mg/kg at rate of 2.5 mg/kg/hr.

Empiric treatment for fungal infection in patients with febrile neutropenia; for aspergillus, candida, or cryptococcus infections unresponsive to Fungizone; or for patients with renal impairment or toxicity from Fungizone (AmBisome)
IV Infusion
Adults, Children. 3-5 mg/kg over 1 hr.

Invasive aspergillus in patients with renal impairment, renal toxicity, or treatment failure with Fungizone (Amphotec)
IV Infusion
Adults, Children. 3-4 mg/kg over 2-4 hrs.

Cutaneous and mucocutaneous infections caused by Candida albicans, such as paronychia, oral thrush, perlèche, diaper rash, and intertriginous candidiasis (Topical)
Adults, Elderly, Children. Apply liberally to the affected area and rub in 2-4 times/day.

Cryptococcosis; blastomycosis; systemic candidiasis; disseminated forms of moniliasis, coccidioidomycosis, and histoplasmosis; zygomycosis; sporotrichosis; and aspergillosis (Fungizone)
IV Infusion
Adults, Elderly. Dosage based on pt tolerance, severity of infection. Initially, 1-mg test dose is given over 20-30 min. If test dose is tolerated, 5-mg dose may be given the same day. Subsequently, increases of 5 mg/dose are made q12-24h until desired daily dose is reached. Alternatively, if test dose is tolerated, a dose of 0.25 mg/kg is given same day; increased to 0.5 mg/kg the second day. Dose increased until desired daily dose reached. Total daily dose: 1 mg/kg/day up to 1.5 mg/kg every other day. Do not exceed maximum total daily dose of 1.5 mg/kg.

Children. Test dose: 0.1 mg/kg/dose (maximum 1 mg) infused over 20-60 min. If tolerated, then initial dose: 0.4 mg/kg same day; Dose may be increased in 0.25 mg/kg increments. Maintenance dose: 0.25-1 mg/kg/day.

$ AVAILABLE FORMS/COST
ABLC
• Sol, Inj-IV: 5 mg/ml, 10 ml: **$134.66**
Amphotericin B
• Powder, Inj-IV: 50 mg vial, 1's: **$10.00-$20.45**
Amphotericin B Cholesteryl Sulfate
• Powder, Inj-IV: 50 mg vial, 1's: **$93.33**; 100 mg vial, 1's: **$160.00**
Amphotericin B Liposomal
• Powder, Inj-IV: 50 mg vial, 1's: **$196.25**
CONTRAINDICATIONS: Hypersensitivity to amphotericin B, sulfite
PREGNANCY AND LACTATION: Pregnancy category B; excretion in human milk unknown; due to the potential toxicity, consider discontinuing nursing
SIDE EFFECTS
Frequent (greater than 10%)
Abelcet: Chills, fever, increased serum creatinine, multiple organ failure
AmBisome: Hypokalemia, hypomagnesemia, hyperglycemia, hypocalcemia, edema, abdominal pain, back pain, chills, chest pain, hypotension, diarrhea, nausea, vomiting, headache, fever, rigors, insomnia, dyspnea, epistaxis, increased liver/renal function test results
Amphotec: Chills, fever, hypotension, tachycardia, increased creatinine, hypokalemia, bilirubinemia
Fungizone: Fever, chills, headache, anemia, hypokalemia, hypomagnesemia, anorexia, malaise, generalized pain, nephrotoxicity
Topical: Local irritation, dry skin

Rare
Topical: Skin rash
SERIOUS REACTIONS
• Cardiovascular toxicity as evidenced by hypotension and ventricular fibrillation and anaphylaxis occur rarely.
• Vision and hearing alterations, seizures, liver failure, coagulation defects, multiple organ failure, and sepsis may be noted.
INTERACTIONS
Drugs
▣ *Aminoglycosides:* Synergistic nephrotoxicity
▣ *Cyclosporine:* Increased nephrotoxicity of both drugs
▣ *Neuromuscular blocking agents:* Prolonged muscle relaxation due to hypokalemia
Labs
• *Increase:* Serum bilirubin, serum conjugated bilirubin, serum cholesterol
• *Decrease:* Serum unconjugated bilirubin

SPECIAL CONSIDERATIONS
PATIENT/FAMILY EDUCATION
• Long-term therapy may be needed to clear infection (2 wk-3 mo depending on type of infection)
MONITORING PARAMETERS
• BUN, serum creatinine; if BUN exceeds 40 mg/dl or serum creatinine exceeds 3 mg/dl, discontinue the drug or reduce dosage until renal function improves
• Regular monitoring of CBC, K, Na, Mg, LFTs
• Total dosage

ampicillin

(am'pi-sill-in)

Rx: Marcillin, Principen, Totacillin

Combinations

Rx: with probenecid (Polycillin PRB, Probampin)

Chemical Class: Penicillin derivative, aminopenicillin

Therapeutic Class: Antibiotic

CLINICAL PHARMACOLOGY

Mechanism of Action: A penicillin that inhibits cell wall synthesis in susceptible microorganisms. *Therapeutic Effect:* Produces bactericidal effect.

Pharmacokinetics

Moderately absorbed from the gastrointestinal (GI) tract. Protein binding: 28%. Widely distributed. Partially metabolized in liver. Primarily excreted in urine. Removed by hemodialysis. **Half-life:** 1-1.9 hrs (half-life increased in impaired renal function).

INDICATIONS AND DOSAGES

Respiratory tract, skin/skin-structure infections

PO

Adults, Elderly, Children weighing more than 20 kg. 250-500 mg q6h.

Children weighing less than 20 kg. 50 mg/kg/day in divided doses q6h.

IM/IV

Adults, Elderly, Children weighing more than 40 kg. 250-500 mg q6h.

Children weighing less than 40 kg. 25-50 mg/kg/day in divided doses q6-8h. Bacterial meningitis, septicemia

IM/IV

Adults, Elderly. 2 g q4h or 3 g q6h. Children. 100-200 mg/kg/day in divided doses q4h. Gonococcal infections

PO

Adults. 3.5 g one time with 1 g probenecid. Perioperative prophylaxis

IM/IV

Adults, Elderly. 2 g 30 min before procedure. May repeat in 8 hrs.

Children. 50 mg/kg using same dosage regimen. Usual neonate dosage

IM/IV

Neonates 7-28 days old. 75 mg/kg/day in divided doses q8h up to 200 mg/kg/day in divided doses q6h.

Neonates 0-7 days old. 50 mg/kg/day in divided doses q12h up to 150 mg/kg/day in divided doses q8h.

$ AVAILABLE FORMS/COST

• Cap, Gel—Oral: 250 mg, 100's: **$7.43-$23.46**; 500 mg, 100's: **$16.04-$37.89**

• Powder, Inj-IM, IV: 125 mg/vial, 1's: **$1.35-$1.58**; 250 mg/vial, 1's: **$0.79-$1.62**; 500 mg/vial, 1's: **$1.04-$4.31**; 1 g/vial, 1's: **$1.49-$8.89**; 2 g/vial, 1's: **$2.43-$16.24**

• Powder, Reconst—Oral: 125 mg/5 ml, 100, 200 ml: **$3.96-$9.69**/200 ml; 250 mg/5 ml, 100, 200 ml: **$6.50-$15.64**/200 ml

CONTRAINDICATIONS: Hypersensitivity to any penicillin, infectious mononucleosis

PREGNANCY AND LACTATION: Pregnancy category B; excreted into breast milk in low concentrations; no adverse effects have been observed

SIDE EFFECTS

Frequent

Pain at IM injection site, GI disturbances, including mild diarrhea, nausea, or vomiting, oral or vaginal candidiasis

Occasional

Generalized rash, urticaria, phlebitis, thrombophlebitis with IV administration, headache

Rare

Dizziness, seizures, especially with IV therapy

SERIOUS REACTIONS

• Altered bacterial balance may result in potentially fatal superinfections and antibiotic-associated colitis as evidenced by abdominal cramps, watery or severe diarrhea, and fever.

• Severe hypersensitivity reactions, including anaphylaxis and acute interstitial nephritis occur rarely.

INTERACTIONS

Drugs

▣ *Atenolol:* Reduced serum concentration of atenolol

▣ *Chloramphenicol:* Inhibited antibacterial activity of ampicillin; administer ampicillin 3 hr before chloramphenicol

▣ *Macrolide antibiotics:* Inhibited antibacterial activity of ampicillin; administer amoxicillin 3 hr before macrolides

▣ *Methotrexate:* Increased serum methotrexate concentrations

▣ *Oral contraceptives:* Occasional impairment of oral contraceptive efficacy; consider use of supplemental contraception during cycles in which ampicillin is used

▣ *Tetracyclines:* Inhibited antibacterial activity of ampicillin; administer ampicillin 3 hr before tetracycline

Labs

• *False positive:* Urine amino acids

• *Increase:* Urine glucose (Clinitest method), plasma phenyldanine (dried blood spot method), CSF protein (Ektachem method), serum protein (Biuret method), serum theophylline (3M Diagnostics TheoFast method), serum uric acid

• *Decrease:* Serum cholesterol (CHOD-iodide method only), serum folate (bioassay method only), urine glucose (Clinistix and Diastix methods)

SPECIAL CONSIDERATIONS

PATIENT/FAMILY EDUCATION

• Administer on an empty stomach

• Administer at even intervals

• Shake oral suspensions well before administering, discard after 14 days

• High rates of rash in patients on allopurinol, with mononucleosis, lymphatic leukemia

• Amoxicillin is better oral choice given greater ease of dosing and lower incidence of diarrhea

---

ampicillin/sulbactam

(am′pi-sill-in/sul-bac′tam)

Rx: Unasyn

Chemical Class: Penicillin derivative, aminopenicillin; penicillinate (sulbactam)

Therapeutic Class: Antibiotic

CLINICAL PHARMACOLOGY

Mechanism of Action: Ampicillin inhibits bacterial cell wall synthesis, while sulbactam inhibits bacterial beta-lactamase. *Therapeutic Effect:* Ampicillin is bactericidal in susceptible microorganisms. Sulbactam protects ampicillin from enzymatic degradation

Pharmacokinetics

Protein binding: 28%-38%. Widely distributed. Partially metabolized in the liver. Primarily excreted in urine. Removed by hemodialysis. **Half-life:** 1 hr (increased in impaired renal function).

INDICATIONS AND DOSAGES

Skin/skin-structure, intraabdominal, and gynecologic infections

IV, IM

Adults, Elderly. 1.5 g (1 g ampicillin/500 mg sulbactam) to 3 g (2 g ampicillin/1 g sulbactam) q6h.

Skin and skin-structure infections

IV

Children 1-12 yr. 150-300 mg/kg/day in divided doses q6h.

Dosage in renal impairment

Dosage and frequency are modified based on creatinine clearance and the severity of the infection.

Creatinine Clearance	*Dosage*
greater than 30 ml/min	0.5-3 g q6-8h
15-29 ml/min	1.5-3 g q12h
5-14 ml/min	1.5-3 g q24h
less than 5 ml/min	Not recommended

$ **AVAILABLE FORMS/COST**

• Powder, Inj-IM, IV: 1.5 g, (1 g ampicillin + 0.5 g sulbactam) 1's: **$7.81-$9.43**; 3.0 g, (2 g ampicillin + 1 g sulbactam) 1's: **$14.74-$16.24**

CONTRAINDICATIONS: Hypersensitivity to any penicillin, infectious mononucleosis

PREGNANCY AND LACTATION: Pregnancy category B; animal studies at doses 10× the human dose reveal no evidence of harm; low concentrations excreted in breast milk

SIDE EFFECTS

Frequent

Diarrhea and rash (most common), urticaria, pain at IM injection site, thrombophlebitis with IV administration, oral or vaginal candidiasis

Occasional

Nausea, vomiting, headache, malaise, urine retention

SERIOUS REACTIONS

• Severe hypersensitivity reactions, including anaphylaxis, acute interstitial nephritis, and blood dyscrasias may occur.

• Antibiotic-associated colitis and other superinfections may result from altered bacterial balance.

• Overdose may produce seizures.

INTERACTIONS

Drugs

[3] *Chloramphenicol:* Inhibited antibacterial activity of ampicillin/sulbactam; administer ampicillin/sulbactam 3 hr before chloramphenicol

[3] *Macrolide antibiotics:* Inhibited antibacterial activity of ampicillin/sulbactam; administer ampicillin/sulbactam 3 hr before macrolides

[3] *Methotrexate:* Increased serum methotrexate concentrations

[3] *Oral contraceptives:* Occasional impairment of oral contraceptive efficacy; consider use of supplemental contraception during cycles in which ampicillin/sulbactam is used

[3] *Tetracyclines:* Inhibited antibacterial activity of ampicillin/sulbactam; administer ampicillin/sulbactam 3 hr before tetracyclines

Labs

• *False positive:* Urine amino acids

• *Increase:* Urine glucose (Clinitest method), plasma phenyldanine (dried blood spot method), CSF protein (Ektachem method), serum protein (biuret method) serum theophylline (3M Diagnostics TheoFast method), serum uric acid, serum creatinine

• *Decrease:* Serum cholesterol (CHOD-iodide method only), serum folate (bioassay method only)

SPECIAL CONSIDERATIONS

• Do not reconstitute or administer with aminoglycosides (ampicillin inactivates aminoglycosides, may be administered separately)

• Safety and efficacy established for pediatric skin and soft tissue infections only

amprenavir

(am-prehn'-eh-veer)

Rx: Agenerase

Chemical Class: Protease inhibitor, HIV

Therapeutic Class: Antiretroviral

CLINICAL PHARMACOLOGY

Mechanism of Action: An antiretroviral that inhibits HIV-1 protease by binding to the enzyme's active site, thus preventing processing of viral precursors and resulting in the formation of immature, noninfectious viral particles. *Therapeutic Effect:* Impairs HIV replication and proliferation.

Pharmacokinetics

Rapidly absorbed after PO administration. Protein binding: 90%. Metabolized in the liver. Primarily excreted in feces. **Half-life:** 7.1-10.6 hr.

INDICATIONS AND DOSAGES

HIV-1 infection (in combination with other antiretrovirals)

PO

Adults, Children 13-16 yr. 1,200 mg capsules twice a day.

Children 4-12 yr, and children 13-16 yr weighing less than 50 kg. 20 mg/kg twice a day or 15 mg/kg 3 times a day. Maximum: 2,400 mg/day.

Oral solution

Adults. 1400 mg 2 times/day.

Children 4-12 yr, and children 13-16 yr weighing less than 50 kg). 22.5 mg/kg/day (1.5 ml/kg) oral solution twice a day or 17 mg/kg/day (1.1 ml/kg) 3 times a day. Maximum: 2,800 mg/day.

Dosage in hepatic impairment

Dosage and frequency are modified based on the Child-Pugh score.

Child-Pugh Score	*Capsules*	*Oral Solution*
5–8	450 mg bid	513 mg bid
9–12	300 mg bid	342 mg bid

$ **AVAILABLE FORMS/COST**

• Cap—Oral: 50 mg, 480's: **$235.37**; 150 mg, 240's: **$367.77**

• Liq—Oral: 15 mg/ml, 240 ml: **$36.77**

NOTE: Capsules of amprenavir contain 109 IU of vitamin E; liquid contains 46 IU per ml

CONTRAINDICATIONS: None known

PREGNANCY AND LACTATION: Pregnancy category C; excreted in breast milk of animals

SIDE EFFECTS

Frequent

Diarrhea or loose stools (56%), nausea (38%), oral paresthesia (30%), rash (25%), vomiting (20%)

Occasional

Peripheral paresthesia (12%), depression (4%)

SERIOUS REACTIONS

• Severe hypersensitivity reactions or Stevens-Johnson syndrome as evidenced by blisters, peeling of the skin, loosening of skin and mucous membranes, and fever may occur.

INTERACTIONS

Drugs

3 *Abacavir:* Mild increase in amprenavir plasma level when given with abacavir

⚠ *Astemizole:* Increased plasma levels of astemizole

3 *Barbiturates:* Increased clearance of amprenavir; reduced clearance of barbiturates

2 *Carbamazepine:* Increased clearance of amprenavir; reduced clearance of carbamazepine

⚠ *Cisapride:* Increased plasma levels of cisapride

⚠ *Ergot alkaloids:* Increased plasma levels of ergot alkaloids

3 *Erythromycin:* Reduced clearance of amprenavir; amprenavir reduces clearance of erythromycin

⚠ *Lovastatin:* Amprenavir reduces clearance of lovastatin

⚠ *Midazolam:* Increased plasma levels of midazolam and prolonged effect

3 *Nevirapine:* Reduces plasma amprenavir levels

3 *Oral contraceptives:* Amprenavir may reduce efficacy

3 *Phenytoin:* Increased clearance of amprenavir; reduced clearance of phenytoin

2 *Rifabutin:* Increased clearance of amprenavir; reduced clearance of rifabutin

⚠ *Rifampin:* Increased clearance of amprenavir

3 *Ritonavir:* Decreased clearance of amprenavir

3 *Saquinavir:* Decreased clearance of saquinavir; reduce dose of Fortovase (saquinavir soft gel capsule) to 800 mg tid

3 *Sildenafil:* Decreased clearance of sildenafil

⚠ *Simvastatin:* Amprenavir reduces clearance of simvastatin

⚠ *Terfenadine:* Increased plasma levels of terfenadine

⚠ *Triazolam:* Increased plasma levels of triazolam and prolonged effect

SPECIAL CONSIDERATIONS
PATIENT/FAMILY EDUCATION
• May take with or without food, but do not take with a high-fat meal
• Do not take supplemental vitamin E; capsule and liquid forms have vitamin E in them

MONITORING PARAMETERS
• CBC, metabolic panel, hepatic function panel, CD4 lymphocyte count, HIV RNA level

---

amyl nitrite
(am'il)

Rx: Amyl nitrite
Chemical Class: Nitrate, organic
Therapeutic Class: Antianginal; antidote, cyanide; vasodilator

CLINICAL PHARMACOLOGY
Mechanism of Action: A nitrite vasodilator that relaxes smooth muscles. Reduces afterload and improves vascular supply to the myocardium. *Therapeutic Effect:* Dilates coronary arteries, improves blood flow to ischemic areas within myocardium. Following inhalation, systemic vasodilation occurs.

Pharmacokinetics
The vapors are absorbed rapidly through the pulmonary alveoli and metabolized rapidly. Partially excreted in the urine.

INDICATIONS AND DOSAGES
Acute relief of angina pectoris
Nasal inhalation
Adults, Elderly. Place crushed capsule to nostrils for 0.18-0.3 ml inhalation of vapors. Repeat at 5-10 min intervals. No more than 3 doses in 15-30 min period.

$ **AVAILABLE FORMS/COST**
• Sol—INH: 0.3 ml, 12's: **$3.96-$7.56**

UNLABELED USES: Cyanide toxicity

CONTRAINDICATIONS: Closed-angle glaucoma, severe anemia, head injury, postural hypotension, pregnancy, hypersensitivity to nitrates

PREGNANCY AND LACTATION: Pregnancy category C; markedly reduces systemic blood pressure and blood flow on maternal side of the placenta

SIDE EFFECTS
Frequent
Headache (may be severe) occurs mostly in early therapy, diminishes rapidly in intensity, usually disappears during continued treatment; transient flushing of face and neck; dizziness (especially if patient is standing immobile or is in a warm environment); weakness; postural hypotension
Occasional
Nausea, rash vomiting
Rare
Involuntary passage of urine and feces, restlessness, weakness

SERIOUS REACTIONS
• Large doses may produce hemolytic anemia or methemoglobinemia.
• Severe postural hypotension manifested by fainting, pulselessness, cold or clammy skin, and profuse sweating may occur.
• Tolerance may occur with repeated, prolonged therapy.
• High dose tends to produce severe headache.

INTERACTIONS
Drugs
▣ *Alcohol:* Exaggerated hypotension and cardiac collapse
▣ *Calcium channel blockers:* Exaggerated symptomatic orthostatic hypotension
▣ *Dihydroergotamine:* Increases the bioavailability of dihydroergotamine with resultant increase in mean standing systolic blood pressure; functional antagonism, decreasing effects
▣ *Sildenafil:* Excessive hypotensive effects
Labs
• False decrease in cholesterol via Zlatkis-Zak color reaction

SPECIAL CONSIDERATIONS
• Volatile nitrites abused for sexual stimulation; transient dizziness, weakness, or other signs of cerebral hypoperfusion may develop following inhalation
PATIENT/FAMILY EDUCATION
• Drug should be inhaled while the patient is seated or lying down
• Taking after drinking alcohol may worsen side effects
• Alert to probable headache, dizziness, or flushing side effects
• Amyl nitrite is very flammable
• Tolerance may develop with repeated use

---

anagrelide
(ah-na' greh-lide)
Rx: Agrylin
Chemical Class: Quinazoline derivative
Therapeutic Class: Antiplatelet agent

CLINICAL PHARMACOLOGY
Mechanism of Action: A hematologic agent that reduces platelet production and prevents platelet shape changes caused by platelet aggregating agents. *Therapeutic Effect:* Inhibits platelet aggregation.
Pharmacokinetics
After oral administration, plasma concentration peak within 1 hr. Extensively metabolized. Primarily excreted in urine. **Half-life:** About 3 days.

INDICATIONS AND DOSAGES
Thrombocythemia
PO
Adults, Elderly. Initially, 0.5 mg 4 times a day or 1 mg twice a day. Adjust to lowest effective dosage, increasing by up to 0.5 mg/day or less in any 1 wk. Maximum: 10 mg/day or 2.5 mg/dose.

AVAILABLE FORMS/COST
• Cap-Oral: 0.5 mg, 100's: **$651.48**;
1 mg, 100's: **$1,302.93**
CONTRAINDICATIONS: None known
PREGNANCY AND LACTATION:
Pregnancy category C; not recommended in women who are or may become pregnant; excretion into breast milk unknown
SIDE EFFECTS
Frequent (5% or more)
Headache, palpitations, diarrhea, abdominal pain, nausea, flatulence, bloating, asthenia, pain, dizziness
Occasional (less than 5%)
Tachycardia, chest pain, vomiting, paresthesia, peripheral edema, anorexia, dyspepsia, rash
Rare
Confusion, insomnia
SERIOUS REACTIONS
• Angina, heart failure, and arrhythmias occur rarely.
SPECIAL CONSIDERATIONS
MONITORING PARAMETERS
• Platelet count q2 days during first wk, then weekly thereafter until maintenance dose reached

---

anakinra
(an-a-kin'ra)
Rx: Kineret
Chemical Class: Recombinant interleukin receptor antagonist (IL-1Ra)
Therapeutic Class: Disease-modifying antirheumatic drug (DMARD); immunomodulatory agent

CLINICAL PHARMACOLOGY
Mechanism of Action: An interleukin-1 (IL-1) receptor antagonist that blocks the binding of IL-1, a protein that is a major mediator of joint disease and is present in excess amounts in patients with rheumatoid arthritis. *Therapeutic Effect:* Inhibits the inflammatory response.
Pharmacokinetics
No accumulation of anakinra in tissues or organs was observed after daily subcutaneous doses. Excreted in urine. **Half-life:** 4–6 hr.
INDICATIONS AND DOSAGES
Rheumatoid arthritis
Subcutaneous
Adults, Children older than 18 yr, Elderly. 100 mg/day, given at same time each day.
AVAILABLE FORMS/COST
• Sol, Inj-SC: 100 mg/0.67 ml: **$41.25**
CONTRAINDICATIONS: Known hypersensitivity to *Escherichia coli*–derived proteins, serious infection
PREGNANCY AND LACTATION:
Pregnancy category B; excretion into breast milk unknown; use caution in nursing mothers
SIDE EFFECTS
Occasional
Injection site ecchymosis, erythema, and inflammation
Rare
Headache, nausea, diarrhea, abdominal pain
SERIOUS REACTIONS
• Infections, including upper respiratory tract infection, sinusitis, flu-like symptoms, and cellulitis, have been noted.
• Neutropenia may occur, particularly when anakinra is used in combination with tumor necrosis factor-blocking agents.
INTERACTIONS
Drugs
❷ *Etanercept:* increased rate of serious infections, neutropenia
SPECIAL CONSIDERATIONS
• Currently recommended for management of rheumatoid arthritis after failure of other DMARD agents

PATIENT/FAMILY EDUCATION
• Signs and symptoms of allergic reactions, injection site reactions, and infections and advised of appropriate actions
• Proper disposal of needles, syringes

MONITORING PARAMETERS
• Patient reported outcomes (disability index, patient global assessment), physician assessments (tender/painful/swollen joints, physician's global assessment), objective measures (ESR, CRP); neutrophil counts baseline, q3mo, then quarterly qyr

---

anastrozole
Rx: Arimidex
Chemical Class: Benzyltriazole derivative
Therapeutic Class: Antineoplastic

CLINICAL PHARMACOLOGY
Mechanism of Action: Decreases the circulating estrogen level by inhibiting aromatase, the enzyme that catalyzes the final step in estrogen production. *Therapeutic Effect:* Inhibitis the growth of breast cancers that are stimulated by estrogens.
Pharmacokinetics
Well absorbed into systemic circulation (absorption not affected by food). Protein binding: 40%. Extensively metabolized in the liver. Eliminated by biliary system and, to a lesser extent, kidneys. **Mean half-life:** 50 hr in postmenopausal women. Steady-state plasma levels reached in about 7 days.

INDICATIONS AND DOSAGES
Breast cancer
PO
Adults, Elderly. 1 mg once a day.

$ AVAILABLE FORMS/COST
• Tab-Oral: 1 mg, 30's: **$234.39**
CONTRAINDICATIONS: None known
PREGNANCY AND LACTATION: Pregnancy category D; excretion into breast milk unknown
SIDE EFFECTS
Frequent (16%-8%)
Asthenia, nausea, headache, hot flashes, back pain, vomiting, cough, diarrhea
Occasional (6%-4%)
Constipation, abdominal pain, anorexia, bone pain, pharyngitis, dizziness, rash, dry mouth, peripheral edema, pelvic pain, depression, chest pain, paresthesia
Rare (2%-1%)
Weight gain, diaphoresis
SERIOUS REACTIONS
• Thrombophlebitis, anemia, leukopenia, and vaginal hemorrhage occur rarely.
• Vaginal hemorrhage occurs rarely (2%).

SPECIAL CONSIDERATIONS
• No difference between doses of 1-10 mg qday
• Objective response in 10% of patients
• Usually ineffective in estrogen receptor negative patients and those unresponsive to prior tamoxifen

MONITORING PARAMETERS
• Body weight, edema
• Thromboembolic events
• CBC, blood chemistry, LFTs, serum lipids

anthralin
(anth-rah'lin)
Rx: Dritho-Scalp,
Drithocreme, Micanol
Chemical Class: Anthratriol
derivative
Therapeutic Class: Antipsoriatic; keratolytic

CLINICAL PHARMACOLOGY
Mechanism of Action: A topical agent that binds DNA, inhibiting synthesis of nucleic protein, and reduces mitotic activity. *Therapeutic Effect:* Results in damage to DNA sugar and enhances membrane lipid peroxidation, which may play a critical role in the antipsoriatic action.

Pharmacokinetics
Poorly absorbed systemically, but excellent epidermal absorption. Auto-oxidized to inactive metabolites – danthrone and dianthrone. Rapid urinary excretion, so significant levels do not accumulate in the blood or other tissues. **Half-life:** 6 hrs.

INDICATIONS AND DOSAGES
Psoriasis
Topical
Adults, Elderly. Apply in a thin layer to affected areas q12h or q24h.

$ AVAILABLE FORMS/COST
• Cre—Top: 0.1%, 50 g: **$38.35-$65.49**; 0.5%, 50 g: **$46.15**; 1%, 50 g: **$47.23-$73.29**
• Oint-Top: 0.1%, 45 g: **$29.39**; 0.25%, 45 g: **$30.85**; 0.5%, 42 g: **$33.65**; 1%, 45 g: **$34.89**
UNLABELED USES: Inflammatory linear verrucous epidermal nevus
CONTRAINDICATIONS: Acute psoriasis where inflammation is present, erythroderma, hypersensitivity to anthralin

PREGNANCY AND LACTATION:
Pregnancy category C; excretion into human milk unknown; because of the potential for tumorigenicity shown in animal studies, use with caution in nursing mothers

SIDE EFFECTS
Frequent
Irritation
Rare
Neutrophilia, proteinuria, staining of the skin

SERIOUS REACTIONS
• Patients with renal disease should have routine urine tests for albuminuria.
• Hypersensitivity reaction, such as burning, erythema, and dermatitis, may occur.

SPECIAL CONSIDERATIONS
PATIENT/FAMILY EDUCATION
• Use plastic gloves for application and wear a plastic cap over treated scalp at bedtime to avoid staining
• Apply a protective film of petrolatum to areas surrounding plaque
• May stain fabrics

aprepitant
Rx: Emend, Emend 3-Day
Chemical Class: Triazolone
derivative
Therapeutic Class: Antiemetic

CLINICAL PHARMACOLOGY
Mechanism of Action: A selective human substance P and neurokinin-1 (NK_1) receptor antagonist that inhibits chemotherapy-induced nausea and vomiting centrally in the chemoreceptor trigger zone. *Therapeutic Effect:* Prevents the acute and delayed phases of chemotherapy-induced emesis, including vomiting caused by high-dose cisplatin.

Pharmacokinetics

Crosses the blood-brain barrier. Extensively metabolized in the liver. Eliminated primarily by liver metabolism (not excreted renally). **Half-life:** 9–13 hr.

INDICATIONS AND DOSAGES

Prevention of chemotherapy-induced nausea and vomiting

PO

Adults, Elderly: 125 mg 1 hr before chemotherapy on day 1 and 80 mg once a day in the morning on days 2 and 3.

Ⓢ AVAILABLE FORMS/COST

• Cap-Oral: 80 mg, 30's: **$3,037.50**; 125 mg, 30's: **$3,300.00**; Unit-of-use tri-fold pack containing one 125 mg capsule and two 80 mg capsules:

CONTRAINDICATIONS: Breast-feeding, concurrent use of pimozide (Orap)

PREGNANCY AND LACTATION: Pregnancy category B; excretion into breast milk unknown, use caution in nursing mothers

SIDE EFFECTS

Frequent (17%–10%)

Fatigue, nausea, hiccups, diarrhea, constipation, anorexia

Occasional (8%–4%)

Headache, vomiting, dizziness, dehydration, heartburn

Rare (3% or less)

Abdominal pain, epigastric discomfort, gastritis, tinnitus, insomnia

SERIOUS REACTIONS

• Neutropenia and mucous membrane disorders occur rarely.

INTERACTIONS

Drugs

⚠ *Pimozide, terfenadine, astemizole, cisapride:* Increased risk of fatal cardiac dysrhythmia through CYP 3A4 inhibition

▣ *Antineoplastics (docetaxel, paclitaxel, etoposide, irinotecan, ifosfamide, imatinib, vinorelbine, vinblastine, vincristine):* Increased concentrations of these drugs through CYP 3A4 inhibition

▣ *Benzodiazepines (midazolam, alprazolam, triazolam):* Increased concentrations of these drugs through CYP 3A4 inhibition

▣ *Warfarin:* Increased hypoprothrombinemic response to warfarin

▣ *Oral contraceptives:* Reduced contraceptive effectiveness

▣ *Dexamethasone:* Oral dexamethasone doses should be reduced by approximately 50% when coadministered with aprepitant to achieve exposures of dexamethasone similar to those obtained when it is given without aprepitant

▣ *Methylprednisolone:* IV methylprednisolone doses should be reduced by approximately 25%, and oral methylprednisolone doses should be reduced by approximately 50% when coadministered with aprepitant to achieve exposures of methylprednisolone similar to those obtained when it is given without aprepitant

▣ *Tolbutamide:* Reduced effect of this drug

▣ *CYP 3A4 inhibitors (ketoconazole, itraconazole, nefazodone, troleandomycin, clarithromycin, ritonavir, nelfinavir, diltiazem, paroxetine):* Increased plasma concentrations of aprepitant

▣ *CYP 3A4 inducers (rifampin, carbamazepine, phenytoin):* Reduced plasma concentrations of aprepitant

SPECIAL CONSIDERATIONS

• Augments the antiemetic activity of the 5-HT₃-receptor antagonist ondansetron and the corticosteroid dexamethasone and inhibits both the acute and delayed phases of cisplatin-induced emesis

argatroban
(ar-gat'tro-ban)
Rx: Acova
Chemical Class: L-arginine derivative; thrombin inhibitor
Therapeutic Class: Anticoagulant; direct thrombin inhibitor

CLINICAL PHARMACOLOGY
Mechanism of Action: A direct thrombin inhibitor that reversibly binds to thrombin-active sites. Inhibits thrombin-catalyzed or thrombin-induced reactions, including fibrin formation, activation of coagulant factors V, VIII, and XIII; also inhibits protein C formation; and platelet aggregation. *Therapeutic Effect:* Produces anticoagulation.

Pharmacokinetics
Following IV administration, distributed primarily in extracellular fluid. Protein binding: 54%. Metabolized in the liver. Primarily excreted in the feces, presumably through biliary secretion. **Half-life:** 39–51 min.

INDICATIONS AND DOSAGES
To prevent and treat heparin-induced thrombocytopenia
IV infusion
Adults, Elderly. Initially, 2 mcg/kg/min administered as a continuous infusion. After initial infusion, dose may be adjusted until steady state aPTT is 1.5–3 times initial baseline value, not to exceed 100 sec.

Percutaneous coronary intervention
IV Infusion
Adults, Elderly. Initially, 25 mcg/kg/min and administer bolus of 350 mcg/kg over 3-5 min. ACT checked in 5-10 min following bolus. If ACT is less than 300 sec, give additional bolus 150 mcg/kg, increase infusion to 30 mcg/kg/min. If ACT is greater than 450 sec, decrease infusion to 15 mcg/kg/min. Once ACT of 300-450 sec achieved, proceed with procedure.

Dosage in hepatic impairment
Adults, Elderly. Initially, 0.5 mcg/kg/min.

💲 AVAILABLE FORMS/COST
• Sol, Inj-IV: 100 mg/ml, 2.5 ml: **$896.31**

CONTRAINDICATIONS: Overt major bleeding

PREGNANCY AND LACTATION: Pregnancy category B; excretion into human milk unknown, use caution in nursing mothers

SIDE EFFECTS
Frequent (8%–3%)
Dyspnea, hypotension, fever, diarrhea, nausea, pain, vomiting, infection, cough

SERIOUS REACTIONS
• Ventricular tachycardia and atrial fibrillation occur occasionally.
• Major bleeding and sepsis occur rarely.

INTERACTIONS
Drugs
▣ *Antiplatelet agents:* Increased bleeding risk
▣ *Heparin:* Allow heparin's effect on the aPTT to decrease prior to initiation of argatroban; co-administration is unlikely since heparin is contraindicated in patients with HIT
▣ *Warfarin:* Increased prolongation of prothrombin time and INR (see SPECIAL CONSIDERATIONS)

Labs
• *Increased:* aPTT, PT, INR, activated clotting time, thrombin time

SPECIAL CONSIDERATIONS
• Discontinue all parenteral anticoagulants prior to administration
• Recognize the potential for combined effects on INR with co-administration of argatroban and war-

[A]

farin; an INR should be measured daily while argatroban and warfarin are co-administered; in general, with doses of argatroban up to 2 mcg/kg/min, argatroban can be discontinued when the INR is >4 on combined therapy; after argatroban is discontinued, repeat the INR measurement in 4-6 hr; resume the argatroban infusion if the repeat INR is below the desired therapeutic range; repeat this procedure daily until the desired therapeutic range on warfarin alone is reached; for argatroban doses greater than 2 mcg/kg/min, temporarily reduce the dose of argatroban to a dose of 2 mcg/kg/min; repeat the INR on argatroban and warfarin 4-6 hr after reduction of the argatroban dose and follow the process outlined above for administering argatroban at doses up to 2 mcg/kg/min

MONITORING PARAMETERS

• aPTT, hemoglobin, hematocrit, platelet count

aripiprazole

(ara-pip′rah-zole)

Rx: Abilify

Chemical Class: Quinolinone derivative

Therapeutic Class: Antipsychotic

CLINICAL PHARMACOLOGY

Mechanism of Action: An antipsychotic agent that provides partial agonist activity at dopamine and serotonin (5-HT_{1A}) receptors and antagonist activity at serotonin (5-HT_{2A}) receptors. *Therapeutic Effect:* Diminishes schizophrenic behavior.

Pharmacokinetics

Well absorbed through the GI tract. Protein binding: 99% (primarily albumin). Reaches steady levels in 2 wks. Metabolized in the liver. Eliminated primarily in feces and, to a lesser extent, in urine. Not removed by hemodialysis. **Half-life:** 75 hr.

INDICATIONS AND DOSAGES

Schizophrenia

PO

Adults, Elderly. Initially, 10–15 mg once a day. May increase up to 30 mg/day.

[$] **AVAILABLE FORMS/COST**

• Tab—Oral: 5 mg, 10 mg, 15 mg, 30's; all: **$316.07**; 20 mg, 30 mg, 30's; all: **$446.98**

UNLABELED USES: Schizoaffective disorder

CONTRAINDICATIONS: None known.

PREGNANCY AND LACTATION: Pregnancy category C; excreted in milk of rats during lactation; no human information

SIDE EFFECTS

Frequent (11%–5%)

Weight gain, headache, insomnia, vomiting

Occasional (4%–3%)

Light-headedness, nausea, akathisia, somnolence

Rare (2% or less)

Blurred vision, constipation, asthenia or loss of energy and strength, anxiety, fever, rash, cough, rhinitis, orthostatic hypotension

SERIOUS REACTIONS

• Extrapyramidal symptoms and neuroleptic malignant syndrome occur rarely.

INTERACTIONS

Drugs

[3] *Alcohol:* Additive CNS depression and psychomotor depression

3 *α-blockers (doxazocin, prazocin, terazocin):* Potential for enhanced blood pressure lowering effect

2 *Amiodarone:* Hepatic metabolism inhibition; consider decreasing aripiprazole dose

2 *Azole antifungals (fluconazole, itraconazole, ketoconazole, miconazole, variconazole):* Increased aripiprazole and metabolite concentrations via CYP3A4 inhibition; reduce dose of aripiprazole

3 *Bosentan:* Hepatic metabolism induced; consider doubling aripirazole dose

2 *Carbamazepine, oxcarbazepine:* Reductions in aripiprazole and metabolite concentrations via CYP3A4 induction; double dose of aripiprazole

3 *Centrally acting agents (i.e., opiates, antidepressants, antihistamines, sedative/hypnotics):* Additive CNS depression and psychomotor depression

3 *Cimetidine:* Hepatic metabolism inhibition; consider reducing aripiprazole dose or use alternate H_2 receptor blocker

3 *Cyclosporine:* Hepatic metabolism inhibition; consider reducing aripiprazole dose

3 *Danazole:* Hepatic metabolism inhibition; consider reducing aripiprazole dose

3 *Delavirdine:* Hepatic metabolism inhibition; consider reducing aripiprazole dose

3 *Dexamethasone:* Hepatic metabolism induced; consider doubling aripirazole dose

3 *Diltiazem:* Hepatic metabolism inhibition; consider reducing aripiprazole dose

3 *Droperidol:* Increased risk of extrapyrimidal reactions, CNS depression, QT prolongation with similar drug (ziprasidone)

2 *Efavirenz:* Hepatic metabolism induced; consider doubling aripiprazole dose

2 *Estrogen:* Hepatic metabolism inhibition; consider reducing aripiprazole dose

3 *Grapefruit juice:* Increased aripiprazole and metabolite concentrations via CYP3A4 inhibition

2 *Griseofulvin:* Hepatic metabolism induced; consider doubling aripiprazole dose

2 *Isoniazid:* Hepatic metabolism induced; consider doubling aripiprazole dose

3 *Macrolide antibiotics (erythromycin, clairithromycin):* Increased aripiprazole and metabolite concentrations via CYP3A4 inhibition

2 *Protease inhibitors (indinivir, saquinivir, ritonavir, nelfinavir, amprenivir, lopinavir):* Hepatic metabolism inhibition; consider reducing aripiprazole dosage

2 *Quinidine:* Increased aripiprazole and metabolite concentrations via CYP2D6 inhibition; reduce dose of aripiprazole by approximately 50%

2 *SSRI's (Fluoxetine, fluvoxamine, paroxetine):* Increased aripiprazole and metabolite concentrations via CYP2D6 inhibition; reduce dose of aripiprazole by approximately 50%

SPECIAL CONSIDERATIONS
• Reports of efficacy in acutely relapsed schizophrenia and schizoaffective disorder, and has an improved tolerability profile compared to haloperidol

PATIENT/FAMILY EDUCATION
• Understanding of potential interference with cognitive and motor performance, potential for drug interactions, and risk factors for neuroleptic malignant syndrome (overheating, dehydration)

MONITORING PARAMETERS
• Improvement of both positive and negative schizophrenic symptoms; periodic BP and heart rate; abnormal movement monitoring

---

ascorbic acid (vitamin C)

(a-skor'bic)

Rx: injection: Cenolate, CEE-500, Mega-C/A Plus, Ortho/CS
OTC: Ascorbicap, Cecon, Cevi-Bid, Ce-Vi-Sol, C-Crystals, Cebid Timecelles, Dull-C, Flavorcee, N'ice Vitamin C Drops
Chemical Class: Vitamin, water soluble
Therapeutic Class: Acidifier, urinary; vitamin

CLINICAL PHARMACOLOGY
Mechanism of Action: Assists in collagen formation and tissue repair and is involved in oxidation reduction reactions and other metabolic reactions. *Therapeutic Effect:* Involved in carbohydrate use and metabolism, as eell as synthesis of carnitine, lipids, and proteins. Preserves blood vessel integrity.
Pharmacokinetics
Readily absorbed from the GI tract. Protein binding: 25%. Metabolized in the liver. Excreted in urine. Removed by hemodialysis.
INDICATIONS AND DOSAGES
Dietary supplement
PO
Adults, Elderly. 50–200 mg/day.
Children. 35–100 mg/day.
Acidification of urine
PO
Adults, Elderly. 4-12 g/day in 3-4 divided doses.
Children. 500 mg q6-8h.

Scurvy
PO
Adults, Elderly. 100-250 mg 1-2 times a day.
Children. 100-300 mg/day in divided doses.
Prevention and reduction of severity of colds
PO
Adults, Elderly. 1-3 g/day in divided doses.

$ AVAILABLE FORMS/COST
• Cap-Oral: 500 mg, 100's: **$2.54-$19.24**
• Sol, Inj-IM, IV, SC: 250 mg/ml, 2 ml: **$2.40**; 500 mg/ml, 2 ml: **$0.63**
• Liq-Oral: 100 mg/ml, 50 ml: **$19.68**; 250 mg/ml, 500 ml: **$33.20**; 500 mg/5ml, 480 ml: **$14.00**
• Tab—Oral: 100 mg, 100's: **$1.29**; 250 mg, 100's: **$1.30-$2.99**; 500 mg, 100's: **$1.54-$6.95**; 1000 mg, 100's: **$3.25-$28.00**; 1500 mg, 60's: **$5.65-$8.70**
• Tab, Chewable-Oral: 25 mg, 125's: **$2.69**; 100 mg, 100's: **$1.30-$1.96**; 250 mg, 100's: **$2.00-$4.60**; 500 mg, 100's: **$3.00-$6.95**
UNLABELED USES: Prevention of common cold, control of idiopathic methemoglobinemia, urine acidifier
CONTRAINDICATIONS: None known.
PREGNANCY AND LACTATION: Pregnancy category A if doses do not exceed the RDA, otherwise pregnancy category C; excreted into breast milk via a saturable process; the RDA during lactation is 90-100 mg; maternal supplementation up to the RDA is needed only in those women with poor nutritional status
SIDE EFFECTS
Rare
Abdominal cramps, nausea, vomiting, diarrhea, increased urination with doses exceeding 1 g

Parenteral: Flushing, headache, dizziness, sleepiness or insomnia, soreness at injection site.

SERIOUS REACTIONS

• Ascorbic acid may acidify urine, leading to crystalluria.

• Large doses of IV ascorbic acid may lead to deep vein thrombosis.

• Abrupt discontinuation after prolonged use of large doses may produce rebound ascorbic acid deficiency.

INTERACTIONS

Drugs

3 *Antacids:* Vitamin C increases the amount of aluminum absorbed from aluminum-containing antacids

Labs

• *False negative:* Amine-dependent stool occult blood, urine bilirubin, blood, leukocyte determinations

• *False positive:* Urine glucose

• *Decrease:* Urine amphetamine, serum AST (Ames Seralyzer method), urine barbiturate (Abbott TDx method) serum bicarbonate (Kodak Ektachem 700 method), serum bilirubin (Jendrassik method), serum cholesterol (Olympus, Abbott TDx, CHOD-PAP methods), serum CK (Kodak Ektachem Systems), serum creatinine (Merck, Wako, Boehringer Mannheim methods), urine glucose (glucose oxidase methods), serum HDL-cholesterol (Kodak Ektachem Systems), urine oxalate (oxalate decarboxylase methods), urine porphobilinogen, serum triglycerides (GPO-PAP, Boehringer Mannheim methods), serum urea nitrogen (Ames Seralyzer), serum uric acid (Ames Seralyzer), urine uric acid (Kodak Ektachem Systems)

• *Increase:* Serum amylase (only at toxic ascorbic acid levels), serum AST (SMA 12/60 method), serum bilirubin (SMA 12/60 method), serum glucose (SMA 12/60 and O-toluidine methods), serum HbAlc (electrophoretic method), urine β-hydroxybutyrate, urine 17-hydroxy corticosteroids, urine iodide, urine 17-ketosteroids, urine oxalate (chromatographic methods), serum phosphate (Boehringer-Mannheim method), CSF and urine protein (Kodak Ektachem Systems), serum uric acid (Klein and phosphotungstate methods)

aspirin
(as´pir-in)

Rx: Aspirin CR, Aspirin Delayed Release, Easprin, ZORprin

OTC: Ascriptin, Aspergum, Bayer, Bayer Children's Aspirin, Ecotrin, Ecotrin Maximum Strength, 8-Hour Bayer Extended Release, Empirin, Maximum Bayer, Norwich

Combinations

Rx: with butalbital (Fiorinal); with codeine (Empirin); with dihydrocodeine and caffeine (Synalgos DC); with dipyridamole (Aggrenox); with oxycodone (Percodan); with propoxyphene (Darvon)

OTC: with antacids (Ascriptin, Bufferin, Magnaprin)

Chemical Class: Salicylate derivative

Therapeutic Class: Antiinflammatory; antiplatelet agent; antipyretic; nonnarcotic analgesic

CLINICAL PHARMACOLOGY

Mechanism of Action: A nonsteroidal salicylate that inhibits prostaglandin synthesis, acts on the hypothalamus heat-regulating center, and interferes with the production of thromboxane A, a substance that stimulates platelet aggregation. *Therapeutic Effect:* Reduces inflammatory response and intensity of pain; decreases fever; inhibits platelet aggregation.

Pharmacokinetics

Route	*Onset*	*Peak*	*Duration*
PO	1 hr	2–4 hr	24 hr

Rapidly and completely absorbed from GI tract; enteric-coated absorption delayed; rectal absorption delayed and incomplete. Protein binding: High. Widely distributed. Rapidly hydrolyzed to salicylate. **Half-life:** 15–20 min (aspirin); 2–3 hr (salicylate at low dose); more than 20 hr (salicylate at high dose).

INDICATIONS AND DOSAGES

Analgesia, fever

PO, Rectal

Adults, Elderly. 325–1,000 mg q4-6h

Children. 10–15 mg/kg/dose q4-6h. Maximum: 4 g/day.

Anti-inflammatory

PO

Adults, Elderly. Initially, 2.4–3.6 g/day in divided doses; then 3.6–5.4 g/day.

Children. Initially, 60–90 mg/kg/day in divided doses; then 80–100 mg/kg/day.

Suspected MI

PO

Adults, Elderly. 162 mg as soon as the MI is suspected, then daily for 30 days after the MI.

Prevention of MI

PO

Adults, Elderly. 75–325 mg/day.

Prevention of stroke after transient ischemic attack

PO

Adults, Elderly. 50–325 mg/day.

Kawasaki disease

PO

Children. 80–100 mg/kg/day in divided doses.

[$] **AVAILABLE FORMS/COST**

• Gum Tab, Chewable—Oral: 227.5 mg, 16's: **$2.18**

• Supp—Rect: 60 mg, 12's: **$3.25**; 125 mg, 12's: **$2.00-$4.95**; 300 mg, 12's: **$3.56-$4.05**; 600 mg, 12's: **$2.40-$4.20**; 1200 mg, 12's: **$2.13**

• Tab, Chewable—Oral: 81 mg, 36's: **$0.51-$2.40**

• Tab, Enteric Coated—Oral: 81 mg, 120's: **$1.08-$6.91**; 162 mg, 60's: **$3.76-$4.20**; 300 mg, 1000's: **$17.80**; 325 mg, 100's: **$1.31-$22.30**; 500 mg, 60's: **$2.50-$6.48**; 650 mg, 100's: **$3.95**; 975 mg, 100's: **$8.19-$15.32**

• Tab-Oral: 81 mg, 100's: **$3.75-$3.95**; 325 mg, 100's: **$0.56-$14.04**; 500 mg, 100's: **$1.10-$7.44**; 650 mg, 100's: **$3.50-$13.55**

• Tab, Sus Action—Oral: 800 mg, 100's: **$7.66-$98.49**; 975 mg, 100's: **$13.20-$14.50**

UNLABELED USES: Prevention of thromboembolism, treatment of Kawasaki disease

CONTRAINDICATIONS: Allergy to tartrazine dye, bleeding disorders, chickenpox or flu in children and teenagers, GI bleeding or ulceration, hepatic impairment, history of hypersensitivity to aspirin or NSAIDs

PREGNANCY AND LACTATION: Pregnancy category C (category D if full doses used in 3rd trimester); use in pregnancy should generally be avoided; in pregnancies at risk for the development of pregnancy-induced hypertension and preeclampsia, and in fetuses with intrauterine growth retardation, low-dose aspirin (40-150 mg/day) may be beneficial; excreted into breast milk in low concentrations

SIDE EFFECTS
Occasional
GI distress (including abdominal distention, cramping, heartburn, and mild nausea); allergic reaction (including bronchospasm, pruritus, and urticaria)

SERIOUS REACTIONS
• High doses of aspirin may produce GI bleeding and gastric mucosal lesions.
• Dehydrated, febrile children may experience aspirin toxicity quickly. Reye's syndrome may occur in children with the chickenpox or the flu.
• Low-grade toxicity characterized is by tinnitus, generalized pruritus (possibly severe), headache, dizziness, flushing, tachycardia, hyperventilation, diaphoresis, and thirst.
• Market toxicity is characterized by hyperthermia, restlessness, seizures, abnormal breathing patterns, respiratory failure, and coma.

INTERACTIONS
Drugs
❸ *ACE inhibitors:* Reduced antihypertensive effect
❷ *Acetazolamide:* Increased concentrations of acetazolamide, possibly leading to CNS toxicity
❸ *Antacids:* Decreased serum salicylate concentrations; high dose salicylates only
❸ *Corticosteroids:* Increased incidence and/or severity of GI ulceration; enhanced salicylate excretion
❸ *Diltiazem:* Enhanced antiplatelet effect of aspirin
❸ *Ethanol:* Enhanced aspirin-induced GI mucosal damage and aspirin-induced prolongation of bleeding time
❸ *Griseofulvin:* Reduced serum salicylate level
❸ *Intrauterine contraceptive device:* May reduce contraceptive effectiveness

❷ *Methotrexate:* Increased serum methotrexate concentrations and enhanced methotrexate toxicity
❷ *Oral anticoagulants:* Increased risk of bleeding by inhibiting platelet function and possibly by producing gastric erosions
❸ *Probenecid:* Salicylates inhibit the uricosuric activity of probenecid
❸ *Sulfinpyrazone:* Salicylates inhibit the uricosuric activity of sulfinpyrazone
❸ *Sulfonylureas:* Enhanced hypoglycemic response to sulfonylureas
❷ *Warfarin:* Enhanced hypoprothrombinemic effect of warfarin
❸ *Zafirlukast:* Increased plasma concentrations of zafirlukast
Labs
• *Increase:* Serum acetaminophen (Glynn-Kendal method), urine acetoacetate (Gerhardt ferric chloride procedure), urine glucose (Ames Clinitest method), serum HbAlc (chromatographic and electrophoretic, but not colorimetric methods), urine hippuric acid, urine homogentisic acid, urine homovanillic acid, urine ketones (Gerhardt's test), urine phenyl ketones, CSF and urine protein (Folm-Ciocalteu method), serum and urine uric acid (non-specific methods only)
• *Decrease:* Serum albumin, urine glucose (glucose oxidase methods), total serum phenytoin (but not free serum phenytoin)

SPECIAL CONSIDERATIONS
• 81 mg qday may be as effective as higher doses in primary and secondary MI prevention

PATIENT/FAMILY EDUCATION
• Administer with food
• Do not exceed recommended doses
• Read label on other OTC drugs, many contain aspirin
• Therapeutic response may take 2 wk (arthritis)

- Avoid alcohol ingestion, GI bleeding may occur
- **Not to be given to children with flu-like symptoms or chickenpox; Reye's syndrome may develop**
MONITORING PARAMETERS
- AST, ALT, bilirubin, creatinine, CBC, hematocrit if patient is on long-term therapy

---

atazanavir

Rx: Reyataz
Chemical Class: Protease inhibitor, HIV
Therapeutic Class: Antiretroviral

CLINICAL PHARMACOLOGY
Mechanism of Action: An antiviral that acts as an HIV-1 protease inhibitor, selectively preventing the processing of viral precursors found in cells infected with HIV-1. *Therapeutic Effect:* Prevents the formation of mature HIV cells.

Pharmacokinetics
Rapidly absorbed after PO administration. Protein binding: 86%. Extensively metabolized in the liver. Excreted primarily in urine and, to a lesser extent, in feces. **Half-life:** 5-8 hr.

INDICATIONS AND DOSAGES
HIV-1 infection
PO
Adults, Elderly (antiretroviral-naive). 400 mg (2 capsules) once a day with food.
Adults, Elderly (antiretroviral-experienced). 300 mg and ritonavir (Norvir) 100 mg once a day.

HIV-1 infection (concurrent therapy with efavirenz)
PO
Adults, Elderly. 300 mg atazanavir, 100 mg ritonavir, and 600 mg efavirenz as a single daily dose with food.

HIV-1 infection (concurrent therapy with didanosine)
PO
Adults, Elderly. Give atazanavir with food 2 hours before or 1 hour after didanosine.

HIV-1 infection (concurrent therapy with tenofovir)
PO
Adults, Elderly. 300 mg atazanavir and 100 mg ritonavir and 300 mg tenofovir given as a single daily dose with food.

HIV-1 infection in patients with mild to moderate hepatic impairment
PO
Adults, Elderly. 300 mg once a day with food.

AVAILABLE FORMS/COST
- Cap-Oral: 100 mg, 150 mg, 200 mg, 60's; all: **$828.00**
CONTRAINDICATIONS: Concurrent use with ergot derivatives, midazolam, pimozide, or triazolam; severe hepatic insufficiency
PREGNANCY AND LACTATION: Pregnancy category B; breast milk excretion unknown (breast-feeding not advised for HIV infected women)
SIDE EFFECTS
Frequent (16%-14%)
Nausea, headache
Occasional (9%-4%)
Rash, vomiting, depression, diarrhea, abdominal pain, fever
Rare (3% or less)
Dizziness, insomnia, cough, fatigue, back pain
SERIOUS REACTIONS
- A severe hypersensitivity reaction (marked by angioedema and chest pain) and jaundice may occur.

INTERACTIONS

• **(competitively inhibits CYP1A2, CYP2C9 systems)**

Drugs

❷ *Amiodarone:* Increased plasma levels of amiodarone

❸ *Antacids:* Antacids reduce absorption of atazanavir, take atazanavir 2 hr before or 1 hr after antacids

⚠ *Astemizole:* Increased plasma levels of astemizole

❷ *Atorvastatin:* Atazanavir reduces clearance of atorvastatin

❸ *Barbiturates:* Increased clearance of atazanavir; reduced clearance of barbiturates

⚠ *Bepridil:* Increased plasma levels of bepridil

❸ *Calcium channel blockers:* Atazanavir reduces clearance of calcium channel blockers

❸ *Carbamazepine:* Increased clearance of atazanavir; reduced clearance of carbamazepine

⚠ *Cisapride:* Increased plasma levels of cisapride

❷ *Clarithromycin:* Atazanavir reduces clearance of clarithromycin; reduce clarithromycin dose by 50%

❸ *Cyclosporine:* Atazanavir reduces clearance of cyclosporine, monitor plasma levels

❸ *Desipramine:* Atazanavir increases AUC of desipramine, monitor plasma levels

❷ *Didanosine (buffered formulation):* Didanosine, buffered formulation (but not didanosine EC) reduces absorption of atazanavir, take atazanavir 2 hr before or 1 hr after didanosine, buffered formulation

❷ *Diltiazem:* Atazanavir reduces diltiazem clearance, reduce diltiazem dose by 50%

❷ *Efavirenz:* Efavirenz increases atazanavir clearance, give atazanavir 300 mg qday with ritonavir 100 mg qday, when coadministered with efavirenz; no change in efavirenz dose

⚠ *Ergot alkaloids:* Increased plasma levels of ergot alkaloids

❷ *Flecainide:* Increased plasma levels of flecainide

❷ *H2 receptor antagonists:* H2 receptor antagonists reduce absorption of atazanavir, separate dosing by 12 hrs

⚠ *Indinavir:* Potential for additive hyperbilirubinemia

⚠ *Irinotecan:* Atazanavir increases plasma levels of irinotecan

❷ *Lidocaine:* Increased plasma levels of lidocaine

⚠ *Lovastatin:* Atazanavir markedly reduces clearance of lovastatin

⚠ *Midazolam:* Increased plasma levels of midazolam and prolonged effect

❷ *Oral contraceptives:* Atazanavir increases ethinyl estradiol and norethindrone plasma levels

❸ *Phenytoin:* Increased clearance of atazanavir; reduced clearance of phenytoin

⚠ *Pimozide:* Increased plasma levels of pimozide

⚠ *Proton pump inhibitors:* Marked reduction of atazanavir absorption and lower plasma levels

❷ *Quinidine:* Increased plasma levels of quinidine

❷ *Rifabutin:* Increased clearance of atazanavir; reduced clearance of rifabutin; reduce rifabutin dose to 150 mg qod

⚠ *Rifampin:* Increased clearance of atazanavir

⚠ *Rifapentine:* Increased clearance of atazanavir

❷ *Ritonavir:* Ritonavir decreases clearance of atazanavir, reduce atazanavir does to 300 mg qday

❷ *Saquinavir:* Decreased clearance of saquinavir, dose adjustment may be needed but optimal dose not established

❷ *Sildenafil:* Atazanavir markedly reduces clearance of sildenafil, reduce sildenafil dose to 25 mg q48hrs

❸ *Sirolimus:* Atazanavir reduces clearance of sirolimus, monitor plasma levels

⚠ *St. John's wort:* St. John's wort reduces plasma levels of atazanavir

❸ *Tacrolimus:* Atazanavir reduces clearance of tacrolimus, monitor plasma levels

⚠ *Terfenadine:* Increased plasma levels of terfenadine

⚠ *Triazolam:* Increased plasma levels of triazolam and prolonged effect

❷ *Vardenafil:* Atazanavir reduces clearance of vardenafil, reduce vardenafil dose to 2.5 mg q24hrs

❷ *Warfarin:* Atazanavir increases warfarin effect

SPECIAL CONSIDERATIONS

• Reduced susceptibility to atazanavir is conferred by the following mutations of the HIV protease gene: N88S, I50L, I84V, A71V, and M46I

• In patients with no prior antiretroviral therapy, a randomized trial found atazanavir equivalent to efavirenz when both were part of a 3 drug combination including zidovudine and lamivudine; another trial found atazanavir equivalent to nelfinavir when both were part of a 3 drug combination including lamivudine and stavudine

• In patients with prior antiretroviral therapy, a randomized trial found that viral suppression rates for atazanavir were lower than with lopinavir/ritonavir (HIV RNA <400 copies/ml after 24 weeks of therapy: 54% vs 75%; HIV RNA <50 copies/ml after 24 weeks of therapy:

34% vs 50%; CD4 count change after 24 weeks of therapy: +101 cells/mm^3 vs 121 cells/mm^3

• Always check updated treatment guidelines before initiating or changing antiretroviral therapy (http://AIDSinfo.nih.gov)

PATIENT/FAMILY EDUCATION

• Antacids or buffered medications reduce absorption of atazanavir, take atazanavir 2 hrs before or 1 hr after antacids or buffered medications

• Any medications that reduce stomach acid also reduce absorption of atazanavir; consult prescriber before using

MONITORING PARAMETERS

• CBC, ALT, AST, bilirubin, HIV RNA, CD4 count

---

atenolol

(a-ten'oh-lol)

Rx: Tenormin
Combinations
　Rx: with chlorthalidone (Tenoretic)
Chemical Class: β_1-adrenergic blocker, cardioselective
Therapeutic Class: Antianginal; antihypertensive

CLINICAL PHARMACOLOGY

Mechanism of Action: A beta$_1$-adrenergic blocker that acts as an antianginal, antiarrhythmic, and antihypertensive agent by blocking beta$_1$-adrenergic receptors in cardiac tissue. *Therapeutic Effect:* Slows sinus node heart rate, decreasing cardiac output and blood pressure (BP). Decreases myocardial oxygen demand.

Pharmacokinetics

Route	Onset	Peak	Duration
PO	1 hr	2–4 hr	24 hr

Incompletely absorbed from the GI tract. Protein binding: 6%–16%. Minimal liver metabolism. Primarily excreted unchanged in urine. Removed by hemodialysis. **Half-life:** 6–7 hr (increased in impaired renal function).

INDICATIONS AND DOSAGES

Hypertension

PO

Adults. Initially, 25–50 mg once a day. May increase dose up to 100 mg once a day.

Elderly. Usual initial dose, 25 mg a day.

Children. Initially, 0.8–1 mg/kg/dose given once a day. Range: 0.8-1.5 mg/kg/day. **Maxiumum:** 2 mg/kg/day or 100 mg/day.

Angina pectoris

PO

Adults. Initially, 50 mg once a day. May increase dose up to 200 mg once a day.

Elderly. Usual initial dose, 25 mg a day.

Acute MI

IV

Adults. Give 5 mg over 5 min; may repeat in 10 min. In those who tolerate full 10-mg IV dose, begin 50-mg tablets 10 min after last IV dose followed by another 50-mg oral dose 12 hr later. Thereafter, give 100 mg once a day or 50 mg twice a day for 6–9 days. Or, for those who do not tolerate full IV dose, give 50 mg orally twice a day or 100 mg once a day for at least 7 days.

Dosage in renal impairment

Dosage interval is modified based on creatinine clearance.

Creatinine Clearance	*Dosage interval*
15–35 ml/min	50 mg a day
less than 15 ml/min	50 mg every other day

[$] **AVAILABLE FORMS/COST**

• Sol, Inj-IV, Buffered: 0.5 mg/ml, 10 ml: **$8.37**

• Tab-Oral: 25 mg, 100's: **$5.27-$128.86**; 50 mg, 100's: **$6.28-$137.86**; 100 mg, 100's: **$8.64-$197.23**

UNLABELED USES: Improved survival in diabetics with heart disease; treatment of hypertrophic cardiomyopathy, pheochromocytoma, and syndrome of mitral valve prolapse; prevention of migraine, thyrotoxicosis, tremors

CONTRAINDICATIONS: Cardiogenic shock, overt heart failure, second- or third-degree heart block, severe bradycardia

PREGNANCY AND LACTATION: Pregnancy category D; frequently used in the third trimester for treatment of hypertension (many studies of efficacy and safety of atenolol in pregnancy-induced hypertension); long-term use has been associated with intrauterine growth retardation; excreted into breast milk; observe for signs of β-blockade

SIDE EFFECTS

Atenolol is generally well tolerated, with mild and transient side effects.

Frequent

Hypotension manifested as cold extremities, constipation or diarrhea, diaphoresis, dizziness, fatigue, headache, and nausea

Occasional

Insomnia, flatulence, urinary frequency, impotence or decreased libido, mental depression

Rare

Rash, arthralgia, myalgia, confusion (especially in the elderly), altered taste

SERIOUS REACTIONS

• Overdose may produce profound bradycardia and hypotension.

- Abrupt atenolol withdrawal may result in diaphoresis, palpitations, headache, and tremors.
- Atenolol administration may precipitate CHF or MI in patients with cardiac disease; thyroid storm in those with thyrotoxicosis; and peripheral ischemia in those with existing peripheral vascular disease.
- Hypoglycemia may occur in patients with previously controlled diabetes.
- Thrombocytopenia, manifested as unusual bruising or bleeding, occurs rarely.

INTERACTIONS

Drugs

🔳 *Adenosine:* Bradycardia aggravated

🔳 *α₁-adrenergic blockers:* Potential enhanced first dose response (marked initial drop in blood pressure, particularly on standing [especially prazosin])

🔳 *Amoxicillin, Ampicillin:* Reduced atenolol bioavailability

🔳 *Antacids:* Reduced atenolol absorption

🔳 *Calcium channel blockers:* Enhanced effects of both drugs, particularly AV node conduction slowing; reduced atenolol clearance

🔳 *Clonidine:* Exacerbation of rebound hypertension upon discontinuation of clonidine

🔳 *Digoxin:* Additive prolongation of atrioventricular (AV) conduction time

🔳 *Dipyridamole:* Bradycardia aggravated

🔳 *Disopyramide:* Additive decreases in cardiac output

🔳 *Lidocaine:* Increased serum lidocaine concentrations possible

🔳 *Neostigmine:* Increased bradycardia aggravated

🔳 *NSAIDs:* Reduced antihypertensive effects of atenolol

🔳 *Physostigmine:* Increased bradycardia aggravated

🔳 *Tacrine:* Increased bradycardia aggravated

② *Theophylline:* Antagonistic pharmacodynamic effects

SPECIAL CONSIDERATIONS

- Properties of low lipid solubility and competitive cardioselectivity yield less CNS and bronchospastic adverse effects than propranolol

PATIENT/FAMILY EDUCATION

- Do not discontinue abruptly, may precipitate angina
- Report bradycardia, dizziness, confusion, depression, fever, shortness of breath, swelling of the extremities
- Take pulse at home, notify clinician if <50 beats/min
- Avoid hazardous activities if dizziness, drowsiness, lightheadedness are present
- May mask the symptoms of hypoglycemia, except for sweating, in diabetic patients

MONITORING PARAMETERS

- Blood pressure, heart rate

---

atomoxetine

(auto-mox'eh-teen)

Rx: Strattera

Chemical Class: Propylamine derivative

Therapeutic Class: Selective norepinephrine transporter inhibitor

---

CLINICAL PHARMACOLOGY

Mechanism of Action: A norepinephrine reuptake inhibitor that enhances noradrenergic function by selective inhibition of the presynaptic norepinephrine transporter. *Therapeutic Effect:* Improves symptoms of attention-deficit hyperactivity disorder (ADHD).

Pharmacokinetics

Rapidly absorbed after PO administration. Protein binding: 98% (primarily to albumin). Eliminated primarily in urine and, to a lesser extent, in feces. Not removed by hemodialysis. **Half-life:** 4–5 hr in general population, 22 hr in 7% of Caucasians and 2% of African-Americans; (increased in moderate to severe hepatic insufficiency).

INDICATIONS AND DOSAGES

ADHD

PO

Adults, children weighing 70 kg and more. 40 mg once a day. May increase after at least 3 days to 80 mg as a single daily dose or in divided doses. Maximum: 100 mg.

Children weighing less than 70 kg. Initially, 0.5 mg/kg/day. May increase after at least 3 days to 1.2 mg/kg/day. Maximum: 1.4 mg/kg/day or 100 mg.

Dosage in hepatic impairment

Expect to administer 50% of normal atomoxetine dosage to patients with moderate hepatic impairment and 25% of normal dosage to those with severe hepatic impairment.

💲 AVAILABLE FORMS/COST

• Cap-Oral: 10 mg, 18 mg, 25 mg, 40 mg, 60 mg, 30's; all: **$94.50**

UNLABELED USES: Treatment of depression.

CONTRAINDICATIONS: Angle-closure glaucoma, use within 14 days of MAOIs

PREGNANCY AND LACTATION: Pregnancy category C; excretion into breast milk unknown; use caution in nursing mothers

SIDE EFFECTS

Frequent

Headache, dyspepsia, nausea, vomiting, fatigue, decreased appetite, dizziness, altered mood

Occasional

Tachycardia, hypertension, weight loss, delayed growth in children, irritability

Rare

Insomnia, sexual dysfunction in adults, fever

SERIOUS REACTIONS

• Urine retention or urinary hesitance may occur.

• In overdose, gastric emptying and repeated use of activated charcoal may prevent systemic absorption.

INTERACTIONS

Drugs

② *MAOIs:* Hypertensive crisis

③ *Albuterol, other β-agonists:* Potentiated effects on the cardiovascular system

③ *CYP2D6 inhibitors (fluoxetine, paroxetine, quinidine):* Increased levels of atomoxetine

SPECIAL CONSIDERATIONS

• Promoted as a "milder" but equally efficacious agent; inadequate comparisons available – should not be considered over conventional therapy

MONITORING PARAMETERS

• Pretreatment blood samples for PCR-CYP2D6 genotyping (poor-metabolizer alleles) in selected patients (e.g., those with a history of super sensitivity/marked clinical response to other medications)

• History: Improvement of ADHD symptoms such as inattentiveness, hyperactivity, anxiety, impaired academic/social functioning; interviewing via ADHD Rating Scale-IV (parent version); routine blood chemistry periodically during prolonged administration; BP, pulse rate, body weight periodically during prolonged administration; signs and symptoms of toxicity

atorvastatin
(a-tor'va-sta-tin)

Rx: Lipitor
Combinations
  Rx: with amlodipine (Caduet); with benazepril (Lotrel)
Chemical Class: Substituted hexahydronaphthalene
Therapeutic Class: HMG-CoA reductase inhibitor; antilipemic

CLINICAL PHARMACOLOGY
Mechanism of Action: An antihyperlipidemic that inhibits HMG-CoA reductase, the enzyme that catalyzes the early step in cholesterol synthesis. *Therapeutic Effect:* Decreases LDL and VLDL cholesterol, and plasma triglyceride levels; increases HDL cholesterol concentration.
Pharmacokinetics
Poorly absorbed from the GI tract. Protein binding: greater than 98%. Metabolized in the liver. Minimally eliminated in urine. Plasma levels are markedly increased in chronic alcoholic hepatic disease, but are unaffected by renal disease. **Half-life:** 14 hr.

INDICATIONS AND DOSAGES
Hyperlipidemia, Reduction of risk of myocardial infarction (MI), angina revascularization procedures
PO
Adults, Elderly. Initially, 10–40 mg a day given as a single dose. Dose range: Increase at 2- to 4-wk intervals to maximum of 80 mg/day.
Children 10-17 yr. Initially, 10 mg/day, may increase to 20 mg/day.
Familial hypercholesterolemia
PO
Children 10-17 yr. Initially, 10 mg/day. May increase to 20 mg/day.

$ AVAILABLE FORMS/COST
• Tab, Film-Coated—Oral: 10 mg, 90's: **$222.43**; 20 mg, 40 mg, 80 mg, 90's; all: **$327.93**

CONTRAINDICATIONS: Active hepatic disease, lactation, pregnancy, unexplained elevated hepatic function test results

PREGNANCY AND LACTATION: Pregnancy category X; not recommended for nursing mothers

SIDE EFFECTS
Atorvastatin is generally well tolerated. Side effects are usually mild and transient.
Frequent (16%)
Headache
Occasional (5%–2%)
Myalgia, rash or pruritus, allergy
Rare (2%-1%)
Flatulence, dyspepsia

SERIOUS REACTIONS
• Cataracts may develop, and photosensitivity may occur.

INTERACTIONS
Drugs
▣ *Azole antifungals (fluconazole, itraconazole, ketoconazole, miconazole):* Increased atorvastatin levels; increased risk of rhabdomyolysis

▣ *Bile acid sequestrants (cholestyramine, colestipol):* 25% reduction in atorvastatin plasma levels if coadministered

▣ *Cyclosporine:* Concomitant administration increases risk of severe myopathy or rhabdomyolysis

▣ *Digoxin:* Elevation of digoxin level (approximately 20%)

▣ *Erythromycin:* Increased atorvastatin concentrations (approximately 40%); increased risk of rhabdomyolysis

▣ *Fibric acid:* Increased risk of severe myopathy, especially with high statin doses

◼ *Nefazodone:* Increased atorvastatin levels; increased risk of rhabdomyolyisis

◼ *Niacin:* Concomitant administration increases risk of severe myopathy or rhabdomyolysis

◼ *Oral contraceptives:* Coadministration increases AUC for norethindrone and ethinyl estradiol by approximately 30% and 20%, respectively

SPECIAL CONSIDERATIONS

• Base statin selection on lipid-lowering prowess, cost, and availability
• Potency and ability to lower serum triglycerides is unique among the HMG-CoA reductase inhibitors. However, no outcome data available

PATIENT/FAMILY EDUCATION

• Report symptoms of myalgia, muscle tenderness, or weakness
• Take daily doses in the evening for increased effect

MONITORING PARAMETERS

• Cholesterol (max therapeutic response 4-6 wk)
• LFT's (AST, ALT) at baseline and at 12 wk of therapy: if no change, no further monitoring necessary (discontinue if elevations persist at >3 × upper limit of normal)
• CPK in patients complaining of diffuse myalgia, muscle tenderness, or weakness

---

atovaquone
(a-toe′va-kwone)
Rx: Mepron
Combinations
   Rx: with proguanil (Malarone)
Chemical Class: Hydroxynapthoquinone derivative
Therapeutic Class: Antiprotozoal

CLINICAL PHARMACOLOGY

Mechanism of Action: A systemic anti-infective that inhibits the mitochondrial electron-transport system at the cytochrome bc1 complex (Complex III), which interrupts nucleic acid and adenosine triphosphate synthesis. *Therapeutic Effect:* Antiprotozoal and antipneumocystic activity.

Pharmacokinetics

Absorption increased with a high-fat meal. Protein binding: greater than 99%. Metabolized in liver. Primarily excreted in feces. **Half-life:** 2-3 days.

INDICATIONS AND DOSAGES

Pneumocystis carinii pneumonia (PCP)

PO

Adults. 750 mg twice a day with food for 21 days.

Children. 40 mg/kg/day in 2 divided doses. Maximumum: 1500 mg/day.

Prevention of PCP

PO

Adults. 1,500 mg once a day with food.

Children 4-24 mos. 45 mg/kg/day as single dose. Maximumum: 1500 mg/day.

Children 1-3 mos and older than 24 mos. 30 mg/kg/day as single dose. Maximumum: 1500 mg/day.

Usual pediatric dosage
PO
Children. 40 mg/kg/day with food.
S **AVAILABLE FORMS/COST**
• Susp—Oral: 750 mg/5 ml, 210 ml: **$738.64**
• Tab—Oral: 62.5 mg atovaquone-25 mg proguanil, 100's: **$174.00**; 250 mg atovaquone-100 mg proguanil, 100's: **$470.40**

CONTRAINDICATIONS: Development or history of potentially life-threatening allergic reaction to the drug

PREGNANCY AND LACTATION: Pregnancy category C; human breast milk studies not available; in rats, concentrations in milk 30% of maternal serum

SIDE EFFECTS
Frequent (greater than 10%)
Rash, nausea, diarrhea, headache, vomiting, fever, insomnia, cough
Occasional (less than 10%)
Abdominal discomfort, thrush, asthenia, anemia, neutropenia

SERIOUS REACTIONS
• None known.

SPECIAL CONSIDERATIONS
• Plasma concentrations have been shown to correlate with the likelihood of successful treatment and survival

---

atropine
(a'troe-peen)
Rx: Atropine Care, Atropen Autoinjector, Atropisol, Atrosulf-1, Isopto Atropine, Ocu-Tropine, Sal-Tropine
Chemical Class: Belladonna alkaloid
Therapeutic Class: Antiasthmatic; anticholinergic; antispasmodic; bronchodilator; gastrointestinal; mydriatic; ophthalmic anticholinergic

CLINICAL PHARMACOLOGY
Mechanism of Action: An acetylcholine antagonist that inhibits the action of acetylcholine by competing with acetylcholine for common binding sites on muscarinic receptors, which are located on exocrine glands, cardiac and smooth-muscle ganglia, and intramural neurons. This action blocks all muscarinic effects. *Therapeutic Effect:* Decreases GI motility and secretory activity, and GU muscle tone (ureter, bladder); produces ophthalmic cycloplegia, and mydriasis.

INDICATIONS AND DOSAGES
Asystole, slow pulseless electrical activity
IV
Adults, Elderly. 1 mg; may repeat q3-5min up to total dose of 0.04 mg/kg.
Pre-anesthetic
IV/IM/Subcutaneous
Adults, Elderly. 0.4-0.6 mg 30-60 min pre-op.
Children weighing 5 kg or more. 0.01-0.02 mg/kg/dose to maximum of 0.4 mg/dose.
Children weighing less than 5 kg. 0.02 mg/kg/dose 30-60 min pre-op.

Bradycardia
IV
Adults, Elderly. 0.5-1 mg q5min not to exceed 2 mg or 0.04 mg/kg.
Children. 0.02 mg/kg with a minimum of 0.1 mg to a maximum of 0.5 mg in children and 1 mg in adolescents. May repeat in 5 min. Maximum total dose: 1 mg in children, 2 mg in adolescents.

$ AVAILABLE FORMS/COST
• Sol, Inj—IM, IV, SC: 0.05 mg/ml, 5 ml: **$6.25-$7.50**; 0.1 mg/ml, 5 ml: **$3.24-$12.35**; 0.4 mg/ml, 1 ml: **$0.44-$1.80**; 0.5 mg/ml, 1 ml: **$2.38**; 1 mg/ml, 1 ml: **$0.49-$1.98**
• Sol, Inj (Pen injector)—IM: 0.5 mg, 1 mg, 2 mg: *cost not available*
• Oint—Ophth: 1%, 3.5 g: **$1.35-$3.30**
• Sol—Ophth: 1%, 5 ml: **$2.52-$19.00**; 2%, 2 ml: **$4.76**
• Tab—Oral: 0.4 mg, 100's: **$29.95**

CONTRAINDICATIONS: Bladder neck obstruction due to prostatic hypertrophy, cardiospasm, intestinal atony, myasthenia gravis in those not treated with neostigmine, narrow-angle glaucoma, obstructive disease of the GI tract, paralytic ileus, severe ulcerative colitis, tachycardia secondary to cardiac insufficiency or thyrotoxicosis, toxic megacolon, unstable cardiovascular status in acute hemorrhage

PREGNANCY AND LACTATION: Pregnancy category C; passage into breast milk still controversial; neonates particularly sensitive to anticholinergic agents; compatible with breast-feeding

SIDE EFFECTS
Frequent
Dry mouth, nose, and throat that may be severe; decreased sweating, constipation, irritation at subcutaneous or IM injection site

Occasional
Swallowing difficulty, blurred vision, bloated feeling, impotence, urinary hesitancy

Rare
Allergic reaction, including rash and urticaria; mental confusion or excitement, particularly in children, fatigue

SERIOUS REACTIONS
• Overdosage may produce tachycardia, palpitations, hot, dry or flushed skin, absence of bowel sounds, increased respiratory rate, nausea, vomiting, confusion, somnolence, slurred speech, dizziness and CNS stimulation.
• Overdosage may also produce psychosis as evidenced by agitation, restlessness, rambling speech, visual hallucinations, paranoid behavior, and delusions, followed by depression.

INTERACTIONS
Drugs
▣ *Amantadine:* Enhanced anticholinergic effect of atropine; enhanced CNS effect of amantadine
▣ *Neuroleptics:* Reduced neuroleptic effect
▣ *Rimantadine:* Enhanced anticholinergic effect of atropine; enhanced CNS effect of rimantadine
▣ *Tacrine:* May reduce anticholinergic effect of atropine; atropine may reduce CNS effect of tacrine

auranofin
(ah-ran'-oh-fin)
Rx: Ridaura
Chemical Class: Gold compound
Therapeutic Class: Disease-modifying antirheumatic drug (DMARD)

CLINICAL PHARMACOLOGY
Mechanism of Action: Gold compounds that alter cellular mechanisms, collagen biosynthesis, enzyme systems, and immune responses. *Therapeutic Effect:* Suppress synovitis in the active stage of rheumatoid arthritis.
Pharmacokinetics
Auranofin (29% gold): Moderately absorbed from the GI tract. Protein binding: 60%. Rapidly metabolized. Primarily excreted in urine. **Half-life:** 21–31 days. Aurothioglucose (50% gold): Slowly and erratically absorbed after IM administration. Protein binding: 95%–99%. Primarily excreted in urine. **Half-life:** 3–27 days (increased with increased number of doses).

INDICATIONS AND DOSAGES
Rheumatoid arthritis
PO
Adults, Elderly. 6 mg/day as a single or 2 divided doses. If there is no response in 6 mo, may increase to 9 mg/day in 3 divided doses. If response is still inadequate, discontinue.
Children. 0.1 mg/kg/day as a single or 2 divided doses. Maintenance: 0.15 mg/kg/day. Maximum: 0.2 mg/kg/day.
IM
Adults, Elderly. Initially, 10 mg, followed by 25 mg for 2 doses, then 50 mg weekly until total dose of 0.8–1 g has been given. If patient has im-proved and shows no signs of toxicity, may give 50 mg q3-4wk for many months.
Children. 0.25 mg/kg; may increase by 0.25 mg/kg each week. Maintenance: 0.75–1 mg/kg/dose. Maximum: 25 mg/dose for 20 doses, then repeated q2–4wk.

$\boxed{\text{S}}$ AVAILABLE FORMS/COST
• Cap, Gel—Oral: 3 mg, 60's: **$170.26-$224.50**
UNLABELED USES: Treatment of pemphigus, psoriatic arthritis
CONTRAINDICATIONS: Bone marrow aplasia, history of gold-induced pathologies (including blood dyscrasias, exfoliative dermatitis, necrotizing enterocolitis, and pulmonary fibrosis), severe blood dyscrasias
PREGNANCY AND LACTATION: Pregnancy category C; nursing not recommended; gold appears in breast milk
SIDE EFFECTS
Frequent
Auranofin: Diarrhea (50%), pruritic rash (26%), abdominal pain (14%), stomatitis (13%), nausea (10%)
Aurothioglucose: Rash (39%), stomatitis (19%), diarrhea (13%).
Occasional
Aurothioglucose: Nausea, vomiting, anorexia, abdominal cramps
SERIOUS REACTIONS
• Signs and symptoms of gold toxicity, the primary serious reaction, include decreased Hgb level, decreased granulocyte count (less than 150,000/mm^3), proteinuria, hematuria, stomatitis, blood dyscrasias (anemia, leukopenia [WBC count less than 4,000/mm^3], thrombocytopenia, and eosinophilia), glomerulonephritis, nephrotic syndrome, and cholestatic jaundice.
SPECIAL CONSIDERATIONS
• Pruritus is a warning sign for development of cutaneous reactions

• Metallic taste may be a warning sign of stomatitis development

MONITORING PARAMETERS
• CBC, platelet count, urinalysis, renal function, and LFTs before treatment
• CBC, platelet count, urinalysis every month during therapy
• Gold toxicity

---

aurothioglucose/gold sodium thiomalate

Rx: Solganol (aurothioglucose); Aurolate, Myochrysine (gold sodium thiomalate)
Chemical Class: Heavy metal, active gold compound (50%)
Therapeutic Class: Disease-modifying antirheumatic drug (DMARD)

CLINICAL PHARMACOLOGY
Mechanism of Action: Aurothioglucose: A gold compound that alters cellular mechanisms, collagen biosynthesis, enzyme systems, and immune responses. *Therapeutic Effect:* Suppresses synovitis of the active stage of rheumatoid arthritis.
Gold sodium thiomalate: A gold compound whose mechanism of action is unknown. May decrease prostaglandin synthesis or alter cellular mechanisms by inhibiting sulfhydryl systems. *Therapeutic Effect:* Decreases synovial inflammation, retards cartilage and bone destruction, suppresses or prevents but does not cure, arthritis, synovitis.

Pharmacokinetics
Aurothioglucose (50% gold): Slow, erratic absorption after IM administration. Protein binding: 95%-99%. Primarily excreted in urine. **Half-life:** 3- 27 days (half-life increased with increased number of doses).

Gold sodium thiomalate: Well absorbed. Protein binding: 95%. Widely distributed. Metabolized in liver. Excreted in urine and feces. Not removed my hemodialysis. **Half-life:** 5 days.

INDICATIONS AND DOSAGES
Rheumatoid arthritis (Aurothioglucose)
IM
Adults, Elderly. Initially, 10 mg, then 25 mg for 2 doses, then 50 mg weekly thereafter until total dose of 0.8- 1 g given. If patient is improved and there are no signs of toxicity, may give 50 mg at 3- to 4-wk intervals for many months.
Children. 0. 25 mg/kg, may increase by 0. 25 mg/kg each week. Maintenance: 0.75- 1 mg/kg/dose. Maximum: 25-mg dose for total of 20 doses, then q2-4wks.

Rheumatoid arthritis (Gold sodium thiomalate)
IM
Adults, Elderly. Initially, 10 mg, then 25 mg for second dose. Follow with 25- 50 mg/wk until improvement noted or total of 1 g administered. Maintenance: 25- 50 mg q2wks for 2- 20 wks; if stable, may increase to q3-4wk intervals.
Children. Initially, 10 mg, then 1 mg/kg/wk. Maximum single dose: 50 mg. Maintenance: 1 mg/kg/dose at 2- to 4-wk intervals.

Dosage in renal impairment

Creatinine Clearance	Dosage
50-80 ml/min	50% of usual dosage
less than 50 ml/min	not recommended

S   AVAILABLE FORMS/COST
Aurothioglucose
• Inj, Susp in Oil—IM: 50 mg/ml, 10 ml: **$167.70-$182.24**
Gold Sodium Thiomalate
• Sol, Inj-IM: 50 mg/ml, 10 ml: **$118.11-$156.86**

UNLABELED USES: Treatment of pemphigus, psoriatic arthritis

CONTRAINDICATIONS:

Aurothioglucose

Bone marrow aplasia, history of gold-induced pathologies, including blood dyscrasias, exfoliative dermatitis, necrotizing enterocolitis, and pulmonary fibrosis, serious adverse effects with previous gold therapy, severe blood dyscrasias

Gold sodium thiomalate

Colitis, concurrent use of antimalarials, immunosuppressive agents, penicillamine, or phenylbutazone, congestive heart failure (CHF), exfoliative dermatitis, history of blood dyscrasias, severe liver or renal impairment, systemic lupus erythematosus

PREGNANCY AND LACTATION: Pregnancy category C; gold has been demonstrated in breast milk and in the serum and red blood cells of a nursing infant; the slow excretion and persistence of gold in the mother, even after discontinuing therapy, must also be considered

SIDE EFFECTS

Frequent

Aurothioglucose: Rash, stomatitis, diarrhea

Gold sodium thiomalate: Pruritic dermatitis, stomatitis, marked by erythema, redness, shallow ulcers of oral mucous membranes, sore throat, and difficulty swallowing, diarrhea or loose stools, abdominal pain, nausea

Occasional

Aurothioglucose: Nausea, vomiting, anorexia, abdominal cramps

Gold sodium thiomalate: Vomiting, anorexia, flatulence, dyspepsia, conjunctivitis, photosensitivity

Rare

Gold sodium thiomalate: Constipation, urticaria, rash

SERIOUS REACTIONS

• Gold toxicity is the primary serious reaction. Signs and symptoms of gold toxicity include decreased hemoglobin, leukopenia (WBC count less than $4,000/mm^3$), reduced granulocyte counts (less than $150,000/mm^3$), proteinuria, hematuria, stomatitis (sores, ulcers and white spots in the mouth and throat), blood dyscrasias (anemia, leukopenia, thrombocytopenia and eosinophilia), glomerulonephritis, nephritic syndrome, and cholestatic jaundice.

SPECIAL CONSIDERATIONS

• Pruritus is a warning sign for development of cutaneous reactions

• Metallic taste may be a warning sign of stomatitis development

MONITORING PARAMETERS

• CBC, platelet count, urinalysis, renal function, and LFTs before treatment

• CBC, platelet count, urinalysis every month during therapy

• Gold toxicity

---

azathioprine
(ay-za-thye′oh-preen)
Rx: Imuran
Chemical Class: 6-mercaptopurine derivative; purine analog
Therapeutic Class: Immunosuppressant

CLINICAL PHARMACOLOGY

Mechanism of Action: An immunologic agent that antagonizes purine metabolism and inhibits DNA, protein, and RNA synthesis. *Therapeutic Effect:* Suppresses cell-mediated hypersensitivities; alters antibody production and immune response in transplant recipients; reduces the severity of arthritis symptoms.

INDICATIONS AND DOSAGES
Adjunct in prevention of renal allograft rejection
PO, IV

Adults, Elderly, Children. 2–5 mg/kg/day on day of transplant, then 1–3 mg/kg/day as maintenance dose.

Rheumatoid arthritis
PO

Adults. Initially, 1 mg/kg/day as a single dose or in 2 divided doses. May increase by 0.5 mg/kg/day after 6–8 wk at 4-wk intervals up to maximum of 2.5 mg/kg/day. Maintenance: Lowest effective dosage. May decrease dose by 0.5 mg/kg or 25 mg/day q4wk (while other therapies, such as rest, physiotherapy, and salicylates, are maintained).

Elderly. Initially, 1 mg/kg/day (50–100 mg); may increase by 25 mg/day until response or toxicity.

Dosage in renal impairment
Dosage is modified based on creatinine clearance.

Creatinine Clearance	Dose
10–50 ml/min	75% of usual dose
less than 10 ml/min	50% of usual dose

§ AVAILABLE FORMS/COST
• Powder, Inj-IV: 100 mg/vial: **$62.99-$113.59**
• Tab-Oral: 50 mg, 100's: **$130.93-$249.63**; 75 mg, 100's: **$294.70**; 100 mg, 100's: **$392.94**

UNLABELED USES: Treatment of biliary cirrhosis, chronic active hepatitis, glomerulonephritis, inflammatory bowel disease, inflammatory myopathy, multiple sclerosis, myasthenia gravis, nephrotic syndrome, pemphigoid, pemphigus, polymyositis, systemic lupus erythematosus

CONTRAINDICATIONS: Pregnant patients with rheumatoid arthritis

PREGNANCY AND LACTATION:
Pregnancy category D

SIDE EFFECTS
Frequent
Nausea, vomiting, anorexia (particularly during early treatment and with large doses)
Occasional
Rash
Rare
Severe nausea and vomiting with diarrhea, abdominal pain, hypersensitivity reaction

SERIOUS REACTIONS
• Azathioprine use increases the risk of developing neoplasia (new abnormal-growth tumors).
• Significant leukopenia and thrombocytopenia may occur, particularly in those undergoing kidney transplant rejection.
• Hepatotoxicity occurs rarely.

INTERACTIONS
Drugs
❷ *Allopurinol:* Allopurinol may increase toxicity of azathioprine; dosage adjustment is necessary
❸ *Warfarin:* Reduced warfarin effect

SPECIAL CONSIDERATIONS
• Severe leukopenia and/or thrombocytopenia may occur as well as macrocytic anemia and bone marrow depression; fungal, viral, bacterial, and protozoal infections may be fatal; may increase the patient's risk of neoplasia via mutagenic and carcinogenic properties (skin cancer and reticulum cell or lymphomatous tumors); temporary depression in spermatogenesis

MONITORING PARAMETERS
• Hgb, WBC, platelets monthly
• D/C if leukocytes are <3000/mm^3
• Therapeutic response may take 3-4 mo in rheumatoid arthritis

A

azelaic acid
(a-zuh-lay'ick)

Rx: Azelex, Finacea Ge
Chemical Class: Dicarboxylic acid
Therapeutic Class: Antiacne agent

CLINICAL PHARMACOLOGY
Mechanism of Action: A hypopigmentation agent that possesses antimicrobial action by inhibiting cellular protein synthesis in aerobic and anaerobic microorganisms. *Therapeutic Effect:* Improves acne vulgaris, normalizing keratin process.

Pharmacokinetics
Minimal absorption after topical administration. Metabolized in liver. Excreted in urine as unchanged drug. **Half-life:** 12 hrs.

INDICATIONS AND DOSAGES
Antiacne, hypopigmentation
Topical
Adults, Adolescents. Apply topically to affected area 2 times/day (morning and evening).

S AVAILABLE FORMS/COST
• Cre-Top: 15%, 30 g: **$48.94**; 20%, 30, 50 g: **$40.44-$50.95**/30 g

CONTRAINDICATIONS: Hypersensitivity to azelaic acid or any component of the formulation

PREGNANCY AND LACTATION: Pregnancy category B; distributed in breast milk but little absorbed systemically and unlikely that concentrations of this normal dietary consituent would exceed baseline endogenous concentrations

SIDE EFFECTS
Occasional
Pruritus, stinging, burning, tingling
Rare
Erythema, dryness, rash, peeling, irritation, contact dermatitis

SERIOUS REACTIONS
• None reported.

SPECIAL CONSIDERATIONS
• Wash hands after application; avoid contact with mucous membranes; if drug gets into eyes, wash with large quantities of water
• If skin irritation occurs, decrease frequency of application or temporarily discontinue treatment
• Azelaic acid is a naturally occurring substance found in the human diet

azelastine
(a'zel-ah-steen)

Rx: Astelin (nasal), Optivar (ophthalmic)
Chemical Class: Phthalazinone derivative
Therapeutic Class: Antihistamine

CLINICAL PHARMACOLOGY
Mechanism of Action: An antihistamine that competes with histamine for histamine receptor sites on cells in the blood vessels, GI tract, and respiratory tract. *Therapeutic Effect:* Relieves symptoms associated with seasonal allergic rhinitis such as increased mucus production and sneezing and symptoms associated with allergic conjunctivitis, such as redness, itching, and excessive tearing.

Pharmacokinetics

Route	Onset	Peak	Duration
Nasal spray	0.5–1 hr	2–3 hr	12 hr
Ophthalmic	N/A	3 min	8 hr

Well absorbed through nasal mucosa. Primarily excreted in feces. **Half-life:** 22 hrs

INDICATIONS AND DOSAGES
Allergic rhinitis
Nasal

Adults, Elderly, Children 12 yr and older. 2 sprays in each nostril twice a day.

Children 5–11 yr. 1 spray in each nostril twice a day.

Allergic conjunctivitis
Ophthalmic

Adults, Elderly, Children 3 yr or older. 1 drop into affected eye twice a day.

$ AVAILABLE FORMS/COST
• Spray, Nasal—INH: 137 mcg/spray, 34 ml (2 x 17 ml bottles), 100 sprays/bottle: **$59.57-$62.24**

• Sol—Ophth: 0.05%, 3, 6, 10 ml: **$46.51**/3 ml

CONTRAINDICATIONS: Breast-feeding women, history of hypersensitivity to antihistamines, neonates or premature infants, third trimester of pregnancy

PREGNANCY AND LACTATION: Pregnancy category C, excretion into breast milk unknown

SIDE EFFECTS
Frequent (20%–15%)
Headache, bitter taste

Rare
Nasal burning, paroxysmal sneezing

Ophthalmic: Transient eye burning or stinging, bitter taste, headache

SERIOUS REACTIONS
• Epistaxis occurs rarely.

SPECIAL CONSIDERATIONS
• Low sedating antihistamine nasal spray with first-dose activity; note: onset of action not as fast as decongestant nasal sprays, but appropriate for prn use

PATIENT/FAMILY EDUCATION
• Advise caution with use concomitant with activities that require concentration or while operating machinery; may cause drowsiness

• Preservative in ophth sol, benzlkonium chloride, may be absorbed by soft contact lenses, wait at least 10 min after instilling ophth sol before inserting soft contacts

---

azithromycin
(ay-zi-thro-mye'sin)
Rx: Zithromax
Chemical Class: Macrolide derivative
Therapeutic Class: Antibiotic

CLINICAL PHARMACOLOGY
Mechanism of Action: A macrolide antibiotic that binds to ribosomal receptor sites of susceptible organisms, inhibiting RNA-dependent protein synthesis. *Therapeutic Effect:* Bacteriostatic or bactericidal, depending on the drug dosage.

Pharmacokinetics
Rapidly absorbed from the GI tract. Protein binding: 7%-50%. Widely distributed. Eliminated primarily unchanged by biliary excretion. *Half-life:* 68 hr.

INDICATIONS AND DOSAGES
Respiratory tract, skin, and skin-structure infections
PO

Adults, Elderly. 500 mg once, then 250 mg/day for 4 days.

Children 6 mo and older. 10 mg/kg once (maximum 500 mg) then 5 mg/kg/day for 4 days (maximum 250 mg).

Acute bacterial exacerbations of COPD
PO

Adults. 500 mg/day for 3 days.

Otitis media
PO

Children 6 mo and older. 10 mg/kg once (maximum 500 mg) then 5 mg/kg/day for 4 days (maximum 250 mg). Single dose: 30 mg/kg.

Maximum: 1500 mg. Three day regimen: 10 mg/kg/day as single daily dose. Maximum: 500 mg/day.

Pharyngitis, tonsillitis

PO

Children older than 2 yr. 12 mg/kg/day (maximum 500 mg) for 5 days.

Chancroid

PO

Adults, Elderly: 1 g as single dose.

Children: 20 mg/kg as single dose. Maximum: 1 g.

Treatment of Mycobacterium avium complex (MAC)

PO

Adults, Elderly. 500 mg/day in combination.

Children. 5 mg/kg/day (maximum 250 mg) in combination.

Prevention of MAC

PO

Adults, Elderly. 1,200 mg/wk alone or with rifabutin.

Children. 5 mg/kg/day (maximum 250 mg) or 20 mg/kg/wk (maximum 1,200 mg) alone or with rifabutin.

Nongonococcal urethritis and cervicitis due to Chlamydia trachomatis

PO

Adults. 1 g as a single dose.

Usual pediatric dosage

PO

Children older than 6 mo. 10 mg/kg once (maximum: 500 mg) then 5 mg/kg/day for 4 days (maximum 250 mg).

Usual parenteral dosage (Community Acquired Pneumonia, PID)

IV

Adults. 500 mg/day, followed by oral therapy.

[$] **AVAILABLE FORMS/COST**

- Cap-Oral: 250 mg, 6's: **$37.32-$46.38**
- Powder, Inj-IV: 500 mg/vial: **$24.44-$27.83**
- Sachet—Oral: 1 g: **$22.75**
- Susp—Oral: 100 mg/5 ml, 15 ml: **$31.01-$34.73**; 200 mg/5 ml, 15, 22.5, 30 ml: **$31.01-$38.26**/15 ml
- Tab—Oral: 250 mg, 30's: **$235.35**; 500 mg, 30's: **$470.69**; 600 mg, 30's: **$564.84**

UNLABELED USES: Chlamydial infections, gonococcal pharyngitis, uncomplicated gonococcal infections of the cervix, urethra, and rectum

CONTRAINDICATIONS: Hypersensitivity to azithromycin or other macrolide antibiotics

PREGNANCY AND LACTATION: Pregnancy category B; excretion into breast milk unknown

SIDE EFFECTS

Occasional

Nausea, vomiting, diarrhea, abdominal pain

Rare

Headache, dizziness, allergic reaction

SERIOUS REACTIONS

- Antibiotic-associated colitis and other superinfections may result from altered bacterial balance.
- Acute interstitial nephritis and hepatotoxicity occur rarely.

INTERACTIONS

Drugs

[3] *Penicillins:* Azithromycin may inhibit antibacterial activity of penicillins

Labs

- *Increase:* Serum 17 Hydroxycorticosteroids, 17 ketosteroids
- *Decrease:* Serum folate (bioassay only)

SPECIAL CONSIDERATIONS

- Otitis media: single dose and 3d therapy similar efficacy but fewer side effects than amoxicillin/clavulanate × 10d
- Group A strep pharyngitis; 12 mg/kg/d × 5d shown to have superior cure rate to PCN × 10d but no data on rheumatic fever prophylaxis

PATIENT/FAMILY EDUCATION
• Tablet may be taken without regard to food. Suspension and capsule should be taken on an empty stomach

---

aztreonam
(az-tree'oo-nam)
Rx: Azactam
Chemical Class: Monobactam
Therapeutic Class: Antibiotic

CLINICAL PHARMACOLOGY
Mechanism of Action: A monobactam antibiotic that inhibits bacterial cell wall synthesis. *Therapeutic Effect:* Bactericidal.
Pharmacokinetics
Completely absorbed after IM administration. Protein binding: 56%-60%. Partially metabolized by hydrolysis. Primarily excreted unchanged in urine. Removed by hemodialysis. **Half-life:** 1.4-2.2 hr (increased in impaired renal or hepatic function).
INDICATIONS AND DOSAGES
UTIs
IV, IM
Adults, Elderly. 500 mg-1 g q8-12h.
Moderate to severe systemic infections
IV, IM
Adults, Elderly. 1-2 g q8-12h.
Severe or life-threatening infections
IV
Adults, Elderly. 2 g q6-8h.
Cystic Fibrosis
IV
Children. 50 mg/kg/dose q6-8h up to 200 mg/kg/day. Maximum: 8g/d.
Mild to severe infections in children
IV
Children. 30 mg/kg q6-8h. Maximum: 120 mg/kg/day.

Neonates. 60-120 mg/kg/day q6-12h.
Dosage in renal impairment
Dosage and frequency are modified based on creatinine clearance and the severity of the infection:

Creatinine Clearance	Dosage
10-30 ml/min	1-2 g initially, then ½ usual dose at usual intervals
less than 10 ml/min	1-2 g initially; then ¼ usual dose at usual intervals

$ **AVAILABLE FORMS/COST**
• Powder, Inj-IM, IV: 500 mg/vial: **$11.64**; 1 g/vial: **$21.61**; 2 g/vial: **$43.13**
UNLABELED USES: Treatment of bone and joint infections
CONTRAINDICATIONS: None known.
PREGNANCY AND LACTATION: Pregnancy category B; excreted in breast milk in concentrations <1% of maternal serum concentrations
SIDE EFFECTS
Occasional (less than 3%)
Discomfort and swelling at IM injection site, nausea, vomiting, diarrhea, rash
Rare (less than 1%)
Phlebitis or thrombophlebitis at IV injection site, abdominal cramps, headache, hypotension
SERIOUS REACTIONS
• Antibiotic-associated colitis and other superinfections may result from altered bacterial balance.
• Severe hypersensitivity reactions, including anaphylaxis, occur rarely.
INTERACTIONS
Drugs
▣ *Aminoglycosides:* Potential increased nephrotoxicity, ototoxicity
▣ *Cephalosporins, imipenem:* Antagonism secondary to antibiotic-induced high levels of β-lactamase

SPECIAL CONSIDERATIONS
• Minimal cross-reactivity between aztreonam and penicillins and cephalosporins; aztreonam and aminoglycosides have been shown to be synergistic *in vitro* against most strains of *P. aeruginosa,* many strains of *Enterobacteriaceae,* and other gram-negative aerobic bacilli

---

bacitracin
(bass-i-tray′sin)
Rx: Ak-Tracin, Baci-Rx, Bacticin, Ocu-Tracin, Spectro-Bacitracin
Combinations
Rx: with neomycin, poly-mixin, and hydrocortisone (Cortisporin)
OTC: with neomycin and polymixin (Neosporin); with polymixin (Polysporin)
Chemical Class: Bacillus subtilis derivative
Therapeutic Class: Antibacterial; ophthalmic antibiotic

CLINICAL PHARMACOLOGY
Mechanism of Action: An antibiotic that interferes with plasma membrane permeability and inhibits bacterial cell wall synthesis in susceptible bacteria. *Therapeutic Effect:* Bacteriostatic.
INDICATIONS AND DOSAGES
Superficial ocular infections
Ophthalmic
Adults. ½-inch ribbon in conjunctival sac q3-4h.
Skin abrasions, superficial skin infections
Topical
Adults, Children. Apply to affected area 1-5 times a day.
Surgical treatment and prophylaxis
Irrigation

Adults, Elderly. 50,000-150,000 units, as needed.
AVAILABLE FORMS/COST
• Powder, Inj—IM: 50,000 U/vial: **$5.00-$11.88**
• Oint—Ophth: 500 unit/g, 3.5 g: **$1.30-$11.96**
• Oint—Top: 500 unit/g, 15, 30, 60, 120, 144, 454, 480 g: **$0.95-$17.60**/30 g
CONTRAINDICATIONS: None known
PREGNANCY AND LACTATION: Pregnancy category C
SIDE EFFECTS
Rare
Ophthalmic: Burning, itching, redness, swelling, pain
Topical: Hypersensitivity reaction (allergic contact dermatitis, burning, inflammation, pruritus)
SERIOUS REACTIONS
• Severe hypersensitivity reactions, including apnea and hypotension, occur rarely.
SPECIAL CONSIDERATIONS
• Administer IM in deep muscle mass; rotate injection site; do *not* give IV/SC

---

baclofen
(bak′loe-fen)
Rx: Lioresal, Lioresal Intrathecal
Chemical Class: GABA chlorophenyl derivative
Therapeutic Class: Skeletal muscle relaxant

CLINICAL PHARMACOLOGY
Mechanism of Action: A direct-acting skeletal muscle relaxant that inhibits transmission of reflexes at the spinal cord level. *Therapeutic Effect:* Relieves muscle spasticity.

Pharmacokinetics
Well absorbed from the GI tract. Protein binding: 30%. Partially metabolized in the liver. Primarily excreted in urine. **Half-life:** 2.5–4 hr; intrathecal: 1.5 hr.

INDICATIONS AND DOSAGES
Spasticity
PO
Adults. Initially, 5 mg 3 times a day. May increase by 15 mg/day at 3-day intervals. Range: 40–80 mg/day. Maximum: 80 mg/day.
Elderly. Initially, 5 mg 2–3 times a day. May gradually increase dosage.
Children. Initially, 10–15 mg/day in divided doses q8h. May increase by 5-15 mg/day at 3-day intervals. Maximum: 40 mg/day (children 2-7 yr); 60 mg/day (children 8 yr and older).
Usual intrathecal dosage
Adults, Elderly, Children older than 12 yr. 300–800 mcg/day.
Children 12 yr and younger. 100–300 mcg/day.

$ AVAILABLE FORMS/COST
• Kit—Intrathecal: 0.05 mg/ml, 20 ml: **$78.00-$84.00**; 0.5 mg/ml, 20 ml: **$208.00**; 2 mg/ml, 5 ml: **$213.50-$226.75**
• Tab—Oral: 10 mg, 100's: **$31.75-$64.90**; 20 mg, 100's: **$56.90-$118.85**

UNLABELED USES: Treatment of trigeminal neuralgia
CONTRAINDICATIONS: Skeletal muscle spasm due to cerebral palsy, Parkinson's disease, rheumatic disorders, CVA
PREGNANCY AND LACTATION: Pregnancy category C; present in breast milk, 0.1% of mother's dose; compatible with breast-feeding
SIDE EFFECTS
Frequent (greater than 10%)
Transient somnolence, asthenia, dizziness, light-headedness, nausea, vomiting

Occasional (10%–2%)
Headache, paresthesia, constipation, anorexia, hypotension, confusion, nasal congestion
Rare (less than 1%)
Paradoxical CNS excitement or restlessness, slurred speech, tremor, dry mouth, diarrhea, nocturia, impotence

SERIOUS REACTIONS
• Abrupt discontinuation of baclofen may produce hallucinations and seizures.
• Overdose results in blurred vision, seizures, myosis, mydriasis, severe muscle weakness, strabismus, respiratory depression, and vomiting.

SPECIAL CONSIDERATIONS
• Abrupt discontinuation may lead to hallucinations, spasticity, tachycardia; drug should be tapered off over 1-2 wk

balsalazide

(ball-sal'a-zide)
Rx: Colazal
Chemical Class: 5-amino derivative of salicylic acid
Therapeutic Class: Gastrointestinal antiinflammatory

CLINICAL PHARMACOLOGY
Mechanism of Action: A 5-aminosalicylic acid derivative that changes intestinal microflora, altering prostaglandin production and inhibiting function of natural killer cells, mast cells, neutrophils, and macrophages. *Therapeutic Effect:* Diminishes inflammatory effect in colon.

INDICATIONS AND DOSAGES
Ulcerative colitis
PO
Adults, Elderly. Three 750-mg capsules 3 times a day for 8 wk.

§ **AVAILABLE FORMS/COST**
• Cap—Oral: 750 mg, 280's: **$320.00**

CONTRAINDICATIONS: Hypersensitivity to salicylates

PREGNANCY AND LACTATION: Pregnancy category B; excretion into breast milk unknown, mesalamine has produced adverse effects in a nursing infant and should be used with caution during breastfeeding; observe nursing infant closely for changes in stool consistency

SIDE EFFECTS
Frequent (8%–6%)
Headache, abdominal pain, nausea, diarrhea
Occasional (4%–2%)
Vomiting, arthralgia, rhinitis, insomnia, fatigue, flatulence, coughing, dyspepsia

SERIOUS REACTIONS
• Liver toxicity occurs rarely.

INTERACTIONS
Drugs
③ *Orally administered antibiotics:* Theoretical interference with the release of mesalamine in the colon

SPECIAL CONSIDERATIONS
• The recommended dose of 6.75 g/day provides approximately 2.4 g of free mesalamine to the colon

---

becaplermin
(beh-cap-lear-min)
Rx: Regranex
Chemical Class: Recombinant human platelet-derived growth factor (rhPDGF-BB)
Therapeutic Class: Diabetic neuropathic ulcer agent

B

CLINICAL PHARMACOLOGY
Mechanism of Action: A platelet-derived growth factor that heals open wounds. *Therapeutic Effect:* Stimulates body to grow new tissue.
Pharmacokinetics
None reported.

INDICATIONS AND DOSAGES
Ulcers
Topical
Adults, Elderly. Apply once daily (spread evenly; cover with saline-moistened gauze dressing). After 12 hrs, rinse ulcer, re-cover with saline gauze.

§ **AVAILABLE FORMS/COST**
• Gel—Top: 0.01%, 15 g: **$533.15**

CONTRAINDICATIONS: Neoplasms at site of application, hypersensitivity to becaplermin or any component of the formulation

PREGNANCY AND LACTATION: Pregnancy category C; excretion into breast milk is unknown but would be expected to be low given the systemic bioavailability of the drug

SIDE EFFECTS
Occasional
Local rash near ulcer

SERIOUS REACTIONS
• None reported.

SPECIAL CONSIDERATIONS
PATIENT/FAMILY EDUCATION
• Refrigerate
• Wash hands before applying

MONITORING PARAMETERS
• If the ulcer does not decrease in size by approximately 30% after 10 wk of treatment or complete healing has not occurred in 20 wk, continued treatment should be reassessed

---

beclomethasone
(be-kloe-meth'a-sone)
Rx: *INH:* Qvar
Rx: *NASAL:* Beconase AQ, Beconase, Vancenase, Vancenase AQ, Vancenase AQ 84 mcg
Chemical Class: Glucocorticoid, synthetic
Therapeutic Class: Corticosteroid, antiinflammatory

CLINICAL PHARMACOLOGY
Mechanism of Action: An adrenocorticosteroid that prevents or controls inflammation by controlling the rate of protein synthesis; decreasing migration of polymorphonuclear leukocytes and fibroblasts; and reversing capillary permeability. *Therapeutic Effect:* Inhalation: Inhibits bronchoconstriction, produces smooth muscle relaxation, decreases mucus secretion. Intranasal: Decreases response to seasonal and perennial rhinitis.
Pharmacokinetics
Rapidly absorbed from pulmonary, nasal, and GI tissue. Undergoes extensive first-pass metabolism in the liver. Protein binding: 87%. Primarily eliminated in feces. **Half-life:** 15 hr.
INDICATIONS AND DOSAGES
Long-term control of bronchial asthma, reduces need for oral corticosteriod therapy for asthma
Oral inhalation

Adults, Elderly Children 12 yr and older. 40-160 mcg twice a day. Maxiumum: 320 mcg twice a day.
Children 5–11 yr. 40 mcg twice a day. Maximum: 80 mcg twice a day.
Relief of seasonal or perennial rhinitis, prevention of nasal polyp recurrence after surgical removal, treatment of nonallergic rhinitis
Nasal Inhalation
Adults, Children older than 12 yr. 1–2 sprays in each nostril twice a day.
Children 6–12 yr. 1 spray in each nostril twice a day. May increase up to 2 sprays in each nostril twice a day.
S **AVAILABLE FORMS/COST**
• MDI Aer—INH: 40 mcg/inh, 7.3 g: **$52.69**; 42 mcg/INH, 6.7 g: **$17.23-$24.70**; 42 mcg/INH, 16.8 g: **$32.78-$54.75**; 80 mcg/INH, 7.3 g: **$66.39**
• MDI Aer—Nasal INH: 42 mcg/INH, 7 g: **$40.15-$45.55**; 42 mcg/INH, 16.8 g: **$32.78-$53.54**
• MDI Double Strength Aer—INH: 84 mcg/INH; 12.2 g: **$53.33**
• Spray—Nasal: 42 mcg/spray, 25 g: **$37.55-$68.23**; 84 mcg/INH, 19 g: **$55.78-$60.26**
UNLABELED USES: Prevention of seasonal rhinitis (nasal form)
CONTRAINDICATIONS: Hypersensitivity to beclomethasone, status asthmaticus
PREGNANCY AND LACTATION: Pregnancy category C; breast milk excretion unknown; other corticosteroids excreted in low concentrations with systemic administration; compatible with breast-feeding
SIDE EFFECTS
Frequent
Inhalation (14%–4%): Throat irritation, dry mouth, hoarseness, cough
Intranasal: Nasal burning, mucosal dryness

Occasional

Inhalation (3%–2%): Localized fungal infection (thrush)

Intranasal: Nasal-crusting epistaxis, sore throat, ulceration of nasal mucosa

Rare

Inhalation: Transient bronchospasm, esophageal candidiasis

Intranasal: Nasal and pharyngeal candidiasis, eye pain

SERIOUS REACTIONS

• An acute hypersensitivity reaction, as evidenced by urticaria, angioedema, and severe bronchospasm, occurs rarely.

• A transfer from systemic to local steroid therapy may unmask previously suppressed bronchial asthma condition.

SPECIAL CONSIDERATIONS

PATIENT/FAMILY EDUCATION

• Rinse mouth with water following INH to decrease possibility of fungal infections, dysphonia

• Review proper MDI administration technique regularly

• Systemic corticosteroid effects from inhaled and nasal steroids inadequate to prevent adrenal insufficiency in patients withdrawn from corticosteroids abruptly

• Response to nasal steroids seen in 3 days-2 wk; discontinue if no improvement in 3 wk

• For prophylactic use, no role in acute treatment of asthma/allergy

---

belladonna alkaloids
(bell-a-don-a al-kuh-loydz)
Rx: Belladonna Tincture
Combinations
Rx: with butalbital (Butibel); with ergotamine and phenobarbital (Bellergal-S, Phenerbel-S); with phenobarbital (Donnatal, Donnatal Extentabs)
Chemical Class: Belladonna alkaloid
Therapeutic Class: Anticholinergic; antispasmodic; gastrointestinal

CLINICAL PHARMACOLOGY

Mechanism of Action: Competitive inhibitors of the muscarinic actions of acetylcholine, acting at receptors located in exocrine glands, smooth and cardiac muscle and intramural neurons. Composed of 3 main constituents atropine, scopolamine and hyoscyamine. Scopolamine exerts greater effects on the CNS, eye and secretory glands than the constituents atropine and hyoscyamine. Atropine exerts more activity on the heart, intestine and bronchial muscle and exhibits a more prolonged duration of action compared to scopolamine. Hyoscyamine exerts similar actions to atropine but has more potent central and peripheral nervous system effects. *Therapeutic effect:* Peripheral anticholinergic and antispasmodic action, mild sedation.

Pharmacokinetics

None known.

INDICATIONS AND DOSAGES

Irritable bowel syndrome, acute enterocolitis

PO

Adults: 1-2 tablets or capsules 3-4 times daily or 1-2 teaspoonfuls of elixir 3-4 times daily according to conditions and severity of symptoms.

Children: Dosage varies depending on body weight and may be dosed every 4 or 6 hours.

$ AVAILABLE FORMS/COST

• Tincture—Oral: 27-33 mg/100 ml, 120 ml: **$8.52**

CONTRAINDICATIONS: Glaucoma, obstructive uropathy, obstructive disease of gastrointestinal tract, paralytic ileus, intestinal atony of the elderly or debilitated patient, unstable cardiovascular status in acute hemorrhage, severe ulcerative colitis especially if complicated by toxic megacolon, myasthenia gravis, hiatal hernia associated with reflux esophagitis, hypersensitivity to any component of the formulation, acute intermittent porphyria.

PREGNANCY AND LACTATION: Pregnancy category C; excretion into breast milk is controversial; neonates may be particularly sensitive to anticholinergic agents; use caution in nursing mothers

SIDE EFFECTS

Frequent

Dry mouth, urinary retention, flushing, pupillary dilation, constipation, confusion, redness of the skin, flushing, dry skin, allergic contact dermatitis, headache, excitement, agitation, dizziness, lightheadedness, drowsiness, unsteadiness, confusion, slurred speech, sedation, hyperreflexia, convulsions, vertigo, coma, mydriasis, photophobia, blurred vision, dilation of pupils

Rare

Hallucinations, acute psychosis, Stevens-Johnson Syndrome, photosensitivity

SERIOUS REACTIONS

• Signs and symptoms of overdose include headache, nausea, vomiting, blurred vision, dilated pupils; hot and dry skin, dizziness, dryness of the mouth, difficulty in swallowing and CNS stimulation.

• Treatment should consist of gastric lavage, emetics, and activated charcoal. If indicated, parenteral cholinergic agents such as physostigmine or bethanechol chloride should be added.

INTERACTIONS

Drugs

▣ *Amantadine:* Enhanced anticholinergic effect; enhanced CNS effect of amantadine

▣ *Neuroleptics:* Reduced neuroleptic effect

▣ *Rimantadine:* Enhanced anticholinergic effect; enhanced CNS effect of rimantadine

▣ *Tacrine:* May reduce anticholinergic effect of atropine; belladonna may reduce CNS effect of tacrine

SPECIAL CONSIDERATIONS

• Product contains hyoscyamine, atropine, and scopolamine

PATIENT/FAMILY EDUCATION

• Avoid hot environments, heat stroke may occur

• Use sunglasses when outside to prevent photophobia

belladonna and opium
(bell-a-don'a)
Rx: B & O Supprettes
Chemical Class: Belladonna alkaloid; opiate
Therapeutic Class: Antispasmodic; narcotic analgesic
DEA Class: Schedule II

CLINICAL PHARMACOLOGY
Mechanism of Action: Anticholinergic alkaloids that inhibits the action of acetylcholine at post-ganglionic (muscarinic) receptor sites. Morphine (10% of opium) depresses cerebral cortex, hypothalamus, and medullary centers. *Therapeutic Effect:* Decreases digestive secretions, increases GI muscle tone, reduces GI force, alters pain perception and emotional response to pain.

Pharmacokinetics
Onset of action occurs within 30 minutes Absorption is dependent on body hydration. Metabolized in liver to form glucuronide metabolites.

INDICATIONS AND DOSAGES
Analgesic, antispasmodic
Rectal
Adults, Elderly. 1 suppository 1-2 times/day. Maximum: 4 doses/day.

S AVAILABLE FORMS/COST
• Supp—Rect: 16.2 mg-30 mg, 12's: **$31.90-$37.38**; 16.2 mg-60 mg, 12's: **$38.60-$40.13**

UNLABELED USES: Glaucoma, severe renal or hepatic disease, bronchial asthma, respiratory depression, convulsive disorders, acute alcoholism, premature labor, hypersensitivity to belladonna or opium or its components

CONTRAINDICATIONS: None known.

PREGNANCY AND LACTATION: Pregnancy category C; excretion of belladonna into breast milk is controversial; neonates may be particularly sensitive to anticholinergic agents, therefore use caution in nursing mothers

SIDE EFFECTS
Frequent
Dry mouth, nose, skin and throat, decreased sweating, constipation, irritation at site of administration, drowsiness, urinary retention, dizziness
Occasional
Blurred vision, decreased flow of breast milk, bloated feeling, drowsiness, headache, intolerance to light, nervousness, flushing
Rare
Dizziness, faintness, pruritis, urticaria

SERIOUS REACTIONS
• Respiratory depression, increased intraocular pain, loss of memory, orthostatic hypotension, tachycardia, and ventricular fibrillation rarely occur.
• Tolerance to the drug's analgesic effect and physical dependence may occur with repeated use.

INTERACTIONS
Drugs
▣ *Amantadine:* Enhanced anticholinergic effect; enhanced CNS effect of amantadine
▣ *Neuroleptics:* Reduced neuroleptic effect
▣ *Rimantadine:* Enhanced anticholinergic effect; enhanced CNS effect of rimantadine
▣ *Tacrine:* May reduce anticholinergic effect; belladonna may reduce CNS effect of tacrine

SPECIAL CONSIDERATIONS
PATIENT/FAMILY EDUCATION
• Moisten finger and suppository with water before inserting

• May cause drowsiness, dry mouth, and blurred vision

• Store at room temperature; DO NOT refrigerate

---

benazepril

(be-naze′a-pril)

Rx: Lotensin

Combinations

   Rx: with hydrochlorothiazide (Lotensin HCT)

   Rx: with amlodipine (Lotrel)

Chemical Class: Angiotensin-converting enzyme (ACE) inhibitor, nonsulfhydryl

Therapeutic Class: Antihypertensive

CLINICAL PHARMACOLOGY

Mechanism of Action: An ACE inhibitor that decreases the rate of conversion of angiotensin I to angiotensin II, a potent vasoconstrictor. Reduces peripheral arterial resistance. *Therapeutic Effect:* Lowers blood pressure (BP).

Pharmacokinetics

Route	Onset	Peak	Duration
PO	1 hr	2–4 hr	24 hr

Partially absorbed from the GI tract. Protein binding: 97%. Metabolized in the liver to active metabolite. Primarily excreted in urine. Minimal removal by hemodialysis. **Half-life:** 35 min; metabolite 10–11 hr.

INDICATIONS AND DOSAGES

Hypertension (monotherapy)

PO

Adults. Initially, 10 mg/day. Maintenance: 20–40 mg/day as single in 2 divided doses. Maximum: 80 mg/day.

Elderly. Initially, 5–10 mg/day. Range: 20–40 mg/day.

Hypertension (combination therapy)

PO

Adults. Discontinue diuretic 2-3 days prior to initiating benazepril, then dose as noted above. If unable to discontinue diuretic, begin benazepril at 5 mg/day.

Dosage in renal impairment

For adult patients with creatinine clearance less than 30 ml/min, initially, 5 mg/day titrated up to maximum of 40 mg/day.

S   **AVAILABLE FORMS/COST**

• Tab—Oral: 5 mg, 10 mg, 20 mg, 40 mg, 100's; all: **$116.79**

UNLABELED USES: Treatment of CHF

CONTRAINDICATIONS: History of angioedema from previous treatment with ACE inhibitors

PREGNANCY AND LACTATION: Pregnancy category C (1st trimester), category D (2nd and 3rd trimesters); ACE inhibitors can cause fetal and neonatal morbidity and death when administered to pregnant women; detectable in breast milk in trace amounts, a newborn would receive <0.1% of the mg/kg maternal dose; effect on nursing infant has not been determined

SIDE EFFECTS

Frequent (6%–3%)

Cough, headache, dizziness

Occasional (2%)

Fatigue, somnolence or drowsiness, nausea

Rare (less than 1%)

Rash, fever, myalgia, diarrhea, loss of taste

SERIOUS REACTIONS

• Excessive hypotension ('first-dose syncope') may occur in patients with CHF and in those who are severely salt or volume depleted.

• Angioedema (swelling of the face and lips) and hyperkalemia occur rarely.

• Agranulocytosis and neutropenia may be noted in those with collagen vascular disease, including scleroderma and systemic lupus erythematosus, and impaired renal function.

• Nephrotic syndrome may be noted in patients with history of renal disease.

INTERACTIONS

Drugs

➋ *Allopurinol:* Combination may predispose to hypersensitivity reactions

➌ *α-adrenergic blockers:* Exaggerated first dose hypotensive response when added to benazepril

➌ *Aspirin:* May reduce hemodynamic effects of benazepril; less likely at doses under 236 mg; less likely with nonacetylated salicylates

➌ *Azathioprine:* Increased myelosuppression

➌ *COX-2 inhibitors:* May reduce hemodynamic effects of benazepril

➌ *Cyclosporine:* Combination may cause renal insufficiency

➌ *Insulin:* Benazepril may enhance insulin sensitivity

➌ *Iron:* Benazepril may increase chance of systemic reaction to IV iron

➌ *Lithium:* Reduced lithium clearance

➌ *Loop diuretics:* Initiation of benazepril may cause hypotension and renal insufficiency in patients taking loop diuretics

➌ *NSAIDs:* May reduce hemodynamic effects of benazepril

➌ *Potassium-sparing diuretics:* Increased risk of hyperkalemia

➌ *Trimethoprim:* Additive risk of hyperkalemia, especially in patient predisposed to renal insufficiency

Labs

• ACE inhibition can account for approximately 0.5 mEq/L rise in serum potassium

SPECIAL CONSIDERATIONS

PATIENT/FAMILY EDUCATION

• Caution with salt substitutes containing potassium chloride

• Rise slowly to sitting/standing position to minimize orthostatic hypotension

• Dizziness, fainting, lightheadedness may occur during 1st few days of therapy

• May cause altered taste perception or cough; persistent dry cough usually does not subside unless medication is stopped

MONITORING PARAMETERS

• BUN, creatinine, potassium within 2 wk after initiation of therapy (increased levels may indicate acute renal failure)

---

bentoquatam

(ben'-toe-kwa-tam)

Rx: Ivy Block
Chemical Class: Organoclay compound
Therapeutic Class: Rhus dermatitis protectant

CLINICAL PHARMACOLOGY

Mechanism of Action: An organoclay substance that absorbs and binds to urushiol, the active principle in poison oak, ivy, and sumac. *Therapeutic Effect:* Blocks urushiol skin contact and absorption.

Pharmacokinetics

None reported.

INDICATIONS AND DOSAGES

Contact dermatitis prophylaxis caused by poison oak, ivy, or sumac

Topical

Adults, Elderly, Children 6 yrs and older. Apply thin film over skin at least 15 minutes before potential exposure. Re-apply q4h or sooner if needed.

§ **AVAILABLE FORMS/COST**

• Lotion—Top: 5%, 120 ml: **$11.95**

CONTRAINDICATIONS: Hypersensitivity to bentoquatam or any of its components such as methylparabens

SIDE EFFECTS

Occasional

Erythema

SERIOUS REACTIONS

• None reported.

SPECIAL CONSIDERATIONS

PATIENT/FAMILY EDUCATION

• To be used prior to exposure only

---

benzocaine

(ben′zoe-kane)

Rx: Americaine

OTC: Anbesol, Bicozene, Boil-ease, Chigger-tox, Dermoplast, Foille, Hurricaine, Orajel, Orabase, Solarcaine

Combinations

   Rx: with antipyrine (Allergen, Auralgan, Auroto); with benzethonium chloride (Americaine, Otocain); with phenylephrine (Tympagesic)

Chemical Class: Benzoic acid derivative

Therapeutic Class: Anesthetic, local

CLINICAL PHARMACOLOGY

Mechanism of Action: A local anesthetic that blocks nerve conduction in the autonomic, sensory, and motor nerve fibers. Competes with calcium ions for membrane binding. Reduces permeability of resting nerves to potassium and sodium ions. *Therapeutic Effect:* Produces local analgesic effect.

Pharmacokinetics

Poorly absorbed by topical administration. Well absorbed from mucous membranes and traumatized skin. Metabolized in liver and by hydrolysis with cholinesterase. Minimal excretion in urine.

INDICATIONS AND DOSAGES

Canker sores

Topical

Adults, Elderly, Children older than 2 yrs. Apply gel, liquid, or ointment to affected area. Maximum: 4 times/day.

Denture irritation
Topical
Adults, Elderly. Apply thin layer of gel to affected area up to 4 times/day or until pain is relieved.
General lubrication
Topical
Adults, Elderly, Children older than 2 yrs. Apply gel to exterior of tube or instrument prior to use.
Otitis externa, otitis media
Otic
Adults, Elderly, Children older than 1 yr. Instill 4-5 drops into external ear canal of affected ears. Repeat q1-2h as needed.
Pain and itching associated with sunburn, insect bites, minor cuts, scrapes, minor burns, minor skin irritations
Topical
Adults, Elderly, Children older than 2 yrs. Apply to affected area 3-4 times/day.
Pharyngitis
PO
Adults, Elderly. 1 lozenge q2h. Maximum 8 lozenges/day.
Toothache/teething pain
Topical
Adults, Elderly, Children older than 2 yrs. Apply gel, liquid, or ointment to affected areas. Maximum: 4 times/day.
Anesthesia
Topical
Adults, Elderly. Apply aerosol, gel, ointment, liquid q4-12h as needed.
S **AVAILABLE FORMS/COST**
• Cre—Top: 5%, 10, 30 g: **$1.00**/30 g
• Gel—Top: 10%, 5, 10, 30 g: **$3.17-$4.17**/10 g; 20%, 2, 5, 20, 30, 120 g: **$8.50**/30 g; 6.3%, 7.5 g: **$4.52**; 7.5%, 10, 15 g: **$3.32**/15 g
• Liq—Top: 20%, 30 ml: **$8.50**
• Oint—Rect: 20%, 30 g: **$3.63-$4.36**
• Oint—Top: 10%, 30 g: **$11.25**

• Paste—Top: 20%, 5, 15 g: **$6.38**/15 g
• Sol—Otic: (with antipyrine) 10 ml-15 ml: **$1.24-$12.27**/15 ml
• Spray/Aerosol—Top: 20%, 60, 120 ml: **$3.46-$39.99**/60 ml
UNLABELED USES: Obesity, spasticity
CONTRAINDICATIONS: Hypersensitivity to benzocaine or ester-type local anesthetics, perforated tympanic membrane or ear discharge (otic preparations)
PREGNANCY AND LACTATION: Pregnancy category C; excretion in breast milk unknown; use caution in nursing mothers
SIDE EFFECTS
Occasional
Burning, stinging, angioedema, contact dermatitis, taste disorders
SERIOUS REACTIONS
• Methemoglobinermia occurs rarely in infants and young children.
SPECIAL CONSIDERATIONS
PATIENT/FAMILY EDUCATION
• Protect the solution from light and heat, do not use if it is brown or contains a precipitate
• Discard this product 6 mo after dropper is first placed in the drug solution

---

benzonatate
(ben-zoe′na-tate)
Rx: Tessalon Perles
Chemical Class: Tetracaine derivative
Therapeutic Class: Antitussive

CLINICAL PHARMACOLOGY
Mechanism of Action: A non-narcotic antitussive that anesthetizes stretch receptors in respiratory passages, lungs, and pleura. *Therapeutic Effect:* Reduces cough production.

INDICATIONS AND DOSAGES
Antitussive
PO

Adults, Elderly, Children older than 10 yr. 100 mg 3 times a day or every 4 hours up to 600 mg/day.

$ **AVAILABLE FORMS/COST**
• Cap, Elastic—Oral: 100 mg, 100's: **$76.45-$113.22**

CONTRAINDICATIONS: None known.

PREGNANCY AND LACTATION: Pregnancy category C; excretion into breast milk unknown; use with caution in nursing mothers

SIDE EFFECTS
Occasional

Mild somnolence, mild dizziness, constipation, GI upset, skin eruptions, nasal congestion

SERIOUS REACTIONS
• A paradoxical reaction, including restlessness, insomnia, euphoria, nervousness, and tremor, has been noted.

SPECIAL CONSIDERATIONS
PATIENT/FAMILY EDUCATION
• Avoid driving, other hazardous activities until stabilized on this medication
• Do not chew or break capsules, will anesthetize mouth

---

benzoyl peroxide
(ben'zoe-ill per-ox'ide)

Rx: Benzac, Benzagel, Benzashave, Benzox, Brevoxyl, Delaqua, Desquam-E, Desquam-X, Pan-Oxyl, Persa-Gel

OTC: Acetoxyl, Acne-10, Acnomel, Advanced Formula Oxy Sensitive, Ambi-10, Benoxyl, Clearasil, Clear by Design, Dermoxyl, Dryox, Exact, Fostex, Loroxide, Neutrogena, Oxyderm, Oxy-10, Perfectoderm, Solugel

Chemical Class: Benzoic acid derivative
Therapeutic Class: Antiacne agent

CLINICAL PHARMACOLOGY
Mechanism of Action: A keratolytic agent that releases free-radical oxygen which oxidizes bacterial proteins in the sebaceous follicles decreasing the number of anaerobic bacteria and decreasing irritating-type free fatty acids. *Therapeutic Effect:* Bactericidal action against Propionbacterium acnes and Staphlococcus epidermidis.

Pharmacokinetics
Minimal absorption through skin. Gel is more penetrating than cream. Metabolized to benzoic acid in skin. Excreted in urine as benzoate.

INDICATIONS AND DOSAGES
Acne
Topical

Adults. Apply 2.5%-10% concentration 1-2 times/day.

$ **AVAILABLE FORMS/COST**
• Bar—Top: 5%, 10%, 4 oz: **$4.67-$9.34**/10%

• Cre—Top: 5%, 45, 60, 120 g: **$1.73-$2.24**/45 g; 10%, 30, 45, 120, 450 g: **$2.48-$4.91**/30 g
• Gel—Top: 2.5%, 45, 60, 90 g: **$4.93**/45 g; 4%, 42, 90 g: **$72.45**/90 g; 5%, 30, 45, 60, 90 g: **$5.68-$25.51**/45 g; 10%, 45, 60, 90 g: **$5.89-$30.75**/45 g
• Liq—Top: 2.5%, 240 ml: **$23.67-$29.81**; 5%, 30, 90, 120, 150, 240 ml: **$26.71-$34.94**/240 ml; 10%, 30, 60, 90, 120, 150, 240 ml: **$14.59-$38.69**/240 ml
• Lotion—Top: 5%, 30, 60 ml: **$2.00-$5.61**/30 ml; 10%, 30, 60, 90, 360 ml: **$8.71-$21.42**/60 ml
• Pad—Top: 3%, 6%, 30's: **$55.63**
UNLABELED USES: Dermal ulcers, seborrheic dermatitis, surgical wounds, tinea pedis, tinea versicolor
CONTRAINDICATIONS: Hypersensitivity to benzoyl peroxide or any component of the formulation
PREGNANCY AND LACTATION: Pregnancy category C; excretion into milk unknown
SIDE EFFECTS
Occasional
Irritation, dryness, burning, peeling, stinging, contact dermatitis, bleaching of hair
SERIOUS REACTIONS
• Hypersensitivity reactions have been reported with benzoyl peroxide use.
INTERACTIONS
Drugs
■ *Tretinoin:* Excess skin irritation
SPECIAL CONSIDERATIONS
PATIENT/FAMILY EDUCATION
• Keep away from eyes, mouth, inside of nose and other mucous membranes
• May cause transitory feeling of warmth or slight stinging
• Expect dryness and peeling, discontinue use if rash or irritation develops. Use lower concentration in fair-skinned individuals

• Water-based cosmetics may be used over drug; don't counter-treat dryness with emollients

---

benztropine
(benz′troe-peen)
Rx: Cogentin
Chemical Class: Tertiary amine
Therapeutic Class: Anti-Parkinson's agent; anticholinergic

CLINICAL PHARMACOLOGY
Mechanism of Action: An antiparkinson agent that selectively blocks central cholinergic receptors, helping to balance cholinergic and dopaminergic activity. *Therapeutic Effect:* Reduces the incidence and severity of akinesia, rigidity, and tremor.

INDICATIONS AND DOSAGES
Parkinsonism
PO
Adults. 0.5–6 mg/day as a single dose or in 2 divided doses. Titrate by 0.5 mg at 5–6 day intervals.
Elderly. Initially, 0.5 mg once or twice a day. Titrate by 0.5 mg at 5–6 day intervals. Maximum: 4 mg/day.
Drug-induced extrapyramidal symptoms
PO, IM
Adults. 1–4 mg once or twice a day.
Children older than 3 yr. 0.02-0.05 mg/kg/dose once or twice a day.
Acute dystonic reactions
IM, IV
Adults. Initially, 1–2 mg; then 1–2 mg PO twice a day to prevent recurrence.

$ AVAILABLE FORMS/COST
• Sol, Inj—IM, IV: 1 mg/ml, 2 ml: **$8.22**
• Tab—Oral: 0.5 mg, 100's: **$6.51-$22.06**; 1 mg, 100's: **$6.88-$17.75**; 2 mg, 100's: **$9.38-$30.34**

CONTRAINDICATIONS: Angle-closure glaucoma, benign prostatic hyperplasia, children younger than 3 years, GI obstruction, intestinal atony, megacolon, myasthenia gravis, paralytic ileus, severe ulcerative colitis

PREGNANCY AND LACTATION: Pregnancy category C; an inhibitory effect on lactation may occur; infants may be particularly sensitive to anticholinergic effects

SIDE EFFECTS

Frequent

Somnolence, dry mouth, blurred vision, constipation, decreased sweating or urination, GI upset, photosensitivity

Occasional

Headache, memory loss, muscle cramps, anxiety, peripheral paresthesia, orthostatic hypotension, abdominal cramps

Rare

Rash, confusion, eye pain

SERIOUS REACTIONS

• Overdose may produce severe anticholinergic effects, such as unsteadiness, somnolence, tachycardia, dyspnea, skin flushing, and severe dryness of the mouth, nose, or throat.

• Severe paradoxical reactions, marked by hallucinations, tremor, seizures, and toxic psychosis, may occur.

INTERACTIONS

Drugs

▣ *Anticholinergics:* Excess anticholinergic side effects

▣ *Amantadine:* Potentiates CNS side effects of amantadine

▣ *Neuroleptics:* Inhibition of therapeutic response to neuroleptics; excessive anticholinergic effects

▣ *Tacrine:* Reduced therapeutic effects of both drugs

PATIENT/FAMILY EDUCATION

• Do not discontinue abruptly

• Administer with or after meals to prevent GI upset

• Drug may increase susceptibility to heat stroke

---

benzylpenicilloyl-polylysine

(ben'zil-pen-i-sil'oyl-pol-i-lie-'seen)

Rx: Pre-Pen
Chemical Class: Penicillin derivative
Therapeutic Class: Penicillin allergy skin test

CLINICAL PHARMACOLOGY

Mechanism of Action: A diagnostic agent that invokes immunoglobulin E which produce type I accelerated urticarial reactions to penicillins. *Therapeutic Effect:* A positive reaction will suggest penicillin sensitivity.

Pharmacokinetics

Not known.

INDICATIONS AND DOSAGES

Penicillin sensitivity

Intradermal

Adults, Children. Use a tuberculin syringe with a 26 to 30 gauge, short bevel needle. A dose of 0.01 to 0.02 ml is injected intradermally. A control of 0.9% sodium chloride should be injected about 1½ inches from the test site. Skin response usually occurs within 5 to 15 minutes.

Scratch test

Adults, Children. Use a 20 gauge needle to make 3 to 5 mm nonbleeding scratch of the epidermis. Apply a small drop of solution to scratch and rub gently with applicator or toothpick. A positive reaction consists of a pale wheal surrounding the scratch site develops within 10 minutes and ranges from 5 to 15 mm in diameter.

S **AVAILABLE FORMS/COST**
• Sol, Inj—Intradermal: 0.25 ml: **$19.42-$29.35**

CONTRAINDICATIONS: Systemic or marked local reaction to its previous administration or hypersensitivity to penicillin

PREGNANCY AND LACTATION: Pregnancy category C

SIDE EFFECTS
Frequent
Skin rash
Occasional
Nausea

SERIOUS REACTIONS
• None significant.

SPECIAL CONSIDERATIONS
• Does not identify those patients who react to a minor antigenic determinant (i.e., anaphylaxis); does not reliably predict the occurrence of late reactions; patients with a negative skin test may still have allergic reactions to therapeutic penicillin

---

bepridil
(beh′prih-dill)
Rx: Vascor
Chemical Class: Diarylamino-propylamine ether
Therapeutic Class: Antianginal; calcium channel blocker

CLINICAL PHARMACOLOGY
Mechanism of Action: A calcium channel blocker that inhibits calcium ion entry across cell membranes of cardiac and vascular smooth muscle; decreases heart rate, myocardial contractility, slows SA and AV conduction. *Therapeutic Effect:* Dilates coronary arteries, peripheral arteries/arterioles.

Pharmacokinetics
Rapidly, completely absorbed from GI tract. Undergoes first-pass metabolism in liver to active metabolite. Primarily excreted in urine. Not removed by hemodialysis. **Half-life:** less than 24 hrs.

INDICATIONS AND DOSAGES
Chronic stable angina
PO
Adults, Elderly: Initially, 200 mg/day; after 10 days, dosage may be adjusted. Maintenance: 200–400 mg/day.

S **AVAILABLE FORMS/COST**
• Tab, Plain Coated—Oral: 200 mg, 90's: **$380.38**; 300 mg, 90's: **$438.21**; 400 mg, 30's: **$105.13**

CONTRAINDICATIONS: Sick sinus syndrome/second- or third-degree AV block (except in presence of pacemaker), severe hypotension (<90 mm Hg, systolic), history of serious ventricular arrhythmias, uncompensated cardiac insufficiency, congenital QT interval prolongation, use with other drugs prolonging QT interval

PREGNANCY AND LACTATION: Pregnancy category C; excreted in breast milk; use caution in nursing mothers

SIDE EFFECTS
Frequent
Dizziness, lightheadedness, nervousness, headache, asthenia (loss of strength), hand tremor, nausea, diarrhea
Occasional
Drowsiness, insomnia, tinnitus, abdominal discomfort, palpitations, dry mouth, shortness of breath, wheezing, anorexia, constipation
Rare
Peripheral edema, anxiety, flatulence, nasal congestion, paresthesia.

SERIOUS REACTIONS
• CHF, second- and third-degree AV block occur rarely.

• Serious arrhythmias can be induced.

• Overdosage produces nausea, drowsiness, confusion, slurred speech, profound bradycardia.

INTERACTIONS

Drugs

▪ *β-blockers:* Additive depressant effects on myocardial contractility or AV conduction

▪ *Digitalis glycosides:* Reduced clearance; increased digitalis levels; potential toxicity

SPECIAL CONSIDERATIONS

PATIENT/FAMILY EDUCATION

• ECGs will be necessary during initiation of therapy and after dosage changes

• Notify provider immediately for irregular heartbeat, shortness of breath, pronounced dizziness, constipation, or hypotension

• May be taken with food or meals

MONITORING PARAMETERS

• Blood pressure, pulse, respiration, ECG intervals (PR, QRS, QT) at initiation of therapy and again after dosage increases prologation of QT interval by >0.52 sec predisposes to proarrythmia

• Serum potassium (normalize before initiation)

---

betamethasone

(bay-ta-meth'a-sone)

Rx: *Systemic:* Celestone, Celstone Soluspan

Rx: *Topical:* Alphatrex, Betatrex, Diprolene, Diprosone, Luxiq Qualisone, Maxivate, Valisone

Combinations

Rx: with clotrimazole (Lotrisone)

Chemical Class: Glucocorticoid, synthetic

Therapeutic Class: Corticosteroid, systemic; corticosteroid, topical

---

CLINICAL PHARMACOLOGY

Mechanism of Action: An adrenocortical steroid that controls the rate of protein synthesis, depresses the migration of polymorphonuclear leukocytes and fibroblasts, reduces capillary permeability and prevents or controls inflammation. *Therapeutic Effect:* Decreases tissue response to inflammatory process.

INDICATIONS AND DOSAGES

Anti-inflammation, immunosuppression, corticosteroid replacement therapy

PO

Adults, Elderly. 0.6–7.2 mg/day.

Children. 0.063–0.25 mg/kg/day in 3–4 divided doses.

Relief of inflamed and pruritic dermatoses

Topical

Adults, Elderly. 1-3 times a day. Foam: Apply twice a day.

$ AVAILABLE FORMS/COST

• Cre (dipropionate)—Top: 0.05%, 15, 45, 60 g: **$7.03-$59.37**/45 g

• Cre (valerate)—Top: 0.1%, 15, 45 g: **$2.88-$25.00**/45 g

• Cre, Augmented (dipropionate)—Top: 0.05%, 15, 45 g, 50 g: **$9.07-$62.19**/45 g
• Gel, (dipropionate)—Top: 0.05%, 15, 45, 50 g: **$51.30**/45 g
• Foam, (valerate)—Top: 0.12%, 50, 100 g: **$59.96**/50 g
• Susp, Inj (sodium phosphate)—Intra-articular, Intradermal, IM: 4 mg/ml, 5 ml: **$7.45-$20.47**
• Lotion (dipropionate)—Top: 0.05%, 20, 60 ml: **$11.55-$72.33**/60 ml
• Lotion (valerate)—Top: 0.1%, 20, 60 ml: **$6.01-$21.78**/60 ml
• Lotion, Augmented (dipropionate)—Top: 0.05%, 30, 60 ml: **$48.64**/30 ml
• Oint (dipropionate)—Top: 0.05%, 15, 45 g: **$6.42-$59.37**/45 g
• Oint (valerate)—Top: 0.1%, 15, 45 g: **$4.09-$25.00**/45 g
• Oint, Augmented (dipropionate)—Top: 0.05%, 15, 50 g: **$10.75-$94.83**/50 g
• Syr—Oral: 0.6 mg/5 ml, 120 ml: **$41.22**
• Tab—Oral: 0.6 mg, 100's: **$186.54**

CONTRAINDICATIONS: Hypersensitivity to betamethasone, systemic fungal infections

PREGNANCY AND LACTATION: Pregnancy category C; used in patients with premature labor at about 24-36 wk gestation to stimulate fetal lung maturation (see dosage); excreted in breast milk, could suppress infant's growth and interfere with endogenous corticosteroid production

SIDE EFFECTS
Frequent
Systemic: Increased appetite, abdominal distention, nervousness, insomnia, false sense of well-being
Topical: Burning, stinging, pruritus

Occasional
Systemic: Dizziness, facial flushing, diaphoresis, decreased or blurred vision, mood swings
Topical: Allergic contact dermatitis, purpura or blood-containing blisters, thinning of skin with easy bruising, telangiectases or raised dark red spots on skin

SERIOUS REACTIONS
• Overdose may cause systemic hypercorticism and adrenal suppression.

INTERACTIONS
Drugs
▨ *Aminoglutethamide:* Enhanced elimination of corticosteroids; marked reduction in corticosteroid response; increased clearance of prednisone; doubling of dose may be necessary
▨ *Antidiabetics:* Increased blood glucose
▨ *Barbiturates, carbamazepine:* Reduced serum concentrations of corticosteroids; increased clearance of prednisone
▨ *Cholestyramine, colestipol:* Possible reduced absorption of corticosteroids
▨ *Cyclosporine:* Possible increased concentration of both drugs, seizures
▨ *Erythromycin, troleandomycin, clarithromycin, ketoconazole:* Possible enhanced steroid effect
▨ *Estrogens, oral contraceptives:* Enhanced effects of corticosteroids
▨ *Isoniazid:* Reduced plasma concentrations of isoniazid
▨ *IUDs:* Inhibition of inflammation may decrease contraceptive effect
▨ *NSAIDs:* Increased risk GI ulceration
▨ *Rifampin:* Reduced therapeutic effect of corticosteroids; may reduce hepatic clearance of prednisone

3 *Salicylates:* Subtherapeutic salicylate concentrations possible
Labs
• *False negative:* Skin allergy tests
SPECIAL CONSIDERATIONS
• Recommend single daily doses in AM
• Signs of adrenal insufficiency include fatigue, anorexia, nausea, vomiting, diarrhea, weight loss, weakness, dizziness and low blood sugar; drug-induced secondary adrenocorticoid insufficiency may be minimized by gradual systemic dosage reduction; relative insufficiency may exist for up to 1 yr after discontinuation of therapy; be prepared to supplement in situations of stress
• May mask infections
• Do not give live virus vaccines to patients on prolonged therapy
• Patients on chronic steroid therapy should wear medic alert bracelet
• Do not use topical products on weeping, denuded, or infected areas
MONITORING PARAMETERS
• Serum K and glucose
• Growth of children on prolonged therapy

---

betaxolol
(bay-tax'oh-lol)
Rx: Betoptic, Betoptic S, Kerlone
Chemical Class: β$_1$-adrenergic blocker, cardioselective
Therapeutic Class: Antianginal; antihypertensive

CLINICAL PHARMACOLOGY
Mechanism of Action: An antihypertensive and antiglaucoma agent that blocks beta$_1$-adrenergic receptors in cardiac tissue. Reduces aqueous humor production. *Therapeutic Effect:* Slows sinus heart rate, decreases BP and reduces intraocular pressure (IOP).
INDICATIONS AND DOSAGES
Hypertension
PO
Adults. Initially, 5-10 mg/day. May increase to 20 mg/day after 7-14 days.
Elderly. Initially, 5 mg/day.
Chronic open-angle glaucoma and ocular hypertension
Eye drops
Adults, Elderly. 1 drop twice a day.
Dosage in renal impairment
For adult and elderly patients who are on dialysis, initially give 5 mg/day; increase by 5 mg/day q2wk. Maximum: 20 mg/day.
S AVAILABLE FORMS/COST
• Sol—Ophth: 0.5%, 2.5, 5, 10, 15 ml: **$23.03-$26.75/5 ml**
• Susp—Ophth: 0.25%, 2.5, 5, 10, 15 ml: **$26.94-$40.00/5 ml**
• Tab, Plain Coated—Oral: 10 mg, 100's: **$104.90**; 20 mg, 100's: **$116.18**
UNLABELED USES: Treatment of angle-closure glaucoma during or after iridectomy, malignant glaucoma, secondary glaucoma; with miotics, to decrease IOP in acute and chronic angle-closure glaucoma
CONTRAINDICATIONS: Cardiogenic shock, overt cardiac failure, second- or third-degree heart block, sinus bradycardia
PREGNANCY AND LACTATION: Pregnancy category C; excretion into breast milk unknown; use caution in nursing mothers
SIDE EFFECTS
Betaxolol is generally well tolerated, with mild and transient side effects.

Frequent
Systemic: Hypotension manifested as dizziness, nausea, diaphoresis, headache, fatigue, constipation or diarrhea, dyspnea

Ophthalmic: Eye irritation, visual disturbances

Occasional
Systemic: Insomnia, flatulence, urinary frequency, impotence or decreased libido, bradycardia, bronchospasm

Ophthalmic: Increased light sensitivity, watering of eye

Rare
Systemic: Rash, arrhythmias, arthralgia, myalgia, confusion, altered taste, increased urination

Ophthalmic: Dry eye, conjunctivitis, eye pain

SERIOUS REACTIONS
• Overdose may produce profound bradycardia, hypotension, and bronchospasm.

• Abrupt withdrawal may result in diaphoresis, palpitations, headache, and tremors.

• Betaxolol administration may precipitate CHF or MI in patients with cardiac disease; thyroid storm in those with thyrotoxicosis; and peripheral ischemia in those with existing peripheral vascular disease.

• Hypoglycemia may occur in patients with previously controlled diabetes.

• Ophthalmic overdose may produce bradycardia, hypotension, bronchospasm, and acute cardiac failure.

INTERACTIONS
Drugs
③ *α₁-adrenergic blockers:* Potential enhanced first dose response (marked initial drop in blood pressure, particularly on standing [especially prazosin])

③ *Amiodarone:* Bradycardia/ventricular dysrhythmia

③ *Anesthetics, local:* Enhanced sympathomimetic effects, hypertension due to unopposed α-receptor stimulation

③ *Antacids:* May reduce β-blocker absorption

③ *Antidiabetics:* Delayed recovery from hypoglycemia, hyperglycemia, attenuated tachycardia during hypoglycemia, hypertension during hypoglycemia

③ *Clonidine:* Rebound hypertension; discontinue β-blocker prior to clonidine withdrawl

③ *Digoxin:* Additive prolongation of atrioventricular (AV) conduction time

③ *Dihydropyridine calcium channel blockers:* Severe hypotension or impaired cardiac performance; most prevalent with impaired left ventricular function, cardiac arrhythmias, or aortic stenosis

③ *Dipyridamole:* Bradycardia

③ *Disopyramide:* Additive decreases in cardiac output

③ *Epinephrine:* Enhanced pressor response resulting in hypertension

③ *Neostigmine:* Bradycardia

③ *Neuroleptics:* Increased serum levels of both resulting in accentuated pharmacologic response to both drugs

③ *NSAIDs:* Reduced hypotensive effects

③ *Phenylephrine:* Acute hypertensive episodes

③ *Tacrine:* Additive bradycardia

② *Theophylline:* Antagonist pharmacodynamics

SPECIAL CONSIDERATIONS
• Do not discontinue oral drug abruptly, may precipitate angina or MI

• Anaphylactic reactions may be more severe and not be as responsive to usual doses of epinephrine

• Transient stinging/discomfort is relatively common with ophthalmic preparations, notify clinician if severe

MONITORING PARAMETERS
• Blood pressure, pulse, intraocular pressure (ophth)

---

bethanechol
(be-than'e-kole)
Rx: Duvoid, Urecholine
Chemical Class: Choline ester
Therapeutic Class: Cholinergic stimulant

CLINICAL PHARMACOLOGY
Mechanism of Action: A cholinergic that acts directly at cholinergic receptors in the smooth muscle of the urinary bladder and GI tract. Increases detrusor muscle tone. *Therapeutic Effect:* May initiate micturition and bladder emptying. Improves gastric and intestinal motility.

INDICATIONS AND DOSAGES
Postoperative and postpartum urine retention, atony of bladder
PO
Adults, Elderly. 10–50 mg 3–4 times a day. Minimum effective dose determined by giving 5–10 mg initially, then repeating same amount at 1-hr intervals until desired response is achieved, or maximum of 50 mg is reached.
Children. 0.6 mg/kg/day in 3–4 divided doses.

ⓢ AVAILABLE FORMS/COST
• Sol, Inj—SC: 5 mg/ml, 1 ml: **$5.62**
• Tab—Oral: 5 mg, 100's: **$4.01-$71.32**; 10 mg, 100's: **$3.75-$149.53**; 25 mg, 100's: **$4.50-$199.34**; 50 mg, 100's: **$9.00-$285.46**

UNLABELED USES: Treatment of congenital megacolon, gastroesophageal reflux, postoperative gastric atony

CONTRAINDICATIONS: Active or latent bronchial asthma, acute inflammatory GI tract conditions, anastomosis, bladder wall instability, cardiac or coronary artery disease, epilepsy, hypertension, hyperthyroidism, hypotension, GI or urinary tract obstruction, parkinsonism, peptic ulcer, pronounced bradycardia, recent GI resection, vasomotor instability

PREGNANCY AND LACTATION: Pregnancy category C; abdominal pain and diarrhea have been reported in a nursing infant exposed to bethanechol in milk; use caution in nursing mothers

SIDE EFFECTS
Occasional
Belching, blurred or changed vision, diarrhea, urinary urgency

SERIOUS REACTIONS
• Overdosage produces CNS stimulation (including insomnia, anxiety, and orthostatic hypotension), and cholinergic stimulation (such as headache, increased salivation diaphoresis, nausea, vomiting, flushed skin, abdominal pain, and seizures).

INTERACTIONS
Drugs
▨ *β-blockers:* Additive bradycardia
▨ *Tacrine:* Increased cholinergic effects

SPECIAL CONSIDERATIONS
• Recommend taking on an empty stomach to avoid nausea and vomiting

B

biperiden
(bye-per'i-den)
Rx: Akineton
Chemical Class: Tertiary amine
Therapeutic Class: Anti-Parkinson's agent; anticholinergic

CLINICAL PHARMACOLOGY
Mechanism of Action: A weak anticholinergic that exhibits competitive antagonism of acetylcholine at cholinergic receptors in the corpus striatum, which restores balance. *Therapeutic Effect:* Antiparkinson activity.

Pharmacokinetics
Well absorbed from gastrointestinal (GI) tract. Protein binding: 23%-33%. Widely distributed. **Half-life:** 18-24 hrs.

INDICATIONS AND DOSAGES
Extrapyramidal symptoms
PO

Adults, Elderly. 2 mg 3-4 times/day. Dosage in renal impairment.

Parkinsonism
PO

Adults, Elderly. 2 mg 1-3 times/day.

$ **AVAILABLE FORMS/COST**
• Tab—Oral: 2 mg, 100's: **$46.90**
UNLABELED USES: Adjunct to methadone maintenance
CONTRAINDICATIONS: None known.
PREGNANCY AND LACTATION: Pregnancy category C; breast milk excretion not known; nursing infants particularly sensitive to anticholinergic effects

SIDE EFFECTS
Frequent
Orthostatic hypotension, anorexia, headache, blurred vision, urinary retention, dry mouth or nose
Occasional
Insomnia, agitation, euphoria
Rare
Vomiting, depression, irritation or swelling of eyes, rash

SERIOUS REACTIONS
• Overdosage may vary from severe anticholinergic effects, such as unsteadiness, severe drowsiness, dryness of mouth, nose, or throat, tachycardia, shortness of breath, and skin flushing.
• Also produces severe paradoxical reaction, marked by hallucinations, tremor, seizures, and toxic psychosis.

INTERACTIONS
Drugs
◧ *Amantadine:* Potentiates CNS side effect of amantadine
◧ *Anticholinergics:* Increased anticholinergic effects
◧ *Neuroleptics:* Inhibition of therapeutic response to neuroleptics; excessive anticholinergic effects
◧ *Tacrine:* Reduced therapeutic effects of both drugs

SPECIAL CONSIDERATIONS
• Give parenteral dose with patient recumbent to prevent postural hypotension

PATIENT/FAMILY EDUCATION
• May increase susceptibility to heatstroke
• Do not discontinue drug abruptly; taper off over 1 wk

bisacodyl

(bis-a-koe′dill)

OTC: Bisac-Evac, Bisco-Lax, Dulagen, Dulcolax, Fleet Bisacodyl

Chemical Class: Diphenylmethane derivative

Therapeutic Class: Laxative, stimulant

CLINICAL PHARMACOLOGY

Mechanism of Action: A GI stimulant that has a direct effect on colonic smooth musculature by stimulating the intramural nerve plexi. *Therapeutic Effect:* Promotes fluid and ion accumulation in the colon increasing peristalsis and producing a laxative effect.

Pharmacokinetics

Route	Onset	Peak	Duration
PO	6–12 hr	N/A	N/A
Rectal	15–60 min	N/A	N/A

Minimal absorption following oral and rectal administration. Absorbed drug is excreted in urine; remainder is eliminated in feces.

INDICATIONS AND DOSAGES

Treatment of constipation

PO

Adults, Children older than 12 yr. 5–15 mg as needed. Maxiumum: 30 mg.

Children 3–12 yr. 5–10 mg or 0.3 mg/kg at bedtime or after breakfast.

Elderly. Initially, 5 mg/day.

Rectal

Adults, Children 12 yr and older. 10 mg to induce bowel movement.

Children 2–11 yr. 5–10 mg as a single dose.

Children younger than 2 yr. 5 mg.

Elderly. 5–10 mg/day.

$ **AVAILABLE FORMS/COST**

• Liq—Rect: 10 mg/37.5 ml: **$1.24**

• Supp—Rect: 10 mg, 12's: **$1.66-$8.37**

• Tab, Enteric Coated—Oral: 5 mg, 100's: **$1.78-$32.61**

CONTRAINDICATIONS: Abdominal pain, appendicitis, intestinal obstruction, nausea, undiagnosed rectal bleeding, vomiting

PREGNANCY AND LACTATION: Pregnancy category B; excreted in breast milk

SIDE EFFECTS

Frequent

Some degree of abdominal discomfort, nausea, mild cramps, faintness

Occasional

Rectal administration: burning of rectal mucosa, mild proctitis

SERIOUS REACTIONS

• Long-term use may result in laxative dependence, chronic constipation, and loss of normal bowel function.

• Prolonged use or overdose may result in electrolyte or metabolic disturbances (such as hypokalemia, hypocalcemia, and metabolic acidosis or alkalosis), as well as persistent diarrhea, vomiting, muscle weakness, malabsorption, and weight loss.

INTERACTIONS

Labs

• *False decrease:* glucose (Clinistix, Diastix); no effect with Tes-tape

SPECIAL CONSIDERATIONS

PATIENT/FAMILY EDUCATION

• Do not take within 1 hr of antacids or milk

bismuth subsalicylate

OTC: Pepto-Bismol, Pink Bismuth

Combinations

Rx: with metronidazole, tetracycline (Helidac)

Chemical Class: Salicylate derivative

Therapeutic Class: Antidiarrheal; antiulcer agent; gastrointestinal

CLINICAL PHARMACOLOGY

Mechanism of Action: An antinauseant and antiulcer agent that absorbs water and toxins in the large intestine and forms a protective coating in the intestinal mucosa. Also possesses antisecretory and antimicrobial effects. *Therapeutic Effect:* Prevents diarrhea. Helps treat *Helicobacter-pylori*-associated peptic ulcer disease.

INDICATIONS AND DOSAGES

Diarrhea, gastric distress

PO

Adults, Elderly. 2 tablets (30 ml) q30–60min. Maximum: 8 doses in 24 hr.

Children 9–12 yr. 1 tablet or 15 ml q30–60min. Maximum: 8 doses in 24 hr.

Children 6–8 yr. Two-thirds of a tablet or 10 ml q30–60min. Maximum: 8 doses in 24 hr.

Children 3–5 yr. One-third of a tablet or 5 ml q30–60min. Maximum: 8 doses in 24 hr.

H. pylori–associated duodenal ulcer, gastritis

PO

Adults, Elderly. 525 mg 4 times a day, with 500 mg amoxicillin and 500 mg metronidazole, 3 times a day after meals, for 7–14 days.

Chronic infant diarrhea

PO

Children 2-24 mo. 2.5 ml q4h.

[$] **AVAILABLE FORMS/COST**

• Susp—Oral: 262 mg/15 ml, 30, 120, 240, 360, 480 ml: **$1.66-$4.21/** 240 ml; 524 mg/15 ml, 120, 240, 360 ml: **$1.65-$4.03**; 690 mg/30 ml, 240, 480 ml: **$1.51-$4.08**/240 ml

• Susp—Oral: 262 mg/15 ml, 120, 240, 360, 480 ml: **$2.29-$9.40**/240 ml; 524 mg/15 ml, 120, 240, 360 ml: **$4.03**/240 ml

• Tab, Chewable—Oral: 262 mg, 30's: **$1.85-$3.75**

UNLABELED USES: Prevention of traveler's diarrhea

CONTRAINDICATIONS: Bleeding ulcers, gout, hemophilia, hemorrhagic states, renal impairment

PREGNANCY AND LACTATION: Pregnancy category C; salicylate excreted in breast milk

SIDE EFFECTS

Frequent

Grayish black stools

Rare

Constipation

SERIOUS REACTIONS

• Debilitated patients and infants may develop impaction.

INTERACTIONS

Drugs

[2] *Tetracyclines:* Decreased absorption of tetracyclines

Labs

• *Color:* Blackens or discolors stool

• *Glucose (urine):* Interferes with Benedict's reaction

SPECIAL CONSIDERATIONS

PATIENT/FAMILY EDUCATION

• Chew or dissolve in mouth; do not swallow whole

• Shake suspension before using

• Stop use if symptoms do not improve within 2 days or become worse, or if diarrhea is accompanied by high fever or severe abdominal pain

bisoprolol

(bis-ope'pro-lal)

Rx: Zebeta
Combinations
  Rx: with hydrochlorothiazide: (Ziac)
Chemical Class: β_1-adrenergic blocker, cardioselective
Therapeutic Class: Antihypertensive

CLINICAL PHARMACOLOGY

Mechanism of Action: An antihypertensive that blocks beta$_1$-adrenergic receptors in cardiac tissue. *Therapeutic Effect:* Slows sinus heart rate and decreases BP.

Pharmacokinetics

Well absorbed from the GI tract. Protein binding: 26%–33%. Metabolized in the liver. Primarily excreted in urine. Not removed by hemodialysis. **Half-life:** 9–12 hr (increased in impaired renal function).

INDICATIONS AND DOSAGES

Hypertension

PO

Adults. Initially, 5 mg/day. May increase up to 20 mg/day.

Elderly. Initially, 2.5–5 mg/day. May increase by 2.5–5 mg/day. Maximum: 20 mg/day.

Dosage in hepatic impairment

For adults and elderly patients with cirrhosis or hepatitis whose creatinine clearance is less than 40 ml/minute, initially give 2.5 mg.

AVAILABLE FORMS/COST

• Tab, Plain Coated—Oral: 5 mg, 30's: **$36.58-$42.70**; 10 mg, 30's: **$36.58-$42.70**

• Tab, Plain Coated—Oral - with hydrochlorothiazide: 2.5 mg-6.25 mg, 100's: **$95.12-$142.38**; 5 mg-6.25 mg, 100's: **$95.12-$142.38**; 10 mg-6.25 mg, 100's: **$85.50-$114.15**

UNLABELED USES: Angina pectoris, premature ventricular contractions, supraventricular arrhythmias,

CONTRAINDICATIONS: Cardiogenic shock, overt cardiac failure, second- or third-degree heart block

PREGNANCY AND LACTATION: Pregnancy category C; similar drug, atenolol frequently used in the third trimester for treatment of hypertension (many studies of efficacy and safety of atenolol in pregnancy-induced hypertension); long-term use has been associated with intrauterine growth retardation; excreted into breast milk; observe for signs of β-blockade

SIDE EFFECTS

Frequent

Hypotension manifested as dizziness, nausea, diaphoresis, headache, cold extremities, fatigue, constipation or diarrhea

Occasional

Insomnia, flatulence, urinary frequency, impotence or decreased libido

Rare

Rash, arthralgia, myalgia, confusion (especially in the elderly), altered taste

SERIOUS REACTIONS

• Overdose may produce profound bradycardia and hypotension.

• Abrupt withdrawal may result in diaphoresis, palpitations, headache, and tremulousness.

• Bisoprolol administration may precipitate CHF and MI in patients with heart disease; thyroid storm in those with thyrotoxicosis; and peripheral ischemia in those with existing peripheral vascular disease.

• Hypoglycemia may occur in patients with previously controlled diabetes.

• Thrombocytopenia, including unusual bruising and bleeding, occurs rarely.

INTERACTIONS
Drugs

③ *Adenosine:* Additive bradycardia

③ *α₁-adrenergic blockers:* Potential enhanced first dose response [marked initial drop in blood pressure, particularly on standing (especially prazosin)]

③ *Amiodarone:* Increased bradycardic effect of bisoprolol

③ *Antidiabetics:* Reduced response to hypoglycemia (sweating persists)

③ *Barbiturates:* Enhanced bisoprolol metabolism

③ *Cimetidine:* Plasma levels of β-blocker may be elevated

③ *Clonidine:* Rebound hypertension; discontinue beta blocker prior to clonidine withdrawal

③ *Cocaine:* Bisoprolol potentiates cocaine-induced coronary vasoconstriction

③ *Contrast media:* Increased risk for anaphylaxis

③ *Digoxin, digitoxin:* Potentiation of bradycardia; additive prolongation of atrioventricular (AV) conduction time

③ *Dipyridamole:* Additive bradycardia

③ *Disopyramide:* Additive decreases in cardiac output

③ *Fluoxetine:* Fluoxetine inhibits CYPD26, partially responsible for bisoprolol metabolism; increased β-blocker effects

③ *Lidocaine:* β-blocker-induced reductions in cardiac output and hepatic blood flow may yield increased lidocaine concentrations

③ *Neostigmine:* Additive bradycardia

③ *Neuroleptics:* Decreased bisoprolol metabolism; decreased neuroleptic metabolism

③ *NSAIDs:* Reduced antihypertensive effect

③ *Physostigmine:* Additive bradycardia

③ *Rifampin:* Increases clearance by 51%, reduced β-blocker effects

③ *Tacrine:* Additive bradycardia

② *Theophylline:* Bisoprolol reduces clearance of theophylline; antagonistic pharmacodynamics

SPECIAL CONSIDERATIONS
• Property of competitive cardioselectivity yields less bronchospastic adverse effects

MONITORING PARAMETERS
• Heart rate, blood pressure

---

bitolterol
(bye-tole′ter-ol)
Chemical Class: Sympathomimetic amine; β₂-adrenergic agonist
Therapeutic Class: Antiasthmatic; bronchodilator

CLINICAL PHARMACOLOGY
Mechanism of Action: An antiadrenergic, sympatholytic agent that stimulates beta2-adrenergic receptors in lungs. *Therapeutic Effect:* Relaxes bronchial smooth muscle, relieves bronchospasm, reduces airway resistance.

Pharmacokinetics
Onset of action is rapid with duration of 4-8 hrs. Rapidly absorbed following aerosol administration. Primarily distributed to lungs. Metabolized in liver. Excreted in urine and feces. **Half-life:** 3 hrs.

INDICATIONS AND DOSAGES
Brochospasm
Inhalation
Adults, Elderly, Children 12 yrs and older. Use 2 inhalations, separated by 1–3 minute interval. A third inhalation may be required.

Prevention of bronchospasm
Inhalation

Adults, Elderly, Children 12 yrs and older. Use 2 inhalations q8h. Do not exceed 3 inhalations q6h, or 2 inhalations q4h.

💲 AVAILABLE FORMS/COST
• MDI—INH: 0.37 mg/puff, 15 ml in metered dose inhaler: **$35.23**
• Sol—INH: 0.2%, 30 ml: **$16.54**; 0.2%, 60 ml: **$31.34**

UNLABELED USES: Chronic obstructive pulmonary disease

CONTRAINDICATIONS: History of hypersensitivity to sympathomimetics, bitolterol, or any of its components.

PREGNANCY AND LACTATION: Pregnancy category C; excretion into breast milk unknown

SIDE EFFECTS
Frequent

Tremor

Occasional

Cough, dry or irritated mouth/throat, headache, nausea, vomiting

Rare

Dizziness, vertigo, palpitations, insomnia

SERIOUS REACTIONS
• Although tolerance to the bronchodilating effect has not been observed, prolonged or too frequent use may lead to tolerance.
• Severe paradoxical bronchoconstriction may occur with excessive use.

INTERACTIONS
Drugs

② β-*blockers:* Decreased action of bitolterol, cardioselective β-blockers preferable if concurrent use necessary

③ *Furosemide:* Potential for additive hypokalemia

• No real clinical advantage over less expensive agents (e.g., albuterol, metaproterenol)

PATIENT/FAMILY EDUCATION
• Wash inhaler in warm water and dry qday
• If previously effective dosage regimen fails to provide usual relief, seek medical advice immediately

---

bivalirudin
(bye-va-leer′u-din)

Rx: Angiomax
Chemical Class: Hirudin derivative; thrombin inhibitor
Therapeutic Class: Anticoagulant; direct thrombin inhibitor

CLINICAL PHARMACOLOGY
Mechanism of Action: An anticoagulant that specifically and reversibly inhibits thrombin by binding to its receptor sites. *Therapeutic Effect*: Decreases acute ischemic complications in patients with unstable angina pectoris.

Pharmacokinetics

Route	Onset	Peak	Duration
IV	Immediate	N/A	1 hr

Primarily eliminated by kidneys. Twenty-five percent removed by hemodialysis. **Half-life:** 25 min (increased in moderate to severe renal impairment).

INDICATIONS AND DOSAGES
Anticoagulant in patients with unstable angina who are undergoing percutaneous transluminal coronary angioplasty (PTCA) in conjunction with aspirin
IV

Adults, Elderly. 1 mg/kg as IV bolus followed by 4-hr IV infusion at rate of 2.5 mg/kg/hr. After initial 4-hr infusion is completed, give additional IV infusion at rate of 0.2 mg/ kg/hr for 20 hr or less, if necessary.

Dosage in renal impairment

GFR	Dosage Reduced by
30–59 ml/min	20%
10–29 ml/min	60%
Dialysis	90%

$ AVAILABLE FORMS/COST
• Powder, Inj—IV: 250 mg/vial: **$456.25**

CONTRAINDICATIONS: Active major bleeding

PREGNANCY AND LACTATION: Pregnancy category B; because of possible adverse effects on the neonate and the potential for increased maternal bleeding, particularly during the third trimester, should be used during pregnancy only if clearly needed; excretion into breast milk unknown, use caution in nursing mothers

SIDE EFFECTS
Frequent (42%)
Back pain
Occasional (15%–12%)
Nausea, headache, hypotension, generalized pain
Rare (8%–4%)
Injection site pain, insomnia, hypertension, anxiety, vomiting, pelvic or abdominal pain, bradycardia, nervousness, dyspepsia, fever, urine retention

SERIOUS REACTIONS
• A hemorrhagic event occurs rarely and is characterized by a fall in BP or Hct.

INTERACTIONS
Drugs
③ *Heparin, thrombolytics, warfarin:* Increased risk of major bleeding

SPECIAL CONSIDERATIONS
• Safety and effectiveness have not been established in patients with unstable angina who are not undergoing PTCA or in patients with other acute coronary syndromes
• In comparative studies of PTCA in unstable angina, incidence of major bleeding lower than heparin (4% vs 9%)
• Safety and efficacy with platelet inhibitors other than aspirin (e.g., glycoprotein IIb/IIIa inhibitors) not established

MONITORING PARAMETERS
• In clinical trials, the dose of bivalirudin was not titrated according to the activated clotting time (ACT)

---

bosentan
(bo'sen-tan)
Rx: Tracleer
Chemical Class: Pyrimidine derivative
Therapeutic Class: Endothelin receptor antagonist

CLINICAL PHARMACOLOGY
Mechanism of Action: An endothelin receptor antagonist that blocks endothelin-1, the neurohormone that constricts pulmonary arteries. *Therapeutic Effect:* Improves exercise ability and slows clinical worsening of pulmonary arterial hypertension (PAH).

Pharmacokinetics
Highly bound to plasma proteins, mainly albumin. Metabolized in the liver. Eliminated by biliary excretion. **Half-life:** Approximately 5 hr.

INDICATIONS AND DOSAGES
PAH in those with World Health Organization Class III or IV symptoms
PO
Adults, Elderly. 62.5 mg twice a day for 4 wks; then increase to mainte-

nance dosage of 125 mg twice a day. *Children weighing less than 40 kg.* 62.5 mg twice a day.

S   AVAILABLE FORMS/COST
• Tab—Oral: 62.5, 125 mg, 60's; all: **$2,970.00**

CONTRAINDICATIONS: Administration with cyclosporine or glyburide, pregnancy

PREGNANCY AND LACTATION: Pregnancy category X; expected to cause fetal harm if administered to pregnant women; excretion into human breast milk unknown

SIDE EFFECTS
Occasional
Headache, nasopharyngitis, flushing
Rare
Dyspepsia (heartburn, epigastric distress), fatigue, pruritus, hypotension

SERIOUS REACTIONS
• Abnormal hepatic function, lower extremity edema, and palpitations occur rarely.

INTERACTIONS
Drugs
▣ *Hormonal contraceptives:* Induction of CYP3A4 by bosentan may increase metabolism of contraceptive with possible failure
▲ *Cyclosporine A:* Increased bosentan trough concentrations of 3-30 fold and decreased cyclosporine A levels by 50% with concomitant administration
② *Glyburide:* Increased risk of liver enzyme elevations
▣ *Ketoconazole:* Ketoconazole is a potent CYP3A4 inhibitor; concurrent administration increases bosentan levels 2 fold
▣ *Simvastatin and other statins:* Concurrent administration decreased simvastatin and metabolites by 50%

▣ *Warfarin:* Concurrent administration reduces both S-warfarin (CYP2C9 substrate) and R-warfarin (CYP3A4 substrate) by 29% and 38% respectively, but without clinical changes in INR

SPECIAL CONSIDERATIONS
• Because of potential liver injury and in an effort to decrease the risk of fetal exposure, the drug may only be prescribed through the TRACLEER Access Program by calling 1-866-228-3546

MONITORING PARAMETERS
• Blood pressure, blood chemistries to include transaminases, monthly pregnancy test, hemoglobin levels at 1 and 3 months

---

bretylium
(bre-til'ee-um)
Rx: Bretylium Tosylate-Dextrose
Chemical Class: Bromobenzyl quaternary ammonium compound
Therapeutic Class: Antiarrhythmic, class III

CLINICAL PHARMACOLOGY
Mechanism of Action: An antiarrhythmic that directly affects myocardial cell membranes. *Therapeutic Effect:* Contributes to suppression of ventricular tachycardia.
Pharmacokinetics
Absorption is not expected to be present in peripheral blood at recommended doses. Protein binding: 1-6%. Not metabolized. Excreted unchanged in urine. Removed by hemodialysis. **Half-life:** 6-13.5 hrs.

INDICATIONS AND DOSAGES
Ventricular arrhythmias, immediate, life threatening
IV
Adults, Elderly. 5 mg/kg undiluted by rapid IV injection. May increase

to 10 mg/kg, repeat as needed. Maintenance: 5–10 mg/kg diluted over 8 minutes or longer, q6h or IV infusion at 1–2 mg/minute.

Children. 5 mg/kg, then 10 mg/kg at 15–30 minute intervals. Maximum: 30 mg/kg total dose. Maintenance: 5–10 mg/kg q6h.

Ventricular arrhythmias, other

IM

Adults, Elderly. 5–10 mg/kg undiluted, may repeat at 1–2 hour intervals. Maintenance: 5–10 mg/kg q6–8h

IV

Adults, Elderly. 5–10 mg/kg diluted over 8 minutes or longer, may repeat at 1–2 hour intervals. Maintenance: 5–10 mg/kg q6h or IV infusion at 1–2 mg/minute.

Children. 5–10 mg/kg/dose diluted q6h.

[$] **AVAILABLE FORMS/COST**

• Sol, Inj—IM, IV: 50 mg/ml, 10 ml: **$2.31-$35.86**

UNLABELED USES: Treatment of cervical dystonia in patients who have developed resistance to botulinum toxin type A.

CONTRAINDICATIONS: Hypersensitivity to bretylium or any component of the formulation

PREGNANCY AND LACTATION: Pregnancy category C

SIDE EFFECTS

Frequent

Transitory hypertension followed by postural and supine hypotension in 50% of pts observed as dizziness, lightheadedness, faintness, vertigo

Occasional

Diarrhea, loose stools, nausea, vomiting

Rare

Angina, bradycardia

SERIOUS REACTIONS

• Respiratory depression from possible neuromuscular blockade.

INTERACTIONS

Drugs

[3] *Catecholamines:* Enhanced pressor effects

[3] *Digoxin:* Digitalis toxicity may be aggravated by the initial norepinephrine release

SPECIAL CONSIDERATIONS

MONITORING PARAMETERS

• ECG, electrolytes, BP

bromocriptine

(broe-moe-krip'teen)

Rx: Parlodel

Chemical Class: Ergot alkaloid derivative

Therapeutic Class: Anti-Parkinson's agent; dopaminergic; ovulation stimulant

CLINICAL PHARMACOLOGY

Mechanism of Action: A dopamine agonist that directly stimulates dopamine receptors in the corpus striatum and inhibits prolactin secretion. Also suppresses secretion of growth hormone. *Therapeutic Effect:* Improves symptoms of parkinsonism, suppresses galactorrhea, and reduces serum growth hormone concentrations in acromegaly.

Pharmacokinetics

Indication	*Onset*	*Peak*	*Duration*
Prolactin lowering	2 hr	8 hr	24 hr
Antiparkinson	0.5–1.5 hr	2 hr	N/A
Growth hormone suppressant	1–2 hr	4–8 wk	4–8 hr

Minimally absorbed from the GI tract. Protein binding: 90%–96%. Metabolized in the liver. Excreted in feces by biliary secretion. **Half-life:** 15 hr.

INDICATIONS AND DOSAGES

Hyperprolactinemia

PO

Adults, Elderly. Initially, 1.25–2.5 mg/day. May increase by 2.5 mg/day at 3-to 7-day intervals. Range: 2.5 mg 2–3 times a day.

Parkinson's disease

PO

Adults, Elderly. Initially, 1.25 mg twice a day. May increase by 2.5 mg/day every 14–28 days. Range: 30–90 mg/day.

Acromegaly

PO

Adults, Elderly. Initially, 1.25–2.5 mg. May increase at 3-7 day intervals. Usual dose 20-30 mg/day.

[$] **AVAILABLE FORMS/COST**

• Cap, Gel—Oral: 5 mg, 100's: **$306.06-$476.20**

• Tab—Oral: 2.5 mg, 100's: **$157.70-$312.06**

UNLABELED USES: Treatment of cocaine addiction, hyperprolactinemia associated with pituitary adenomas, neuroleptic malignant syndrome

CONTRAINDICATIONS: Hypersensitivity to ergot alkaloids, peripheral vascular disease, pregnancy, severe ischemic heart disease, uncontrolled hypertension

PREGNANCY AND LACTATION: Pregnancy category D; since it prevents lactation, should not be administered to mothers who elect to breast-feed infants

SIDE EFFECTS

Frequent

Nausea (49%), headache (19%), dizziness (17%)

Occasional (7%–3%)

Fatigue, lightheadedness, vomiting, abdominal cramps, diarrhea, constipation, nasal congestion, somnolence, dry mouth

Rare

Muscle cramps, urinary hesitancy

SERIOUS REACTIONS

• Visual or auditory hallucinations have been noted in patients with Parkinson's disease.

• Long-term, high-dose therapy may produce continuing rhinorrhea, syncope, GI hemorrhage, peptic ulcer, and severe abdominal pain.

INTERACTIONS

Drugs

[3] *Erythromycin:* Marked elevations in bromocriptine levels

⚠ *Isometheptene:* Case report of hypertension and ventricular tachycardia with combination

[3] *Neuroleptics:* Neuroleptic drugs probably inhibit the ability of bromocriptine to lower serum prolactin concentrations in patients with pituitary adenomas; theoretically, bromocriptine should inhibit the antipsychotic effects of neuroleptic agents, but clinical evidence suggests that this may be uncommon

⚠ *Phenylpropanolamine:* Increased risk of hypertension and seizures

SPECIAL CONSIDERATIONS

• Routine use for suppression of lactation not recommended

PATIENT/FAMILY EDUCATION

• Use measures to prevent orthostatic hypotension

brompheniramine

(brome-fen-ir'a-meen)

Rx: Colhist, ND Stat,
Nasahist-B

OTC: Dimetane Extentabs
Combinations

  Rx: with phenylpropanolamine, codeine (Bromanate DC, Bromphen DC with Codeine, Dimetane-DC Cough, Myphetane DC Cough, Polyhistine CS); with pseudoephedrine, dextromethorphan (Bromadine-DM, Bromarest DX, Bromatane DX, Bromfed DM, Bromphen DX, Dimetane DX, Myphetane DX)

  OTC: with phenylpropanolamine (Bromaline, Bromanate, Dimaphen, Dimetane Decongestant, Dimetapp, Vicks DayQuil Allergy); with pseudoephedrine (Bromfed, Drixoral)

Chemical Class: Alkylamine derivative
Therapeutic Class: Antihistamine

CLINICAL PHARMACOLOGY
Mechanism of Action: An alklamine that competes with histamine at histaminic receptor sites. Inhibits central acetylcholine. *Therapeutic Effect:* Results in anticholinergic, antipruritic, antitussive, antiemetic effects. Produces antidyskinetic, sedative effect.

Pharmacokinetics
Rapidly absorbed after PO administration. Widely distributed. Metabolized in liver. Primarily excreted in urine. **Half-life:** 25 hrs.

INDICATIONS AND DOSAGES
Allergic rhinitis, anaphylaxis, urticarial transfusion reactions, urticaria
PO
Adults, Elderly, Children 12 yrs and older. 4 mg q4-6h or 8-12 mg extended/timed-release q12h.
Children younger than 12 yrs. 1-2 mg q4-6h.

Amelioration of allergic reactions to blood or plasma, anaphylaxis as an adjunct to epinephrine and other standard measures after the acute symptoms have been controlled, other uncomplicated allergic conditions of the immediate type when oral therapy is impossible or contraindicated
IM/IV/SC
Adults, Elderly, Children 12 yrs and older. 5-20 mg/day in 2 divided doses. Maximum: 40 mg/day.
Children younger than 12 yrs. 0.125 mg/kg/day or 3.75 mg/m2 in 3-4 divided doses.

AVAILABLE FORMS/COST
• Cap—Oral: 4 mg, 24's: **$4.39**
• Elixir—Oral: 2 mg/5 ml, 120, 480 ml: **$1.78-$4.60**/120 ml
• Sol, Inj—IM, IV, SC: 10 mg/ml, 10 ml: **$5.50-$16.65**
• Susp—Oral: 12 mg/5 ml, 118 ml: **$104.00**
• Tab, Sus Action—Oral: 12 mg, 100's: **$24.38**
• Tab—Oral: 4 mg, 100's: **$2.95**
• Tab, Chewable—Oral: 12 mg, 60's: **$79.95**

CONTRAINDICATIONS: Concurrent MAOI therapy, focal CNS lesions, newborn or premature infants, hypersensitivity to brompheniramine or related drugs

PREGNANCY AND LACTATION: Pregnancy category C; an association between 1st trimester exposure and congenital defects has been found in humans; excreted into breast milk, compatible with breast-feeding

SIDE EFFECTS

Frequent

Drowsiness, dizziness, dry mouth, nose, or throat, urinary retention, thickening of bronchial secretions Elderly: Sedation, dizziness, hypotension

Occasional

Epigastric distress, flushing, blurred vision, tinnitus, paresthesia, sweating, chills

SERIOUS REACTIONS

• Children may experience dominant paradoxical reactions, including restlessness, insomnia, euphoria, nervousness, and tremors.

• Overdosage in children may result in hallucinations, seizures, and death.

• Hypersensitivity reaction, such as eczema, pruritus, rash, cardiac disturbances, and photosensitivity, may occur.

INTERACTIONS

Labs

• *Aminoacids:* Urine, increase; on thin-layer chromatography

• *Amphetamine:* Urine, increase; false positives

• *False negative:* Skin allergy tests

SPECIAL CONSIDERATIONS

PATIENT/FAMILY EDUCATION

• Do not crush or chew sustained release forms

• Use hard candy, gum, frequent rinsing of mouth for dryness

---

budesonide
(bu-dess′ah-nide)

Rx: *Powder INH:* Pulmicort Turbuhaler

Rx: *Suspension INH:* Pulmicort Respules

Rx: *Nasal:* Rhinocort Aqua

Chemical Class: Glucocorticoid, synthetic

Therapeutic Class: Antiasthmatic; corticosteroid, antiinflammatory

---

CLINICAL PHARMACOLOGY

Mechanism of Action: A glucocorticoid that inhibits the accumulation of inflammatory cells and decreases and prevents tissues from responding to the inflammatory process. *Therapeutic Effect:* Relieves symptoms of allergic rhinitis or Crohn's disease.

Pharmacokinetics

Minimally absorbed from nasal tissue; moderately absorbed from inhalation. Protein binding: 88%. Primarily metabolized in the liver. **Half-life:** 2–3 hr.

INDICATIONS AND DOSAGES

Rhinitis

Intranasal (Rhinocort Aqua)

Adults, Elderly, Children 6 yr and older. 1 spray in each nostril once a day. Maximum: 8 sprays/day for adults and children 12 yr and older; 4 sprays/day for children younger than 12 yr.

Bronchial asthma

Nebulization

Children 6 mo–8 yr. 0.25–1 mg/day titrated to lowest effective dosage. Inhalation

Adults, Elderly, Children 6 yr and older. Initially, 200–400 mcg twice a day. Maximum: Adults: 800 mcg twice a day. Children: 400 mcg twice a day.

Crohn's disease
PO
Adults, Elderly. 9 mg once a day for up to 8 wk.

$ AVAILABLE FORMS/COST
• Cap, Sus Action—Oral: 3 mg, 100's: **$237.44**
• MDI—INH: 200 mcg/inh, 4 g (200 doses): **$151.00**
• MDI—Nasal: 32 mcg/inh, 7 g (200 doses): **$46.15**
• Susp—INH: 0.25 mg/2 ml, 0.5 mg/2 ml; all: **$4.75**
• Spray—Nasal: 32 mcg/inh, 8.6 g: **$68.46**

UNLABELED USES: Treatment of vasomotor rhinitis

CONTRAINDICATIONS: Hypersensitivity to any corticosteroid or its components, persistently positive sputum cultures for *Candida albicans*, primary treatment of status asthmaticus, systemic fungal infections, untreated localized infection involving nasal mucosa

SIDE EFFECTS
Frequent (greater than 3%)
Nasal: Mild nasopharyngeal irritation, burning, stinging, or dryness; headache; cough
Inhalation: Flu-like symptoms, headache, pharyngitis
Occasional (3%–1%)
Nasal: Dry mouth, dyspepsia, rebound congestion, rhinorrhea, loss of taste
Inhalation: Back pain, vomiting, altered taste, voice changes, abdominal pain, nausea, dyspepsia

SERIOUS REACTIONS
• An acute hypersensitivity reaction marked by urticaria, angioedema, and severe bronchospasm, occurs rarely.

SPECIAL CONSIDERATIONS
• May allow discontinuation of chronic systemic corticosteroids in many patients with asthma

• 3-7 days required for maximum benefit (nasal)

PATIENT/FAMILY EDUCATION
• To be used on regular basis, not for acute symptoms
• Use bronchodilators before oral inhaler (for patients using both)
• Nasal vehicle may cause rhinitis

MONITORING PARAMETERS
• Monitor children for growth as well as for effects on the HPA axis during chronic therapy
• Monitor patients switched from chronic systemic corticosteroids to avoid acute adrenal insufficiency in response to stress

---

bumetanide
(byoo-met'a-nide)
Rx: Bumex
Chemical Class: Sulfonamide derivative
Therapeutic Class: Diuretic, loop

CLINICAL PHARMACOLOGY
Mechanism of Action: A loop diuretic that enhances excretion of sodium, chloride, and to lesser degree, potassium, by direct action at the ascending limb of the loop of Henle and in the proximal tubule. *Therapeutic Effect:* Produces diuresis.

Pharmacokinetics

Route	Onset	Peak	Duration
PO	30–60 min	60–120 min	4–6 hr
IV	Rapid	15–30 min	2–3 hr
IM	40 min	60–120 min	4–6 hr

Completely absorbed from the GI tract (absorption decreased in CHF and nephrotic syndrome). Protein binding: 94%–96%. Partially metabolized in the liver. Primarily excreted in urine. Not removed by hemodialysis. **Half-life:** 1–1.5 hr.

INDICATIONS AND DOSAGES

Edema

PO

Adults, Children older than 18 yr. 0.5–2 mg as a single dose in the morning. May repeat at q4-5hr.

Elderly. 0.5 mg/day, increased as needed.

IV, IM

Adults, Elderly. 0.5–2 mg/dose; may repeat in 2–3 hr. Or 0.5–1 mg/hr by continuous IV infusion.

Hypertension

PO

Adults, Elderly. Initially, 0.5 mg/day. Range: 1–4 mg/day. Maximum: 5 mg/day. Larger doses may be given 2–3 doses/day.

Usual pediatric dosage

PO, IV, IM

Children. 0.015–0.1 mg/kg/dose q6–24h.

AVAILABLE FORMS/COST

• Sol, Inj—IM, IV: 0.25 mg/ml, 2 ml: **$1.63-$2.15**
• Tab—Oral: 0.5 mg, 100's: **$27.25-$45.21**; 1 mg, 100's: **$38.15-$63.49**; 2 mg, 100's: **$64.53-$107.31**

UNLABELED USES: Treatment of hypercalcemia, hypertension

CONTRAINDICATIONS: Anuria, hepatic coma, severe electrolyte depletion

PREGNANCY AND LACTATION: Pregnancy category C; cardiovascular disorders such as pulmonary edema, severe hypertension, or CHF are probably the only valid indications for loop diuretics during pregnancy; excretion into breast milk unknown

SIDE EFFECTS

Expected

Increased urinary frequency and urine volume

Frequent

Orthostatic hypotension, dizziness

Occasional

Blurred vision, diarrhea, headache, anorexia, premature ejaculation, impotence, dyspepsia

Rare

Rash, urticaria, pruritus, asthenia, muscle cramps, nipple tenderness

SERIOUS REACTIONS

• Vigorous diuresis may lead to profound water and electrolyte depletion, resulting in hypokalemia, hyponatremia, dehydration, coma, and circulatory collapse.

• Ototoxicity -- manifested as deafness, vertigo, or tinnitus -- may occur, especially in patients with severe renal impairment and those taking other ototoxic drugs.

• Blood dyscrasias and acute hypotensive episodes have been reported.

INTERACTIONS

Drugs

3 *Aminoglycosides (gentamicin, kanamycin, neomycin, streptomycin):* Additive ototoxicity (ethacrynic acid > furosemide, torsemide, bumetanide)

3 *Angiotensin converting enzyme inhibitors:* Initiation of ACEI with intensive diuretic therapy may result in precipitous fall in blood pressure; ACEIs may induce renal insufficiency in the presence of diuretic-induced sodium depletion

3 *Barbiturates (phenobarbital):* Reduced diuretic response

3 *Bile acid-binding resins (cholestyramine, colestipol):* Resins markedly reduce the bioavailability and diuretic response of furosemide

3 *Carbenoxolone:* Severe hypokalemia from coadministration

3 *Cephalosporins (cephaloridine, cephalothin):* Enhanced nephrotoxicity with coadministration

❷ *Cisplatin:* Additive ototoxicity (ethacrynic acid > furosemide, torsemide, bumetanide)

❸ *Clofibrate:* Enhanced effects of both drugs, especially in hypoalbuminemic patients

❸ *Corticosteroids:* Concomitant loop diuretic and corticosteroid therapy can result in excessive potassium loss

❸ *Digitalis glycosides (digoxin, digitoxin):* Diuretic-induced hypokalemia may increase risk of digitalis toxicity

❸ *Nonsteroidal antiinflammatory drugs (flurbiprofen, ibuprofen, indomethacin, naproxen, piroxicam, sulindac):* Reduced diuretic and antihypertensive effects

❸ *Phenytoin:* Reduced diuretic response

❸ *Serotonin-reuptake inhibitors (fluoxetine, paroxetine, sertraline):* Case reports of sudden death; enhanced hyponatremia proposed; causal relationships not established

❸ *Terbutaline:* Additive hypokalemia

❸ *Tubocurarine:* Prolonged neuromuscular blockade

Labs
• *Cortisol:* False increases
• *Glucose:* Falsely low urine tests with Clinistix and Diastix
• *Thyroxine:* Increased serum concentration
• *T_3 uptake:* Interference causes increased serum values

SPECIAL CONSIDERATIONS
• Cross-sensitivity with furosemide rare; may substitute bumetanide at a 1:40 ratio with furosemide in patients allergic to furosemide; may show cross-hypersensitivity to sulfonamides

PATIENT/FAMILY EDUCATION
• Take early in the day

MONITORING PARAMETERS
• *Frequent:* electrolyte, calcium, glucose, uric acid, CO_2, BUN, creatinine during 1st months, then periodically
• *Consider:* CBC, LFTs
• Monitor for tinnitus, hearing loss (IV doses >120 mg; concomitant ototoxic drugs, renal disease)

bupivacaine

(byoo-piv′a-caine)

Rx: Marcaine, Marcaine Spinal, Sensorcaine, Sensorcaine-MPF
Combinations
Rx: with epinephrine (Marcaine with Epinephrine, Sensorcaine with Epinephrine, Sensorcaine-MPF with Epinephrine)
Chemical Class: Amide derivative
Therapeutic Class: Anesthetic, local

CLINICAL PHARMACOLOGY
Mechanism of Action: An amide-type anesthetic that stabilizes neuronal membranes and prevents initiation and transmission of nerve impulses thereby effecting local anesthetic actions. *Therapeutic Effect:* Produces local analgesia.

Pharmacokinetics
Onset of action occurs within 4-10 minutes depending on route of administration. Duration is 1.5- 8.5 hrs. Well absorbed. Protein binding: 95%. Metabolized in liver. Excreted in urine. **Half life:** 1.5-5.5 hrs (Adults), 8.1 hrs. (Neonates)

INDICATIONS AND DOSAGES: Dose varies with procedure, depth of anesthesia, vascularity of tissues, duration of anesthesia and condition of patient.

Analgesic, epidural (partial to moderate motor blockade)

IV

Adults, Elderly. 10-20 ml (25-50 mg) of a 0.25% solution. Repeat once q3h as needed.

Children more than 10 kg. 1-2.5 mg/kg single dose as a 0.125% or 0.25% solution or 0.2-0.4 mg/kg/hr continuous infusion as a 0.1%, 0.125%, or 0.25% solution. Maximum: 0.4 mg/kg/hr.

Children less than 10 kg. 1-1.25 mg/kg single dose as a 0.125% or 0.25% solution or 0.1-0.2 mg/kg/hr continuous infusion as a 0.1%, 0.125%, or 0.25% solution. Maximum: 0.2 mg/kg/hr.

Analgeisic, epidural (moderate to complete motor blockade)

IV

Adults, Elderly. 10-20 ml (50-100 mg) as a 0.5% solution. Repeat once q3h as needed.

Children more than 10 kg. 1-2.5 mg/kg single dose as a 0.125% or 0.25% solution or 0.2-0.4 mg/kg/hr continuous infusion as a 0.1%, 0.125%, or 0.25% solution. Maximum: 0.4 mg/kg/hr.

Children less than 10 kg. 1-1.25 mg/kg single dose as a 0.125% or 0.25% solution or 0.1-0.2 mg/kg/hr continuous infusion as a 0.1%, 0.125%, or 0.25% solution. Maximum: 0.2 mg/kg/hr.

Analgesic, epidural (complete motor blockade)

IV

Adults. 10-20 ml (75-150 mg) as a 0.75% solution. Repeat once q3h as needed.

Children more than 10 kg. 1-2.5 mg/kg single dose as a 0.125% or 0.25% solution or 0.2-0.4 mg/kg/hr continuous infusion as a 0.1%, 0.125%, or 0.25% solution. Maximum: 0.4 mg/kg/hr.

Children less than 10 kg. 1-1.25 mg/kg single dose as a 0.125% or 0.25% solution or 0.1-0.2 mg/kg/hr continuous infusion as a 0.1%, 0.125%, or 0.25% solution. Maximum: 0.2 mg/kg/hr.

Analgesic, intrapleural

IV

Adults, Elderly. 10-30 ml bolus of 0.25%, 0.375%, or 0.5% q4-8h or 0.375% solution with epinephrine continuous infusion at 6 ml/hr after 20 ml loading dose.

Analgesic, caudal (moderate to complete blockade)

IV

Adults, Elderly. 15-30 mL of 0.5% solution (75-150 mg) OR 0.25% solution (37.5-75 mg), repeated once every 3 hr as needed

Children more than 10 kg. 1-2.5 mg/kg single dose as a 0.125% or 0.25% solution or 0.2-0.4 mg/kg/hr continuous infusion as a 0.1%, 0.125%, or 0.25% solution. Maximum: 0.4 mg/kg/hr.

Children less than 10 kg. 1-1.25 mg/kg single dose as a 0.125% or 0.25% solution or 0.1-0.2 mg/kg/hr continuous infusion as a 0.1%, 0.125%, or 0.25% solution. Maximum: 0.2 mg/kg/hr.

Analgesic, dental

IV

Adults, Elderly. 1.8-3.6 ml of 0.5% solution (9-18 mg) with epinephrine. A second dose of 9 mg may be administered. Maximum: 90 mg total dose.

Analgesic, peripheral nerve block (moderate to complete motor blockade)

IV

Adults, Elderly. 5-37.5 ml (25-175 mg) of 0.5% solution or 5-70 ml (12.5-175 mg) of 0.25% solution.

Repeat q3h as needed. Maximum: up to 400 mg/day.

Children 12 years and older. 0.3-2.5 mg/kg as a 0.25% or 0.5% solution. Maximum: 1 ml/kg of 0.25% solution or 0.5 ml/kg of 0.5% solution.

Analgesic, retrobulbar (complete motor blockade)

IV

Adults, Elderly. 2-4 ml (15-30 mg) of 0.75% solution.

Analgesic, sympathetic blockade

IV

Adults, Elderly. 20-50 ml (50-125 mg) of 0.25% (no epinephrine) solution. Repeat once q3h as needed.

Analgesic, hyperbaric spinal (obstetrical, normal vaginal delivery)

IV

Adults, Elderly. 0.8 ml (6 mg) bupivacaine in dextrose as 0.75% solution

Analgesic, hyperbaric spinal (obstetrical, cesarean section)

IV

Adults, Elderly. 1-1.4 ml (7.5-10.5 mg) bupivacaine in dextrose as 0.75% solution.

Anesthesia, hyperbaric spinal (surgical, lower extremity and perineal procedures)

IV

Adults, Elderly. 1 ml (7.5 mg) bupivacaine in dextrose as 0.75% solution

Children 12 years and older. 0.3-0.6 mg/kg bupivacaine in dextrose as a 0.75% solution

Anesthesia, spinal (surgical, lower abdominal procedures)

IV

Adults, Elderly. 1.6 ml (12 mg) bupivacaine in dextrose as 0.75% solution.

Children 12 years and older. 0.3-0.6 mg/kg bupivacaine in dextrose as a 0.75% solution

Anesthesia, spinal (surgical, hyperbaric, upper abdominal procedures)

IV

Adults, Elderly. 2 ml (15 mg) bupivacaine in dextrose administered in horizontal position

Children 12 years and older. 0.3-0.6 mg/kg bupivacaine in dextrose as a 0.75% solution

Analgesic, local infiltration

IV

Adults, Elderly. 0.25% solution. Maximum: 225 mg with epinephrine or 175 mg without epinephrine.

Children 12 years and older. 0.5-2.5 mg/kg as a 0.25% or 0.5% solution. Maximum: 1 ml/kg of 0.25% solution or 0.5 ml/kg of 0.5% solution.

$ AVAILABLE FORMS/COST

• Sol, Inj—Caudal Block, Epidural: 0.25%, 10 ml: **$3.20**; 0.5%, 10 ml: **$2.63**; 0.75%, 10 ml: **$3.74**

CONTRAINDICATIONS: Local infection at the site of proposed lumbar puncture (spinal anesthesia), obstetrical paracervical block anesthesia, septicemia (spinal anesthesia), severe hemorrhage, severe hypotension or shock, arrhythmias such as complete heart block, which severely restrict cardiac output (spinal anesthesia), sulfite allergy (epinephrine containing solutions only), hypersensitivity to bupivacaine products or to other amide-type anesthetics

PREGNANCY AND LACTATION: Pregnancy category C; excretion into breast milk unknown; regional use may prolong labor and delivery

SIDE EFFECTS

Occasional

Hypotension, bradycardia, palpitations, respiratory depression, dizziness, headache, vomiting, nausea, restlessness, weakness, blurred vision, tinnitus, apnea

SERIOUS REACTIONS

• Arterial hypotension, bradycardia, ventricular arrhythmias, central nervous system (CNS) depression and excitation, convulsions, respiratory arrest, tinnitus have been reported.

• Solutions with epinephrine contain metabisulfite, a sulfite that may cause allergic-type reactions, including anaphylaxis.

INTERACTIONS
Drugs

▣ β-*blockers:* Hypertensive reactions possible, especially with local anesthetics containing epinephrine; acute discontinuation of β-blockers before local anesthesia may increase the risk of side effects due to anesthetic

SPECIAL CONSIDERATIONS

• Amide-type local anesthetic

MONITORING PARAMETERS

• Blood pressure, pulse, respiration during treatment, ECG

• Fetal heart tones if drug is used during labor

---

buprenorphine
(byoo-pre-nor′feen)
Rx: Buprenex, Subutex (sublingual)
Combinations
   Rx: with naloxone (Suboxone)
Chemical Class: Opiate derivative; thebaine derivative
Therapeutic Class: Narcotic agonist-antagonist analgesic
DEA Class: Schedule V

CLINICAL PHARMACOLOGY
Mechanism of Action: An opioid agonist-antagonist that binds with opioid receptors in the CNS. *Therapeutic Effect:* Alters the perception of and emotional response to pain; blocks the effects of herion and produces minimal opioid withdrawal symptoms.

INDICATIONS AND DOSAGES
Analgesia
IV, IM
Adults, Children older than 12 yr. 0.3 mg q6-8h as needed. May repeat once in 30–60 min. Range: 0.15–0.6 mg q4-8h as needed.
Children 2–12 yr. 2–6 mcg/kg q4-6h as needed.
Elderly. 0.15 mg q6h as needed.

Opioid dependence
Sublingual
Adults, Elderly, Children older than 16 yr. Initially, 12–16 mg/day, beginning at least 4 hr after last use of heroin or short-acting opioid. Maintenance: 16 mg/day. Range: 4–24 mg/day. Patients should be switched to buprenorphine and naloxone combination, is preferred for maintenance treatment.

▣ AVAILABLE FORMS/COST

• Sol, Inj—IM, IV: 0.3 mg/ml; 1 ml: **$2.98-$3.23**

• Tab—SL: 2 mg, 30's: **$93.75**; 8 mg, 30's: **$175.00**

• Tab—SL (with naloxone): 2 mg-0.5 mg, 30's: **$81.25**; 8 mg-2 mg, 30's: **$143.75**

CONTRAINDICATIONS: Hypersensitivity to buprenorphine; hypersensitivity to naloxone for those receiving the fixed combination product containing naloxone (Suboxone)

PREGNANCY AND LACTATION: Pregnancy category C; safe use in labor and delivery has not been established; excretion into breast milk unknown

SIDE EFFECTS
Frequent
Tablet: Headache, pain, insomnia, anxiety, depression, nausea, ab-

dominal pain, constipation, back pain, weakness, rhinitis, withdrawal syndrome, infection, diaphoresis Injection (more than 10%): Sedation
Occasional
Injection: Hypotension, respiratory depression, dizziness, headache, vomiting, nausea, vertigo
SERIOUS REACTIONS
• Overdose results in cold and clammy skin, weakness, confusion, severe respiratory depression, cyanosis, pinpoint pupils, and extreme somnolence progressing to seizures, stupor, and coma.

SPECIAL CONSIDERATIONS
• Effective long-acting opioid agonist-antagonist; unconfirmed reported lower physical dependence; no significant advantages
• Use of SL tabs restricted to physicians licensed to treat opiod dependence
• In opiod dependence use Subutex during induction and Suboxone for unsupervised administration
PATIENT/FAMILY EDUCATION
• Do not swallow SL tablets
MONITORING PARAMETERS
• Respiration rate

---

bupropion
(byoo-proe'pee-on)
Rx: Wellbutrin, Wellbutrin SR, Zyban
Chemical Class: Aminoketone derivative
Therapeutic Class: Antidepressant

CLINICAL PHARMACOLOGY
Mechanism of Action: An aminoketone that blocks the reuptake of neurotransmitters, including serotonin and norepinephrine at CNS presynaptic membranes, increasing their availability at postsynaptic re-

ceptor sites. Also reduces the firing rate of noradrenergic neurons. *Therapeutic Effect:* Relieves depression and nicotine withdrawal symptoms.
Pharmacokinetics
Rapidly absorbed from the GI tract. Protein binding: 84%. Crosses the blood-brain barrier. Undergoes extensive first-pass metabolism in the liver to active metabolite. Primarily excreted in urine. **Half-life:** 14 hr.
INDICATIONS AND DOSAGES
Depression
PO (Immediate-Release)
Adults. Initially, 100 mg twice a day. May increase to 100 mg 3 times a day no sooner than 3 days after beginning therapy. Maximum: 450 mg/day.
Elderly. 37.5 mg twice a day. May increase by 37.5 mg q3–4 days. Maintenance: Lowest effective dosage.
PO (Sustained-Release)
Adults. Initially, 150 mg/day as a single dose in the morning. May increase to 150 mg twice a day as early as day 4 after beginning therapy. Maximum: 400 mg/day.
Elderly. 50–100 mg/day. May increase by 50–100 mg/day q3–4 days. Maintenance: Lowest effective dosage.
PO (Extended-Release)
Adults. 150 mg once a day. May increase to 300 mg once a day. Maximum: 450 mg a day.
Smoking cessation
PO
Adults. Initially, 150 mg a day for 3 days; then 150 mg twice a day for 7–12 wk.
$ AVAILABLE FORMS/COST
• Tab, Coated—Oral: 75 mg, 100's: **$72.00-$108.33**; 100 mg, 100's: **$96.06-$144.49**

• Tab, Sus Action—Oral: 100 mg, 60's: **$101.23-$112.60**; 150 mg, 60's: **$108.99-$125.13**; 200 mg, 60's: **$224.13**

UNLABELED USES: Treatment of attention deficit hyperactivity disorder in adults and children

CONTRAINDICATIONS: Current or prior diagnosis of anorexia nervosa or bulimia, seizure disorder, use within 14 days of MAOIs.

PREGNANCY AND LACTATION: Pregnancy category B; excretion into breast milk unknown

SIDE EFFECTS

Frequent (32%–18%)

Constipation, weight gain or loss, nausea, vomiting, anorexia, dry mouth, headache, diaphoresis, tremor, sedation, insomnia, dizziness, agitation

Occasional (10%–5%)

Diarrhea, akinesia, blurred vision, tachycardia, confusion, hostility, fatigue

SERIOUS REACTIONS

• The risk of seizures increases in patients taking more than 150 mg/dose of bupropion, in patients with a history of bulimia or seizure disorders and in patients discontinuing drugs that may lower the seizure threshold.

SPECIAL CONSIDERATIONS

• Equal efficacy as tricyclic antidepressants; advantages include minimal anticholinergic effects, lack of orthostatic hypotension, no cardiac conduction problems, absence of weight gain, no sedation

• Fewer sexual side effects than TCAs or SSRIs

• Prescribe in equally divided doses of 3 or 4 times daily to minimize risk of seizures

PATIENT/FAMILY EDUCATION

• Ability to perform tasks requiring judgment or motor and cognitive skills may be impaired

• Therapeutic effects may take 2-4 wk

• Do not discontinue medication quickly after long-term use

---

buspirone
(byoo-spir'own)
Rx: BuSpar
Chemical Class: Azaspirodecanedione
Therapeutic Class: Anxiolytic

CLINICAL PHARMACOLOGY

Mechanism of Action: Although its exact mechanism of action is unknown, this nonbarbiturate is thought to bind to serotonin and dopamine receptors in the CNS. The drug may also increase norepinephrine metabolism in the locus ceruleus. *Therapeutic Effect:* Produces anxiolytic effect.

Pharmacokinetics

Rapidly and completely absorbed from the GI tract. Protein binding: 95%. Undergoes extensive first-pass metabolism. Metabolized in the liver to active metabolite. Primarily excreted in urine. Not removed by hemodialysis. **Half-life**: 2–3 hr.

INDICATIONS AND DOSAGES

Short-term management (up to 4 weeks) of anxiety disorders

PO

Adults. 5 mg 2–3 times a day or 7.5 mg 2 twice a day. May increase by 5 mg/day every 2–4 days. Maintenance: 15–30 mg/day in 2–3 divided doses. Maximum: 60 mg/day.

Elderly. Initially, 5 mg twice a day. May increase by 5 mg/day every 2–3 days. Maximum: 60 mg/day.

Children. Initially, 5 mg/day. May increase by 5 mg/day at weekly intervals. Maximum: 60 mg/day.

§ AVAILABLE FORMS/COST

• Tab—Oral: 5 mg, 100's: **$68.94-$90.70**; 7.5 mg, 100's: **$106.32**; 10 mg, 100's: **$134.50-$162.80**; 15 mg, 60's: **$176.64-$212.49**; 30 mg, 60's: **$218.10-$255.27**

UNLABELED USES: Management of panic attack, premenstrual syndrome (aches, pain, fatigue, irritability)

CONTRAINDICATIONS: Concurrent use of MAOIs, severe hepatic or renal impairment

PREGNANCY AND LACTATION: Pregnancy category B; excretion into breast milk unknown; use caution in nursing mothers

SIDE EFFECTS

Frequent (12%–6%)

Dizziness, somnolence, nausea, headache

Occasional (5%–2%)

Nervousness, fatigue, insomnia, dry mouth, lightheadedness, mood swings, blurred vision, poor concentration, diarrhea, paresthesia

Rare

Muscle pain and stiffness, nightmares, chest pain, involuntary movements

SERIOUS REACTIONS

• Buspirone does not appear to cause drug tolerance, psychological or physical dependence, or withdrawal syndrome.

• Overdose may produce severe nausea, vomiting, dizziness, drowsiness, abdominal distention, and excessive pupil contraction.

INTERACTIONS

Drugs

§ *Fluoxetine:* Reduced therapeutic response to both drugs

⚠ *MAOIs:* Elevated blood pressure, don't give concomitantly

§ *Haloperidol:* Increased serum conc. of haloperidol

§ *CYP3A4 inhibitors: Diltiazem, verapamil, erythromycin, itraconazole, nefazodone, ketoconazole, ritonavir, grapefruit juice;* plasma buspirone concentration increased, adverse events likely, may need to adjust dose

§ *CYP3A4 inducers: Rifampin, dexamethasone, phenytoin, phenobarbital, carbamazepine;* plasma buspirone concentration decreased, may need to adjust dose to maintain anxiolytic effect

SPECIAL CONSIDERATIONS

• Advantages include less sedation (preferable in elderly), less effect on psychomotor and psychologic function, minimal propensity to interact with ethanol and other CNS depressants

• Will not prevent benzodiazepine withdrawal

PATIENT/FAMILY EDUCATION

• Optimal results may take 3-4 wk of treatment, some improvement may be seen after 7-10 days

butalbital compound

(byoo-tal-bi-tal)
Rx: *Butalbital/
acetaminophen/caffeine:*
Amaphen, Americet,
Endolor, Esgic, Ezol, Fioricet,
Fiorpap, Geone, Medigesic,
Repan, Tencet
Rx: *Butalbital/
acetaminophen/caffeine
with codeine:* Ezol III, Fioricet
w/codeine
Rx:
Butalbital/acetaminophen:
Bancap, Phrenilin, Phrenilin
Forte, Sedapap-10, Triaprin
Rx:
Butalbital/aspirin/caffeine:
Farbital, Fiorgen PF, Fiorinal,
Fiormor Fiortal Fortabs
Rx:
*Butalbital/aspirin/caffeine
with codeine:* Fiorinal
w/codeine
Chemical Class: Barbituric
acid derivative
Therapeutic Class: Nonnar-
cotic analgesic

CLINICAL PHARMACOLOGY
Mechanism of Action: A barbiturate that depresses the central nervous system. *Therapeutic Effect:*
Pain relief and sedation.
Pharmacokinetics
Well absorbed from the gastroin tes-
tinal (GI) tract. Widely distributed to
most tissues in the body. Protein
binding: varies. Excreted in the
urine as unchanged drug or metabolites. **Half-life:** 35 hrs (butalbital).
INDICATIONS AND DOSAGES
*Relief of mild to moderate pain,
tension headaches*
PO

Adults, Elderly. 1-2 tablets/capsules
q4h. Maximum: 6 tablets/capsules
daily.

AVAILABLE FORMS/COST
Butalbital/Acetaminophen/Caf-
feine
• Cap, Gel—Oral: 50 mg/325 mg/40
mg, 100's: **$7.95-$156.65**
• Tab, Uncoated—Oral: 50 mg/325
mg/40 mg, 30's: **$8.00-$164.98**
• With Codeine Cap, Gel—Oral: 50
mg/325 mg/40 mg/30 mg, 100's:
$124.50-$163.56
Butalbital/Aspirin/Caffeine
• Cap, Gel—Oral: 50 mg/325 mg/40
mg, 100's: **$37.13-$78.04**
• Tab, Uncoated—Oral: 325 mg/50
mg/40 mg, 100's: **$4.46-$79.40**
• With Codeine Cap, Gel—Oral: 50
mg/325 mg/ 40 mg/ 30 mg, 100's:
$93.61-$163.56

CONTRAINDICATIONS: Hypersensitivity to butalbital or any component of the formulation, porphyria
PREGNANCY AND LACTATION:
Pregnancy category C (category D if
used for prolonged periods or in
high doses at term); excretion into
breast milk unknown (see also aspirin, acetaminophen, and caffeine)
SIDE EFFECTS
Frequent
Drowsiness, excitation, confusion,
excitement, mental depression,
lightheadedness, dizziness, stomach upset, nausea, sleep disturbances
Rare
Rapid/irregular heartbeat, rash,
itching, swelling, severe dizziness,
trouble breathing, toxic epidermal
necrolysis
SERIOUS REACTIONS
• Symptoms of overdose may include vomiting, unusual drowsi-

ness, lack of feeling alert, slow or shallow breathing, cold or clammy skin, loss of consciousness, dark urine, stomach pain, and extreme fatigue.

INTERACTIONS
Drugs

Oral anticoagulants: Barbiturates inhibit the hypoprothrombinemic response to oral anticoagulants; fatal bleeding episodes have occurred when barbiturates were discontinued in patients stabilized on an anticoagulant (see also aspirin, acetaminophen, and caffeine)

SPECIAL CONSIDERATIONS

PATIENT/FAMILY EDUCATION
• May cause psychological and/or physical dependence
• May cause drowsiness, use caution driving or operating machinery
• Avoid alcohol and other CNS depressants

---

butenafine

(byoo-ten'a-feen)
Rx: Mentax
OTC: Lotrimin Ultra
Chemical Class: Benzylamine derivative
Therapeutic Class: Antifungal

CLINICAL PHARMACOLOGY
Mechanism of Action: An antifungal agent that locks biosynthesis of ergosterol, essential for fungal cell membrane. Fungicidal. *Therapeutic Effect:* Relieves athletes foot.
Pharmacokinetics

Total amount absorbed into systemic circulation has not been determined. Metabolized in liver. Excreted in urine. **Half-life:** 35 hrs.

INDICATIONS AND DOSAGES
Tinea pedis, tinea corporis, tinea cruris, tinea versicolor
Topical
Adults, Elderly, Children 12 yrs and older. Apply to affected area and immediate surrounding skin daily for 4 wks.

AVAILABLE FORMS/COST
• Cre—Top: 1%, 15, 30 g: **$40.27**/15 g

UNLABELED USES: Onychomycosis, seborrheic dermatitis
CONTRAINDICATIONS: Hypersensitivity to butenafine or any component of the formulation
PREGNANCY AND LACTATION: Pregnancy category B
SIDE EFFECTS
Occasional (2%)
Contact dermatitis, burning/stinging, worsening of the condition
Rare (less than 2%)
Erythema, irritation, pruritus
SERIOUS REACTIONS
• *None known.*
SPECIAL CONSIDERATIONS

• Good cutaneous absorption, prolonged skin retention, and fungicidal activity are potential advantages. Comparative trials with other agents necessary

---

butoconazole

(byoo-toe-ko'na-zole)
OTC: Femstat-3
Chemical Class: Imidazole derivative
Therapeutic Class: Antifungal

CLINICAL PHARMACOLOGY
Mechanism of Action: An antifungal similar to imidazole derivatives that inhibits the steroid synthesis, a vital component of fungal cell formation, thereby damaging the fun-

gal cell membrane. *Therapeutic Effect:* Fungistatic.

Pharmacokinetics

Not known.

INDICATIONS AND DOSAGES

Treatment of candidiasis

Topical

Adults, Elderly. Insert 1 applicatorful intravaginally at bedtime for up to 3 or 6 days.

AVAILABLE FORMS/COST

• Cre—Vag: 2%, 3 × 5 g applicators: **$10.81**

CONTRAINDICATIONS: Hypersensitivity to butoconazole or any of its components

PREGNANCY AND LACTATION: Pregnancy category C; excretion into breast milk unknown

SIDE EFFECTS

Occasional

Vaginal itching, burning, irritation

SERIOUS REACTIONS

• Soreness, swelling, pelvic pain or cramping rarely occurs.

---

butorphanol

(byoo-tor'fa-nole)

Rx: Stadol

Chemical Class: Morphinian congener; opiate derivative
Therapeutic Class: Narcotic agonist-antagonist analgesic
DEA Class: Schedule IV

CLINICAL PHARMACOLOGY

Mechanism of Action: An opioid that binds to opiate receptor sites in the central nervous system (CNS). Reduces intensity of pain stimuli incoming from sensory nerve endings. *Therapeutic Effect:* Alters pain perception and emotional response to pain.

Pharmacokinetics

Route	Onset	Peak	Duration
IM	10-30 min	30-60 min	3-4 hr
IV	less than 1 min	30 min	2-4 hr
Nasal	15 min	1-2 hr	4-5 hr

Rapidly absorbed after IM injection. Protein binding: 80%. Extensively metabolized in the liver. Primarily excreted in urine. **Half-life:** 2.5-4 hr.

INDICATIONS AND DOSAGES

Analgesia

IM

Adults. 1-4 mg q3-4h as needed.
Elderly. 1 mg q4-6h as needed.

IV

Adults. 0.5-2 mg q3-4h as needed.
Elderly. 1 mg q4-6h as needed.

Migraine

Nasal

Adults. 1 mg or 1 spray in one nostril. May repeat in 60-90 min. May repeat 2-dose sequence q3-4h as needed. Alternatively, 2 mg or 1 spray each nostril if patient remains recumbent, may repeat in 3-4 hrs.

AVAILABLE FORMS/COST

• Aer, Spray—Nasal: 10 mg/ml, 2.5 ml: **$75.25-$102.65**

• Sol, Inj—IM, IV: 1 mg/ml, 1 ml: **$4.63-$8.73**; 2 mg/ml, 1 ml: **$7.25-$26.60**

CONTRAINDICATIONS: CNS disease that affects respirations, physical dependence on other opioid analgesics, preexisting respiratory depression, pulmonary disease

PREGNANCY AND LACTATION: Pregnancy category B; crosses placenta; excreted in breast milk, though probably clinically insignificant

SIDE EFFECTS

Frequent

Parenteral: Somnolence (43%), dizziness (19%)

Nasal: Nasal congestion (13%), insomnia (11%)

Occasional

Parenteral (3%-9%): Confusion, diaphoresis, clammy skin, lethargy, headache, nausea, vomiting, dry mouth

Nasal (3%-9%): Vasodilation, constipation, unpleasant taste, dyspnea, epistaxis, nasal irritation, upper respiratory tract infection, tinnitus

Rare

Parenteral: Hypotension, pruritus, blurred vision, sensation of heat, CNS stimulation, insomnia

Nasal: Hypertension, tremor, ear pain, paresthesia, depression, sinusitis

SERIOUS REACTIONS

• Abrupt withdrawal after prolonged use may produce symptoms of narcotic withdrawal, such as abdominal cramping, rhinorrhea, lacrimation, anxiety, increased temperature, and piloerection or goose bumps.

• Overdose results in severe respiratory depression, skeletal muscle flaccidity, cyanosis, and extreme somnolence progressing to seizures, stupor, and coma.

• Tolerance to analgesic effect and physical dependence may occur with chronic use.

INTERACTIONS

Drugs

• *Nasal vasoconstrictors:* Slower onset of action of butorphanol (nasal spray)

SPECIAL CONSIDERATIONS

• Chronic use can precipitate withdrawal symptoms of anxiety, agitation, mood changes, hallucinations, dysphoria, weakness, and diarrhea

• Although not classified as a controlled substance by the FDA, prolonged use can result in habituation and drug-seeking behavior

• 2 mg=1 spray in each nostril

---

cabergoline
(cab-err-go-leen)

Rx: Dostinex

Chemical Class: Ergoline derivative

Therapeutic Class: Anti-Parkinson's agent; dopaminergic

CLINICAL PHARMACOLOGY

Mechanism of Action: Agonist at dopamine D2 receptors suppressing prolactin secretion. *Therapeutic effects:* Shrinks prolactinomas, restores gonadal function.

Pharmacokinetics

Cabergoline is administered orally and undergoes significant first-pass metabolism following systemic absorption. Extensively metabolized in the liver. Elimination is primarily in the feces. **Half-life:** 80 hours.

INDICATIONS AND DOSAGES

Hyperprolactemia (idiopathic or primary pituitary adenomas)

PO

Adults, elderly. 0.25 mg 2 times per week, titrate by 0.25 mg/dose no more than every 4 weeks up to 1 mg 2 times per week

PV

Adults. 0.5 mg 2 to five times per week

Parkinson's disease

PO

Adults. 0.5 mg/day and titrate to response. Mean effective dose is 3 mg/day and ranges from 0.5 – 6 mg/day.

Restless leg syndrome (RLS)

PO

Adults. 0.5 mg once daily at bedtime, slowly titrate up until symptoms resolve or drug-intolerance limits further adjustment. Mean effective dose is 2 mg/day and ranges from 1-4 mg/day.

• Tab—Oral: 0.5 mg, 8's: **$262.95**
UNLABELED USES: Parkinson's disease, restless leg syndrome (RLS)
CONTRAINDICATIONS: Hypersensitivity to cabergoline, ergot alkaloids or any one of its components.
Uncontrolled hypertension.
PREGNANCY AND LACTATION:
Pregnancy category B; unknown if excreted in breast milk
SIDE EFFECTS
Frequent
Nausea, orthostatic hypotension, confusion, dyskinesia, hallucinations, peripheral edema
Occasional
Headache, vertigo, dizziness, dyspepsia, postural hypotension, constipation, asthenia, fatigue, abdominal pain, drowsiness
Rare
Vomiting, dry mouth, diarrhea, flatulence, anxiety, depression, dysmenorrheal, dyspepsia, mastalgia, paresthesias, vertigo, visual impairment, pleuropulmonary changes, pleural effusion, pulmonary fibrosis, heart failure, peptic ulcer
SERIOUS REACTIONS
• Overdosage may produce nasal congestion, syncope, or hallucinations.

SPECIAL CONSIDERATIONS
• More potent with longer half-life than bromocriptine or pergolide, allowing for less frequent dosing
• Initial treatment produces dramatic response; as disease progresses response duration decreases

---

caffeine
OTC: Caffedrine, No-Doz, QuickPep, StayAwake, Vivarin
Chemical Class: Xanthine derivative
Therapeutic Class: Analeptic; central nervous system stimulant

---

CLINICAL PHARMACOLOGY
Mechanism of Action: A methylxanthine and competitive inhibitor of phosphodiesterase that blocks antagonism of adenosine receptors. *Therapeutic Effect:* Stimulates respiratory center, increases minute ventilation, decreases threshold of or increases response to hypercapnia, increases skeletal muscle tone, decreases diaphragmatic fatigue, increases metabolic rate, and increases oxygen consumption.
Pharmacokinetics
Protein binding: 36%. Widely distributed through the tissues and CSF. Metabolized in lever. Excreted in urine. **Half-life:** 3-7 hrs.
INDICATIONS AND DOSAGES
Drowsiness, fatigue
Adults, Elderly. 200 mg no sooner than every 3-4 hours, as needed.
§ **AVAILABLE FORMS/COST**
• Sol, Inj-IM, IV: 125 mg/ml, 2 ml: **$9.70-$24.38** (Rx only)
• Tab—Oral: 100 mg, 12's: **$2.32**; 200 mg, 30's: **$1.85**
CONTRAINDICATIONS: Hypersensitivity to caffeine, xanthines or any other component of the formulation
PREGNANCY AND LACTATION:
Pregnancy category B; amounts in breast milk after maternal ingestion of caffeinated beverages not clinically significant; accumulation can occur in heavy-using mothers

SIDE EFFECTS
Occasional

Agitation, insomnia, nervousness, restlessness, GI irritation

SERIOUS REACTIONS

• At high doses, caffeine can cause arrhythmias, palpitations, and tachycardia.

INTERACTIONS
Drugs

▧ *β-adrenergic agents:* Enhanced β-adrenergic stimulating effects

▧ *Cimetidine:* Impairs caffeine metabolism resulting in excessive CNS or cardiovascular effects

▧ *Clozapine:* Caffeine inhibits CYP1A2, with elevations of clozapine levels

▧ *Contraceptives, oral:* Impair caffeine metabolism resulting in excessive CNS or cardiovascular effects

▧ *Disulfiram:* Impairs caffeine metabolism resulting in excessive CNS or cardiovascular effects

▧ *Fluroquinolone antibiotics:* Increases caffeine concentrations and may enhance its side effects

▧ *Fluconazole:* Increased caffeine concentrations

▧ *Mexiletine:* 30%-50% reduction in caffeine clearance; potentially increased risk of CNS or cardiovascular effects

▧ *Phenylpropanolamine:* Additive effects

▧ *Phenytoin:* Induced hepatic metabolism of caffeine; decreased caffeine effects

▧ *Pipemidic acid:* Produces a large increase in caffeine concentrations and may increase side effects

▧ *Terbinafine:* Impairs caffeine metabolism resulting in excessive CNS or cardiovascular effects

▧ *Theophylline:* Caffeine reduces theophylline clearance by 30%; may affect serum theophylline levels

Labs

• *False positive elevations:* Serum uric acid levels, urine levels of VMA, catecholamines, 5-hydroxy-indoleacetic acid

SPECIAL CONSIDERATIONS
PATIENT/FAMILY EDUCATION

• Gradual taper if used long-term to prevent withdrawal syndrome, especially headache

• Most authorities believe caffeine and other analeptics should not be used in overdose with CNS depressants and recommend other supportive therapy

---

calcipotriene
(kal-sip'oh-tri-een)
Rx: Dovonex
Chemical Class: Vitamin D analog
Therapeutic Class: Antipsoriatic

CLINICAL PHARMACOLOGY
Mechanism of Action: A synthetic vitamin D_3 analogue that regulates skin cell (keratinocyte) production and development. *Therapeutic Effect:* preventing abnormal growth and production of psoriasis (abnormal keratinocyte growth).

Pharmacokinetics

Minimal absorption through intact skin. Metabolized in liver.

INDICATIONS AND DOSAGES
Psoriasis

Topical

Adults, Elderly, Children 12 yrs and older. Apply thin layer to affected skin twice daily (morning and evening); rub in gently and completely.

Scalp psoriasis

Topical Solution

Adults, Elderly, Children 12 yrs and older. Apply to lesions after combing hair.

AVAILABLE FORMS/COST
- Cre—Top: 0.005%, 30, 60, 100, 120 g: **$46.73**/30 g
- Oint—Top: 0.005%, 30, 60, 100, 120 g: **$46.73**/30 g
- Sol—Top: 0.005%, 60 ml: **$104.25**

CONTRAINDICATIONS: Hypercalcemia or evidence of vitamin D toxicity, use on face, hypersensitivity to calcipotriene or any component of the formulation

PREGNANCY AND LACTATION: Pregnancy category C

SIDE EFFECTS

Frequent

Burning, itching, skin irritation

Occasional

Erythema, dry skin, peeling, rash, worsening of psoriasis, dermatititis

Rare

Skin atrophy, hyperpigmentation, folliculitis

SERIOUS REACTIONS
- Potential for hypercalcemia may occur.

SPECIAL CONSIDERATIONS

MONITORING PARAMETERS
- Serum calcium (if elevated discontinue therapy until normal calcium levels are restored); topical administration can yield systemic effects with excessive use

calcitonin
(kal-si-toe'nin)

Rx: Salmon: Calcimar, Salmonine, Osteocalein, Miacalcin (nasal)

Rx: Human: Cibacalcin (orphan drug)

Chemical Class: Polypeptide hormone

Therapeutic Class: Antidote, hypercalcemia; antiosteoporotic

CLINICAL PHARMACOLOGY

Mechanism of Action: A synthetic hormone that decreases osteoclast activity in bones, decreases tubular reabsorption of sodium and calcium in the kidneys, and increases absorption of calcium in the GI tract. *Therapeutic Effect:* Regulates serum calcium concentrations.

Pharmacokinetics

Injection form rapidly metabolized (primarily in kidneys); primarily excreted in urine. Nasal form rapidly absorbed. **Half-life:** 70–90 min (injection); 43 min (nasal).

INDICATIONS AND DOSAGES

Skin testing before treatment in patients with suspected sensitivity to calcitonin-salmon

Adults, Elderly. Prepare a 10-international units/ml dilution; withdraw 0.05 ml from a 200-international units/ml vial in a tuberculin syringe; fill up to 1 ml with 0.9% NaCl. Take 0.1 ml and inject intracutaneously on inner aspect of forearm. Observe after 15 min; a positive response is the appearance of more than mild erythema or wheal.

Paget's disease

IM, Subcutaneous

Adults, Elderly. Initially, 100 international units/day. Maintenance: 50 international units/day or 50–100 international units every 1-3 days.
Intranasal
Adults, Elderly. 200–400 international units/day.

Osteoporosis imperfecta
IM, Subcutaneous
Adults. 2 international units/kg 3 times a week.

Postmenopausal osteoporosis
IM, Subcutaneous
Adults, Elderly. 100 international units/day with adequate calcium and vitamin D intake.
Intranasal
Adults, Elderly. 200 international units/day as a single spray, alternating nostrils daily.

Hypercalcemia
IM, Subcutaneous
Adults, Elderly. Initially, 4 international units/kg q12h; may increase to 8 international units/kg q12h if no response in 2 days; may further increase to 8 international units/kg q6h if no response in another 2 days.

§ **AVAILABLE FORMS/COST**
• Sol, Inj-IM, SC: 200 IU/ml, 2 ml: **$31.35-$42.11** (salmon)
• Spray-Nasal: 200 IU/metered dose, 14 doses/2 ml: **$78.16**

UNLABELED USES: Treatment of secondary osteoporosis due to drug therapy or hormone disturbance
CONTRAINDICATIONS: Hypersensitivity to gelatin desserts or salmon protein
PREGNANCY AND LACTATION: Pregnancy category C; inhibits lactation in animals
SIDE EFFECTS
Frequent
IM, Subcutaneous (10%): Nausea (may occur 30 min after injection, usually diminishes with continued therapy), inflammation at injection site

Nasal (12%–10%): Rhinitis, nasal irritation, redness, sores
Occasional
IM, Subcutaneous (5%–2%): Flushing of face or hands
Nasal (5%–3%): Back pain, arthralgia, epistaxis, headache
Rare
IM, Subcutaneous: Epigastric discomfort, dry mouth, diarrhea, flatulence
Nasal: Itching of earlobes, edema of feet, rash, diaphoresis
SERIOUS REACTIONS
• Patients with a protein allergy may develop a hypersensitivity reaction.
SPECIAL CONSIDERATIONS
PATIENT/FAMILY EDUCATION
• Before first dose of new bottle of nasal spray pump must be activated by holding upright and pumping nozzle 6 times until a faint spray is emitted

---

calcitriol
(kal-si-trye´ole)
Rx: Calcijex, Rocaltrol
Chemical Class: Vitamin D analog
Therapeutic Class: Antiosteoporotic; vitamin D analog

CLINICAL PHARMACOLOGY
Mechanism of Action: A fat-soluble vitamin that is essential for absorption, utilization of calcium phosphate, and normal calcification of bone. *Therapeutic Effect:* Stimulates calcium and phosphate absorption from small intestine, promotes secretion of calcium from bone to blood, promotes renal tubule phosphate resorption, acts on bone cells to stimulate skeletal growth and on parathyroid gland to suppress hormone synthesis and secretion.

Pharmacokinetics

Rapidly absorbed from small intestine. Extensive metabolism in kidneys. Primarily excreted in feces; minimal excretion in urine. **Half-life:** 5- 8 hrs.

INDICATIONS AND DOSAGES

Renal failure

PO

Adults, Elderly. 0.25 mcg/day or every other day.

Children. 0.25-2 mcg/day with hemodialysis; 0.014-0.41 mcg/kg/day without hemodialysis.

IV

Adults, Elderly. 0.5 mcg/day (0.01 mcg/kg) 3 times/week. Dose range: 0.5-3 mcg (0.01-0.05 mcg/kg) 3 times/week.

Children. 0.01-0.05 mcg/kg 3 times/week with hemodialysis.

Hypoparathyroidism/pseudohypoparathyroidism

PO

Adults, Elderly. 0.5-2 mcg/day

Children 6 yrs and older. 0.5-2 mcg once daily.

Children 5-1 yrs. 0.25-0.75 mcg once daily

Children less than 1 yr. 0.04-0.08 mcg/kg once daily.

Vitamin D-dependent rickets

PO

Adults, Elderly, Children. 1 mcg once daily.

Vitamin D-resistant rickets

PO

Adults, Elderly, Children. 0.015-0.02 mcg/kg once daily. Maintenance: 0.03-0.06 mcg/kg once daily. Maximum: 2 mcg once daily.

Ⓢ AVAILABLE FORMS/COST

• Cap, Elastic—Oral: 0.25 mcg, 100's: **$120.95-$139.99**; 0.5 mcg, 100's: **$193.38-$223.83**

• Sol, Inj-IV: 1 mcg/ml, 1 ml: **$13.09-$15.31**; 2 mcg/ml, 1 ml: **$26.18**

• Sol-Oral: 1 mcg/15 ml: **$179.00**

CONTRAINDICATIONS: Hypercalcemia, malabsorption syndrome, vitamin D toxicity, hypersensitivity to other vitamin D products or analogs

PREGNANCY AND LACTATION: Pregnancy category C; may be excreted in breast milk

SIDE EFFECTS

Occasional

Hypercalcemia, headache, irritability, constipation, metallic taste, nausea, polyuria

SERIOUS REACTIONS

• Early signs of overdosage are manifested as weakness, headache, somnolence, nausea, vomiting, dry mouth, constipation, muscle and bone pain, and metallic taste sensation.

• Later signs of overdosage are evidenced by polyuria, polydipsia, anorexia, weight loss, nocturia, photophobia, rhinorrhea, pruritus, disorientation, hallucinations, hyperthermia, hypertension, and cardiac arrhythmias.

INTERACTIONS

Drugs

③ *Thiazide diuretics:* Increased risk of hypercalcemia

③ *Verapamil:* Hypercalcemia may inhibit the activity of verapamil

SPECIAL CONSIDERATIONS

PATIENT/FAMILY EDUCATION

• Adequate dietary calcium is necessary for clinical response to vitamin D therapy

MONITORING PARAMETERS

• Blood Ca^{2+} and phosphate determinations must be made every week until stable, or more frequently if necessary

• Vitamin D levels also helpful, although less frequently

• Height and weight in children

calcium salts

Rx: Calcium acetate: PhosLo
OTC: *Calcium carbonate:* Amitone, Cal-Carb Forte, Calci-Chew, Calci-Mix, Caltrate 600, Chooz, Florical, Maalox, Mallamint, Mylanta, Nephro-Calci, Os-Cal 500, Oysco 500, Oyst-Cal 500, Oyster Calcium, Rolaids, Titralac, Tums, Tums Ex; *Calcium citrate:* Citracal; *Calcium glubionate:* Neo-Calglucon; *Tricalcium phosphate:* Posture
Combinations
  Rx: with cholecalciferol (Os-Cal-D)
  OTC: with sodium fluoride (Caltrate, Florical)
Chemical Class: Divalent cation
Therapeutic Class: Antacid; antiosteoporotic; phosphate adsorbent (acetate)

CLINICAL PHARMACOLOGY

Mechanism of Action: An electrolyte that is essential for the function and integrity of the nervous, muscular, and skeletal systems. Calcium plays an important role in normal cardiac and renal function, respiration, blood coagulation, and cell membrane and capillary permeability. It helps regulate the release and storage of neurotransmitters and hormones, and it neutralizes or reduces gastric acid (increase pH). Calcium acetate combines with dietary phosphate to form insoluble calcium phosphate. *Therapeutic Effects:* Replaces calcium in deficiency states; controls hyperphosphatemia in end-stage renal disease.

Pharmacokinetics
Moderately absorbed from the small intestine (absorption depends on presence of vitamin D metabolites and patient's pH). Primarily eliminated in feces.

INDICATIONS AND DOSAGES

Hyperphosphatemia
PO (calcium acetate)
Adults, Elderly. 2 tablets 3 times a day with meals.

Hypocalcemia
PO (calcium carbonate)
Adults, Elderly. 1–2 g/day in 3–4 divided doses.
Children. 45–65 mg/kg/day in 3–4 divided doses.
PO (calcium glubionate)
Adults, Elderly. 16-18 g/day in 4-6 divided doses.
Children, Infants. 0.6-2 g/kg/day in 4 divided doses.
Neonates. 1.2 g/kg/day in 4-6 divided doses.
IV (calcium chloride)
Adults, Elderly. 0.5–1 g repeated q4–6h as needed.
Children. 2.5–5 mg/kg/dose q4–6h.
IV (calcium gluconate)
Adults, Elderly. 2–15 g/24 hr.
Children. 200–500 mg/kg/day.

Antacid
PO (calcium carbonate)
Adults, Elderly. 1–2 tabs (5–10 ml) q2h as needed.

Osteoporosis
PO (calcium carbonate)
Adults, Elderly. 1200 mg/day.

Cardiac arrest
IV (calcium chloride)
Adults, Elderly. 2–4 mg/kg. May repeat q10min.
Children. 20 mg/kg. May repeat in 10 min.

Hypocalcemia tetany
IV (calcium chloride)
Adults, Elderly. 1 g may repeat in 6 hours.

C

Children. 10 mg/kg over 5–10 min. May repeat in 6–8 hr.

IV (calcium gluconate)

Adults, Elderly. 1–3 g until therapeutic response achieved.

Children. 100–200 mg/kg/dose q6–8h.

§ **AVAILABLE FORMS/COST**

Calcium Acetate

• Sol, Inj-IV: 0.5 mEq/ml, 10 ml: **$0.90**

• Tab-Oral: 667 mg, 200's: **$16.41**

Calcium Carbonate (mg of calcium)

• Susp—Oral: 1250 mg (500 mg Ca)/5 ml, 500 ml: **$12.37**

• Tab, Chewable-Oral: 500 mg, 100's: **$2.73**; 600 mg, 85's: **$5.52**; 750 mg (300 mg Ca), 96's: **$2.78-$4.88**; 1000 mg, 72's: **$2.78-$4.00**; 1250 mg (500 mg Ca), 100's: **$5.99-$11.66**

• Tab-Oral: 650 mg (260 mg Ca), 100's: **$3.98**; 1250 mg (500 mg Ca), 60's: **$1.25-$7.11**

Calcium Chloride

• Sol, Inj-IV: 10%, 10 ml: **$2.71-$13.45**

Calcium Citrate (mg of calcium)

• Tab-Oral: 950 mg (200 mg Ca), 100's: **$3.00-$6.88**

Calcium Glubionate (mg of calcium)

• Syr—Oral: 1800 mg (115 mg Ca)/5 ml, 480 ml: **$17.95-$24.95**

Calcium Gluconate (mg of calcium)

• Sol, Inj-IV: 10%, 10 ml: **$0.50-$1.45**

• Tab—Oral: 500 mg (45 mg Ca), 100's: **$13.68-$16.45**; 650 mg (58.5 mg Ca), 100's: **$4.25**; 1000 mg (90 mg Ca), 100's: **$26.70**

Calcium Lactate (mg of calcium)

• Tab—Oral: 325 mg (42.25 mg Ca), 100's: **$1.50-$2.25**; 650 mg (84.5 mg Ca), 100's: **$0.99-$7.30**

Tribasic Calcium Phosphate (mg of calcium)

• Tab—Oral: 1565.2 mg (600 mg Ca), 60's: **$7.97**

UNLABELED USES: Treatment of hyperphosphatemia (calcium carbonate)

CONTRAINDICATIONS: Calcium renal calculi, digoxin toxicity, hypercalcemia, hypercalciuria, sarcoidosis, ventricular fibrillation

Calcium acetate: Decreased renal function, hypoparathyroidism

PREGNANCY AND LACTATION: Pregnancy category C; some oral supplemental calcium may be excreted in breast milk (chloride, gluconate, unknown); concentrations not sufficient to produce an adverse effect in neonates

SIDE EFFECTS

Frequent

PO: Chalky taste

Parenteral: Hypotension; flushing; feeling of warmth; nausea; vomiting; pain, rash, redness, or burning at injection site; diaphoresis

Occasional

PO: Mild constipation, fecal impaction, peripheral edema, metabolic alkalosis (muscle pain, restlessness, slow breathing, altered taste)

Calcium carbonate: Milk-alkali syndrome (headache, decreased appetite, nausea, vomiting, unusual tiredness)

Rare

Difficult or painful urination

SERIOUS REACTIONS

• Hypercalcemia is a serious adverse effect of calcium acetate use. Early signs include constipation, headache, dry mouth, increased thirst, irritability, decreased appetite, metallic taste, fatigue, weakness, and depression. Later signs include confusion, somnolence, hypertension, photosensitivity, arrhythmias, nausea, vomiting, and increased painful urination.

INTERACTIONS
Drugs
■ *Calcium channel blockers:* Calcium administration (especially parenteral) may inhibit calcium channel blocker activity

■ *Digoxin, digitoxin:* Elevated calcium concentrations associated with acute digitalis toxicity

■ *Doxycycline, Tetracycline:* Cotherapy with a tetracycline and a divalent or trivalent cation can reduce the serum concentration and efficacy of tetracyclines

■ *Iron:* Some calcium antacids reduce the GI absorption of iron; inhibition of the hematological response to iron has been reported

■ *Itraconazole, Ketoconazole:* Antacids containing calcium may reduce antifungal concentrations

■ *Quinidine:* Calcium antacids capable of increasing urine pH may increase serum quinidine concentrations

■ *Quinolones:* Reduced bioavailability of quinolone antibiotics

■ *Sodium polystyrene sulfonate resin:* Combined use with calcium-containing antacid may result in systemic alkalosis

■ *Thiazides:* Large doses of calcium with thiazides may lead to milk-alkali syndrome

Labs
• *False increase:* Chloride, green color, benzodiazepine (false positive)

• *False decrease:* Magnesium, oxylate, lipase

SPECIAL CONSIDERATIONS
• Percentage elemental calcium content of various calcium salts: calcium acetate (25%), calcium carbonate (40%), calcium chloride (27.2%), calcium citrate (21%), calcium glubionate (6.5%), calcium glucceptate (8.2%), calcium gluconate (9.3%), calcium lactate (13%), tricalcium phosphate, (39%)

MONITORING PARAMETERS
• Serum calcium or serum ionized calcium concentrations (ionized calcium concentrations are preferable to determine free and bound calcium, especially with concurrent low serum albumin)

• Alternatively, ionized calcium can be estimated using the following rule: Total serum calcium will fall by 0.8 mg/dL for each 1.0 g/dL decrease in serum albumin concentration

---

(kan-de-sar′-tan)
Rx: Atacand
Chemical Class: Angiotensin II receptor antagonist
Therapeutic Class: Antihypertensive

CLINICAL PHARMACOLOGY
Mechanism of Action: An angiotensin II receptor, type AT_1, antagonist that blocks the vasoconstrictor and aldosterone-secreting effects of angiotensin II, inhibiting the binding of angiotensin II to the AT_1 receptors. *Therapeutic Effect:* Causes vasodilation, decreases peripheral resistance, and decreases BP.
Pharmacokinetics

Route	Onset	Peak	Duration
PO	2–3 hr	6–8 hr	Greater than 24 hr

Rapidly, completely absorbed. Protein binding: greater than 99%. Undergoes minor hepatic metabolism to inactive metabolite. Excreted unchanged in urine and in the feces through the biliary system. Not removed by hemodialysis. **Half-life:** 9 hr.

INDICATIONS AND DOSAGES
Hypertension alone or in combination with other antihypertensives
PO
Adults, Elderly, Patients with mildly impaired liver or renal function. Initially, 16 mg once a day in those who are not volume depleted. Can be given once or twice a day with total daily doses of 8–32 mg. Give lower dosage in those treated with diuretics or with severely impaired renal function.

$ AVAILABLE FORMS/COST
• Tab-Oral: 4 mg, 8 mg, 16 mg, 30's; all: **$44.45**; 32 mg, 30's: **$60.14**
UNLABELED USES: Treatment of heart failure
CONTRAINDICATIONS: Hypersensitivity to candesartan
PREGNANCY AND LACTATION: Pregnancy category C (1st trimester) and D (2nd and 3rd trimester); use caution in nursing mothers
SIDE EFFECTS
Occasional (6%–3%)
Upper respiratory tract infection, dizziness, back and leg pain
Rare (2%–1%)
Pharyngitis, rhinitis, headache, fatigue, diarrhea, nausea, dry cough, peripheral edema
SERIOUS REACTIONS
• Overdosage may manifest as hypotension and tachycardia. Bradycardia occurs less often. Institute supportive measures.
INTERACTIONS
Drugs
❸ *Cimetidine:* Increased levels of candesartan
❸ *Fluconazole:* Decreased conversion to active metabolite (CYP2C9 inhibition), loss of antihypertensive effects

❷ *Lithium:* Increased renal lithium reabsorption at the proximal tubular site due to the natriuresis associated with the inhibition of aldosterone secretion; increased risk of lithium toxicity
❸ *Potassium-sparing diuretics, salt substitutes, potassium supplements:* Increased risk of hyperkalemia
❸ *Phenobarbital:* Decreased levels of candesartan
❸ *Rifampin:* Induced metabolism resulting in a decrease in the area under the concentration-time curve (AUC) and half-life and reduced efficacy of candesartan

SPECIAL CONSIDERATIONS
• Potentially as or more effective than angiotensin-converting enzyme inhibitors, without cough; no evidence for reduction in morbidity and mortality as first-line agents in hypertension yet; whether they provide the same cardiac and renal protection also still tentative; like ACE inhibitors, less effective in black patients

PATIENT/FAMILY EDUCATION
• Call your clinician immediately if the following side effects are noted: wheezing; lip, throat or face swelling; hives or rash

MONITORING PARAMETERS
• Baseline electrolytes, urinalysis, blood urea nitrogen and creatinine with recheck at 2-4 wk after initiation (sooner in volume-depleted patients); monitor sitting BP; watch for symptomatic hypotension, particularly in volume-depleted patients

capreomycin

(kap-ree-oh-mye′sin)
Rx: Capastat
Chemical Class: Polypeptide antibiotic
Therapeutic Class: Antituberculosis agent

CLINICAL PHARMACOLOGY

Mechanism of Action: A cyclic polypeptide antimicrobial but the mechanism of action is not well understood. *Therapeutic Effect:* Suppresses mycobacterial multiplication.

Pharmacokinetics

Not well absorbed from the gastrointestinal (GI) tract. Undergoes little metabolism. Primarily excreted unchanged in urine. **Half-life:** 4-6 hrs (half-life is increased with impaired renal function).

INDICATIONS AND DOSAGES

Tuberculosis

IM

Adults, Elderly, Children. 15-20 mg/kg/day for 60-120 days, followed by 1 g 2-3 times/wk. Maximum: 1 g/day.

AVAILABLE FORMS/COST

• Sol, Inj-IM: 1 g/vial: **$25.54**

UNLABELED USES: Treatment of atypical mycobacterial infections

CONTRAINDICATIONS: Concurrent use of other ototoxic or nephrotoxic drugs, hypersensitivity to capreomycin

PREGNANCY AND LACTATION: Pregnancy category C; breast milk excretion is unknown; however, problems in humans have not been documented (poorly absorbed from GI tract)

SIDE EFFECTS

Frequent

Ototoxicity, nephrotoxicity

Occasional

Eosinophilia

Rare

Rash, fever, urticaria, hypokalemia, thrombocytopenia, vertigo

SERIOUS REACTIONS

• Renal failure, ototoxicity, and thrombocytopenia can occur.

INTERACTIONS

Drugs

■ *Amphotericin B, Cephalosporins, Cyclosporine, Methoxyflurane:* Additive nephrotoxicity risk

■ *Carboplatin:* Additive ototoxicity

② *Ethacrynic acid:* Additive ototoxicity

② *Neuromuscular blocking agents:* Potentiate the respiratory suppression produced by neuromuscular blocking agents

■ *Oral anticoagulants:* Enhanced hypoprothrombinemic response

SPECIAL CONSIDERATIONS

• When used in renal insufficiency or pre-existing auditory impairment, risks of additional 8th-nerve impairment or renal injury should be weighed against the benefits of therapy

MONITORING PARAMETERS

• Electrolytes, BUN, creatinine weekly
• Blood levels of drug
• Audiometric testing before, during, after treatment

capsaicin

(cap-say'sin)

OTC: Zostrix, Zostrix HP

Chemical Class: Alkaloid derivative of solanaceae plant family

Therapeutic Class: Topical analgesic

CLINICAL PHARMACOLOGY

Mechanism of Action: A topical analgesic that depletes and prevents reaccumulation of the chemomediator of pain impulses (substance P) from peripheral sensory neurons to CNS. *Therapeutic Effect:* Relieves pain.

Pharmacokinetics

None reported.

INDICATIONS AND DOSAGES

Treatment of neuralgia, osteoarthritis, rheumatoid arthritis

Topical

Adults, Elderly, Children older than 2 yrs. Apply directly to affected area 3–4 times/day. Continue for 14 to 28 days for optimal clinical response.

[$] **AVAILABLE FORMS/COST**

• Cre—Top: 0.025%, 20, 45, 60 g: **$3.60-$12.44**/60 g; 0.075%, 30, 45, 60 g: **$8.05-$26.95**/60 g

• Lot—Top: 0.025%, 30 ml: **$5.40**; 0.075% 30 ml: **$6.00**

UNLABELED USES: Treatment of neurogenic pain

CONTRAINDICATIONS: Hypersensitivity to capsaicin or any component of the formulation

SIDE EFFECTS

Frequent

Burning, stinging, erythema at site of application

SERIOUS REACTIONS

• None known.

SPECIAL CONSIDERATIONS

• Pretreatment with topical lidocaine 5% ointment may relieve burning

PATIENT/FAMILY EDUCATION

• Wash hands following use

captopril

(cap-toe-pril)

Rx: Capoten

Combinations

Rx: with hydrochlorothiazide (Capozide)

Chemical Class: Angiotensin-converting enzyme (ACE) inhibitor, nonsulfhydryl

Therapeutic Class: Antihypertensive

CLINICAL PHARMACOLOGY

Mechanism of Action: An ACE inhibitor that suppresses the renin-angiotensin-aldosterone system and prevents conversion of angiotensin I to angiotensin II, a potent vasoconstrictor; may also inhibit angiotensin II at local vascular and renal sites. Decreases plasma angiotensin II, increases plasma renin activity, and decreases aldosterone secretion. *Therapeutic Effect:* Reduces peripheral arterial resistance, pulmonary capillary wedge pressure; improves cardiac output and exercise tolerance.

Pharmacokinetics

Route	*Onset*	*Peak*	*Duration*
PO	0.25 hr	0.5–1.5 hr	Dose related

Rapidly, well absorbed from the GI tract (absorption is decreased in the presence of food). Protein binding: 25%–30%. Metabolized in the liver. Primarily excreted in urine. Removed by hemodialysis. **Half-life:** less than 3 hrs (increased in those with impaired renal function).

INDICATIONS AND DOSAGES

Hypertension

PO

Adults, Elderly. Initially, 12.5–25 mg 2–3 times a day. After 1–2 wk, may increase to 50 mg 2–3 times a day. Diuretic may be added if no response in additional 1–2 wk. If taken in combination with diuretic, may increase to 100–150 mg 2–3 times a day after 1–2 wk. Maintenance: 25–150 mg 2–3 times a day. Maximum: 450 mg/day.

CHF

PO

Adults, Elderly. Initially, 6.25–25 mg 3 times a day. Increase to 50 mg 3 times a day. After at least 2 wk, may increase to 50–100 mg 3 times a day. Maximum: 450 mg/day.

Post-myocardial infarction, impaired liver function

PO

Adults, Elderly. 6.25 mg a day, then 12.5 mg 3 times a day. Increase to 25 mg 3 times a day over several days up to 50 mg 3 times a day over several weeks.

Diabetic nephropathy prevention of kidney failure

PO

Adults, Elderly. 25 mg 3 times a day.
Children. Initially 0.3–0.5 mg/kg/dose titrated up to a maximum of 6 mg/kg/day in 2–4 divided doses.
Neonates. Initially, 0.05–0.1 mg/kg/dose q8-24h titrated up to 0.5 mg/kg/dose given q6-24h.

Dosage in renal impairment

Creatinine clearance 10-50 ml/min. 75% of normal dosage.
Creatinine clearance less than 10 ml/min. 50% of normal dosage.

$ **AVAILABLE FORMS/COST**
• Tab-Oral: 12.5 mg, 100's: **$54.95-$120.94**; 25 mg, 100's: **$63.93-$128.37**; 50 mg, 100's: **$100.50-$220.12**; 100 mg, 100's: **$129.95-$293.14**

UNLABELED USES: Diagnosis of anatomic renal artery stenosis, hypertensive crisis, rheumatoid arthritis

CONTRAINDICATIONS: History of angioedema from previous treatment with ACE inhibitors

PREGNANCY AND LACTATION: Pregnancy category C (1st trimester) and D (2nd and 3rd trimesters—fetal and neonatal hypotension, neonatal skull hypoplasia, anuria, reversible or irreversible renal failure, death, oligohydramnios); excreted into breast milk in small amounts; compatible with breast-feeding

SIDE EFFECTS

Frequent (7%–4%)
Rash
Occasional (4%–2%)
Pruritus, dysgeusia (change in sense of taste)
Rare (less than 2%–0.5%)
Headache, cough, insomnia, dizziness, fatigue, paresthesia, malaise, nausea, diarrhea or constipation, dry mouth, tachycardia

SERIOUS REACTIONS
• Excessive hypotension (first-dose syncope) may occur in patients with CHF and in those who are severely salt and volume depleted.
• Angioedema (swelling of face and lips) and hyperkalemia occur rarely.
• Agranulocytosis and neutropenia may be noted in those with collagen vascular disease, including scleroderma and systemic lupus erythematosus, and impaired renal function.
• Nephrotic syndrome may be noted in those with history of renal disease.

INTERACTIONS
Drugs
❷ *Allopurinol:* Increased risk of hypersensitivity reactions including Stevens-Johnson syndrome, skin eruptions, fever, and arthralgias

❸ *α-blockers:* Possible exaggerated "first dose" response

❸ *Aspirin:* Reduced hemodynamic effects of captopril; less likely at doses <236 mg qday

❸ *Azathioprine:* Increased risk of myelosuppression

❸ *Cyclosporine:* Increased risk of nephrotoxicity

❸ *Indomethacin:* Inhibits the antihypertensive response to ACE inhibition; other NSAIDs probably have similar effect

❸ *Insulin:* ACE inhibitors enhance insulin sensitivity; hypoglycemia possible

❸ *Iron:* Increased risk of systemic reaction (GI symptoms, hypotension) with parenteral iron

❸ *Lithium:* Increased risk of lithium toxicity

❸ *Loop diuretics:* Initiation of ACE inhibition therapy with concurrent intensive diuretic therapy may cause significant hypotension, renal insufficiency

❸ *Mercaptopurine:* Increased risk of neutropenia

❸ *Potassium, Potassium-sparing diuretics:* ACE inhibition tends to increase potassium; increased risk of hyperkalemia in predisposed patients

❸ *Trimethoprim:* Additive risk of hyperkalemia, especially in patient predisposed to renal insufficiency

Labs
• ACE inhibition can account for approximately 0.5mEq/L rise in serum potassium

• Blood in urine: Decreased reactivity with occult blood test

• Fructosamine: Captopril interferes with assay increasing serum fructosamine

• Ketones in urine: False positive dip-sticks

• *False positive:* Urine acetone

SPECIAL CONSIDERATIONS
PATIENT/FAMILY EDUCATION
• Caution with salt substitutes containing potassium chloride

• Rise slowly to sitting/standing position to minimize orthostatic hypotension

• Dizziness, fainting, lightheadedness may occur during 1st few days of therapy

• May cause altered taste perception or cough; persistent dry cough usually does not subside unless medication is stopped; notify clinician if these symptoms persist

MONITORING PARAMETERS
• BUN, creatinine, potassium within 2 wk after initiation of therapy (increased levels may indicate acute renal failure)

---

carbamazepine
(kar-ba-maz′e-peen)
Rx: Atretol, Carbatrol, Epitol, Tegretol, Tegretol-XR
Chemical Class: Iminostilbene derivative
Therapeutic Class: Anticonvulsant; antimanic; antineuralgic; antipsychotic

---

CLINICAL PHARMACOLOGY
Mechanism of Action: An iminostilbene derivative that decreases sodium and calcium ion influx into neuronal membranes, reducing post-tetanic potentiation at synapses. *Therapeutic Effect:* Reduces seizure activity.

Pharmacokinetics

Slowly and completely absorbed from the GI tract. Protein binding: 75%. Metabolized in the liver to active metabolite. Primarily excreted in urine. Not removed by hemodialysis. **Half-life:** 25-65 hr (decreased with chronic use).

INDICATIONS AND DOSAGES
Seizure control

PO

Adults, Children older than 12 yr. Initially, 200 mg twice a day. May increase dosage by 200 mg/day at weekly intervals. Range: 400-1200 mg/day in 2-4 divided doses. Maximum: 1.6-2.4 g/day.

Children 6-12 yr. Initially, 100 mg twice a day. May increase by 100 mg/day at weekly intervals. Range: 20-30 mg/kg/day. Maxiumum: 1000 mg/day.

Children younger than 6 yr. Initially 5 mg/kg/day. May increase at weekly intervals to 10 mg/kg/day up to 20 mg/kg/day.

Elderly. Initially 100 mg 1-2 times a day. May increase by 100 mg/day at weekly intervals. Usual dose 400-1000 mg/day.

Trigeminal neuralgia, diabetic neuropathy

PO

Adults. Initially, 100 mg twice a day. May increase by 100 mg twice a day up to 400-800 mg/day. Maxiumum: 1200 mg/day.

Elderly. Initially 100 mg 1-2 times a day. May increase by 100 mg/day at weekly intervals. Usual dose 400-1000 mg/day.

Ⓢ AVAILABLE FORMS/COST
• Cap, Sus Action—Oral: 200 mg, 300 mg, 120's; all: **$122.08**
• Susp—Oral: 100 mg/5 ml, 450 ml: **$31.10-$38.55**
• Tab-Oral: 200 mg, 100's: **$9.76-$60.45**
• Tab, Chewable—Oral: 100 mg, 100's: **$16.77-$39.81**
• Tab, Sus Action—Oral: 100 mg, 100's: **$29.98**; 200 mg, 100's: **$59.86**; 400 mg, 100's: **$119.64**

UNLABELED USES: Treatment of alcohol withdrawal, bipolar disorder, diabetes insipidus, neurogenic pain, psychotic disorders

CONTRAINDICATIONS: Concomitant use of MAOIs, history of myelosuppression, hypersensitivity to tricyclic antidepressants

PREGNANCY AND LACTATION: Pregnancy category C; concentration in milk approximately 60% of maternal plasma concentration; compatible with breast-feeding

SIDE EFFECTS
Frequent

Drowsiness, dizziness, nausea, vomiting

Occasional

Visual abnormalities (spots before eyes, difficulty focusing, blurred vision), dry mouth or pharynx, tongue irritation, headache, fluid retention, diaphoresis, constipation or diarrhea, behavioral changes in children

SERIOUS REACTIONS
• Toxic reactions may include blood dyscrasias (such as aplastic anemia, agranulocytosis, thrombocytopenia, leukopenia, leukocytosis, and eosinophilia), cardiovascular disturbances (such as CHF, hypotension or hypertension, thrombophlebitis and arrhythmias), and dermatologic effects (such as rash, urticaria, pruritus, and photosensitivity).
• Abrupt withdrawal may precipitate status epilepticus.

INTERACTIONS
Drugs

③ *Acetaminopen:* Enhanced hepatotoxic potential; reduced acetaminophen response

◼ *Antidepressants, tricyclic:* Carbamazepine reduces serum concentrations of imipramine and probably other cyclic antidepressants

◼ *Benzodiazepines (alprazolam, diazepam, midazolam, triazolam):* Metabolized by CYP3A4; enzyme induced by carbamazepine; reduced benzo effect

❷ *Calcium channel blockers:* Verapamil and diltiazem reduce the metabolism of carbamazepine leading to increased carbamazepine toxicity when these CCBs are added to chronic carbamazepine therapy; enzyme induction by carbamazepine can reduce the bioavailability of CCBs that undergo extensive 1st-pass hepatic clearance, like felodipine (94% reduction)

◼ *Cimetidine:* Transient (1 week) increases in carbamazepine levels

◼ *Corticosteroids:* Carbamazepine reduces levels and therapeutic effect

◼ *Cyclosporine:* Carbamazepine reduces cyclosporine blood levels

❷ *Danazol:* Increases carbamazepine levels with toxicity expected

◼ *Doxycycline:* Carbamazepine reduces doxycycline levels and antibiotic effects

◼ *Erythromycin, clarithromycin:* Increased carbamazepine levels

◼ *Ethinyl Estradiol, Oral contraceptives:* Carbamazepine-induced metabolic induction may lead to menstrual irregularities and unplanned pregnancies

◼ *Felbamate:* Reductions in carbamazepine levels and increases in 10,11-epoxide metabolite, along with decreased felbamate concentrations

◼ *Fluoxetine, fluvoxamine:* Inhibits carbamazepine metabolism, increased levels and risk of toxicity

◼ *Isoniazid:* Increases carbamazepine levels with increased risk of toxicity

◼ *Isotretinoin:* Reduced carbamazepine bioavailability

◼ *Lamotrigine:* Increased carbamazepine metab and risk of toxicity; carbamazepine reduces lamotrigine levels

◼ *Lithium:* Increased potential for neurotoxicity with normal lithium concentrations; reverses carbamazepine-induced leukopenia; additive antithyroidal effects

◼ *Mebendazole:* Carbamazepine decreases mebendazole levels, significant only when large doses given

◼ *Methadone:* Carbamazepine reduces levels and therapeutic effect

◼ *Metronidazole:* Increases carbamazepine concentrations with toxicity

◼ *Neuroleptics:* Reduced concentration of and therapeutic response to these agents when used with carbamazepine

◼ *Omeprazole:* May increase carbamazepine concentrations

◼ *Oral anticoagulants:* Decreased prothrombin time

◼ *Phenytoin:* Concurrent use reduces serum concentrations of both

❷ *Propoxyphene:* Increases carbamazepine levels

◼ *Theophylline:* Carbamazepine reduces levels and therapeutic effect

◼ *Thyroid:* Carbamazepine reduces levels and therapeutic effect

◼ *Valproic acid:* Valproic acid can increase, decrease, or have no effect on carbamazepine, monitor serum levels; carbamazepine decreases levels of valproic acid

Labs
• *Chloride, serum:* falsely elevated at elevated carbamazepine concentrations

• *Thyroxine (T₄), free serum:* Falsely elevated by certain test methods

• *Tri-iodothyronine (T₃), free serum:* Falsely decreased by certain test methods

• *T₃ uptake:* Carbamazepine interference falsely increases assay

• *Uric acid, serum:* High carbamazepine levels falsely decrease uric acid

SPECIAL CONSIDERATIONS
PATIENT/FAMILY EDUCATION
• Caution about driving and other activities that require alertness, at least initially
• Drug may turn urine pink to brown
MONITORING PARAMETERS
• CBC—aplastic anemia and agranulocytosis have been reported 5-8× greater than in the general public
• Liver function test
• Serum drug levels (therapeutic 4-12 mcg/ml) during initial treatment

---

carbamide peroxide
OTC: *Otic:* Debrox, Murine Ear Drops
OTC: *Oral:* Gly-Oxide Liquid, Orajel Perioseptic, Proxigel
Chemical Class: Urea compound and hydrogen peroxide
Therapeutic Class: Cerumenolytic; topical oral antiinflammatory

CLINICAL PHARMACOLOGY
Mechanism of Action: A cerumenolytic that releases oxygen on contact with moist mouth tissues to provide cleansing effects, reduce inflammation, relieve pain, and inhibit odor-forming bacteria. In the ear, oxygen is released and hydrogen peroxide is reduced to water which enables the chemical reaction. *Ther-apeutic Effect:* Relieves inflammation of gums and lips. Emulsifies and disperses ear wax.
Pharmacokinetics
Not known.

INDICATIONS AND DOSAGES
Earwax removal
Topical, solution
Adults, Elderly, Children 12 yrs or older. Tilt head and administer 5-10 drops twice a day for up to 4 days.
Children 12 years or younger. Tilt head and administer 1-5 drops twice a day for up to 4 days.

Oral lesions
Topical, gel
Adults, Elderly, Children. Apply to affected area 4 times a day.
Topical, solution
Adults, Elderly, Children. Apply several drops undiluted on affected area 4 times a day after meals and at bedtime.

Ⓢ AVAILABLE FORMS/COST
• Gel-Oral Topical: 10%, 36 g: **$11.09**
• Liq-Oral Topical: 10%, 15, 60 ml: **$3.36-$8.03**/60 ml; 15%, 13.3 ml: **$3.98**
• Sol—Otic: 6.5%, 15, 30 ml: **$1.01-$8.68**/15 ml

UNLABELED USES: Dental whitener

CONTRAINDICATIONS: Dizziness, ear discharge or drainage, ear injury, ear pain, irritation, or rash, hypersensitivity to carbamide peroxide or any one of its components

PREGNANCY AND LACTATION: Pregnancy category C

SIDE EFFECTS
Occasional
Oral: Gingival sensitivity

SERIOUS REACTIONS
• Opportunistic infections caused by organisms like Candida albicans is possible with prolonged use.

carbenicillin
(kar-ben-ih-sill'in)
Rx: Geocillin
Chemical Class: Penicillin derivative, extended-spectrum
Therapeutic Class: Antibiotic

CLINICAL PHARMACOLOGY
Mechanism of Action: A penicillin that inhibits cell wall synthesis in susceptible microorganisms. *Therapeutic Effect:* Produces bactericidal effect.
Pharmacokinetics
Moderately absorbed from the gastrointestinal (GI) tract. Protein binding: 50%. Widely distributed. Partially metabolized in liver. Primarily excreted in urine. Removed by hemodialysis. **Half-life:** 1-1.5 hrs (half-life increased in impaired renal function).

INDICATIONS AND DOSAGES
Prostatitis
PO
Adults, Elderly. 764 mg q6h.
Urinary tract infection
PO
Adults, Elderly. 382-764 mg q6h.
$ **AVAILABLE FORMS/COST**
• Tab-Oral: 382 mg, 100's: **$236.64**
UNLABELED USES: Perioperative prophylaxis
CONTRAINDICATIONS: Hypersensitivity to any penicillin
PREGNANCY AND LACTATION: Pregnancy category B
SIDE EFFECTS
Frequent
GI disturbances, including mild diarrhea, nausea, or vomiting, oral or vaginal candidiasis
Occasional
Generalized rash, urticaria, phlebitis, headache
Rare
Dizziness, seizures

SERIOUS REACTIONS
• Altered bacterial balance may result in potentially fatal superinfections and antibiotic-associated colitis as evidenced by abdominal cramps, watery or severe diarrhea, and fever.
• Severe hypersensitivity reactions, including seizures, occur rarely.
INTERACTIONS
Drugs
▣ *Aminoglycosides:* Chemically inactivated by carbenicillin
▣ *Gentamicin:* 25% increase in serum gentamicin concentration
▣ *Methotrexate:* Increased methotrexate serum concentration
▣ *Probenecid:* Increased carbenicillin concentrations
Labs
• *Albumin:* Decreased serum concentrations
• *Amino acids:* Increased urine concentrations
• *Bilirubin:* Increased serum bilirubin levels
• *Glucose:* False positive using Clinitest
• *Protein:* Increased serum levels
• *Triglycerides:* Increased serum levels
SPECIAL CONSIDERATIONS
NOTE: When high and rapid blood and urine levels of antibiotic are indicated, alternative parenteral therapy should be used

carbidopa and levodopa

(kar-bee-doe'pa; lee-voe-doe'pa)

Rx: Parcopa, Sinemet, Sinemet CR

Chemical Class: Catecholamine precursor

Therapeutic Class: Anti-Parkinson's agent; antidyskinetic

CLINICAL PHARMACOLOGY

Mechanism of Action: Levodopa is converted to dopamine in the basal ganglia thus increasing dopamine concentration in brain and inhibiting hyperactive cholinergic activity. Carbidopa prevents peripheral breakdown of levodopa, allowing more levodopa to be available for transport into the brain. *Therapeutic Effect:* Reduces tremor.

Pharmacokinetics

Carbidopa is rapidly and completely absorbed from the GI tract. Widely distributed. Excreted primarily in urine. Levodopa is converted to dopamine. Excreted primarily in urine. **Half-life:** 1-2 hr (carbidopa); 1–3 hr (levodopa).

INDICATIONS AND DOSAGES

Parkinsonism

PO

Adults. Initially, 25/100 mg 2–4 times a day. May increase up 200/2,000 mg daily.

Elderly. Initially, 25/100 mg twice a day. May increase as necessary.

When converting a patient from Sinemet to Sinemet CR (50 mg/200 mg), dosage is based on the total daily dose of levodopa, as follows:

Sinemet	Sinemet CR
300–400 mg	1 tablet twice a day
500–600 mg	1.5 tablet twice a day or 1 tab 3 times a day
700–800 mg	4 tablets in 3 or more divided doses
900–1,000 mg	5 tablets in 3 or more divided doses

Intervals between doses of Sinemet CR should be 4–8 hr while awake.

AVAILABLE FORMS/COST

• Tab-Oral: 10 mg-100 mg, 100's: **$32.34-$82.69**; 25 mg-100 mg, 100's: **$26.05-$93.36**; 25 mg-250 mg, 100's: **$41.16-$118.96**

• Tab, Sus Action—Oral: 25 mg-100 mg, 100's: **$93.10-$104.59**; 50 mg-200 mg, 100's: **$180.85-$201.16**

CONTRAINDICATIONS: Angle-closure glaucoma, use within 14 days of MAOIs

PREGNANCY AND LACTATION: Pregnancy category C; should not be given to nursing mothers

SIDE EFFECTS

Frequent (90%–10%)

Uncontrolled movements of face, tongue, arms, or upper body; nausea and vomiting (80%); anorexia (50%)

Occasional

Depression, anxiety, confusion, nervousness, urine retention, palpitations, dizziness, light-headedness, decreased appetite, blurred vision, constipation, dry mouth, flushed skin, headache, insomnia, diarrhea, unusual fatigue, darkening of urine and sweat

Rare

Hypertension, ulcer, hemolytic anemia (marked by fatigue)

SERIOUS REACTIONS

• Patients on long-term therapy have a high incidence of involuntary choreiform, dystonic, and dyskinetic movements.

• Numerous mild to severe CNS and psychiatric disturbances may occur, including reduced attention span, anxiety, nightmares, daytime somnolence, euphoria, fatigue, paranoia, psychotic episodes, depression, and hallucinations.

INTERACTIONS

Drugs

🔳 *Antipsycotics (haloperidol, olanzapine, phenothiazines, quetiapine, risperidone, ziprasidone):* Inhibition of the antiparkinsonian effect of levodopa through dopamine receptor antagonism

🔳 *Benzodiazepines:* May exacerbate Parkinsonism in patients receiving levodopa; inhibits antiparkinsonian effects of levodopa

🔳 *Buproprion:* Increased risk of adverse effects

🔳 *Food:* High protein diets inhibit the efficacy of levodopa

🔳 *Iron (oral):* Reduces levodopa bioavailability by 50%

🔳 *Isoniazid:* May inhibit the clinical response to levodopa through dopamine receptor antagonism

🔳 *MAOIs:* May result in hypertensive response, do not use levodopa until MAOIs have been discontinued for 2 wks

🔳 *Methionine:* Inhibits the clinical response to levodopa

🔳 *Metoclopramide:* May inhibit the clinical response to levodopa through dopamine receptor antagonism, may increase the bioavailability of levodopa through delayed gastric emptying

🔳 *Phenytoin:* May inhibit the antiparkinsonian effect of levodopa

🔳 *Pyridoxine:* Inhibits the antiparkinsonian effect of levodopa; concurrent carbidopa negates the interaction

🔳 *Spiramycin:* Reduces the plasma concentration of levodopa, with reduction of antiparkinsonian efficacy

🔳 *Tacrine:* May inhibit the effect of levodopa in Parkinsons patients; dosage adjustments may be required

🔳 *Tricyclic antidepressants:* Increased risk of adverse effects, hypertension and dyskinesias

Labs

• *Acid phosphatase:* Increased serum acid phosphatase

• *Amino acids:* Increased urine amino acids

• *Aspartate aminotransferase:* Increased serum aspartate aminotransferase

• *Bilirubin:* Decreased serum bilirubin at concentrations of 15 mg/dL (Kodak Ektachem systems 2083); increased bilirubin at concentrations above 80 mg/dL (methods of Jendrassik and Grof) and below 5 mg/dL (Kodak Ektachem systems 2083)

• *Bilirubin, conjugated:* Decreased serum levels by 0.3 mg/dL at therapeutic levels of levodopa; minimally increased serum levels at markedly elevated levodopa concentrations (i.e., >60 mg/dL)

• *Catecholamines:* Increased plasma catecholamines, reported as epinephrine and norepinephrine

• *Cholinesterase:* Increased serum cholinesterase activity

• *Sputum:* Brown discoloration reported

• *Creatinine:* Increased serum creatinine

• *Creatinine clearance:* Increased urinary creatinine clearance (Jaffe method)

• *Ferric chloride test:* False positive

• *Glucose:* Decreases serum glucose as measured by GODPERID method, Ames Seralyzer, and glucose oxidase method; increased serum glucose by alkaline ferricyanide procedure, Technicon SMA method, and glucokinase method of Scott; false negative urine glucose (inhibits glucose oxidase method)

• *Guaiacols Spot test:* False negative

• *Hydroxy-methoxymandelic acid:* Increased urinary levels
• *Lithium:* Positive bias on serum lithium levels measured with Kodak Ektachem systems 2083
• *Triglycerides:* Lowered triglyceride levels measured by GPOPAP method
• *Urea nitrogen:* Decreases BUN
• *Uric acid:* Lowers serum urate levels as measured by uricase PAP method

SPECIAL CONSIDERATIONS
• If previously on levodopa, discontinue for at least 12 hr before change to carbidopa-levodopa combination

PATIENT/FAMILY EDUCATION
• Limit protein taken with drug
• Arise slowly from a reclining position
• Wearing off effect may occur at end of dosing interval
• Saliva, urine, or sweat may turn dark color (red, brown, or black)
• Delayed onset up to 1 hr with controlled release formulation possible compared to immediate release formulation

---

carboprost
(kar'boe-prost)
Rx: Hemabate
Chemical Class: Prostaglandin F_2-alpha analog
Therapeutic Class: Abortifacient; antihemorrhagic, uterine; uterine stimulant

CLINICAL PHARMACOLOGY
Mechanism of Action: A prostaglandin similar to prostaglandin F2 alpha (dinoprost) that directly acts on myometrium and stimulates contraction in gravid uterus. *Therapeutic Effect:* Produces cervical dilation and softening.

Pharmacokinetics
None reported.

INDICATIONS AND DOSAGES
Abortion
IM
Adults. Initially, 100–250 mcg, may repeat at 1.5–3.5 hour intervals. May increase up to 500 mcg if uterine contractility inadequate. Maximum: 12 mg total dose or continuous administration for more than 2 days.

Postpartum hemorrhage
IM
Adults. Initially, 250 mcg, may repeat at 15–90 minute intervals. Maximum: 2 mg total dose.

AVAILABLE FORMS/COST
• Sol, Inj-IM: 0.25 mg/ml, 1 ml: **$59.43**

UNLABELED USES: Treatment of incomplete abortion, benign hydatiform mole, induction of labor, ripening of cervix prior to abortion.

CONTRAINDICATIONS: Acute pelvic inflammatory disease, active cardiac disease, pulmonary disease, renal disease, hepatic disease, pregnancy, hypersensitivity to carboprost or other prostaglandins

PREGNANCY AND LACTATION: Pregnancy category C; any dose which produces increased uterine tone could put the embryo or fetus at risk.

SIDE EFFECTS
Frequent
Nausea
Occasional
Facial flushing
Rare
Vomiting, diarrhea

SERIOUS REACTIONS
• Excessive dosing may cause uterine hypertonicity with spasm and tetanic contraction, leading to cervical laceration/perforation and uterine rupture and hemorrhage.

SPECIAL CONSIDERATIONS

• Antiemetic, analgesic, and antidiarrheal medications should be considered concurrently to counter adverse GI effects
• In the treatment of uterine atony, IV oxytocin, uterine massage and IM methylergonovine (unless contraindicated) should be used before carboprost

carisoprodol

(kar'i-so-pro'dol)

Rx: Soma

Combinations

Rx: with aspirin (Soma Compound); with aspirin and codeine (Soma Compound with Codeine)

Chemical Class: Meprobamate congener

Therapeutic Class: Skeletal muscle relaxant

CLINICAL PHARMACOLOGY

Mechanism of Action: A centrally-acting skeletal muscle relaxant whose exact mechanism is unknown. Effects may be due to its CNS depressant actions. *Therapeutic Effect:* Relieves muscle spasms and pain.

INDICATIONS AND DOSAGES

Adjunct to rest, physical therapy, analgesics, and other measures for relief of discomfort from acute, painful musculoskeletal conditions

PO

Adults, Elderly. 350 mg 4 times a day.

[$] **AVAILABLE FORMS/COST**

• Tab-Oral: 350 mg, 100's: **$5.94-$389.35**

CONTRAINDICATIONS: Acute intermittent porphyria, sensitivity to meprobamate

PREGNANCY AND LACTATION: Pregnancy category C; crosses placenta; excreted in breast milk (2-4× maternal plasma)

SIDE EFFECTS

Frequent (greater than 10%)

Somnolence

Occasional (10%–1%)

Tachycardia, facial flushing, dizziness, headache, lightheadedness, dermatitis, nausea, vomiting, abdominal cramps, dyspnea

SERIOUS REACTIONS

• Overdose may cause CNS and respiratory depression, shock, and coma.

SPECIAL CONSIDERATIONS

• Caution when used in addiction-prone individuals
• Abused on the street in conjunction with narcotics

PATIENT/FAMILY EDUCATION

• Abrupt cessation may precipitate mild withdrawal symptoms such as abdominal cramps, insomnia, chills, headache, and nausea

carteolol

(kar-tee'oh-lole)

Rx: Cartrol; Ocupress (ophthal)

Chemical Class: β-adrenergic blocker, nonselective

Therapeutic Class: Antiglaucoma agent; antihypertensive

CLINICAL PHARMACOLOGY

Mechanism of Action: An antihypertensive that blocks beta1-adrenergic receptor at normal doses and beta2- adrenergic receptors at large doses. Predominantly blocks beta1-adrenergic receptors in cardiac tissue. Reduces aqueous humor production. *Therapeutic Effect:* Slows sinus heart rate, decreases cardiac output, decreases blood pressure (BP), increases airway resistance, decreases intraocular pressure.

Pharmacokinetics

Well absorbed from the gastrointestinal (GI) tract. Protein binding: unknown. Minimally metabolized in liver. Primarily excreted unchanged in urine. Not removed by hemodialysis. **Half-life:** 6 hrs (increased in decreased renal function).

INDICATIONS AND DOSAGES

Hypertension

PO

Adults, Elderly. Initially, 2.5 mg/day as single dose either alone or in combination with diuretic. May increase gradually to 5–10 mg/day as a single dose. Maintenance: 2.5–5 mg/day.

Dosage in renal impairment

Creatinine Clearance	*Dosage Interval*
>60 ml/min	24 hrs
20-60 ml/min	48 hrs
<20 ml/min	72 hrs

Open-angle glaucoma, ocular hypertension

Ophthalmic

Adults, Elderly. 1 drop 2 times/day.

$ **AVAILABLE FORMS/COST**

• Sol—Ophth: 1%, 5, 10, 15 ml: **$37.06-$61.71**/10 ml

• Tab-Oral: 2.5 mg, 100's: **$106.88**; 5 mg, 100's: **$136.93**

UNLABELED USES: Combination with miotics decreases IOP in acute/chronic angle closure glaucoma, treatment of secondary glaucoma, malignant glaucoma, angle closure glaucoma during/after iridectomy

CONTRAINDICATIONS: Bronchial asthma, COPD, bronchospasm, overt cardiac failure, cardiogenic shock, heart block greater than first degree, persistently severe bradycardia

PREGNANCY AND LACTATION: Pregnancy category C; excreted in breast milk

SIDE EFFECTS

Frequent

Oral: Hypotension manifested as dizziness, nausea, diaphoresis, headache, cold extremities, fatigue, constipation/diarrhea

Ophthalmic: Redness of eye or inside of eyelids, decreased night vision

Occasional

Oral: Insomnia, flatulence, urinary frequency, impotence or decreased libido

Ophthalmic: Blepharoconjunctivitis, edema, droopy eyelid, staining of cornea, blurred vision, brow ache, increased light sensitivity, burning, stinging

Rare

Rash, arthralgia, myalgia, confusion (especially elderly), taste disturbances

SERIOUS REACTIONS

• Abrupt withdrawal (particularly in those with coronary artery disease) may produce angina or precipitate MI.

• May precipitate thyroid crisis in those with thyrotoxicosis.

• Beta-blockers may mask signs and symptoms of acute hypoglycemia (tachycardia, BP changes) in diabetic patients.

INTERACTIONS

Drugs

[3] *Adenosine:* Increased risk of bradycardic response

[3] *Amiodarone:* Increased bradycardic effect of carteolol

[3] *Antacids:* Decreased absorption of oral carteolol

[3] *Antidiabetics:* Carteolol reduces response to hypoglycemia (sweating excepted)

3 *Antipyrine:* Many β-blockers increase serum concentrations of antipyrine; though antipyrine is not used therapeutically, this interaction has implications for other drugs whose metabolism is similarly inhibited

3 *Barbiturates, Rifampin:* Enhanced carteolol metabolism

3 *Bupivacaine:* Potentiates cardiodepression and heart block

3 *Cimetidine, Propafenone, Propoxyphene, Quinidine:* Decreased carteolol metabolism

3 *Cocaine:* β-Blockade increases angina-inducing potential of cocaine

3 *Contrast media:* Increased risk of anaphylaxis

3 *Digoxin, digitoxin:* Bradycardia potentiated

3 *Dipyridamole:* Bradycardia potentiated

3 *Epinepherine:* Enhanced pressor response resulting in hypertension and bradycardia

3 *Fluoxetine:* Fluoxetine may reduce hepatic metabolism; increased β-blocking activity

3 *Isoproterenol:* Reduced effectiveness of isoproterenol in the treatment of asthma

3 *Neuroleptics:* Decreased carteolol metabolism; decreased neuroleptic metabolism

3 *Nonsteroidal anti-inflammatory drugs:* Reduced antihypertensive effect of carteolol

3 *Physostigmine:* Additive bradycardia

3 *Prazosin, Terazosin:* Enhanced 1st-dose response to α-blockers

3 *Tacrine:* Additive bradycardia

3 *Theophylline:* Decreased metabolism of theophylline

SPECIAL CONSIDERATIONS

• Does not alter serum cholesterol or triglycerides

PATIENT/FAMILY EDUCATION

• Do not stop drug abruptly; taper over 2 wk

• Do not use OTC products containing α-adrenergic stimulants (nasal decongestants, cold remedies) unless directed by physician

---

carvedilol
(kar-vea'die-lole)
Rx: Coreg
Chemical Class: α-adrenergic blocker, peripheral; β-adrenergic blocker, nonselective
Therapeutic Class: Antihypertensive

CLINICAL PHARMACOLOGY
Mechanism of Action: An antihypertensive that possesses nonselective beta-blocking and alpha-adrenergic blocking activity. Causes vasodilation. *Therapeutic Effect:* Reduces cardiac output, exercise-induced tachycardia, and reflex orthostatic tachycardia; reduces peripheral vascular resistance.
Pharmacokinetics

Route	Onset	Peak	Duration
PO	30 min	1–2 hr	24 hr

Rapidly and extensively absorbed from the GI tract. Protein binding: 98%. Metabolized in the liver. Excreted primarily via bile into feces. Minimally removed by hemodialysis. **Half-life:** 7–10 hr. Food delays rate of absorption.

INDICATIONS AND DOSAGES
Hypertension
PO
Adults, Elderly. Initially, 6.25 mg twice a day. May double at 7-to 14-day intervals to highest tolerated dosage. Maximum: 50 mg/day.

CHF
PO
Adults, Elderly. Initially, 3.125 mg twice a day. May double at 2-wk intervals to highest tolerated dosage. Maximum: For patients weighing more than 85 kg, give 50 mg twice a day, for those weighing 85 kg or less, give 25 mg twice a day.

Left ventricular dysfunction
PO
Adults, Elderly. Initially, 3.125-6.25 mg twice a day. May increase at intervals of 3-10 days up to 25 mg twice a day.

$ **AVAILABLE FORMS/COST**
- Tab, Coated—Oral: 3.125, 6.25, 12.5, 25 mg, 100's; all: **$179.99**

UNLABELED USES: Treatment of angina pectoris, idiopathic cardiomyopathy

CONTRAINDICATIONS: Bronchial asthma or related bronchospastic conditions, cardiogenic shock, pulmonary edema, second- or third-degree AV block, severe bradycardia

PREGNANCY AND LACTATION: Pregnancy category C; increased spontaneous abortion in animal studies; highly lipophilic with a large volume of distribution, may accumulate in human breast milk; monitor infant closely

SIDE EFFECTS
Carvedilol is generally well tolerated, with mild and transient side effects.

Frequent (6%–4%)
Fatigue, dizziness

Occasional (2%)
Diarrhea, bradycardia, rhinitis, back pain

Rare (less than 2%)
Orthostatic hypotension, somnolence, UTI, viral infection

SERIOUS REACTIONS
- Overdose may produce profound bradycardia, hypotension, bronchospasm, cardiac insufficiency, cardiogenic shock, and cardiac arrest.
- Abrupt withdrawal may result in diaphoresis, palpitations, headache, and tremors.
- Carvedilol administration may precipitate CHF and MI in patients with heart disease; thyroid storm in those with thyrotoxicosis; and peripheral ischemia in those with existing peripheral vascular disease.
- Hypoglycemia may occur in patients with previously controlled diabetes.

INTERACTIONS
Drugs

3 *α_1-adrenergic blockers:* Potential enhanced first dose response (marked initial drop in blood pressure, particularly on standing)

3 *Amiodarone:* Symptomatic bradycardia and sinus arrest; AV node refractory period prolonged and sinus node automaticity decreased, especially patients with bradycardia, sick sinus syndrome, or partial AV block

3 *Benzodiazepines:* Increased benzodiazepine activity

3 *Catecholamine-depleting agents (reserpine, MAOIs):* Hypotension or bradycardia possible

3 *Cimetidine:* Via inhibition of hepatic metabolism, cimetidine increases β-blocker serum concentrations

3 *Clonidine:* Withdrawal of clonidine abruptly may exaggerate the hypertension due to unopposed alpha stimulation; safer than other β-blockers, however

3 *Cyclosporin:* Increased trough cyclosporin concentrations

CYP2D6 inhibitors (quinidine, fluoxetine, paroxetine, propafenone): Increased levels of carvedilol

Digoxin: Additive prolongation of AV conduction time

Dihydropyridine calcium channel blockers: Severe hypotension or impaired cardiac performance; most prevalent with impaired left ventricular function, cardiac arrhythmias, or aortic stenosis

Diltiazem: Potentiates β-adrenergic effects; hypotension, left ventricular failure, and AV conduction disturbances problematic in elderly, patients with left ventricular dysfunction, aortic stenosis, or with large doses of either drug

Hypoglycemic agents: Masked hypoglycemia, hyperglycemia

Nonsteroidal antiinflammatory drugs: Reduced antihypertensive effect

Rifampin: 70% decrease in carvedilol concentrations

Verapamil: Potentiates β-adrenergic effects; hypotension, left ventricular failure, and AV conduction disturbances problematic in elderly, patients with left ventricular dysfunction, aortic stenosis, or with large doses of either drug

SPECIAL CONSIDERATIONS
• Response less in African-Americans

PATIENT/FAMILY EDUCATION
• Do not discontinue abruptly; may require taper; rapid withdrawal may produce rebound hypertension or angina
• Careful monitoring essential when initiating therapy to detect and correct worsening symptoms of heart failure
• If heart rate drops below 55 beats per minute, reduce dosage
• Take with food

• Avoid driving, hazardous tasks during initiation of therapy

MONITORING PARAMETERS
• Congestive heart failure: Functional status, cough, dyspnea on exertion, paroxysmal nocturnal dyspnea, exercise tolerance, and ventricular function
• Hypertension: Blood pressure

---

cascara sagrada
OTC: Aromatic Cascara Fluid extract, Cascara Sagrada, Cascara Aromatic
Chemical Class: Anthraquinone derivative
Therapeutic Class: Laxative, stimulant

CLINICAL PHARMACOLOGY
Mechanism of Action: A GI stimulant that has a direct effect on colonic smooth musculature, by stimulating intramural nerve plexi. *Therapeutic Effect:* Promotes fluid and ion accumulation in the colon, increasing peristalsis and promoting a laxative effect.

INDICATIONS AND DOSAGES
Treatment of constipation
PO
Adults, Elderly. 5 ml at bedtime.
Children 2-11 yr. 2.5 ml, 1–3 ml as a single dose.
Infant. 1.25 ml, 0.5–2 ml as a single dose.

AVAILABLE FORMS/COST
• Sol (fluid extract)—Oral: 120, 480 ml: **$6.99**/480 ml
• Tab—Oral: 325 mg, 100's: **$4.20**

CONTRAINDICATIONS: Abdominal pain, appendicitis, intestinal obstruction, nausea, vomiting

PREGNANCY AND LACTATION: Pregnancy category C; excreted in breast milk

SIDE EFFECTS
Frequent
Pink-red, red-violet, red-brown, or yellow-brown discoloration of urine
Occasional
Some degree of abdominal discomfort, nausea, mild cramps, faintness
SERIOUS REACTIONS
• Long-term use may result in laxative dependence, chronic constipation, and loss of normal bowel function.
• Prolonged use or overdose may result in electrolyte or metabolic disturbances (such as hypokalemia, hypocalcemia, and metabolic acidosis or alkalosis), as well as persistent diarrhea, vomiting, muscle weakness, malabsorption, and weight loss.
INTERACTIONS
Labs
• *Increase:* Color of urine (brown-acid; yellow-pink-alkaline); porphobilinogen; urobiligen
SPECIAL CONSIDERATIONS
• Stimulant laxatives are habit forming
• Long term use may lead to colonic atony

---

castor oil
OTC: Emulsoil, Purge, Neoloid
Chemical Class: Fatty acid ester
Therapeutic Class: Laxative, stimulant

CLINICAL PHARMACOLOGY
Mechanism of Action: A laxative prepared from the bean of the castor plant but the exact mechanism of action is unknown. Acts primarily in the small intestine. May be hydrolyzed to ricinoleic acid which reduces net absorption of fluid and electrolytes and stimulates peristalsis. *Therapeutic Effect:* Increases peristalsis, promotes laxative effect.
Pharmacokinetics
Minimal absorption by the gastrointestinal (GI) tract. May be metabolized like other fatty acids.
INDICATIONS AND DOSAGES
Constipation
PO
Adults, Elderly, Children 12 yrs and older. 15-60 ml as a single dose.
Children 2- 12 yrs. 5-15 ml as a single dose.
Children less than 2 yrs. 1-2 ml as a single dose. Maximum: 5 ml as a single dose.
ⓢ AVAILABLE FORMS/COST
• Liq-Oral: 30, 60, 120, 480 ml: **$0.76-$2.13**/60 ml
• Susp-Oral: 95%, 30, 60 ml: **$2.55-$3.00**/60 ml
CONTRAINDICATIONS: Abdominal pain, appendicitis, intestinal obstruction, nausea, vomiting
PREGNANCY AND LACTATION: Pregnancy category X; excreted in breast milk
SIDE EFFECTS
Occasional
Some degree of abdominal discomfort, nausea, mild cramps, griping, faintness
SERIOUS REACTIONS
• Long-term use may result in laxative dependence, chronic constipation, and loss of normal bowel function.
• Chronic use or overdosage may result in electrolyte disturbances, such as hypokalemia, hypocalcemia, and metabolic acidosis or alkalosis, persistent diarrhea, malabsorption, and weight loss. Electrolyte disturbance may produce vomiting and muscle weakness.
SPECIAL CONSIDERATIONS
• Stimulant laxatives are habit forming

• Long-term use may lead to colonic atony

---

cefaclor
(sef'a-klor)
Rx: Ceclor, Ceclor CD
Chemical Class: Cephalosporin (2nd generation)
Therapeutic Class: Antibiotic

CLINICAL PHARMACOLOGY
Mechanism of Action: A second-generation cephalosporin that binds to bacterial cell membranes and inhibits cell wall synthesis. *Therapeutic Effect:* Bactericidal.
Pharmacokinetics
Well absorbed from the GI tract. Protein binding: 25%. Widely distributed. Primarily excreted unchanged in urine. Moderately removed by hemodialysis. **Half-life:** 0.6-0.9 hr (increased in impaired renal function).

INDICATIONS AND DOSAGES
Bronchitis
PO
Adults, Elderly (extended-release). 500 mg q12h for 7 days.
Lower respiratory tract infections
PO
Adults, Elderly. 250-500 mg q8h.
Otitis media
PO
Children. 20-40 mg/kg/day in 2-3 divided doses. Maximum: 1 g/day.
Pharyngitis, skin/skin structure infections, tonsillitis
PO
Adults, Elderly (extended-release). 375 mg q12h.
Adults, Elderly (regular-release). 250-500 mg q8h.
Children. 20-40 mg/kg/day in 2-3 divided doses. Maxiumum: 1 g/day.

Urinary tract infections
PO
Adults, Elderly. 250-500 mg q8h.
Children. 20-40 mg/kg/day in 2-3 divided doses q8h. Maximum: 1 g/day.
PO (Extended-Release Tablets)
Adults, Children older than 16 yr. 375-500 mg q12h.
Otitis media
PO
Children older than 1 mo. 40 mg/kg/day in divided doses q8h. Maximum: 1 g/day.
Dosage in renal impairment
Decreased dosage may be necessary in patients with creatinine clearance less than 40 ml/min.

S AVAILABLE FORMS/COST
• Cap, Gel—Oral: 250 mg, 100's: **$50.82-$233.15**; 500 mg, 100's: **$100.89-$439.47**
• Powder, Reconst—Oral: 125 mg/5 ml, 75, 150 ml: **$11.54-$37.20**/150 ml; 187 mg/5 ml, 50, 100 ml: **$26.65-$41.28**/100 ml; 250 mg/5 ml, 75, 150 ml: **$17.85-$68.53**/150 ml; 375 mg/5 ml, 50, 100 ml: **$23.29-$56.92**/100 ml
• Tab, Sus Action—Oral: 375 mg, 500 mg, 100's; all: **$379.30**

CONTRAINDICATIONS: History of anaphylactic reaction to penicillins or hypersensitivity to cephalosporins

PREGNANCY AND LACTATION: Pregnancy category B; excreted in breast milk

SIDE EFFECTS
Frequent
Oral candidiasis, mild diarrhea, mild abdominal cramping, vaginal candidiasis
Occasional
Nausea, serum sickness-like reaction (marked by fever and joint pain; usually occurs after the second course of therapy and resolves after the drug is discontinued)

Rare

Allergic reaction (pruritus, rash, and urticaria)

SERIOUS REACTIONS

• Antibiotic-associated colitis and other superinfections may result from altered bacterial balance.

• Nephrotoxicity may occur, especially in patients with pre-existing renal disease.

• Patients with a history of allergies, especially to penicillin, are at increased risk for developing a severe hypersensitivity reaction, marked by severe pruritus, angioedema, bronchospasm, and anaphylaxis.

INTERACTIONS

Drugs

▪ *Aminoglycosides:* Additive nephrotoxicity

▪ *Loop diuretics:* Increased nephrotoxicity

❷ *Warfarin:* Hypoprothrombinemic response enhanced

Labs

• *Creatinine:* Analytical increases and decreases depending on assay

SPECIAL CONSIDERATIONS

• Last choice 2nd generation cephalosporin given relative decreased activity against *S. pneumonia* and increased side effects

---

cefadroxil
(sef-a-drox′ill)
Rx: Duricef
Chemical Class: Cephalosporin (1st generation)
Therapeutic Class: Antibiotic

CLINICAL PHARMACOLOGY
Mechanism of Action: A first-generation cephalosporin that binds to bacterial cell membranes and inhibits cell wall synthesis. *Therapeutic Effect:* Bactericidal.

Pharmacokinetics

Well absorbed from the GI tract. Protein binding: 15%-20%. Widely distributed. Primarily excreted unchanged in urine. Removed by hemodialysis. **Half-life:** 1.2-1.5 hr (increased in impaired renal function).

INDICATIONS AND DOSAGES

UTIs

PO

Adults, Elderly. 1-2 g/day as a single dose or in 2 divided doses.

Children. 30 mg/kg/day in 2 divided doses. Maximum: 2 g/day.

Skin and skin-structure infections, group A beta-hemolytic streptococcal pharyngitis, tonsillitis

PO

Adults, Elderly. 1-2 g in 2 divided doses.

Children. 30 mg/kg/day in 2 divided doses. Maximum: 2 g/day.

Impetigo

PO

Children. 30 mg/kg/day as a single or in 2 divided doses. Maximum: 2 g/day.

Dosage in renal impairment

After an initial 1-g dose, dosage and frequency are modified based on creatinine clearance and the severity of the infection.

Creatinine Clearance	Dosage Interval
25-50 ml/min	500 mg q12h
10-25 ml/min	500 mg q24h
0-10 ml/min	500 mg q36h

AVAILABLE FORMS/COST

• Cap—Oral: 500 mg, 100's: **$319.95-$703.38**

• Powder, Reconst—Oral: 125 mg/5 ml, 100 ml: **$17.11**; 250 mg/5 ml, 50, 100 ml: **$32.14-$49.26**/100 ml; 500 mg/5 ml, 75, 100 ml: **$54.08-$68.18**/100 ml

• Tab-Oral: 1 g, 100's: **$697.11**

CONTRAINDICATIONS: History of anaphylactic reaction to penicillins or hypersensitivity to cephalosporins

PREGNANCY AND LACTATION: Pregnancy category B; low concentrations in milk

SIDE EFFECTS

Frequent

Oral candidiasis, mild diarrhea, mild abdominal cramping, vaginal candidiasis

Occasional

Nausea, unusual bruising or bleeding, serum sickness-like reaction (marked by fever and joint pain; usually occurs after the second course of therapy and resolves after the drug is discontinued)

Rare

Allergic reaction (rash, pruritus, urticaria), thrombophlebitis (pain, redness, swelling at injection site)

SERIOUS REACTIONS

• Antibiotic-associated colitis and other superinfections may result from altered bacterial balance.

• Nephrotoxicity may occur, especially in patients with pre-existing renal disease.

• Patients with a history of allergies, especially to penicillin, are at increased risk for developing a severe hypersensitivity reaction, marked by severe pruritus, angioedema, bronchospasm, and anaphylaxis.

INTERACTIONS

Drugs

3 *Aminoglycosides:* Additive nephrotoxicity

3 *Loop diuretics:* Increased nephrotoxicity

SPECIAL CONSIDERATIONS

• No clinical advantage over less expensive cephalexin

cefamandole

(sef-a-man'dole)

Rx: Mandol
Chemical Class: Cephalosporin (2nd generation)
Therapeutic Class: Antibiotic

CLINICAL PHARMACOLOGY

Mechanism of Action: A second-generation cephalosporin that binds to bacterial cell membranes. *Therapeutic Effect:* Inhibits synthesis of bacterial cell wall. Bactericidal.

Pharmacokinetics

Well absorbed from the gastrointestinal (GI) tract. Protein binding: 56%-78%. Widely distributed. Primarily excreted unchanged in urine and high concentrations in feces. Moderately removed by hemodialysis. **Half-life:** 0.5-1 hrs (half-life is increased with impaired renal function).

INDICATIONS AND DOSAGES

Severe infections

IV/IM

Adults, Elderly. 500-1000 mg q4-8h. Maximum: 2 g q4h.

Children older than 1 mo. 50-150 mg/kg/day in divided doses q4-8h.

Creatinine Clearance	Dosage
25-50 ml/min	1-2 g q8h
10-25 ml/min	1 g q8h
10 ml/min or less	1 g q12h

S AVAILABLE FORMS/COST

• Powder, Inj—IM, IV: 1 g/vial: **$0.90-$9.73**; 2 g/vial: **$18.13-$18.80**

UNLABELED USES: None known.

CONTRAINDICATIONS: Hypersensitivity to cephalosporins, any component of the formulation, or other cephalosporins

PREGNANCY AND LACTATION:
Pregnancy category B; low milk concentrations

SIDE EFFECTS

Frequent

Diarrhea, thrombophlebitis (pain, redness, swelling at injection site)

Occasional

Nausea, fever, vomiting

Rare

Allergic reaction as evidenced by pruritus, rash, and urticaria

SERIOUS REACTIONS

• Antibiotic-associated colitis manifested as severe abdominal pain and tenderness, fever, and watery and severe diarrhea, and other superinfections, may result from altered bacterial balance.

• Nephrotoxicity may occur, especially in patients with preexisting renal disease.

• Severe hypersensitivity reaction including severe pruritus, angioedema, bronchospasm, and anaphylaxis, particularly in patients with a history of allergies, especially to penicillin, may occur.

INTERACTIONS

Drugs

③ *Aminoglycosides:* Potential additive nephrotoxicity

③ *Ethanol:* Disulfiram-like reactions secondary to acetaldehyde accumulation

③ *Loop diuretics:* Increased nephrotoxicity

② *Oral anticoagulants:* Additive hypoprothrombinemia

Labs

• *Creatinine:* Increases and decreases depending on assay

• *Erythromycin:* False positive

• *Metronidazole:* Interferes with assay

---

cefazolin

(sef-a′zoe-lin)

Rx: Ancef, Kefzol, Zolicef
Chemical Class: Cephalosporin (1st generation)
Therapeutic Class: Antibiotic

CLINICAL PHARMACOLOGY

Mechanism of Action: A first-generation cephalosporin that binds to bacterial cell membranes and inhibits its cell wall synthesis. *Therapeutic Effect:* Bactericidal.

Pharmacokinetics

Widely distributed. Protein binding: 85%. Primarily excreted unchanged in urine. Moderately removed by hemodialysis. **Half-life:** 1.4-1.8 hr (increased in impaired renal function).

INDICATIONS AND DOSAGES

Uncomplicated UTIs

IV, IM

Adults, Elderly. 1 g q12h.

Mild to moderate infections

IV, IM

Adults, Elderly. 250-500 mg q8-12h.

Severe infections

IV, IM

Adults, Elderly. 0.5-1 g q6-8h.

Life-threatening infections

IV, IM

Adults, Elderly. 1-1.5 g q6h. Maximum: 12 g/day.

Perioperative prophylaxis

IV, IM

Adults, Elderly. 1 g 30-60 min before surgery, 0.5-1 g during surgery, and q6-8h for up to 24 hrs postoperatively.

Usual pediatric dosage

Children. 50-100 mg/kg/day in divided doses q8h. Maximum: 6 g/day.

Neonates older than 7 days. 40-60 mg/kg/day in divided doses q8-12h.

Neonates 7 days and younger. 40 mg/kg/day in divided doses q12h.

Dosage in renal impairment

Dosing frequency is modified based on creatinine clearance.

Creatinine Clearance	Dosage Interval
10-30 ml/min	Usual dose q12h
less than 10 ml/min	Usual dose q24h

S AVAILABLE FORMS/COST

• Powder, Inj—IM, IV: 500 mg/vial: **$1.50-$4.50**; 1 g/vial: **$1.90-$13.32**

CONTRAINDICATIONS: History of anaphylactic reaction to penicillins or hypersensitivity to cephalosporins

PREGNANCY AND LACTATION: Pregnancy category B; low milk concentrations

SIDE EFFECTS

Frequent

Discomfort with IM administration, oral candidiasis, mild diarrhea, mild abdominal cramping, vaginal candidiasis

Occasional

Nausea, serum sickness-like reaction (marked by fever and joint pain; usually occurs after the second course of therapy and resolves after the drug is discontinued)

Rare

Allergic reaction (rash, pruritus, urticaria), thrombophlebitis (pain, redness, swelling at injection site)

SERIOUS REACTIONS

• Antibiotic-associated colitis and other superinfections may result from altered bacterial balance.

• Nephrotoxicity may occur, especially in patients with pre-existing renal disease.

• Patients with a history of allergies, especially to penicillin, are at increased risk for developing a severe hypersensitivity reaction, marked by severe pruritus, angioedema, bronchospasm, and anaphylaxis.

INTERACTIONS

Drugs

▨ *Aminoglycosides:*   Additive nephrotoxicity

▨ *Chloramphenicol:* Inhibits antibacterial activity of cefazolin

▨ *Loop diuretics:* Increased nephrotoxicity

❷ *Oral Anticoagulants:* Additive hypoprothrombinemia

---

cefdinir

(sef' di-neer)

Rx: Omnicef

Chemical Class: Cephalosporin (3rd generation)

Therapeutic Class: Antibiotic

CLINICAL PHARMACOLOGY

Mechanism of Action: A third-generation cephalosporin that binds to bacterial cell membranes and inhibits cell wall synthesis. *Therapeutic Effect:* Bactericidal.

Pharmacokinetics

Moderately absorbed from the GI tract. Protein binding: 60%-70%. Widely distributed. Not appreciably metabolized. Primarily excreted unchanged in urine. Minimally removed by hemodialysis. **Half-life:** 1-2 hr (increased in impaired renal function).

INDICATIONS AND DOSAGES

Community-acquired pneumonia

PO

Adults, Elderly, Children 13 yr and older. 300 mg q12h for 10 days.

Acute exacerbation of chronic bronchitis

PO

Adults, Elderly. 300 mg q12h for 5-10 days.

Acute maxillary sinusitis
PO

Adults, Elderly, Children 13 yr and older. 300 mg q12h or 600 mg q24h for 10 days.

Children 6 mo-12 yr. 7 mg/kg q12h or 14 mg/kg q24h for 10 days.

Pharyngitis or tonsillitis
PO

Adults, Elderly, Children 13 yr and older. 300 mg q12h for 5-10 days or 600 mg q24h for 10 days.

Children 6 mos-12 yrs. 7 mg/kg q12h for 5-10 days or 14 mg/kg q24h for 10 days.

Uncomplicated skin or skin-structure infections
PO

Adults, Elderly, Children 13 yr and older. 300 mg q12h for 10 days.

Children 6 mo-12 yr. 7 mg/kg q12h for 10 days.

Acute bacterial otitis media
PO (Capsules)

Children 6 mo-12 yr. 7 mg/kg q12h or 14 mg/kg q24h for 10 days.

Usual pediatric dosage for oral suspension
Children weighing 81-95 lb (37-43 kg). 12.5 ml (2.5 tsp) q12h or 25 ml (5 tsp) q24h.

Children weighing 61-80 lb (28-36 kg). 10 ml (2 tsp) q12h or 20 ml (4 tsp) q24h.

Children weighing 41-60 lb (19-27 kg). 7.5 ml (1 tsp) q12h or 15 ml (3 tsp) q24h.

Children weighing 20-40 lb (9-18 kg). 5 ml (1 tsp) q12h or 10 ml (2 tsp) q24h.

Infants weighing less than 20 lb (9 kg). 2.5 ml (½ tsp) q12h or 5 ml (1 tsp) q24h.

Dosage in renal impairment
For patients with creatinine clearance less than 30 ml/min, dosage is 300 mg/day as single daily dose. For hemodialysis patients, dosage is 300 mg or 7 mg/kg/dose every other day.

$ AVAILABLE FORMS/COST
• Cap—Oral: 300 mg, 60's: **$272.34**
• Susp—Oral: 125 mg/5 ml, 60, 100 ml: **$71.70**/100 ml

CONTRAINDICATIONS: History of anaphylactic reaction to penicillins or hypersensitivity to cephalosporins

PREGNANCY AND LACTATION: Pregnancy category B, not detected in human milk after administration of single 600 mg dose

SIDE EFFECTS
Frequent
Oral candidiasis, mild diarrhea, mild abdominal cramping, vaginal candidiasis
Occasional
Nausea, serum sickness-like reaction (marked by fever and joint pain; usually occurs after the second course of therapy and resolves after the drug is discontinued)
Rare
Allergic reaction (rash, pruritus, urticaria)

SERIOUS REACTIONS
• Antibiotic-associated colitis and other superinfections may result from altered bacterial balance.
• Nephrotoxicity may occur, especially in patients with pre-existing renal disease.
• Patients with a history of allergies, especially to penicillin, are at increased risk for developing a severe hypersensitivity reaction, marked by severe pruritus, angioedema, bronchospasm, and anaphylaxis.

INTERACTIONS
Drugs
3 *Antacids, iron:* Interference with cefdinir absorption, take antibiotic 2 hr before or after (can be administered with iron fortified infant formula)
3 *Probenecid:* Inhibits cefdinir excretion

3 *Live typhoid vaccine:* Interference with immune response to vaccine, give vaccine at least 24 hr after last dose
Labs
• *False positive:* Urine ketones using nitroprusside method, urine glucose using Clinitest, Benedict's or Fehling's solution, direct Coomb's
SPECIAL CONSIDERATIONS
• May be taken without regard to food
• More active *in vitro* against *S. aureus* and *Enterococcus faecalis* than cefixime, but less active against some enterobacteraceae

---

cefditoren
(seff-di-tore'en)
Rx: Spectracef
Chemical Class: Cephalosporin
(3rd generation)
Therapeutic Class: Antibiotic

CLINICAL PHARMACOLOGY
Mechanism of Action: A third-generation cephalosporin that binds to bacterial cell membranes and inhibits cell wall synthesis. *Therapeutic effect:* Bactericidal.
Pharmacokinetics
Moderately absorbed from the gastrointestinal (GI) tract. Protein binding: 88%. Not metabolized. Excreted in the urine. Minimally removed by hemodialysis. **Half-life:** 1.6 hrs (half-life increased with impaired renal function).
INDICATIONS AND DOSAGES
Pharyngitis, tonsillitis, skin infections
PO
Adults, Elderly, Children older than 12 yr. 200 mg twice a day for 10 days.

Acute exacerbation of chronic bronchitis
PO
Adults, Elderly, Children older than 12 yr. 400 mg twice a day for 10 days.
Community-acquired pneumonia
PO
Adults, Elderly, Children older than 12 yr. 400 mg 2 twice a day for 14 days.
Dosage in renal impairment
Dosage and frequency are modified based on creatinine clearance.

Creatinine Clearance	Dosage
50-80 ml/min	No adjustment necessary.
30-49 ml/min	200 mg twice a day
less than 30 ml/min	200 mg once a day

S **AVAILABLE FORMS/COST**
• Tab, Coated—Oral: 200 mg, 60's: **$113.25**
CONTRAINDICATIONS: Carnitine deficiency, inborn errors of metabolism, known allergy to cephalosporins, hypersensitivity to milk protein
PREGNANCY AND LACTATION: Pregnancy category B; excreted into breast milk
SIDE EFFECTS
Occasional (11%)
Diarrhea
Rare (4%-1%)
Nausea, headache, abdominal pain, vaginal candidiasis, dyspepsia, vomiting
SERIOUS REACTIONS
• · Antibiotic-associated colitis and other superinfections may occur.
• Patients with a history of allergies, especially to penicillin, are at increased risk for developing a severe hypersensitivity reaction, marked by severe pruritus, angioedema, bronchospasm, and anaphylaxis.

INTERACTIONS
Drugs
③ *Antacids, H_2 blockers:* Reduced absorption of cefditoren
③ *Probenecid:* Decreased cefditoren excretion
Labs
• *False positive:* Urine glucose (Benedict's or Fehling's solution or Clinitest tablets)
• *False negative:* Urine, plasma glucose (glucose oxidase or hexokinase methods)

SPECIAL CONSIDERATIONS
• Older oral cephalosporins preferred; no more efficacious than 2nd generation oral cephalosporins, no advantage over penicillin in strep pharyngitis
• Not recommended for prolonged therapy as carnitine deficiency may result

PATIENT/FAMILY EDUCATION
• Take with meals

---

cefepime

(sef'e-peem)

Rx: Maxipime
Chemical Class: Cephalosporin (4th generation)
Therapeutic Class: Antibiotic

CLINICAL PHARMACOLOGY
Mechanism of Action: A fourth-generation cephalosporin that binds to bacterial cell membranes and inhibits cell wall synthesis. *Therapeutic Effect:* Bactericidal.
Pharmacokinetics
Well absorbed after IM administration. Protein binding: 20%. Widely distributed. Primarily excreted unchanged in urine. Removed by hemodialysis. **Half-life:** 2-2.3 hr (increased in impaired renal function, and in the elderly).

INDICATIONS AND DOSAGES
Pneumonia
IV
Adults, Elderly. 1-2 g q12h for 7-10 days.
Children 2 mo and older. 50 mg/kg q12h. Maximum: 2 g/dose.
Intraabdominal infections
IV
Adults, Elderly. 2 g q12h for 10 days.
Skin and skin structure infections
IV
Adults, Elderly. 2 g q12h for 10 days.
Children 2 mo and older. 50 mg/kg q12h. Maximum: 2 g/dose.
UTIs
IV
Adults, Elderly. 0.5-2 g q12h for 7-10 days.
Children 2 mo and older. 50 mg/kg q12h. Maximum: 2 g/dose.
Febrile neutropenia
IV
Adults, Elderly. 2 g q8h.
Children 2 mo and older. 50 mg/kg q8h. Maximum: 2 g/dose.
Dosage in renal impairment
Dosage and frequency are modified based on creatinine clearance and the severity of the infection.

Creatinine Clearance	Dose
30-60 ml/min	0.5-2 g q24h
11-29 ml/min	0.5-1 g q24h
10 ml/min or less	0.25-0.5 g q24h

Ⓢ **AVAILABLE FORMS/COST**
• Powder, Inj—IV/IM: 500 mg/vial: **$8.56**; 1 g/ml vial: **$15.30-$18.79**; 2 g/ml vial: **$30.36-$36.59**
CONTRAINDICATIONS: History of anaphylactic reaction to penicillins or hypersensitivity to cephalosporins
PREGNANCY AND LACTATION: Pregnancy category B; excreted into breast milk in very low concentrations (0.5 mcg/ml)

SIDE EFFECTS
Frequent

Discomfort with IM administration, oral candidiasis, mild diarrhea, mild abdominal cramping, vaginal candidiasis

Occasional

Nausea, serum sickness-like reaction (marked by fever and joint pain; usually occurs after the second course of therapy and resolves after the drug is discontinued)

Rare

Allergic reaction (rash, pruritus, urticaria), thrombophlebitis (pain, redness, swelling at injection site)

SERIOUS REACTIONS

• Antibiotic-associated colitis manifested and other superinfections may result from altered bacterial balance.

• Nephrotoxicity may occur, especially in patients with pre-existing renal disease.

• Patients with a history of allergies, especially to penicillin, are at increased risk for developing a severe hypersensitivity reaction, marked by severe pruritus, angioedema, bronchospasm, and anaphylaxis.

INTERACTIONS
Drugs

3 *Aminoglycosides:* Additive nephrotoxicity

3 *Loop diuretics:* Increased nephrotoxicity

2 *Oral anticoagulants:* Potential increase in hypoprothrombinemic response to oral anticoagulants

Labs

• *False positive:* Positive direct Coombs test, positive urine glucose test (copper reduction method, i.e., Clinitest)

SPECIAL CONSIDERATIONS

• Broad spectrum, 4th generation cephalosporin demonstrating a low potential for resistance due to lack of β-lactamase induction and low potential for selection of resistant mutant strains; as effective as ceftazidime and cefotaxime in comparative trials; twice daily dosing may add economic advantage

---

cefixime
(sef-ix'ime)
Chemical Class: Cephalosporin (3rd generation)
Therapeutic Class: Antibiotic

CLINICAL PHARMACOLOGY
Mechanism of Action: A third-generation cephalosporin that binds to bacterial cell membranes and inhibits cell wall synthesis. *Therapeutic Effect:* Bactericidal.

Pharmacokinetics

Moderately absorbed from the GI tract. Protein binding: 65%-70%. Widely distributed. Primarily excreted unchanged in urine. Minimally removed by hemodialysis. **Half-life:** 3-4 hr (increased in renal impairment).

INDICATIONS AND DOSAGES
Otitis media, acute bronchitis, acute exacerbations of chronic bronchitis, pharyngitis, tonsillitis, and uncomplicated UTIs
PO

Adults, Elderly, Children weighing more than 50 kg. 400 mg/day as a single dose or in 2 divided doses.

Children 6 mo-12 yr weighing less than 50 kg. 8 mg/kg/day as a single dose or in 2 divided doses. Maximum: 400 mg.

Uncomplicated gonorrhea
PO

Adults. 400 mg as a single dose.

Dosage in renal impairment

Dosage is modified based on creatinine clearance.

Creatinine Clearance	% of Usual Dose
21-60 ml/min	75%
Less than 20 ml/min	50%

AVAILABLE FORMS/COST

• Susp—Oral: 100 mg/5 ml, 50. 75, 100 ml: **$36.51-$39.70**/50 ml
• Tab, Plain Coated—Oral: 200 mg, 100's: **$408.61**; 400 mg, 100's: **$800.81**

CONTRAINDICATIONS: History of anaphylactic reaction to penicillins, hypersensitivity to cephalosporins

PREGNANCY AND LACTATION: Pregnancy category B; excreted in breast milk

SIDE EFFECTS

Frequent

Oral candidiasis, mild diarrhea, mild abdominal cramping, vaginal candidiasis

Occasional

Nausea, serum sickness–like reaction (marked by arthralgia and fever; usually occurs after second course of therapy and resolves after drug is discontinued)

Rare

Allergic reaction (rash, pruritus, urticaria)

SERIOUS REACTIONS

• Antibiotic-associated colitis and other superinfections may result from altered bacterial balance.

• Nephrotoxicity may occur, especially in patients with pre-existing renal disease.

• Patients with a history of allergies, especially to penicillin, are at increased risk for developing a severe hypersensitivity reaction, marked by severe pruritus, angioedema, bronchospasm, and anaphylaxis.

INTERACTIONS

Drugs

3 *Aminoglycosides:* Additive nephrotoxicity

3 *Loop diuretics:* Increased nephrotoxicity

2 *Oral anticoagulants:* Enhanced hypoprothrombinemia

Labs

• *Cefotaxime:* Interferes with assay
• *Creatinine:* Increases or decreases depending on assay

SPECIAL CONSIDERATIONS

• No *S. aureus* coverage

---

cefoperazone

(sef-oh-per'a-zone)

Rx: Cefobid
Chemical Class: Cephalosporin (3rd generation)
Therapeutic Class: Antibiotic

CLINICAL PHARMACOLOGY

Mechanism of Action: A third-generation cephalosporin that binds to bacterial cell membranes. *Therapeutic Effect:* Inhibits synthesis of bacterial cell wall. Bactericidal.

Pharmacokinetics

Widely distributed, including cerebrospinal fluid (CSF). Protein binding: 82%-93%. Metabolized and excreted in kidney and urine. Removed by hemodialysis. **Half-life:** 1.6-2.4 hrs (half-life is increased with impaired renal function).

INDICATIONS AND DOSAGES

Mild to moderate infections

IM/IV

Adults, Elderly. 2-4 g/day in 2 divided doses q12h.

Severe or life-threatening infections

IM/IV

Adults, Elderly. Total daily dose and/or frequency may be increased to 6-12 g/day divided into 2, 3, or 4 equal doses of 1.5-4 g per dose.

Dosage in renal and/or hepatic impairment

Do not exceed 4 g/day in those with liver disease and/or biliary obstruction. Modification of dose usually not necessary in those with renal impairment. Dose should not exceed 1-2 g/day in those with both hepatic and substantial renal impairment.

$ AVAILABLE FORMS/COST
• Powder, Inj—IM, IV: 1 g: **$18.00**; 2 g: **$35.99**; 10 g: **$157.28**

UNLABELED USES: Treatment of Lyme disease

CONTRAINDICATIONS: Anaphylactic reaction to penicillins, history of hypersensitivity to cephalosporins or any one of its components.

PREGNANCY AND LACTATION: Pregnancy category B; low concentrations excreted in human milk

SIDE EFFECTS

Frequent

Discomfort with IM administration, oral candidiasis, mild diarrhea, mild abdominal cramping, vaginal candidiasis

Occasional

Nausea, unusual bruising/bleeding, serum sickness reaction

Rare

Allergic reaction, rash, pruritus, urticaria, thrombophlebitis (pain, redness, swelling at injection site)

SERIOUS REACTIONS

• Antibiotic-associated colitis manifested as severe abdominal pain and tenderness, fever, and watery and severe diarrhea, and other superinfections may result from altered bacterial balance.

• Nephrotoxicity may occur, especially in patients with preexisting renal disease. Severe hypersensitivity reaction including severe pruritus, angioedema, bronchospasm, and anaphylaxis, particularly in patients with a history of allergies, especially to penicillins, may occur.

INTERACTIONS

Drugs

▣ *Aminoglycosides:* Increased risk of nephrotoxicity

▣ *Ethanol:* Disulfiram-like reactions

▣ *Loop diuretics:* Increased nephrotoxicity

② *Oral anticoagulants:* Via hypoprothrombinemia, may enhance anticoagulant effects

Labs

• *Creatinine:* Increased serum values

SPECIAL CONSIDERATIONS

• No dose adjustment necessary in renal failure when usual doses are administered

PATIENT/FAMILY EDUCATION

• Avoid alcohol during and for 3 days after use

---

cefotaxime

(sef-oh-taks´eem)

Rx: Claforan

Chemical Class: Cephalosporin (3rd generation)

Therapeutic Class: Antibiotic

CLINICAL PHARMACOLOGY

Mechanism of Action: A third-generation cephalosporin that binds to bacterial cell membranes and inhibits cell wall synthesis. *Therapeutic Effect:* Bactericidal.

Pharmacokinetics

Widely distributed, including to CSF. Protein binding: 30%-50%. Partially metabolized in the liver to active metabolite. Primarily excreted in urine. Moderately removed by hemodialysis. **Half-life:** 1 hr (increased in impaired renal function).

INDICATIONS AND DOSAGES
Uncomplicated infections
IV, IM
Adults, Elderly. 1 g q12h.
Mild to moderate infections
IV, IM
Adults, Elderly. 1-2 g q8h.
Severe infections
IV, IM
Adults, Elderly. 2 g q6-8h.
Life-threatening infections
IV, IM
Adults, Elderly. 2 g q4h.
Children: 2 g q4h. Maximum: 12 g/day.
Gonorrhea
IM
Adults. (Male): 1 g as a single dose. (Female): 0.5 g as a single dose.
Perioperative prophylaxis
IV, IM
Adults, Elderly. 1 g 30-90 min before surgery.
Cesarean section
IV
Adults. 1 g as soon as umbilical cord is clamped, then 1 g 6 and 12 hr after first dose.
Usual pediatric dosage
Children weighing 50 kg or more. 1-2 g q6-8h.
Children 1 mo-12 yr weighing less than 50 kg. 100-200 mg/kg/day in divided doses q6-8h.
Dosage in renal impairment
For patients with creatinine clearance less than 20 ml/min give half of dose at usual dosing intervals.

§ AVAILABLE FORMS/COST
• Powder, Inj—IM, IV: 0.5 g/vial: **$7.20**; 1 g/vial: **$10.60-$14.05**; 2 g/vial: **$22.24-$26.39**

UNLABELED USES: Treatment of Lyme disease

CONTRAINDICATIONS: History of anaphylactic reaction to penicillins or hypersensitivity to cephalosporins

PREGNANCY AND LACTATION:
Pregnancy category B; low milk concentrations

SIDE EFFECTS
Frequent
Discomfort with IM administration, oral candidiasis, mild diarrhea, mild abdominal cramping, vaginal candidiasis
Occasional
Nausea, serum sickness-like reaction (marked by fever and joint pain; usually occurs after the second course of therapy and resolves after the drug is discontinued)
Rare
Allergic reaction (rash, pruritus, urticaria), thrombophlebitis (pain, redness, swelling at injection site)

SERIOUS REACTIONS
• Antibiotic-associated colitis and other superinfections may result from altered bacterial balance.
• Nephrotoxicity may occur, especially in patients with pre-existing renal disease.
• Patients with a history of allergies, especially to penicillin, are at increased risk for developing a severe hypersensitivity reaction, marked by severe pruritus, angioedema, bronchospasm, and anaphylaxis.

INTERACTIONS
Drugs
③ *Aminoglycosides:* Additive nephrotoxicity
③ *Chloramphenicol:* Inhibits antibacterial activity of cefotaxime
② *Oral anticoagulants:* Hypoprothrombinemia
Labs
• *False serum increases:* Albumin, alkaline phosphatase, calcium ceftriaxone, cholesterol, creatine kinase, creatinine, glucose, iron, iron saturation, metronidazole, potassium, sodium, tetracycline, trimethoprim

• *False serum decreases:* Ammonia, amylase, chloride, γ-glutamyltransferase (GGT), lactate dehydrogenase, magnesium, phosphate, potassium, urea nitrogen, uric acid
• *False positive:* Clindamycin, colistin, erythromycin, polymyxin

---

cefotetan
(sef'oh-tee-tan)
Rx: Cefotan
Chemical Class: Cephamycin
Therapeutic Class: Antibiotic

CLINICAL PHARMACOLOGY
Mechanism of Action: A second-generation cephalosporin that binds to bacterial cell membranes and inhibits cell wall synthesis. *Therapeutic Effect:* Bactericidal.
Pharmacokinetics
Protein binding: 78%-91%. Primarily excreted unchanged in urine. Minimally removed by hemodialysis. **Half-life:** 3-4.6 hr (increased in impaired renal function).
INDICATIONS AND DOSAGES
UTIs
IV, IM
Adults, Elderly. 1-2 g in divided doses q12-24h.
Mild to moderate infections
IV, IM
Adults, Elderly. 1-2 g q12h.
Severe infections
IV, IM
Adults, Elderly. 2 g q12h.
Life-threatening infections
IV, IM
Adults, Elderly. 3 g q12h.
Perioperative prophylaxis
IV
Adults, Elderly. 1-2 g 30-60 min before surgery.
Cesarean section
IV

Adults. 1-2 g as soon as umbilical cord is clamped.
Usual pediatric dosage
Children. 40-80 mg/kg/day in divided doses q12h. Maximum: 6 g/day.
Dosage in renal impairment
Dosing frequency is modified based on creatinine clearance and the severity of the infection.

Creatinine Clearance	Dosage Interval
10-30 ml/min	Usual dose q24h
less than 10 ml/min	Usual dose q48h

$ AVAILABLE FORMS/COST
• Powder, Inj—IM, IV: 10 g: **$118.32**; 1 g/vial: **$11.62-$13.70**; 2 g/vial: **$21.90-$28.09**
CONTRAINDICATIONS: History of anaphylactic reaction to penicillins or hypersensitivity to cephalosporins
PREGNANCY AND LACTATION: Pregnancy category B; small amounts excreted into breast milk
SIDE EFFECTS
Frequent
Discomfort with IM administration, oral candidiasis, mild diarrhea, mild abdominal cramping, vaginal candidiasis
Occasional
Nausea, unusual bleeding or bruising, serum sickness-like reaction (marked by fever and joint pain; usually occurs after the second course of therapy and resolves after the drug is discontinued)
Rare
Allergic reaction (rash, pruritus, urticaria), thrombophlebitis (pain, redness, swelling at injection site)
SERIOUS REACTIONS
• Antibiotic-associated colitis and other superinfections may result from altered bacterial balance.

- Nephrotoxicity may occur, especially in patients with pre-existing renal disease.
- Patients with a history of allergies, especially to penicillin, are at increased risk for developing a severe hypersensitivity reaction, marked by severe pruritus, angioedema, bronchospasm, and anaphylaxis.

INTERACTIONS
Drugs
■ *Aminoglycosides:* Additive nephrotoxicity

■ *Ethanol:* Disulfiram-like reaction

■ *Chloramphenicol:* Inhibits antibacterial activity of cefotetan

❷ *Oral anticoagulants:* Additive hypoprothrombinemia; enhanced anticoagulant effects

SPECIAL CONSIDERATIONS
PATIENT/FAMILY EDUCATION
- Avoid alcohol during and for 3 days after use

---

cefoxitin
(se-fox'i-tin)
Rx: Mefoxin
Chemical Class: Cephamycin
Therapeutic Class: Antibiotic

CLINICAL PHARMACOLOGY
Mechanism of Action: A second-generation cephalosporin that binds to bacterial cell membranes and inhibits cell wall synthesis. *Therapeutic Effect:* Bactericidal.

INDICATIONS AND DOSAGES
Mild to moderate infections
IV, IM

Adults, Elderly. 1-2 g q6-8h.

Severe infections
IV, IM

Adults, Elderly. 1 g q4h or 2 g q6-8h up to 2 g q4h.

Uncomplicated gonorrhea
IM

Adults. 2 g one time with 1 g probenecid.

Perioperative prophylaxis
IV, IM

Adults, Elderly. 2 g 30-60 min before surgery, then q6h for up to 24 hr after surgery.

Children older than 3 mo. 30-40 mg/kg 30-60 min before surgery, then q6h for up to 24 hr after surgery.

Cesarean section
IV

Adults. 2 g as soon as umbilical cord is clamped, then 2 g 4 and 8 hr after first dose, then q6h for up to 24 hr.

Usual pediatric dosage
Children older than 3 mo. 80-160 mg/kg/day in 4-6 divided doses. Maximum: 12 g/day.

Neonates. 90-100 mg/kg/day in divided doses q6-8h.

Dosage in renal impairment
After a loading dose of 1-2 g, dosage and frequency are modified based on creatinine clearance and the severity of the infection.

Creatinine Clearance	Dosage
30-50 ml/min	1-2 g q8-12h
10-29 ml/min	1-2 g q12-24h
5-9 ml/min	500 mg-1 g q12-24h
less than 5 ml/min	500 mg-1 g q24-48h

🅂 **AVAILABLE FORMS/COST**
- Powder, Inj—IM, IV: 1 g: **$10.90-$11.98**; 2 g: **$16.94-$23.87**; 10 g: **$112.25**

CONTRAINDICATIONS: History of anaphylactic reaction to penicillins or hypersensitivity to cephalosporins

PREGNANCY AND LACTATION: Pregnancy category B; low milk concentrations

SIDE EFFECTS
Frequent
Discomfort with IM administration, oral candidiasis, mild diarrhea, mild abdominal cramping, vaginal candidiasis
Occasional
Nausea, serum sickness-like reaction (marked by fever and joint pain; usually occurs after the second course of therapy and resolves after the drug is discontinued).
Rare
Allergic reaction (pruritus, rash, urticaria), thrombophlebitis (pain, redness, swelling at injection site)

SERIOUS REACTIONS
• Antibiotic-associated colitis and other superinfections may result from altered bacterial balance.
• Nephrotoxicity may occur, especially in patients with pre-existing renal disease.
• Patients with a history of allergies, especially to penicillin, are at increased risk for developing a severe hypersensitivity reaction, marked by severe pruritus, angioedema, bronchospasm, and anaphylaxis.

INTERACTIONS
Drugs
☒ *Aminoglycosides:* Additive nephrotoxicity
☒ *Chloramphenicol:* Inhibits antibacterial activity of cefoxitin
② *Oral anticoagulants:* Additive hypoprothrombinemia, enhanced anticoagulant effects
Labs
• *False serum increases:* Creatinine (serum and urine), cefuroxime, gentamicin, metronidazole, potassium, tetracycline
• *False urine increases:* 17-hydroxycorticosteroids
• *False serum decreases:* Creatine clearance
• *False positive:* Polymyxin

cefpodoxime
(sef-pod'ox-ime)
Rx: Vantin
Chemical Class: Cephalosporin (2nd generation)
Therapeutic Class: Antibiotic

CLINICAL PHARMACOLOGY
Mechanism of Action: A third-generation cephalosporin that binds to bacterial cell membranes and inhibits cell wall synthesis. *Therapeutic Effect:* Bactericidal.
Pharmacokinetics
Well absorbed from the GI tract (food increases absorption). Protein binding: 21%-40%. Widely distributed. Primarily excreted unchanged in urine. Partially removed by hemodialysis. **Half-life:** 2.3 hr (increased in impaired renal function and elderly patients).

INDICATIONS AND DOSAGES
Chronic bronchitis, pneumonia
PO
Adults, Elderly, Children older than 13 yr. 200 mg q12h for 10-14 days.
Gonorrhea, rectal gonococcal infection (female patients only)
PO
Adults, Children older than 13 yr. 200 mg as a single dose.
Skin and skin-structure infections
PO
Adults, Elderly, Children older than 13 yr. 400 mg q12h for 7-14 days.
Pharyngitis, tonsillitis
PO
Adults, Elderly, Children older than 13 yr. 100 mg q12h for 5-10 days.
Children 6 mo-13 yr. 5 mg/kg q12h for 5-10 days. Maximum: 100 mg/dose.
Acute maxillary sinusitis
PO
Adults, Children older than 13 yr. 200 mg twice a day for 10 days.

Children 2 mos-13 yr. 5 mg/kg q12h for 10 days. Maximum: 400 mg/day.
UTIs
PO
Adults, Elderly, Children older than 13 yr. 100 mg q12h for 7 days.
Acute otitis media
PO
Children 6 mos-13 yr. 5 mg/kg q12h for 5 days. Maximum: 400 mg/dose.
Dosage in renal impairment
For patients with creatinine clearance less than 30 ml/min, usual dose is given q24h. For patients on hemodialysis, usual dose is given 3 times/wk after dialysis.

$ AVAILABLE FORMS/COST
• Susp—Oral: 50 mg/5 ml, 50, 100 ml: **$48.31**/100 ml; 100 mg/5 ml, 50, 100 ml: **$91.91**/100 ml
• Tab—Oral: 100 mg, 100's: **$407.80**; 200 mg, 100's: **$538.48**
CONTRAINDICATIONS: History of anaphylactic reaction to penicillins or hypersensitivity to cephalosporins
PREGNANCY AND LACTATION: Pregnancy category B; excreted into breast milk; average 2% of serum levels at 4 hr following 200 mg dose
SIDE EFFECTS
Frequent
Oral candidiasis, mild diarrhea, mild abdominal cramping, vaginal candidiasis
Occasional
Nausea, serum sickness-like reaction (marked by fever and joint pain; usually occurs after the second course of therapy and resolves after the drug is discontinued)
Rare
Allergic reaction (pruritus, rash, urticaria)
SERIOUS REACTIONS
• Antibiotic-associated colitis and other superinfections may result from altered bacterial balance.

• Nephrotoxicity may occur, especially in patients with pre-existing renal disease.
• Patients with a history of allergies, especially to penicillin, are at increased risk for developing a severe hypersensitivity reaction, marked by severe pruritus, angioedema, bronchospasm, and anaphylaxis.
INTERACTIONS
Drugs
③ *Aminoglycosides:* Additive nephrotoxicity
③ *Antacids:* Reduced bioavailability and serum cefpodoxime levels
③ *H_2-blockers (cimetidine, famotidine, nizatidine, ranitidine), Proton pump inhibitors (lansoprazole, omeprazole):* Reduced bioavailability and serum cefpodoxime levels
③ *Loop diuretics:* Increased nephrotoxicity
SPECIAL CONSIDERATIONS
• Reserve use for otitis media to infections that fail to respond to less expensive agents (e.g., amoxicillin, co-trimoxazole)
• Suspension tastes very bitter

---

cefprozil
(sef-pro'zil)
Rx: Cefzil
Chemical Class: Cephalosporin (2nd generation)
Therapeutic Class: Antibiotic

CLINICAL PHARMACOLOGY
Mechanism of Action: A second-generation cephalosporin that binds to bacterial cell membranes and inhibits cell wall synthesis. *Therapeutic Effect:* Bactericidal.
Pharmacokinetics
Well absorbed from the GI tract. Protein binding: 36%-45%. Widely distributed. Primarily excreted un-

changed in urine. Moderately removed by hemodialysis. **Half-life:** 1.3 hr (increased in impaired renal function).

INDICATIONS AND DOSAGES
Pharyngitis, tonsillitis
PO
Adults, Elderly. 500 mg q24h for 10 days.
Children 2-12 yr. 7.5 mg/kg q12h for 10 days.

Acute bacterial exacerbation of chronic bronchitis, secondary bacterial infection of acute bronchitis
PO
Adults, Elderly. 500 mg q12h for 10 days.

Skin and skin-structure infections
PO
Adults, Elderly. 250-500 mg q12h for 10 days.
Children. 20 mg/kg q24h for 10 days.

Acute sinusitis
PO
Adults, Elderly. 250-500 mg q12h for 10 days.
Children 6 mo-12 yr. 7.5-15 mg/kg q12h for 10 days.

Otitis media
PO
Children 6 mo-12 yr. 15 mg/kg q12h for 10 days. Maximum: 1 g/day.

Dosage in renal impairment
Patients with creatinine clearance less than 30 ml/min receive 50% of usual dose at usual interval.

$ AVAILABLE FORMS/COST
• Susp—Oral: 125 mg/5 ml, 50, 75, 100 ml: **$35.05-$42.63**/100 ml; 250 mg/5 ml, 50, 75, 100 ml: **$59.63-$77.24**/100 ml
• Tab—Oral: 250 mg, 100's: **$446.09**; 500 mg, 100's: **$908.66**

CONTRAINDICATIONS: History of anaphylactic reaction to penicillins or hypersensitivity to cephalosporins

PREGNANCY AND LACTATION: Pregnancy category B; excreted into breast milk in low concentratons

SIDE EFFECTS
Frequent
Oral candidiasis, mild diarrhea, mild abdominal cramping, vaginal candidiasis
Occasional
Nausea, serum sickness reaction (marked by fever and joint pain; usually occurs after the second course of therapy and resolves after the drug is discontinued)
Rare
Allergic reaction (pruritus, rash, urticaria)

SERIOUS REACTIONS
• Antibiotic-associated colitis and other superinfections may result from altered bacterial balance.
• Nephrotoxicity may occur, especially in patients with pre-existing renal disease.
• Patients with a history of allergies, especially to penicillin, are at increased risk for developing a severe hypersensitivity reaction, marked by severe pruritus, angioedema, bronchospasm, and anaphylaxis.

INTERACTIONS
Drugs
▨ *Aminoglycosides:* Additive nephrotoxicity
▨ *Loop diuretics:* Increased nephrotoxicity

SPECIAL CONSIDERATIONS
• Reserve use for otitis media to infections that fail to respond to less expensive agents (e.g., amoxicillin, co-trimoxazole)
• Suspension contains phenylalanine 28 mg/5 ml

ceftazidime
(sef-taz′i-deem)
Rx: Ceptaz, Fortaz, Tazicef, Tazidime
Chemical Class: Cephalosporin (3rd generation)
Therapeutic Class: Antibiotic

CLINICAL PHARMACOLOGY
Mechanism of Action: A third-generation cephalosporin that binds to bacterial cell membranes and inhibits cell wall synthesis. *Therapeutic Effect:* Bactericidal.
Pharmacokinetics
Widely distributed (including to CSF). Protein binding: 5%-17%. Primarily excreted unchanged in urine. Removed by hemodialysis. **Half-life:** 2 hr (increased in impaired renal function).

INDICATIONS AND DOSAGES
UTIs
IV, IM
Adults. 250-500 mg q8-12h.
Mild to moderate infections
IV, IM
Adults. 1 g q8-12h.
Uncomplicated pneumonia, skin and skin-structure infections
IV, IM
Adults. 0.5-1 g q8h.
Bone and joint infections
IV, IM
Adults. 2 g q12h.
Meningitis, serious gynecologic and intraabdominal infections
IV, IM
Adults. 2 g q8h.
Pseudomonal pulmonary infections in patients with cystic fibrosis
IV
Adults. 30-50 mg/kg q8h. Maximum: 6 g/day.
Usual elderly dosage
Elderly (normal renal function). 500 mg-1 g q12h.

Usual pediatric dosage
Children 1 mo-12 yr. 100-150 mg/kg/day in divided doses q8h. Maximum: 6 g/day.
Neonates 0-4 wk. 100-150 mg/kg/day in divided doses q8-12h.
Dosage in renal impairment
After an initial 1-g dose, dosage and frequency are modified based on creatinine clearance and the severity of the infection.

Creatinine Clearance	Dosage
30-50 ml/min	1 g q12h
16-30 ml/min	1 g q24h
6-15 ml/min	500 mg q24h
less than 5 ml/min	500 mg q48h

AVAILABLE FORMS/COST
• Powder, Inj—IV, IM: 500 mg/vial: **$7.11**; 1 g/vial: **$1.42-$18.48**; 2 g/vial: **$28.45-$43.31**; 6 g/vial: **$82.91-$86.25**

CONTRAINDICATIONS: History of anaphylactic reaction to penicillins or hypersensitivity to cephalosporins
PREGNANCY AND LACTATION: Pregnancy category B; excreted in human milk in low concentrations
SIDE EFFECTS
Frequent
Discomfort with IM administration, oral candidiasis, mild diarrhea, mild abdominal cramping, vaginal candidiasis
Occasional
Nausea, serum sickness-like reaction (marked by fever and joint pain; usually occurs after the second course of therapy and resolves after the drug is discontunued)
Rare
Allergic reaction (pruritus, rash, urticaria), thrombophlebitis (pain, redness, swelling at injection site)

SERIOUS REACTIONS

- Antibiotic-associated colitis and other superinfections may result from altered bacterial balance.
- Nephrotoxicity may occur, especially in patients with pre-existing renal disease.
- Patients with a history of allergies, especially to penicillin, are at increased risk for developing a severe hypersensitivity reaction, marked by severe pruritus, angioedema, bronchospasm, and anaphylaxis.

INTERACTIONS

Drugs

[3] *Aminoglycosides:* Additive nephrotoxicity

[3] *Chloramphenicol:* Inhibition of the antibacterial activity of ceftazidime

[3] *Loop diuretics:* Increased nephrotoxicity

SPECIAL CONSIDERATIONS

- Especially useful for infections due to *Pseudomonas aeruginosa* (with or without an aminoglycoside)

ceftibuten

(cef′ te-bute-in)

Rx: Cedax

Chemical Class: Cephalosporin (3rd generation)

Therapeutic Class: Antibiotic

CLINICAL PHARMACOLOGY

Mechanism of Action: A third-generation cephalosporin that binds to bacterial cell membranes and inhibits its cell wall synthesis. *Therapeutic Effect:* Bactericidal.

Pharmacokinetics

Rapidly absorbed from the gastrointestinal tract. Excreted primarily in urine. **Half-Life:** 2-3h.

INDICATIONS AND DOSAGES

Chronic bronchitis

PO

Adults, Elderly. 400 mg/day once a day for 10 days.

Pharyngitis, tonsillitis

PO

Adults, Elderly. 400 mg once a day for 10 days.

Children older than 6 mo. 9 mg/kg once a day for 10 days. Maximum: 400 mg/day.

Otitis media

PO

Children older than 6 mo. 9 mg/kg once a day for 10 days. Maximum: 400 mg/day.

Dosage in renal impairment

Dosage is modified based on creatinine clearance.

Creatinine Clearance	*Dosage*
50 ml/min and higher	400 mg or 9 mg/kg q24h
30-49 ml/min	200 mg or 4.5 mg/kg q24h
less than 30 ml/min	100 mg or 2.25 mg/kg q24h

[$] **AVAILABLE FORMS/COST**

- Cap, Gel—Oral: 400 mg, 100's: **$854.19**
- Powder, Reconst—Oral: 90 mg/5 ml, 30, 60, 90, 120 ml: **$45.47**/60 ml

CONTRAINDICATIONS: History of anaphylactic reaction to penicillins or hypersensitivity to cephalosporins

PREGNANCY AND LACTATION: Pregnancy category B; excreted into breast milk in negligible concentrations

SIDE EFFECTS

Frequent

Oral candidiasis, mild diarrhea (discharge, itching)

Occasional

Nausea, serum sickness-like reaction (marked by fever and joint pain; usually occurs after the second course of therapy and resolves after the drug is discontinued)

Rare

Allergic reaction (rash, pruritus, urticaria)

SERIOUS REACTIONS

• Antibiotic-associated colitis and other superinfections may result from altered bacterial balance.

• Nephrotoxicity may occur, especially in patients with pre-existing renal disease.

• Patients with a history of allergies, especially to penicillin, are at increased risk for developing a severe hypersensitivity reaction, marked by severe pruritus, angioedema, bronchospasm, and anaphylaxis.

INTERACTIONS

Drugs

▣ *Aminoglycosides:* Additive nephrotoxicity

▣ *Loop diuretics:* Increased nephrotoxicity

SPECIAL CONSIDERATIONS

• Comparable to many other oral cephalosporins; may produce higher serum levels and better penetration, but unsubstantiated

• Clinical application as alternative in respiratory tract infections

• Recommend empty stomach administration for the suspension

---

ceftizoxime

(sef-ti-zox'eem)

Rx: Cefizox

Chemical Class: Cephalosporin (3rd generation)

Therapeutic Class: Antibiotic

CLINICAL PHARMACOLOGY

Mechanism of Action: A third-generation cephalosporin that binds to bacterial cell membranes and inhibits cell wall synthesis. *Therapeutic Effect:* Bactericidal.

Pharmacokinetics

Widely distributed (including to CSF). Protein binding: 30%. Primarily excreted unchanged in urine. Moderately removed by hemodialysis. **Half-life:** 1.7 hr (increased in impaired renal function).

INDICATIONS AND DOSAGES

Uncomplicated UTIs

IV, IM

Adults, Elderly. 500 mg q12h.

Mild, moderate, or severe infections of the biliary, respiratory, and GU tracts; skin, bone, and intraabdominal infections; meningitis; and septicemia

IV, IM

Adults, Elderly. 1-2 g q8-12h.

Life-threatening infections of the biliary, respiratory, and GU tracts; skin, bone and intraabdominal infections; meningitis; and septicemia

IV

Adults, Elderly. 3-4 g q8h, up to 2 g q4h.

Pelvic inflammatory disease (PID)

IV

Adults. 2 g q4-8h.

Uncomplicated gonorrhea

IM

Adults. 1 g one time.

Usual pediatric dosage

Children older than 6 mo: 50 mg/kg q6-8h. Maximum: 12 g/day.

Dosage in renal impairment

After a loading dose of 0.5-1 g, dosage and frequency are modified based creatinine clearance and the severity of the infection.

Creatinine Clearance	Dosage
50-79 ml/min	0.5 g-1.5 g q8h
5-49 ml/min	0.25 g-1 g q12h
less than 5 ml/min	0.25-0.5 g q24h or 0.5 g-1 g q48h

[$] **AVAILABLE FORMS/COST**
• Powder, Inj—IV: 1 g/vial: **$12.81**; 2 g/vial: **$24.00**
CONTRAINDICATIONS: History of anaphylactic reaction to penicillins or hypersensitivity to cephalosporins
PREGNANCY AND LACTATION: Pregnancy category B; excreted in human milk in low concentrations
SIDE EFFECTS
Frequent
Discomfort with IM administration, oral candidiasis, mild diarrhea, mild abdominal cramping, vaginal candidiasis
Occasional
Nausea, serum sickness-like reaction (fever, joint pain; usually occurs after the second course of therapy and resolves after the drug is discontinued)
Rare
Allergic reaction (rash, pruritus, urticaria), thrombophlebitis (pain, redness, swelling at injection site)
SERIOUS REACTIONS
• Antibiotic-associated colitis manifested and other superinfections may result from altered bacterial balance.
• Nephrotoxicity may occur, especially in patients with pre-existing renal disease.
• Patients with a history of allergies, especially to penicillin, are at increased risk for developing a severe hypersensitivity reaction, marked by severe pruritus, angioedema, bronchospasm, and anaphylaxis.
INTERACTIONS
Drugs
[3] *Aminoglycosides:* Additive nephrotoxicity
[3] *Loop diuretics:* Increased nephrotoxicity

ceftriaxone
(sef-try-ax'one)
Rx: Rocephin
Chemical Class: Cephalosporin (3rd generation)
Therapeutic Class: Antibiotic

CLINICAL PHARMACOLOGY
Mechanism of Action: A third-generation cephalosporin that binds to bacterial cell membranes and inhibits cell wall synthesis. *Therapeutic Effect:* Bactericidal.
Pharmacokinetics
Widely distributed (including to CSF). Protein binding: 83%-96%. Primarily excreted unchanged in urine. Not removed by hemodialysis. **Half-life:** 4.3-4.6 hr IV; 5.8-8.7 hr IM (increased in impaired renal function).
INDICATIONS AND DOSAGES
Mild to moderate infections
IV, IM
Adults, Elderly. 1-2 g as a single dose or in 2 divided doses.
Serious infections
IV, IM
Adults, Elderly. Up to 4 g/day in 2 divided doses.
Children. 50-75 mg/kg/day in divided doses q12h. Maximum: 2 g/day.
Skin and skin-structure infections
IV, IM
Children. 50-75 mg/kg/day as a single dose or in 2 divided doses. Maximum: 2 g/day.
Meningitis
IV
Children. Initially, 75 mg/kg, then 100 mg/kg/day as a single dose or in divided doses q12h. Maximum: 4 g/day.

Lyme disease
IV
Adults, Elderly. 2-4 g a day for 10-14 days.
Acute bacterial otitis media
IM
Children. 50 mg/kg once a day for 3 days. Maximum: 1 g/day.
Perioperative prophylaxis
IV, IM
Adults, Elderly. 1 g 0.5-2 hrs before surgery.
Uncomplicated gonorrhea
IM
Adults. 250 mg plus doxycycline one time.
Dosage in renal impairment
Dosage modification is usually unnecessary but liver and renal function test results should be monitored in those with both renal and liver impairment or severe renal impairment.

[$] **AVAILABLE FORMS/COST**
• Powder, Inj—IM, IV: 250 mg/vial: **$15.70-$16.48**; 500 mg/vial: **$28.50-$29.87**; 1 g/vial: **$50.58-$52.76**; 2 g/vial: **$91.98-$104.21**

CONTRAINDICATIONS: History of anaphylactic reaction to penicillins or hypersensitivity to cephalosporins

PREGNANCY AND LACTATION: Pregnancy category B; excreted in breast milk

SIDE EFFECTS
Frequent
Discomfort with IM administration, oral candidiasis, mild diarrhea, mild abdominal cramping, vaginal candidiasis
Occasional
Nausea, serum sickness-like reaction (marked by fever and joint pain; usually occurs after the second course of therapy and resolves after the drug is discontinued)
Rare
Allergic reaction (rash, pruritus, urticaria), thrombophlebitis (pain, redness, swelling at injection site)

SERIOUS REACTIONS
• Antibiotic-associated colitis and other superinfections may result from altered bacterial balance.
• Nephrotoxicity may occur, especially in patients with pre-existing renal disease.
• Patients with a history of allergies, especially to penicillin, are at increased risk for developing a severe hypersensitivity reaction, marked by severe pruritus, angioedema, bronchospasm, and anaphylaxis.

INTERACTIONS
Drugs
[3] *Aminoglycosides:* Additive nephrotoxicity
[3] *Loop diuretics:* Increased nephrotoxicity
[2] *Warfarin:* Hypoprothrombinemic response enhanced

SPECIAL CONSIDERATIONS
• Meningitis the only indication requiring bid dosing; qday sufficient for all other indications in adults
• Often administered in acute care settings for dubious indications due to long $t_{1/2}$, avoid overuse

cefuroxime
(sef-yoor-ox'eem)
Rx: Zinacef, Kefurox (as sodium), Ceftin (as axetil)
Chemical Class: Cephalosporin (2nd generation)
Therapeutic Class: Antibiotic

CLINICAL PHARMACOLOGY
Mechanism of Action: A second-generation cephalosporin that binds to bacterial cell membranes and inhibits cell wall synthesis. *Therapeutic Effect:* Bactericidal.

Pharmacokinetics
Rapidly absorbed from the GI tract. Protein binding: 33%-50%. Widely distributed (including to CSF). Primarily excreted unchanged in urine. Moderately removed by hemodialysis. **Half-life:** 1.3 hr (increased in impaired renal function).

INDICATIONS AND DOSAGES
Ampicillin-resistant influenza; bacterial meningitis; early Lyme disease; GU tract, gynecologic, skin, and bone infections; septicemia; gonorrhea, and other gonococcal infections
IV, IM
Adults, Elderly. 750 mg-1.5 g q8h.
Children. 75-100 mg/kg/day divided q8h. Maximum: 8 g/day.
Neonates. 50-100 mg/kg/day divided q12h.
PO
Adults, Elderly. 125-500 mg twice a day, depending on the infection.

Pharyngitis, tonsillitis
PO
Children 3 mo-12 yr. 125 mg (tablets) q12h or 20 mg/kg/day (suspension) in 2 divided doses.

Acute otitis media, acute bacterial maxillary sinusitis, impetigo
PO
Children 3 mo-12 yr. 250 mg (tablets) q12h or 30 mg/kg/day (suspension) in 2 divided doses.

Bacterial meningitis
IV
Children 3 mo-12 yr. 200-240 mg/kg/day in divided doses q6-8h.

Perioperative prophylaxis
IV
Adults, Elderly. 1.5 g 30-60 min before surgery and 750 mg q8h after surgery.

Usual neonatal dosage
IV, IM
Neonates. 20-100 mg/kg/day in divided doses q12h.

Dosage in renal impairment
Adult dosage and frequency are modified based on creatinine clearance and the severity of the infection.

Creatinine Clearance	Dosage
greater than 20 ml/min	750 mg-1 g q8h
10-20 ml/min	750 mg q12h
less than 10 ml/min	750 mg q24h

AVAILABLE FORMS/COST
• Powder, Inj—IM; IV: 750 mg/vial: **$6.54-$7.38**; 1.5 g/vial: **$12.63-$13.94**
• Powder, Reconst—Oral: 250 mg/5 ml, 50, 100 ml: **$74.99/100 ml**
• Tab, Coated—Oral: 250 mg, 60's: **$263.95**; 500 mg, 60's: **$588.56**

CONTRAINDICATIONS: History of anaphylactic reaction to penicillins or hypersensitivity to cephalosporins

PREGNANCY AND LACTATION: Pregnancy category B; excreted in breast milk

SIDE EFFECTS
Frequent
Discomfort with IM administration, oral candidiasis, mild diarrhea, mild abdominal cramping, vaginal candidiasis
Occasional
Nausea, serum sickness-like reaction (marked by fever and joint pain; usually occurs after the second course of therapy and resolves after the drug is discontinued)
Rare
Allergic reaction (rash, pruritus, urticaria), thrombophlebitis (pain, redness, swelling at injection site)

SERIOUS REACTIONS
• Antibiotic-associated colitis and other superinfections may result from altered bacterial balance.

• Nephrotoxicity may occur, especially in patients with pre-existing renal disease.

• Patients with a history of allergies, especially to penicillin, are at increased risk for developing a severe hypersensitivity reaction, marked by severe pruritus, angioedema, bronchospasm, and anaphylaxis.

INTERACTIONS
Drugs

3 *Aminoglycosides:* Additive nephrotoxicity

3 *Antacids, H$_2$-blockers, omeprazole, lansoprazole:* Decreased absorption of cefuroxime axetil

3 *Loop diuretics:* Increased nephrotoxicity

SPECIAL CONSIDERATIONS
• Oral tabs and oral susp not bioequivalent

• Take with food

• Alternative to amoxicillin or co-trimoxazole for resistant upper respiratory pathogens; expensive, but bid dosing

---

celecoxib
(sel-eh-cox'ib)
Rx: Celebrex
Chemical Class: Cyclooxyge-nase-2 (COX-2) inhibitor
Therapeutic Class: COX-2 specific inhibitor; NSAID; non-narcotic analgesic

CLINICAL PHARMACOLOGY
Mechanism of Action: An NSAID that inhibits cyclo-oxygenase-2, the enzyme responsible for prostaglandin synthesis. Mechanism of action in treating familial adenomatous polyposis is unknown. *Therapeutic Effect:* Reduces inflammation and relieves pain.

Pharmacokinetics
Widely distributed. Protein binding: 97%. Metabolized in the liver. Primarily eliminated in feces. **Half-life:** 11.2 hr.

INDICATIONS AND DOSAGES
Osteoarthritis
PO
Adults, Elderly. 200 mg/day as a single dose or 100 mg twice a day.
Rheumatoid arthritis
PO
Adults, Elderly. 100–200 mg twice a day.
Acute pain
PO
Adults, Elderly. Initially, 400 mg with additional 200 mg on day 1, if needed. Maintenance: 200 mg twice a day as needed.
Familial adenomatous polyposis
PO
Adults, Elderly. 400 mg twice daily (with food).

AVAILABLE FORMS/COST
• Cap—Oral: 100 mg, 100's: **$180.83**; 200 mg, 100's: **$296.59**; 400 mg, 60's: **$266.93**

CONTRAINDICATIONS: Hypersensitivity to aspirin, NSAIDs, or sulfonamides

PREGNANCY AND LACTATION: Pregnancy category C; breast milk secretion unknown

SIDE EFFECTS
Frequent (greater than 5%)
Diarrhea, dyspepsia, headache, upper respiratory tract infection
Occasional (5%–1%)
Abdominal pain, flatulence, nausea, back pain, peripheral edema, dizziness, rash

SERIOUS REACTIONS
• None known.

INTERACTIONS
Drugs

3 *Diuretics:* Potential reduction of both diuretic and antihypertensive effects of loop and thiazide diuretics

3 *ACE-inhibitors:* May reduce antihypertensive effect of ACE-inhibitors

3 *Fluconazole:* Two-fold increase in celecoxib plasma concentration due to inhibition of CYP2C9

3 *Lithium:* Steady-state lithium plasma levels increased 18%

3 *Warfarin:* Bleeding events reported, predominantly in elderly; increases in PT possible

SPECIAL CONSIDERATIONS
• COX-2 specific inhibition good choice for patients with inflammatory conditions who are at high risk of gastrointestinal adverse effects (e.g., older than 60 years, history of peptic ulcer disease, prolonged, high-dose NSAID therapy, concurrent use of corticosteroids or anticoagulants)

MONITORING PARAMETERS
• Rheumatoid arthritis—Decreased acute phase reactants (ESR, C-reactive protein), pain relief, reduction in number of swollen joints, improved range of motion, less fatigue, functional capacity, structural damage, maintenance of normal lifestyle
• Osteoarthritis—Decreased pain and stiffness of affected joints
• Toxicity—Initial hemogram, fecal occult blood, then q6-12 mo; electrolytes and renal function tests q6-12 mo; LFT's q6-12 mo in high-risk patients; query patient for dyspepsia, nausea, vomiting, right upper abdominal pain, anorexia, fatigue, jaundice, edema, weight gain, decreased urine output

cellulose sodium phosphate

Rx: Calcibind
Chemical Class: Phosphorylated cellulose
Therapeutic Class: Hypercalciuria

CLINICAL PHARMACOLOGY
Mechanism of Action: A nonabsorbable compound that alters urinary composition of calcium, magnesium, phosphate, and oxalate. Calcium binds to cellulose sodium phosphate therefore preventing intestinal absorption of it. *Therapeutic Effect:* Prevents the formation of kidney stones.
Pharmacokinetics
Not absorbed from gastrointestinal (GI) tract. Eliminated in the feces.

INDICATIONS AND DOSAGES
Absorptive hypercalciuria Type I
Acute bleeding
PO
Adults, Elderly. Initially, 15 g/day (5 g with each meal). Decrease dosage to 10 g/day when urinary calcium is less than 150 mg/day.

S AVAILABLE FORMS/COST
• Powder, Reconst—Oral: 2.5 g/scoop, 300 g: **$103.13**

UNLABELED USES: Absorptive hypercalciuria Type II

CONTRAINDICATIONS: Primary or secondary hyperparathyroidism, including renal hypercalciuria (renal calcium leak), hypomagnesemic states (serum magnesium <1.5 mg/dl), bone disease (osteoporosis, osteomalacia, osteitis), hypocalcemic states (e.g. hypoparathyroidism, intestinal malabsorption), normal or low intestinal absorption and renal excretion of calcium, enteric hyperoxaluria, and patients with high fasting urinary calcium or hypophosphatemia.

PREGNANCY AND LACTATION: Pregnancy category C

SIDE EFFECTS

Occasional

GI disturbance, manifested by poor taste of the drug, loose bowel movements, diarrhea, dyspepsia.

SERIOUS REACTIONS

- Hyperoxaluria and hypomagnesiuria, which negate the beneficial effect of hypocalciuria on new stone formation, magnesium depletion, and depletion of trace metals (copper, zinc, iron) may occur.

SPECIAL CONSIDERATIONS

PATIENT/FAMILY EDUCATION

- Suspend each dose of CSP powder in glass of water, soft drink or fruit juice
- Ingest within 30 min of a meal

MONITORING PARAMETERS

- Serum Ca, Mg, copper, zinc, iron, parathyroid hormone, CBC every 3 to 6 mo
- Serum parathyroid hormone should be obtained at least once between the 1st 2 wk to 3 mo of treatment

cephalexin

(sef-a-lex'in)

Rx: Biocef, Keflex

Chemical Class: Cephalosporin (1st generation)

Therapeutic Class: Antibiotic

CLINICAL PHARMACOLOGY

Mechanism of Action: A first-generation cephalosporin that binds to bacterial cell membranes and inhibits its cell wall synthesis. *Therapeutic Effect:* Bactericidal.

Pharmacokinetics

Rapidly absorbed from the GI tract. Protein binding: 10%-15%. Widely distributed. Primarily excreted unchanged in urine. Moderately removed by hemodialysis. **Half-life:** 0.9-1.2 hr (increased in impaired renal function).

INDICATIONS AND DOSAGES

Bone infections, prophylaxis of rheumatic fever, follow-up to parenteral therapy

PO

Adults, Elderly. 250-500 mg q6h up to 4 g/day.

Streptococcal pharyngitis, skin and skin-structure infections, uncomplicated cystitis

PO

Adults, Elderly. 500 mg q12h.

Usual pediatric dosage

Children. 25-100 mg/kg/day in 2-4 divided doses.

Otitis media

PO

Children. 75-100 mg/kg/day in 4 divided doses.

Dosage in renal impairment

After usual initial dose, dosing frequency is modified based on creatinine clearance and the severity of the infection.

Creatinine Clearance	*Dosage Interval*
10-40 ml/min	Usual dose q8-12h
less than 10 ml/min	Usual dose q12-24h

[$] **AVAILABLE FORMS/COST**

- Cap, Gel—Oral: 250 mg, 100's: **$12.62-$180.87**; 500 mg, 100's: **$27.18-$323.71**
- Powder, Reconst—Oral: 125 mg/5 ml, 100, 200 ml: **$4.53-$21.00**/100 ml; 250 mg/5 ml, 100, 200 ml: **$6.19-$32.99**/100 ml
- Tab—Oral: 250 gm, 100's: **$37.50-$57.00**; 500 mg, 100's: **$62.85-$225.02**

CONTRAINDICATIONS: History of anaphylactic reaction to penicillins or hypersensitivity to cephalosporins

PREGNANCY AND LACTATION: Pregnancy category B; excreted in breast milk

SIDE EFFECTS

Frequent

Oral candidiasis, mild diarrhea, mild abdominal cramping, vaginal candidiasis

Occasional

Nausea, serum sickness-like reaction (marked by fever and joint pain; ususally occurs after the second course of therapy and resolves after the drug is discontinued)

Rare

Allergic reaction (rash, pruritus, urticaria)

SERIOUS REACTIONS

• Antibiotic-associated colitis and other superinfections may result from altered bacterial balance.

• Nephrotoxicity may occur, especially in patients with pre-existing renal disease.

• Patients with a history of allergies, especially to penicillin, are at increased risk for developing a severe hypersensitivity reaction, marked by severe pruritus, angioedema, bronchospasm, and anaphylaxis.

INTERACTIONS

Drugs

▨ *Aminoglycosides:* Additive nephrotoxicity

▨ *Loop diuretics:* Increased nephrotoxicity

Labs

• *Increase:* Urinary amino acids

• *False positive:* Urine glucose with Benedict's, Fehlings, Clinitest

• *Decrease:* Urine leukocytes

SPECIAL CONSIDERATIONS

• 1st generation oral cephalosporin of choice

cephradine
(sef'ra-deen)
Rx: Velosef
Chemical Class: Cephalosporin (1st generation)
Therapeutic Class: Antibiotic

CLINICAL PHARMACOLOGY

Mechanism of Action: A first-generation cephalosporin that binds to bacterial cell membranes. Inhibits synthesis of bacterial cell wall. *Therapeutic Effect:* Bactericidal.

Pharmacokinetics

Well absorbed from the gastrointestinal (GI) tract. Protein binding: 18%-20%. Widely distributed. Primarily excreted unchanged in urine. Removed by hemodialysis. **Half-life:** 1-2 hrs (half-life is increased with impaired renal function).

INDICATIONS AND DOSAGES

Mild, moderate, or severe infections of the respiratory, and genitourinary (GU) tracts; bone, joint, and skin infections; prostatitis; otitis media

PO

Adults, Elderly. 250-500 mg q6h. Maximum: 8 g/day.

Children older than 9 mo. 25-50 mg/kg/day in divided doses q6-12h. Maximum: 4 g/day.

Dosage in renal impairment

Dosage and frequency are based on the degree of renal impairment and the severity of infection. After initial 1-g dose:

Creatinine Clearance	Dosage Interval
10-50 ml/min	250 mg q6h
0-10 ml/min	125 mg q6h

▨ **AVAILABLE FORMS/COST**

• Cap, Gel—Oral: 250 mg, 100's: **$35.00-$98.81**; 500 mg, 100's: **$65.00-$209.05**

• Powder, Reconst—Oral: 125 mg/5 ml, 100 ml: **$6.90-$10.14**/100 ml; 250 mg/5 ml, 100, 200 ml: **$12.90-$20.33**/100 ml

CONTRAINDICATIONS: History of hypersensitivity to penicillins and cephalosporins

PREGNANCY AND LACTATION: Pregnancy category B; excreted into breast milk in low concentrations; no adverse effects have been observed

SIDE EFFECTS
Frequent
Diarrhea, mild abdominal cramping, vaginal candidiasis (discharge, itching)
Occasional
Nausea, headache, unusual bruising or bleeding, serum sickness reaction (fever, joint pain)
Rare
Allergic reaction (rash, pruritus, urticaria)

SERIOUS REACTIONS
• Antibiotic-associated colitis as evidenced by severe abdominal pain and tenderness, fever, and watery and severe diarrhea, and other superinfections may result from altered bacterial balance.
• Nephrotoxicity may occur, especially in patients with preexisting renal disease.
• Severe hypersensitivity reaction including severe pruritus, angioedema, bronchospasm, and anaphylaxis, particularly in patients with history of allergies, especially penicillin, may occur.

INTERACTIONS
Drugs
3 *Aminoglycosides:* Additive nephrotoxicity
3 *Loop diuretics:* Increased nephrotoxicity

SPECIAL CONSIDERATIONS
• No advantage over cephalexin; cost should be major consideration for selection of first generation cephalosporins

---

cetirizine
(si-tear'a-zeen)
Rx: Zyrtec
Combinations
Rx: with pseudoephedrine (Zyrtec-D 12 Hour Tablets)
Chemical Class: Piperazine derivative
Therapeutic Class: Antihistamine

CLINICAL PHARMACOLOGY
Mechanism of Action: A second-generation piperazine that competes with histamine for H_1-receptor sites on effector cells in the GI tract, blood vessels, and respiratory tract. *Therapeutic Effect:* Prevents allergic response, produces mild bronchodilation, blocks histamine-induced bronchitis.

Pharmacokinetics

Route	Onset	Peak	Duration
PO	less than 1 hr	4–8 hr	less than 24 hr

Rapidly and almost completely absorbed from the GI tract (absorption not affected by food). Protein binding: 93%. Undergoes low first-pass metabolism; not extensively metabolized. Primarily excreted in urine (more than 80% as unchanged drug). **Half-life:** 6.5–10 hr.

INDICATIONS AND DOSAGES
Allergic rhinitis, urticaria
PO
Adults, Elderly, Children older than 5 yr. Initially, 5–10 mg/day as a single or in 2 divided doses.

Children 2–5 yr. 2.5 mg/day. May increase up to 5 mg/day as a single or in 2 divided doses.
Children 12-23 mo. Initially, 2.5 mg/day. May increase up to 5 mg/day in 2 divided doses.
Children 6-11 mo. 2.5 mg once a day.
Dosag in renal or hepatic impairment
For adult and elderly patients with renal impairment (creatinine clearance of 11–31 ml/min), those receiving hemodialysis (creatinine clearance of less than 7 ml/min), and those with hepatic impairment, dosage is decreased to 5 mg once a day.

[$] **AVAILABLE FORMS/COST**
- Syrup—Oral: 5 mg/5 ml,120, 473 ml: **$123.30**/473
- Tab, Coated—Oral: 5, 10 mg, 100's; all: **$210.95**
- Tab, Sus Action—Oral: 5mg-120 mg, 100's: **$105.48**

UNLABELED USES: Treatment of bronchial asthma

CONTRAINDICATIONS: Hypersensitivity to cetirizine or hydroxyzine

PREGNANCY AND LACTATION: Pregnancy category B; excreted into breast milk

SIDE EFFECTS
Occasional (10%–2%)
Pharyngitis; dry mucous membranes, nose, or throat; nausea and vomiting; abdominal pain; headache; dizziness; fatigue; thickening of mucus; somnolence; photosensitivity; urine retention

SERIOUS REACTIONS
- Children may experience paradoxical reactions, including restlessness, insomnia, euphoria, nervousness, and tremor.
- Dizziness, sedation, and confusion are more likely to occur in elderly patients.

SPECIAL CONSIDERATIONS
- H_1 antagonist with minimal effect on CNS; no affinity for other receptors
- Very potent antihistamine
- Kinetics allow qday dosing and do not have cytochrome P-450 drug interactions
- Effective against itching

cevimeline
(sev-im′el-ine)
Rx: Evoxac
Chemical Class: Oxathiolane derivative
Therapeutic Class: Salivation stimulant

CLINICAL PHARMACOLOGY
Mechanism of Action: A cholinergic agonist that binds to muscarinic receptors of effector cells, thereby increasing secretion of exocrine glands, such as salivary glands. *Therapeutic Effect:* Relieves dry mouth.

INDICATIONS AND DOSAGES
Dry mouth
PO
Adults. 30 mg 3 times a day.

[$] **AVAILABLE FORMS/COST**
- Cap, Gel—Oral: 30 mg, 100's: **$155.94**

CONTRAINDICATIONS: Acute iritis, angle-closure glaucoma, uncontrolled asthma

PREGNANCY AND LACTATION: Pregnancy category C; excretion into breast milk unknown; use caution in nursing mothers

SIDE EFFECTS
Frequent (19%–11%)
Diaphoresis, headache, nausea, sinusitis, rhinitis, upper respiratory tract infection, diarrhea
Occasional (10%–3%)

Dyspepsia, abdominal pain, cough, UTI, vomiting, back pain, rash, dizziness, fatigue

Rare (2%–1%)

Skeletal pain, insomnia, hot flashes, excessive salivation, rigors, anxiety

SERIOUS REACTIONS

• Cevimeline use may result in decreased visual acuity, especially at night, and impaired depth perception.

INTERACTIONS

Drugs

③ *β-blockers:* Increased possibility of cardiac conduction disturbances

③ *Parasympathomimetics:* Additive pharmacologic effects

③ *Antimuscarinics:* Potential interference with desirable antimuscarinic effects

SPECIAL CONSIDERATIONS

PATIENT/FAMILY EDUCATION

• May cause visual disturbance, use caution driving at night or performing hazardous activities in reduced lighting

• Ensure adequate fluid intake to prevent dehydration, especially if drug causes excessive sweating

charcoal, activated

OTC: *Oral caps:* CharcoCaps

OTC: *Oral tablets:* Charco Plus DS

OTC: *Oral Suspensions (activated):* Actidose-Aqua, Liqui-Char, CharcoAide

Combinations

  OTC: with simethicone (Charcoal Plus, Flatulex); with sorbitol (Actidose with sorbitol)

Chemical Class: Carbon

Therapeutic Class: Antidiarrheal; antidote; antiflatulent

CLINICAL PHARMACOLOGY

Mechanism of Action: An antidote that adsorbs (detoxifies) ingested toxic substances, irritants, intestinal gas. *Therapeutic Effect:* Inhibits gastrointestinal (GI) absorption and absorbs intestinal gas.

Pharmacokinetics

Not orally absorbed from the GI tract. Not metabolized. Excreted in feces as charcoal. **Half-life:** Unknown.

INDICATIONS AND DOSAGES

Acute poisoning

PO

Adults, Elderly, Children 12 yrs and older. Give 30-100 g as slurry (30 g in at least 8 oz H_2O) or 12.5-50 g in aqueous or sorbitol suspension. Usually given as single dose.

Children more than 1 yr and less than 12 yrs. 25-50 g as a single dose. Smaller doses (10-25 g) may be used in children 1-5 yrs due to smaller gut lumen capacity.

Ⓢ **AVAILABLE FORMS/COST**

• Cap—Oral: 260 mg, 50's: **$3.40**

• Susp (activated)—Oral: 25 g/120 ml: **$6.17-$11.85**; 50 g/240 ml: **$9.43-$76.50**

• Tab, enteric coated—Oral: 250 mg, 125's: **$11.53**

CONTRAINDICATIONS: Intestinal obstruction, GI tract not anatomically intact; patients at risk of hemorrhage or GI perforation, if use would increase risk and severity of aspiration, not effective for cyanide, mineral acids, caustic alkalis, organic solvents, iron, ethanol, methanol poisoning, lithium, do not use charcoal with sorbitol in patients with fructose intolerance, charcoal with sorbitol not recommended in children <1 year of age, hypersensitivity to charcoal or any component of the formation

SIDE EFFECTS
Occasional
Diarrhea, GI discomfort, intestinal gas

SERIOUS REACTIONS
• Hypernatremia, hypokalemia, and hypermagnesemia may occur with coadministration of cathartics.

INTERACTIONS
Drugs
❷ *Digitalis glycosides:* Reduced digoxin levels; less effect on digitoxin

SPECIAL CONSIDERATIONS
• Administer activated charcoal for adsorption in emergency management of poisonings as a slurry with water, a saline cathartic, or sorbitol

---

chloral hydrate
(klor-al hye′drate)
Rx: Aquachloral
Chemical Class: Halogenated alcohol
Therapeutic Class: Sedative/hypnotic
DEA Class: Schedule IV

CLINICAL PHARMACOLOGY
Mechanism of Action: A nonbarbiturate chloral derivative that produces CNS depression. *Therapeutic Effect:* Induces quiet, deep sleep, with only a slight decrease in respiratory rate and BP.

INDICATIONS AND DOSAGES
Premedication for dental or medical procedures
PO, Rectal
Adults. 0.5–1 g.
Children. 75 mg/kg up to 1 g total.
Premedication for EEG
PO, Rectal
Adults. 0.5–1.5 g.
Children. 25–50 mg/kg/dose 30-60 min prior to EEG. May repeat in 30 min. Maximum: 1 g for infants, 2 g for children.

▣ AVAILABLE FORMS/COST
• Cap, Gel—Oral: 500 mg, 100's: **$7.31-$13.60**
• Supp—Rect: 325 mg, 12's: **$32.31**; 500 mg, 100's: **$213.50**; 650 mg, 12's: **$39.75**
• Syr—Oral: 500 mg/5 ml, 480 ml: **$3.07-$13.43**

CONTRAINDICATIONS: Gastritis, marked hepatic or renal impairment, severe cardiac disease

PREGNANCY AND LACTATION: Pregnancy category C; excreted into breast milk; may cause mild drowsiness in infant, otherwise compatible with breast-feeding

SIDE EFFECTS
Occasional
Gastric irritation (nausea, vomiting, flatulence, diarrhea), rash, sleepwalking
Rare
Headache, paradoxical CNS hyperactivity or nervousness in children, excitement or restlessness in the elderly (particularly in patients with pain).

SERIOUS REACTIONS
• Overdose may produce somnolence, confusion, slurred speech, severe incoordination, respiratory depression, and coma.

INTERACTIONS
Drugs
▣ *Ethanol:* Additive CNS-depressant effects
▣ *Warfarin:* Transient increase in the hypoprothrombinemic response to warfarin
Labs
• *Interference:* Urine catecholamines, urinary 17-hydroxycorticosteroids
• *False positive:* Urine glucose (Benedict's reagent)
• *False increase:* Serum urea nitrogen, vitamin B_{12}

SPECIAL CONSIDERATIONS
• Not as effective as benzodiazepines, loses much of effectiveness for inducing and maintaining sleep after 2 weeks of use
• Frequently used preoperatively or preprocedurally in children because less paradoxical excitement (not confirmed by well-controlled studies)

PATIENT/FAMILY EDUCATION
• May cause GI upset, recommend administration with full glass of water or fruit juice, dilute syrup in a half glass of water or fruit juice

---

chloramphenicol
(klor-am-fen'i-kole)
Rx: *Systemic:* Chloromycetin
Rx: *Ophthalmic:*
Chloromycetin Ophthalmic, Chloroptic
Rx: *Otic:* Chloromycetin Otic
Combinations
  Rx: Ophthalmic: Hydrocortisone acetate and polymixin B sulfate (Opthocort); hydrocortisone acetate (Chloromycetin Hydrocortisone)
Chemical Class: Dichloroacetic acid derivative
Therapeutic Class: Antibiotic

CLINICAL PHARMACOLOGY
Mechanism of Action: A dichloroacetic acid derivative that inhibits bacterial protein synthesis by binding to bacterial ribosomal receptor sites. *Therapeutic Effect:* Bacteriostatic (may be bactericidal in high concentrations).

INDICATIONS AND DOSAGES
Mild to moderate infections caused by organisms resistant to other less toxic antibiotics
IV
Adults, Elderly. 50-100 mg/kg/day in divided doses q6h. Maximum: 4 g/day.
Children older than 1 mo. 50-75 mg/kg/day in divided doses q6h. Maximum: 4 g/day
Meningitis
IV
Children older than 1 mo. 50-100 mg/kg/day in divided doses q6h.
Usual ophthalmic dosage
Adults, Elderly, Children. 1-2 drops 4-6 times/day.

Ⓢ AVAILABLE FORMS/COST
• Powder, Inj-IV: 1 g/vial: **$7.60-$12.38**

• Oint—Ophth: 1%, 3.5 g: **$1.65-$20.52**

• Sol—Ophth: 0.5%, 2.5, 7.5, 15 ml: **$2.70-$7.60**/15 ml

CONTRAINDICATIONS: Hypersensitivity to chloramphenicol

PREGNANCY AND LACTATION: Pregnancy category C; use caution at term due to potential for "gray baby syndrome" toxicity; excreted into breast milk; milk levels are too low to precipitate the "gray baby syndrome," but a theoretical risk does exist for bone marrow depression

SIDE EFFECTS

Occasional

Systemic: Nausea, vomiting, diarrhea

Ophthalmic: Blurred vision, burning, stinging, hypersensitivity reaction

Otic: Hypersensitivity reaction

Rare

"Gray baby" syndrome in neonates (abdominal distention, blue-gray skin color, cardiovascular collapse, unresponsiveness), rash, shortness of breath, confusion, headache, optic neuritis (blurred vision, eye pain), peripheral neuritis (numbness and weakness in feet and hands)

SERIOUS REACTIONS

• Superinfection due to bacterial or fungal overgrowth may occur.

• There is a narrow margin between effective therapy and toxic levels producing blood dyscrasias.

• Myelosuppression, with resulting aplastic anemia, hypoplastic anemia, and pancytopenia, may occur weeks or months later.

INTERACTIONS

Drugs

3 *Barbiturates:* Increased serum barbiturate concentrations; reduced serum chloramphenicol concentrations

3 *Ceftazidime:* Inhibited antibacterial activity

3 *Cimetidine:* Increased risk of myelosuppression

3 *Penicillins:* Inhibited antibacterial activity of penicillins

3 *Phenytoin:* Predictable increases in serum phenytoin concentrations, toxicity has occurred

3 *Rifampin:* Reduced chloramphenicol concentrations

3 *Sulfonylureas:* Increased hypoglycemic effects of tolbutamide and chlorpropamide

2 *Warfarin:* Enhanced hypoprothrombinemic response to warfarin and possibly other oral anticoagulants

Labs

• *False positive:* Urine glucose (copper reduction)

• *False decrease:* Serum folate, serum urea nitrogen, serum uric acid

• *False increase:* 17-ketosteroids, CSF protein, serum protein, serum urea nitrogen

SPECIAL CONSIDERATIONS

• Because of severe adverse effects (e.g. aplastic anemia) not indicated for less serious infections; aplastic anemia reported with topical use

MONITORING PARAMETERS

• CBC with platelets and reticulocytes before and frequently during therapy (discontinue drug if bone marrow depression occurs); serum iron and iron-binding globulin saturation may also be useful

• Serum drug level (peak 10-20 mcg/ml, trough 5-10 mcg/ml) weekly (more often in impaired hepatic, renal systems)

• Early signs of "gray baby syndrome" (cyanosis, abdominal distension, irregular respiration, failure to feed), ***drug should be discontinued immediately***

chlordiazepoxide
(klor-dye-az-e-pox'ide)
Rx: Libritabs, Librium, Mitran, Reposaus-10
Combinations
  Rx: with amitriptyline (Limbitrol DS 10-25); with clidinium (Clindex, Librax)
Chemical Class: Benzodiazepine
Therapeutic Class: Anxiolytic
DEA Class: Schedule IV

CLINICAL PHARMACOLOGY
Mechanism of Action: A benzodiazepine that enhances the action of the inhibitory neurotransmitter gamma- aminobutyric acid in the CNS. *Therapeutic Effect:* Produces anxiolytic effect.

INDICATIONS AND DOSAGES
Alcohol withdrawal symptoms
PO
Adults, Elderly. 50–100 mg. May repeat q2–4h. Maximum: 300 mg/24 hr.

Anxiety
PO
Adults. 15–100 mg/day in 3–4 divided doses.
Elderly. 5 mg 2–4 times a day.

AVAILABLE FORMS/COST
• Cap, Gel—Oral: 5 mg, 100's: **$0.94-$66.41**; 10 mg, 100's: **$1.11-$96.54**; 25 mg, 100's: **$1.34-$165.56**
• Inj, Conc, w/buf—IM, IV: 100 mg/ampul, 5 ml: **$26.31**

UNLABELED USES: Treatment of panic disorder, tension headache, tremors

CONTRAINDICATIONS: Acute alcohol intoxication, acute angle-closure glaucoma

PREGNANCY AND LACTATION: Pregnancy category D; excreted into breast milk; drug and metabolites may accumulate to toxic levels in nursing infant

SIDE EFFECTS
Frequent
Pain at IM injection site; somnolence, ataxia, dizziness, confusion with oral dose (particularly in elderly or debilitated patients)
Occasional
Rash, peripheral edema, GI disturbances
Rare
Paradoxical CNS reactions, such as hyperactivity or nervousness in children and excitement or restlessness in the elderly (generally noted during first 2 weeks of therapy, particularly in presence of uncontrolled pain)

SERIOUS REACTIONS
• IV administration may produce pain, swelling, thrombophlebitis, and carpal tunnel syndrome.
• Abrupt or too rapid withdrawal may result in pronounced restlessness, irritability, insomnia, hand tremors, abdominal or muscle cramps, diaphoresis, vomiting, and seizures.
• Overdose results in somnolence, confusion, diminished reflexes, and coma.

INTERACTIONS
Drugs
 Cimetidine: Increased plasma levels of chlordiazepoxide and/or active metabolites
 Disulfiram: Increased serum chlordiazepoxide concentrations
 Ethanol: Enhanced adverse psychomotor side effects of benzodiazepines
 Fluconazole, itraconazole, ketoconazole: Increased chlordiazepoxide concentrations

3 *Levodopa:* Potential for exacerbation of Parkinsonism in patients taking levodopa

Labs
• *False increase:* Urine 5-HIAA, urine 17-ketogenic steroids
• *False decrease:* Urine 17-ketogenic steroids
• *False positive:* Urine pregnancy tests

SPECIAL CONSIDERATIONS
• No advantage over diazepam; poor choice for elderly patients
• Do not use for everyday stress or use longer than 4 mo
• Do not discontinue medication abruptly after long-term use

---

chloroquine / chloroquine phosphate
(klor′oh-kwin)
Rx: Aralen
Chemical Class: 4-amino-quinoline derivative
Therapeutic Class: Amebicide; antimalarial

CLINICAL PHARMACOLOGY
Mechanism of Action: An amebecide that concentrates in parasite acid vesicles and may interfere with parasite protein synthesis. *Therapeutic Effect:* Increases pH and inhibits parasite growth.

Pharmacokinetics
Rate of absorption is variable. Chloroquine is almost completely absorbed from the gastrointestinal (GI) tract. Protein binding: 50%-65%. Widely distributed into body tissues such as eyes, heart, kidneys, liver, and lungs. Partially metabolized to active de-ethylated metabolites (principle metabolite is

desethylchloroquine). Excreted in urine. Removed by hemodialysis.
Half-life: 1-2 mos.

INDICATIONS AND DOSAGES
Chloroquine Phosphate
Treatment of malaria (acute attack): Dose (mg base)

Dose	Time	Adults	Children
Initial	Day 1	600 mg	10 mg/kg
Second	6 hrs later	300 mg	5 mg/kg
Third	Day 2	300 mg	5 mg/kg
Fourth	Day 3	300 mg	5 mg/kg

Suppression of malaria
PO
Adults. 300 mg (base)/wk on same day each week beginning 2 wks before exposure; continue for 6-8 wks after leaving endemic area.
Children. 5 mg (base)/kg/wk.

Malaria prophylaxis
PO
Adults. 600 mg base initially given in 2 divided doses 6 hrs apart.
Children. 10 mg base/kg.

Amebiasis
PO
Adults. 1 g (600 mg base) daily for 2 days; then, 500 mg (300 mg base)/day for at least 2-3 wks.

Chloroquine HCL
Treatment of malaria
IM
Adults. Initially, 160-200 mg base (4-5 ml), repeat in 6 hrs. Maximum: 800 mg base in first 24 hrs. Begin oral therapy as soon as possible and continue for 3 days until approximately 1.5 g base given.
Children. Initially, 5 mg base/kg, repeat in 6 hrs. Do not exceed 10 mg base/ kg/24 hrs.

Amebiasis
IM
Adults. 160-200 mg base (4-5 ml) daily for 10-12 days. Change to oral therapy as soon as possible.

AVAILABLE FORMS/COST
• Sol, Inj-IV, IM (Hydrochloride): 50 mg/ml, 5 ml: **$20.72**
• Tab-Oral (Phosphate): 250 mg (150 mg base), 100's: **$17.50-$189.75**; 500 mg (300 mg base), 100's: **$101.25-$151.05**

UNLABELED USES: Treatment of sarcoid-associated hypercalcemia, juvenile arthritis, rheumatoid arthritis, systemic lupus erythematosus, solar urticaria, chronic cutaneous vasculitis

CONTRAINDICATIONS: Hypersensitivity to 4-aminoquinoline compounds, retinal or visual field changes

PREGNANCY AND LACTATION: Pregnancy category C; excreted into breast milk; average infant consumption, considered safe;
NOTE: Doesn't protect infant against malaria

SIDE EFFECTS
Frequent
Discomfort with IM administration, mild transient headache, anorexia, nausea, vomiting
Occasional
Visual disturbances (blurring, difficulty focusing); nervousness, fatigue, pruritus esp. of palms, soles, scalp; bleaching of hair, irritability, personality changes, diarrhea, skin eruptions
Rare
Phlebitis or thrombophlebitis at IV injection site, abdominal cramps, headache, hypotension

SERIOUS REACTIONS
• Ocular toxicity and ototoxicity have been reported.
• Prolonged therapy: peripheral neuritis and neuromyopathy, hypotension, ECG changes, agranulocytosis, aplastic anemia, thrombocytopenia, convulsions, psychosis.

• Overdosage includes symptoms of headache, vomiting, visual disturbance, drowsiness, convulsions, hypokalemia followed by cardiovascular collapse, and death.

INTERACTIONS
Drugs
③ *Chlorpromazine:* Increased chlorpromazine concentrations
③ *Cyclosporine:* Elevates cyclosporine levels, toxicity possible
③ *Methotrexate:* Decreased methotrexate levels
③ *Praziquantel:* Decreased praziquantel absorption

SPECIAL CONSIDERATIONS
• Certain strains of *P. falciparum* have become resistant to chloroquine

MONITORING PARAMETERS
• Ophthalmic examinations (visual acuity, slit lamp, funduscopic, visual fields) and CBC if long-term treatment or drug dosage >150 mg/day

---

chlorothiazide
(klor-oh-thye'a-zide)
Rx: Aralen
Combinations
  Rx: with methyldopa (Aldoclor); with reserpine (Chloroserp, Diaserp, Diupres)
Chemical Class: Sulfonamide derivative
Therapeutic Class: Antihypertensive; diuretic, thiazide

CLINICAL PHARMACOLOGY
Mechanism of Action: A sulfonamide derivative that acts as a thiazide diuretic and antihypertensive. As a diuretic blocks reabsorption of water, the electrolytes sodium and potassium at cortical diluting segment of distal tubule. As an antihy-

pertensive reduces plasma, extracellular fluid volume, decreases peripheral vascular resistance (PVR) by direct effect on blood vessels. *Therapeutic Effect:* Promotes diuresis, reduces blood pressure (BP).

Pharmacokinetics

Poorly absorbed from the gastrointestinal (GI) tract. Not metabolized. Primarily excreted unchanged in urine. Not removed by hemodialysis. **Half-life:** 45 -120 min.

INDICATIONS AND DOSAGES

Edema, hypertension

PO

Adults. 0.5 -1 g 1-2 times/day. May give every other day or 3-5 days/wk.

Children 12 years and older. 10-20 mg/kg/dose in divided doses q8-12h. Maximum: 2g/day.

Children 2- 12 yrs. 1 g/day.

Children 6 mos- 2 yrs. 10-20 mg/kg/day in divided doses q12-24h. Maximum: 375 mg/day.

Children younger than 6 mos. 20-30 mg/kg/day in divided doses q12h. Maximum: 375 mg/day.

Hypertension

IV

Adults. 0.5 -1 g in divided doses q12-24h.

$ **AVAILABLE FORMS/COST**

• Powder, Inj-IV: 500 mg/vial: **$11.04**

• Susp—Oral: 250 mg/5 ml, 237 ml: **$12.26**

• Tab-Oral: 250 mg, 100's: **$4.00-$14.07**; 500 mg, 100's: **$25.25-$26.50**

UNLABELED USES: Treatment of diabetes insipidus, prevention of calcium-containing renal stones

CONTRAINDICATIONS: Anuria, history of hypersensitivity to sulfonamides or thiazide diuretics, renal decompensation

PREGNANCY AND LACTATION: Pregnancy category C; therapy for preexisting hypertension can be continued throughout pregnancy with minimal risk; initiating for simple edema not recommended; few unequivocal indications for diuretic therapy in pregnancy except for pulmonary edema or congestive heart failure; excreted in low concentrations in breast milk; compatible with breast-feeding

SIDE EFFECTS

Expected

Increase in urine frequency and volume

Frequent

Potassium depletion

Occasional

Postural hypotension, headache, gastrointestinal (GI) disturbances, photosensitivity reaction, muscle spasms, alopecia, rash, urticaria

SERIOUS REACTIONS

• Vigorous diuresis may lead to profound water loss and electrolyte depletion, resulting in hypokalemia, hyponatremia, and dehydration.

• Acute hypotensive episodes may occur.

• Hyperglycemia may be noted during prolonged therapy.

• GI upset, pancreatitis, dizziness, paresthesias, headache, blood dyscrasias, pulmonary edema, allergic pneumonitis, and dermatologic reactions occur rarely.

• Overdosage can lead to lethargy and coma without changes in electrolytes or hydration.

INTERACTIONS

Drugs

[2] *Angiotensin-converting enzyme inhibitors:* Risk of postural hypotension when added to ongoing diuretic therapy; more common with loop diuretics; first-dose hypotension possible in patients with sodium depletion or hypovolemia

caused by diuretics or sodium restriction; hypotensive response is usually transient; hold diuretic day of first dose

🔳 *Calcium (high doses):* Risk of milk-alkali syndrome; monitor for hypercalcemia

🔳 *Carbenoxolone:* Additive potassium wasting; severe hypokalemia

🔳 *Cholestyramine/colestipol:* Reduced serum concentrations of thiazide diuretics

🔳 *Corticosteroids:* Concomitant therapy may result in excessive potassium loss

🔳 *Diazoxide:* Hyperglycemia

🔳 *Digitalis glycosides:* Diuretic-induced hypokalemia may increase the risk of digitalis toxicity

🔳 *Hypoglycemic agents:* Thiazide diuretics tend to increase blood glucose, may increase dosage requirements of antidiabetic drugs

🔳 *Lithium:* Increases serum lithium concentrations; toxicity may occur

🔳 *Methotrexate:* Increased bone marrow suppression

🔳 *Nonsteroidal antiinflammatory drugs:* Concurrent use may reduce diuretic and antihypertensive effects

Labs
• *Interference:* Urine 17-hydroxycorticosteroids
• False decrease: urine estriol

SPECIAL CONSIDERATIONS
• Doses above 250 mg provide no further blood pressure reduction, but are more likely to induce metabolic disturbance (i.e., hypokalemia, hyperuricemia, etc.)
• May protect against osteoporotic hip fractures
• Loop diuretics or metolazone more effective if CrCl <40-50 ml/min

PATIENT/FAMILY EDUCATION
• Will increase urination temporarily (approximately 3 wk); take early in the day to prevent sleep disturbance
• May cause sensitivity to sunlight; avoid prolonged exposure to the sun and other ultraviolet light
• May cause gout attacks; notify clinician if sudden joint pain occurs

MONITORING PARAMETERS
• Weight, urine output, serum electrolytes, BUN, creatinine, CBC, uric acid, glucose, lipids

---

chloroxine
(klor-ox'ine)
Rx: Capitrol
Chemical Class: Hydroxyquinoline derivative
Therapeutic Class: Antiseborrheic

CLINICAL PHARMACOLOGY
Mechanism of Action: An antifungal that reduces scaling of the epidermis by slowing down mitotic activity. *Therapeutic Effect:* Reduces the excess scaling in patients with dandruff or seborrheic dermatitis.

Pharmacokinetics
No studies have investigated the absorption/pharmacokinetics of chloroxine.

INDICATIONS AND DOSAGES
Dandruff, seborrheic dermatitis
Adults. Shampoo affected area twice weekly.

🟦 **AVAILABLE FORMS/COST**
• Shampoo—Top: 110 ml: **$22.26**

UNLABELED USES: Not known.

CONTRAINDICATIONS: Acutely inflamed lesions, hypersensitivity to chloroxine or any one of its components.

PREGNANCY AND LACTATION:
Pregnancy category C; excretion into breast milk unknown

SIDE EFFECTS
Discoloration of light hair, skin irritation, burning

SERIOUS REACTIONS
• None known.

SPECIAL CONSIDERATIONS

PATIENT/FAMILY EDUCATION
• Improvement may not occur for 14 days

---

chlorpheniramine
(klor-fen-ir´a-meen)
Rx: Chlor-Phen, Prohist-8
OTC: Aller-Chlor,
Chlo-Amine, Chlorate,
Chlor-Trimeton, Pfeiffer's
Allergy, Teldrin
Combinations
  Rx: with codeine (Codeprex);
    with hydrocodone (Tussionex); with phenylephrine
    and pyrilamine (Rynaton);
    with phenylpropanolamine
    (Ornade, Resaid S.R.); with
    pseudoephedrine (Deconamine, Fedahist)
  OTC: with pseudoephedrine
    (Chlor-Trimeton, Dorcol
    Children's Cold Formula
    Liquid, Fedahist)
Chemical Class: Alkylamine
derivative
Therapeutic Class: Antihistamine

CLINICAL PHARMACOLOGY
Mechanism of Action: A propylamine derivative antihistamine that competes with histamine for histamine receptor sites on cells in the blood vessels, gastrointestinal (GI) tract, and respiratory tract. *Therapeutic Effect:* Inhibits symptoms associated with seasonal allergic rhinitis such as increased mucus production and sneezing.

Pharmacokinetics
Well absorbed after PO and parenteral administration. Food delays absorption. Widely distributed. Metabolized in liver. Primarily excreted in urine. Not removed by dialysis. **Half-life:** 20 hrs.

INDICATIONS AND DOSAGES
Allergic rhinitis, common cold
PO
Adults, Elderly. 4 mg q6-8h or 8-12 mg (sustained-release) q8-12h. Maximum: 24 mg/day.
Children 12 yrs and older. 4 mg q6-8h or 8 mg (sustained-release) q12h. Maximum: 24 mg/day.
Children 6-11 yrs. 2 mg q4-6h. Maximum: 12 mg/day.
IM/IV/SC
Adults, Elderly. 5-40 mg as a single dose. Maximum: 40 mg/day.
SC
Children 6 yrs and older. 87.5 mcg/kg or 2.5 mg/m2 4 times/day.

AVAILABLE FORMS/COST
• Cap, Gel, Sus Action—Oral: 8 mg, 100's: **$6.25-$10.95**; 12 mg, 100's: **$4.20-$14.60**
• Sol, Inj-IV: 10 mg/ml, 1 ml: **$0.40**
• Syr—Oral: 2 mg/5 ml, 120, 480 ml: **$2.49-$3.60**/120 ml
• Tab-Oral: 4 mg, 100's: **$0.68-$13.20**
• Tab, Chewable—Oral: 2 mg, 96's: **$14.80**
• Tab, Sus Action—Oral: 8 mg, 100's: **$11.53-$22.31**; 12 mg, 100's: **$35.78**; 16 mg, 12's: **$6.77**

CONTRAINDICATIONS: Hypersensitivity to chlorpheniramine or its components

PREGNANCY AND LACTATION:
Pregnancy category B

SIDE EFFECTS
Frequent

Drowsiness, dizziness, muscular weakness, hypotension, dry mouth, nose, throat, and lips, urinary retention, thickening of bronchial secretions

Elderly: Sedation, dizziness, hypotension

Occasional

Epigastric distress, flushing, visual or hearing disturbances, paresthesia, diaphoresis, chills

SERIOUS REACTIONS

• Children may experience dominant paradoxical reactions, including restlessness, insomnia, euphoria, nervousness, and tremors.

• Overdosage in children may result in hallucinations, seizures, and death.

• Hypersensitivity reaction, such as eczema, pruritus, rash, cardiac disturbances, and photosensitivity, may occur.

• Overdosage may vary from CNS depression, including sedation, apnea, hypotension, cardiovascular collapse, or death to severe paradoxical reaction, such as hallucinations, tremor, and seizures.

SPECIAL CONSIDERATIONS

• More potent antihistamine than nonsedating agents (e.g., fexofenidine), good first-line choice for allergic rhinitis

PATIENT/FAMILY EDUCATION

• Tolerance develops to sedation with chronic use

chlorpromazine
(klor-proe'ma-zeen)

Rx: Thorazine

Chemical Class: Aliphatic phenothiazine derivative

Therapeutic Class: Antiemetic; antipsychotic

CLINICAL PHARMACOLOGY

Mechanism of Action: A phenothiazine that blocks dopamine neurotransmission at postsynaptic dopamine receptor sites. Possesses strong anticholinergic, sedative, and antiemetic effects; moderate extrapyramidal effects; and slight antihistamine action. *Therapeutic Effect:* Relieves nausea and vomiting; improves psychotic consitions; controls intractable hiccups and porphyria.

Pharmacokinetics

Rapidly absorbed after oral or IM administration. Protein binding: 92%-97%. Metabolized in the liver. Excreted in urine. **Half-life:** 6 hr.

INDICATIONS AND DOSAGES
Severe nausea or vomiting

PO

Adults, Elderly. 10–25 mg q4–6h.

Children. 0.5–1 mg/kg q4–6h.

IM, IV

Adults, Elderly. 25–50 mg q4–6h.

Children. 0.5–1 mg/kg q6–8h.

Rectal

Adults, Elderly. 50–100 mg q6–8h.

Children. 1 mg/kg q6–8h.

Psychotic disorders

PO

Adults, Elderly. 30–800 mg/day in 1–4 divided doses.

Children older than 6 mo. 0.5–1 mg/kg q4–6h.

IM, IV

Adults, Elderly. Initially, 25 mg; may repeat in 1–4 hr. May gradually increase to 400 mg q4–6h. Maximum: 300–800 mg/day.

Children older than 6 mo. 0.5–1 mg/kg q6–8h. Maximum: 75 mg/day for children 5–12 yr; 40 mg/day for children younger than 5 yr.

Intractable hiccups
PO, IV, IM

Adults. 25–50 mg 3 times a day.

Porphyria
PO

Adults. 25-50 mg 3-4 times a day.

IM

Adults, Elderly. 25 mg 3-4 times a day.

$ AVAILABLE FORMS/COST
• Conc—Oral: 30 mg/ml, 120 ml: **$5.31-$17.66**; 100 mg/ml, 240 ml: **$20.12-$192.20**
• Sol, Inj-IM, IV: 25 mg/ml, 1 ml: **$1.80-$4.18**
• Supp—Rect: 25 mg, 100's: **$5.91**; 100 mg, 12's: **$59.75**
• Syrup-Oral: 10 mg/5 ml, 120 ml: **$15.95**
• Tab-Oral: 10 mg, 100's: **$5.34-$29.94**; 25 mg, 100's: **$3.00-$62.81**; 50 mg, 100's: **$4.00-$75.40**; 100 mg, 100's: **$7.00-$97.00**; 200 mg, 100's: **$10.00-$100.00**

UNLABELED USES: Treatment of choreiform movement of Huntington's disease

CONTRAINDICATIONS: Comatose states, myelosuppression, severe cardiovascular disease, severe CNS depression, subcortical brain damage

PREGNANCY AND LACTATION: Pregnancy category C; enters breast milk in small concentrations; report of drowsy and lethargic infant who consumed milk with 92 ng/ml concentration

SIDE EFFECTS

Frequent

Somnolence, blurred vision, hypotension, color vision or night vision disturbances, dizziness, decreased sweating, constipation, dry mouth, nasal congestion

Occasional

Urinary retention, photosensitivity, rash, decreased sexual function, swelling or pain in breasts, weight gain, nausea, vomiting, abdominal pain, tremors

SERIOUS REACTIONS

• Extrapyramidal symptoms appear to be dose related and are divided into three categories: akathisia (including inability to sit still, tapping of feet), parkinsonian symptoms (such as masklike face, tremors, shuffling gait, hypersalivation), and acute dystonias (including torticollis, opisthotonos, and oculogyric crisis). A dystonic reaction may also produce diaphoresis and pallor.

• Tardive dyskinesia, including tongue protrusion, puffing of the cheeks, and puckering of the mouth is a rare reaction that may be irreversible.

• Abrupt discontinuation after long-term therapy may precipitate nausea, vomiting, gastritis, dizziness, and tremors.

• Blood dyscrasias, particularly agranulocytosis and mild leukopenia, may occur.

• Chlorpromazine may lower the seizure threshold.

INTERACTIONS

Drugs

▣ *Amodiaquine, chloroquine, sulfadoxine-pyrimethamine:* Increased chlorpromazine concentrations

▣ *Anticholinergics:* May inhibit neuroleptic response; excess anticholinergic effects

3 *Antidepressants:* Potential for increased therapeutic and toxic effects from increased levels of both drugs

3 *Barbiturates:* Decreased neuroleptic levels

3 *Clonidine, guanadrel, guanethidine:* Severe hypotensive episodes possible

3 *Epinephrine:* Blunted pressor response to epinephrine

3 *Ethanol:* Additive CNS depression

2 *Levodopa:* Inhibited antiparkinsonian effect of levodopa

3 *Lithium:* Lowered levels of both drugs, rarely neurotoxicity in acute mania

3 *Narcotic analgesics:* Hypotension and increased CNS depression

3 *Orphenadrine:* Lower neuroleptic concentrations, excessive anticholinergic effects

3 *Propranolol:* Increased plasma levels of both drugs with accentuated responses

Labs

• *False decrease:* 5-HIAA, vitamin B$_{12}$
• *Interference:* 17-ketogenic steroids
• *False increase:* Urine bilirubin, cholesterol, urine porphobilinogen, CSF protein, urine protein
• *False positive:* Ferric chloride test, guiacols spot test, phenylketones

SPECIAL CONSIDERATIONS
PATIENT/FAMILY EDUCATION

• Orthostasis on rising, especially in elderly
• Avoid hot tubs; hot showers; tub baths
• Meticulous oral hygiene; frequent rinsing of mouth, sugarless gum for dry mouth
• Use a sunscreen and sunglasses
• Urine may turn pink or red

---

chlorpropamide
(klor-pro′pa-mide)
Rx: Diabinese
Chemical Class: Sulfonylurea (1st generation)
Therapeutic Class: Antidiabetic; hypoglycemic

CLINICAL PHARMACOLOGY
Mechanism of Action: A first-generation sulfonylurea that promotes release of insulin from beta cells of pancreas. *Therapeutic Effect:* Lowers blood glucose concentration.

Pharmacokinetics
Rapidly absorbed from the gastrointestinal (GI) tract. Protein binding: 60%-90%. Extensively metabolized in liver. Excreted primarily urine. Removed by hemodialysis. **Half-life:** 30-42 hrs.

INDICATIONS AND DOSAGES
Diabetes mellitus, combination therapy
PO
Adults. Initially, 250 mg once a day. Maintenance: 250-500 mg once a day. Maximum: 750 mg/day.
Elderly. Initially, 100-125 mg once a day. Maintenance: 100-250 mg once a day. Increase or decrease by 50-125 mg a day for 3-5 day intervals.

Renal function impairment
Not recommended.

$ AVAILABLE FORMS/COST
• Tab-Oral: 100 mg, 100's: **$4.50-$46.60**; 250 mg, 100's: **$13.40-$98.46**

UNLABELED USES: Neurogenic diabetes insipidus
CONTRAINDICATIONS: Diabetic complications, such as ketosis, aci-

dosis, and diabetic coma, severe liver or renal impairment, sole therapy for type 1 diabetes mellitus, or hypersensitivity to sulfonylureas

PREGNANCY AND LACTATION: Pregnancy category D; inappropriate for use during pregnancy due to inadequate blood glucose control, potential for prolonged neonatal hypoglycemia, and risk of congenital abnormalities; insulin is the drug of choice for control of blood sugars during pregnancy; breast milk reported at 17% of plasma; the potential for neonatal hypoglycemia dictates caution in nursing mothers

SIDE EFFECTS

Frequent

Headache, upper respiratory tract infection

Occasional

Sinusitis, myalgia (muscle aches), pharyngitis, aggravated diabetes mellitus

SERIOUS REACTIONS

• Possible increased risk of cardiovascular mortality with this class of drugs.

• Overdosage can cause severe hypoglycemia prolonged by extended half-life.

INTERACTIONS

Drugs

⬛ *Anabolic steroids, Chloramphenicol, Fibric acid derivatives, MAOIs, Salicylates, Sulfonamides:* Enhanced hypoglycemic effect

⚠ *Ethanol:* Altered glycemic control, most commonly hypoglycemia; disulfiram-like reaction may occur

⬛ *Halofenate:* Increased sulfonylurea concentrations

➋ *NSAIDs:* Enhanced hypoglycemic effect

⬛ *Thiazide diuretics:* Increased glucose concentrations, may increase dose requirements

Labs

• *False increase:* Serum calcium

• Due to potential for prolonged hypoglycemia, other sulfonylureas should be considered before trying chlorpropamide (especially in the elderly)

PATIENT/FAMILY EDUCATION

• Multiple drug interactions, including alcohol and salicylates

• Symptoms of hypoglycemia: tingling lips/tongue, nausea, confusion, fatigue, sweating, hunger, visual changes (spots)

MONITORING PARAMETERS

• Self-monitored blood glucose; glycosolated hemoglobin q3-6 mo

---

chlorthalidone
(klor-thal′i-doan)

Rx: Hygroton, Thalitone
Combinations
  Rx: with atenolol (Tenoretic); with clonidine (Combipres, Chlorpres); with reserpine (Demi-Regroton, Regroton)
Chemical Class: Phthalimidine derivative
Therapeutic Class: Antihypertensive; diuretic, thiazide

CLINICAL PHARMACOLOGY

Mechanism of Action: A thiazide diuretic that blocks reabsorption of sodium, potassium, and water at the distal convoluted tubule; also decreases plasma and extracellular fluid volume and peripheral vascular resistance. *Therapeutic Effect:* Produces diuresis; lowers BP.

Pharmacokinetics

Route	Onset	Peak	Duration
PO (diuretic)	2 hr	2–6 hr	Up to 36 hr

Rapidly absorbed from the GI tract. Excreted unchanged in urine. **Half-life:** 35–50 hr. Onset of antihypertensive effect: 3–4 days; optimal therapeutic effect: 3–4 wk.

INDICATIONS AND DOSAGES
Hypertension, edema
PO
Adults. 25–100 mg/day or 100 mg 3 times a week.
Elderly. Initially, 12.5–25 mg/day or every other day.

AVAILABLE FORMS/COST
• Tab-Oral: 15 mg, 100's: **$84.78**; 25 mg, 100's: **$5.50-$23.40**; 50 mg, 100's: **$6.45-$24.55**; 100 mg, 100's: **$8.45-$148.86**

CONTRAINDICATIONS: Anuria, history of hypersensitivity to sulfonamides or thiazide diuretics, renal decompensation

PREGNANCY AND LACTATION: Pregnancy category B; therapy for preexisting hypertension can be continued throughout pregnancy with minimal risk; initiating for simple edema not recommended; few unequivocal indications for diuretic therapy in pregnancy except for pulmonary edema or congestive heart failure; compatible with breast-feeding

SIDE EFFECTS
Expected
Increase in urinary frequency and urine volume
Frequent
Potassium depletion (rarely produces symptoms)
Occasional
Anorexia, impotence, diarrhea, orthostatic hypotension, GI disturbances, photosensitivity
Rare
Rash

SERIOUS REACTIONS
• Vigorous diuresis may lead to profound water and electrolyte depletion, resulting in hypokalemia, hyponatremia, and dehydration.
• Acute hypotensive episodes may occur.
• Hyperglycemia may occur during prolonged therapy.
• Overdose can lead to lethargy and coma without changes in electrolytes or hydration.

INTERACTIONS
Drugs
❷ *Angiotensin-converting enzyme inhibitors:* Risk of postural hypotension when added to ongoing diuretic therapy; more common with loop diuretics; first dose hypotension possible in patients with sodium depletion or hypovolemia due to diuretics or sodium restriction; hypotensive response is usually transient; hold diuretic day of first dose
❸ *Calcium:* Increased risk of milk-alkali syndrome
❸ *Carbenoxolone:* Additive potassium wasting, severe hypokalemia
❸ *Cholestyramine, Colestipol:* Reduced absorption
❸ *Corticosteroids:* Concomitant therapy may result in excessive potassium loss
❸ *Diazoxide:* Hyperglycemia
❸ *Digitalis glycosides:* Diuretic-induced hypokalemia increases risk of digitalis toxicity
❸ *Hypoglycemic agents:* Increased dosage requirements due to increased glucose levels
❸ *Lithium:* Increased lithium levels, potential toxicity
❸ *Methotrexate:* Increased risk of bone marrow depression
❸ *Nonsteroidal antiinflammatory drugs:* Concurrent use may reduce diuretic and antihypertensive effects

Labs
• False decrease: urine esriol

SPECIAL CONSIDERATIONS
• Doses above 25 mg provide no further blood pressure reduction, but are more likely to induce metabolic disturbance (i.e., hypokalemia, hyperuricemia, etc.)
• May protect against osteoporotic hip fractures
• Loop diuretics or metolazone more effective if CrCl <40-50 ml/min

PATIENT/FAMILY EDUCATION
• Will increase urination temporarily (approximately 3 wk); take early in the day to prevent sleep disturbance
• May cause sensitivity to sunlight; avoid prolonged exposure to the sun and other ultraviolet light
• May cause gout attacks; notify clinician if sudden joint pain occurs

MONITORING PARAMETERS
• Weight, urine output, serum electrolytes, BUN, creatinine, CBC, uric acid, glucose, lipids

---

chlorzoxazone
(klor-zox'a-zone)
Rx: Parafon Forte DSC, Remular-S, Paraflex
Chemical Class: Benzoxazole derivative
Therapeutic Class: Skeletal muscle relaxant

CLINICAL PHARMACOLOGY
Mechanism of Action: A skeletal muscle relaxant that inhibits transmission of reflexes at the spinal cord level. *Therapeutic Effect:* Relieves muscle spasticity.

Pharmacokinetics
Readily absorbed from the gastrointestinal (GI) tract. Metabolized in liver. Primarily excreted in urine. **Half-life:** 1.1 hrs.

INDICATIONS AND DOSAGES
Musculoskeletal pain
PO
Adults, Elderly. 250-500 mg 3-4 times/day. Maximum: 750 mg 3-4 day.
Children. 20 mg/kg/day in 3- 4 divided doses.

AVAILABLE FORMS/COST
• Tab-Oral: 250 mg, 100's: **$5.25-$30.00**; 500 mg, 100's: **$9.75-$171.35**

CONTRAINDICATIONS: Hypersensitivity to chlorzoxazone or any one of its components.

PREGNANCY AND LACTATION: Pregnancy category C

SIDE EFFECTS
Frequent
Drowsiness, fever, headache
Occasional
Nausea, vomiting, stomach cramps, rash

SERIOUS REACTIONS
• Overdosage results in nausea, vomiting, diarrhea, and hypotension.

SPECIAL CONSIDERATIONS
PATIENT/FAMILY EDUCATION
• Potential for psychologic dependency

cholestyramine
(koe-less-tir'a-meen)

Rx: Questran, Questran Light, LoCHOLEST, LoCHOLEST Light, Preva Lite
Chemical Class: Bile acid sequestrant
Therapeutic Class: Antilipemic; bile acid sequestrant

CLINICAL PHARMACOLOGY
Mechanism of Action: An antihyperlipoproteinemic that binds with bile acids in the intestine, forming an insoluble complex. Binding results in partial removal of bile acid from enterohepatic circulation. *Therapeutic Effect:* Removes LDL cholesterol from plasma.

Pharmacokinetics
Not absorbed from the GI tract. Decreases in serum LDL apparent in 5 to 7 days and in serum cholesterol in 1 mo. Serum cholesterol returns to baseline levels about 1 mo after drug is discontinued.

INDICATIONS AND DOSAGES
Primary hypercholesterolemia
PO
Adults, Elderly. 3–4 g 3–4 times a day. Maximum: 16–32 g/day in 2–4 divided doses.
Children older than 10 yr. 2 g/day. Maximum: 8 g/day in 2 or more divided doses.
Children 10 yr and younger. Initially, 2 g/day. Range: 1–4 g/day.
Pruritis
PO
Adults, Elderly. 4 g 1-2 times a day. Maintenance: Up to 24 g/day in divided doses.

Ⓢ AVAILABLE FORMS/COST
• Powder—Oral: 4 g/9 g, 60 pkts: **$48.68-$167.46**; 4 g/9 g, 378 g: **$46.58-$73.34** (Questran)

• Powder, Reconst—Oral: 4 g/5 g, 60 pkts: **$79.49-$168.38**; 4 g/5 g, 210 and 231 g: **$46.68-$55.45**/210 g (Questran Light)

UNLABELED USES: Treatment of diarrhea (due to bile acids), hyperoxaluria

CONTRAINDICATIONS: Complete biliary obstruction, hypersensitivity to cholestyramine or tartrazine (frequently seen in aspirin hypersensitivity)

PREGNANCY AND LACTATION: Pregnancy category C

SIDE EFFECTS
Frequent
Constipation (may lead to fecal impaction), nausea, vomiting, abdominal pain, indigestion
Occasional
Diarrhea, belching, bloating, headache, dizziness
Rare
Gallstones, peptic ulcer disease, malabsorption syndrome

SERIOUS REACTIONS
• GI tract obstruction, hyperchloremic acidosis, and osteoporosis secondary to calcium excretion may occur.
• High dosage may interfere with fat absorption, resulting in steatorrhea.

INTERACTIONS
Drugs
🔳 *Acetaminophen, Amiodarone, Corticosteroids, Diclofenac, Digitalis glycosides, Furosemide, Methotrexate, Metronidazole, Thiazide diuretics, Thyroid hormones, Valproic acid:* Cholestyramine reduces interacting drug concentrations and probably subsequent therapeutic response

🔳 *Oral anticoagulants:* Inhibition of hypoprothrombinemic response; colestipol might be less likely to interact

SPECIAL CONSIDERATIONS
• Avoid use in patients with elevated triglycerides
PATIENT/FAMILY EDUCATION
• Give all other medications 1 hr before or 4 hr after cholestyramine to avoid poor absorption
• Mix drug with applesauce or noncarbonated beverage (2-6 oz), let stand for 2 min; do not take dry

---

choline magnesium trisalicylate

(koe′leen mag-nees′ee-um tri-sal′eh-cye′late)

Rx: Trilisate, Tricosal
Chemical Class: Salicylate derivative
Therapeutic Class: NSAID; nonnarcotic analgesic

CLINICAL PHARMACOLOGY

Mechanism of Action: A nonsteroidal salicylate that inhibits prostaglandin synthesis and acts on the hypothalamus heat-regulating center. *Therapeutic Effect:* Reduces inflammatory response and intensity of pain stimulus reaching sensory nerve endings.

Pharmacokinetics

Rapidly absorbed from gastrointestinal (GI) tract Oral route onset 1 hour, peak 2 hours and duration 9-17 hours. Protein binding: High. Widely distributed. Excreted in the urine. **Half-life:** 2-3 hrs.

INDICATIONS AND DOSAGES

Analgesic, acute painful shoulder, anti-inflammatory, antipyretic
PO
Adults, Elderly. Initially, 500 mg – 1500 mg q8-12h, then 1-4.5 g/day.
Children less than 37 kg. 50 mg/kg/day in divided doses.

§ **AVAILABLE FORMS/COST**
• Liq—Oral: 500 mg/5 ml (293 mg-362 mg), 240 ml: **$28.68-$44.05**
• Tab-Oral: 500 mg (293 mg-362 mg), 100's: **$25.00-$107.91**; 750 mg (440 mg-544 mg), 100's: **$30.00-$128.64**; 1000 mg (587 mg-725 mg), 100's: **$38.00-$133.95**

CONTRAINDICATIONS: Allergy to tartrazine dye, bleeding disorders, GI bleeding or ulceration, history of hypersensitivity to choline magnesium trisalicylate, aspirin, or NSAIDs.

PREGNANCY AND LACTATION: Pregnancy category C; excreted into breast milk

SIDE EFFECTS

Side effects appear less frequently with short-term treatment.

Occasional

Nausea, dyspepsia (heartburn, indigestion, epigastric pain), tinnitus

Rare

Anorexia, headache vomiting, flatulence, dizziness, somnolence, insomnia, fatigue, hearing impairment

SERIOUS REACTIONS

• High doses may produce GI bleeding.
• Overdosage may be characterized by ringing in ears, generalized pruritus (may be severe), headache, dizziness, flushing, tachycardia, hyperventilation, sweating, and thirst.

INTERACTIONS

Labs

• *False increase:* Serum bicarbonate, CSF protein, serum theophylline
• *False decrease:* Urine cocaine, urine estrogen, serum glucose, urine 17-hydroxycorticosteroids, urine opiates
• *False positive:* Ferric chloride test

SPECIAL CONSIDERATIONS
• Consider for patients with GI intolerance to aspirin or patients in whom interference with normal platelet function by aspirin or other NSAIDs is undesirable

PATIENT/FAMILY EDUCATION
• Solution may be mixed with fruit juice just before administration; do not mix with antacid

MONITORING PARAMETERS
• Liver and renal function studies, stool for occult blood and hct if long-term therapy

---

ciclopirox
(sye-kloe-peer' ox)
Rx: Loprox, Penlac, Nail Lacquer
Chemical Class: N-hydroxypyridinone derivative
Therapeutic Class: Antifungal

CLINICAL PHARMACOLOGY
Mechanism of Action: An antifungal that inhibits the transport of essential elements in the fungal cell, thereby interfering with biosynthesis in fungi. *Therapeutic Effect:* Results in fungal cell death.

Pharmacokinetics
Absorbed through intact skin. Distributed to epidermis, dermis, including hair, hair follicles, and sebaceous glands. Protein binding: 98%. Primarily excreted in urine and to a lesser extent in feces. **Half-life:** 1.7 hrs.

INDICATIONS AND DOSAGES
Tinea pedis
Topical
Adults, Elderly, Children 10 yrs and older. Apply 2 times a day until signs and symptoms significantly improve.

Tinea cruris, Tinea corporis
Topical
Adults, Elderly, Children 10 yrs and older. Apply 2 times a day until signs and symptoms significantly improve.

Onychomycosis
Topical (solution)
Adults, Elderly, Children 10 yrs and older. Apply to the affected area (nails) daily. Remove with alcohol every 7 days.

Seborrheic dermatitis
Shampoo
Adults, Elderly, Children 10 yrs and older. Apply to affected scalp areas 2 times a day, in the morning and evening for 4 weeks.

$ AVAILABLE FORMS/COST
• Cre—Top: 0.77%, 15, 30, 90 g: **$47.13**/30 g
• Gel—Top: 0.77%, 30, 45, 100 g: **$47.13**/30 g
• Lotion—Top: 0.77%, 30, 60 ml: **$47.39**/30 ml
• Sol—Top, Nail Laquer: 8%, 3.3, 6.6 ml: **$59.94**/3.3 ml

CONTRAINDICATIONS: Hypersensitivity to ciclopirox or any one of its components

PREGNANCY AND LACTATION: Pregnancy category B; excretion into breast milk unknown

SIDE EFFECTS
Rare
Topical: Irritation, burning, redness, pain at the site of application

SERIOUS REACTIONS
• None known.

SPECIAL CONSIDERATIONS
• Use of nail lacquer requires monthly removal of the unattached, infected nails by a health care professional; in clinical trials <12% of patients achieved a clear or almost clear nail

PATIENT/FAMILY EDUCATION

• *Cream/gel/lotion:*
• Continue medication for several days after condition clears
• Consult prescriber if no improvement after 4 wk of treatment
• *Nail lacquer:*
• 48 weeks of daily applications considered full treatment, may take 6 mo before see improvement

---

cidofovir
(ci-dah'fo-veer)
Rx: Vistide
Chemical Class: Acyclic purine nucleoside analog
Therapeutic Class: Antiviral

CLINICAL PHARMACOLOGY

Mechanism of Action: An anti-infective that inhibits viral DNA synthesis by incorporating itself into the growing viral DNA chain. *Therapeutic Effect:* Suppresses replication of cytomegalovirus (CMV).

Pharmacokinetics

Protein binding: less than 6%. Excreted primarily unchanged in urine. Effect of hemodialysis unknown. Elimination **half-life:** 1.4-3.8 hr.

INDICATIONS AND DOSAGES

CMV retinitis in patients with AIDS (in combination with probenecid)

IV infusion

Adults. Induction: Usual dosage, 5 mg/kg at constant rate over 1 hr once weekly for 2 consecutive wk. Give 2 g of PO probenecid 3 hr before cidofovir dose, and then give 1 g 2 hr and 8 hr after completion of the 1-hr cidofovir infusion (total of 4 g). In addition, give 1 L of 0.9% NaCl over 1-2 hr immediately before the cidofovir infusion. If tolerated, a second liter may be infused over 1-3 hr at the start of the infusion or immediately afterward. Maintenance: 5 mg/kg cidofovir at constant rate over 1 hr once every 2 wk.

Dosage in renal impairment

Dosages are modified based on creatinine clearance.

Creatinine Clearance	Induction Dose	Maintenance Dose
41-55 ml/min	2 mg/kg	2 mg/kg
30-40 ml/min	1.5 mg/kg	1.5 mg/kg
20-29 ml/min	1 mg/kg	1 mg/kg
19 ml/min or less	0.5 mg/kg	0.5 mg/kg

§ AVAILABLE FORMS/COST

• Sol, Inj-IV: 75 mg/ml; 5 ml: **$888.00**

UNLABELED USES: Treatment of ganciclovir-resistant CMV, foscarnet-resistant CMV, adenovirus, and acyclovir-resistant herpes simplex virus or varicella-zoster virus

CONTRAINDICATIONS: Direct intraocular injection, history of clinically severe hypersensitivity to probenecid or other sulfa-containing drugs, hypersensitivity to cidofovir, renal function impairment (serum creatinine level greater than 1.5 mg/dl, creatinine clearance of 55 ml/min or less, or urine protein level greater than 100 mg/dl)

PREGNANCY AND LACTATION: Pregnancy category C

SIDE EFFECTS

Frequent

Nausea, vomiting (65%), fever (57%), asthenia (46%), rash (30%), diarrhea (27%), headache (27%), alopecia (25%), chills (24%), anorexia (22%), dyspnea (22%), abdominal pain (17%)

SERIOUS REACTIONS

• Serious adverse reactions may include proteinuria (80%), nephrotoxicity (53%), neutropenia (31%), elevated serum creatinine levels

(29%), infection (24%), anemia (20%), ocular hypotony (a decrease in intraocular pressure, 12%), and pneumonia (9%).

• Concurrent use of probenecid may produce a hypersensitivity reaction characterized by a rash, fever, chills, and anaphylaxis.

• Acute renal failure occurs rarely.

INTERACTIONS
Drugs
3 *Aminoglycosides:* Additive nephrotoxicity

3 *Amphotericin B:* Additive nephrotoxicity

3 *Foscarnet:* Additive nephrotoxicity

3 *Pentamidine:* Additive nephrotoxicity (IV route only)

SPECIAL CONSIDERATIONS
• Concurrent high-dose PO probenecid plus saline hydration reduces nephrotoxicity; procedure: probenecid 2 g 3 hr prior to INF, then 1 g at 2 and 8 hr after INF; normal saline 1000 ml over 1 hr immediately prior to INF

MONITORING PARAMETERS
• Renal function, urinalysis (especially serum creatinine and urine protein prior to each dose), and blood chemistry (to include serum uric acid, phosphate, and bicarbonate), white counts with differential during intravenous therapy

---

cilostazol
(sil-os'tah-zol)
Rx: Pletal
Chemical Class: Quinolinone derivative
Therapeutic Class: Hemorrheologic agent

CLINICAL PHARMACOLOGY
Mechanism of Action: A phosphodiesterase III inhibitor that inhibits platelet aggregation. Dilates vascular beds with greatest dilation in femoral beds. *Therapeutic Effect:* Improves walking distance in patients with intermittent claudication.

Pharmacokinetics
Moderately absorbed from the GI tract. Protein binding: 95%–98%. Extensively metabolized in the liver. Excreted primarily in the urine and, to a lesser extent, in the feces. Not removed by hemodialysis. **Half-life:** 11–13 hr. Therapeutic effect is usually noted in 2–4 wk but may take as long as 12 wk.

INDICATIONS AND DOSAGES
Intermittent claudication
PO
Adults, Elderly. 100 mg twice a day at least 30 min before or 2 hr after meals.

AVAILABLE FORMS/COST
• Tab, Coated—Oral: 50 mg, 100 mg, 60's; all: **$112.60**

CONTRAINDICATIONS: CHF of any severity

PREGNANCY AND LACTATION: Pregnancy category C; excreted in breast milk

SIDE EFFECTS
Frequent (34%–10%)
Headache, diarrhea, palpitations, dizziness, pharyngitis

Occasional (7%–3%)
Nausea, rhinitis, back pain, peripheral edema, dyspepsia, abdominal pain, tachycardia, cough, flatulence, myalgia
Rare (2%–1%)
Leg cramps, paresthesia, rash, vomiting

SERIOUS REACTIONS
• Signs and symptoms of overdose are noted by severe headache, diarrhea, hypotension, and cardiac arrhythmias.

INTERACTIONS
Drugs
▣ *Diltiazem:* Increase cilostazol concentrations
▣ *Erythromycin, azole antifungals, fluoxetine, nefazadone, and sertraline:* as CYP3A4 or CYP2C19 inhibitors, may increase cilostazol levels; clinical effects unknown
▣ *Omeprazole:* Increase cilostazol concentrations
▣ *Foods: Grapefruit juice:* Increases cilostazol levels; *High fat:* increases absorption of cilostazol (80% increase of Cmax, 25% increase of AUC)

SPECIAL CONSIDERATIONS
• Cilostazol has been shown, in a multicenter, randomized, double-blind study (DPPARA2), to be superior to pentoxifylline for treatment of claudication symptoms

PATIENT/FAMILY EDUCATION
• Take ½ hr before meal or 2 hr after meal

MONITORING PARAMETERS
• Beneficial effects usually seen in 2 to 4 wk, may take up to 12 wk

---

cimetidine
(sye-met'i-deen)
Rx: Tagamet
OTC: Tagamet HB
Chemical Class: Imidazole derivative
Therapeutic Class: Antiulcer agent

CLINICAL PHARMACOLOGY
Mechanism of Action: An antiulcer agent and gastric acid secretion inhibitor that inhibits histamine action at histamine 2 receptor sites of parietal cells. *Therapeutic Effect:* Inhibits gastric acid secretion during fasting, at night, or when stimulated by food, caffeine, or insulin.

Pharmacokinetics
Well absorbed from the GI tract. Protein binding: 15%–20%. Widely distributed. Metabolized in the liver. Primarily excreted in urine. Not removed by hemodialysis. **Half-life:** 2 hrs; increased with impaired renal function.

INDICATIONS AND DOSAGES
Active ulcer
PO
Adults, Elderly. 300 mg 4 times a day or 400 mg twice a day or 800 mg at bedtime.
IM, IV
Adults, Elderly. 300 mg q6h or 150 mg as single dose followed by 37.5 mg/hr continuous infusion.
Prevention of duodenal ulcer
PO
Adults, Elderly. 400–800 mg at bedtime.
Gastric hypersecretory secretions
PO, IV, IM
Adults, Elderly. 300–600 mg q6h. Maximum: 2,400 mg/day.
Children. 20–40 mg/kg/day in divided doses q6h.

Infants. 10–20 mg/kg/day in divided doses q6–12h.
Neonates. 5–10 mg/kg/day in divided doses q8–12h.

Gastrointestinal reflux disease
PO
Adults, Elderly. 800 mg twice a day or 400 mg 4 times a day for 12 wks.

OTC use
PO
Adults, Elderly. 100 mg up to 30 min before meals. Maximum: 2 doses/day.

Prevention of upper GI bleeding
IV infusion
Adults, Elderly. 50 mg/hr.

Dosage in renal impairment
Dosage is based on a 300-mg dose in adults. Dosage interval is modified based on creatinine clearance.

Creatinine Clearance	Dosage Interval
greater than 40 ml/min	q6h
20–40 ml/min	q8h or decrease dose by 25%
less than 20 ml/min	q12h or decrease dose by 50%

Give after hemodialysis and q12h between dialysis sessions.

[$] **AVAILABLE FORMS/COST**
• Sol, Inj-IM, IV: 150 mg/2 ml: **$1.49-$3.32**
• Sol, Inj-IV: 300 mg/50 ml, 50 ml: **$3.12**
• Liq—Oral: 300 mg/5 ml, 240, 480 ml: **$79.80-$170.56**/480 ml
• Tab, Coated-Oral: 200 mg, 100's: **$9.90-$96.55** (OTC); 300 mg, 100's: **$76.00-$119.31**; 400 mg, 100's: **$126.86-$167.66**; 800 mg, 100's: **$158.95-$394.43**

UNLABELED USES: Prevention of aspiration pneumonia; treatment of acute urticaria, chronic warts, upper GI bleeding

CONTRAINDICATIONS: None known

PREGNANCY AND LACTATION: Pregnancy category B; excreted into breast milk and may accumulate; theoretically, adversely affects the nursing infant's gastric acidity, inhibits drug metabolism, and produces CNS stimulation—all not reported; compatible with breast-feeding

SIDE EFFECTS
Occasional (4%–2%)
Headache
Elderly and severely ill patients, patients with impaired renal function: Confusion, agitation, psychosis, depression, anxiety, disorientation, hallucinations. Effects reverse 3 to 4 days after discontinuance.
Rare (less than 2%)
Diarrhea, dizziness, somnolence, nausea, vomiting, gynecomastia, rash, impotence

SERIOUS REACTIONS
• Rapid IV administration may produce cardiac arrhythmias and hypotension.

INTERACTIONS
Drugs
[3] *Amiodarone, benzodiazepines; calcium channel blockers; amiodarone; cyclic antidepressants; carbamazepine; carmustine; chloramphenicol; cisapride; citalopram; clozapine; diltiazem; femoxidine; flecanide; glyburide; glipizide; labetolol; lidocaine; lomustine; melphalan; metoprolol; narcotic analgesics; moricizine; N-acetylprocainamide; nicotine; phenytoin; peridolol; praziquantel; procainamide; propafinone; propranolol; quinidine; tacrine; theophylline; tolbutamide:* Increased concentrations of interacting drugs with potential for toxicity

[3] *Ketoconazole, cefpodoxime, cefuroxime:* Reduced concentrations of interacting drugs

❷ *Warfarin:* Increased concentrations of interacting drugs with potential for toxicity
Labs
• *False positive:* Hemoccult
SPECIAL CONSIDERATIONS
• Generic formulations offer less costly alternative for patients not at risk for drug interactions
PATIENT/FAMILY EDUCATION
• Stagger doses of cimetidine and antacids

---

cinacalcet
(sin-a-cal'set)
Rx: Sensipar
Chemical Class: Calcimimetic agent
Therapeutic Class: Hyperparathyroidism (secondary)

CLINICAL PHARMACOLOGY
Mechanism of Action: A calcium receptor agonist that increases the sensitivity of the calcium-sensing receptor on the parathyroid gland to extracellular calcium, thus lowering the parathyroid hormone (PTH) level. *Therapeutic Effect:* Decreases serum calcium and PTH levels.
Pharmacokinetics
Extensively distributed after PO administration. Protein binding: 93%-97%. Rapidly and extensively metabolized by multiple enzymes. Primarily eliminated in urine with a lesser amount excreted in feces.
Half-life: 30-40 hr.
INDICATIONS AND DOSAGES
Hypercalcemia in parathyroid carcinoma
PO
Adults, Elderly. Initially, 30 mg twice a day. Titrate dosage sequentially (60 mg twice a day, 90 mg twice a day, and 90 mg 3-4 times a day) every 2-4 wk as needed to normalize serum calcium levels.

Secondary hyperparathyroidism in patients on dialysis
PO
Adults, Elderly. Initially, 30 mg once a day. Titrate dosage sequentially (60, 90, 120, and 180 mg once a day) every 2-4 wk.
CONTRAINDICATIONS: None known.
PREGNANCY AND LACTATION: Pregnancy category C; unknown if excreted into human milk, but excreted with high mild-to-plasma ratio in rats; not recommended in breast-feeding
SIDE EFFECTS
Frequent (31%-21%)
Nausea, vomiting, diarrhea
Occasional (15%-10%)
Myalgia, dizziness
Rare (7%-5%)
Asthenia, hypertension, anorexia, non-cardiac chest pain
SERIOUS REACTIONS
• Overdose may lead to hypocalcemia.
INTERACTIONS
Drugs
❸ *Flecainide, vinblastine, thioridazine, tricyclic antidepressants:* Inhibited metabolism by cinacalcet inhibition of CYP2D6, may require dosage reduction
❸ *Ketoconazole:* Increased cinacalcet levels by ketoconazole inhibition of CYP3A4, monitor PTH and calcium levels to determine if dosage adjustment indicated
SPECIAL CONSIDERATIONS
• Can be used alone or in combination with vitamin D sterols and/or phosphate binders
PATIENT/FAMILY EDUCATION
• Take with food or shortly after a meal. Do not divide tablets
MONITORING PARAMETERS
• Serum calcium and phosphorus within 1 week

• iPTH 1-4 weeks after initiation or dose adjustment
• Once maintenance dose established, serum calcium and phosphorus q month, iPTH q 1-3 months to target of 150-300 pg/mL

---

ciprofloxacin
(sip-ro-floks'a-sin)
Rx: Ciloxan (ophthalmic), Cipro, Cipro XR
Chemical Class: Fluoroquinolone derivative
Therapeutic Class: Antibiotic

CLINICAL PHARMACOLOGY
Mechanism of Action: A fluoroquinolone that inhibits the enzyme DNA gyrase in susceptible bacteria, interfering with bacterial cell replication. *Therapeutic Effect:* Bactericidal.
Pharmacokinetics
Well absorbed from the GI tract (food delays absorption). Protein binding: 20%-40%. Widely distributed (including to CSF). Metabolized in the liver to active metabolite. Primarily excreted in urine. Minimal removal by hemodialysis.
Half-life: 4-6 hr (increased in impaired renal function and the elderly).

INDICATIONS AND DOSAGES
Mild to moderate UTIs
PO
Adults, Elderly. 250 mg q12h.
IV
Adults, Elderly. 200 mg q12h.
Complicated UTIs, mild to moderate respiratory tract, bone, joint, skin and skin-structure infections; infectious diarrhea
PO
Adults, Elderly. 500 mg q12h.
IV
Adults, Elderly. 400 mg q12h.

Severe, complicated infections
PO
Adults, Elderly. 750 mg q12h.
IV
Adults, Elderly. 400 mg q12h.
Prostatitis
PO
Adults, Elderly. 500 mg q12h for 28 days.
Uncomplicated bladder infection
PO
Adults. 100 mg twice a day for 3 days.
Acute sinusitis
PO
Adults. 500 mg q12h.
Uncomplicated gonorrhea
PO
Adults. 250 mg as a single dose.
Cystic fibrosis
IV
Children. 30 mg/kg/day in 2-3 divided doses. Maximum: 1.2 g/day.
PO
Children. 40 mg/kg/day. Maximum: 2 g/day.
Corneal ulcer
Ophthalmic
Adults, Elderly. 2 drops q15min for 6 hr, then 2 drops q30min for the remainder of first day, 2 drops q1h on second day, and 2 drops q4h on days 3-14.
Conjunctivitis
Ophthalmic
Adults, Elderly. 1-2 drops q2h for 2 days, then 2 drops q4h for next 5 days.
Dosage in renal impairment
Dosage and frequency are modified based on creatinine clearance and the severity of the infection.

Creatinine Clearance	Dosage Interval
less than 30 ml/min	Usual dose q18-24h

Hemodialysis
250-500 mg q24h (after dialysis).

Peritoneal Dialysis

250-500 mg q24h (after dialysis).

$ **AVAILABLE FORMS/COST**

• Sol, Inj-IV: 200 mg/100 ml, 1's: **$15.61**; 400 mg/200 ml, 1's: **$30.01**
• Oint—Ophth: 0.3%, 3.5 g: **$54.00**
• Sol—Ophth: 0.3%, 2.5, 5, 10 ml: **$32.95-$53.78**/5 ml
• Powder, Reconst-Oral: 250 mg/5 ml, 100 ml: **$104.96**; 500 mg/5 ml, 100 ml: **$122.89**
• Tab-Oral: 100 mg, 6's: **$22.59**; 250 mg, 100's: **$495.59**; 500 mg, 100's: **$580.10**; 750 mg, 100's: **$432.70**
• Tab, Sus Action—Oral: 500 mg, 100's: **$866.25**; 1000 mg, 100's: **$986.25**

UNLABELED USES: Treatment of chancroid

CONTRAINDICATIONS: Hypersensitivity to ciprofloxacin or other quinolones; for ophthalmic administration: vaccinia, varicella, epithelial herpes simplex, keratitis, mycobacterial infection, fungal disease of ocular structure, use after uncomplicated removal of a foreign body.

PREGNANCY AND LACTATION: Pregnancy category C; appears in breast milk at levels similar to serum; allow 48 hr to elapse after last dose before resuming breastfeeding

SIDE EFFECTS

Frequent (5%-2%)

Nausea, diarrhea, dyspepsia, vomiting, constipation, flatulence, confusion, crystalluria

Ophthalmic: Burning, crusting in corner of eye

Occasional (less than 2%)

Abdominal pain or discomfort, headache, rash

Ophthalmic: Bad taste, sensation of something in eye, eyelid redness or itching

Rare (less than 1%)

Dizziness, confusion, tremors, hallucinations, hypersensitivity reaction, insomnia, dry mouth, paresthesia

SERIOUS REACTIONS

• Superinfection (especially enterococcal or fungal), nephropathy, cardiopulmonary arrest, chest pain, and cerebral thrombosis may occur.

• Hypersensitivity reactions, including photosensitivity (as evidenced by rash, pruritus, blisters, edema, and burning skin), have occurred in patients receiving fluoroquinolones.

• Arthropathy may occur if the drug is given to children younger than 18 years.

• Sensitization to the ophthalmic form of the drug may contraindicate later systemic use of ciprofloxacin.

INTERACTIONS

Drugs

🔳 *Aluminum:* Reduced absorption of ciprofloxacin; do not take within 4 hr of dose

🔳 *Antacids:* Reduced absorption of ciprofloxacin; do not take within 4 hr of dose

🔳 *Antipyrine:* Inhibits metabolism of antipyrine; increased plasma antipyrine level

🔳 *Caffeine:* Inhibits metabolism of caffeine; increased plasma caffeine level

🔳 *Calcium:* Reduced absorption of ciprofloxacin; do not take within 4 hr of dose

🔳 *Diazepam:* Inhibits metabolism of diazepam; increased plasma diazepam level

🔳 *Didanosine:* Markedly reduced absorption of ciprofloxacin; take ciprofloxacin 2 hr before didanosine

🔳 *Foscarnet:* Coadministration increases seizure risk

🔳 *Iron:* Reduced absorption of ciprofloxacin; do not take within 4 hr of dose

3 *Magnesium:* Reduced absorption of ciprofloxacin; do not take within 4 hr of dose

3 *Metoprolol:* Inhibits metabolism of metoprolol; increased plasma metoprolol level

3 *Pentoxifylline:* Inhibits metabolism of pentoxifylline; increased plasma pentoxifylline level

3 *Phenytoin:* Inhibits metabolism of phenytoin; increased plasma phenytoin level

3 *Propranolol:* Inhibits metabolism of propranolol; increased plasma propranolol level

3 *Ropinirole:* Inhibits metabolism of ropinirole; increased plasma ropinirole level

3 *Sodium bicarbonate:* Reduced absorption of ciprofloxacin; do not take within 4 hr of dose

3 *Sucralfate:* Reduced absorption of ciprofloxacin; do not take within 4 hr of dose

3 *Theobromine:* Inhibits metabolism of theobromine; increased plasma theobromine level

3 *Theophylline:* Inhibits metabolism of theophylline; cut maintenance theophylline dose in half during therapy with ciprofloxacin

3 *Warfarin:* Inhibits metabolism of warfarin; increases hypoprothrombinemic response to warfarin

3 *Zinc:* Reduced absorption of ciprofloxacin; do not take within 4 hr of dose

Labs

• *False increase:* Urine coproporphyrin I, coproporphyrin III, urine porphyrins

SPECIAL CONSIDERATIONS

• Reserve use for UTI to documented pseudomonal infection or complicated UTI

• Considered 1st-line therapy for otitis externa in diabetic patients

citalopram
(sy-tal'oh-pram)
Rx: Celexa
Chemical Class: Bicyclic phthalane derivative
Therapeutic Class: Antidepressant, selective serotonin reuptake inhibitor (SSRI)

CLINICAL PHARMACOLOGY
Mechanism of Action: A selective serotonin reuptake inhibitor that blocks the uptake of the neurotransmitter serotonin at CNS presynaptic neuronal membranes, increasing its availability at postsynaptic receptor sites. *Therapeutic Effect:* Relieves depression.

Pharmacokinetics
Well absorbed after PO administration. Protein binding: 80%. Primarily metabolized in the liver. Primarily excreted in feces with a lesser amount eliminated in urine. **Half-life:** 35 hr.

INDICATIONS AND DOSAGES
Depression
PO
Adults. Initially, 20 mg once a day in the morning or evening. May increase in 20-mg increments at intervals of no less than 1 wk. Maximum: 60 mg/day.
Elderly, Patients with hepatic impairment. 20 mg/day. May titrate to 40 mg/day only for nonresponding patients.

AVAILABLE FORMS/COST
• Sol—Oral: 10 mg/5 ml, 240 ml: **$119.63**
• Tab, Coated—Oral: 10 mg, 100's: **$250.18**; 20 mg, 100's: **$260.75**; 40 mg, 100's: **$272.10**

UNLABELED USES: Treatment of alcohol abuse, dementia, diabetic neuropathy, obsessive-compulsive disorder, smoking cessation

CONTRAINDICATIONS: Sensitivity to citalopram, use within 14 days of MAOIs

PREGNANCY AND LACTATION: Pregnancy category C; breast-feeding: unknown, 2 cases of infants experiencing excessive somnolence, decreased feeding, and weight loss have been reported

SIDE EFFECTS

Frequent (21%–11%)

Nausea, dry mouth, somnolence, insomnia, diaphoresis

Occasional (8%–4%)

Tremor, diarrhea, abnormal ejaculation, dyspepsia, fatigue, anxiety, vomiting, anorexia

Rare (3%–2%)

Sinusitis, sexual dysfunction, menstrual disorder, abdominal pain, agitation, decreased libido

SERIOUS REACTIONS

• Overdose is manifested as dizziness, drowsiness, tachycardia, somnolence, confusion, and seizures.

INTERACTIONS

Drugs

❷ *Buspirone:* Increased risk of serotonin syndrome

❸ *Cimetidine:* Increased levels of desmethylcitalopram via inhibition of CYP2D6 by cimetidine

❸ *Imipramine:* Increased bioavailability and half-life of desipramine (the major metabolite of imipramine) via inhibition of CYP2D6 by citalopram

⚠ *MAOIs, dexfenfluramine, sibutramine:* increased risk of sertonin syndrome

❸ *Metoprolol:* May increase levels of metoprolol, but no clinically significant changes in blood pressure or heart rate have been observed

❸ *Naratriptan, rizatriptan, sumatriptan, zolmatriptan:* Increased risk of weakness, hyperreflexia, and incoordination

• No clinical advantage over other SSRIs

PATIENT/FAMILY EDUCATION

• Therapeutic response may take 5 to 6 wk; most commonly taken once daily in the afternoon or evening

---

clarithromycin

(clare-i-thro-mye'sin)

Rx: Biaxin, Biaxin XL

Chemical Class: Macrolide derivative

Therapeutic Class: Antibiotic

CLINICAL PHARMACOLOGY

Mechanism of Action: A macrolide that binds to ribosomal receptor sites of susceptible organisma, inhibiting protein synthesis of the bacterial cell wall. *Therapeutic Effect:* Bacteriostatic; may be bactericidal with high dosages or very susceptible microorganisms.

Pharmacokinetics

Well absorbed from the GI tract. Protein binding: 65%-75%. Widely distributed. Metabolized in the liver to active metabolite. Primarily excreted in urine. Not removed by hemodialysis. **Half-life:** 3-7 hr; metabolite 5-7 hr (increased in impaired renal function).

INDICATIONS AND DOSAGES

Bronchitis

PO

Adults, Elderly. 500 mg q12h for 7-14 days.

Skin, soft tissue infections

PO

Adults, Elderly. 250 mg q12h for 7-14 days.

Children. 7.5 mg/kg q12h for 10 days.

MAC prophylaxis

PO

Adults, Elderly. 500 mg 2 times/day.

Children. 7.5 mg/kg q12h. Maximum: 500 mg 2 times/day.

MAC treatment

PO

Adults, Elderly. 500 mg 2 times/day in combination.

Children. 7.5 mg/kg q12h in combination. Maximum: 500 mg 2 times/day.

Pharyngitis, tonsillitis

PO

Adults, Elderly. 250 mg q12h for 10 days.

Children. 7.5 mg/kg q12h for 10 days.

Pneumonia

PO

Adults, Elderly. 250 mg q12h for 7-14 days.

Children. 7.5 mg/kg q12h.

Maxillary sinusitis

PO

Adults, Elderly. 500 mg q12h for 14 days.

Children. 7.5 mg/kg q12h. Maximum: 500 mg 2 times/day.

H. pylori

PO

Adults, Elderly. 500 mg q12h for 10-14 days in combination.

Acute otitis media

PO

Children. 7.5 mg/kg q12h for 10 days.

Dosage in renal impairment

For patients with creatinine clearance less than 30 ml/min, reduce dose by 50% and administer once or twice a day.

[$] AVAILABLE FORMS/COST

- Powder, Reconst—Oral: 125 mg/5 ml, 50, 100 ml: **$39.84**/100 ml; 250 mg/5 ml, 50, 100 ml: **$75.93**/100 ml
- Tab, Coated—Oral: 250, 500 mg, 60's: **$271.35**
- Tab, Coated, Sust Action—Oral: 500 mg, 60's: **$285.81**

CONTRAINDICATIONS: Hypersensitivity to clarithromycin or other macrolide antibiotics

PREGNANCY AND LACTATION: Pregnancy category C; excretion into breast milk unknown; use caution in nursing mothers

SIDE EFFECTS

Occasional (6%-3%)

Diarrhea, nausea, altered taste, abdominal pain

Rare (2%-1%)

Headache, dyspepsia

SERIOUS REACTIONS

- Antibiotic-associated colitis and other superinfections may result from altered bacterial balance.
- Hepatotoxicity and thrombocytopenia occur rarely.

INTERACTIONS

Drugs

[3] *Alfentanil:* Prolonged anesthesia and respiratory depression

[3] *Alprazolam:* Increased plasma alprazolam concentration

[3] *Amprenavir:* Plasma concentrations of clarithromycin may be increased by amprenavir; plasma concentrations of amprenavir may be increased by clarithromycin

[3] *Atorvastatin:* Increased plasma atorvastatin concentration with risk of rhabdomyolysis

[3] *Bromocriptine:* Increased bromocriptine concentration with toxicity

[3] *Buspirone:* Increased plasma buspirone concentration

[3] *Carbamazepine:* Markedly increased plasma carbamazepine concentrations

⚠ *Cisapride:* QT prolongation and life-threatening dysrhythmia

[2] *Clozapine:* Increased plasma clozapine concentrations

[3] *Colchicine:* Potential colchicine toxicity

[3] *Cyclosporine:* Increased plasma cyclosporine concentrations

3 *Diazepam:* Increased plasma concentration of diazepam

3 *Digoxin:* Reduced bacterial flora may increase plasma digoxin concentrations

3 *Disopyramide:* Increased plasma disopyramide concentrations

2 *Ergotamine:* Potential for ergotism

3 *Ethanol:* Ethanol reduces plasma clarithromycin concentration

3 *Felodipine:* Increased plasma felodipine concentrations

3 *Food:* Food may increase or decrease the bioavailability of clarithromycin

3 *Indinavir:* Plasma concentrations of clarithromycin may be increased by indinavir; plasma concentrations of indinavir may be increased by clarithromycin

3 *Itraconazole:* Increased plasma itraconazole concentration

3 *Lovastatin:* Increased plasma lovastatin concentration with risk of rhabdomyolysis

3 *Methylprednisolone:* Increased plasma methylprednisolone concentrations

3 *Midazolam:* Increased plasma concentration of midazolam

3 *Nelfinavir:* Plasma concentrations of clarithromycin may be increased by nelfinavir; plasma concentrations of nelfinavir may be increased by clarithromycin

3 *Penicillin:* Decreased activity of penicillin

⚠ *Pimozide:* QT prolongation and life-threatening dysrhythmia

3 *Phenytoin:* Increased plasma phenytoin concentrations

3 *Quinidine:* Increased plasma concentration of quinidine

3 *Rifabutin:* Increased plasma rifabutin concentrations

3 *Ritonavir:* Plasma concentrations of clarithromycin may be increased by ritonavir, plasma concentrations of ritonavir may be increased by clarithromycin

3 *Saquinavir:* Plasma concentrations of clarithromycin may be increased by saquinavir; plasma concentrations of saquinavir may be increased by clarithromycin

3 *Sildenafil:* Increased plasma sildenafil concentration

2 *Simvastatin:* Increased plasma simvastatin concentration with risk of rhabdomyolysis

3 *Tacrolimus:* Increased plasma tacrolimus concentration

⚠ *Terfenadine:* QT prolongation and life-threatening dysrhythmia

3 *Theophylline:* Increased plasma theophylline concentration

3 *Triazolam:* Increased plasma triazolam concentration

3 *Valproic acid:* Increased plasma valproic acid concentration

3 *Warfarin:* Increased hypoprothrombinemic response to warfarin

3 *Zafirlukast:* Reduced plasma zafirlukast concentration probably by reducing bioavailability

3 *Zopiclone:* Increased plasma zopiclone concentration

SPECIAL CONSIDERATIONS
PATIENT/FAMILY EDUCATION

• Take Sus Action TAB with food, immediate release and granules without regard to food

• Do NOT refrigerate suspension

clemastine

(klem'as-teen)
Rx: Clemastine
OTC: Dayhist-1, Tavist
Combinations
    OTC: with pseudoephedrine
    and acetaminophen (Tavist
    Allergy/Sinus/Headache
    Tablets)
Chemical Class: Ethanolamine
derivative
Therapeutic Class: Antihista-
mine

CLINICAL PHARMACOLOGY

Mechanism of Action: An ethanolamine that competes with histamine on effector cells in the gastrointestinal (GI) tract, blood vessels, and respiratory tract. *Therapeutic Effect:* Relieves allergy
symptoms, including urticaria,
rhinitis, and pruritus.

Pharmacokinetics

Route	Onset	Peak	Dura-tion
PO	15–60 min	5–7 hrs	10–12 hr

Well absorbed from the GI tract.
Metabolized in the liver. Excreted
primarily in urine.

INDICATIONS AND DOSAGES

Allergic rhinitis, urticaria
PO
Adults, Children older than 11 yr.
1.34 mg twice a day up to 2.68 mg 3
times a day. Maximum: 8.04
mg/day.
Children 6–11 yr. 0.67–1.34 mg
twice a day. Maximum: 4.02
mg/day.
Children younger than 6 yr. 0.05
mg/kg/day divided into 2–3 doses
per day. Maximum: 1.34 mg/day.
Elderly. 1.34 mg 1-2 times a day.

ⓢ AVAILABLE FORMS/COST

• Syr—Oral: 0.67 mg/5 ml, 120, 480
ml: **$16.50-$31.44**/120 ml
• Tab-Oral: 1.34 mg, 16's:
$3.73-$6.88; 2.68 mg, 100's:
$25.01-$86.08 (OTC)
CONTRAINDICATIONS: Angle-
closure glaucoma, hypersensitivity
to clemastine, use within 14 days of
MAOIs
*Drug: Alcohol, other CNS depres-
sants:* May increase CNS depression.
MAOIs: May increase the anticholinergic and CNS depressant effects
of clemastine.
Herbal
None known.
Food
None known.
PREGNANCY AND LACTATION:
Pregnancy category C; excreted into
breast milk; may cause drowsiness
and irritability in nursing infant; use
with caution during breast-feeding
SIDE EFFECTS
Frequent
Somnolence, dizziness, urine retention, thickening of bronchial secretions, dry mouth, nose, or throat; in
elderly, sedation, dizziness, hypotension
Occasional
Epigastric distress, flushing, blurred
vision, tinnitus, paresthesia, diaphoresis, chills
SERIOUS REACTIONS
• A hypersensitivity reaction,
marked by eczema, pruritus, rash,
cardiac disturbances, angioedema,
and photosensitivity, may occur.
• Overdose symptoms may vary
from CNS depression, including sedation, apnea, cardiovascular collapse, and death to severe paradoxical reaction, such as hallucinations,
tremor, and seizures.

• Children may experience paradoxical reactions, such as restlessness, insomnia, euphoria, nervousness, and tremors.

• Overdose in children may result in hallucinations, seizures, and death.

SPECIAL CONSIDERATIONS

• No advantage over loratadine or cetirizine; lower doses associated with less sedation and efficacy

---

clindamycin
(klin-da-mye'sin)
Rx: Cleocin, Cleocin T, Cleocin vaginal cream, Cleocin vaginal ovules, Clinda-Derm
Chemical Class: Lincomycin derivative
Therapeutic Class: Antibiotic

CLINICAL PHARMACOLOGY
Mechanism of Action: A lincosamide antibiotic that inhibits protein synthesis of the bacterial cell wall by binding to bacterial ribosomal receptor sites. Topically, it decreases fatty acid concentration on the skin. *Therapeutic Effect:* Bacteriostatic. Prevents outbreaks of acne vulgaris.
Pharmacokinetics
Rapidly absorbed from the GI tract. Protein binding: 92%-94%. Widely distributed. Metabolized in the liver to some active metabolites. Primarily excreted in urine. Not removed by hemodialysis. **Half-life:** 2.4-3 hr (increased in impaired renal function and premature infants).

INDICATIONS AND DOSAGES
Chronic bone and joint, respiratory tract, skin and soft-tissue, intraabdominal, and female GU infections; endocarditis; septicemia
PO
Adults, Elderly. 150-450 mg/dose q6-8h.

Children. 10-30 mg/kg/day in 3-4 divided doses. Maximum: 1.8 g/day.
IV, IM
Adults, Elderly. 1.2-1.8 g/day in 2-4 divided doses.
Children. 25-40 mg/kg/day in 3-4 divided doses. Maximum: 4.8 g/day.
Bacterial vaginosis
PO
Adults, Elderly. 300 mg twice a day for 7 days.
Intravaginal
Adults. One applicatorful at bedtime for 3-7 days or 1 suppository at bedtime for 3 days.
Acne vulgaris
Topical
Adults. Apply thin layer to affected area twice a day.

AVAILABLE FORMS/COST
• Cap, Gel—Oral: 75 mg, 100's: **$119.90**; 150 mg, 100's: **$96.43-$250.88**; 300 mg, 100's: **$371.71-$500.01**
• Cre—Vag: 2%, 40 g: **$49.78**
• Gel—Top: 1%, 30, 60 g: **$21.23-$42.60**/30 g
• Granule, Reconst—Oral: 75 mg/5 ml, 100 ml: **$25.26**
• Sol, Inj-IM, IV: 150 mg/ml, 2 ml: **$3.74-$4.85**
• Lotion—Top: 1%, 60 ml: **$45.12-$59.28**
• Sol—Top: 1%, 30, 60 ml: **$6.10-$48.39**/60 ml
• Supp—Vag: 100 mg, 3's: **$46.54**
• Swab-Top: 1%, 60's: **$29.88-$56.16**

UNLABELED USES: Treatment of malaria, otitis media, *Pneumocystis carinii* pneumonia, toxoplasmosis
CONTRAINDICATIONS: History of antibiotic-associated colitis, regional enteritis, or ulcerative colitis; hypersensitivity to clindamycin or lincomycin; known allergy to tartrazine dye

PREGNANCY AND LACTATION:
Pregnancy category B; excreted into breast milk; compatible with breast-feeding

SIDE EFFECTS
Frequent
Systemic: Abdominal pain, nausea, vomiting, diarrhea
Topical: Dry scaly skin
Vaginal: Vaginitis, pruritus
Occasional
Systemic: Phlebitis or thrombophlebitis with IV administration, pain and induration at IM injection site, allergic reaction, urticaria, pruritus
Topical: Contact dermatitis, abdominal pain, mild diarrhea, burning or stinging
Vaginal: Headache, dizziness, nausea, vomiting, abdominal pain
Rare
Vaginal: Hypersensitivity reaction

SERIOUS REACTIONS
• Antibiotic-associated colitis and other superinfections may occur during and several weeks after clindamycin therapy (including the topical form).
• Blood dyscrasias (leukopenia, thrombocytopenia) and nephrotoxicity (proteinuria, azotemia, oliguria) occur rarely.

INTERACTIONS
Drugs
🔳 *Food:* Decreased clindamycin concentrations with diet foods containing sodium cyclamate
② *Kaolin-pectin:* Decreased clindamycin concentrations
Labs
• *False increase:* Serum theophylline

SPECIAL CONSIDERATIONS
• Most active antibiotic against anaerobes

• Preferred topical antiacne antibiotic

PATIENT/FAMILY EDUCATION
• Avoid intercourse and use of vaginal products (tampons, douches) when using the vag cream or suppositories
• Vag cream contains mineral oil and vag suppositories contain an oleaginous base which may weaken rubber or latex products such as condoms or diaphragms, avoid use within 72 hr following treatment with vag cream or suppositories

---

clioquinol
(klee-oh-kwee′nole)
OTC: Clioquinol
Combinations
   Rx: with hydrocortisone (Ala-Quin, Corque, Dek-Quin); with hydrocortisone and pramoxine (1 + 1 − F)
Chemical Class: Hydroxyquinoline derivative
Therapeutic Class: Topical anti-infective

CLINICAL PHARMACOLOGY
Mechanism of Action: Clioquinol is a broad-spectrum antibacterial agent but the mechanism of action is unknown. Hydrocotisone is a corticosteroid that diffuses across cell membranes, forms complexes with specific receptors and further binds to DNA and stimulates transcription of mRNA (messenger RNA) and subsequent protein synthesis of various enzymes thought to be ultimately responsible for the anti-inflammatory effects of corticosteroids applied topically to the skin. *Therapeutic Effect:* Alters membrane function and produces antibacterial activity.

Pharmacokinetics

Clioquinol may be absorbed through the skin in sufficient amounts.

INDICATIONS AND DOSAGES

Antibacterial, antifungal skin conditions

Topical

Adults, Elderly, Children 12 yrs and older. Apply to skin 3-4 times/day.

$ AVAILABLE FORMS/COST

Clioquinol/Hydrocortisone

• Cre—Top: 3%-0.5%, 15, 30 g: **$2.75**/15 g; 3%-1%, 20, 30 g: **$2.43-$6.20**/20 g

• Oint—Top: 3%-1%, 20, 30 g: **$1.44**/20 g

CONTRAINDICATIONS: Lesions of the eye, tuberculosis of skin, diaper rash, hypersensitivity to clioquinol or hydrocortisone or any other component of the formulation

PREGNANCY AND LACTATION: Pregnancy category C; excretion into breast milk unknown

SIDE EFFECTS

Occasional

Blistering, burning, itching, peeling, skin rash, redness, swelling

SERIOUS REACTIONS

• Thinning of skin with easy bruising may occur with prolonged use.

SPECIAL CONSIDERATIONS

• Potential neurotoxicity with absorption (with occlusion); since other agents without this toxicity exist, questionable utility

clobetasol

(klo-bet′a-sol)

Rx: Cormax, Embeline E, Temovate, Temovate Emolliant, Olux

Chemical Class: Corticosteroid, synthetic

Therapeutic Class: Corticosteroid, topical

CLINICAL PHARMACOLOGY

Mechanism of Action: A corticosteroid that inhibits accumulation of inflammatory cells at inflammation sites, phagocytosis, lysosomal enzyme release and synthesis or release of mediators of inflammation. *Therapeutic Effect:* Decreases or prevents tissue response to inflammatory process.

Pharmacokinetics

May be absorbed from intact skin. Metabolized in liver. Excreted in the urine.

INDICATIONS AND DOSAGES

Anti-inflammatory, corticosteroid replacement therapy

Topical

Adults, Elderly, Children more than 12 yrs and older. Apply 2 times/day for 2 weeks.

Foam

Adults, Elderly, Children more than 12 yrs and older. Apply 2 times/day for 2 wks.

$ AVAILABLE FORMS/COST

• Cre—Top: 0.05%, 15, 30, 45, 60 g: **$19.57-$52.60**/30 g

• Foam—Top: 0.05%, 50, 100 g: **$90.11**/50 g

• Gel—Top: 0.05%, 15, 30, 60 g: **$39.89-$40.69**/30 g

• Oint—Top: 0.05%, 15, 30, 45, 60 g: **$19.57-$41.04**/30 g

• Sol—Top: 0.05%, 25, 50 ml: **$39.60-$72.49**/50 ml

CONTRAINDICATIONS: Hypersensitivity to clobetasol or other corticosteroids.

PREGNANCY AND LACTATION: Pregnancy category C; unknown whether top application could result in sufficient systemic absorption to produce detectable amounts in breast milk (systemic corticosteroids are secreted into breast milk in quantities not likely to have detrimental effects on infant)

SIDE EFFECTS

Frequent

Local irritation, dry skin, itching, redness

Occasional

Allergic contact dermatitis

Rare

Cushing's syndrome, numbness of fingers, skin atrophy

SERIOUS REACTIONS

• Overdosage can occur from topically applied clobetasol propionate absorbed in sufficient amounts to produce systemic effects producing reversible adrenal suppression, manifestations of Cushing's syndrome, hyperglycemia, and glucosuria in some patients.

SPECIAL CONSIDERATIONS

• No demonstrated superiority over other high-potency agents; cost should govern use

PATIENT/FAMILY EDUCATION

• Apply sparingly only to affected area

• Avoid contact with the eyes

• Do not put bandages or dressings over treated area unless directed by clinician

• Do not use on weeping, denuded, or infected areas

• Discontinue drug, notify clinician if local irritation or fever develops

---

clocortolone

(klo-kort′o-lone)

Rx: Cloderm

Chemical Class: Corticosteroid, synthetic

Therapeutic Class: Corticosteroid, topical

CLINICAL PHARMACOLOGY

Mechanism of Action: A topical corticosteroid that inhibits accumulation of inflammatory cells at inflammation sites, suppresses mitotic activity, and cause vasoconstriction. *Therapeutic Effect:* Decreases or prevents tissue response to inflammatory process.

Pharmacokinetics

Absorption is variable and dependent upon many factors including integrity of skin, dose, vehicle used, and use of occlusive dressings. Small amounts may be absorbed from the skin. Metabolized in liver. Excreted in the urine and feces.

INDICATIONS AND DOSAGES

Dermatoses

Topical

Adults, Elderly, Children 12 yrs and older. Apply 1-4 times/day.

$ AVAILABLE FORMS/COST

• Cre—Top: 0.1%, 15, 45, 90 g: **$21.56**/15 g

CONTRAINDICATIONS: Hypersensitivity to clocortolone pivalate or other corticosteroids; viral, fungal, or tubercular skin lesions

PREGNANCY AND LACTATION: Pregnancy category C; unknown whether top application could result in sufficient systemic absorption to produce detectable amounts in breast milk (systemic corticosteroids are secreted into breast milk in quantities not likely to have detrimental effects on infant)

SIDE EFFECTS

Occasional

Local irritation, burning, itching, redness

Allergic contact dermatitis

Rare

Hypertrichosis, hypopigmentation, maceration of skin, miliaria, perioral dermatitis, skin atrophy, striae

SERIOUS REACTIONS

• Overdosage can occur from topically applied clocortolone pivalate absorbed in sufficient amounts to produce systemic effects in some patients.

SPECIAL CONSIDERATIONS

• No demonstrated superiority over other low-potency agents; cost should govern use

PATIENT/FAMILY EDUCATION

• Apply sparingly only to affected area

• Avoid contact with the eyes

• Do not put bandages or dressings over treated area unless directed by clinician

• Discontinue drug, notify clinician if local irritation or fever develops

• Do not use on weeping, denuded, or infected areas

clofazimine

(kloe-faz'i-meen)

Rx: Lamprene

Chemical Class: Iminophenazine dye

Therapeutic Class: Leprostatic; mycobacterium avium complex

CLINICAL PHARMACOLOGY

Mechanism of Action: An antibiotic that binds to mycobacterial DNA. *Therapeutic Effect:* Inhibits mycobacterial growth and produces anti-inflammatory action.

INDICATIONS AND DOSAGES

Leprosy

PO

Adults, Elderly. 100 mg/day in combination with dapsone and rifampin for 3 yr then 100 mg/day as monotherapy.

Children. 1 mg/kg/day in combination with dapsone and rifampin.

Erythema nodosum

PO

Adults, Elderly. 100-200 mg/day for up to 3 mo, then 100 mg/day.

[$] **AVAILABLE FORMS/COST**

• Cap-Oral: 50 mg, 100's: **$20.58**

CONTRAINDICATIONS: None significant.

PREGNANCY AND LACTATION: Pregnancy category C; excreted into breast milk; do not administer to nursing mother unless clearly indicated

SIDE EFFECTS

Frequent (greater than 10%)

Dry skin, abdominal pain, nausea, vomiting, diarrhea, skin discoloration (pink to brownish-black)

Occasional (10%-1%)

Rash; pruritus; eye irritation; discoloration of sputum; sweat and urine

SERIOUS REACTIONS

• None significant.

INTERACTIONS

Labs

• *Increase:* Albumin, bilirubin, AST

SPECIAL CONSIDERATIONS

• Use in conjunction with other antileprosy agents to prevent development of resistance

PATIENT/FAMILY EDUCATION

• May discolor skin from pink to brownish black, as well as discoloring the conjunctivae, lacrimal fluid, sweat, sputum, urine, and feces; skin discoloration may take several mo or yr to disappear after discontinuation of therapy

clomiphene
(kloe'mi-feen)
Rx: Clomid, Milophene, Serophene
Chemical Class: Estrogen agonist-antagonist; triarylethylene compound
Therapeutic Class: Ovulation stimulant

CLINICAL PHARMACOLOGY
Mechanism of Action: An ovulation stimulator that promotes release of pituitary gonadotropins. *Therapeutic Effect:* Stimulates ovulation.
Pharmacokinetics
Readily absorbed. Time to peak occurs within 6.5 hrs. Undergoes enterohepatic recirculation. Primarily excreted in feces. **Half-life:** 5-7 days.

INDICATIONS AND DOSAGES
Ovulatory failure, females
PO
Adults. 50 mg/day for 5 days (first course); start the regimen on the fifth day of cycle. Increase dose only if unresponsive to cyclic 50 mg. Maximum: 100 mg/day for 5 days.

S **AVAILABLE FORMS/COST**
• Tab-Oral: 50 mg, 30's: **$75.23-$313.63**
UNLABELED USES: Infertility in males
CONTRAINDICATIONS: Liver dysfunction, abnormal uterine bleeding, enlargement or development of ovarian cyst, uncontrolled thyroid or adrenal dysfunction in the presence of an organic intracranial lesion such as pituitary tumor, pregnancy, hypersensitivity to clomiphene
PREGNANCY AND LACTATION: Pregnancy category X; each new course of drug should be started only after pregnancy has been excluded

SIDE EFFECTS
Frequent (13%-10%)
Hot flashes, ovarian enlargement
Occasional (5%-2%)
Abdominal/pelvic discomfort, bloating, nausea, vomiting, breast discomfort (females)
Rare (less than 1%)
Vision disturbances, abnormal menstrual flow, breast enlargement (males), headache, mental depression, ovarian cyst formation, thromboembolism, uterine fibroid enlargement

SERIOUS REACTIONS
• Thrombophlebitis, alopecia, and polyuria occurs rarely.

SPECIAL CONSIDERATIONS
• Though gonadotropin therapy is more effective for inducing ovulation, expense and time requirements warrant clomiphene trial

PATIENT/FAMILY EDUCATION
• Risk of multiple births increased—is approx 8% (7% twins, <1% triplets or greater)
• Record basal body temperature to determine whether ovulation has occurred; if ovulation can be determined (there is a slight decrease in temperature, then a sharp increase for ovulation), attempt coitus 3 days before and qod until after ovulation
• Prolonged use may increase the risk of ovarian cancer

clomipramine
(klom-ip'ra-meen)
Rx: Anafranil
Chemical Class: Dibenzocyclo-heptene derivative; tertiary amine
Therapeutic Class: Antidepressant, tricyclic; antiobsessional

CLINICAL PHARMACOLOGY
Mechanism of Action: A tricyclic antidepressant that blocks the reuptake of neurotransmitters, such as norepinephrine and serotonin, at CNS presynaptic membranes, increasing their availability at postsynaptic receptor sites. *Therapeutic Effect:* Reduces obsessive-compulsive behavior.

INDICATIONS AND DOSAGES
Obsessive-compulsive disorder
PO

Adults, Elderly. Initially, 25 mg/day. May gradually increase to 100 mg/day in the first 2 wk. Maximum: 250 mg/day.

Children 10 yr and older. Initially, 25 mg/day. May gradually increase up to maximum of 200 mg/day.

$ AVAILABLE FORMS/COST
• Cap, Gel—Oral: 25 mg, 100's: **$35.28-$329.46**; 50 mg, 100's: **$46.63-$442.04**; 75 mg, 100's: **$60.13-$561.00**

UNLABELED USES: Treatment of bulimia nervosa, cataplexy associated with narcolepsy, mental depression, neurogenic pain, panic disorder

CONTRAINDICATIONS: Acute recovery period after MI, use within 14 days of MAOIs

PREGNANCY AND LACTATION: Pregnancy category C; withdrawal symptoms, including jitteriness, tremor, and seizures have been reported in neonates whose mothers had taken clomipramine until delivery; has been found in human milk; use caution in nursing mothers

SIDE EFFECTS
Frequent

Somnolence, fatigue, dry mouth, blurred vision, constipation, sexual dysfunction (42%), ejaculatory failure (20%), impotence, weight gain (18%), delayed micturition, orthostatic hypotension, diaphoresis, impaired concentration, increased appetite, urine retention

Occasional

GI disturbances (such as nausea, GI distress, and metallic taste), asthenia, aggressiveness, muscle weakness

Rare

Paradoxical reactions (agitation, restlessness, nightmares, insomnia), extrapyramidal symptoms, (particularly fine hand tremor), laryngitis, seizures

SERIOUS REACTIONS
• Overdose may produce seizures; cardiovascular effects, such as severe orthostatic hypotension, dizziness, tachycardia, palpitations, and arrhythmias; and altered temperature regulation, including hyperpyrexia or hypothermia.

• Abrupt discontinuation after prolonged therapy may produce headache, malaise, nausea, vomiting, and vivid dreams.

• Anemia and agranulocytosis have been noted.

INTERACTIONS
Drugs

🔢 *Barbiturates:* Reduced serum concentrations of cyclic antidepressants

② *Bethanidine:* Reduced antihypertensive effect of bethanidine

🔢 *Carbamazepine:* Reduced cyclic antidepressant serum concentrations

❷ *Clonidine:* Reduced antihypertensive response to clonidine; enhanced hypertensive response with abrupt clonidine withdrawal

❸ *Debrisoquin:* Inhibited antihypertensive response of debrisoquin

❷ *Epinephrine:* Markedly enhanced pressor response to IV epinephrine

❸ *Ethanol:* Additive impairment of motor skills; abstinent alcoholics may eliminate cyclic antidepressants more rapidly than nonalcoholics

❸ *Fluoxetine, fluvoxamine, grapefruit juice:* Marked increases in cyclic antidepressant plasma concentrations

❸ *Guanethidine:* Inhibited antihypertensive response to guanethidine

⚠ *MAOIs:* Excessive sympathetic response, mania, or hyperpyrexia possible

❷ *Moclobemide:* Potential association with fatal or non-fatal serotonin syndrome

❸ *Neuroleptics:* Increased therapeutic and toxic effects of both drugs

❷ *Norepinephrine:* Markedly enhanced pressor response to norepinephrine

❷ *Phenylephrine:* Enhanced pressor response to IV phenylephrine

❸ *Propoxyphene:* Enhanced effect of cyclic antidepressants

❸ *Quinidine:* Increased cyclic antidepressant serum concentrations

SPECIAL CONSIDERATIONS
PATIENT/FAMILY EDUCATION
• Beneficial effects may take 2-3 wk
• Use caution while driving or during other activities requiring alertness; may cause drowsiness
• Avoid alcohol and other CNS depressants
• Do not discontinue abruptly

clonazepam
(kloe-na′zi-pam)
Rx: Klonopin
Chemical Class: Benzodiazepine
Therapeutic Class: Anticonvulsant; anxiolytic
DEA Class: Schedule IV

CLINICAL PHARMACOLOGY
Mechanism of Action: A benzodiazepine that depresses all levels of the CNS; inhibits nerve impulse transmission in the motor cortex and suppresses abnormal discharge in petit mal seizures. *Therapeutic Effect:* Produces anxiolytic and anticonvulsant effects.

Pharmacokinetics
Well absorbed from the GI tract. Protein binding: 85%. Metabolized in the liver. Excreted in urine. Not removed by hemodialysis. **Half-life:** 18-50 hr.

INDICATIONS AND DOSAGES
Adjunctive treatment of Lennox-Gastaut syndrome (petit mal variant) and akinetic, myoclonic, and absence (petit mal) seizures
PO

Adults, Elderly, Children 10 yrs and older. 1.5 mg/day; may be increased in 0.5- to 1-mg increments every 3 days until seizures are controlled. Do not exceed maintenance dosage of 20 mg/day.

Infants, Children younger than 10 yr or weighing less than 30 kg. 0.01-0.03 mg/kg/day in 2-3 divided doses; may be increased by up to 0.5 mg every 3 days until seizures are controlled. Do not exceed maintenance dosage of 0.2 mg/kg/day.

Panic disorder
PO

Adults, Elderly. Initially, 0.25 mg twice a day; increased in increments of 0.125-0.25 mg twice a day every 3 days. Maximum: 4 mg/day.

§ **AVAILABLE FORMS/COST**
• Tab-Oral: 0.5 mg, 100's: **$13.92-$110.05**; 1 mg, 100's: **$11.82-$125.53**; 2 mg, 100's: **$21.51-$173.93**
• Tab, Disintegrating-Oral: 0.125 mg, 0.25 mg, 60's; all: **$64.50**; 0.5 mg, 60's: **$66.15**; 1 mg, 60's: **$75.60**; 2 mg, 60's: **$104.74**

UNLABELED USES: Adjunctive treatment of seizures; treatment of simple, complex partial, and tonic-clonic seizures

CONTRAINDICATIONS: Narrow-angle glaucoma, significant hepatic disease

PREGNANCY AND LACTATION: Pregnancy category D; increased risk of congenital malformations, episodes of prolonged apnea, hypothermia in newborn reported; excreted into breast milk, breast-feeding not recommended

SIDE EFFECTS
Frequent
Mild, transient drowsiness; ataxia; behavioral disturbances (aggression, irritability, agitation), especially in children
Occasional
Rash, ankle or facial edema, nocturia, dysuria, change in appetite or weight, dry mouth, sore gums, nausea, blurred vision
Rare
Paradoxical CNS reactions, including hyperactivity or nervousness in children and excitement or restlessness in the elderly — (particularly in the presence of uncontrolled pain).

SERIOUS REACTIONS
• Abrupt withdrawal may result in pronounced restlessness, irritability, insomnia, hand tremors, abdominal or muscle cramps, diaphoresis, vomiting, and status epilepticus.

• Overdose results in somnolence, confusion, diminished reflexes, and coma.

INTERACTIONS
Drugs
▨ *CNS depressants:* Alcohol, narcotics, barbiturates, anxiolytics, phenothiazine, thioxanthene and butyrophenone antipsychotics, MAOIs, tricyclic antidepressants; CNS depression potentiated
▨ *CYP3A inducers:* Phenytoin, carbamazepine, phenobarbital; decreased serum clonazepam concentrations
▨ *Disulfiram:* Increased serum clonazepam concentrations
▨ *Oral antifungals:* Increased serum clonazepam concentrations, use cautiously
▨ *Valproic acid:* Increased occurrence of absence seizures

SPECIAL CONSIDERATIONS
• Up to 30% of patients have shown a loss of anticonvulsant activity, often within 3 mo of administration; dosage adjustment may reestablish efficacy

PATIENT/FAMILY EDUCATION
• Do not take more than prescribed amount, may be habit-forming
• Avoid driving, activities that require alertness; drowsiness may occur
• Avoid alcohol ingestion or other CNS depressants
• Do not discontinue medication abruptly after long-term use

MONITORING PARAMETERS
• Although relationship between serum concentrations and seizure control is not well established, proposed therapeutic concentrations are 20-80 ng/ml; potentially toxic concentrations >80 ng/ml
• Close attention to seizure frequency is important in order to detect the emergence of tolerance

clonidine

(klon'ih-deen)

Rx: Catapres, Catapres-TTS, Duraclon

Combinations

Rx: with chlorthalidone (Chlorpres, Combipress)

Chemical Class: Imidazoline derivative

Therapeutic Class: Antihypertensive; centrally acting sympathoplegic

CLINICAL PHARMACOLOGY

Mechanism of Action: An antiadrenergic, sympatholytic agent that prevents pain signal transmission to the brain and produces analgesia at pre- and post-alpha-adrenergic receptors in the spinal cord. *Therapeutic Effect:* Reduces peripheral resistance; decreases BP and heart rate.

Pharmacokinetics

Route	*Onset*	*Peak*	*Duration*
PO	0.5–1 hr	2–4 hr	Up to 8 hr

Well absorbed from the GI tract. Transdermal best absorbed from the chest and upper arm; least absorbed from the thigh. Protein binding: 20%–40%. Metabolized in the liver. Primarily excreted in urine. Minimally removed by hemodialysis. **Half-life:** 12–16 hr (increased with impaired renal function).

INDICATIONS AND DOSAGES

Hypertension

PO

Adults. Initially, 0.1 mg twice a day. Increase by 0.1–0.2 mg q2–4 days. Maintenance: 0.2–1.2 mg/day in 2–4 divided doses up to maximum of 2.4 mg/day.

Elderly. Initially, 0.1 mg at bedtime. May increase gradually.

Children. 5–25 mcg/kg/day in divided doses q6h. Increase at 5- to 7-day intervals. Maximum: 0.9 mg/day.

Transdermal

Adults, Elderly. System delivering 0.1 mg/24 hr up to 0.6 mg/24 hr q7 days.

Attention deficit hyperactivity disorder (ADHD)

PO

Children. Initially 0.05 mg/day. May increase by 0.05 mg/day q3–7 days. Maximum: 0.3–0.4 mg/day.

Severe pain

Epidural

Adults, Elderly. 30–40 mcg/hr.

Children. Initially, 0.5 mcg/kg/hr, not to exceed adult dose.

[$] **AVAILABLE FORMS/COST**

- Film, cont rel—Percutaneous: 0.1 mg/24 hr, 12's: **$168.60**; 0.2 mg/24 hr, 12's: **$283.83**; 0.3 mg/24 hr, 4's: **$131.25**
- Sol-Intrathecal: 100 mcg/ml, 10 ml: **$58.06**
- Tab-Oral: 0.1 mg, 100's: **$3.25-$90.83**; 0.2 mg, 100's: **$4.25-$138.95**; 0.3 mg, 100's: **$4.75-$174.36**

UNLABELED USES: ADHD, diagnosis of pheochromocytoma, opioid withdrawal, prevention of migraine headaches, treatment of dysmenorrhea or menopausal flushing

CONTRAINDICATIONS: Epidural contraindicated in those patients with bleeding diathesis or infection at the injection site, and in those receiving anticoagulation therapy

PREGNANCY AND LACTATION: Pregnancy category C; secreted into breast milk; hypotension has not been observed in nursing infants, although clonidine was found in the serum of the infants

SIDE EFFECTS
Frequent
Dry mouth (40%), somnolence (33%), dizziness (16%), sedation, constipation (10%)
Occasional (5%–1%)
Tablets, injection: Depression, swelling of feet, loss of appetite, decreased sexual ability, itching eyes, dizziness, nausea, vomiting, nervousness
Transdermal: Itching, reddening or darkening of skin
Rare (less than 1%)
Nightmares, vivid dreams, cold feeling in fingers and toes

SERIOUS REACTIONS
• Overdose produces profound hypotension, irritability, bradycardia, respiratory depression, hypothermia, miosis (pupillary constriction), arrhythmias, and apnea.
• Abrupt withdrawal may result in rebound hypertension associated with nervousness, agitation, anxiety, insomnia, hand tingling, tremor, flushing, and diaphoresis.

INTERACTIONS
Drugs
3 *β-blockers:* Rebound hypertension from clonidine withdrawal exacerbated by noncardioselective β-blockers
2 *Cyclic antidepressants:* Cyclic antidepressants may inhibit the antihypertensive response to clonidine
3 *Cyclosporine, tacrolimus:* Increased cyclosporine or tacrolimus concentrations
3 *Insulin:* Diminished symptoms of hypoglycemia
3 *Neuroleptics, nitroprusside:* Severe hypotension possible

SPECIAL CONSIDERATIONS
PATIENT/FAMILY EDUCATION
• Avoid hazardous activities, since drug may cause drowsiness
• Do not discontinue oral drug abruptly or withdrawal symptoms may occur (anxiety, increased BP, headache, insomnia, increased pulse, tremors, nausea, sweating)
• Response may take 2-3 days if drug is given transdermally
• Do not use OTC (cough, cold, or allergy) products unless directed by clinician
• Rise slowly to sitting or standing position to minimize orthostatic hypotension, especially elderly
• Dizziness, fainting, lightheadedness may occur during 1st few days of therapy
• May cause dry mouth; use hard candy, saliva product, or frequent rinsing of mouth

MONITORING PARAMETERS
• Blood pressure (posturally), blood glucose in patients with diabetes mellitus, confusion, mental depression

---

clopidogrel
(clo-pid′o-grill)
Rx: Plavix
Chemical Class: Thienopyridine derivative
Therapeutic Class: Antiplatelet agent

CLINICAL PHARMACOLOGY
Mechanism of Action: A thienopyridine derivative that inhibits binding of the enzyme adenosine phosphate (ADP) to its platelet receptor and subsequent ADP-mediated activation of a glycoprotein complex. *Therapeutic Effect:* Inhibits platelet aggregation.

Pharmacokinetics

Route	Onset	Peak	Duration
PO	1 hr	2 hr	N/A

Rapidly absorbed. Protein binding: 98%. Extensively metabolized by the liver. Eliminated equally in the urine and feces. **Half-life:** 8 hr.

INDICATIONS AND DOSAGES
Myocardial infarction (MI), stroke reduction
PO
Adults, Elderly. 75 mg once a day.
Acute coronary syndrome
PO
Adults, Elderly. Initially, 300 mg loading dose, then 75 mg once a day (in combination with aspirin).

§ AVAILABLE FORMS/COST
• Tab, Film-Coated—Oral: 75 mg, 90's: **$260.28**

CONTRAINDICATIONS: Active bleeding, coagulation disorders, severe hepatic disease

PREGNANCY AND LACTATION: Pregnancy category B; excreted into breast milk in rats

SIDE EFFECTS
Frequent (15%)
Skin disorders
Occasional (8%–6%)
Upper respiratory tract infection, chest pain, flu-like symptoms, headache, dizziness, arthralgia
Rare (5%–3%)
Fatigue, edema, hypertension, abdominal pain, dyspepsia, diarrhea, nausea, epistaxis, dyspnea, rhinitis

SERIOUS REACTIONS
• None known.

INTERACTIONS
Drugs
■ *Fluvastatin:* Inhibition of hepatic metabolism (CYP2C9) of fluvastatin with increased risk of myositis; *in vitro* data
■ *Nonsteroidal antiinflammatory agents:* Increased bleeding risk
■ *Phenytoin:* Inhibition of hepatic metabolism (CYP2C9) of phenytoin and increased risk of toxicity; *in vitro* data

■ *Tamoxifen:* Inhibition of hepatic metabolism (CYP2C9) and increased tamoxifen effects; *in vitro* data
■ *Tolbutamide:* Inhibition of hepatic metabolism (CYP2C9) of tolbutamide with increased risk of hypoglycemia; *in vitro* data
■ *Torsemide:* Inhibition of hepatic metabolism (CYP2C9) of torsemide with enhanced diuretic effects; *in vitro* data; increased bleeding risk
■ *Warfarin:* Inhibition of hepatic metabolism (CYP2C9) of warfarin with enhanced hypoprothrombinemic effects; *in vitro* data; increased bleeding risk

SPECIAL CONSIDERATIONS
• Comparative studies indicate that the drug is at least effective as aspirin; comparisons with ticlopidine lacking, however, no frequent CBC monitoring necessary
• Should probably replace ticlopidine as an aspirin alternative
• 28 × the cost of an equivalent supply of aspirin

PATIENT/FAMILY EDUCATION
• Inform clinician of signs and symptoms of bleeding, prior to surgery, dental work; inform clinician of sore throat, fever, etc. (consider neutropenia)

---

clorazepate
(klor-az′e-pate)
Rx: Gen-Xene, Tranxene, Tranxene-SD
Chemical Class: Benzodiazepine
Therapeutic Class: Anxiolytic
DEA Class: Schedule IV

CLINICAL PHARMACOLOGY
Mechanism of Action: A benzodiazepine that depresses all levels of the CNS, including limbic and re-

ticular formation, by binding to benzodiazepine receptor sites on the gamma-aminobutyric acid (GABA) receptor complex. Modulates GABA, a major inhibitory neurotransmitter in the brain. *Therapeutic Effect:* Produces anxiolytic effect, suppresses seizure activity.

INDICATIONS AND DOSAGES
Anxiety
PO

Adults, Elderly.(Regular release): 7.5-15 mg 2-4 times a day. (Sustained release): 11.25 mg or 22.5 mg once a day at bedtime.

Anticonvulsant
PO

Adults, Elderly, Children older than 12 yr. Initially, 7.5 mg 2-3 times a day. May increase by 7.5 mg at weekly intervals. Maximum: 90 mg/day.

Children 9–12 yr. Initially, 3.75–7.5 mg twice a day. May increase by 2.75 mg at weekly intervals. Maximum: 60 mg/day.

Alcohol withdrawal
PO

Adults, Elderly. Initially, 30 mg, then 15 mg 2–4 times a day on first day. Gradually decrease dosage over subsequent days. Maximum: 90 mg/day.

$ AVAILABLE FORMS/COST
• Tab-Oral: 3.75 mg, 100's: **$22.31-$242.05**; 7.5 mg, 100's: **$28.03-$301.15**; 15 mg, 100's: **$40.46-$408.55**
• Tab, Sus Action-Oral: 11.25 mg, 100's: **$634.34**; 22.5 mg, 100's: **$812.41**

CONTRAINDICATIONS: Acute narrow-angle glaucoma

PREGNANCY AND LACTATION: Pregnancy category D; excreted into breast milk; drug and metabolites may accumulate to toxic levels in nursing infant

SIDE EFFECTS
Frequent
Somnolence
Occasional
Dizziness, GI disturbances, nervousness, blurred vision, dry mouth, headache, confusion, ataxia, rash, irritability, slurred speech
Rare
Paradoxical CNS reactions, such as hyperactivity or nervousness in children and excitement or restlessness in the elderly or debilitated (generally noted during first 2 weeks of therapy, particularly in presence of uncontrolled pain)

SERIOUS REACTIONS
• Abrupt or too-rapid withdrawal may result in pronounced restlessness, irritability, insomnia, hand tremors, abdominal or muscle cramps, diaphoresis, vomiting, and seizures.
• Overdose results in somnolence, confusion, diminished reflexes, and coma.

INTERACTIONS
Drugs
▣ *Cimetidine:* Increased plasma levels of clorazepate and/or active metabolites
▣ *Disulfiram:* Increased serum clorazepate concentrations
▣ *Ethanol:* Enhanced adverse psychomotor side effects of benzodiazepines
▣ *Rifampin:* Reduced serum clorazepate concentrations

SPECIAL CONSIDERATIONS
• Do not use for everyday stress or for longer than 4 mo
• No advantage over diazepam

PATIENT/FAMILY EDUCATION
• Do not discontinue medication abruptly after long-term use

clotrimazole

(kloe-try-mah-zole)
Rx: *Topical:* Lotrimin, Fungoid
Rx: *Oral:* Mycelex
Rx: *Vaginal:* Mycelex-G, Mycelex Twin Pack
OTC: *Topical:* Cruex, Lotrimin AF, Desenex
OTC: *Vaginal:* Gynelotrimin 3, Gynelotrimin 7, Mycelex 7
Combinations
   Rx: with betamethasone dipropionate (Lotrisone)
Chemical Class: Imidazole derivative
Therapeutic Class: Topical antifungal

CLINICAL PHARMACOLOGY
Mechanism of Action: An antifungal that binds with phospholipids in fungal cell membrane. The altered cell membrane permeability. *Therapeutic Effect:* Inhibits yeast growth.
Pharmacokinetics
Poorly, erratically absorbed from GI tract. Bound to oral mucosa. Absorbed portion metabolized in liver. Eliminated in feces. Topical: Minimal systemic absorption (highest concentration in stratum corneum). Intravaginal: Small amount systemically absorbed. **Half-life:** 3.5-5 hrs.

INDICATIONS AND DOSAGES
Oropharyngeal candidiasis treatment
PO
Adults, Elderly. 10 mg 5 times/day for 14 days.
Oropharyngeal candidiasis prophylaxis
PO
Adults, Elderly. 10 mg 3 times/day.

Dermatophytosis, cutaneous candidiasis
Topical
Adults, Elderly. 2 times/day. Therapeutic effect may take up to 8 wks.
Vulvovaginal candidiasis
Vaginal (Tablets)
Adults, Elderly. 1 tablet (100 mg) at bedtime for 7 days; 2 tablets (200 mg) at bedtime for 3 days; or 500 mg tablet one time.
Vaginal (Cream)
Adults, Elderly. 1 applicatorful at bedtime for 7-14 days.

$\boxed{\$}$ AVAILABLE FORMS/COST
• Cre—Top: 1%, 15, 30, 45 g: **$6.42-$32.17**/30 g
• Cre—Vag: 1%, 45, 90 g: **$5.00-$23.69**/45 g
• Lotion—Top: 1%, 30 ml: **$31.06**
• Sol—Top: 1%, 10, 30 ml: **$2.97-$19.86**/30 ml
• Tab, Sus Action-Vag: 100 mg, 7's: **$7.20-$17.12**; 200 mg, 3's: **$9.00-$10.26**; 500 mg, 1's: **$13.88-$15.40**
• Troche—Buccal: 10 mg, 70's: **$73.26-$118.08**

UNLABELED USES: Topical: Treatment of paronychia, tinea barbae, tinea capitas.
CONTRAINDICATIONS: Hypersensitivity to clotrimazole or any component of the formulation, children <3 yrs
PREGNANCY AND LACTATION: Pregnancy category B; excretion in breast milk unknown
SIDE EFFECTS
Frequent
Oral: Nausea, vomiting, diarrhea, abdominal pain
Occasional
Topical: Itching, burning, stinging, erythema, urticaria
Vaginal: Mild burning (tablets/cream); irritation, cystitis (cream)
Rare
Vaginal: Itching, rash, lower abdominal cramping, headache

SERIOUS REACTIONS
• None reported.
INTERACTIONS
Drugs
3 *Cyclosporine, Tacrolimus:* Clotrimazole troche administration may increase cyclosporine or tacrolimus concentrations

---

clozapine
(klo′za-peen)
Rx: Clozaril
Chemical Class: Dibenzodiazepine derivative
Therapeutic Class: Antipsychotic

CLINICAL PHARMACOLOGY
Mechanism of Action: A dibenzodiazepine derivative that interferes with the binding of dopamine at dopamine receptor sites; binds primarily at nondopamine receptor sites. *Therapeutic Effect:* Diminishes schizophrenic behavior.
INDICATIONS AND DOSAGES
Schizophrenic disorders, reduce suicidal behavior
PO
Adults. Initially, 25 mg once or twice a day. May increase by 25–50 mg/day over 2 wk until dosage of 300–450 mg/day is achieved. May further increase by 50–100 mg/day no more than once or twice a week, Range: 200–600 mg/day. Maximum: 900 mg/day.
Elderly. Initially, 25 mg/day. May increase by 25 mg/day. Maximum: 450 mg/day.
S AVAILABLE FORMS/COST
• Tab-Oral: 12.5 mg, 100's: **$43.38**; 25 mg, 100's: **$131.94-$146.77**; 100 mg, 100's: **$341.86-$380.27**
NOTE: Available only through patient management system, combining WBC testing, patient monitoring, pharmacy and drug distribution services, all linked to compliance with required safety monitoring (1-800-448-5938)
CONTRAINDICATIONS: Coma, concurrent use of other drugs that may suppress bone marrow function, history of clozapine-induced agranulocytosis or severe granulocytopenia, myeloproliferative disorders, severe CNS depression
PREGNANCY AND LACTATION: Pregnancy category B; may be excreted in breast milk; avoid breastfeeding during clozapine therapy
SIDE EFFECTS
Frequent
Somnolence (39%), salivation (31%), tachycardia (25%), dizziness (19%), constipation (14%)
Occasional
Hypotension (9%); headache (7%); tremor, syncope, diaphoresis, dry mouth (6%); nausea, visual disturbances (5%); nightmares, restlessness, akinesia, agitation, hypertension, abdominal discomfort or heartburn, weight gain (4%)
Rare
Rigidity, confusion, fatigue, insomnia, diarrhea, rash
SERIOUS REACTIONS
• Seizures occur in about 3% of patients.
• Overdose produces CNS depression (including sedation, coma, and delirium), respiratory depression, and hypersalivation.
• Blood dyscrasias, particularly agranulocytosis; and mild leukopenia, may occur.
INTERACTIONS
Drugs
3 *Carbamazepine, phenytoin, primadone, valproic acid:* Considerable reduction in plasma clozapine concentrations

3 *Cimetidine, clarithromycin, tro-leandomycin:* Increased serum clozapine concentrations

3 *Digitoxin:* Increased serum digitoxin concentrations due to protein-binding displacement

3 *Diazepam:* Isolated cases of cardiorespiratory collapse have been reported

3 *Epinephrine:* Reversed pressor effects of epinephrine

2 *Erythromycin:* Increased serum clozapine concentrations

3 *Fluoxetine:* Modest elevation of serum clozapine concentrations

2 *Fluvoxamine:* Marked increase in plasma clozapine concentrations and side effects; increased risk of leukocytosis

3 *Paroxetine:* Modest elevation of serum clozapine concentrations

3 *Quinidine:* Increased serum clozapine concentrations possible

3 *Sertraline:* Modest elevation of serum clozapine concentrations

3 *Type 1C antiarrhythmics:* Propafenone, flecainide, encainide; increased serum clozapine concentration possible

3 *Warfarin:* Increased serum warfarin concentrations due to protein-binding displacement

SPECIAL CONSIDERATIONS

• The risk of agranulocytosis and seizures limits use to patients who have failed to respond or were unable to tolerate treatment with appropriate courses of standard antipsychotics

• Advise patients to report immediately the appearance of lethargy, weakness, fever, sore throat, malaise, mucous membrane ulceration, or other possible signs of infection

• Patients cannot be reinitiated on clozapine if WBC counts fall below 2000/mm^3 or ANC falls below 1000/mm^3 during clozapine therapy

MONITORING PARAMETERS

• WBC at baseline and then qwk for first 6 mo, every other week thereafter if WBC counts maintained (WBC ≥3000/mm^3, ANC ≥1500/mm^3); WBC counts qwk for at least 4 weeks after discontinuation

• Blood pressure, LFTs

---

codeine
(koe'deen)

Rx: Codeine Sulfate

Combinations

  Rx: with acetaminophen (Tylenol no. 2, Tylenol no. 3, Tylenol no. 4); with aspirin (Empirin no. 3, Empirin no. 4); with chlorpheniramine (Codeprex); with guaifenesin (Robitussin AC); with APAP (Capital, Aceta); with APAP butalbital, caffeine (Fioricet, Phenaphen); with aspirin (Fiorinal)

Chemical Class: Natural opium alkaloid; phenanthrene derivative

Therapeutic Class: Antitussive; narcotic analgesic

DEA Class: Schedule II

CLINICAL PHARMACOLOGY

Mechanism of Action: An opioid agonist that binds to opioid receptors at many cites in the CNS, particularly in the medulla. This action inhibits the ascending pain pathways. *Therapeutic Effect:* Alters the perception of and emotional response to pain, suppresses cough reflex.

INDICATIONS AND DOSAGES

Analgesia

PO, IM, Subcutaneous

Adults, Elderly. 30 mg q4–6h. Range: 15–60 mg.

Children. 0.5–1 mg/kg q4–6h. Maximum: 60 mg/dose.

Cough
PO

Adults, Elderly, Children 12 yr and older. 10–20 mg q4–6h.
Children 6–11 yr. 5–10 mg q4–6h.
Children 2–5 yr. 2.5–5 mg q4–6h.

Dosage in renal impairment
Dosage is modified based on creatinine clearance.

Creatinine Clearance	Dosage
10–50 ml/min	75% of usual dose
less than 10 ml/min	50% of usual dose

$ AVAILABLE FORMS/COST
• Sol, Inj-IM, SC: 15 mg/ml, 2 ml: **$0.93**; 30 mg/ml, 2 ml: **$1.18**; 60 mg/ml, 1 ml: **$1.26**
• Sol—Oral: 15 mg/5 ml, 500 ml: **$35.78**
• Tab-Oral (phosphate): 30 mg, 100's: **$58.94-$80.50**; 60 mg, 100's : **$112.62-$148.93**
• Tab-Oral (sulfate): 15 mg, 100's: **$43.37**; 30 mg, 100's: **$46.69-$51.69**; 60 mg, 100's: **$85.52**

UNLABELED USES: Treatment of diarrhea

CONTRAINDICATIONS: None known.

PREGNANCY AND LACTATION: Pregnancy category C (category D if used for prolonged periods or in high doses at term); use during labor produces neonatal respiratory depression; passes into breast milk in very small amounts; compatible with breast-feeding

SIDE EFFECTS
Frequent

Constipation, somnolence, nausea, vomiting

Occasional

Paradoxical excitement, confusion, palpitations, facial flushing, decreased urination, blurred vision, dizziness, dry mouth, headache, hypotension (including orthostatic hypotension), decreased appetite, injection site redness, burining, or pain

Rare

Hallucinations, depression, abdominal pain, insomnia

SERIOUS REACTIONS
• Too-frequent use may result in paralytic ileus.

• Overdose may produce cold and clammy skin, confusion, seizures, decreased BP, restlessness, pinpoint pupils, bradycardia, respiratory depression, decreased LOC, and severe weakness.

• The patient sho uses codeine repeatedly may develop a tolerance to the drug's analgesic effect as well as physical dependence.

INTERACTIONS
Drugs

▣ *Barbiturates:* Additive respiratory and CNS depressant effects

▣ *Antihistamines, chloral hydrate, glutethimide, methocarbamol:* Enhanced depressant effects

▣ *Cimetidine:* Increased respiratory and CNS depression

▣ *Ethanol:* Additive CNS effects

➋ *Quinidine:* Inhibited analgesic effect of codeine

Labs

• *Increase:* Urine morphine
• False elevatons of amylase and lipase

SPECIAL CONSIDERATIONS
PATIENT/FAMILY EDUCATION
• Minimize nausea by administering with food and remain lying down following dose

• Do not administer agonist/antagonist analgesics (i.e., pentazocine, nalbuphine, butorphanol, dezocine, buprenorphine) to patient who has received a prolonged course of codeine (a pure agonist). In opioid-dependent patients, mixed agonist/antagonist analgesics may precipitate withdrawal symptoms

---

colchicine
(kol'chi-seen)
Combinations
Rx: with probenicid
(Proben-C, Colbenemid)
Chemical Class: Colchicum autumnale alkaloid
Therapeutic Class: Antigout agent

CLINICAL PHARMACOLOGY
Mechanism of Action: An alkaloid that decreases leukocyte motility, phagocytosis, and lactic acid production. *Therapeutic Effect:* Decreases urate crystal deposits and reduces inflammatory process.

Pharmacokinetics
Rapidly absorbed from the GI tract. Highest concentration is in the liver, spleen, and kidney. Protein binding: 30%–50%. Reenters the intestinal tract by biliary secretion and is reabsorbed from the intestines. Partially metabolized in the liver. Eliminated primarily in feces.

INDICATIONS AND DOSAGES
Acute gouty arthritis
PO

Adults, Elderly. 0.6–1.2 mg; then 0.6 mg q1–2h or 1–1.2 mg q2h, until pain is relieved or nausea, vomiting, or diarrhea occurs. Total dose: 4–8 mg.
IV

Adults, Elderly. Initially, 2 mg; then 0.5 mg q6h until satisfactory response. Maximum: 4 mg/wk or 4 mg/one course of treatment. If pain recurs, may give 1–2 mg/day for several days but no sooner than 7 days after a full course of IV therapy (total of 4 mg).

Chronic gouty arthritis
PO

Adults, Elderly. 0.5–0.6 mg once weekly up to once a day, depending on number of attacks per year.

⬛ AVAILABLE FORMS/COST
• Sol, Inj-IV: 1 mg/2 ml, 2 ml: **$7.75**
• Tab-Oral: 0.5 mg, 30's: **$16.92**; 0.6 mg, 100's: **$3.95-$31.93**

UNLABELED USES: To reduce frequency of recurrence of familial Mediterranean fever; treatment of acute calcium pyrophosphate deposition, amyloidosis, biliary cirrhosis, recurrent pericarditis, sarcoid arthritis

CONTRAINDICATIONS: Blood dyscrasias; severe cardiac, GI, hepatic, or renal disorders

PREGNANCY AND LACTATION: Pregnancy category D (known teratogen)

SIDE EFFECTS
Frequent
PO: Nausea, vomiting, abdominal discomfort
Occasional
PO: Anorexia
Rare
Hypersensitivity reaction, including angioedema
Parenteral: Nausea, vomiting, diarrhea, abdominal discomfort, pain or redness at injection site, neuritis in injected arm

SERIOUS REACTIONS
• Bone marrow depression, including aplastic anemia, agranulocytosis, and thrombocytopenia, may occur with long-term therapy.
• Overdose initially causes a burning feeling in the skin or throat, severe diarrhea, and abdominal pain. The patient then experiences fever, seizures, delirium, and renal impairment, marked by hematuria and oliguria. The third stage of overdose causes hair loss, leukocytosis, and stomatitis.

INTERACTIONS
Drugs

▪ *Cyclosporine, tacrolimus:* Increased serum level of cyclosporine or tacrolimus

▪ *Erythromycin, clarithromycin, troleandomycin:* Potential for severe colchicine toxicity

Labs

• *Interference:* Urinary 17-hydroxycorticosteroids

SPECIAL CONSIDERATIONS
MONITORING PARAMETERS
• CBC, platelets, reticulocytes before and during therapy (q3mo)

---

colesevelam
(koh-le-sev′e-lam)
Rx: WelChol
Chemical Class: Hydrophilic nonabsorbed polymer
Therapeutic Class: Antilipemic; bile acid sequestrant

CLINICAL PHARMACOLOGY
Mechanism of Action: A bile acid sequestrant and nonsystemic polymer that binds with bile acids in the intestines, preventing their reabsorption and removing them from the body. *Therapeutic Effect:* Decreases LDL cholesterol.

INDICATIONS AND DOSAGES: To decrease LDL cholesterol level in primary hypercholesterolemia (Fredrickson type IIa)

PO

Adults, Elderly. 3 tablets with meals twice a day or 6 tablets once a day with a meal. May increase daily dose to 7 tablets a day.

$ **AVAILABLE FORMS/COST**
• Tab-Oral: 625 mg, 180's: **$159.46**

CONTRAINDICATIONS: Complete biliary obstruction, hypersensitivity to colesevelam

PREGNANCY AND LACTATION:
Pregnancy category B (no harm in animal studies, but no adequate and well-controlled studies in pregnant women; no expected excretion into breast milk

SIDE EFFECTS
Frequent (12%–8%)

Flatulence, constipation, infection, dyspepsia (heartburn, epigastric distress)

SERIOUS REACTIONS
• GI tract obstruction may occur.

INTERACTIONS
Drugs

• Although no drug interactions have been documented, binding to drugs given concomitantly may be significantly impacted; drug where small differences in serum level may be significant should be monitored closely

SPECIAL CONSIDERATIONS
• Combination colesevelam and an HMG-CoA reductase inhibitor is effective in further lowering serum total cholesterol and LDL-cholesterol levels beyond that achieved by either agent alone

PATIENT/FAMILY EDUCATION
• Tablets should be taken with a liquid, and with a meal

MONITORING PARAMETERS
• Plasma lipids

---

colestipol
(koe-les′ti-pole)
Rx: Colestid
Chemical Class: Bile acid sequestrant
Therapeutic Class: Antilipemic; bile acid sequestrant

CLINICAL PHARMACOLOGY
Mechanism of Action: An antihyperlipoproteinemic that binds with bile acids in the intestine, forming an

insoluble complex. Binding results in partial removal of bile acid from enterohepatic circulation. *Therapeutic Effect:* Removes low-density lipoproteins (LDL) and cholesterol from plasma.

Pharmacokinetics

Not absorbed from the gastrointestinal (GI) tract. Excreted in the feces.

INDICATIONS AND DOSAGES

Primary hypercholesterolemia

PO, granules

Adults, Elderly. Initially, 5 g 1-2 times/day. Range: 5-30 g/day once or in divided doses.

PO, tablets

Adults, Elderly. Initially, 2 g 1-2 times/day. Range: 2-16 g/day.

[$] **AVAILABLE FORMS/COST**

• Granule, Reconst-Oral: 5 g/scoop, 500 g: **$112.33**; 5 g/pkt, 90's: **$166.32**; 5 g/7.5 g pkt, 60's: **$132.85**

• Tab-Oral: 1 g, 120's: **$69.09**

UNLABELED USES: Treatment of diarrhea (due to bile acids); hyperoxaluria

CONTRAINDICATIONS: Complete biliary obstruction, hypersensitivity to bile acid sequestering resins

PREGNANCY AND LACTATION: Pregnancy category B

SIDE EFFECTS

Frequent

Constipation (may lead to fecal impaction), nausea, vomiting, stomach pain, indigestion

Occasional

Diarrhea, belching, bloating, headache, dizziness

Rare

Gallstones, peptic ulcer, malabsorption syndrome

SERIOUS REACTIONS

• GI tract obstruction, hyperchloremic acidosis, and osteoporosis secondary to calcium excretion may occur.

• High dosage may interfere with fat absorption, resulting in steatorrhea.

INTERACTIONS

Drugs

[3] *Acetaminophen, Amiodarone, Corticosteroids, Diclofenac, Digitalis glycosides, Furosemide, Methotrexate, Metronidazole, Thiazide diuretics, Thyroid hormones, Valproic acid:* Cholestyramine reduces interacting drug concentrations and probably subsequent therapeutic response

[3] *Oral anticoagulants:* Inhibition of hypoprothrombinemic response; colestipol might be less likely to interact

SPECIAL CONSIDERATIONS

• Bile acid sequestrant choice should be based on cost and patient acceptability

• Give all other medications 1 hr before colestipol or 4 hr after colestipol to avoid poor absorption

cortisone

(kor'ti-sone)

Rx: Cortone

Chemical Class: Glucocorticoid

Therapeutic Class: Corticosteroid, systemic

CLINICAL PHARMACOLOGY

Mechanism of Action: An adrenocortical steroid that inhibits the accumulation of inflammatory cells at inflammation sites, phagocytosis, lysosomal enzyme release and synthesis, and release of mediators of inflammation. *Therapeutic Effect:* Prevents or suppresses cell-mediated immune reactions. Decreases or prevents tissue response to inflammatory process.

INDICATIONS AND DOSAGES: Dosage is dependent on the condition being treated and patient response.

Anti-inflammation, immunosuppression

PO

Adults, Elderly. 25–300 mg/day in divided doses q12-24h.

Children. 2.5–10 mg/kg/day in divided doses q6-8h.

Physiologic replacement

PO

Adults, Elderly. 25–35 mg/day.

Children. 0.5–0.75 mg/kg/day in divided doses q8h.

[$] **AVAILABLE FORMS/COST**

- Susp, Inj-IM: 50 mg/ml: **$0.95**
- Tab-Oral: 25 mg, 100's: **$3.34-$50.48**

CONTRAINDICATIONS: Hypersensitivity to corticosteroids, administration of live virus vaccine, peptic ulcers (except in life-threatening situations), systemic fungal infection

PREGNANCY AND LACTATION: Pregnancy category C; excreted in breast milk

SIDE EFFECTS

Frequent

Insomnia, heartburn, anxiety, abdominal distention, increased diaphoresis, acne, mood swings, increased appetite, facial flushing, delayed wound healing, increased susceptibility to infection, diarrhea or constipation

Occasional

Headache, edema, change in skin color, frequent urination

Rare

Tachycardia, allergic reaction (such as rash and hives), psychological changes, hallucinations, depression

SERIOUS REACTIONS

- Long-term therapy may cause hypocalcemia, hypokalemia, muscle wasting in arms and legs, osteoporosis, spontaneous fractures, amenorrhea, cataracts, glaucoma, peptic ulcer disease, and CHF.
- Abrupt withdrawal following long-term therapy may cause anorexia, nausea, fever, headache, joint pain, rebound inflammation, fatigue, weakness, lethargy, dizziness, and orthostatic hypotension.

INTERACTIONS

Drugs

[3] *Aminoglutethamide:* Enhanced elimination of corticosteroids; marked reduction in corticosteroid response; doubling of dose may be necessary

[3] *Antidiabetics:* Increased blood glucose

[3] *Barbiturates, carbamazepine:* Reduced serum concentrations of corticosteroids

[3] *Cholestyramine, colestipol:* Possible reduced absorption of corticosteroids

[3] *Cyclosporine:* Possible increased concentration of both drugs, seizures

[3] *Erythromycin, troleandomycin, clarithromycin, ketoconazole:* Possible enhanced steroid effect

[3] *Estrogens, oral contraceptives:* Enhanced effects of corticosteroids

[3] *Isoniazid:* Reduced plasma concentrations of isoniazid

[3] *IUDs:* Inhibition of inflammation may decrease contraceptive effect

[3] *NSAIDs:* Increased risk GI ulceration

[3] *Rifampin:* Reduced therapeutic effect of corticosteroids

[3] *Salicylates:* Subtherapeutic salicylate concentrations possible

SPECIAL CONSIDERATIONS

- Increased dose of rapidly acting corticosteroids may be necessary in patient subjected to unusual stress
- May mask infections

• Do not give live virus vaccines to patients on prolonged therapy
• Patients on chronic steroid therapy should wear medical bracelet
• Drug-induced adrenocorticoid insufficiency may be minimized by gradual systemic dosage reduction; relative insufficiency may exist for up to 1 yr after discontinuation
• Symptoms of adrenal insufficiency include: nausea, fatigue, anorexia, hypotension, hypoglycemia, fever

MONITORING PARAMETERS
• Serum K and glucose
• Growth in children on prolonged therapy
• Edema, blood pressure, CHF, mental status, weight

---

cosyntropin
(kos-syn-troe′pin)
Rx: Cortrosyn
Chemical Class: ACTH derivative
Therapeutic Class: Corticosteroid, adrenal

CLINICAL PHARMACOLOGY
Mechanism of Action: A glucocorticoid that stimulates initial reaction in synthesis of adrenal steroids from cholesterol. *Therapeutic Effect:* Increases endogenous corticoid synthesis.
Pharmacokinetics
None reported.
INDICATIONS AND DOSAGES
Screening test for adrenal function
IM
Adults, Elderly, Children 2 yrs and older. 0.25-0.75 mg one time.
Children less than 2 yrs. 0.125 mg one time.
Neonates. 0.015 mg/kg/dose.
IV infusion

Adults. 0.25 mg in D5W or 0.9% NaCl infused at rate of 0.04 mg/hr.

$ **AVAILABLE FORMS/COST**
• Powder, Inj-IM, IV: 0.25 mg: **$85.09**
CONTRAINDICATIONS: Hypersensitivity to cosyntropin or corticotropin
PREGNANCY AND LACTATION:
Pregnancy category C
SIDE EFFECTS
Occasional
Nausea, vomiting
Rare
Hypersensitivity reaction (fever, pruritus)
SERIOUS REACTIONS
• None reported.
SPECIAL CONSIDERATIONS
MONITORING PARAMETERS
• Check plasma cortisol levels at baseline and 30-60 min after drug is administered; normal adrenal function indicated by an increase of at least 70 mcg/L or a measured level of 20 mcg

---

co-trimoxazole (sulfamethoxazole and trimethoprim)
(koe-trye-mox′a-zole)
Rx: Bactrim, Bethaprim, Cotrim, Comoxol, Septra, Sulfatrim, Uroplus
Chemical Class: Dihydrofolate reductase inhibitor (trimethoprim); sulfonamide derivative (sulfamethoxazole)
Therapeutic Class: Antibiotic

CLINICAL PHARMACOLOGY
Mechanism of Action: A sulfonamide and folate antagonist that blocks bacterial synthesis of essential nucleic acids. *Therapeutic Effect:* Bactericidal in susceptible microorganisms.

Pharmacokinetics

Rapidly and well absorbed from the GI tract. Protein binding: 45%-60%. Widely distributed. Metabolized in the liver. Excreted in urine. Minimally removed by hemodialysis. **Half-life:** sulfamethoxazole 6-12 hr, trimethoprim 8-10 hr (increased in impaired renal function).

INDICATIONS AND DOSAGES
Mild to moderate infections
PO, IV
Adults, Elderly, Children older than 2 mo. 6-12 mg/kg/day in divided doses q12h.
Serious infections, Pneumocystis Carinii pneumonia (PCP)
PO, IV
Adults, Elderly, Children older than 2 mo. 15-20 mg/kg/day in divided doses q6-8 h.
Prevention of PCP
PO
Adults. One double-strength tablet each day.
Children. 150 mg/m^2/day on 3 consecutive days/wk.
Traveler's diarrhea
PO
Adults, Elderly. One double-strength tablet q12h for 5 days.
Acute exacerbation of chronic bronchitis
PO
Adults, Elderly. One double-strength tablet q12h for 14 days.
Prevention of UTIs
PO
Adults, Elderly, children older than 2 mo. 2 mg/kg/dose once a day.
Dosage in renal impairment
Dosage and frequency are modified based on creatinine clearance, the severity of the infection and the serum concentration of the drug. For those with creatinine clearance of 15-30 ml/min, a 50% dosage reduction is recommended.

$ **AVAILABLE FORMS/COST**
• Sol-Conc, Inj-IV: 80 mg SMX/16 mg TMP/5 ml: **$4.13-$10.38**
• Susp—Oral: 200 mg SMX/40 mg TMP/5 ml, 100, 150, 200, 480 ml: **$6.33-$9.26/200 ml**
• Tab-Oral: 400 mg SMX/80 mg TMP, 100's: **$11.04-$110.69**; 800 mg SMX/160 mg TMP, 100's: **$9.09-$185.04**

UNLABELED USES: Treatment of bacterial endocarditis; gonorrhea; meningitis; septicemia; sinusitis; and biliary tract, bone, joint, chancroid, chlamydial, intraabdominal, skin and soft-tissue infections

CONTRAINDICATIONS: Hypersensitivity to trimethoprim or any sulfonamides, infants younger than 2 months old, megaloblastic anemia due to folate deficiency.

PREGNANCY AND LACTATION: Pregnancy category C; **do not use at term,** may cause kernicterus in the neonate; not recommended in the neonatal nursing period because sulfonamides excreted in breast milk may cause kernicterus

SIDE EFFECTS
Frequent
Anorexia, nausea, vomiting, rash (generally 7-14 days after therapy begins), urticaria
Occasional
Diarrhea, abdominal pain, pain or irritation at the IV infusion site
Rare
Headache, vertigo, insomnia, seizures, hallucinations, depression

SERIOUS REACTIONS
• Rash, fever, sore throat, pallor, purpura, cough, and shortness of breath may be early signs of serious adverse reactions.
• Fatalities have occasionally occurred after Stevens-Johnson syndrome, toxic epidermal necrolysis, fulminant hepatic necrosis, agranu-

locytosis, aplastic anemia, and other blood dyscrasias in patients taking sulfonamides.

• Myelosuppression, decrased platelet count and severe dermatologic reactions may occur, especially in the elderly.

INTERACTIONS
Drugs

3 *Dapsone:* Increased dapsone and trimethoprim concentrations

3 *Disulfiram, metronidazole:* Cotrimoxazole contains 10% ethanol, disulfiram reaction possible

3 *Methotrexate:* Elevated methotrexate concentrations and toxicity

3 *Oral anticoagulants:* Enhanced hypoprothrombinemic response to warfarin and possibly other oral anticoagulants

3 *Oral hypoglycemics:* Increased potential for hypoglycemia

3 *Phenytoin:* Increased phenytoin concentrations

Labs

• *False increase:* Creatinine (due to interference with assay), urobilinogen, urine protein, plasma α-aminonitrogen

• *False positive:* Urinary glucose test

• *False decrease:* Serum creatine kinase

SPECIAL CONSIDERATIONS

• Pay special attention to complaints of skin rash, especially those involving mucous membranes (could signify early Stevens-Johnson syndrome), sore throat, mouth sores, fever, or unusual bruising or bleeding

MONITORING PARAMETERS

• Baseline and periodic CBC for patients on long-term or high-dose therapy

---

cromolyn
(kroe'moe-lin)
Rx: *Inhalation:* Intal
Rx: *Opthalmic:* Crolom, Opticrom
Rx: *Oral:* Gastrocrom
Rx: *Nasal:* Nasalcrom
Chemical Class: Mast cell stabilizer
Therapeutic Class: Antiasthmatic; inhaled antiinflammatory; nasal antiinflammatory; ophthalmic antiinflammatory

---

CLINICAL PHARMACOLOGY

Mechanism of Action: An antiasthmatic and antiallergic agent that prevents mast cell release of histamine, leukotrienes, and slow-reacting substances of anaphylaxis by inhibiting degranulation after contact with antigens. *Therapeutic Effect:* Helps prevent symptoms of asthma, allergic rhinitis, mastocytosis, and exercise-induced bronchospasm.

Pharmacokinetics

Minimal absorption after PO, inhalation, or nasal administration. Absorbed portion excreted in urine or by biliary system. **Half-life:** 80–90 min.

INDICATIONS AND DOSAGES
Asthma

Inhalation (nebulization)

Adults, Elderly, Children older than 2 yr. 20 mg 3–4 times a day.

Aerosol spray

Adults, Elderly, Children 12 yrs and older. Initially, 2 sprays 4 times a day. Maintenance: 2–4 sprays 3–4 times a day.

Children 5–11 yr. Initially, 2 sprays 4 times a day, then 1–2 sprays 3–4 times a day.

Prevention of bronchospasm

Inhalation (nebulization)

Adults, Elderly, Children older than 2 yr. 20 mg within 1 hr before exercise or exposure to allergens.

Aerosol spray

Adults, Elderly, Children older than 5 yr. 2 sprays within 1 hr before exercise or exposure to allergens.

Food allergy, inflammatory bowel disease

PO

Adults, Elderly, Children older than 12 yr. 200–400 mg 4 times a day.

Children 2–12 yr. 100–200 mg 4 times a day. Maximum: 40 mg/kg/day.

Allergic rhinitis

Intranasal

Adults, Elderly, Children older than 6 yr. 1 spray each nostril 3–4 times a day. May increase up to 6 times a day.

Systemic mastocytosis

PO

Adults, Elderly, Children older than 12 yr. 200 mg 4 times a day.

Children 2–12 yr. 100 mg 4 times a day. Maximum: 40 mg/kg/day.

Children younger than 2 yr. 20 mg/kg/day in 4 divided doses. Maximum: 30 mg/kg/day (children 6 mo–2 yr).

Conjunctivitis

Ophthalmic

Adults, Elderly, Children older than 4 yr. 1–2 drops in both eyes 4–6 times a day.

§ AVAILABLE FORMS/COST

• Aer, Spray—INH: 800 mcg/spray, 8.1 g, 112 sprays: **$53.59**; 800 mcg/spray, 14.2 g, 200 sprays: **$85.26**

• Sol—INH: 10 mg/ml, 2 ml 60's: **$42.00-$49.80**

• Spray-Nasal: 5.2 mg/spray, 13, 26 ml: **$8.74/13 ml**

• Sol—Ophth: 4%, 10 ml: **$36.47-$44.56**

• Sol—Oral: 20 mg/ml, 5 ml: **$2.28**

CONTRAINDICATIONS: Status asthmaticus

PREGNANCY AND LACTATION: Pregnancy category B; excretion in breast milk unknown

SIDE EFFECTS

Frequent

PO: Headache, diarrhea

Inhalation: Cough, dry mouth and throat, stuffy nose, throat irritation, unpleasant taste

Nasal: Nasal burning, stinging, or irritation; increased sneezing

Ophthalmic: Eye burning or stinging

Occasional

PO: Rash, abdominal pain, arthralgia, nausea, insomnia

Inhalation: Bronchospasm, hoarseness, lacrimation

Nasal: Cough, headache, unpleasant taste, postnasal drip

Ophthalmic: Lacrimation and itching of eye

Rare

Inhalation: Dizziness, painful urination, arthralgia, myalgia, rash

Nasal: Epistaxis, rash

Ophthalmic: Chemosis or edema of conjunctiva, eye irritation

SERIOUS REACTIONS

• Anaphylaxis occurs rarely when cromolyn is given by the inhalation, nasal, or oral route.

SPECIAL CONSIDERATIONS

PATIENT/FAMILY EDUCATION

• Therapeutic effect in asthma may take up to 4 wk

crotamiton

(kroe-tam'i-ton)

Rx: Eurax
Chemical Class: Chloroformate salt
Therapeutic Class: Scabicide

CLINICAL PHARMACOLOGY

Mechanism of Action: A scabicidal agent whose exact mechanism is unknown. *Therapeutic Effect:* Scabicidal activity against Sarcoptes scabiei.

Pharmacokinetics
Not known.

INDICATIONS AND DOSAGES

Treatment of scabies
Topical
Adults, Elderly, Children. Wash and scrub away loose scales and towel dry. Apply a thin layer and massage into skin over the entire body with special attention to skin folds, creases, and interdigital spaces. Repeat application in 24 hours. Take a cleansing bath 48 hours after the final application. Treatment may be repeated after 7-10 days if live mites are still present.

Pruritus
Topical
Adults, Elderly, Children. Massage into affected areas until medication is completely absorbed. Repeat as needed.

Ⓢ AVAILABLE FORMS/COST

• Cre—Top: 10%, 60 g: **$13.36**
• Lotion—Top: 10%, 60, 454 ml: **$14.24**/60 ml
UNLABELED USES: Folliculitis, pediculosis
CONTRAINDICATIONS: Hypersensitivity to crotamiton or any one of its components
PREGNANCY AND LACTATION: Pregnancy category C

SIDE EFFECTS

Occasional
Itching, burning, irritation, warm sensation, contact dermatitis
SERIOUS REACTIONS
• None known.

SPECIAL CONSIDERATIONS

PATIENT/FAMILY EDUCATION
• 60 g is sufficient for 2 applications/adult
• Reapply locally during 48 hr treatment period after handwashing, etc.
• A cleansing bath should be taken 48 hr after the last application
• After treatment, use topical corticosteroids to decrease contact dermatitis, antihistamines for pruritus; pruritus may continue for 4-6 wk

cyanocobalamin (vitamin B$_{12}$)

(sye-an-oh-koe-bal'a-min)

Rx: Cyanoject, Cyomin
Chemical Class: Vitamin B complex
Therapeutic Class: Hematinic; vitamin

CLINICAL PHARMACOLOGY

Mechanism of Action: Acts as a coenzyme for various metabolic functions, including fat and carbohydrate metabolism and protein synthesis. *Therapeutic Effect:* Necessary for cell growth and replication, hematopoiesis, and myelin synthesis.

Pharmacokinetics
In the presence of calcium, absorbed systemically in lower half of ileum. Initially, bound to intrinsic factor; this complex passes down intestine, binding to receptor sites on ileal mucosa. Protein binding: High. Metabolized in the liver. Primarily eliminated unchanged in urine. **Half-life:** 6 days.

INDICATIONS AND DOSAGES
Pernicious anemia
IM, Subcutaneous
Adults, Elderly. 100 mcg/day for 7 days, then every other day for 7 days, then every 3-4 days for 2-3 wk. Maintenance: 100 mcg/mo (oral 1000-2000 mcg/day).
Children. 30-50 mcg/day for 2 or more wk. Maintenance: 100 mcg/mo.
Neonates. 1000 mcg/day for 2 or more wk. Maintenance: 50 mcg/mo.
Uncomplicated vitamin B₁₂ deficiency
PO
Adults, Elderly.   1,000–2,000 mcg/day
IM, Subcutaneous
Adults, Elderly. 100 mcg/day for 5–10 days, followed by 100–200 mcg/mo.
Complicated vitamin B₁₂ deficiency
IM, Subcutaneous
Adults, Elderly. 1000 mcg (with Im or IV folic acid 15 mg) as a single dose, then 1000 mcg/day plus oral folic acid 5 mg/day for 7 days.
§ AVAILABLE FORMS/COST
• Gel-Nasal: 500 mcg/0.1 ml, 2.3 ml: **$149.50**
• Sol, Inj-IM, IV, SC: 1000 mcg/ml: **$0.11-$10.00**
• Tab—Oral: 100   mcg,   100's: **$1.55-$4.50**;   250   mcg,   100's: **$2.55-$3.90**;   500   mcg,   100's: **$3.00-$5.85**;   1000   mcg,   100's: **$5.02-$10.50**
• Tab—SL: 2500 mcg, 50's: **$5.76**
CONTRAINDICATIONS: Folic acid deficiency anemia, hereditary optic nerve atrophy, history of allergy to cobalamins
PREGNANCY AND LACTATION: Pregnancy category C; excreted in breast milk in concentrations that approximate the mother's serum; compatible with breast-feeding

SIDE EFFECTS
Occasional
Diarrhea, pruritus
SERIOUS REACTIONS
• Impurities in preparation may cause a rare allergic reaction.
• Peripheral vascular thrombosis, pulmonary edema, hypokalemia, and CHF may occur.
SPECIAL CONSIDERATIONS
• Recommended dietary allowance: 0.5-2.6 mcg/day depending on age and status (i.e., more during pregnancy and lactation)
• Nutritional sources: egg yolks, fish, organ meats, dairy products, clams, oysters
MONITORING PARAMETERS
• CBC with reticulocyte count after 1st wk of therapy

⊸cyclobenzaprine
(sye-kloe-ben'za-preen)
⊸ Rx: Flexeril
Chemical Class: Tricyclic amine
⊸Therapeutic Class: Skeletal muscle relaxant

CLINICAL PHARMACOLOGY
Mechanism of Action: A centrally acting skeletal muscle relaxant that reduces tonic somatic muscle activity at the level of the brainstem. *Therapeutic Effect:* Relieves local skeletal muscle spasm.
Pharmacokinetics

Route	Onset	Peak	Dura-tion
PO	1 hr	3–4 hr	12–24 hr

Well but slowly absorbed from the GI tract. Protein binding: 93%. Metabolized in the GI tract and the liver. Primarily excreted in urine. **Half-life:** 1–3 days.

INDICATIONS AND DOSAGES
Acute, painful musculoskeletal conditions
PO

Adults. Initially, 5 mg 3 times a day. May increase to 10 mg 3 times a day.
Elderly. 5 mg 3 times a day.
Dosage in hepatic impairment
Mild: 5 mg 3 times a day.
Moderate and severe: Not recommended.

$ AVAILABLE FORMS/COST
• Tab, Coated—Oral: 5 mg, 100's: **$124.06**; 10 mg, 100's: **$7.33-$137.81**
UNLABELED USES: Treatment of fibromyalgia
CONTRAINDICATIONS: Acute recovery phase of MI, arrhythmias, CHF, heart block, conduction disturbances, hyperthyroidism, use within 14 days of MAOIs
PREGNANCY AND LACTATION: Pregnancy category B; no data available, but closely related tricyclic antidepressants are excreted into breast milk

SIDE EFFECTS
Frequent
Somnolence (39%), dry mouth (27%), dizziness (11%)
Rare (3%–1%)
Fatigue, asthenia, blurred vision, headache, nervousness, confusion, nausea, constipation, dyspepsia, unpleasant taste

SERIOUS REACTIONS
• Overdose may result in visual hallucinations, hyperactive reflexes, muscle rigidity, vomiting, and hyperpyrexia.

INTERACTIONS
Drugs
3 *Droperidol, fluoxetine:* A patient receiving cyclobenzaprine and fluoxetine developed ventricular tachycardia and fibrillation after droperidol was added; relative contribution of each drug to the adverse effect unclear
2 *MAOIs:* Hyperpyretic crisis, severe convulsions, and deaths have occurred in patients receiving closely related tricyclic antidepressants and MAOIs; separate use by 14 days
Labs
• *Interference:* Serum amitriptyline assay

SPECIAL CONSIDERATIONS
• Avoid use in elderly due to anticholinergic side effects

PATIENT/FAMILY EDUCATION
• Use caution with alcohol, other CNS depressants
• Avoid with hazardous activities if drowsiness or dizziness occur

cyclophosphamide
(sye-kloe-foss'fa-mide)
Rx: Cytoxan, Neosar
Chemical Class: Nitrogen mustard, synthetic
Therapeutic Class: Antineoplastic

CLINICAL PHARMACOLOGY
Mechanism of Action: An alkylating agent that inhibits DNA and RNA protein synthesis by cross-linking with DNA and RNA strands, preventing cell growth. Cell cycle-phase nonspecific. *Therapeutic Effect:* Potent immunosuppressant.
Pharmacokinetics
Well absorbed from the GI tract. Protein binding: Low. Crosses the blood-brain barrier. Metabolized in the liver to active metabolites. Primarily excreted in urine. Removed by hemodialysis. **Half-life:** 3-12 hr.

INDICATIONS AND DOSAGES
Ovarian adenocarcinoma, breast carcinoma, Hodgkin's disease, non-Hodgkin's lymphoma, multiple myeloma, leukemia (acute lymphoblastic, acute myelogenous, acute monocytic, chronic granulocytic, chronic lymphocytic), mycosis fungoides, disseminated neuroblastoma, retinoblastoma
PO
Adults. 1-5 mg/kg/day.
Children. Initially, 2-8 mg/kg/day. Maintenance: 2-5 mg/kg twice a week.
IV
Adults. 40-50 mg/kg in divided doses over 2-5 days; or 10-15 mg/kg every 7-10 days or 3-5 mg/kg twice a week.
Children. 2-8 mg/kg/day for 6 days or total dose for 7 days once a week.
Biopsy-proven   minimal-change nephrotic syndrome
PO
Adults, Children. 2.5-3 mg/kg/day for 60-90 days.

$ AVAILABLE FORMS/COST
• Powder, Inj-IV: 1, 2 g/vial: **$22.03**/1 g; 100, 200 mg/vial: **$6.19**/100 mg
• Tab-Oral: 25 mg, 100's: **$203.22-$213.38**; 50 mg, 100's: **$341.68-$414.47**

UNLABELED USES: Treatment of carcinoma of bladder, cervix, endometrium, lung, prostate, or testicles; germ cell ovarian tumors; osteosarcoma; rheumatoid arthritis; systemic lupus erythematosus

CONTRAINDICATIONS: None known.

PREGNANCY AND LACTATION: Pregnancy category D; excreted in breast milk; contraindicated because of potential for adverse effects relating to immune suppression, growth, and carcinogenesis

SIDE EFFECTS
Expected
Marked leukopenia 8-15 days after initial therapy
Frequent
Nausea, vomiting (beginning about 6 hr after administration and lasting about 4 hr); alopecia (33%)
Occasional
Diarrhea, darkening of skin and fingernails, stomatitis, headache, diaphoresis
Rare
Pain or redness at injection site

SERIOUS REACTIONS
• Cyclophosphamide's major toxic effect is myelosuppression resulting in blood dyscrasias, such as leukopenia, anemia, thrombocytopenia, and hypoprothrombinemia.
• Expect leukopenia to resolve in 17 to 28 days. Anemia generally occurs after large doses or prolonged therapy. Thrombocytopenia may occur 10-15 days after drug initiation.
• Hemorrhagic cystitis occurs commonly in long-term therapy, especially in pediatric patients.
• Pulmonary fibrosis and cardiotoxicity have been noted with high doses.
• Amenorrhea, azoospermia, and hyperkalemia may also occur.

INTERACTIONS
Drugs
▣ *Allopurinol:* Increased cyclophosphamide toxicity
▣ *Digoxin:* Decreased digoxin absorption from tablets; Lanoxicaps and elixir not affected
▣ *Succinylcholine:* Prolonged neuromuscular blockade
▣ *Warfarin:* Inhibited hypoprothrombinemic response to warfarin

SPECIAL CONSIDERATIONS
MONITORING PARAMETERS
- CBC, differential, platelet count qwk; withhold drug if WBC is <4000 or platelet count is <75,000
- Renal function studies: BUN, UA, serum uric acid; urine CrCl before, during therapy
- I&O; report fall in urine output ≤30 ml/hr

Creatinine Clearance	Dosage Interval
10-50 ml/min	q24h
less than 10 ml/min	q36-48h

AVAILABLE FORMS/COST
- Cap, Gel—Oral: 250 mg, 40's: **$167.40**

UNLABELED USES: Gaucher's disease, acute urinary tract infections

CONTRAINDICATIONS: Epilepsy, depression, severe anxiety, psychosis, severe renal insufficiency, excessive concurrent use of alcohol, history of hypersensitivity reactions with previous cycloserine therapy

PREGNANCY AND LACTATION: Pregnancy category C; excreted into breast milk (72% of serum levels); compatible with breast-feeding

SIDE EFFECTS
Occasional

Drowsiness, headache, dizziness, vertigo, seizures, confusion, psychosis, paresis, tremor, vitamin B_{12} deficiency, folate deficiency, cardiac arrhythmias, increased liver enzymes

SERIOUS REACTIONS
- Neurotoxicity, as evidenced by confusion, agitation, CNS depression, psychosis, coma, and seizures, occur rarely.
- Neurotoxic effects of cycloserine may be treated and prevented with the administration of 200 to 300 mg of pyridoxine daily.

INTERACTIONS
Drugs

3 *Isoniazid:* Increased risk of CNS toxicity

SPECIAL CONSIDERATIONS
- L-enantiomer (1-cycloserine) in Gaucher's disease (Orphan Drug)
- Pyridoxine may prevent neurotoxicity (200-300 mg/day)

---

cycloserine
(sye-kloe-ser'een)

Rx: Seromycin
Chemical Class: Streptomyces orchidaceus product
Therapeutic Class: Antituberculosis agent

CLINICAL PHARMACOLOGY
Mechanism of Action: An antitubercular that inhibits cell wall synthesis by competing with the amino acid, D-alanine, for incorporation into the bacterial cell wall. *Therapeutic Effect:* Causes disruption of bacterial cell wall. Bactericidal or bacteriostatic.

Pharmacokinetics
Readily absorbed from the gastrointestinal (GI) tract. No protein binding. Widely distributed (including cerebrospinal fluid [CSF]). Metabolized in liver. Primarily excreted in urine. Removed by hemodialysis. **Half-life:** 10 hrs.

INDICATIONS AND DOSAGES
Tuberculosis

Adults, Elderly. 250 mg q12h for 14 days, then 500 mg to 1g/day in 2 divided doses for 18-24 months. Maximum: 1 g as a single daily dose.
Children. 10-20 mg/kg/day in 2 divided doses. Maximum: 1000 mg/day for 18-24 months.

Dosage in renal impairment

PATIENT/FAMILY EDUCATION
• Avoid concurrent alcohol
MONITORING PARAMETERS
• Mental status closely and liver function tests qwk

---

cyclosporine
(sye-kloe-spor'in)
Rx: Neoral, Sandimmune, SangCya, Restasis (ophth)
Chemical Class: Cyclic peptide
Therapeutic Class: Immuno-suppressant

CLINICAL PHARMACOLOGY
Mechanism of Action: A cyclic polypeptide that inhibits both cellular and humoral immune responses by inhibiting interleukin-2, a proliferative factor needed for T-cell activity. *Therapeutic Effect:* Prevents organ rejection and relieves symptoms of psoriasis and arthritis.
Pharmacokinetics
Variably absorbed from the GI tract. Protein binding: 90%. Widely distributed. Metabolized in the liver. Eliminated primarily by biliary or fecal excretion. Not removed by hemodialysis. **Half-life:** Adults, 10–27 hr; children, 7–19 hr.

INDICATIONS AND DOSAGES
Transplantation, prevention of organ rejection
PO
Adults, Elderly, Children. 10-18 mg/kg/dose given 4-12 hr prior to organ transplantation. Maintenance: 5–15 mg/kg/day in divided doses then tapered to 3-10 mg/kg/day.
IV
Adults, Elderly, Children. Initially, 5–6 mg/kg/dose given 4–12 hr prior to organ transplantation. Maintenance: 2-10 mg/kg/day in divided doses.

Rheumatoid arthritis
PO
Adults, Elderly. Initially, 2.5 mg/kg a day in 2 divided doses. May increase by 0.5-0.75 mg/kg/day. Maximum: 4 mg/kg/day.
Psoriasis
PO
Adults, Elderly. Initially, 2.5 mg/kg/day in 2 divided doses. May increase by 0.5 mg/kg/day. Maximum: 4 mg/kg/day.
Dry eye
Ophthalmic
Adults, Elderly. Instill 1 drip in each affected eye q12h.

AVAILABLE FORMS/COST
Neoral
• Cap—Oral, for microemulsion: 25 mg, 30's: **$46.82**; 100 mg, 30's: **$186.97**
• Liq—Oral, for microemulsion: 100 mg/ml, 50 ml: **$332.83**
Restasis
• Emulsion—Ophth: 0.05%, 0.4 ml: **$2.93**
Sandimmune
• Cap—Oral: 25 mg, 30's: **$52.09**; 100 mg, 30's: **$207.98**
• Sol, Inj-IV: 50 mg/ml, 5 ml: **$27.50-$29.16**
• Sol—Oral: 100 mg/ml, 50 ml: **$299.53-$336.64**
Seromycin
• Cap—Oral: 250 mg, 40's: **$167.40**
UNLABELED USES: Treatment of alopecia areata, aplastic anemia, atopic dermatitis, Behçet's disease, biliary cirrhosis, prevention of corneal transplant rejection
CONTRAINDICATIONS: History of hypersensitivity to cyclosporine or polyoxyethylated castor oil
PREGNANCY AND LACTATION: Pregnancy category C; excreted into breast milk; avoid nursing

SIDE EFFECTS
Frequent
Mild to moderate hypertension (26%), hirsutism (21%), tremor (12%)
Occasional (4%–2%)
Acne, leg cramps, gingival hyperplasia (marked by red, bleeding, and tender gums), paresthesia, diarrhea, nausea, vomiting, headache
Rare (less than 1%)
Hypersensitivity reaction, abdominal discomfort, gynecomastia, sinusitis

SERIOUS REACTIONS
• Mild nephrotoxicity occurs in 25% of renal transplant patients, 38% of cardiac transplant patients, and 37% of liver transplant patients, generally 2 to 3 months after transplantation (more severe toxicity is generally occurs soon after transplantation). Hepatotoxicity occurs in 4% of renal transplant patients, 7% of cardiac transplant patients, and 4% of liver transplant patients, generally within the first month after transplantation. Both toxicities usually respond to dosage reduction.
• Severe hyperkalemia and hyperuricemia occur occasionally.

INTERACTIONS
Drugs
③ Allopurinol, amiodarone, chloroquine, clarithromycin, clonidine, clotrimazole, oral contraceptives, erythromycin, fluconazole, griseofulvin, itraconazole, ketoconazole, miconazole, ticlopidine: Increased cyclosporine levels, potential for toxicity
③ Aminoglycosides, amphotericin B, colchicine, enalapril, melphalan, sulfonamides: Additive nephrotoxicity with cyclosporine
② Anabolic steroids: Increased cyclosporine levels, potential for toxicity
③ Barbiturates, carbamazepine, nafcillin, pyrazinamide, phenytoin, sulfonamides: Reduced cyclosporine levels, potential for therapeutic failure
③ Calcium channel blockers: Diltiazem, verapamil increase cyclosporine levels; isradipine, nifedipine, nitrendipine do not interact
③ Cisapride, metoclopramide: Increased bioavailability and serum levels of single-dose cyclosporine
③ Digitalis glycosides: Cyclosporine in patients stabilized on digitalis leads to increased levels and potential toxicity
③ Doxorubicin, imipenem: CNS toxicity
③ HMG-CoA reductase inhibitors: Increased risk of reversible myopathy
③ Methotrexate: Increased toxicity of both agents
③ NSAIDs: Increased risk of cyclosporine nephrotoxicity
② Rifampin: Reduced cyclosporine levels, potential for therapeutic failure

SPECIAL CONSIDERATIONS
• Neoral has increased bioavailability compared to Sandimmune (do NOT use interchangeably)

PATIENT/FAMILY EDUCATION
• Oral sol may be mixed with milk, chocolate milk, or orange juice to improve palatability. Do not mix with grapefruit juice (increased cyclosporine levels)
• Ophthalmic product may be used with artificial tears — allow 15 min interval between products

MONITORING PARAMETERS
• Renal function studies: BUN, creatinine qmo during treatment, 3 mo after treatment
• Liver function studies and serum levels during treatment

• Blood level monitoring: maintenance of 24-hr trough levels of 250-800 ng/ml (whole blood, RIA) or 50-300 ng/ml (plasma, RIA) should minimize side effects and rejection events

---

cyproheptadine
(si-proe-hep'ta-deen)
Rx: Cyprohetadine
Chemical Class: Piperidine derivative
Therapeutic Class: Antihistamine

CLINICAL PHARMACOLOGY
Mechanism of Action: An antihistamine that competes with histamine at histaminic receptor sites. Anticholinergic effects cause drying of nasal mucosa. *Therapeutic Effect:* Relieves allergic conditions (urticaria, pruritus).
Pharmacokinetics
Well absorbed from GI tract. Metabolized in liver. Primarily eliminated in feces. **Half-life:** 16 hrs.
INDICATIONS AND DOSAGES
Allergic condition
PO
Adults, Children older than 15 yrs. 4 mg 3 times/day. May increase dose but do not exceed 0.5 mg/kg/day.
Children 7-14 yrs. 4 mg 2-3 times/day, or 0.25 mg/kg daily in divided doses.
Children 2-6 yrs. 2 mg 2-3 times/day, or 0.25 mg/kg daily in divided doses.
Usual elderly dosage
PO
Initially, 4 mg 2 times/day.
[S] AVAILABLE FORMS/COST
• Syr—Oral: 2 mg/5 ml, 480 ml: **$9.00-$10.75**
• Tab-Oral: 4 mg, 100's: **$3.55-$50.89**

CONTRAINDICATIONS: Acute asthmatic attack, patients receiving MAO inhibitors, history of hypersensitivity to antihistamines
PREGNANCY AND LACTATION: Pregnancy category B; excreted in breast milk
SIDE EFFECTS
Frequent
Drowsiness, dizziness, muscular weakness, dry mouth/nose/throat/lips, urinary retention, thickening of bronchial secretions
Elderly
Frequent
Sedation, dizziness, hypotension
Occasional
Epigastric distress, flushing, visual disturbances, hearing disturbances, paresthesia, sweating, chills
SERIOUS REACTIONS
• Children may experience dominant paradoxical reaction (restlessness, insomnia, euphoria, nervousness, tremors).
• Overdosage in children may result in hallucinations, convulsions, death.
• Hypersensitivity reaction (eczema, pruritus, rash, cardiac disturbances, angioedema, photosensitivity) may occur.
• Overdosage may vary from CNS depression (sedation, apnea, cardiovascular collapse, death) to severe paradoxical reaction (hallucinations, tremor, seizures).
INTERACTIONS
Drugs
[3] *Fluoxetine:* Potential for worsening of depression when cyproheptodine added to fluoxetine therapy
Labs
• *False positive:* Urine tricyclic antidepressant assay

dalteparin

(doll'teh-pare-in)

Rx: Fragmin

Chemical Class: Heparin derivative, depolymerized; low-molecular weight heparin

Therapeutic Class: Anticoagulant

CLINICAL PHARMACOLOGY

Mechanism of Action: An antithrombin that inhibits factor Xa and thrombin in the presence of low-molecular-weight heparin. Only slightly influences platelet aggregation, PT, and aPTT. *Therapeutic Effect:* Produces anticoagulation.

Pharmacokinetics

Route	*Onset*	*Peak*	*Duration*
Subcutaneous	N/A	4 hr	N/A

Protein binding: less than 10%. **Half-life:** 3–5 hr.

INDICATIONS AND DOSAGES

Low- to moderate-risk abdominal surgery

Subcutaneous

Adults, Elderly. 2,500 international units 1–2 hr before surgery, then daily for 5–10 days.

High-risk abdominal surgery

Subcutaneous

Adults, Elderly. 5,000 international units 1–2 hr before surgery, then daily for 5–10 days.

Total hip surgery

Subcutaneous

Adults, Elderly. 2,500 international units 1–2 hr before surgery, then 2,500 units 6 hrs after surgery, then 5,000 units/day for 7–10 days.

Unstable angina, non–Q-wave MI

Subcutaneous

Adults, Elderly. 120 international units/kg q12h (maximum: 10,000 international units/dose) given with aspirin until clinically stable.

Prevention of DVT or PE in the acutely ill patient

Subcutaneous

Adults, Elderly. 5,000 international units once a day.

[$] **AVAILABLE FORMS/COST**

- Sol—SC: 2500 anti-Factor Xa/0.2 ml: **$17.21**; 5000 anti-Factor Xa/0.2 ml: **$27.93**; 10,000 anti-Factor Xa/1 ml: **$55.85**

CONTRAINDICATIONS: Active major bleeding; concurrent heparin therapy; hypersensitivity to dalteparin, heparin, or pork products; thrombocytopenia associated with positive in vitro test for antiplatelet antibody

PREGNANCY AND LACTATION: Pregnancy category B

SIDE EFFECTS

Occasional (7%–3%)

Hematoma at injection site

Rare (less than 1%)

Hypersensitivity reaction (chills, fever, pruritus, urticaria, asthma, rhinitis, lacrimation, headache); mild, local skin irritation

SERIOUS REACTIONS

- Overdose may lead to bleeding complications ranging from local ecchymoses to major hemorrhage.
- Thrombocytopenia occurs rarely.

INTERACTIONS

Drugs

[3] *Aspirin:* Increased risk of hemorrhage

[3] *Oral anticoagulants:* Additive anticoagulant effects

SPECIAL CONSIDERATIONS

- Cannot be used interchangeably (unit for unit) with unfractionated heparin or other low molecular weight heparins

MONITORING PARAMETERS

• CBC with platelets, stool occult blood, urinalysis
• Monitoring aPTT is not required

---

danazol

(da'-na-zole)
Rx: Danocrine
Chemical Class: Androgen; ethisterone derivative
Therapeutic Class: Androgen

CLINICAL PHARMACOLOGY

Mechanism of Action: A testosterone derivative that suppresses the pituitary-ovarian axis by inhibiting the output of pituitary gonadotropins. Causes atrophy of both normal and ectopic endometrial tissue in endometriosis. Follicle-stimulating hormone (FSH) and luteinizing hormone (LH) are depressed in fibrocystic breast disease. Inhibits steroid synthesis and binding of steroids to their receptors in breast tissues. Increases serum levels of esterase inhibitor. *Therapeutic Effect:* Produces anovulation and amenorrhea, reduces the production of estrogen, corrects biochemical deficiency as seen in hereditary angioedema.

Pharmacokinetics
Well absorbed from gastrointestinal (GI) tract. Metabolized in liver, primarily to 2-hydroxymethylethisterone. Excreted in urine. **Half-life:** 4.5 hrs.

INDICATIONS AND DOSAGES

Endometriosis
PO
Adults. 200-800 mg/day in 2 divided doses for 3-9 mos.

Fibrocystic breast disease
PO
Adults. 100-400 mg/day in 2 divided doses.

Hereditary angioedema
PO
Adults. Initially, 200 mg 2-3 times/day. Decrease dose by 50% or less at 1-3 mo intervals. If attack occurs, increase dose by up to 200 mg/day.

$ **AVAILABLE FORMS/COST**
• Cap, Gel—Oral: 50 mg, 100's: **$158.60-$159.86**; 100 mg, 100's: **$237.96-$286.45**; 200 mg, 100's: **$396.50-$477.08**

UNLABELED USES: Treatment of gynecomastia, menorrhagia, precocious puberty

CONTRAINDICATIONS: Cardiac impairment, hypercalcemia, pregnancy, prostatic or breast cancer in males, severe liver or renal disease

PREGNANCY AND LACTATION: Pregnancy category X; may result in androgenic effects in the fetus; initiate therapy during menstruation or rule out pregnancy prior to initiating therapy in women of child-bearing potential; contraindicated during breast-feeding

SIDE EFFECTS

Frequent
Females: Amenorrhea, breakthrough bleeding/spotting, decreased breast size, increased weight, irregular menstrual period.

Occasional
Males/females: Edema, rhabdomyolysis (muscle cramps, unusual fatigue), virilism (acne, oily skin), flushed skin, altered moods

Rare
Males/females: Hematuria, gingivitis, carpal tunnel syndrome, cataracts, severe headache, vomiting, rash, photosensitivity
Females: Enlarged clitoris, hoarseness, deepening voice, hair growth, monilial vaginitis
Males: Decreased testicle size.

SERIOUS REACTIONS
• Jaundice may occur in those receiving 400 mg/day or more. Liver dysfunction, eosinophilia, thrombocytopenia, pancreatitis occur rarely.
INTERACTIONS
Drugs
❷ *Carbamazepine:* Predictably increases serum carbamazepine concentrations, toxicity possible
❷ *Cyclosporine:* Increased serum cyclosporine concentrations, toxicity possible
❸ *HMG-CoA reductase inhibitors (lovastatin, pravastatin):* Myositis risk increased
❷ *Oral anticoagulants:* Enhanced hypoprothrombinemic response
❷ *Tacrolimus:* Increased tacrolimus concentrations, toxicity possible
Labs
• *False decrease:* Plasma cortisol, serum testosterone, serum thyroxine
• *False increase:* Plasma cortisol, serum testosterone
SPECIAL CONSIDERATIONS
• Useful for palliative treatment of moderate to severe endometriosis or infertility due to endometriosis and for those whom alternative hormonal therapy is ineffective, intolerable, or contraindicated
• Drug of choice for treating all types of hereditary angioedema except for children or pregnant women where fibrolytic inhibitors (aminocaproic acid) may be preferred
• Breast pain should be treated conservatively (analgesics, supportive bra). Hormonal therapy is not innocuous. Symptoms usually return after discontinuation
• Ovarian function usually returns within 60-90 days after discontinuation

PATIENT/FAMILY EDUCATION
• Use nonhormonal contraceptive measures during therapy; discontinue use if pregnancy is suspected
MONITORING PARAMETERS
• Potassium, blood sugar, urine glucose during long-term therapy

D

dantrolene
(dan'troe-leen)
Rx: Dantrium
Chemical Class: Hydantoin derivative
Therapeutic Class: Antidote, malignant hyperthermia; skeletal muscle relaxant

CLINICAL PHARMACOLOGY
Mechanism of Action: A skeletal muscle relaxant that reduces muscle contraction by interfering with release of calcium ion. Reduces calcium ion concentration. *Therapeutic Effect:* Dissociates excitation-contraction coupling. Interferes with catabolic process associated with malignant hyperthermic crisis.
Pharmacokinetics
Poorly absorbed from the gastrointestinal (GI) tract. Protein binding: High. Metabolized in the liver. Primarily excreted in urine. **Half-life:** IV: 4-8 hrs; PO: 8.7 hrs.
INDICATIONS AND DOSAGES
Spasticity
PO
Adults, Elderly. Initially, 25 mg/day. Increase to 25 mg 2-4 times a day, then by 25-mg increments up to 100 mg 2-4 times a day.
Children. Initially, 0.5 mg/kg twice a day. Increase to 0.5 mg/kg 3- 4 times a day, then in increments of 0. 5 mg/kg/day up to 3 mg/kg 2-4 times a day. Maximum: 400 mg/day.

Prevention of malignant hyperthermic crisis

PO

Adults, Elderly, Children. 4-8 mg/kg/day in 3-4 divided doses 1-2 days before surgery; give last dose 3-4 hr before surgery.

IV

Adults, Elderly, Children. 2.5 mg/kg about 1.25 hr before surgery.

Management of malignant hyperthermic crisis

IV

Adults, Elderly, Children. Initially a minimum of 1 mg/kg rapid IV; may repeat up to total cumulative dose of 10 mg/kg. May follow with 4-8 mg/kg/day PO in 4 divided doses up to 3 days after crisis.

§ AVAILABLE FORMS/COST

• Cap, Gel—Oral: 25 mg, 100's: **$114.50**; 50 mg, 100's: **$171.53**; 100 mg, 100's: **$213.36**

• Powder, Inj-IV: 20 mg, 1's: **$71.10**

UNLABELED USES: Relief of exercise-induced pain in patients with muscular dystrophy, treatment of flexor spasms and neuroleptic malignant syndrome

CONTRAINDICATIONS: Active hepatic disease

PREGNANCY AND LACTATION: Pregnancy category C; do not use in nursing women

SIDE EFFECTS

Frequent

Drowsiness, dizziness, weakness, general malaise, diarrhea (mild)

Occasional

Confusion, diarrhea (may be severe), headache, insomnia, constipation, urinary frequency

Rare

Paradoxical CNS excitement or restlessness, paresthesia, tinnitus, slurred speech, tremor, blurred vision, dry mouth, nocturia, impotence, rash, pruritus

SERIOUS REACTIONS

• There is a risk of liver toxicity, most notably in females, those 35 years of age and older, and those taking other medications concurrently.

• Overt hepatitis noted most frequently between 3rd and 12th month of therapy.

• Overdosage results in vomiting, muscular hypotonia, muscle twitching, respiratory depression, and seizures.

INTERACTIONS

Drugs

◪ *Calcium channel blockers:* Rare cases of CV collapse with concomitant use of dantrolene and verapamil; calcium channel blockers and dantrolene use not recommended during management of malignant hyperthermia

◪ *CNS depressants:* Increased drowsiness

◪ *Estrogen:* Possible increased hepatotoxicity in females >35 yr on estrogen therapy

◪ *Vecuronium:* Dantrium may potentiate vecuronium-induced neuromuscular block

SPECIAL CONSIDERATIONS

• Use carefully where spasticity is utilized to sustain upright posture and balance in locomotion or to obtain or maintain increased function

• Discontinue after 6 wk if improvement does not occur

• Use lowest dose possible (hepatotoxicity dose-related)

PATIENT/FAMILY EDUCATION

• IV therapy may decrease grip strength and increase weakness of leg muscles, especially walking down stairs

• Caution driving or operating hazardous machinery

MONITORING PARAMETERS

• Baseline and periodic LFTs (AST, ALT, alk phosphatase, total bilirubin)

dapsone

(dap′sone)
Rx: Dapsone
Chemical Class: Sulfone
Therapeutic Class: Antiprotozoal; leprostatic

CLINICAL PHARMACOLOGY
Mechanism of Action: An antibiotic that is a competitive antagonist of para-aminobenzoic acid (PABA); it prevents normal bacterial utilization of PABA for synthesis of folic acid. *Therapeutic effect:* Inhibits bacterial growth.

INDICATIONS AND DOSAGES
Leprosy
PO
Adults, Elderly. 50-100 mg/day for 3-10 yr.
Children. 1-2 mg/kg/24 hr. Maximum: 100 mg/day.
Dermatitis herpetiformis
PO
Adults, Elderly. Initially, 50 mg/day. May increase up to 300 mg/day.
Pneumocystis carinii pneumonia (PCP)
PO
Adults, Elderly. 100 mg/day in combination with trimethoprim for 21 days.
Prevention of PCP
PO
Adults, Elderly. 100 mg/day.
Children older than 1 mo. 2 mg/kg/day. Maximum: 100 mg/day.

[$] **AVAILABLE FORMS/COST**
• Tab-Oral: 25 mg, 100's: **$18.90**; 100 mg, 100's: **$19.75**

UNLABELED USES: Treatment of inflammatory bowel disorders, malaria

CONTRAINDICATIONS: None significant.

PREGNANCY AND LACTATION: Pregnancy category C; extensive, but uncontrolled, experience and 2 published surveys in pregnant women have not shown increases in the risk for fetal abnormalities if administered during all trimesters; excreted in breast milk, hemolytic reactions can occur in neonates, discontinue nursing or discontinue drug; alternatively, some authors have suggested infants should be kept with mothers infected with leprosy, and breast-feeding during drug therapy encouraged

SIDE EFFECTS
Frequent (greater than 10%)
Hemolytic anemia, methemoglobinemia, rash
Occasional (10%-1%)
Hemolysis, photosensitivity reaction

SERIOUS REACTIONS
• Agranulocytosis and blood dyscrasias may occur.

INTERACTIONS
Drugs
[3] *Didanosine:* Higher failure rate in pneumocystis infections, possibly due to inhibited dissolution of dapsone in stomach; administer dapsone 2-3 hr before didanosine
[3] *Probenecid:* Increased serum dapsone concentrations, clinical importance not established
[3] *Rifampin:* Reduced serum dapsone concentrations; increased methemoglobin concentrations
[3] *Trimethoprim:* Increased serum dapsone concentrations; increased trimethoprim concentrations

SPECIAL CONSIDERATIONS
• Use in conjunction with either rifampin or clofazimine to prevent development of drug resistance and reduce infectiousness of patient with leprosy more quickly

PATIENT/FAMILY EDUCATION
• Full therapeutic effects on leprosy may not occur for several mo; compliance with dosage schedule, duration is necessary
MONITORING PARAMETERS
• CBC weekly for the 1st mo, qmo for 6 mo, and semiannually thereafter
• Periodic LFTs

---

daptomycin

Rx: Cubicin
Chemical Class: Lipopeptide, cyclic
Therapeutic Class: Antibiotic

CLINICAL PHARMACOLOGY
Mechanism of Action: A lipopeptide antibacterial agent that binds to bacterial membranes and causes a rapid depolarization of the membrane potential. The loss of membrane potential leads to inhibition of protein, DNA, and RNA synthesis. *Therapeutic Effect:* Bactericidal.
Pharmacokinetics
Widely distributed. Protein binding: 90%. Primarily excreted unchanged in urine. Moderately removed by hemodialysis. **Half-life:** 7-8 hr (increased in impaired renal function).
INDICATIONS AND DOSAGES
Complicated skin and skin-structure infections
IV
Adults, Elderly. 4 mg/kg every 24 hr for 7-14 days.
Dosage in renal impairment
For patients with creatinine clearance of less than 30 ml/min, dosage is 4 mg/kg q48h for 7-14 days.
Ⓢ **AVAILABLE FORMS/COST**
• Powder, Inj-IV: 500 mg/vial: **$161.39**
CONTRAINDICATIONS: None known

PREGNANCY AND LACTATION: Pregnancy category B, breast milk excretion unknown
SIDE EFFECTS
Frequent (6%-5%)
Constipation, nausea, peripheral injection site reactions, headache, diarrhea
Occasional (4%-3%)
Insomnia, rash, vomiting
Rare (less than 3%)
Pruritus, dizziness, hypotension
SERIOUS REACTIONS
• Skeletal muscle myopathy, characterized by muscle pain and weakness, particularly of the distal extremities, occurs rarely.
• Antibiotic-associated colitis and other superinfections may result from altered bacterial balance.
SPECIAL CONSIDERATIONS
• Experience with coadministration of HMG-CoA reductase inhibitors and daptomycin is limited; consider holding HMG-CoA reductase inhibitors in patients receiving daptomycin
• **Not** effective for pneumonia even due to susceptible organisms
MONITORING PARAMETERS
• CPK (weekly; discontinue in symptomatic patients with CPK elevation >1000 U/L (~5× ULN), or in asymptomatic patients with CPK >10× ULN

darbepoetin alfa

(dar-beh-poe'ee-tin)
Rx: Aranesp
Chemical Class: Amino acid glycoprotein
Therapeutic Class: Hematopoietic agent

CLINICAL PHARMACOLOGY
Mechanism of Action: A glycoprotein that stimulates formation of RBCs in bone marrow; increases serum half-life of epoetin. *Therapeutic Effect:* Induces erythropoiesis and release of reticulocytes from bone marrow.
Pharmacokinetics
Well absorbed after subcutaneous administration. **Half-life:** 48.5 hr.

INDICATIONS AND DOSAGES
Anemia in chronic renal failure
IV bolus, Subcutaneous
Adults, Elderly. Initially, 0.45 mcg/kg once weekly. Adjust dosage to achieve and maintain a target Hgb not to exceed 12 g/dl. Do not increase dosage more frequently than once monthly. Limit increases in Hgb by less than 1 g/dl over any 2-week period.
Anemia associated with chemotherapy
IV, Subcutaneous
Adults, Elderly. 2.25 mcg/kg/dose once a week.

ⓢ AVAILABLE FORMS/COST
• Sol, Inj-IV, SC: 200 mcg/vial: **$997.50**; 100 mcg/vial: **$498.75**; 60 mcg/vial: **$299.25**; 40 mcg/vial: **$199.50**; 25 mcg/vial: **$124.69**

CONTRAINDICATIONS: History of sensitivity to mammalian cell-derived products or human albumin, uncontrolled hypertension

PREGNANCY AND LACTATION: Pregnancy category C, unknown if excreted in human milk

SIDE EFFECTS
Frequent
Myalgia, hypertension or hypotension, headache, diarrhea
Occasional
Fatigue, edema, vomiting, reaction at administration site, asthenia, dizziness

SERIOUS REACTIONS
• Vascular access thrombosis, CHF, sepsis, arrhythmias, and anaphylactic reaction occur rarely.

SPECIAL CONSIDERATIONS
• Two formulations available, one containing polysorbate 80, the other containing human albumin; a theoretical risk for Creutzfeldt-Jakob disease exists with the albumin formulation but is considered extremely remote
• Advantage over erythropoietin is decreased frequency of dosing

PATIENT/FAMILY EDUCATION
• Educate about blood pressure monitoring
• Proper instruction for home administration if deemed appropriate

MONITORING PARAMETERS
• Hematocrit/hemoglobin weekly for 4 weeks or until stable; if Hb increases >1.0 g/dL in any 2 week period, decrease dose (possible increased seizure risk); target Hb level to not exceed 12 g/L
• Serum ferritin, transferrin saturation; supplemental iron recommended if ferritin <100 mcg/L or transferrin saturation <20%
• If lack of response or failure to maintain response occur, check for causative factors (e.g., folate or vitamin B_{12} deficiency, occult blood loss, malignancy)
• Blood pressure

deferoxamine
(de-fer-ox′a-meen)
Rx: Desferal
Chemical Class: Siderochrome
Therapeutic Class: Antidote,
heavy metal

CLINICAL PHARMACOLOGY
Mechanism of Action: An antidote
that binds with iron to form complex. *Therapeutic Effect:* Promotes
urine excretion of acute iron poisoning.
Pharmacokinetics
Well absorbed after IM, SC administration. Widely distributed. Rapidly metabolized in tissues, plasma.
Excreted in urine, eliminated in feces via biliary excretion. Removed
by hemodialysis. **Half-life:** 6 hrs.

INDICATIONS AND DOSAGES
Acute iron intoxication
IM
Adults: Initially, 90 mg/kg, then 45
mg/kg up to 1 g q4-12h. Maximum:
6 g/day.
IV
Adults: 15 mg/kg/hr up to 90 mg/kg
q8hrs. Maximum: 6 g/day.
Children: 15 mg/kg/hr.
Chronic iron overload
Subcutaneous
Adults. 1-2 g/day (20-40 mg/kg)
over 8-24 hrs.
Children: 10 mg/kg/day.
IM
Adults. 0.5-1 g/day. In addition to
IM, 2 g infused at rate not to exceed
15 mg/kg/hr.

AVAILABLE FORMS/COST
• Powder, Inj-IM, IV, SC: 500 mg:
$12.48-$18.66; 2 g: **$48.06-$72.54**

CONTRAINDICATIONS: Severe renal disease, anuria, primary hemochromatosis, hypersensitivity to deferoxamine mesylate or any component of the formulation

PREGNANCY AND LACTATION:
Pregnancy category C; excretion
into breast milk unknown; use caution in nursing mothers

SIDE EFFECTS
Frequent
Pain, induration at injection site,
urine color change (to orange-rose)
Occasional
Abdominal discomfort, diarrhea,
leg cramps, impaired vision

SERIOUS REACTIONS
• Neurotoxicity, including high-frequency hearing loss, has been reported.

SPECIAL CONSIDERATIONS
• Acute iron intoxication
• Deferoxamine indicated if:
  • Free serum iron present
  • Patient symptomatic
  • Serum iron >350 mcg/dL

PATIENT/FAMILY EDUCATION
• May turn urine red

MONITORING PARAMETERS
• Visual acuity tests, slit-lamp examinations, funduscopy, and audiometry are recommended periodically in patients treated for prolonged periods of time
• BUN, creatinine, CrCl
• Serum iron levels

delavirdine
(deh-la′ver-deen)
Rx: Rescriptor
Chemical Class: Arylpiperazine derivative; non-nucleoside
reverse transcriptase inhibitor
Therapeutic Class: Antiretroviral

CLINICAL PHARMACOLOGY
Mechanism of Action: A nonnucleoside reverse transcriptase inhibitor that binds directly to HIV-1
reverse transcriptase and blocks
RNA- and DNA-dependent DNA

polymerase activities. *Therapeutic Effect:* Interrupts HIV replication, slowing the progression of HIV infection.

Pharmacokinetics

Rapidly absorbed after PO administration. Protein binding: 98%. Primarily distributed in plasma. Metabolized in the liver. Eliminated in feces and urine. **Half-life:** 2-11 hr.

INDICATIONS AND DOSAGES

HIV infection (in combination with other antiretrovirals)

PO

Adults. 400 mg 3 times a day.

S AVAILABLE FORMS/COST

• Tab-Oral: 100 mg, 360's: **$316.35**; 200 mg, 180's: **$316.35**

CONTRAINDICATIONS: None known.

PREGNANCY AND LACTATION: Pregnancy category C, teratogenic in rats; excreted in breast milk at high concentrations

SIDE EFFECTS

Frequent (18%)

Rash, pruritus

Occasional (greater than 2%)

Headache, nausea, diarrhea, fatigue, anorexia

SERIOUS REACTIONS

• None known.

INTERACTIONS

Drugs

🟦 *Aluminum:* Antacids reduce GI absorption of delavirdine by 50% if taken at same time; separate doses by at least 1 hr

🟦 *Antacids:* Antacids reduce GI absorption of delavirdine by 50% if taken at same time; separate doses by at least 1 hr

🟦 *Barbiturates:* Barbiturates decrease plasma delavirdine levels

🟦 *Benzodiazepines:* Delavirdine increases benzodiazepine plasma levels by inhibiting hepatic metabolism

🟦 *Calcium:* Antacids reduce GI absorption of delavirdine by 50% if taken at same time; separate doses by at least 1 hr

🟦 *Carbamazepine:* Carbamazepine decreases plasma delavirdine levels

② *Cimetidine:* Cimetidine reduces GI absorption of delavirdine; coadministration not recommended

② *Cisapride:* Delavirdine increases cisapride plasma level; coadministration not recommended

🟦 *Clarithromycin:* Delavirdine increases clarithromycin plasma levels; clarithromycin increases delavirdine plasma levels

🟦 *Dapsone:* Delavirdine increases dapsone plasma level

🟦 *Didanosine:* Delavirdine reduces didanosine absorption; didanosine reduces delavirdine absorption; separate doses by at least 1 hr

② *Ergotamines:* Delavirdine increases ergotamine plasma level; coadministration not recommended

② *Famotidine:* Famotidine reduces GI absorption of delavirdine; coadministration not recommended

🟦 *Fluoxetine:* Fluoxetine increases delavirdine levels by inhibiting hepatic metabolism

🟦 *Indinavir:* Delavirdine increases indinavir AUC by 40%; reduce indinavir dose to 600 mg tid

② *Lansoprazole:* Lansoprazole reduces GI absorption of delavirdine; coadministration not recommended

② *Lovastatin:* Delavirdine increases lovastatin plasma level; coadministration not recommended

🟦 *Magnesium:* Antacids reduce GI absorptioin of delavirdine by 50% if taken at same time; separate doses by at least 1 hr

② *Midazolam:* Delavirdine increases midazolam plasma level; coadministration not recommended

3 *Nelfinavir:* Delavirdine increases nelfinavir AUC by 100%; nelfinavir reduces delavirdine AUC by 50%; no data on dose adjustment

2 *Nizatidine:* Nizatidine reduces GI absorption of delavirdine; coadministration not recommended

3 *Nifedipine:* Delavirdine increases nifedipine plasma level

2 *Omeprazole:* Omeprazole reduces GI absorption of delavirdine; coadministration not recommended

3 *Phenytoin:* Phenytoin decreases plasma delavirdine level

2 *Quinidine:* Delavirdine increases quinidine plasma level

2 *Ranitidine:* Ranitidine reduces GI absorption of delavirdine; coadministration not recommended

2 *Rifabutin:* Rifabutin decreases plasma delavirdine level; coadministration not recommended

⚠ *Rifampin:* Rifampin decreases plasma delavirdine level; coadministration contraindicated

3 *Ritonavir:* Delavirdine increases ritonavir AUC by 70%; no data on dose adjustment

2 *Saquinavir:* Delavirdine increases saquinavir AUC by 5-fold; additive hepatic toxicity possible; adjust Fortovase dose to 800 mg tid

2 *Simvastatin:* Delavirdine increases simvastatin plasma level; coadministration not recommended

3 *Sodium bicarbonate:* Antacids reduce GI absorption of delavirdine by 50% if taken at same time; separate doses by at least 1 hr

⚠ *Terfenadine:* Delavirdine increases terfenadine plasma level; coadministration contraindicated

2 *Triazolam:* Delavirdine increases triazolam plasma level; coadministration not recommended

3 *Warfarin:* Delavirdine increases warfarin effect

SPECIAL CONSIDERATIONS
PATIENT/FAMILY EDUCATION
• May take without regard to food; patients with achlorhydria should take with acidic beverage (orange or cranberry juice); may cause alcohol intolerance

MONITORING PARAMETERS
• CBC, hepatic, and renal function

---

demeclocycline
(dem-e-kloe-sye′kleen)
Rx: Declomycin
Chemical Class: Tetracycline derivative
Therapeutic Class: Antibiotic

CLINICAL PHARMACOLOGY
Mechanism of Action: A tetracycline antibiotic that inhibits bacterial protein synthesis by binding to ribosomal receptor sites; also inhibits ADH-induced water reabsorption. *Therapeutic Effect:* Bacteriostatic; also produces water diuresis.

INDICATIONS AND DOSAGES
Mild to moderate infections, including acne, pertussis, chronic bronchitis, and UTIs
PO
Adults, Elderly. 150 mg 4 times a day or 300 mg 2 times a day.
Children older than 8 yr. 8-12 mg/kg/day in 2-4 divided doses.

Uncomplicated gonorrhea
PO
Adults. Initially, 600 mg, then 300 mg q12h for 4 days for total of 3 g.

Syndrome of inappropriate ADH secretion (SIADH)
PO
Adults, Elderly. Initially, 900-1200 mg/day in 3-4 divided doses, then decrease dose to 600-900 mg/day in divided doses.

💲 AVAILABLE FORMS/COST
• Tab-Oral: 150 mg, 100's: **$1,049.38**; 300 mg, 48's: **$911.88**

CONTRAINDICATIONS: Children 8 years and younger, last half of pregnancy

PREGNANCY AND LACTATION: Pregnancy category D; problems associated with use of the tetracyclines during or around pregnancy include adverse effects on fetal teeth and bones, maternal liver toxicity, and congenital defects; excreted into breast milk in low concentrations; use caution in nursing mothers

SIDE EFFECTS
Frequent
Anorexia, nausea, vomiting, diarrhea, dysphagia, possibly severe photosensitivity, (with moderate to high demeclocycline dosage).
Occasional
Urticaria, rash; diabetes insipidus syndrome, marked by polydipsia, polyuria, and weakness (with long-term therapy).

SERIOUS REACTIONS
• Superinfection (especially fungal), anaphylaxis, and benign intracranial hypertension occur rarely.
• Bulging fontanelles occur rarely in infants.

INTERACTIONS
Drugs
3 *Antacids:* Reduced serum concentration of demeclocycline; take 2 hr before or 6 hr after antacids containing aluminum, calcium, or magnesium

2 *Bismuth:* Reduced serum concentration of demeclocycline; do not coadminister

3 *Calcium:* See antacids

3 *Cholestyramine:* Reduced serum concentration of demeclocycline; take 2 hr before or 3 hr after cholestyramine

3 *Colestipol:* Reduced serum concentration of demeclocycline; take 2 hr before or 3 hr after colestipol

3 *Digoxin:* Demeclocycline may increase serum digoxin levels

3 *Food:* Reduced serum concentration of demeclocycline; take 2 hr before or 3 hr after food

3 *Iron:* Reduced serum concentration of demeclocycline; take 2 hr before or 3 hr after iron

3 *Magnesium:* See antacids

2 *Methoxyflurane:* Demeclocycline enhances nephrotoxicity of methoxyflurane

3 *Oral contraceptives:* Contraceptive failure may occur rarely; mechanism unknown

3 *Penicillins:* Demeclocycline may reduce penicillin efficacy

3 *Warfarin:* Demeclocycline may increase effect of warfarin

3 *Zinc:* Reduced serum concentration of demeclocycline; take 2 hr before or 3 hr after zinc

Labs
• *False increase:* Urinary catecholamines

SPECIAL CONSIDERATIONS
• No advantages over other tetracyclines as anti-infective; higher incidence of phototoxicity; active against water intoxication and SIADH

PATIENT/FAMILY EDUCATION
• Sunscreen does not seem to decrease photosensitivity
• Avoid milk products; take with full glass of water on an empty stomach 1 hr before meals or 2 hr after meals

MONITORING PARAMETERS
• LFTs during prolonged administration

desipramine

(dess-ip'ra-meen)

Rx: Norpramin

Chemical Class: Dibenza-zepine derivative; secondary amine

Therapeutic Class: Antidepressant, tricyclic

CLINICAL PHARMACOLOGY

Mechanism of Action: A tricyclic antidepressant that blocks the reuptake of neurotransmitters, such as norepinephrine and serotonin, at presynaptic membranes, increasing their availability at postsynaptic receptor sites. Also has strong anticholinergic activity. *Therapeutic Effect:* Relieves depression.

Pharmacokinetics

Rapidly, and well absorbed from the GI tract. Protein binding: 90%. Metabolized in the liver. Primarily excreted in urine. Minimally removed by hemodialysis. **Half-life:** 12-27 hr.

INDICATIONS AND DOSAGES

Depression

PO

Adults. 75 mg/day. May gradually increase to 150-200 mg/day. Maximum: 300 mg/day.

Elderly. Initially, 10-25 mg/day. May gradually increase to 75-100 mg/day. Maximum: 300 mg/day.

Children older than 12 yr. Initially, 25-50 mg/day. May gradually increase to 100 mg/day. Maximum: 150 mg/day.

Children 6-12 yr. 1-3 mg/kg/day. Maximum: 5 mg/kg/day.

$ AVAILABLE FORMS/COST

• Tab-Oral: 10 mg, 100's: **$15.90-$120.00**; 25 mg, 100's: **$23.61-$85.44**; 50 mg, 100's: **$19.24-$160.84**; 75 mg, 100's: **$53.15-**$190.80; 100 mg, 100's: **$74.40-$269.00**; 150 mg, 50's: **$53.90-$194.89**

UNLABELED USES: Treatment of attention deficit hyperactivity disorder, bulimia nervosa, cataplexy associated with narcolepsy, cocaine withdrawal, neurogenic pain, panic disorder

CONTRAINDICATIONS: Angle-closure glaucoma, use within 14 days of MAOIs

PREGNANCY AND LACTATION: Pregnancy category C; excreted into breast milk; effect on the nursing infant unknown, but may be of concern

SIDE EFFECTS

Frequent

Somnolence, fatigue, dry mouth, blurred vision, constipation, delayed micturition, orthostatic hypotension, diaphoresis, impaired concentration, increased appetite, urine retention

Occasional

GI disturbances (such as nausea, GI distress, metallic taste)

Rare

Paradoxical reactions (agitation, restlessness, nightmares, insomnia), extrapyramidal symptoms (particularly fine hand tremor)

SERIOUS REACTIONS

Overdose may produce confusion, seizures, somnolence, arrhythmias, fever, hallucinations, dyspnea, vomiting, and unusual fatigue or weakness.

Abrupt discontinuation after prolonged therapy may produce severe headache, malaise, nausea, vomiting, and vivid dreams.

INTERACTIONS

Drugs

🔳 *Barbiturates:* Reduced serum concentrations of cyclic antidepressants

② *Bethanidine:* Reduced antihypertensive effect of bethanidine

③ *Carbamazepine:* Reduced serum concentrations of cyclic antidepressants

③ *Cimetidine:* Increased serum concentrations of cyclic antidepressants

② *Clonidine:* Reduced antihypertensive effect of clonidine; enhanced hypertensive response with abrupt clonidine withdrawal

③ *Debrisoquin:* Reduced antihypertensive effect of debrisoquin

③ *Diltiazem:* Increased serum concentrations of cyclic antidepressants

② *Epinephrine:* Markedly enhanced pressor response to IV epinephrine

③ *Ethanol:* Additive impairment of motor skills; abstinent alcoholics may eliminate cyclic antidepressants faster than nonalcoholics

③ *Fluoxetine:* Marked increases in serum concentrations of cyclic antidepressants

③ *Fluvoxamine:* Marked increases in serum concentrations of cyclic antidepressants

② *Guanabenz, guanethidine:* Reduced antihypertensive effect

③ *Guanadrel, guanfacine:* Reduced antihypertensive effect

③ *Indinavir:* Increase in serum concentrations of cyclic antidepressants

③ *Lithium:* Increased risk of neurotoxicity

② *Moclobemide:* Potential association with fatal or nonfatal serotonin syndrome

② *MAOIs:* Excessive sympathetic response, manias, or hyperpyrexia possible

③ *Neuroleptics:* Increased therapeutic and toxic effects of both drugs

② *Norepinephrine:* Markedly enhanced pressor response to IV norepinephrine

③ *Paroxetine:* Marked increases in serum concentrations of cyclic antidepressants

③ *Propoxyphene:* Increased serum concentrations of cyclic antidepressants

③ *Quinidine:* Increased serum concentrations of cyclic antidepressants

③ *Rifampin:* Reduced serum concentrations of cyclic antidepressants

③ *Ritonavir:* Marked increases in serum concentrations of cyclic antidepressants

③ *Sulfonylureas:* Cyclic antidepressants may increase hypoglycemic effect

SPECIAL CONSIDERATIONS

• Equally effective as other tricyclic antidepressants for depression; fewer anticholinergic effects than tertiary amines, less orthostasis, and mild stimulatory property

PATIENT/FAMILY EDUCATION

• Therapeutic effects may take 4-6 wk

• Use caution in driving or other activities requiring alertness

• Avoid alcohol and other CNS depressants

• Do not discontinue abruptly after long-term use

MONITORING PARAMETERS

• Determination of desipramine plasma concentrations is not routinely recommended but may be useful in identifying toxicity, drug interactions, or noncompliance (adjustments in dosage should be made according to clinical response not plasma concentrations); therapeutic level is 50-200 ng/ml

desirudin

Rx: Iprivask

Chemical Class: Hirudin derivative; thrombin inhibitor

Therapeutic Class: Anticoagulant

CLINICAL PHARMACOLOGY

Mechanism of Action: An anticoagulant that binds specifically and directly to thrombin, inhibiting free circulating and clot-bound thrombin. *Therapeutic Effect:* Prolongs the clotting time of human plasma.

Pharmacokinetics

Completely absorbed. Distributed in extracellular space. Metabolized and eliminated by the kidney. **Half-life:** 2–3 hr.

INDICATIONS AND DOSAGES

Prevention of deep vein thrombosis in patients undergoing hip replacement surgery

Subcutaneous

Adults, Elderly. Initially, 15 mg q12h given 5–15 min before surgery but following induction of regional block anesthesia, if used. May administer up to 12 days post surgery.

Moderate renal impairment (creatinine clearance 31–60 ml/min or higher)

Subcutaneous

Adults, Elderly. 5 mg q12h.

Severe renal impairment (creatinine clearance less than 31 ml/min)

Subcutaneous

Adults, Elderly. 1.7 mg q12h.

[$] **AVAILABLE FORMS/COST**

• Powder, Inj-IV, SC: 15.75 mg/0.6 ml: *cost not available*

CONTRAINDICATIONS: Hypersensitivity to natural or recombinant hirudins (anticoagulation factors), active bleeding, irreversible coagulation disorders

PREGNANCY AND LACTATION: Pregnancy category C; teratogenic in animal studies; excretion into breast milk unknown, use caution in nursing mothers

SIDE EFFECTS

Frequent (6%)

Hematoma

Occasional (4%–2%)

Injection site mass, wound secretion, nausea, hypersensitivity reaction

SERIOUS REACTIONS

• Serious or major hemorrhage and anaphylactic reaction occur rarely.

INTERACTIONS

Drugs

[3] *Dextran 40, systemic glucocorticoids, thrombolytics, and anticoagulants:* Increased risk of bleeding

[3] *Salicylates, NSAIDS, aspirin, ticlopidine, dipyridamole, sulfinpyrazone, clopidogrel, glycoprotein IIb/IIIa antagonists:* Increased risk of bleeding

SPECIAL CONSIDERATIONS

MONITORING PARAMETERS

• If CRCL <60 ml/min monitor aPTT and serum Cr at least daily; if aPTT exceeds 2× control: interrupt therapy until the value returns to less than 2× control and then resume therapy at a reduced dose guided by the initial degree of aPTT abnormality

desloratidine
(des-loer-at'ah-deen)
Rx: Clarinex, Clarinex
RediTabs
Chemical Class: Piperidine
derivative
Therapeutic Class: Antihistamine

CLINICAL PHARMACOLOGY
Mechanism of Action: A nonsedating antihistamine that exhibits selective peripheral histamine H_1 receptor blocking action. Competes with histamine at receptor sites. *Therapeutic Effect:* Prevents allergic responses mediated by histamine, such as rhinitis and urticaria.
Pharmacokinetics
Rapidly and almost completely absorbed from the GI tract. Distributed mainly in liver, lungs, GI tract, and bile. Metabolized in the liver to active metabolite and undergoes extensive first-pass metabolism. Eliminated in urine and feces. **Half-life:** 27 hr (increased in the elderly and in renal or hepatic impairment).

INDICATIONS AND DOSAGES
Allergic rhinitis, urticaria
PO
Adults, Elderly, Children older than 12 yr. 5 mg once a day.
Dosage in hepatic or renal impairment
Dosage is decreased to 5 mg every other day.

S **AVAILABLE FORMS/COST**
• Tab, Film-Coated—Oral: 5 mg, 100's: **$242.20**
CONTRAINDICATIONS: None known.
PREGNANCY AND LACTATION: Pregnancy category C; passes into breast milk, use caution in nursing mothers

SIDE EFFECTS
Frequent (12%)
Headache
Occasional (3%)
Dry mouth, somnolence
Rare (less than 3%)
Fatigue, dizziness, diarrhea, nausea
SERIOUS REACTIONS
• None known.
SPECIAL CONSIDERATIONS
• No advantage over loratidine (parent compound) which is now available OTC
• Intranasal corticosteroids are preferred therapy unless allergy symptoms are mild and infrequent
• Reserve for patients unable to tolerate sedating antihistamines like chlorpheniramine
PATIENT/FAMILY EDUCATION
• May be taken without regard to meals
• Take orally-disintegrating tabs immediately after opening the blister packet

desmopressin
(des-moe-press'in)
Rx: DDAVP, Stimate
Chemical Class: Arginine vasopressin analog
Therapeutic Class: Antidiuretic; antihemophilic; hemostatic

CLINICAL PHARMACOLOGY
Mechanism of Action: A synthetic pituitary hormone that increases reabsorption of water by increasing permeability of collecting ducts of the kidneys. Also serves as a plasminogen activator. *Therapeutic Effect:* Increases plasma factor VIII (antihemophilic factor). Decreases urinary output.

Pharmacokinetics

Route	Onset	Peak	Duration
PO	1 hr	2–7 hr	6–8 hr
IV	15–30 min	1.5–3 hr	N/A
Intranasal	15 min–1 hr	1–5 hr	5–21 hr

Poorly absorbed after oral or nasal administration. Metabolism: Unknown. **Half-life:** Oral: 1.5– 2.5 hr. Intranasal: 3.3–3.5 hr. IV: 0.4–4 hr.

INDICATIONS AND DOSAGES

Primary nocturnal enuresis

PO

Children 12 yr and older. 0.2–0.6 mg once before bedtime.

Intranasal

Children 6 yr and older. Initially, 20 mcg (0.2 ml) at bedtime; use one-half dose in each nostril. Adjust to maximum of 40 mcg/day.

Central cranial diabetes insipidus

PO

Adults, Elderly, Children 12 yr and older. Initially, 0.05 twice a day. Range: 0.1–1.2 mg/day in 2–3 divided doses.

Children younger than 12 yr. Initially, 0.05 mg; then twice a day. Range: 0.1–0.8 mg daily.

Intranasal

Adults, Elderly, Children older than 12 yr. 5–40 mcg (0.05–0.4 ml) in 1–3 doses/day.

Children 3 mo–12 yr. Initially, 5 mcg (0.05 ml)/day. Range: 5–30 mcg (0.05–0.3 ml)/day.

IV, Subcutaneous

Adults, Elderly, Children older than 12 yr. 2–4 mcg/day in 2 divided doses or 1/10 of maintenance intranasal dose.

Hemophilia A, Von Willebrand's Disease (Type I)

IV infusion

Adults, Elderly, Children weighing 10 kg or more. 0.3 mcg/kg diluted in 50 ml 0.9% NaCl.

Children weighing less than 10 kg. 0.3 mcg/kg diluted in 10 ml 0.9% NaCl.

Intranasal

Adults, Elderly, Children 12 yr and older weighing 50 kg or more. 300 mcg; use 1 spray in each nostril.

Adults, Elderly, Children 12 yrsand older weighing less than 50 kg. 150 mcg as a single spray.

$ AVAILABLE FORMS/COST

• Sol, Inj-IV; SC: 4 mcg/ml: **$8.34-$27.48**

• Sol—Nasal: 0.1 mg/ml, 2 ml: **$87.61**

• Spray—Nasal: 10 mcg/inh, 5 ml: **$120.80-$165.90**; 0.15 mg/inh, 2 ml: **$643.75**

• Tab—Oral: 0.1 mg, 100's: **$253.90**; 0.2 mg, 100's: **$365.70**

CONTRAINDICATIONS: Hemophilia A with factor VIII levels less than 5%; hemophilia B; severe type I, type IIB, or platelet-type von Willebrand's disease

PREGNANCY AND LACTATION: Pregnancy category B (no uterotonic action at antidiuretic doses); compatible with breast-feeding

SIDE EFFECTS

Occasional

IV: Pain, redness, or swelling at injection site; headache; abdominal cramps; vulval pain; flushed skin; mild BP elevation; nausea with high dosages

Nasal: Rhinorrhea, nasal congestion, slight BP elevation

SERIOUS REACTIONS

• Water intoxication or hyponatremia, marked by headache, somnolence, confusion, decreased urination, rapid weight gain, seizures, and coma, may occur in overhydration. Children, elderly patients, and infants are especially at risk.

SPECIAL CONSIDERATIONS

• Though useful in the treatment of children with enuresis, relapse following discontinuation is common; conservative therapy preferred long-term; desmopressin best used intermittently (e.g., overnight with friend)

PATIENT/FAMILY EDUCATION

• Nasal tube delivery system is supplied with a flexible calibrated plastic tube (rhinyle); draw sol into the rhinyle, insert 1 end of tube into nostril, blow on the other end to deposit sol deep into nasal cavity

• Ingest only enough water to satisfy thirst (especially elderly and children)

MONITORING PARAMETERS

• Diabetes insipidus: Urine volume and osmolality, plasma osmolality

• Hemophilia A: Determine factor VIII coagulant activity before injecting desmopressin for hemostasis; if activity is <5% of normal, do not rely on desmopressin

• Von Willebrand's disease: Assess levels of factor VIII coagulant, factor VIII antigen, and ristocetin cofactor; skin bleeding time may also be helpful

---

desonide

(dess'oh-nide)

Rx: Delomide, DesOwen, Tridesilon

Chemical Class: Corticosteroid, synthetic

Therapeutic Class: Corticosteroid, topical

CLINICAL PHARMACOLOGY

Mechanism of Action: A topical corticosteroid that has anti-inflammatory, antipruritic, and vasoconstrictive properties. The exact mechanism of the anti-inflammatory process is unclear. *Therapeutic Effect:* Reduces or prevents tissue response to the inflammatory process.

Pharmacokinetics

Large variation in absorption determined by many factors. Metabolized in the liver. Primarily excreted by the kidneys and small amounts in the bile.

INDICATIONS AND DOSAGES

Dermatoses

Topical

Adults, Elderly. Apply sparingly 2-3 times/day.

Otitis externa

Aural

Adults, Elderly, Children. Instill 3 to 4 drops into the ear 3-4 times/day.

Ⓢ **AVAILABLE FORMS/COST**

• Cre—Top: 0.05%, 15, 60, 90 g: **$8.55-$28.75**/15 g

• Lotion—Top: 0.05%, 60, 120 ml: **$32.83-$33.89**/60 ml

• Oint—Top: 0.05%, 15, 60 g: **$12.95-$24.94**/15 g

CONTRAINDICATIONS: Perforated eardrum, history of hypersensitivity to desonide or other corticosteroids

PREGNANCY AND LACTATION: Pregnancy category C; unknown whether top application could result in sufficient systemic absorption to produce detectable amounts in breast milk (systemic corticosteroids are secreted into breast milk in quantities not likely to have detrimental effects on infant)

SIDE EFFECTS

Occasional

Burning and stinging at site of application, dryness, skin peeling, contact dermatitis

SERIOUS REACTIONS

• The serious reactions of long-term therapy and the addition of occlusive dressings are reversible hypothalamic-pituitary-adrenal (HPA)

axis suppression, manifestations of Cushing's syndrome, hyperglycemia and glucosuria.

SPECIAL CONSIDERATIONS
PATIENT/FAMILY EDUCATION

• Apply sparingly only to affected area
• Avoid contact with the eyes
• Do not put bandages or dressings over treated area unless directed by clinician
• Discontinue drug and notify clinician if local irritation or fever develops
• Do not use on weeping, denuded, or infected areas

---

desoximetasone
(des-ox-i-met′a-sone)
Rx: Topicort, Topicort LP
Chemical Class: Corticosteroid, synthetic
Therapeutic Class: Corticosteroid, topical

CLINICAL PHARMACOLOGY
Mechanism of Action: A high potency, fluoronated topical corticosteroid that has anti-inflammatory, antipruritic, and vasoconstrictive properties. The exact mechanism of the anti-inflammatory process is unclear. *Therapeutic Effect:* Reduces tissue response to the inflammatory process.

Pharmacokinetics
Large variation in absorption among sites. Protein binding in varying degrees. Metabolized in liver. Primarily excreted in urine.

INDICATIONS AND DOSAGES
Dermatoses
Topical
Adults, Elderly. Apply sparingly 2 times/day.
Children. Apply sparingly 1-2 times/day.

§ **AVAILABLE FORMS/COST**
• Cre—Top: 0.05%, 15, 60 g: **$9.90-$18.80**/15 g; 0.25%, 15, 60 g: **$13.33-$34.26**/15 g
• Gel—Top: 0.05%, 15, 60 g: **$18.44-$29.75**/15 g
• Oint—Top: 0.25%, 15, 60 g: **$15.41-$42.83**/15 g

UNLABELED USES: Eczema, psoriasis vulgaris

CONTRAINDICATIONS: History of hypersensitivity to desoximetasone or other corticosteroids

PREGNANCY AND LACTATION: Pregnancy category C; it is unknown whether topical application could result in sufficient systemic absorption to produce detectable amounts in breast milk (systemic corticosteroids are secreted into breast milk in quantities not likely to have any detrimental effects on infant)

SIDE EFFECTS
Frequent
Itching, redness, irritation, burning at site of application
Occasional
Dryness, folliculitis, hypertrichosis, acneiform eruptions, hypopigmentation, perioral dermatitis
Rare
Allergic contact dermatitis, adrenal suppression, atrophy, striae, miliaria, photosensitivity

SERIOUS REACTIONS
• Serious reactions of long-term therapy and addition of occlusive dressings are reversible hypothalamic-pituitary-adrenal (HPA) axis suppression, manifestations of Cushing's syndrome, hyperglycemia, and glucosuria.
• Abruptly withdrawing the drug after long-term therapy may require supplemental systemic corticosteroids.

SPECIAL CONSIDERATIONS

• Potent, fluorinated topical corticosteroid with comparable efficacy to fluocinonide, diflorasone, amcinonide, betamethasone, dipropionate, and halcinonide; cost should govern use

PATIENT/FAMILY EDUCATION

• Apply sparingly only to affected area
• Avoid contact with the eyes
• Do not put bandages or dressings over treated area unless directed by clinician
• Discontinue drug, notify clinician if local irritation or fever develops
• Do not use on weeping, denuded, or infected areas

D

dexamethasone

(dex-a-meth'a-sone)
Rx: *Ophthalmic:* Ak-Dex Ophthalmic, Maxidex, Ocumed
Rx: *Systemic:* Cortastat, Dalalone D.P., Decadron, Decaject, Dexasone L.A., Dexone LA, Solurex, Dalalone, Dexasone, Dexone
Combinations
  Rx: with neomycin, (Neo-Decadron, Ak-Neo-Dex); with neomycin and poly-mixin B (Dexacidin, Maxitrol, Dexasporin); with tobramycin (Tobradex); with lidocaine (Decadron with Xylocaine)
Chemical Class: Glucocorticoid, synthetic
Therapeutic Class: Corticosteroid, ophthalmic; corticosteroid, systemic

CLINICAL PHARMACOLOGY

Mechanism of Action: A long-acting glucocorticoid that inhibits accumulation of inflammatory cells at inflammation sites, phagocytosis, lysosomal enzyme release and synthesis, and release of mediators of inflammation. *Therapeutic Effect:* Prevents and suppresses cell and tissue immune reactions and inflammatory process.

Pharmacokinetics

Rapidly, completely absorbed from the GI tract after oral administration. Widely distributed. Protein binding: High. Metabolized in the liver. Primarily excreted in urine. Minimally removed by hemodialysis. **Half-life:** 3-4.5 hr.

INDICATIONS AND DOSAGES

Anti-inflammatory

PO/IV/IM

Adults, Elderly. 0.75-9 mg/day in divided doses q6-12h.

Children. 0.08-0.3 mg/kg/day in divided doses q6-12h.

Cerebral edema

IV

Adults, Elderly. Initially, 10 mg, then 4 mg (IM/IV) q6h.

PO/IV/IM

Children. Loading dose of 1-2 mg/kg, then 1-1.5 mg/kg/day in divided doses q4-6h.

Nausea and vomiting in chemotherapy patients

IV

Adults, Elderly. 8–20 mg once, then 4 mg (PO) q4–6h or 8 mg q8h.

Children. 10 mg/m^2/dose (Maximum: 20 mg), then 5 mg/m^2/dose q6h.

Physiologic replacement

PO/IV/IM

Children. 0.03-0.15 mg/kg/day in divided doses q6-12h.

Usual ophthalmic dosage, ocular inflammatory conditions

Ointment

Adults, Elderly, Children. Thin coating 3-4 times/day.

Suspension

Adults, Elderly, Children. Initially, 2 drops q1h while awake and q2h at night for 1 day, then reduce to 3-4 times/day.

S AVAILABLE FORMS/COST

• Elixir—Oral: 0.5 mg/5 ml, 100, 240, 500 ml: **$7.45-$17.50**/100 ml
• Sol, Inj-IM, IV (sod phos): 4 mg/ml, 5 ml: **$2.45-$29.54**; 10 mg/ml, 10 ml: **$4.94-$51.10**
• Susp, Inj-Intraarticular; IM (acetate): 8 mg/ml, 5 ml: **$9.95-$29.95**; 16 mg/ml, 5 ml: **$25.00**
• Oint-Ophth (sod phos): 0.05%, 3.5 g: **$1.65-$7.25**
• Sol-Ophth (sod phos): 0.1%, 5 ml: **$1.95-$21.10**
• Sol—Oral: 1 mg/ml, 30 ml: **$19.05**
• Susp—Ophth: 0.1%, 5, 15 ml: **$36.60**/5 ml
• Tab-Oral: 0.25 mg, 100's: **$4.05-$11.05**; 0.5 mg, 100's: **$6.75-$64.90**; 0.75 mg, 100's: **$2.05-$81.14**; 1 mg, 100's: **$31.82**; 1.5 mg, 100's: **$9.85-$76.00**; 2 mg, 100's: **$62.31**; 4 mg, 100's: **$12.96-$214.00**; 6 mg, 100's: **$51.36-$193.80**

CONTRAINDICATIONS: Active untreated infections, fungal, tuberculosis, or viral diseases of the eye

PREGNANCY AND LACTATION: Pregnancy category C; used in patients with premature labor at about 24-36 wk gestation to stimulate fetal lung maturation; excreted in breast milk; could suppress infant's growth and interfere with endogenous corticosteroid production

SIDE EFFECTS

Frequent

Inhalation: Cough, dry mouth, hoarseness, throat irritation

Intranasal: Burning, mucosal dryness

Ophthalmic: Blurred vision

Systemic: Insomnia, facial swelling or cushingoid appearance, moderate abdominal distention, indigestion, increased appetite, nervousness, facial flushing, diaphoresis

Occasional

Inhalation: Localized fungal infection, such as thrush

Intranasal: Crusting inside nose, nosebleed, sore throat, ulceration of nasal mucosa.

Ophthalmic: Decreased vision, watering of eyes, eye pain, burning, stinging, redness of eyes, nausea, vomiting

Systemic: Dizziness, decreased or blurred vision

Topical: Allergic contact dermatitis, purpura or blood-containing blisters, thinning of skin with easy bruising, telangiectasis or raised dark red spots on skin

Rare

Inhalation: Increased bronchospasm, esophageal candidiasis

Intranasal: Nasal and pharyngeal candidiasis, eye pain

Systemic: General allergic reaction (such as rash and hives); pain, redness, or swelling at injection site; psychological changes; false sense of well-being; hallucinations; depression

SERIOUS REACTIONS

• Long-term therapy may cause muscle wasting (especially in the arms and legs), osteoporosis, spontaneous fractures, amenorrhea, cataracts, glaucoma, peptic ulcer disease, and CHF.

• The ophthalmic form may cause glaucoma, ocular hypertension, and cataracts.

• Abrupt withdrawal following long-term therapy may cause severe joint pain, severe headache, anorexia, nausea, fever, rebound inflammation, fatigue, weakness, lethargy, dizziness, and orthostatic hypotension.

INTERACTIONS

Drugs

◻ *Aminoglutethamide:* Enhanced elimination of corticosteroids; marked reduction in corticosteroid response; increased clearance of dexamethasone; doubling of dose may be necessary

◻ *Antidiabetics:* Increased blood glucose

◻ *Barbiturates, carbamazepine:* Reduced serum concentrations of corticosteroids; increased clearance of dexamethasone

◻ *Cholestyramine, colestipol:* Possible reduced absorption of corticosteroids

◻ *Cyclosporine:* Possible increased concentration of both drugs, seizures

◻ *Erythromycin, troleandomycin, clarithromycin, ketoconazole:* Possible enhanced steroid effect

◻ *Estrogens, oral contraceptives:* Enhanced effects of corticosteroids

◻ *Isoniazid:* Reduced plasma concentrations of isoniazid

◻ *IUDs:* Inhibition of inflammation may decrease contraceptive effect

◻ *NSAIDs:* Increased risk GI ulceration

◻ *Rifampin:* Reduced therapeutic effect of corticosteroids

◻ *Salicylates:* Subtherapeutic salicylate concentrations possible

Labs

• *False negative:* Skin allergy tests

SPECIAL CONSIDERATIONS

• Signs of adrenal insufficiency include fatigue, anorexia, nausea, vomiting, diarrhea, weight loss, weakness, dizziness, and low blood sugar; drug induced secondary adrenocorticoid insufficiency and low blood sugar; drug-induced adrenocorticoid insufficiency may be minimized by gradual systemic dosage reduction; relative insufficiency may exist for up to 1 yr after discontinuation, therefore, be prepared to supplement in situations of stress

• May mask infections

• Do not give live virus vaccines to patients on prolonged therapy

• Patients on chronic steroid therapy should wear medical alert bracelet

MONITORING PARAMETERS

• Potassium and blood sugar during long-term therapy

• Observe growth and development of children on prolonged therapy
• Check lens and intraocular pressure frequently during prolonged use of ophthalmic preparations

dexchlorpheniramine

(dex'klor-fen-eer'a-meen)
Rx: Polaramine
Combinations
Rx: with guaifenesin, pseudoephedrine (Polaramine Expectorant)
Chemical Class: Alkylamine derivative
Therapeutic Class: Antihistamine

CLINICAL PHARMACOLOGY
Mechanism of Action: A propylamine derivative that competes with histamine for H1-receptor sites on effector cells in the gastrointestinal (GI) tract, blood vessels, and respiratory tract. Dexchlorpheniramine is the dextro-isomer of chlorpheniramine and is approximately two times more active. *Therapeutic Effect:* Prevents allergic response, produces mild bronchodilation, blocks histamine-induced bronchitis.
Pharmacokinetics

Route	Onset	Peak	Duration
PO	0.5 hr	1-2 hr	3-6 hr

Well absorbed from the gastrointestinal (GI) tract. Protein binding: 70%. Widely distributed. Metabolized in liver to active metabolite, undergoes extensive first-pass metabolism. Excreted primarily in urine. Not removed by hemodialysis. **Half-life:** 20 hrs.

INDICATIONS AND DOSAGES
Allergic rhinitis, common cold
PO
Adults, Elderly, Children 12 yrs or older. 2 mg q4-6h or 4-6 mg timed release at bedtime or q8-10h.
Children 6-11 yrs. 4 mg timed release at bedtime or 1 mg q4-6h.
Children 2-5 yrs. 0.5 mg q4-6h. Do not use timed release.
[$] **AVAILABLE FORMS/COST**
• Syr—Oral: 2 mg/5ml, 480 ml: **$13.15-$42.36**
• Tab-Oral: 2 mg, 100's: **$55.02**
• Tab, Sus Action—Oral: 4 mg, 100's: **$22.13-$82.97**; 6 mg, 100's: **$44.25-$115.96**
UNLABELED USES: Asthma, chemotherapy-induced stomatitis, dermographia, familial immunodeficiency disease, malaria, mastocytosi, Meniere's disease, nausea, neurocysticercosis, otitis media, psoriasis, radiocontrast media reactions, urticaria
CONTRAINDICATIONS: History of hypersensitivity to antihistamines, newborn or premature infants, nursing mothers, third trimester of pregnancy
PREGNANCY AND LACTATION: Pregnancy category B
SIDE EFFECTS
Frequent
Drowsiness, dizziness, headache, dry mouth, nose, or throat, urinary retention, thickening of bronchial secretions, sedation, hypotension
Occasional
Epigastric distress, flushing, blurred vision, tinnitus, paresthesia, sweating, chills
SERIOUS REACTIONS
• Children may experience dominant paradoxical reactions, including restlessness, insomnia, euphoria, nervousness, and tremors.

• Hypersensitivity reaction, such as eczema, pruritus, rash, cardiac disturbances, and photosensitivity, may occur.

• Overdosage may vary from CNS depression, including sedation, apnea, hypotension, cardiovascular collapse, or death to severe paradoxical reaction, such as hallucinations, tremor, and seizures.

INTERACTIONS
Labs

• *False negative:* Skin allergy tests

SPECIAL CONSIDERATIONS

• Active dextro-isomer of chlorpheniramine

---

dexmethylphenidate
(dex-meth-ill-fen'i-date)
Rx: Focalin
Chemical Class: Piperidine derivative of amphetamine
Therapeutic Class: Central nervous system stimulant

CLINICAL PHARMACOLOGY
Mechanism of Action: A CNS stimulant that blocks the reuptake of norepinephrine and dopamine into presynaptic neurons, increasing the release of these neurotransmitters into the synaptic cleft. *Therapeutic Effect:* Decreases motor restlessness and fatigue; increases motor activity, mental alertness, and attention span; elevates mood.

Pharmacokinetics

Route	Onset	Peak	Dura-tion
PO	N/A	N/A	4–5 hr

Readily absorbed from the GI tract. Plasma concentrations increase rapidly. Metabolized in the liver. Excreted unchanged in urine. **Half-life:** 2.2 hr.

INDICATIONS AND DOSAGES
Attention deficit hyperactivity disorder (ADHD)
PO
Patients new to dexmethylphenidate or methylphenidate. 2.5 mg twice a day (5 mg/day). May adjust dosage in 2.5- to 5-mg increments. Maximum: 20 mg/day.
Patients currently taking methylphenidate. Half the methylphenidate dosage. Maximum: 20 mg/day.

$ **AVAILABLE FORMS/COST**
• Tab-Oral: 2.5 mg, 100's: **$49.21**; 5 mg, 100's: **$70.15**; 10 mg, 100's: **$100.88**

CONTRAINDICATIONS: Diagnosis or family history of Tourette syndrome; glaucoma; history of marked agitation, anxiety, or tension; motor tics; use within 14 days of MAOIs

PREGNANCY AND LACTATION: Pregnancy category C; excretion into breast milk unknown; use caution in nursing mothers

SIDE EFFECTS
Frequent
Abdominal pain, nausea, anorexia, fever
Occasional
Tachycardia, arrhythmias, palpitations, insomnia, twitching
Rare
Blurred vision, rash, arthralgia, insomnia

SERIOUS REACTIONS
• Withdrawal after prolonged therapy may unmask symptoms of the underlying disorder.

• Dexmethylphenidate may lower the seizure threshold in those with a history of seizures.

• Overdose produces excessive sympathomimetic effects, including vomiting, tremor, hyperreflexia, seizures, confusion, hallucinations, and diaphoresis.

• Prolonged administration to children may delay growth.

INTERACTIONS
Drugs
■ *Clonidine:* Serious adverse effects have been reported but no causality has been established

② *MAOIs:* Hypertensive crisis

■ *Phenytoin, phenobarbital, primidone:* Increased levels and risk of toxicity

■ *SSRIs:* Increased serum concentrations

■ *Tricyclic antidepressants:* Increased serum concentrations

■ *Warfarin:* Increased PT and bleeding risk; inhibits warfarin metabolism

Labs
• *False positive:* Urine amphetamine

SPECIAL CONSIDERATIONS
• No clinical data to support use of this agent over racemic methylphenidate

PATIENT/FAMILY EDUCATION
• Take last dose late afternoon or early evening to prevent insomnia
• Reinforce habit-forming potential of medication; caution against taking more than required dose
• Potential for growth retardation

MONITORING PARAMETERS
• Improvement of clinical symptoms, lack of adverse effects; periodic complete blood count with differential, routine blood chemistry; growth determinations (body weight and height), blood pressure, pulse rate

---

dextroamphetamine
(dex-troe-am-fet′a-meen)
Chemical Class: D-β-phenyl-isopropylamine
Therapeutic Class: Central nervous system stimulant
DEA Class: Schedule II

CLINICAL PHARMACOLOGY
Mechanism of Action: An amphetamine that enhances the action of dopamine and norepinephrine by blocking their reuptake from synapses; also inhibits monoamine oxidase and facilitates the release of catecholamines. *Therapeutic Effect:* Increases motor activity and mental alertness; decreases motor restlessness, drowsiness, and fatigue; suppresses appetite.

INDICATIONS AND DOSAGES
Narcolepsy
PO
Adults, Children older than 12 yr. Initially, 10 mg/day. Increase by 10 mg/day at weekly intervals until therapeutic response is achieved.
Children 6-12 yr. Initially, 5 mg/day. Increase by 5 mg/day at weekly intervals until therapeutic response is achieved. Maximum: 60 mg/day.

Attention deficit hyperactivity disorder (ADHD)
PO
Children 6 yr and older. Initially, 5 mg once or twice a day. Increase by 5 mg/day at weekly intervals until therapeutic response is achieved.
Children 3-5 yr. Initially, 2.5 mg/day. Increase by 2.5 mg/day at weekly intervals until therapeutic response is achieved. Maximum: 40 mg/day.

Appetite suppressant
PO
Adults. 5-30 mg daily in divided doses of 5-10 mg each, given 30-60

min before meals; or 1 extended-release capsule in the morning.

§ **AVAILABLE FORMS/COST**

• Cap, Sus Action-Oral: 5 mg, 100's: **$78.76-$94.91**; 10 mg, 100's: **$98.11-$118.20**; 15 mg, 100's: **$125.46-$151.16**

• Tab-Oral: 5 mg, 100's: **$23.48-$39.69**; 10 mg, 100's: **$41.37-$56.16**

CONTRAINDICATIONS: Advanced arteriosclerosis, agitated states, glaucoma, history of drug abuse, hypersensitivity to sympathomimetic amines, hyperthyroidism, moderate to severe hypertension, symptomatic cardiovascular disease, use within 14 days of MAOIs

PREGNANCY AND LACTATION: Pregnancy category C; excreted in breast milk

SIDE EFFECTS

Frequent

Irregular pulse, increased motor activity, talkativeness, nervousness, mild euphoria, insomnia

Occasional

Headache, chills, dry mouth, GI distress, worsening depression in patients who are clinically depressed, tachycardia, palpitations, chest pain, dizziness, decreased appetite

SERIOUS REACTIONS

• Overdose may produce skin pallor or flushing, arrhythmias, and psychosis.

• Abrupt withdrawal after prolonged use of high doses may produce lethargy lasting for weeks.

• Prolonged administration to children with ADHD may inhibit growth.

INTERACTIONS

Drugs

③ *Antacids:* Decreased urinary excretion of dextroamphetamine

③ *Furazolidone:* Hypertensive reactions

③ *Guanadrel, Guanethidine:* Antihypertensive effect inhibited by dextroamphetamine

⚠ *MAOIs:* Severe hypertensive reactions possible

② *Selegiline:* Severe hypertensive reactions possible

③ *Sodium bicarbonate:* May inhibit dextroamphetamine excretion

Labs

• *False positive:* Urine amino acids

SPECIAL CONSIDERATIONS

• Use for obesity should be reserved for patients failing to respond to alternative therapy; weigh the limited benefit against the substantial risk of addiction and dependence

PATIENT/FAMILY EDUCATION

• Tolerance or dependency is common

• Avoid OTC preparations unless approved by clinician

• Do not crush or chew Sus Action dosage forms

---

dextromethorphan

(dex-troe-meth-or´-fan)

Combinations

OTC: with benzocaine (Spec T, Vicks Formula 44 cough control discs, Vicks cough silencers); with guaifenesin (Robitussin DM)

Chemical Class: Levorphanol derivative

Therapeutic Class: Antitussive

CLINICAL PHARMACOLOGY

Mechanism of Action: A chemical relative of morphine without the narcotic properties that acts on the cough center in the medulla oblongata by elevating the threshold for coughing. *Therapeutic Effect:* Suppresses cough.

Pharmacokinetics

Rapidly absorbed from the gastrointestinal (GI) tract. Distributed into cerebrospinal fluid (CSF). Extensively and poorly metabolized in liver to dextrorphan (active metabolite). Excreted unchanged in urine. **Half-life:** 1.4-3.9 hrs (parent compound), 3.4-5.6 hrs. (dextrorphan).

INDICATIONS AND DOSAGES

Cough

PO

Adults, Elderly, Children 12 years and older. 10-20 mg q4h. Maximum: 120 mg/day.

Children 6- 12 yrs. 5-10 mg q4h. Maximum: 60 mg/day.

Children 2-5 yrs. 2.5-5 mg q4h. Maximum: 30 mg/day.

S AVAILABLE FORMS/COST

• Cap-Oral: 30 mg, 30's: **$11.39**

• Drops, Conc-Oral: 7.5 mg/0.8 ml, 15 ml: **$5.12**

• Susp, Sus Action-Oral: 30 mg/5 ml, 90 ml: **$10.01**

• Loz—Oral: 2.5 mg, 20's: **$1.92**; 5 mg, 16's: **$2.56**

• Syr—Oral: 3.5 mg/5 ml, 120 ml: **$3.66**; 7.5 mg/5 ml, 60 ml: **$1.76-$5.69**; 10 mg/5 ml, 120 ml: **$4.00-$6.51**; 15 mg/5 ml, 120 ml: **$2.51-$4.96**

• Tab, Chewable-Oral: 7.5 mg, 18's: **$4.62**

UNLABELED USES: N-methyl-D-aspartate (NMDA) antagonist in cerebral injury

CONTRAINDICATIONS: Coadministration with monoamine oxidase inhibitors (MAOIs), hypersensitivity to dextromethorphan or its components

PREGNANCY AND LACTATION: Pregnancy category C

SIDE EFFECTS

Rare

Abdominal discomfort, constipation, dizziness, drowsiness, GI upset, nausea

SERIOUS REACTIONS

• Overdosage may result in muscle spasticity, increase or decrease in blood pressure (BP), blurred vision, blue fingernails and lips, nausea, vomiting, hallucinations, and respiratory depression.

INTERACTIONS

Drugs

⚠ *Isocarboxazid, MAOIs, Phenelzine:* Increased risk of toxicity due to dextromethorphan

▪ *Quinidine, terbinafine:* Reduced hepatic metabolism of dextromethorphan

▪ *Fluoxetine:* Case report of a patient on fluoxetine developing visual hallucinations when she began to take dextromethorphan; causality not established

❷ *Sibutramine:* Increased risk of serotonin syndrome

---

diazepam

(dye-az′ e-pam)

Chemical Class: Benzodiazepine

Therapeutic Class: Anesthesia adjunct; anticonvulsant; anxiolytic; sedative/hypnotic; skeletal muscle relaxant

DEA Class: Schedule IV

CLINICAL PHARMACOLOGY

Mechanism of Action: A benzodiazepine that depresses all levels of the CNS by enhancing the action of gamma-aminobutyric acid, a major inhibitory neurotransmitter in the brain. *Therapeutic Effect:* Produces anxiolytic effect, elevates the seizure threshold, produces skeletal muscle relaxation.

Pharmacokinetics

Route	Onset	Peak	Dura-tion
PO	30 min	1-2 hr	2-3 hr
IV	1-5 min	15 min	15-60 min
IM	15 min	30-90 min	30-90 min

Well absorbed from the GI tract. Widely distributed. Protein binding: 98%. Metabolized in the liver to active metabolite. Excreted in urine. Minimally removed by hemodialysis. **Half-life:** 20-70 hr (increased in hepatic dysfunction and the elderly).

INDICATIONS AND DOSAGES
Anxiety, skeletal muscle relaxation
PO
Adults. 2-10 mg 2-4 times a day.
Elderly. 2.5 mg twice a day.
Children. 0.12-0.8 mg/kg/day in divided doses q6-8h.
IV, IM
Adults. 2-10 mg repeated in 3-4 hr.
Children. 0.04-0.3 mg/kg/dose q2-4h. Maximum: 0.5 mg/kg in an 8-hr period.
Preanesthesia
IV
Adults, Elderly. 5-15 mg 5-10 min before procedure.
Children. 0.2-0.3 mg/kg. Maximum: 10 mg.
Alcohol withdrawal
PO
Adults, Elderly. 10 mg 3-4 times during first 24 hr, then reduced to 5-10 mg 3-4 times a day as needed.
IV, IM
Adults, Elderly. Initially, 10 mg, followed by 5-10 mg q3-4h.
Status epilepticus
IV
Adults, Elderly. 5-10 mg q10-15min up to 30 mg/8 hr.
Children 5 yr and older. 0.05-0.3 mg/kg/dose q15-30min. Maximum: 10 mg/dose.

Children 1 mo to younger than 5 yr. 0.05-0.3 mg/kg/dose q15-30min. Maximum: 5 mg/dose.
Control of increased seizure activity in patients with refractory epilepsy who are on stable regimens of anticonvulsants
Rectal gel
Adults, Children 12 yr and older. 0.2 mg/kg; may be repeated in 4-12 hr.
Children 6-11 yr. 0.3 mg/kg; may be repeated in 4-12 hr.
Children 2-5 yr. 0.5 mg/kg; may be repeated in 4-12 hr.

🛡 AVAILABLE FORMS/COST
• Sol, Inj-IM, IV: 5 mg/ml, 2 ml: **$1.44-$7.63**
• Conc-Oral: 5 mg/ml, 30 ml: **$27.27**
• Gel-Rectal: 5 mg/ml, 1, 2, 3, 4, ml; all: **$113.27**
• Sol-Oral: 5 mg/5 ml, 500 ml: **$49.47**
• Tab-Oral: 2 mg, 100's: **$3.82-$80.34**; 5 mg, 100's: **$5.99-$124.94**; 10 mg, 100's: **$5.15-$210.33**

UNLABELED USES: Treatment of panic disorder, tension headache, tremors
CONTRAINDICATIONS: Angle-closure glaucoma, coma, pre-existing CNS depression, respiratory depression, severe, uncontrolled pain
PREGNANCY AND LACTATION: Pregnancy category D; drug and metabolite enter breast milk; lethargy and loss of weight in nursing infant have been reported
SIDE EFFECTS
Frequent
Pain with IM injection, somnolence, fatigue, ataxia
Occasional
Slurred speech, orthostatic hypotension, headache, hypoactivity, constipation, nausea, blurred vision

Rare

Paradoxical CNS reactions, such as hyperactivity or nervousness in children and excitement or restlessness in the elderly or debilitated (generally noted during first 2 weeks of therapy, particularly in presence of uncontrolled pain)

SERIOUS REACTIONS

• IV administration may produce pain, swelling, thrombophlebitis, and carpal tunnel syndrome.

• Abrupt or too-rapid withdrawal may result in pronounced restlessness, irritability, insomnia, hand tremor, abdominal or muscle cramps, diaphoresis, vomiting, and seizures.

• Abrupt withdrawal in patients with epilepsy may produce an increase in the frequency or severity of seizures.

• Overdose results in somnolence, confusion, diminished reflexes, and coma.

INTERACTIONS

Drugs

🔳 *Carbamazepine:* Markedly reduces effect of oral diazepam; parenteral diazepam less affected

🔳 *Cimetidine:* Inhibits hepatic metabolism of diazepam

🔳 *Ciprofloxacin:* Inhibits hepatic metabolism of diazepam; may also competitively inhibit gamma-aminobutyric acid receptors

② *Clarithromycin:* Inhibits hepatic metabolism of diazepam

🔳 *Clozapine:* Additive respiratory and cardiovascular depression

🔳 *Delavirdine:* Inhibits hepatic metabolism of diazepam

🔳 *Disulfiram:* Inhibits hepatic metabolism of diazepam

🔳 *Erythromycin:* Inhibits hepatic metabolism of diazepam

🔳 *Ethanol:* Additive CNS effects

🔳 *Fluconazole:* Inhibits hepatic metabolism of diazepam

🔳 *Fluoxetine:* Inhibits hepatic metabolism of diazepam

🔳 *Fluvoxamine:* Inhibits hepatic metabolism of diazepam

🔳 *Isoniazid:* Inhibits hepatic metabolism of diazepam

🔳 *Itraconazole:* Inhibits hepatic metabolism of diazepam

🔳 *Ketoconazole:* Inhibits hepatic metabolism of diazepam

🔳 *Levodopa:* May reduce anti-Parkinsonian effect

🔳 *Metoprolol:* Inhibits hepatic metabolism of diazepam

🔳 *Omeprazole:* Inhibits hepatic metabolism of diazepam

🔳 *Phenytoin:* Markedly reduces effect of oral diazepam; parenteral diazepam less affected

🔳 *Quinolones:* Inhibits hepatic metabolism of diazepam; may also competitively inhibit gamma-aminobutyric acid receptors

🔳 *Rifampin:* Markedly reduces effect of diazepam

🔳 *Troleandomycin:* Inhibits hepatic metabolism of diazepam

Labs

• *Increase:* Urine 5-HIAA

SPECIAL CONSIDERATIONS

• Flumazenil (Mazicon), a benzodiazepine receptor antagonist is indicated for complete or partial reversal of the sedative effects of benzodiazepines

PATIENT/FAMILY EDUCATION

• Avoid driving, activities that require alertness; drowsiness may occur

• Avoid alcohol, other psychotropic medications unless prescribed by clinician

diclofenac

(dye-kloe'fen-ak)

Combinations

Rx: with misoprostol (Arthotec)

Chemical Class: Phenylacetic acid derivative

Therapeutic Class: NSAID; antipyretic; nonnarcotic analgesic

CLINICAL PHARMACOLOGY

Mechanism of Action: An NSAID that inhibits prostaglandin synthesis, reducing the intensity of pain. Also constricts the iris sphincter. May inhibit angiogenesis (the formation of blood vessels) by inhibiting substance P or blocking the angiogenic effects of prostaglandin E. *Therapeutic Effect:* Produces analgesic and anti-inflammatory effects. Prevents miosis during cataract surgery. May reduce angiogenesis in inflammed tissue.

Pharmacokinetics

Route	Onset	Peak	Duration
PO	30 min	2–3 hr	Up to 8 hr

Completely absorbed from the GI tract; penetrates cornea after ophthalmic administration (may be systemically absorbed). Protein binding: greater than 99%. Widely distributed. Metabolized in the liver. Primarily excreted in urine. Minimally removed by hemodialysis. **Half-life:** 1.2–2 hr.

INDICATIONS AND DOSAGES

Osteoarthritis

PO (Cataflam, Voltaren)

Adults, Elderly. 50 mg 2–3 times a day.

PO (Voltaren XR)

Adults, Elderly. 100 mg/day as a single dose.

Rheumatoid arthritis

PO (Cataflam, Voltaren)

Adults, Elderly. 50 mg 2–4 times a day. Maximum: 225 mg/day.

PO (Voltaren XR)

Adults, Elderly. 100 mg once a day. Maximum: 100 mg twice a day.

Ankylosing spondylitis

PO (Voltaren)

Adults, Elderly. 100–125 mg/day in 4–5 divided doses.

Analgesia, primary dysmenorrhea

PO (Cataflam)

Adults, Elderly. 30 mg 3 times a day.

Usual pediatric dosage

Children. 2–3 mg/kg/day in 2-4 divided doses.

Actinic keratoses

Topical

Adults, Adolescents. Apply twice a day to lesion for 60–90 days.

Cataract surgery

Ophthalmic

Adults, Elderly. Apply 1 drop to eye 4 times a day commencing 24 hr after cataract surgery. Continue for 2 wks afterward.

Pain, relief of photophobia in patients undergoing corneal refractive surgery

Ophthalmic

Adults, Elderly. Apply 1 drop to affected eye 1 hr before surgery, within 15 min after surgery, then 4 times a day for 3 days.

[$] **AVAILABLE FORMS/COST**

Diclofenac Sodium

• Sol—Ophth: 0.1%, 5 ml: **$34.38-$56.96**

• Tab, Sus Action—Oral: 100 mg, 100's: **$244.14-$471.65**

• Tab, Enteric Coated—Oral: 25 mg, 100's: **$44.30-$85.80**; 50 mg, 100's: **$25.75-$194.08**; 75 mg, 100's: **$48.75-$235.03**

• Gel—Topical: 3%, 50 g: **$116.86**

Diclofenac Potassium

• Tab-Oral: 50 mg, 100's: **$155.19-$268.21**

UNLABELED USES: Treatment of vascular headaches (oral); to reduce the occurrence and severity of cystoid macular edema after cataract surgery (ophthalmic form)

CONTRAINDICATIONS: Hypersensitivity to aspirin, diclofenac, and other NSAIDs; porphyria

PREGNANCY AND LACTATION: Pregnancy category B; excreted in breast milk

SIDE EFFECTS

Frequent (9%–4%)

PO: Headache, abdominal cramps, constipation, diarrhea, nausea, dyspepsia

Ophthalmic: Burning or stinging on instillation, ocular discomfort

Occasional (3%–1%)

PO: Flatulence, dizziness, epigastric pain

Ophthalmic: Ocular itching or tearing

Rare (less than 1%)

PO: Rash, peripheral edema or fluid retention, visual disturbances, vomiting, drowsiness

SERIOUS REACTIONS

• Overdose may result in acute renal failure.

• Rare reactions with long-term use include peptic ulcer disease, GI bleeding, gastritis, a severe hepatic reaction (jaundice), nephrotoxicity (hematuria, dysuria, proteinuria), and a severe hypersensitivity reaction (bronchospasm or angioedema).

INTERACTIONS

Drugs

3️⃣ *Aminoglycosides:* Reduced clearance with elevated aminoglycoside levels and potential for toxicity (especially indomethacin in premature infants; other NSAIDs probably)

3️⃣ *Anticoagulants:* Excessive hypoprothrombinemia, decreased platelet aggregation with increased risk of GI bleeding

3️⃣ *Antihypertensives (α-blockers, angiotension-converting enzyme inhibitors, angiotensin II receptor blockers, β-blockers, diuretics):* Inhibition of antihypertensive and other favorable hemodynamic effects

3️⃣ *Corticosteroids:* Increased risk of GI ulceration

3️⃣ *Cyclosporine:* Increased nephrotoxicity risk

3️⃣ *Digoxin:* Increased serum digoxin concentrations

3️⃣ *Lithium:* Decreased clearance of lithium (mediated via prostaglandins) resulting in elevated serum lithium levels and risk of toxicity

2️⃣ *Methotrexate:* Decreased renal secretion of methotrexate resulting in elevated methotrexate levels and risk of toxicity

3️⃣ *Phenylpropanolamine:* Possible acute hypertensive reaction

3️⃣ *Potassium-sparing diuretics:* Additive hyperkalemia potential

2️⃣ *Triamterene:* Acute renal failure reported with addition of indomethacin; caution with other NSAIDs

Labs

• *Increase:* Serum AST, plasma cortisol, plasma glucose (oxidase-peroxidase method)

SPECIAL CONSIDERATIONS

• No significant advantage over other NSAIDs; cost should govern use

MONITORING PARAMETERS

• Initial hemogram and fecal occult blood test within 3 mo of starting regular chronic therapy; repeat every 6-12 mo (more frequently in high-risk patients (>65 years, peptic ulcer disease, concurrent steroids or anticoagulants); electrolytes, creatinine, and BUN within 3 mo of starting regular chronic therapy; repeat every 6-12 mo

• Complete healing of actinic keratoses may not be evident for up to 30 days post cessation of therapy

---

dicloxacillin

(dye-klox′a-sill-in)
Chemical Class: Penicillin derivative, penicillinase-resistant
Therapeutic Class: Antibiotic

CLINICAL PHARMACOLOGY

Mechanism of Action: A penicillin that acts as a bactericidal in susceptible microorganisms. *Therapeutic Effect:* Inhibits bacterial cell wall synthesis.

Pharmacokinetics

Well absorbed from gastrointestinal (GI) tract. Rate and extent reduced by food. Distributed throughout body including CSF. Protein binding: 96%. Partially metabolized in liver. Primarily excreted in feces and urine. Not removed by hemodialysis. **Half-life:** 0.7 hrs.

INDICATIONS AND DOSAGES

Respiratory tract infection, staphylococcal and streptococcal infections

PO

Adults, Elderly, Children weighing more than 40 kg. 125-250 mg q6h.
Children weighing less than 40 kg. 12.5-25 mg/kg/day q6h.

AVAILABLE FORMS/COST

• Cap, Gel—Oral: 250 mg, 100's: **$35.25-$93.95**; 500 mg, 100's: **$60.50-$179.00**
• Powder, Reconst—Oral: 62.5 mg/5 ml, 100, 200 ml: **$16.69/200 ml**

CONTRAINDICATIONS: Hypersensitivity to any penicillin

PREGNANCY AND LACTATION: Pregnancy category B; penicillins are excreted into breast milk in low concentrations; compatible with breast-feeding

SIDE EFFECTS

Frequent

Gastrointestinal (GI) disturbances (mild diarrhea, nausea, or vomiting), headache

Occasional

Generalized rash, urticaria

SERIOUS REACTIONS

• Altered bacterial balance may result in potentially fatal superinfections and antibiotic-associated colitis as evidenced by abdominal cramps, watery or severe diarrhea, and fever.

• Severe hypersensitivity reactions, including anaphylaxis and acute interstitial nephritis occur rarely.

INTERACTIONS

Drugs

■ *Macrolide antibiotics, chloramphenicol, tetracyclines:* Possible inhibition of antibacterial activity of penicillins

■ *Methotrexate:* Potentiation of methotrexate toxicity

■ *Oral contraceptives:* Possible impaired contraceptive efficacy

■ *Warfarin:* Reduced hypoprothrombinemic response

Labs

• *False increase:* Nafcillin level

SPECIAL CONSIDERATIONS

PATIENT/FAMILY EDUCATION

• Should be taken with water 1 hr before or 2 hr after meals on an empty stomach

dicyclomine
(dye-sye'kloe-meen)
Chemical Class: Tertiary amine
Therapeutic Class: Anticholinergic; antispasmodic; gastrointestinal

CLINICAL PHARMACOLOGY
Mechanism of Action: A GI antispasmodic and anticholinergic agent that directly acts as a relaxant on smooth muscle. *Therapeutic Effect:* Reduces tone and motility of GI tract.
Pharmacokinetics

Route	Onset	Peak	Duration
PO	1–2 hr	N/A	4 hr

Readily absorbed from the GI tract. Widely distributed. Metabolized in the liver. **Half-life:** 9–10 hr.

INDICATIONS AND DOSAGES
Functional disturbances of GI motility
PO
Adults. 10–20 mg 3–4 times a day up to 40 mg 4 times/day.
Children older than 2 yr. 10 mg 3–4 times a day.
Children 6 mos–2 yr. 5 mg 3–4 times a day.
Elderly. 10–20 mg 4 times a day. May increase up to 160 mg/day.
IM
Adults. 20 mg q4–6h.

$ **AVAILABLE FORMS/COST**
• Cap, Gel—Oral: 10 mg, 100's: **$1.60-$35.01**
• Sol, Inj-IM: 10 mg/ml, 2 ml: **$16.74-$17.96**
• Syr—Oral: 10 mg/5 ml, 480 ml: **$38.90**
• Tab-Oral: 20 mg, 100's: **$1.60-$49.95**

CONTRAINDICATIONS: Bladder neck obstruction due to prostatic hyperplasia, coronary vasospasm, intestinal atony, myasthenia gravis in patients not treated with neostigmine, narrow-angle glaucoma, obstructive disease of the GI tract, paralytic ileus, severe ulcerative colitis, tachycardia secondary to cardiac insufficiency or thyrotoxicosis, toxic megacolon, unstable cardiovascular status in acute hemorrhage

PREGNANCY AND LACTATION:
Pregnancy category B; single case report of apnea in nursing infant; avoid in nursing women

SIDE EFFECTS
Frequent
Dry mouth (sometimes severe), constipation, diminished sweating ability
Occasional
Blurred vision; photophobia; urinary hesitancy; somnolence (with high dosage); agitation, excitement, confusion, or somnolence noted in elderly (even with low dosages); transient light-headedness (with IM route), irritation at injection site (with IM route)
Rare
Confusion, hypersensitivity reaction, increased IOP, nausea, vomiting, unusual fatigue

SERIOUS REACTIONS
• Overdose may produce temporary paralysis of ciliary muscle; pupillary dilation; tachycardia; palpitations; hot, dry, or flushed skin; absence of bowel sounds; hyperthermia; increased respiratory rate; EKG abnormalities; nausea; vomiting; rash over face or upper trunk; CNS stimulation; and psychosis (marked by agitation, restlessness, rambling speech, visual hallucinations, paranoid behavior, and delusions, followed by depression).

INTERACTIONS
Drugs
▣ *Amantadine, Tricyclic antidepressants, MAOIs, H₁-antihistamines:* Increased anticholinergic effects

▣ *Phenothiazines, Levodopa, Ketoconazole:* Decreased therapeutic effects of these drugs

SPECIAL CONSIDERATIONS
• Not for intravenous use

---

didanosine (ddI)
(dye-dan'o-seen)
Chemical Class: Nucleoside analog
Therapeutic Class: Antiretroviral

CLINICAL PHARMACOLOGY
Mechanism of Action: A purine nucleoside analogue that is intracellularly converted into a triphosphate, which interferes with RNA-directed DNA polymerase (reverse transcriptase). *Therapeutic Effect:* Inhibits replication of retroviruses, including HIV.

Pharmacokinetics
Variably absorbed from the GI tract. Protein binding: less than 5%. Rapidly metabolized intracellularly to active form. Primarily excreted in urine. Partially (20%) removed by hemodialysis. **Half-life:** 1.5 hr; metabolite: 8-24 hr.

INDICATIONS AND DOSAGES
HIV infection (in combination with other antiretrovirals)
Tablets (Chewable)
Adults, children 13 yr and older weighing 60 kg or more. 200 mg q12h or 400 mg once a day.
Adults, Children 13 yr and older weighing 60 kg or less. 125 mg q12h or 250 mg once a day.

Children 3 mo to less than 13 yr. 180-300 mg/m²/day in divided doses q12h.
Children younger than 3 mo. 50 mg/m²/day in divided doses q12h.
Delayed-Release Capsules
Adults, Children 13 yr and older, weighing 60 kg or more. 400 mg once a day.
Adults, Children 13 yr and older, weighing 60 kg or less. 250 mg once a day.
Oral solution
Adults, Children 13 yr and older weighing 60 kg or more. 250 mg q12h.
Adults, Children 13 yr and older weighing 60 kig or less. 167 mg q12h.
Pediatric Powder for Oral Solution
Children 3 mo to younger than 13 yr. 180-300 mg/m²/day in divided doses q12h.
Children younger than 3 mo. 50mg/m²/day in divided doses q12h.

Dosage in renal impairment
Patients weighing less than 60 kg:

CrCl	Tablets	Oral Solution	Delayed-Release Capsules
30-59 ml/min	75 mg twice a day	100 mg twice a day	125 mg once a day
10-29 ml/min	100 mg once a day	100 mg once a day	125 mg once a day
less than 10 ml/min	75 mg once a day	100 mg once a day	N/A

CrCl = creatinine clearance

Patients weighing 60 kg or more:

CrCl	Tablets	Oral Solution	Delayed-Release Capsules
30-59 ml/ min	100 mg twice a day	100 mg twice a day	200 mg once a day
10-29 ml/min	150 mg once a day	167 mg once a day	125 mg once a day

less than 10 ml/ min	100 mg once a day	100 mg once a day	125 mg once a day

CrCl = creatinine clearance

§ **AVAILABLE FORMS/COST**

• Cap, Sus Action—Oral: 125 mg, 30's: **$100.78**; 200 mg, 30's: **$161.23**; 250 mg, 30's: **$205.45**; 400 mg, 30's: **$320.89**

• Powder Recon-Oral: 100 mg, 30's: **$65.57**; 167 mg, 30's: **$105.58**; 250 mg, 30's: **$163.95**

• Tab, Chewable—Oral: 25 mg, 60's: **$31.62**; 50 mg, 30's: **$71.14**; 100 mg, 60's: **$118.88–$142.24**; 150 mg, 60's: **$213.39**; 200 mg, 60's: **$284.49**

CONTRAINDICATIONS: Hypersensitivity to didanosine or any of its components

PREGNANCY AND LACTATION: Pregnancy category B; unknown if excreted in breast milk; discontinuation of breast-feeding recommended

SIDE EFFECTS

Frequent

Adults (greater than 10%)

Diarrhea, neuropathy, chills and fever

Children (greater than 25%)

Chills, fever, decreased appetite, pain, malaise, nausea, vomiting, diarrhea, abdominal pain, headache, nervousness, cough, rhinitis, dyspnea, asthenia, rash, pruritus

Occasional

Adults (9%-2%)

Rash, pruritus, headache, abdominal pain, nausea, vomiting, pneumonia, myopathy, decreased appetite, dry mouth, dyspnea

Children (25%-10%)

Failure to thrive, weight loss, stomatitis, oral thrush, ecchymosis, arthritis, myalgia, insomnia, epistaxis, pharyngitis

SERIOUS REACTIONS

• Pneumonia and opportunistic infections occur occasionally.

• Peripheral neuropathy, potentially fatal pancreatitis, retinal changes, and optic neuritis are the major toxic effects.

INTERACTIONS

Drugs

⚠ *Allopurinol:* Increased plasma didanosine concentrations; coadministration not recommended

▣ *Dapsone:* Buffering compound may inhibit dissolution of dapsone in the stomach

▣ *Delavirdine:* Decreased plasma delavirdine concentrations; give ddI 1 hr after delavirdine

▣ *Food:* Reduced bioavailability

▣ *Ganciclovir:* Increased ddI concentrations

▣ *Indinavir:* Decreased plasma indinavir concentrations; give ddI 1 hr after indinavir

▣ *Itraconazole, ketoconazole:* Alkalinization of stomach by didanosine reduces the solubility and absorption of antifungal

▣ *Methadone:* Decreased plasma didanosine concentrations

▣ *Quinolones:* Decreased concentrations after binding to the aluminum and magnesium ions in the didanosine buffering compound

② *Stavudine:* Increased risk of pancreatitis

▣ *Tetracyclines:* Decreased antibiotic concentrations after binding to calcium ions in ddI buffering compound

SPECIAL CONSIDERATIONS

MONITORING PARAMETERS

• Amylase, lipase, ophthalmologic examinations

• Suspend use until pancreatitis excluded if patient develops nausea, abdominal pain

• Tablets contain 264.5 mg sodium, packets 1380 mg sodium

PATIENT/FAMILY EDUCATION

• Administer on empty stomach

diethylpropion
(die-ethyl-prop′ion)
Chemical Class: Phenethyl-
amine derivative
Therapeutic Class: Anorexiant
DEA Class: Schedule IV

CLINICAL PHARMACOLOGY
Mechanism of Action: A sympathomimetic amine that stimulates the
release of norepinephrine and
dopamine. *Therapeutic Effect:* Decreases appetite.
Pharmacokinetics
Rapidly absorbed from the gastrointestinal (GI) tract. Widely distributed. Metabolized in liver to active metabolite and undergoes extensive first-pass metabolism. Excreted in urine. Unknown if removed by hemodialysis. **Half-life:**
4-6 hrs.

INDICATIONS AND DOSAGES
Obesity
PO
Adults. 25 mg 3 times/day before
meals. (Extended-release) 75 mg at
midmorning.

S **AVAILABLE FORMS/COST**
• Tab-Oral: 25 mg, 100's: **$5.60-
$54.39**
• Tab, Sus Action-Oral: 75 mg,
100's: **$48.69-$136.54**
UNLABELED USES: Migraines
CONTRAINDICATIONS: Agitated
states, use of MAOIs within 14 days,
glaucoma, history of drug abuse, hyperthyroidism, advanced arteriosclerosis or severe cardiovascular
disease, severe hypertension, and
hypersensitivity to sympathomimetic amines
PREGNANCY AND LACTATION:
Pregnancy category B; excreted in
breast milk; no reports of adverse effects

SIDE EFFECTS
Frequent
Elevated blood pressure, nervous-
ness, insomnia
Occasional
Dizziness, drowsiness, tremor,
headache, nausea, stomach pain, fe-
ver, rash
Rare
Agranulocytosis, leukopenia,
blurred vision, psychosis, CVA, sei-
zure
SERIOUS REACTIONS
• Overdose may produce agitation,
tachycardia, palpitations, cardiac irregularities, chest pain, psychotic
episode, seizures, and coma.
• Hypersensitivity reactions and
blood dyscrasias occur rarely.
INTERACTIONS
Labs
• *False positive:* Urine cocaine, diazepam, methaqualone, phencyclidine
SPECIAL CONSIDERATIONS
• Tolerance to anorectic effects may
develop within weeks; cross-toler-
ance is almost universal
• Measure the limited usefulness
against the inherent risks (habituation) of this agent
• Most patients will eventually re-
gain weight lost during use of this
product

diflorasone
(die-floor′a-sone)
Chemical Class: Corticosteroid, synthetic
Therapeutic Class: Corticosteroid, topical

CLINICAL PHARMACOLOGY
Mechanism of Action: A high potency, fluorinated corticosteroid that
decreases inflammation by suppression of migration of polymorphonu-

clar leukocytes and reversal of increased capillary permeability. The exact mechanism of the anti-inflammatory process is unclear. *Therapeutic Effect:* Decreases or prevents tissue response to the inflammatory process.

Pharmacokinetics

Poor absorption; occlusive dressings increase absorption. Metabolized in liver. Primarily excreted in urine.

INDICATIONS AND DOSAGES

Dermatoses

Topical

Adults, Elderly. (Cream) Apply sparingly 2- 4 times/day. (Ointment) Apply sparingly 1- 3 times/day.

S AVAILABLE FORMS/COST

• Cre—Top: 0.05%, 15, 30, 60 g: **$43.19-$55.04**/30 g
• Oint—Top: 0.05%, 15, 30, 60 g: **$40.10-$60.72**/30 g

UNLABELED USES: Psoriasis

CONTRAINDICATIONS: History of hypersensitivity to diflorasone or other corticosteroids

PREGNANCY AND LACTATION: Pregnancy category C; unknown whether topical application could result in sufficient systemic absorption to produce detectable amounts in breast milk (systemic corticosteroids are secreted into breast milk in quantities not likely to have detrimental effects on infant)

SIDE EFFECTS

Rare

Itching, redness, dryness, irritation, burning at site of application, arthralgia, folliculitis, maceration, muscle atrophy, secondary infection

SERIOUS REACTIONS

• Overdosage symptoms include moon face, central obesity, hypertension, diabetes, hyperlipidemia, peptic ulcer, increased susceptibility to infection, electrolyte and fluid imbalance, psychosis, and hallucinations.

• The serious reactions of long-term therapy and the addition of occlusive dressings are reversible hypothalamic-pituitary-adrenal (HPA) axis suppression, manifestations of Cushing's syndrome, hyperglycemia, and glucosuria.

SPECIAL CONSIDERATIONS

• No demonstrated superiority over other high-potency agents; cost should govern use

PATIENT/FAMILY EDUCATION

• Apply sparingly only to affected area

• Avoid contact with the eyes

• Do not put bandages or dressings over treated area unless directed by clinician

• Discontinue drug, notify clinician if local irritation or fever develops

• Do not use on weeping, denuded, or infected areas

---

diflunisal

(dye-floo′ni-sal)
Chemical Class: Salicylate derivative
Therapeutic Class: NSAID; antipyretic; nonnarcotic analgesic

CLINICAL PHARMACOLOGY

Mechanism of Action: A nonsteroidal anti-inflammatory that inhibits prostaglandin synthesis, reducing inflammatory response and intensity of pain stimulus reaching sensory nerve endings. *Therapeutic Effect:* Produces analgesic and anti-inflammatory effect.

Pharmacokinetics

Route	Onset	Peak	Duration
PO	1 hr	2-3 hr	8-12 hr

Completely absorbed from the gastrointestinal (GI) tract. Widely distributed. Protein binding: greater than 99%. Metabolized in liver. Primarily excreted in urine. Not removed by hemodialysis. **Half-life:** 8-12 hr.

INDICATIONS AND DOSAGES
Mild to moderate pain
PO

Adults, Elderly. Initially, 0.5-1 g, then 250-500 mg q8-12h. Maximum: 1.5 g/day.

Rheumatoid arthritis, osteoarthritis
PO

Adults, Elderly. 0.5-1 g/day in 2 divided doses. Maximum: 1.5 g/day.

ⓢ AVAILABLE FORMS/COST
• Tab-Oral: 250 mg, 60's: **$46.66-$71.39**; 500 mg, 100's: **$58.33-$129.23**

UNLABELED USES: Treatment of psoriatic arthritis, vascular headache

CONTRAINDICATIONS: Active GI bleeding, factor VII or factor IX deficiencies, hypersensitivity to aspirin or NSAIDs

PREGNANCY AND LACTATION: Pregnancy category C; use during 3rd trimester not recommended due to effects on fetal cardiovascular system (closure of ductus arteriosus); excreted into breast milk in concentrations 2%-7% those in maternal plasma; use caution in nursing mothers

SIDE EFFECTS
Side effects are less common with short-term treatment.

Occasional (9%-3%)
Nausea, dyspepsia (heartburn, indigestion, epigastric pain), diarrhea, headache, rash

Rare (3%-1%)
Vomiting, constipation, flatulence, dizziness, somnolence, insomnia, fatigue, tinnitus

SERIOUS REACTIONS
• Overdosage may produce drowsiness, vomiting, nausea, diarrhea, hyperventilation, tachycardia, diaphoresis, stupor, and coma.
• Peptic ulcer, GI bleeding, gastritis, and severe hepatic reaction, including cholestasis, jaundice occur rarely.
• Nephrotoxicity, including dysuria, hematuria, proteinuria, and nephrotic syndrome, and severe hypersensitivity reaction, marked by bronchospasm and angioedema, occur rarely.

INTERACTIONS
Drugs

▣ *Aminoglycosides:* Reduced clearance with elevated aminoglycoside levels and potential for toxicity

▣ *Anticoagulants:* Excessive hypoprothrombinemia, decreased platelet aggregation with increased risk of GI bleeding

▣ *Antihypertensives (α-blockers, angiotensin-converting enzyme inhibitors, angiotensin II receptor blockers, β-blockers, diuretics):* Inhibition of antihypertensive and other favorable hemodynamic effects

▣ *Corticosteroids:* Increased risk of GI ulceration

▣ *Cyclosporine:* Increased nephrotoxicity risk

▣ *Lithium:* Decreased clearance of lithium (mediated via prostaglandins) resulting in elevated serum lithium levels and risk of toxicity

▣ *Methotrexate:* Decreased renal secretion of methotrexate resulting in elevated methotrexate levels and risk of toxicity

▣ *Phenylpropanolamine:* Possible acute hypertensive reaction

▣ *Potassium-sparing diuretics:* Additive hyperkalemia potential

3 *Triamterene:* Acute renal failure reported with addition of indomethacin; caution with other NSAIDs
Labs
• *False increase:* Serum salicylate
• *False decrease:* T_4, T_3 uptake
SPECIAL CONSIDERATIONS
• No significant advantage over other NSAIDs; cost should govern use
MONITORING PARAMETERS
• Initial hemogram and fecal occult blood test within 3 mo of starting regular chronic therapy; repeat every 6-12 mo (more frequently in high-risk patients (> 65 years, peptic ulcer disease, concurrent steroids or anticoagulants); electrolytes, creatinine, and BUN within 3 mo of starting regular chronic therapy; repeat every 6-12 mo

---

digoxin
(di-jox'in)
Chemical Class: Digitalis glycoside
Therapeutic Class: Antiarrhythmic; cardiac glycoside

CLINICAL PHARMACOLOGY
Mechanism of Action: A cardiac glycoside that increases the influx of calcium from extracellular to intracellular cytoplasm. *Therapeutic Effect:* Potentiates the activity of the contractile cardiac muscle fibers and increases the force of myocardial contraction. Slows the heart rate by decreasing conduction through the SA and AV nodes.
Pharmacokinetics

Route	Onset	Peak	Duration
PO	0.5–2 hr	28 hr	3–4 days
IV	5–30 min	1–4 hr	3–4 days

Readily absorbed from the GI tract. Widely distributed. Protein binding: 30%. Partially metabolized in the liver. Primarily excreted in urine. Minimally removed by hemodialysis. **Half-life:** 36–48 hr (increased with impaired renal function and in the elderly).

INDICATIONS AND DOSAGES
Rapid loading dose for the management and treatment of CHF; control of ventricular rate in patients with atrial fibrillation; treatment and prevention of recurrent paroxysmal atrial tachycardia
PO
Adults, Elderly. Initially, 0.5–0.75 mg, additional doses of 0.125–0.375 mg at 6- to 8-hr intervals. Range: 0.75–1.25 mg.
Children 10 yr and older. 10–15 mcg/kg.
Children 5–9 yr. 20–35 mcg/kg.
Children 2–4 yr. 30–40 mcg/kg.
Children 1–23 mo. 35–60 mcg/kg.
Neonate, full-term. 25–35 mcg/kg.
Neonate, premature. 20–30 mcg/kg.
IV
Adults, Elderly. 0.6–1 mg.
Children 10 yr and older. 8–12 mcg/kg.
Children 5–9 yr. 15–30 mcg/kg.
Children 2–4 yr. 25–35 mcg/kg.
Children 1–23 mo. 30–50 mcg/kg.
Neonates, full-term. 20–30 mcg/kg.
Neonates, premature. 15–25 mcg/kg.
Maintenance dosage for CHF; control of ventricular rate in patients with atrial fibrillation; treatment and prevention of recurrent paroxysmal atrial tachycardia
PO, IV
Adults, Elderly. 0.125–0.375 mg/day.
Children. 25%–35% loading dose (20%–30% for premature neonates)

Dosage in renal impairment

Dosage adjustment is based on creatinine clearance. Total digitalizing dose: decrease by 50% in end-stage renal disease.

Creatinine Clearance	Dosage
10–50 ml/min	25%–75% usual
less than 10 ml/min	10%–25% usual

AVAILABLE FORMS/COST

• Cap, Elastic—Oral: 0.05 mg, 100's: **$14.70-$26.95**; 0.1 mg, 100's: **$29.41**; 0.2 mg, 100's: **$34.21**
• Elixir—Oral: 0.05 mg/ml, 60 ml: **$9.63-$37.53**
• Sol, Inj-IM, IV: 0.1 mg/ml, 1 ml: **$6.68**; 0.25 mg/ml, 2 ml: **$1.50-$3.10**
• Tab-Oral: 0.125 mg, 100's: **$4.44-$34.19**; 0.25 mg, 100's: **$9.63-$30.07**; 0.5 mg, 100's: **$18.50-$25.00**

CONTRAINDICATIONS: Ventricular fibrillation, ventricular tachycardia unrelated to CHF

PREGNANCY AND LACTATION: Pregnancy category C, passes readily to fetus; excreted into breast milk; considered compatible with breast-feeding

SIDE EFFECTS

None known. However, there is a very narrow margin of safety between a therapeutic and toxic result. Long-term therapy may produce mammary gland enlargement in women but is reversible when drug is withdrawn.

SERIOUS REACTIONS

• The most common early manifestations of digoxin toxicity are GI disturbances (anorexia, nausea, vomiting) and neurologic abnormalities (fatigue, headache, depression, weakness, drowsiness, confusion, nightmares).

• Facial pain, personality change, and ocular disturbances (photophobia, light flashes, halos around bright objects, yellow or green color perception) may be noted.

INTERACTIONS

Drugs

3 *Alprazolam, amiodarone, diltiazem, verapamil, bepridil, nitrendipine, quinidine, carvedilol, cyclosporine, erythromycin and tetracyclines (change in bacterial flora causing effect may persist for months), hydroxychloroquine, NSAIDs, azole antifungals, omeprazole, lansoprazole, propafenone, quinine, spironolactone, tacrolimus:* Increased digoxin levels

3 *Amphotericin B diuretics:* Enhanced digitalis toxicity secondary to drug-induced hypokalemia

3 *β-blockers:* Potentiation of bradycardia

3 *Calcium (IV):* Digitalis toxicity

2 *Charcoal:* Reduced digitalis levels

3 *Cholestyramine, Kaolo-pectin (digoxin tablets only) neomycin, penicillamine, rifampin, sulfasalazine:* Reduced digitalis levels

3 *Cyclophosphamide:* Impaired digoxin (especially tablets) absorption; digitoxin not affected

3 *Metoclopramide, cisapride:* Reduced digitalis levels by slowly dissolving digoxin tablets only (Lanoxin tablets and capsules not affected)

3 *Succinylcholine:* Increased arrhythmias

Labs

• *False increase:* Urine 17-hydroxycorticosteroids

SPECIAL CONSIDERATIONS

• Preferred digitalis glycoside
• Rule out digitalis toxicity if nausea, vomiting, arrhythmias develop
• Listed adverse effects are mostly signs of toxicity

MONITORING PARAMETERS

• Heart rate and rhythm, periodic ECGs

• Serum potassium, magnesium, calcium, creatinine

• Serum digoxin levels when compliance, effectiveness, or systemic availability is questioned or toxicity suspected

• Obtain serum drug concentrations at least 8-12 hr after a dose (preferably prior to next scheduled dose); therapeutic range 0.5-2.0 ng/ml

---

digoxin immune Fab

(di-jox′in)

Chemical Class: Antibody fragment

Therapeutic Class: Antidote, digitalis

CLINICAL PHARMACOLOGY

Mechanism of Action: An antidote that binds molecularly to digoxin in the extracellular space. *Therapeutic Effect:* Makes digoxin unavailable for binding at its site of action on cells in the body.

Pharmacokinetics

Route	Onset	Peak	Duration
IV	30 min	N/A	3–4 days

Widely distributed into extracellular space. Excreted in urine. **Half-life:** 15–20 hr.

INDICATIONS AND DOSAGES

Potentially life-threatening digoxin overdose

IV

Adults, Elderly, Children. Dosage varies according to amount of digoxin to be neutralized. Refer to manufacturer's dosing guidelines.

$ AVAILABLE FORMS/COST

• Inj, Conc-Sol—IV: 40 mg/vial, 1's: **$600.00**

CONTRAINDICATIONS: None known

PREGNANCY AND LACTATION:

Pregnancy category C; excretion into breast milk unknown; use caution in nursing mothers

SIDE EFFECTS

None known

SERIOUS REACTIONS

• Hyperkalemia may occur as a result of digitalis toxicity. Signs and symptoms of hyperkalemia include diarrhea, paresthesia of extremities, heaviness of legs, decreased BP, cold skin, grayish pallor, hypotension, mental confusion, irritability, flaccid paralysis, tented T waves, widening QRS interval, and ST depression.

• Hypokalemia may develop rapidly when the effect of digitalis is reversed. Signs and symptoms of hypokalemia include muscle cramping, nausea, vomiting, hypoactive bowel sounds, abdominal distention, difficulty breathing, and orthostatic hypotension.

• Low cardiac output and CHF may occur rarely.

INTERACTIONS

Labs

• *Interference:* Immunoassay digoxin

SPECIAL CONSIDERATIONS

MONITORING PARAMETERS

• Potassium, serum digoxin level prior to therapy

• Continuous ECG monitoring

dihydroergotamine
(dye-hye-droe-er-got'-a-meen)
Rx: D.H.E. 45, Migranal
Chemical Class: Ergot alkaloid
Therapeutic Class: Antimigraine agent

CLINICAL PHARMACOLOGY
Mechanism of Action: An ergotamine derivative, alpha-adrenergic blocker that directly stimulates vascular smooth muscle. May also have antagonist effects on serotonin. *Therapeutic Effect:* Peripheral and cerebral vasoconstriction.

Pharmacokinetics
Slow, incomplete absorption from the gastrointestinal (GI) tract; rate of absorption of intranasal varies. Protein binding: greater than 90%. Undergoes extensive first-pass metabolism in liver. Metabolized to active metabolite. Eliminated in feces via biliary system. **Half-life:** 7-9 hrs.

INDICATIONS AND DOSAGES
Migraine headaches, cluster headaches
IM/Subcutaneous
Adults, Elderly. 1 mg at onset of headache; repeat hourly. Maximum: 3 mg/day; 6 mg/wk.
IV
Adults, Elderly. 1 mg at onset of headache; repeat hourly. Maximum: 2 mg/day; 6 mg/wk.
Intranasal
Adults, Elderly. 1 spray (0.5 mg) into each nostril; repeat in 15 min. Maximum: 4 sprays/day; 8 sprays/wk.

AVAILABLE FORMS/COST
• Inj, Sol-IM, IV: 1 mg/ml, 1 ml: **$35.00-$47.26**
• Spray—Nasal: 0.5 mg/inh, 4 ml: **$33.65**

CONTRAINDICATIONS: Coronary artery disease, hypertension, impaired liver or renal function, malnutrition, peripheral vascular diseases, such as thromboangiitis obliterans, syphilitic arteritis, severe arteriosclerosis, thrombophlebitis, Raynaud's disease, sepsis, severe pruritus

PREGNANCY AND LACTATION: Pregnancy category X; likely excreted into breast milk; ergotamine has caused symptoms of ergotism (e.g., vomiting, diarrhea) in the infant; excessive dosage or prolonged administration may inhibit lactation

SIDE EFFECTS
Occasional
Cough, dizziness, rhinitis, altered taste, throat and nose irritation
Rare
Muscle pain, fatigue, diarrhea, upper respiratory infection, dyspepsia

SERIOUS REACTIONS
• Prolonged administration or excessive dosage may produce ergotamine poisoning manifested as nausea, vomiting, weakness of legs, pain in limb muscles, numbness and tingling of fingers or toes, precordial pain, tachycardia or bradycardia, and hypertension or hypotension.
• Localized edema and itching due to vasoconstriction of peripheral arteries and arterioles may occur.
• Feet or hands will become cold, pale, and numb.
• Muscle pain will occur when walking and later, even at rest.
• Gangrene may occur.
• Occasionally confusion, depression, drowsiness, and seizures appear.

INTERACTIONS
Drugs
❷ *Clarithromycin, erythromycin (not azithromycin or dirithromycin):* Increased ergotism (hypertention and ischemia)
❷ *Nitroglycerin:* Enhanced ergot effect, decreased antianginal effects

❷ *Sibutramine:* Increased risk of serotonin syndrome
SPECIAL CONSIDERATIONS
• Considered alternative abortive acute migraine agent; nasal spray less effective than triptans
PATIENT/FAMILY EDUCATION
• Initiate therapy at first sign of attack
• Prolonged use may lead to withdrawal headaches

---

dihydrotachysterol
(dye-hye-droe-tak-iss′ter-ole)
Chemical Class: Sterol derivative
Therapeutic Class: Antiosteoporotic; vitamin D analog

CLINICAL PHARMACOLOGY
Mechanism of Action: A fat-soluble vitamin that is essential for absorption, utilization of calcium phosphate, and normal calcification of bone. *Therapeutic Effect:* Stimulates calcium and phosphate absorption from small intestine, promotes secretion of calcium from bone to blood, promotes renal tubule phosphate resorption, acts on bone cells to stimulate skeletal growth and on parathyroid gland to suppress hormone synthesis and secretion.
Pharmacokinetics
Well absorbed from small intestine. Metabolized in liver. Eliminated via biliary system; excreted in urine. **Half-life:** Unknown.
INDICATIONS AND DOSAGES
Hypoparathyroidism
PO
Adults, Elderly, Older Children. Initially, 0.8-2.4 mg/day for several days. Maintenance: 0.2-1 mg/day.
Infants, Young Children. Initially, 1-5 mg/day for 4 days, then 0.1-0.5 mg/day.

Nutritional rickets
PO
Adults, Elderly, Children. 0.5 mg as a single dose or 13-50 mcg/day until healing occurs.
Renal osteodystorphy
PO
Adults, Elderly. 0.25-0.6 mg/24 hrs adjusted as necessary to achieve normal serum calcium levels and promote bone healing.
S   AVAILABLE FORMS/COST
• Cap, Gel-Oral: 0.125 mg, 50's: **$176.94**
• Conc-Oral: 0.2 mg/ml, 30 ml: **$44.97**
• Tab-Oral: 0.125 mg, 50's: **$57.22**; 0.2 mg, 100's: **$100.28**; 0.4 mg, 50's: **$104.34**
CONTRAINDICATIONS: Hypercalcemia, malabsorption syndrome, vitamin D toxicity, hypersensitivity to vitamin D products or analogs
PREGNANCY AND LACTATION: Pregnancy category A (category D if used in doses above the recommended daily allowance); excretion into breast milk unknown; vitamin D is excreted into breast milk in limited amounts; considered compatible with breast-feeding, however, serum calcium levels of the infant should be monitored if the mother is receiving pharmacologic doses
SIDE EFFECTS
Occasional
Nausea, vomiting
SERIOUS REACTIONS
• Early signs of overdosage are manifested as weakness, headache, somnolence, nausea, vomiting, dry mouth, constipation, muscle and bone pain, and metallic taste sensation.
• Later signs of overdosage are evidenced by polyuria, polydipsia, anorexia, weight loss, nocturia, photo-

phobia, rhinorrhea, pruritus, disorientation, hallucinations, hyperthermia, hypertension, and cardiac arrhythmias.

SPECIAL CONSIDERATIONS

• Vitamin D analog of choice for prevention and treatment of renal osteodystrophy; less expensive than calcitriol

PATIENT/FAMILY EDUCATION

• Compliance with dosage instructions, diet (evaluate vitamin D ingested in fortified foods, maintain adequate calcium intake) is essential

MONITORING PARAMETERS

• Serum Ca^{++} and phosphate

• If adverse reactions occur rule out hypercalcemia, worsening renal function

---

diltiazem

(dil-tye′a-zem)
Combinations
Rx: with enalapril (Teczem)
Chemical Class: Benzothiazepine
Therapeutic Class: Antianginal; antiarrhythmic, class IV; antihypertensive; calcium channel blocker

---

CLINICAL PHARMACOLOGY
Mechanism of Action: An antianginal, antihypertensive, and antiarrhythmic agent that inhibits calcium movement across cardiac and vascular smooth-muscle cell membranes. This action causes the dilation of coronary arteries, peripheral arteries, and arterioles. *Therapeutic Effect:* Decreases heart rate and myocardial contractility, slows SA and AV conduction and decreases total peripheral vascular resistance by vasodilation.

Pharmacokinetics

Route	Onset	Peak	Duration
PO	0.5–1 hr	N/A	N/A
PO (extended-release)	2–3 hrs	N/A	N/A
IV	3 min	N/A	N/A

Well absorbed from the GI tract. Protein binding: 70%–80%. Undergoes first-pass metabolism in the liver to active metabolite. Primarily excreted in urine. Not removed by hemodialysis. **Half-life:** 3–8 hr.

INDICATIONS AND DOSAGES
Angina related to coronary artery spasm (Prinzmetal's variant), chronic stable angina (effort-associated)
PO
Adults, Elderly. Initially, 30 mg 4 times a day. Increase up to 180–360 mg/day in 3–4 divided doses at 1- to 2-day intervals.
Adults, Elderly (Cardizem LA). Initially, 180 mg/day. May increase at intervals of 7-14 days up to 360 mg/day.
Adults, Elderly (Cardizem CD). Initially, 120–180 mg/day; titrate over 7–14 days. Range: Up to 480 mg/day.
Essential hypertension
PO
Adults, Elderly. (Cardizem CD, Cartia XT): Initially, 180-240 mg once a day. May increase at 2 week intervals. Maintenance 240-360 mg/day. Maximum: 480 mg once a day. (Cardizem SR): Initially, 60-120 mg twice a day. May increase at 2 week intervals. Maintenance: 240-360 mg/day. (Cardizem LA): Initially, 180-240 mg once a day. May increase at 2 week intervals. Maintenance: 120-540 mg/day. (Dilacor XR): 180-240 mg once a day. (Dilacor XT): Initially, 180-240 mg a day. May increase at 2 week intervals.

Maximum: 540 mg once a day. (Taztia XT): Initially, 120-240 mg once a day. May increase at 2 week intervals. Maximum: 540 mg once a day. *Temporary control of rapid ventricular rate in atrial fibrillation or flutter, rapid conversion of paroxysmal supraventricular tachycardia to normal sinus rhythm.*

IV push

Adults, Elderly. Initially, 0.25 mg/kg actual body weight over 2 min. May repeat in 15 min at dose of 0.35 mg/kg actual body weight. Subsequent doses individualized.

IV infusion

Adults, Elderly. After initial bolus injection, may begin infusion at 5–10 mg/hr; may increase by 5 mg/hr up to a maximum of 15 mg/hr. Infusion duration should not exceed 24 hr.

💲 AVAILABLE FORMS/COST

• Cap, Gel, Sus Action—Oral: 60 mg, 100's: **$29.60-$109.51**; 90 mg, 100's: **$79.20-$125.13**; 120 mg, 100's: **$90.01-$153.80**; 180 mg, 100's: **$48.10-$119.08**; 240 mg, 100's: **$112.95-$193.67**; 300 mg, 90's: **$193.38-$287.98**; 360 mg, 90's: **$211.01-$313.26**; 420 mg, 90's: **$245.73**

• Sol, Inj-IV: 5 mg/ml, 5 ml: **$3.93-$10.00**

• Tab-Oral: 30 mg, 100's: **$6.21-$47.27**; 60 mg, 100's: **$8.97-$90.73**; 90 mg, 100's: **$11.75-$131.28**; 120 mg, 100's: **$99.00-$136.40**

CONTRAINDICATIONS: Acute MI, pulmonary congestion, severe hypotension (less than 90 mm Hg, systolic), sick sinus syndrome, second- or third-degree AV block (except in the presence of a pacemaker)

PREGNANCY AND LACTATION: Pregnancy category C; excreted into breast milk in concentrations that may approximate those in maternal serum; use caution in nursing mothers

SIDE EFFECTS

Frequent (10%–5%)

Peripheral edema, dizziness, lightheadedness, headache, bradycardia, asthenia (loss of strength, weakness)

Occasional (5%–2%)

Nausea, constipation, flushing, EKG changes

Rare (less than 2%)

Rash, micturition disorder (polyuria, nocturia, dysuria, frequency of urination), abdominal discomfort, somnolence

SERIOUS REACTIONS

• Abrupt withdrawal may increase frequency or duration of angina.

• CHF and second- and third-degree AV block occur rarely.

• Overdose produces nausea, somnolence, confusion, slurred speech, and profound bradycardia.

INTERACTIONS

Drugs

3️⃣ *α-blockers:* Additive increased antihypertensive effect

3️⃣ *Amiodarone:* Cardiotoxicity with bradycardia and decreased cardiac output

3️⃣ *Antipyrine:* Increased antipyrine concentrations

3️⃣ *Aspirin:* Enhanced antiplatelet activity

3️⃣ *Azole antifungals:* Possible increased calcium channel blocker effects

3️⃣ *β-blockers:* Inhibition of metabolism of propranolol and metoprolol (not atenolol); additive effects on cardiac conduction and hypotension

2️⃣ *Carbamazepine:* Increase in carbamazepine toxicity

③ *Cyclosporine, tacrolimus:* Increased blood concentrations, renal toxicity
③ *Digitalis glycosides:* Reduced elimination, increased digitalis levels, toxicity
③ *Ecainide:* Increased ecainide levels
③ *Erythromycin, troleandomycin:* Increased levels calcium channel blocker
③ *Fentanyl:* Severe hypotension or increased fluid volume requirements
③ *H₂-receptor antagonists:* Serum diltiazem concentrations increased
③ *Lithium:* Neurotoxicity
③ *Neuromuscular blockers:* Prolonged blockade by vecuronium and pancuronium
③ *Nitroprusside:* Enhanced hypotension
③ *Phenobarbital:* Reduced calcium channel blocker concentration
③ *Phenytoin:* Increased phenytoin levels
③ *Rifampin:* Decreased diltiazem concentrations
③ *Tricyclic antidepressants:* Increased TCA levels
Labs
• *False positive:* Urine ketones

---

dimenhydrinate
(dye-men-hye′dri-nate)
Chemical Class: Ethanolamine derivative
Therapeutic Class: Antihistamine; antivertigo agent

CLINICAL PHARMACOLOGY
Mechanism of Action: An antihistamine and anticholinergic that competes for H1 receptor sites on effector cells of the GI tract, blood vessels, and respiratory tract. The anticholinergic action diminishes vestibular stimulation and depresses labyrinthine function. *Therapeutic Effect:* Prevents symptoms of motion sickness.

INDICATIONS AND DOSAGES
Motion sickness
PO
Adults, Elderly, Children older than 12 yr. 50-100 mg q4-6h. Maximum: 400 mg/day.
Children 6–12 yr. 25-50 mg q6-8h. Maximum: 150 mg/day.
Children 2–5 yr. 12.5-25 mg q6-8h. Maximum: 75 mg/day.

💲 AVAILABLE FORMS/COST
• Sol, Inj-IM, IV: 50 mg/ml, 10 ml: **$1.69-$11.40**
• Liq-Oral: 12.5 mg/4 ml, 120, 480 ml: **$12.48**/480 ml
• Tab-Oral: 50 mg, 100's: **$0.77-$21.13**

CONTRAINDICATIONS: None significant.

PREGNANCY AND LACTATION: Pregnancy category B; has been used for the treatment of hyperemesis gravidarum; small amounts are excreted into breast milk; use caution in nursing mothers

SIDE EFFECTS
Frequent
Dry mouth
Occasional
Hypotension, palpitations, tachycardia, headache, somnolence, dizziness, paradoxical stimulation (especially in children), anorexia, constipation, dysuria, blurred vision, tinnitus, wheezing, chest tightness
Rare
Photosensitivity, rash, urticaria

SERIOUS REACTIONS
• None significant.

SPECIAL CONSIDERATIONS
PATIENT/FAMILY EDUCATION
• For prevention of motion sickness administer at least 30 min before exposure to motion

dimercaprol
(dye-mer-kap'-role)
Chemical Class: Dithiol derivative
Therapeutic Class: Antidote, heavy metal

CLINICAL PHARMACOLOGY
Mechanism of Action: A chelating agent that contains two sulfhydryl groups that form a stable, nontoxic chelate 5-membered heterocyclic ring with heavy metals. *Therapeutic Effect:* Prevents the metal from combining with sulfhydryl groups on physiologic proteins and keeps them inactive until they can be excreted.

Pharmacokinetics
Time to peak after IM administration occurs in 30 to 60 minutes. Widely distributed to all tissues including the brain and, mainly, intracellular space. Rapidly metabolized by the liver to inactive metabolites. Excreted in the urine and bile. Removed by hemodialysis. **Half-life:** 4 hrs.

INDICATIONS AND DOSAGES
Poisoning, arsenic (mild)
IM
Adults, Elderly, Children. 2.5 mg/kg 4 times/day for 2 days, 2 times on day 3, then once daily for 10 days or recovery.

Poisoning, arsenic (severe)
IM
Adults, Elderly, Children. 3 mg/kg q4h for 2 days, 4 times on day 3, then twice daily for 10 days or recovery.

Poisoning, gold (mild)
IM
Adults, Elderly, Children. 2.5 mg/kg 4 times/day for 2 days, 2 times on day 3, then once daily for 10 days or recovery.

Adults, Elderly, Children. 2.5 mg/kg 4 times/day for 2 days, 2 times on day 3, then once daily for 10 days or recovery.
IM
Adults, Elderly, Children. 3 mg/kg q4h for 2 days, 4 times on day 3, then twice daily for 10 days or until recovery.

Poisoning, lead (mild)
IM
Adults, Elderly, Children. Initially, 4 mg/kg, then 3 mg/kg q4h for 2-7 days in combination with edetate calcium disodium injection at different injection sites

Poisoning, lead (severe)
IM
Adults, Elderly, Children. 4 mg/kg q4h for 2-7 days in combination with edetate calcium disodium injection at different injection sites

Poisoning, mercury
IM
Adults, Elderly, Children. 5 mg/kg for 1 day, followed by 2.5 mg/kg 1 or 2 times/day for 10 days

Dosage in renal impairment
Adults, Elderly. 2 mg/kg q12h during dialysis.

🔲 AVAILABLE FORMS/COST
• Inj, Sol-IM: 100 mg/ml, 3 ml: **$74.76**

UNLABELED USES: Antimony poisoning, bismuth poisoning, selenium poisoning, silver poisoning, vanadium poisoning

CONTRAINDICATIONS: Acute renal impairment, alkyl mercuring poisoning, G6PD deficiency (unless a life-threatening situation exists), hepatic insufficiency (unless due to arsenic poisoning), use of iron, cadmium or selenium poisoning, hypersensitivity to dimercaprol or any component of the formulations

PREGNANCY AND LACTATION: Pregnancy category D; use only in life-threatening poisoning

SIDE EFFECTS
Frequent
Hypertension, dose-related tachycardia, headache
Occasional
Nausea, vomiting
Rare
Burning eyes, lips, mouth, throat and penis, nervousness, pain at injection site, salivation, fever, dysuria

SERIOUS REACTIONS
• Abscess formation at injection site, blepharospasm, convulsions, thrombocytopenia, and transient neutropenia occur rarely.

SPECIAL CONSIDERATIONS
• Administer by deep IM injection only

MONITORING PARAMETERS
• Blood pressure, pulse
• BUN, Cr, urine pH (alkaline urinary pH decreases renal damage)
• Specific heavy metal levels

---

dinoprostone (PGE2)
(dye-noe-prost′one)
Chemical Class: Prostaglandin E₂
Therapeutic Class: Abortifacient; uterine stimulant

CLINICAL PHARMACOLOGY
Mechanism of Action: A prostaglandin that directly acts on the myometrium, causing softening and dilation effect of the cervix. *Therapeutic Effect:* Stimulates myometrial contractions in gravid uterus.
Pharmacokinetics
Undergoes rapid enzymatic deactivation primarily in maternal lungs. Protein binding: 73%. Primarily excreted in urine. **Half-life:** Less than 5 min.

INDICATIONS AND DOSAGES
Abortifacient
Intravaginal
Adults. 20 mg or one suppository high into vagina. May repeat at 3- to 5-hr intervals until abortion occurs. Do not administer for longer than 2 days.

Ripening of unfavorable cervix
Intracervical
Adults. Initially, 0.5 mg (2.5 ml) (Prepidil); if no cervical or uterine response, may repeat 0.5-mg dose in 6 hr. Maximum: 1.5 mg (7.5 ml) for a 24-hr period. Or 10 mg (Cervidil) over 12-hr period; remove upon onset of active labor or 12 hr after insertion.

§ AVAILABLE FORMS/COST
• Gel—Cervical: 0.5 mg/3 g: **$97.96**
• Insert—Vag: 0.3 mg/hr: **$219.29**
• Supp—Vag: 20 mg, 1's: **$658.04**

CONTRAINDICATIONS: Active cardiac, hepatic, pulmonary or renal disease; acute pelvic inflammatory disease; fetal malpresentation; hypersensitivity to dinoprostone or other prostaglandins; significant cephalopelvic disproportion

PREGNANCY AND LACTATION: Pregnancy category C; complete any failed attempts at pregnancy termination by some other means

SIDE EFFECTS
Frequent
Vomiting (66%), diarrhea (40%), nausea (33%)
Occasional
Headache (10%), chills or shivering (10%), hives, bradycardia, increased uterine pain accompanying abortion, peripheral vasoconstriction
Rare
Flushing, vulvae edema

SERIOUS REACTIONS
• Overdose may cause uterine hypertonicity with spasm and tetanic contraction, leading to cervical laceration or perforation, and uterine rupture or hemorrhage.
INTERACTIONS
Drugs
• *Oxytoxin:* Augmented activity, use sequentially not concurrently (6-12 hr after gel, 30 min after removal of insert)
SPECIAL CONSIDERATIONS
• Do not place gel above level of internal os; use 20 mm endocervical catheter if no effacement present; 10 mm catheter if cervix 50% effaced
• May use small amount water soluble lubricant with insert; do not use insert without retrieval system
PATIENT/FAMILY EDUCATION
• Remain supine for 10-15 min (vag supp), 15-30 min (gel), 2h (insert)
MONITORING PARAMETERS
• Blood pressure, fetal monitor (for cervical ripening)

diphenhydramine
(dye-fen-hye′dra-meen)
Rx: Banaril, Benadryl, Dytuss, Hyrexin, Tusstat, Tuxadryl
OTC: Allermax, Banophen, Banophen Caplets, Belix, Benadryl 25, Benylin Cough, Bydramine Cough, Diphen Cough, Dormarex 2, Genahist, Gen-D-phen, Hydramine Cough, Nidryl, Nordryl Cough, Phendry, Uni-Bent Cough
Combinations
   OTC: with acetaminophen (Excedrin PM, Extra Strength Tylenol PM, Sominex Pain Relief, Unisom with Pain Relief); with calamine (Caladryl)
Chemical Class: Ethanolamine derivative
Therapeutic Class: Anti-Parkinson's agent; antianaphylactic (adjunct); antihistamine; antipruritic; antivertigo agent; hypnotic

CLINICAL PHARMACOLOGY
Mechanism of Action: An ethanolamine that competitively blocks the effects of histamine at peripheral H_1 receptor sites. *Therapeutic Effect:* Produces anticholinergic, antipruritic, antitussive, antiemetic, antidyskinetic, and sedative effects.
Pharmacokinetics

Route	Onset	Peak	Duration
PO	15–30 min	1–4 hr	4–6 hr
IV, IM	less than 15 min	1–4 hr	4–6 hr

Well absorbed after PO or parenteral administration. Protein binding: 98%–99%. Widely distributed. Metabolized in the liver. Primarily excreted in urine. **Half-life:** 1–4 hr.

INDICATIONS AND DOSAGES

Moderate to severe allergic reaction, dystonic reaction

PO, IV, IM

Adults, Elderly. 25–50 mg q4h. Maximum: 400 mg/day.

Children. 5 mg/kg/day in divided doses q6–8h. Maximum: 300 mg/day.

Motion sickness, minor allergic rhinitis

PO, IV, IM

Adults, Elderly, Children 12 yr and older. 25–50 mg q4–6h. Maximum: 300 mg/day.

Children 6–11 yr. 12.5–25 mg q4–6h. Maximum: 150 mg/day.

Children 2–5 yr. 6.25 mg q4–6h. Maximum: 37.5 mg/day.

Antitussive

PO

Adults, Elderly, Children 12 yr and older. 25 mg q4h. Maximum: 150 mg/day.

Children 6–11 yr. 12.5 mg q4h. Maximum: 75 mg/day.

Children 2–5 yr. 6.25 mg q4h. Maximum: 37.5 mg/day.

Nighttime sleep aid

PO

Adults, Elderly, Children 12 yr and older. 50 mg at bedtime.

Children 2–11 yr. 1 mg/kg/dose. Maximum: 50 mg.

Pruritus

Topical

Adults, Elderly, Children 12 yr and older. Apply 1% or 2% cream or spray 3–4 times a day.

Children 2–11 yr. Apply 1% cream or spray 3–4 times a day.

[$] **AVAILABLE FORMS/COST**

- Cap, Gel—Oral: 25 mg, 100's: **$1.04-$21.69**; 50 mg, 100's: **$1.12-$25.93**
- Cream—Top: 2%, 15, 30, 60 g: **$3.16-$11.05**/15 g
- Gel-Top: 2%, 120 g: **$4.57**
- Liq-Oral: 6.25 mg/5 ml, 240 ml: **$4.28**; 12.5 mg/5 ml, 120, 240, 480 ml: **$2.40-$14.02**/480 ml
- Sol, Inj-IM, IV: 10 mg/ml, 30 ml: **$2.00-$8.25**; 50 mg/ml, 1 ml: **$1.03-$2.94**
- Spray-Top: 2%, 60 ml: **$4.57**
- Tab-Oral: 25 mg, 100's: **$2.39-$11.05**; 50 mg, 100's: **$2.00**

CONTRAINDICATIONS: Acute exacerbation of asthma, use within 14 days of MAOIs

PREGNANCY AND LACTATION: Pregnancy category C; excreted into breast milk; although levels are not thought to be sufficiently high after therapeutic doses to affect the infant, the manufacturer considers the drug contraindicated in nursing mothers due to the increased sensitivity of newborn or premature infants to antihistamines

SIDE EFFECTS

Frequent

Somnolence, dizziness, muscle weakness, hypotension, urine retention, thickening of bronchial secretions, dry mouth, nose, throat, or lips; in elderly, sedation, dizziness, hypotension

Occasional

Epigastric distress, flushing, visual or hearing disturbances, paresthesia, diaphoresis, chills

SERIOUS REACTIONS

- Hypersensitivity reactions, such as eczema, pruritus, rash, cardiac disturbances, and photosensitivity, may occur.

• Overdose symptoms may vary from CNS depression, including sedation, apnea, hypotension, cardiovascular collapse, and death, to severe paradoxical reactions, such as hallucinations, tremor, and seizures.

• Children and neonates may experience paradoxical reactions, including restlessness, insomnia, euphoria, nervousness, and tremors.

• Overdosage in children may result in hallucinations, seizures, and death.

INTERACTIONS
Drugs
🔳 *Anticholinergics:* Possible enhanced anticholinergic, CNS effects
Labs
• *False negative:* Skin allergy tests
• *False positive:* Urine methadone, serum and urine tricyclic antidepressant

---

diphenoxylate and atropine
(dye-fen-ox′i-late)
Rx: Lomocot, Lomotil, Lonox. Vi-Atro, Motofen (difenoxin and atropine)
Chemical Class: Meperidine analog
Therapeutic Class: Antidiarrheal
DEA Class: Schedule V

CLINICAL PHARMACOLOGY
Mechanism of Action: A meperidine derivative that acts locally and centrally on gastric mucosa. *Therapeutic Effect:* Reduces intestinal motility.
Pharmacokinetics
Well absorbed from the GI tract. Metabolized in the liver to active metabolite. Primarily eliminated in feces. **Half-life:** 2.5 hr; metabolite, 12–24 hr.

INDICATIONS AND DOSAGES
Diarrhea
PO
Adults, Elderly. Initially, 15–20 mg/day in 3–4 divided doses; then 5–15 mg/day in 2–3 divided doses.
Children 9–12 yr. 2 mg 5 times a day.
Children 6–8 yr. 2 mg 4 times a day.
Children 2–5 yr. 2 mg 3 times a day.

Ⓢ AVAILABLE FORMS/COST
• Sol-Oral: 2.5 mg diphenoxylate/ 0.025 mg atropine/5 ml, 60 ml: **$8.17-$22.30**
• Tab-Oral: 2.5 mg diphenoxylate/ 0.025 mg atropine, 100's: **$3.15-$75.43**; 1 mg difenoxin/0.025 mg atropine, 100's: **$70.31**

CONTRAINDICATIONS: Children younger than 2 years, dehydration, jaundice, narrow-angle glaucoma, severe hepatic disease

PREGNANCY AND LACTATION: Pregnancy category C; excreted in breast milk

SIDE EFFECTS
Frequent
Somnolence, light-headedness, dizziness, nausea
Occasional
Headache, dry mouth
Rare
Flushing, tachycardia, urine retention, constipation, paradoxical reaction (marked by restlessness and agitation), blurred vision

SERIOUS REACTIONS
• Dehydration may predispose to diphenoxylate toxicity.
• Paralytic ileus and toxic megacolon (marked by constipation, decreased appetite, and stomach pain with nausea or vomiting) occur rarely.
• Severe anticholinergic reaction, manifested by severe lethargy, hypotonic reflexes, and hyperthermia, may result in severe respiratory depression and coma.

INTERACTIONS

Drugs

[2] *MAOIs:* Possible hypertensive crisis

[3] *Barbiturates, tranquilizers, narcotics, alcohol:* Potentiation of effects

SPECIAL CONSIDERATIONS

• Equally effective as codeine or loperamide

PATIENT/FAMILY EDUCATION

• Prolonged use not recommended

• Drowsiness or dizziness may occur; use caution when driving or operating dangerous machinery

dipyridamole

(dye-peer-id'a-mole)

Rx: Persantine

Combinations

Rx: with aspirin (Aggrenox)

Chemical Class: Pyrimidine derivative

Therapeutic Class: Antiplatelet agent; coronary vasodilator

CLINICAL PHARMACOLOGY

Mechanism of Action: A blood modifier and platelet aggregation inhibitor that inhibits the activity of adenosine deaminase and phosphodiesterase, enzymes causing accumulation of adenosine and cyclic adenosine monophosphate. *Therapeutic Effect:* Inhibits platelet aggregation; may cause coronary vasodilation.

Pharmacokinetics

Slowly, variably absorbed from the GI tract. Widely distributed. Protein binding: 91%–99%. Metabolized in the liver. Primarily eliminated via biliary excretion. **Half-life:** 10–15 hr.

INDICATIONS AND DOSAGES

Prevention of thromboembolic disorders

PO

Adults, Elderly. 75–400 mg/day in combination with other medications.

Children. 3–6 mg/kg/day in 3 divided doses.

Diagnostic aid

IV

Adults, Elderly (based on weight). 0.142 mg/kg/min infused over 4 min; although a maximum hasn't been determined, doses greater than 60 mg have been determined to be unnecessary for any patient.

[$] AVAILABLE FORMS/COST

• Sol, Inj-IV: 5 mg/ml, 10 ml: **$27.60-$149.63**

• Tab, Coated-Oral: 25 mg, 100's: **$4.75-$55.13**; 50 mg, 100's: **$8.50-$87.99**; 75 mg, 100's: **$11.25-$117.71**

UNLABELED USES: Prevention of myocardial reinfarction, treatment of transient ischemic attacks

CONTRAINDICATIONS: None known.

PREGNANCY AND LACTATION: Pregnancy category C; excreted in breast milk

SIDE EFFECTS

Frequent (14%)

Dizziness

Occasional (6%–2%)

Abdominal distress, headache, rash

Rare (less than 2%)

Diarrhea, vomiting, flushing, pruritus

SERIOUS REACTIONS

• Overdose produces peripheral vasodilation, resulting in hypotension.

INTERACTIONS

Drugs

[3] *Adenosine:* Increased concentrations of adenosine, potentiates adenosine's pharmacologic effects

[3] *β-blockers:* Additive bradycardia

dirithromycin

(die-rith-ro-my'sin)

Rx: Dynabac

Chemical Class: Macrolide derivative

Therapeutic Class: Antibiotic

CLINICAL PHARMACOLOGY

Mechanism of Action: A macrolide that binds to ribosomal receptor sites of susceptible organisms, inhibiting bacterial protein synthesis. *Therapeutic Effect:* Bactericidal or bacteriostatic, depending on drug dosage.

Pharmacokinetics

Rapidly absorbed from the GI tract. Protein binding: 15%-30%.Widely distributed into tissues and within cells. Eliminated primarily unchanged by biliary excretion. Not removed by hemodialysis. **Half-life:** 30-44 hr.

INDICATIONS AND DOSAGES

Pharyngitis, tonsillitis

PO

Adults, Elderly, Children 12 yr and older. 500 mg once a day for 10 days.

Acute or chronic bronchitis, skin and skin-structure infections

PO

Adults, Elderly, Children 12 yr and older. 500 mg once a day for 7 days.

Community-acquired pneumonia

PO

Adults, Elderly, Children 12 yr and older. 500 mg once a day for 14 days.

[$] **AVAILABLE FORMS/COST**

• Tab, Enteric Coated—Oral: 250 mg, 60's: **$261.66**

CONTRAINDICATIONS: Hypersensitivity to dirithromycin or other macrolide antibiotics

PREGNANCY AND LACTATION: Pregnancy category C; excreted into rodent breast milk; no human data

SIDE EFFECTS

Frequent (10%-8%)

Abdominal pain, headache, nausea, diarrhea

Occasional (3%-2%)

Vomiting, dyspepsia, dizziness, nonspecific pain, asthenia

Rare (less than 2%)

Increased cough, flatulence, rash, dyspnea, pruritus and urticaria, insomnia

SERIOUS REACTIONS

• Antibiotic-associated colitis and other superinfections may result from altered bacterial balance.

INTERACTIONS

Drugs

[3] *Penicillins:* Dirithromycin may inhibit antibacterial activity of penicillins

SPECIAL CONSIDERATIONS

• Long $t_{1/2}$ and higher tissue concentrations allow qday dosing; however, the improved antimicrobial activity against *H. influenzae* and lower incidence of GI adverse effects have not been realized with this agent; Azithromycin probably best choice pending further comparisons

PATIENT/FAMILY EDUCATION

• Take with food or within 1 hr of having eaten

disopyramide
(dye-soe-peer'a-mide)
Rx: Norpace, Norpace CR
Chemical Class: Pyramide derivative
Therapeutic Class: Antiarrhythmic, class IA

D

CLINICAL PHARMACOLOGY
Mechanism of Action: An antiarrhythmic that prolongs the refractory period of the cardiac cell by direct effect, decreasing myocardial excitability and conduction velocity. *Therapeutic Effect:* Depresses myocardial contractility. Has anticholinergic and negative inotropic effects.

INDICATIONS AND DOSAGES
Suppression and prevention of ventricular ectopy, unifocal or multifocal premature ventricular contractions, paired ventricular contractions (couplets), and episodes of ventricular tachycardia
PO
Adults, Elderly weighing 50 kg and more. 150 mg q6h (300 mg q12h with extended-release).
Adults, Elderly weighing less than 50 kg. 100 mg q6h (200 mg q12h with extended-release).
Rapid control of arrhythmias
PO
Alert: Do not use extended-release capsules for rapid control.
Adults, elderly weighing 50 kg and more. Initially, 300 mg, then 150 mg q6h or 300 mg (controlled release) q12h.
Adults, elderly weighing less than 50 kg. Initially, 200 mg, then 100 mg q6h or 200 mg (controlled release) q12h.
Severe refractory arrhythmias
PO
Adults, Elderly. Up to 400 mg q6h.

Children 12–18 yr. 6–15 mg/kg/day in divided doses q6h.
Children 4–12 yr. 10–15 mg/kg/day in divided doses q6h.
Children 1–4 yr. 10–20 mg/kg/day in divided doses q6h.
Children younger than 1 yr. 10–30 mg/kg/day in divided doses q6h.
Dosage in renal impairment
With or without loading dose of 150 mg:

Creatinine Clearance	Dosage
40 ml/min and higher	100 mg q6h (extended-release 200 mg q12h)
30–39 ml/min	100 mg q8h
15–29 ml/min	100 mg q12h
less than 15 ml/min	100 mg q24h

Dosage in liver impairment
Adults, Elderly weighing 50 kg and more. 100 mg q6h (200 mg q12h with extended-release).
Dosage in cardiomyopathy, cardiac decompensation
Adults, Elderly weighing 50 kg and more. No loading dose; 100 mg q6–8h with gradual dosage adjustments.

S AVAILABLE FORMS/COST
• Cap-Oral: 100 mg, 100's: **$13.50-$97.23**; 150 mg, 100's: **$27.48-$114.81**
• Cap-Sus Action-Oral: 100 mg, 100's: **$57.56-$117.08**; 150 mg, 100's: **$114.75-$138.39**
UNLABELED USES: Prophylaxis and treatment of supraventricular tachycardia
CONTRAINDICATIONS: Cardiogenic shock, narrow-angle glaucoma (unless patient is undergoing cholinergic therapy), preexisting second- or third-degree atrioventricular (AV) block, preexisting urinary retention

PREGNANCY AND LACTATION:
Pregnancy category C; excreted in breast milk

SIDE EFFECTS

Frequent (greater than 9%)

Dry mouth (32%), urinary hesitancy, constipation

Occasional (9%–3%)

Blurred vision, dry eyes, nose, or throat, urinary retention, headache, dizziness, fatigue, nausea

Rare (less than 1%)

Impotence, hypotension, edema, weight gain, shortness of breath, syncope, chest pain, nervousness, diarrhea, vomiting, decreased appetite, rash, itching

SERIOUS REACTIONS

• May produce or aggravate congestive heart failure (CHF).

• May produce severe hypotension, shortness of breath, chest pain, syncope (especially in patients with primary cardiomyopathy or CHF).

• Hepatotoxicity occurs rarely.

INTERACTIONS

Drugs

☑ *Barbiturates, phenytoin, rifampin:* Reduced disopyramide level via induction

☑ *β-blockers:* Enhanced negative inotropy

☑ *Clarithromycin, erythromycin, troleandromycin:* Macrolide increased disopyramide-serum concentration resulting in dysrhythmias

☑ *Lidocaine:* Arrhythmias or heart failure in predisposed patients

☑ *Potassium, potassium-sparing diuretics:* Increased potassium concentration can enhance disopyramide effects on myocardial conduction

Labs

• *Increase:* Liver enzymes, lipids, BUN, creatinine

• *Decrease:* Hgb/hct, blood glucose

• Due to potential for prodysrhythmic effects, use for asymptomatic PVCs or lesser dysrhythmias should be avoided

MONITORING PARAMETERS

• Monitor ECG closely; if PR, QRS, or QT interval increase by 25%, stop drug

• Therapeutic plasma levels are 2-4 mcg/ml

---

dobutamine
(doe-byoo'ta-meen)
Rx: Dobutrex
Chemical Class: Catecholamine, synthetic
Therapeutic Class: Sympathomimetic; ß-adrenergic agonist

CLINICAL PHARMACOLOGY

Mechanism of Action: A direct-acting inotropic agent acting primarily on beta₁-adrenergic receptors. *Therapeutic Effect:* Decreases preload and afterload, and enhances myocardial contractility, stroke volume, and cardiac output. Improves renal blood flow and urine output.

Pharmacokinetics

Route	Onset	Peak	Duration
IV	1–2 min	10 min	Length of infusion

Metabolized in the liver. Primarily excreted in urine. Not removed by hemodialysis. **Half-life:** 2 min.

INDICATIONS AND DOSAGES

Short-term management of cardiac decompensation

IV infusion

Adults, Elderly, Children. 2.5–15 mcg/kg/min. Rarely, drug can be infused at a rate of up to 40 mcg/kg/min to increase cardiac output.

Neonates. 2–15 mcg/kg/min.

$ AVAILABLE FORMS/COST

• Sol, Inj-IV: 12.5 mg/ml, 20 ml: **$3.13-$16.92**

CONTRAINDICATIONS: Hypovolemia patients, idiopathic hypertrophic subaortic stenosis, sulfite sensitivity

PREGNANCY AND LACTATION: Pregnancy category C; excreted in breast milk

SIDE EFFECTS

Frequent (greater than 5%)

Increased heart rate, increased BP

Occasional (5%–3%)

Pain at injection site

Rare (3%–1%)

Nausea, headache, anginal pain, shortness of breath, fever

SERIOUS REACTIONS

• Overdose may produce a marked increase in heart rate (by 30 beats/minute or higher) marked increase in BP (by 50 mm Hg or higher), anginal pain, and premature ventricular contractions (PVCs).

INTERACTIONS

Drugs

◼ *Sodium bicarbonate:* Alkalinizing substances inactivate dobutamine

SPECIAL CONSIDERATIONS

MONITORING PARAMETERS

• Continuously monitor ECG, BP, and PCWP

---

docusate

(dok'yoo-sate)

OTC: *Sodium;* Colace, Dioeze, Diocto, DOK, DOSS DSS, Modane Soft, Regulax SS

OTC: *Calcium;* Sulfolax, Surfak Stool Softener Combinations

 OTC: with senna concentrate (Senokot-S); with phenolphthalein (Doxidan); with casanthranol (Peri-Colace); with cascara sagrada (Nature's Remedy)

Chemical Class: Anionic surfactant

Therapeutic Class: Laxative, stool softener

CLINICAL PHARMACOLOGY

Mechanism of Action: A bulk-producing laxative that decreases surface film tension by mixing liquid and bowel contents. *Therapeutic Effect:* Increases infiltration of liquid to form a softer stool.

Pharmacokinetics

Minimal absorption from the GI tract. Acts in small and large intestines. Results usually occur 1–2 days after first dose, but may take 3–5 days.

INDICATIONS AND DOSAGES

Stool softener

PO

Adults, Elderly, Children 12 yr and older. 50–500 mg/day in 1–4 divided doses.

Children 6–11 yr. 40–150 mg/day in 1–4 divided doses.

Children 3–5 yr. 20–60 mg/day in 1–4 divided doses.

Children younger than 3 yr. 10–40 mg in 1–4 divided doses.

$ AVAILABLE FORMS/COST
• Cap, Softgel-Oral (sodium): 50 mg, 100's: **$8.85**; 100 mg, 100's: **$1.40-$31.10**; 250 mg, 100's: **$1.83-$8.75**
• Cap, Softgel-Oral (calcium): 240 mg, 100's: **$4.00-$17.63**
• Enema-Rectal (sodium): 283 mg, 30's: **$71.94**
• Liq-Oral (sodium): 150 mg/15 ml, 480 ml: **$5.00-$90.77**
• Syr-Oral (sodium): 60 mg/15 ml, 480 ml: **$2.00-$21.66**

CONTRAINDICATIONS: Acute abdominal pain, concomitant use of mineral oil, intestinal obstruction, nausea, vomiting

PREGNANCY AND LACTATION: Pregnancy category C; no reports linking use of docusate with congenital defects have been located; diarrhea has been reported in 1 infant exposed to docusate while breast-feeding, but relationship between symptom and drug is unknown

SIDE EFFECTS
Occasional
Mild GI cramping, throat irritation (with liquid preparation)
Rare
Rash

SERIOUS REACTIONS
• None known.

SPECIAL CONSIDERATIONS
PATIENT/FAMILY EDUCATION
• Drink plenty of water during administration

dofetilide
(doe-fet′ill-ide)
Rx: Tikosyn
Chemical Class: Methanesulfonanilide derivative
Therapeutic Class: Antiarrhythmic, class III

CLINICAL PHARMACOLOGY
Mechanism of Action: A selective potassium channel blocker that prolongs repolarization without affecting conduction velocity by blocking one or more time-dependent potassium currents. Dofetilide has no effect on sodium channels or adrenergic alpha or beta receptors. *Therapeutic Effect:* Terminates reentrant tachyarrhythmias, preventing reinduction.

INDICATIONS AND DOSAGES
Maintain normal sinus rhythm after conversion from atrial fibrillation or flutter
PO
Adults, Elderly. Individualized using a seven-step dosing algorithm dependent upon calculated creatinine clearance and QT interval measurements.

$ AVAILABLE FORMS/COST
• Cap—Oral: 125 mcg, 250 mcg, 500 mcg, 60's; all: **$121.55**

CONTRAINDICATIONS: Concurrent use of drugs that prolong the QT interva; concurrent use of amiodarone, megestrol, prochlorperazine, or verapamil; congenital or acquired prolonged QT syndrome; paroxysmal atrial fibrillation; severe renal impairment

PREGNANCY AND LACTATION: Pregnancy category C; no information on the presence of dofetilide in breast milk; breast-feeding while on dofetilide not advised

SIDE EFFECTS
Occasional (less than 5%)
Headache, chest pain, dizziness, dyspnea, nausea, insomnia, back and abdominal pain, diarrhea, rash
SERIOUS REACTIONS
• Angioedema, bradycardia, cerebral ischemia, facial paralysis, and serious ventricular arrhythmias or various forms of heart block may be noted.
INTERACTIONS
Drugs
3 *Amiloride:* May compete with dofetilide for renal cationic secretion and subsequently increase dofetilide levels
2 *Cimetidine:* Increases dofetilide levels by 13%-58%, dose dependent
2 *Ketoconazole and other azole antifungals:* Increases dofetilide levels by 53%-97% by inhibition of CYP3A4
3 *Metformin:* May compete with dofetilide for renal cationic secretion and subsequently increase dofetilide levels
2 *Sulfamethoxazole:* Increases dofetilide AUC by 93% and Cmax by 103%
3 *Triamterene:* May compete with dofetilide for renal cationic secretion and subsequently increase dofetilide levels
2 *Trimethoprim:* Increases dofetilide AUC by 93% and Cmax by 103%
2 *Verapamil:* Increases dofetilide levels by 42% and increased risk of torsade de pointes
3 *Other potential drug interactions:* Macrolide antibiotics, protease inhibitors, serotonin reuptake inhibitors, amiodarone, cannabinoids, diltiazem, grapefruit juice, nefazadone, norfloxacin, quinine, zafirlukast: potential to increase dofetilide concentrations via inhibition of CYP3A4

MONITORING PARAMETERS
• ECG, QTc intervals, renal function

---

dolasetron
(doe-lass'eh-tron)
Rx: Anzemat
Chemical Class: Nonbenzamide
Therapeutic Class: Antiemetic

CLINICAL PHARMACOLOGY
Mechanism of Action: A 5-HT$_3$ receptor antagonist that acts centrally in the chemoreceptor trigger zone and peripherally at the vagal nerve terminals. *Therapeutic Effect:* Prevents nausea and vomiting.
Pharmacokinetics
Readily absorbed from the GI tract after PO administration. Protein binding: 69%-77%. Metabolized in the liver. Primarily excreted in urine. Unknown if removed by hemodialysis. **Half-life:** 5-10 hr.
INDICATIONS AND DOSAGES
Prevention of chemotherapy-induced nausea and vomiting
PO
Adults. 100 mg within 1 hr of chemotherapy.
Children 2-16 yr. 1.8 mg/kg within 1 hr of chemotherapy. Maximum: 100 mg.
IV
Adults, Children 1-16 yr. 1.8 mg/kg as a single dose 30 min before chemotherapy. Maximum: 100 mg.
Treatment or prevention of postoperative nausea or vomiting
PO
Adults. 100 mg within 2 hr of surgery.
Children 2-16 yr. . 1.2 mg/kg within 2 hr of surgery. Maximum: 100 mg.

IV

Adults. 12.5 mg 15 min before cessation of anesthesia or as soon as nausea occurs.

Children 2-16 yr. 0.35 mg/kg 15 min before cessation of anesthesia or as soon as nausea occurs. Maximum: 12.5 mg.

$\boxed{S}$ **AVAILABLE FORMS/COST**

• Inj—IV: 100 mg/vial: **$173.16**

• Tab—Oral: 50 mg, 5's: **$249.00-$287.60**; 100 mg, 5's: **$366.54-$381.20**

UNLABELED USES: Radiation therapy induced nausea and vomiting

CONTRAINDICATIONS: None known.

PREGNANCY AND LACTATION: Pregnancy category B; excretion in breast milk unknown, use caution in nursing mothers

SIDE EFFECTS

Frequent (10%-5%)

Headache, diarrhea, fatigue

Occasional (5%-1%)

Fever, dizziness, tachycardia, dyspepsia

SERIOUS REACTIONS

• Overdose may produce a combination of CNS stimulant and depressant effects.

SPECIAL CONSIDERATIONS

• No obvious advantage over other agents in this class (ondansetron, granisetron)

donepezil
(dah-nep'eh-zil)

Rx: Aricept, Aricept ODT
Chemical Class: Cholinesterase inhibitor; piperidine derivative
Therapeutic Class: Antidementia agent; cholinergic

CLINICAL PHARMACOLOGY

Mechanism of Action: A cholinesterase inhibitor that inhibits the enzyme acetylcholinesterase, thus increasing the concentration of acetylcholine at cholinergic synapses and enhancing cholinergic function in the CNS. *Therapeutic Effect:* Slows the progression of Alzheimer's disease.

Pharmacokinetics

Well absorbed after PO administration. Protein binding: 96%. Extensively metabolized. Eliminated in urine and feces. **Half-life:** 70 hr.

INDICATIONS AND DOSAGES

Alzheimer's disease

PO

Adults, Elderly. 5-10 mg/day as a single dose. If initial dose is 5 mg, do not increase to 10 mg for 4-6 wk.

$\boxed{S}$ **AVAILABLE FORMS/COST**

• Tab—Film-coated: 5 mg, 10 mg, 30's; all: **$148.89**

UNLABELED USES: Treatment of autism

CONTRAINDICATIONS: History of hypersensitivity to donepezil or piperidine derivatives

PREGNANCY AND LACTATION: Pregnancy category C

SIDE EFFECTS

Frequent (11%-8%)

Nausea, diarrhea, headache, insomnia, nonspecific pain, dizziness

Occasional (6%-3%)

Mild muscle cramps, fatigue, vomiting, anorexia, ecchymosis

Rare (3%-2%)

Depression, abnormal dreams, weight loss, arthritis, somnolence, syncope, frequent urination

SERIOUS REACTIONS
• Overdose may result in cholinergic crisis, characterized by severe nausea, increased salivation, diaphoresis, bradycardia, hypotension, flushed skin, abdominal pain, respiratory depression, seizures, and cardiorespiratory collapse. Increasing muscle weakness may result in death if respiratory muscles are involved. The antidote is 1-2 mg IV atropine sulfate with subsequent doses based on therapeutic response.

INTERACTIONS
Drugs
■ *Fluvoxamine:* Possible increase in fluvoxamine levels

SPECIAL CONSIDERATIONS
• Clinicians were unable to notice improvement in the majority of patients in clinical trials; advantages over tacrine include qday dosing and apparent lack of liver toxicity

MONITORING PARAMETERS
• Close monitoring for clinical improvement and periodic reassessment of need for continued therapy

---

dopamine
(doe′pa-meen)
Rx: Intropin
Chemical Class: Catecholamine, synthetic
Therapeutic Class: Vasopressor; α- and ß-adrenergic sympathomimetic

---

CLINICAL PHARMACOLOGY
Mechanism of Action: A sympathomimetic (adrenergic agonist) that stimulates adrenergic receptors. Effects are dose dependent. Low dosages (1–5 mcg/kg/min) stimulate dopaminergic receptors, causing renal vasodilation. Low to moderate Dosages (5–15 mcg/kg/min) have a positive inotropic effect by direct action and release of norepinephrine. High dosages (greater than 15 mcg/kg/min) stimulate alpha-receptors. *Therapeutic Effect:* With low dosages, increases renal blood flow, urine flow, and sodium excretion. With low to moderate dosages, increases myocardial contractility, stroke volume, and cardiac output. With high dosages, increases peripheral resistance, renal vasoconstriction, and systolic and diastolic BP.

Pharmacokinetics

Route	Onset	Peak	Dura-tion
IV	1–2 min	N/A	less than 10 min

Widely distributed. Does not cross blood-brain barrier. Metabolized in the liver, kidney, and plasma. Primarily excreted in urine. Not removed by hemodialysis. **Half-life:** 2 min.

INDICATIONS AND DOSAGES
Treatment and prevention of acute hypotension; shock (associated with cardiac decompensation, MI, open heart surgery, renal failure, or trauma), treatment of low cardiac output, treatment of CHF
IV
Adults, Elderly. 1 mcg/kg/min up to 50 mcg/kg/min titrated to desired response.
Children. 1–20 mcg/kg/min. Maximum: 50 mcg/kg/min.
Neonates. 1–20 mcg/kg/min.

S **AVAILABLE FORMS/COST**
• Inj, Conc-Sol—IV: 40 mg/ml, 5 ml: **$3.49-$6.48**; 80 mg/ml, 5 ml: **$4.09-$8.31**; 160 mg/ml, 5 ml: **$8.14-$11.00**

CONTRAINDICATIONS: Pheochromocytoma, sulfite sensitivity, uncorrected tachyarrhythmias, ventricular fibrillation

PREGNANCY AND LACTATION: Pregnancy category C; because dopamine is indicated only in life-threatening situations, chronic use would not be expected; no data available regarding use in breast-feeding

SIDE EFFECTS

Frequent

Headache, ectopic beats, tachycardia, anginal pain, palpitations, vasoconstriction, hypotension, nausea, vomiting, dyspnea

Occasional

Piloerection or goose bumps, bradycardia, widening of QRS complex.

SERIOUS REACTIONS

• High doses may produce ventricular arrhythmias.

• Patients with occlusive vascular disease are at high-risk for further compromise of circulation to the extremities, which may result in gangrene.

• Tissue necrosis with sloughing may occur with extravasation of IV solution.

INTERACTIONS

Drugs

🔟 *Ergot alkaloids:* Gangrene has been reported

🔟 *Phenytoin:* Increased risk of hypotension with IV phenytoin administration

Labs

• *False increase:* Urine amino acids; urine catecholamines; serum creatinine

• *False decrease:* Serum creatinine

SPECIAL CONSIDERATIONS

• *Dilute before use if not prediluted; antidote for extravasation: infiltrate area as soon as possible with 10-15 ml NS containing 5-10 mg phentolamine*

MONITORING PARAMETERS

• Urine flow, cardiac output, blood pressure, pulmonary wedge pressure

dornase alfa

(door'nace al'fa)

Rx: Pulmozyme
Chemical Class: Recombinant human deoxyribonuclease I
Therapeutic Class: Mucolytic

CLINICAL PHARMACOLOGY

Mechanism of Action: An enzyme that selectively splits and hydrolyzes DNA in sputum. *Therapeutic Effect:* Reduces sputum viscosity and elasticity.

INDICATIONS AND DOSAGES

To improve management of pulmonary function in patients with cystic fibrosis

Nebulization

Adults, Children older than 5 yr. 2.5 mg (1 ampule) once daily by recommended nebulizer. May increase to 2.5 mg twice daily.

§ AVAILABLE FORMS/COST

• Sol—INH: 1 mg/ml, 2.5 ml: **$43.87**

CONTRAINDICATIONS: Sensitivity to dornase alfa or epoetin alfa

PREGNANCY AND LACTATION: Pregnancy category B; excretion into breast milk unknown; however, since serum levels of DNase have not been shown to increase above endogenous levels, little drug would be expected to be excreted into breast milk

SIDE EFFECTS

Frequent (greater than 10%)

Pharyngitis, chest pain or discomfort, voice changes

Occasional (10%–3%)

Conjunctivitis, hoarseness, rash

D

SERIOUS REACTIONS
• None significant.
SPECIAL CONSIDERATIONS
• Safety and efficacy have been demonstrated only with the following nebulizers and compressors: disposable jet nebulizer *Hudson T Updraft II,* disposable jet nebulizer *Marquest Acorn II* in conjunction with a *Pulmo-Aide* compressor, and reusable *PARI LC Jet+* nebulizer in conjunction with the *PARI PRONEB* compressor
PATIENT/FAMILY EDUCATION
• Must be stored in refrigerator at 2-8°C and protected from strong light (keep refrigerated when transporting and do not leave at room temp for >24 hr)
• Do not dilute or mix with other drugs in nebulizer

---

doxapram
(dox'a-pram)
Rx: Dopram
Chemical Class: Pyrrolidinone derivative
Therapeutic Class: Analeptic

CLINICAL PHARMACOLOGY
Mechanism of Action: A central nervous system stimulant that directly stimulates the respiratory center in the medulla or indirectly by effects on the carotid. *Therapeutic Effect:* Increases pulmonary ventilation by increasing resting minute ventilation, tidal volume, respiratory frequency, and inspiratory neuromuscular drive, and enhances the ventilatory response to carbon dioxide.
Pharmacokinetics
IV onset 20-40 sec, peak 1-2 min, duration 5-12 min. Metabolized in the liver to metabolites, ketodoxapram (active) and desethyldox-

apram (inactive). Partially excreted in the urine. Not removed by hemodialysis. **Half-life:** 2.4-9.9 hrs.
INDICATIONS AND DOSAGES
Chronic obstructive pulmonary disease (COPD)
IV infusion
Adults, Elderly, Children older than 12 yrs. Initially, 1-2 mg/min. Maximum: 3 g/day for no more than 2 hours.
Drug-induced CNS depression
IV injection
Adults, Elderly, Children older than 12 yrs. Initially, 1-2 mg/kg, repeat after 5 min. May repeat at 1-2 hour intervals, until sustained consciousness. Maximum: 3 g/day.
IV infusion
Adults, Elderly, Children older than 12 yrs. Initially, bolus dose of 2 mg/kg, repeat after 5 min. If no response, wait 1-2 hours and repeat. If stimulation is noted, initiate infusion at 1-3 mg/min. Infusion should not be continued for more than 2 hours. Maximum: 3 g/day.
Respiratory depression
IV injection
Adults, Elderly, Children older than 12 yrs. Initially, 0.5-1 mg/kg. May repeat at 5 minute intervals in patients who demonstrate initial response. Maximum: 2 mg/kg.
IV infusion
Adults, Elderly, Children older than 12 yrs. Initially, 5 mg/min until adequate response or adverse effects are seen. Decrease to 1-3 mg/min. Maximum: 4 mg/kg.
§ AVAILABLE FORMS/COST
• Sol, Inj-IV: 20 mg/ml, 20 ml: **$97.38**

UNLABELED USES: Apnea of prematurity, sleep apnea, congenital central hypoventilation syndrome, obesity-hypoventilation syndrome, post-anesthetic respiratory depression, shivering

CONTRAINDICATIONS: Convulsive disorders, cardiovascular impairment, head injury or cerebral vascular accident, severe hypertension, mechanical ventilation disorders, newborns, hypersensitivity to doxapram.

PREGNANCY AND LACTATION: Pregnancy category B; excretion into breast milk unknown

SIDE EFFECTS

Occasional

Flushing, sweating, pruritus, disorientation, headache, dizziness, hyperactivity, convulsions, dyspnea, cough, tachypnea, hiccough, rebound hypoventilation, phlebitis, variations in heart rate, arrhythmias, chest pain, nausea, vomiting, diarrhea, stimulation of urinary bladder with spontaneous voiding.

SERIOUS REACTIONS

• Overdosage may produce extensions of the pharmacologic effects of the drug. Excessive pressor effect, skeletal muscle hyperactivity, tachycardia, and enhanced deep tendon reflexes may be early signs of overdosage.

INTERACTIONS

Drugs

3 *Anesthetics, inhalation:* Sensitized myocardium at risk of arrhythmia; delay administration of doxapram 10 min

2 *MAO Inhibitors:* Additive pressor effect

SPECIAL CONSIDERATIONS

MONITORING PARAMETERS

• Baseline ABG then q30 min (for use in COPD)

---

doxazosin

(dox-ay′zoe-sin)

Rx: Cardura
Chemical Class: Quinazoline derivative
Therapeutic Class: Antihypertensive; α_1-adrenergic blocker

CLINICAL PHARMACOLOGY

Mechanism of Action: An antihypertensive that selectively blocks alpha$_1$-adrenergic receptors, decreasing peripheral vascular resistance. *Therapeutic Effect:* Causes peripheral vasodilation and lowers of BP. Also relaxes smooth muscle of bladder and prostate.

Pharmacokinetics

Route	Onset	Peak	Duration
PO	N/A	2–6 hr	24 hr

Well absorbed from the GI tract. Protein binding: 98%–99%. Metabolized in the liver. Primarily eliminated in feces. Not removed by hemodialysis. **Half-life:** 19–22 hr.

INDICATIONS AND DOSAGES

Mild to moderate hypertension

PO

Adults. Initially, 1 mg once a day. May increase to a maximum of 16 mg/day.

Elderly. Initially, 0.5 mg once a day.

Benign prostatic hyperplasia, alone or in combination with finasteride (Proscar)

PO

Adults, Elderly. Initially, 1 mg/day. May increase q1–2 wk. Maximum: 8 mg/day.

$ **AVAILABLE FORMS/COST**

• Tab-Oral: 1 mg, 100's: **$92.33-$118.95**; 2 mg, 100's: **$92.33-$123.20**; 4 mg, 100's: **$96.92-$124.85**; 8 mg, 100's: **$101.78-$131.10**

CONTRAINDICATIONS: None known.

PREGNANCY AND LACTATION: Pregnancy category C; may accumulate in breast milk; use caution in nursing mothers

SIDE EFFECTS

Frequent (20%–10%)

Dizziness, asthenia, headache, edema

Occasional (9%–3%)

Nausea, pharyngitis, rhinitis, pain in extremities, somnolence

Rare (3%–1%)

Palpitations, diarrhea, constipation, dyspnea, myalgia, altered vision, dizziness, nervousness

SERIOUS REACTIONS

• First-dose syncope (hypotension with sudden loss of consciousness) may occur 30 to 90 minutes following initial dose of 2 mg or greater, a too rapid increase in dosage, or addition of another antihypertensive agent to therapy. First-dose syncope may be preceded by tachycardia (pulse rate of 120–160 beats/minute).

INTERACTIONS

Drugs

③ *ACE inhibitors:* Increased potential for first dose hypotension

③ *Indomethacin:* Decreased hypotensive effect of doxazosin

③ *Verapamil, nifedipine:* Enhanced hypotensive effects of both drugs

③ *β-adrenergic blockers:* Exaggerated first-dose response

Labs

• False positive urinary metabolites of norepinephrine and VMA

• No effect on prostate specific antigen (PSA)

SPECIAL CONSIDERATIONS

• The doxazosin arm of the ALL-HAT study was stopped early; the doxazosin group had a 25% greater risk of combined cardiovascular disease events which was primarily accounted for by a doubled risk of CHF vs the chlorthalidone group; doxazosin was also found to be less effective at controlling systolic BP an average of 3 mm Hg; may want to consider primary antihypertensives in addition to α-blockers for BPH symptoms

• Use as a single antihypertensive agent limited by tendency to cause sodium and water retention and increased plasma volume

PATIENT/FAMILY EDUCATION

• Alert patient to the possibility of syncopal and orthostatic symptoms, especially with first dose ("first-dose syncope")

• Initial dose should be administered at bedtime in the smallest possible dose

---

doxepin

(dox'eh-pin)

Rx: *Systemic:* Adapin, Sinequan

Rx: *Topical:* Zonalon

Chemical Class: Dibenzoxepin derivative; tertiary amine

Therapeutic Class: Antidepressant, tricyclic; antipruritic, topical

CLINICAL PHARMACOLOGY

Mechanism of Action: A tricyclic antidepressant, antianxiety agent, antineuralgic agent, antipruritic, and antiulcer agent that increases synaptic concentrations of norepinephrine and serotonin. *Therapeutic Effect:* Produces antidepressant and anxiolytic effects.

Pharmacokinetics

Rapidly and well absorbed from the GI tract. Protein binding: 80%-85%. Metabolized in the liver to active metabolite. Primarily excreted in urine. Not removed by hemodialysis. **Half-life:** 6-8 hr. Topical: Absorbed through the skin. Distributed to body tissues. Metabolized to active metabolite. Excreted in urine.

INDICATIONS AND DOSAGES
Depression, anxiety
PO

Adults. 30-150 mg/day at bedtime or in 2-3 divided doses. May increase to 300 mg/day.

Elderly. Initially, 10-25 mg at bedtime. May increase by 10-25 mg/day every 3-7 days. Maximum: 75 mg/day.

Adolescents. Initially, 25-50 mg/day as a single dose or in divided doses. May increase to 100 mg/day.

Children 12 yr and younger. 1-3 mg/kg/day.

Pruritus associated with eczema
Topical

Adults, Elderly. Apply thin film 4 times a day.

Ⓢ AVAILABLE FORMS/COST
• Cre-Top: 5%, 30, 45 g: **$49.34**/30 g
• Cap, Gel-Oral: 10 mg, 100's: **$6.65-$125.62**; 25 mg, 100's: **$7.88-$57.39**; 50 mg, 100's: **$18.90-$80.75**; 75 mg, 100's: **$14.86-$133.96**; 100 mg, 100's: **$13.94-$146.05**; 150 mg, 100's: **$34.93-$59.85**
• Conc-Oral: 10 mg/ml, 120 ml: **$16.81-$33.43**

UNLABELED USES: Treatment of neurogenic pain, panic disorder; prevention of vascular headache, pruritus in idiopathic urticaria

CONTRAINDICATIONS: Angle-closure glaucoma, hypersensitivity to other tricyclic antidepressants, urine retention

PREGNANCY AND LACTATION: Pregnancy category C (top formulation is category B); paralytic ileus has been observed in an infant exposed to doxepin and chlorpromazine at term; excreted into breast milk (as well as active metabolite); effect on nursing infant unknown, but may be of concern

SIDE EFFECTS
Frequent
Oral: Orthostatic hypotension, somnolence, dry mouth, headache, increased appetite, weight gain, nausea, unusual fatigue, unpleasant taste

Topical: Edema, increased itching, eczema, burning, or stinging at application site; altered taste, dizziness, somnolence, dry skin, dry mouth, fatigue, headache, thirst

Occasional
Oral: Blurred vision, confusion, constipation, hallucinations, difficult urination, eye pain, irregular heartbeat, fine muscle tremors, nervousness, impaired sexual function, diarrhea, diaphoresis, heartburn, insomnia

Topical: Anxiety, skin irritation or cracking, nausea

Rare
Oral: Allergic reaction, alopecia, tinnitus, breast enlargement

Topical: Fever, photosensitivity

SERIOUS REACTIONS
• Overdose may produce confusion; seizures; severe somnolence; fast, slow, or irregular heartbeat; fever; hallucinations; agitation; dyspnea; vomiting; and unusual fatigue or weakness.

• Abrupt withdrawal after prolonged therapy may produce headache, malaise, nausea, vomiting, and vivid dreams.

INTERACTIONS
Drugs
③ *Barbiturates:* Reduced serum concentrations of cyclic antidepressants

② *Bethanidine:* Reduced antihypertensive effect of bethanidine

3 *Carbamazepine:* Reduced cyclic antidepressant serum concentrations

2 *Clonidine:* Reduced antihypertensive response to clonidine; enhanced hypertensive response with abrupt clonidine withdrawal

3 *Debrisoquin:* Inhibited antihypertensive response of debrisoquin

2 *Epinephrine:* Markedly enhanced pressor response to IV epinephrine

3 *Ethanol:* Additive impairment of motor skills; abstinent alcoholics may eliminate cyclic antidepressants more rapidly than non-alcoholics

3 *Fluoxetine, fluvoxamine, grapefruit juice:* Marked increases in cyclic antidepressant plasma concentrations

3 *Guanethidine:* Inhibited antihypertensive response to guanethidine

2 *Moclobemide:* Potential association with fatal or non-fatal serotonin syndrome

⚠ *MAOIs:* Excessive sympathetic response, mania, or hyperpyrexia possible

3 *Neuroleptics:* Increased therapeutic and toxic effects of both drugs

2 *Norepinephrine:* Markedly enhanced pressor response to norepinephrine

2 *Phenylephrine:* Enhanced pressor response to IV phenylephrine

3 *Propoxyphene:* Enhanced effect of cyclic antidepressants

3 *Quinidine:* Increased cyclic antidepressant serum concentrations

SPECIAL CONSIDERATIONS
• Equally effective as other tricyclic antidepressants for depression; distinguishing characteristics include: sedative, anxiolytic, antihistaminic properties

PATIENT/FAMILY EDUCATION
• Therapeutic effects may take 4-6 wk

• Do not discontinue abruptly after long-term use
• If drowsiness occurs with top application, decrease surface area being treated or number of daily applications

MONITORING PARAMETERS
• CBC; ECG; mental status: mood, sensorium, affect, suicidal tendencies

---

doxercalciferol
(dox-er-cal-sif′-er-ol)
Chemical Class: Vitamin D analog
Therapeutic Class: Hyperparathyroidism

CLINICAL PHARMACOLOGY
Mechanism of Action: A fat-soluble vitamin that is essential for absorption, utilization of calcium phosphate, and normal calcification of bone. *Therapeutic Effect:* Stimulates calcium and phosphate absorption from small intestine, promotes secretion of calcium from bone to blood, promotes renal tubule phosphate resorption, acts on bone cells to stimulate skeletal growth and on parathyroid gland to suppress hormone synthesis and secretion.
Pharmacokinetics
Readily absorbed from small intestine. Metabolized in liver. Partially eliminated in urine. Not removed by hemodialysis. **Half-life:** up to 96 hrs.

INDICATIONS AND DOSAGES
Secondary hyperparathyroidism, dialysis patients
IV
Adults, Elderly. Titrate dose to lower iPTH to 150-300 pg/ml. Adjust dose at 8-week intervals to a maximum dose of 18 mcg/week. Initially, if

iPTH level is more than 400 pg/ml, give 4 mcg 3 times/week after dialysis, administered as a bolus dose.

Dose titration:

iPTH level decreased by 50% and more than 300 pg/ml: Dose may be increased by 1-2 mcg at 8 week intervals as needed.

iPTH level 150-300 pg/ml: Maintain the current dose.

iPTH level <100 pg/ml: Suspend drug for 1 week and resume at a reduced dose of at least 1 mcg lower.

PO

Adults, Elderly. Dialysis patients: Titrate dose to lower iPTH to 150-300 pg/ml. Adjust dose at 8-week intervals to a maximum dose of 20 mcg 3 times/week. Initially, if iPTH is more than 400 pg/ml, give 10 mcg 3 times/week at dialysis

Dose titration:

iPTH level decreased by 50% and more than 300 pg/ml: Increase dose to 12.5 mcg 3 times/week for 8 more weeks. This titration process may continue at 8 week intervals. Each increase should be by 2.5 mcg/dose.

iPTH level 150-300 pg/ml: Maintain current dose.

iPTH level less than 100 pg/ml: Suspend drug for 1 week and resume at a reduced dose. Decrease each dose by at least 2.5 mcg.

Secondary hyperparathyroidism, predialysis patients

PO

Adults, Elderly. Titrate dose to lower iPTH to 35-70 pg/ml with stage 3 disease or to 70-110 pg/ml with stage 4 disease. Dose may be adjusted at 2-week intervals with a maximum dose of 3.5 mcg/day. Begin with 1 mcg/day.

Dose titration:

iPTH level more than 70 pg/ml with stage 3 disease or more than 110 pg/ml with stage 4 disease: Increase dose by 0.5 mcg every 2 weeks as needed.

iPTH level 35-70 pg/ml with stage 3 disease or 70-110 pg/ml with stage 4 disease: Maintain current dose.

iPTH level is less than 35 pg/ml with stage 3 disease or less than 70 pg/ml with stage 4 disease: Suspend drug for 1 week, then resume at a reduced dose of at least 0.5 mcg lower.

Ⓢ AVAILABLE FORMS/COST

• Cap—Oral: 2.5 mcg, 50's: **$111.85**

• Inj, Sol—IV: 2 {micro} g/ml, 2 ml: **$19.29**

CONTRAINDICATIONS: Hypercalcemia, malabsorption syndrome, vitamin D toxicity, hypersensitivity to doxercalciferol or other vitamin D analogs

PREGNANCY AND LACTATION: Pregnancy category B; excretion into breast milk unknown; use caution in nursing mothers

SIDE EFFECTS

Occasional

Edema, headache, malaise, dizziness, nausea, vomiting, dyspnea

Rare

Bradycardia, sleep disorder, pruritus, anorexia, constipation

SERIOUS REACTIONS

• Early signs of overdosage are manifested as weakness, headache, somnolence, nausea, vomiting, dry mouth, constipation, muscle and bone pain, and metallic taste sensation.

• Later signs of overdosage are evidenced by polyuria, polydipsia, anorexia, weight loss, nocturia, photophobia, rhinorrhea, pruritus, disorientation, hallucinations, hyperthermia, hypertension, and cardiac arrhythmias.

INTERACTIONS
Drugs
3 *Cholestyramine:* Possible impaired intestinal absorption of fat-soluble vitamins

3 *Magnesium:* Possible hypermagnesemia, use not recommended

SPECIAL CONSIDERATIONS
• Do not take Ca supplements; vitamin D, or Mg containing antacids

MONITORING PARAMETERS
• iPTH, serum Ca and serum phosphate qwk during titration
• D/C drug if hypercalcemia, hyperphosphatemia, or serum Ca × serum phosphate product >70, resume when parameters decreased, at a dose ≤2.5 mcg
• Urinary Ca, alkaline phosphatase, renal function tests

---

doxycycline
(dox-i-sye′kleen)
Rx: Atridox, Doryx, Doxy, Doxy Caps, Doxychel Hyclate, Periostat, Vibramycin, Vibra-Tabs
Chemical Class: Tetracycline derivative
Therapeutic Class: Antibiotic

CLINICAL PHARMACOLOGY
Mechanism of Action: A tetracycline antibiotic that inhibits bacterial protein synthesis by binding to ribosomes. *Therapeutic Effect:* Bacteriostatic.

INDICATIONS AND DOSAGES
Respiratory, skin, and soft-tissue infections; UTIs; pelvic inflammatory disease(PID); brucellosis; trachoma; Rocky Mountain spotted fever; typhus; Q fever; rickettsia; severe acne (Adoxa); smallpox; psittacosis; ornithosis; granuloma inguinale; lymphogranuloma venereum; intestinal amebiasis (adjunctive treatment); prevention of rheumatic fever
PO
Adults, Elderly. Initially, 100 mg q12h, then 100 mg/day as single dose or 50 mg q12h for severe infections.
Children 8 yr and older and weighing more than 45 kg. 2-4 mg/kg/day divided q12-24h. Maximum: 200 mg/day.
IV
Adults, Elderly. Initially, 200 mg as 1-2 infusions; then 100-200 mg/day in 1-2 divided doses.
Children 8 yr and older. 2-4 mg/kg/day divided q12-24h. Maximum: 200 mg/day.
Acute gonococcal infections
PO
Adults. Initially, 200 mg, then 100 mg at bedtime on first day; then 100 mg twice a day for 14 days.
Syphilis
PO, IV
Adults. 200 mg/day in divided doses for 14-28 days.
Traveler's diarrhea
PO
Adults, Elderly. 100 mg/day during a period of risk (up to 14 days) and for 2 days after returning home.
Periodontitis
PO
Adults. 20 mg twice a day.
S AVAILABLE FORMS/COST
Doxycycline Calcium
• Syr—Oral: 50 mg/5ml, 480 ml: **$208.79**

Doxycycline Hyclate
• Cap-Oral: 50 mg, 100's: **$19.50-$145.10**; 100 mg, 100's: **$12.71-$91.11**
• Cap, Coated Pellets-Oral: 75 mg, 60's: **$185.50**; 100 mg, 50's: **$102.50-$181.86**
• Powder, Inj-IV: 100 mg/vial: **$14.75**
• Tab-Oral: 20 mg, 100's: **$88.72-$104.69**; 100 mg, 100's: **$88.60-$134.20**

Doxycycline Monohydrate
• Cap, Gel—Oral: 50 mg, 100's: **$118.74-$175.75**; 100 mg, 100's: **$213.23**
• Powder, Reconst—Oral: 25 mg/5 ml, 60 ml: **$14.15**
• Tab-Oral: 50 mg, 100's: **$216.71**; 75 mg, 100's: **$269.06**; 100 mg, 50's: **$176.91**

UNLABELED USES: Treatment of atypical mycobacterial infections, rheumatoid arthritis, gonorrhea and malaria; prevention of Lyme disease; prevention or treatment of traveler's diarrhea.

CONTRAINDICATIONS: Children 8 years and younger, hypersensitivity to tetracyclines or sulfites, last half of pregnancy, severe hepatic dysfunction

PREGNANCY AND LACTATION: Pregnancy category D; excreted into breast milk; theoretical possibility for dental staining seems remote because serum levels in infant undetectable

SIDE EFFECTS
Frequent
Anorexia, nausea, vomiting, diarrhea, dysphagia, possibly severe photosensitivity
Occasional
Rash, urticaria

SERIOUS REACTIONS
• Superinfection (especially fungal) and benign intracranial hypertension (headache, visual changes) may occur.
• Hepatoxicity, fatty degeneration of the liver, and pancreatitis occur rarely.

INTERACTIONS
Drugs
■ *Antacids:* Reduced serum concentration and efficacy of doxycycline
■ *Barbiturates:* Reduced serum doxycycline concentrations
■ *Bismuth:* Reduced bioavailability of doxycycline
■ *Calcium:* See antacids
■ *Carbamazepine:* Reduced serum doxycycline concentrations
■ *Cholestyramine; colestipol:* Reduced serum concentration of doxycycline; take 2 hr before or 3 hr after resin dose
■ *Ethanol:* Chronic ethanol ingestion may reduce the serum concentrations of doxycycline
■ *Iron:* Reduced serum concentration and efficacy of doxycycline
■ *Magnesium:* See antacids
■ *Oral contraceptives:* Potential for decreased efficacy of oral contraceptives
■ *Penicillins:* Doxycycline may reduce penicillin efficacy
■ *Phenytoin:* Reduced serum doxycycline concentrations
■ *Warfarin:* Potential for enhanced hypoprothrombinenic response to warfarin
■ *Zinc:* Reduced serum concentration of doxycycline; take 2 hr before or 3 hr after zinc

SPECIAL CONSIDERATIONS
• Tetracycline of choice due to broad spectrum, long $t_{1/2}$, superior tissue penetration, and excellent oral absorption

PATIENT/FAMILY EDUCATION
• Do not take with antacids, iron products
• Take with food

---

dronabinol
(droe-nab′i-nol)
Rx: Marinol
Chemical Class: Cannabinoid derivative
Therapeutic Class: Antiemetic; appetite stimulant
DEA Class: Schedule II

CLINICAL PHARMACOLOGY
Mechanism of Action: An antiemetic and appetite stimulant that may act by inhibiting vomiting control mechanisms in the medulla oblongata. *Therapeutic Effect:* Inhibits vomiting and stimulates appetite.

INDICATIONS AND DOSAGES
Prevention of chemotherapy-induced nausea and vomiting
PO
Adults, Children. Initially, 5 mg/m^2 1-3 hr before chemotherapy, then q2-4h after chemotherapy for total of 4-6 doses a day. May increase by 2.5 mg/m^2 up to 15 mg/m^2 per dose.
Appetite stimulant
PO
Adults. Initially, 2.5 mg twice a day (before lunch and dinner). Range: 2.5-20 mg/day.

$ AVAILABLE FORMS/COST
• Cap, Elastic—Oral: 2.5 mg, 60's: **$278.31**; 5 mg, 25's: **$241.34**; 10 mg, 60's: **$1,063.72**

CONTRAINDICATIONS: Treatment of nausea and vomiting not caused by chemotherapy

PREGNANCY AND LACTATION: Pregnancy category C; excreted in breast milk

SIDE EFFECTS
Frequent (24%-3%)
Euphoria, dizziness, paranoid reaction, somnolence
Occasional (3%-1%)
Asthenia, ataxia, confusion, abnormal thinking, depersonalization
Rare (less than 1%)
Diarrhea, depression, nightmares, speech difficulties, headache, anxiety, tinnitus, flushed skin

SERIOUS REACTIONS
• Mild intoxication may produce increased sensory awareness (including taste, smell, and sound), altered time perception, reddened conjunctiva, dry mouth, and tachycardia.
• Moderate intoxication may produce memory impairment and urine retention.
• Severe intoxication may produce lethargy, decreased motor coordination, slurred speech, and orthostatic hypotension.

SPECIAL CONSIDERATIONS
• May have additive sedative or behavioral effects with CNS depressants
• Use caution escalating the dose because of increased frequency of adverse reactions at higher doses

---

droperidol
(droe-pear-′ih-dall)
Rx: Inapsine
Combinations
   Rx: with fentanyl (Innovar)
Chemical Class: Butyrophenone derivative
Therapeutic Class: Anesthesia adjunct; antiemetic; sedative

CLINICAL PHARMACOLOGY
Mechanism of Action: A general anesthetic and antiemetic agent that antagonizes dopamine neurotransmission at synapses by blocking

postsynaptic dopamine receptor sites; partially blocks adrenergic receptor binding sites. *Therapeutic Effect:* Produces tranquilization, antiemetic effect.

Pharmacokinetics

Onset of action occurs within 30 minutes. Well absorbed. Metabolized in liver. Excreted in urine and feces. **Half-life:** 2.3 hrs.

INDICATIONS AND DOSAGES

Preoperative

IM/IV

Adults, Elderly, Children 12 yrs and older. 2.5-10 mg 30-60 min before induction of general anesthesia.
Children 2-12 yrs. 0.088-0.165 mg/kg.

Adjunct for induction of general anesthesia

IV

Adults, Elderly, Children 12 yrs and older. 0.22-0.275 mg/kg.
Children 2-12 yrs. 0.088-0.165 mg/kg.

Adjunct for maintenance of general anesthesia

IV

Adults, Elderly. 1.25-2.5 mg.

Diagnostic procedures w/o general anesthesia

IM

Adults, Elderly. 2.5-10 mg 30-60 min before procedure. If needed, may give additional doses of 1.25-2.5 mg (usually by IV injection).

🅢 AVAILABLE FORMS/COST

• Sol, Inj-IM, IV: 2.5 mg/ml, 2 ml: **$1.53-$5.73**

CONTRAINDICATIONS: Known or suspected QT prolongation, hypersensitivity to droperidol or any component of the formulation

PREGNANCY AND LACTATION: Pregnancy category C; has been used to promote analgesia for cesarean section patients without affecting respiration of the newborn; excretion into breast milk unknown, use caution in nursing mothers

NOTE: Has been used as a continuous IV infusion for hyperemesis gravidarum during the 2nd and 3rd trimesters without apparent fetal harm

SIDE EFFECTS

Frequent

Mild to moderate hypotension

Occasional

Tachycardia, postop drowsiness, dizziness, chills, shivering

Rare

Postop nightmares, facial sweating, bronchospasm

SERIOUS REACTIONS

• Extrapyramidal symptoms may appear as akathisia (motor restlessness) and dystonias: torticollis (neck muscle spasm), opisthotonos (rigidity of back muscles), and oculogyric crisis (rolling back of eyes).

• Overdosage includes symptoms of hypotension, tachycardia, hallucinations, and extrapyramidal symptoms.

• Prolonged QT interval, seizures, and arrhythmias have been reported.

INTERACTIONS

Drugs

⚠ *Arrhythmogenic agents:* Any drug known to prolong QT interval should not be used with droperidol; class I or III antiarrhythmics, antimalarials, calcium channel blockers (bepridil, isradipine, nicardipine), neuroleptics (haloperidol, pimozide, thioridazine), antidepressants (desimipramine, venlafaxine)
❷ *Diuretics, laxatives:* Hypokalemia or hypomagnesemia may precipitate QT prolongation
❸ *CNS depressants:* Additive or potentiating effects with droperidol; barbiturates, tranquilizers, opioids

MONITORING PARAMETERS
• QT prolongation has occurred in patients with no known CV disease and with doses at or below recommended doses reserve use for patients who fail to show response to other adequate treatments
• Baseline ECG, blood pressure, heart rate, respiratory rate; if QT >440 msec for males or >450 msec for females, do not use droperidol

drotrecogin alfa
(droh-tree-koh′gen)
Rx: Xigris
Chemical Class: Glycoprotein
Therapeutic Class: Antisepsis syndrome agent

CLINICAL PHARMACOLOGY
Mechanism of Action: A recombinant form of human-activated protein C that exerts an antithrombotic effect by inhibiting Factors Va and VIIIa and may exert an indirect profibrinolytic effect by inhibiting plasminogen activator inhibitor-1 and limiting the generation of activated thrombin-activatable-fibrinolysis-inhibitor. The drug may also exert an anti-inflammatory effect by inhibiting tumor necrosis factor production by monocytes, by blocking leukocyte adhesion to selectins, and by limiting thrombin-induced inflammatory responses. *Therapeutic Effect:* Produces anti-inflammatory, antithrombotic, and profibrinolytic effects.

Pharmacokinetics
Inactivated by endogenous plasma protease inhibitors. Clearance occurs within 2 hr of initiating infusion. **Half-life:** 1.6 hr.

INDICATIONS AND DOSAGES
Severe sepsis
IV infusion
Adults, Elderly. 24 mcg/kg/hr for 96 hr.

§ AVAILABLE FORMS/COST
• Powder, Inj-IV: 5 mg/vial: **$270.38**; 20 mg/vial: **$1,081.50**
CONTRAINDICATIONS: Active internal bleeding, evidence of cerebral herniation, intracranial neoplasm or mass lesion, presence of an epidural catheter, recent (within the past 3 mo) hemorrhagic stroke, recent (within the past 2 mo) intracranial or intraspinal surgery or severe head trauma, trauma with an increased risk of life-threatening bleeding
PREGNANCY AND LACTATION: Pregnancy category C; excretion into breast milk unknown
SIDE EFFECTS
None known.
SERIOUS REACTIONS
• Bleeding (intrathoracic, retroperitoneal, GI, GU, intraabdominal, intracranial) occurs in about 2% of patients.
INTERACTIONS
Labs
• *aPTT:* Drotrecogin alfa affects the aPTT assay, and one-stage coagulation assays based on the aPTT (such as factor VIII, IX, and XI assays); this interference may result in an apparent factor concentration that is less than the true concentration; drotrecogin alfa present in plasma samples does not interfere with one-stage factor assays based on the PT (such as factor II, V, VII, and X assays)
SPECIAL CONSIDERATIONS
• The efficacy of drotrecogin alfa was studied in an international, multi-center, randomized, double-blind, placebo-controlled trial (PROWESS) of 1690 patients with severe sepsis (Bernard GR, et al. Ef-

ficacy and Safety of Recombinant Human Activated Protein C for Severe Sepsis. N Engl J Med. 2001;344:699-709); entry criteria included a systemic inflammatory response presumed due to infection and at least one associated acute organ dysfunction; acute organ dysfunction was defined as one of the following: cardiovascular dysfunction (shock, hypotension, or the need for vasopressor support despite adequate fluid resuscitation); respiratory dysfunction [relative hypoxemia (PaO_2/FiO_2 ratio <250); renal dysfunction (oliguria despite adequate fluid resuscitation); thrombocytopenia (platelet count $<80,000/mm^3$ or 50% decrease from the highest value the previous 3 days); or metabolic acidosis with elevated lactic acid concentrations

• The primary efficacy endpoint was all-cause mortality assessed 28 days after the start of study drug administration; prospectively defined subsets for mortality analyses included groups defined by APACHE II score (a score designed to assess risk of mortality based on acute physiology and chronic health evaluation, see http://www.sfar.org/scores2/ scores2.html); the APACHE II score was calculated from physiologic and laboratory data obtained within the 24 hour period immediately preceding the start of study drug administration irrespective of the preceding length of stay in the Intensive Care Unit; the study was terminated after a planned interim analysis due to significantly decrease mortality in patients on drotrecogin alfa than in patients on placebo (210/850, 25% vs. 259/840, 31% p=0.005); the observed mortality difference between drotrecogin alfa and placebo was limited to the half of patients with higher risk of death, i.e., APACHE II

score >25, the third and fourth quartile APACHE II scores (mortality 31% with treatment, 44% with placebo); the efficacy of drotrecogin alfa has not been established in patients with lower risk of death, e.g., APACHE II score <25

MONITORING PARAMETERS
• CBC with platelets, INR

---

duloxetine
(dual-ox´-ih-teen)
Rx: Cymbalta
Chemical Class: Aryloxypropylamine
Therapeutic Class: Antidepressant (SSNRI or NE/5-HT reuptake inhibitor)

CLINICAL PHARMACOLOGY
Mechanism of Action: An antidepressant that appears to inhibit serotonin and norepinephrine reuptake at neuronal presynaptic membranes; is a less potent inhibitor of dopamine reuptake. *Therapeutic Effect:* Relieves depression.
Pharmacokinetics
Well absorbed from the GI tract. Protein binding: greater than 90%. Extensively metabolized to active metabolites. Excreted primarily in urine and, to a lesser extent, in feces. **Half-life:** 8-17 hr.

INDICATIONS AND DOSAGES
Major depressive disorder
PO
Adults. 20 mg twice a day, increased up to 60 mg/day as a single dose or in 2 divided doses.

CONTRAINDICATIONS: End-stage renal disease (creatinine clearance less than 30 ml/min), severe hepatic impairment, uncontrolled angle-closure glaucoma, use within 14 days of MAOIs

D

PREGNANCY AND LACTATION:

Pregnancy category C; neonates exposed to SSRIs or SNRIs late in the third trimester have developed serious complications, sometimes requiring prolonged hospitalization, respiratory support, and tube feeding: respiratory distress, cyanosis, apnea, seizures, temperature instability, feeding difficulty, vomiting, hypoglycemia, hypotonia, hypertonia, hyperreflexia, tremor jitteriness, irritability, and constant crying. This clinical picture is consistent with a toxic effect of SSRIs and SNRIs or, possibly, a drug discontinuation syndrome. Human breast milk excretion unknown; there is excretion into breast milk of lactating rats; breast-feeding not recommended at this time.

SIDE EFFECTS

Frequent (20%-11%)

Nausea, dry mouth, constipation, insomnia

Occasional (9%-5%)

Dizziness, fatigue, diarrhea, somnolence, anorexia, diaphoresis, vomiting

Rare (4%-2%)

Blurred vision, erectile dysfunction, delayed or failed ejaculation, anorgasmia, anxiety, decreased libido, hot flashes

SERIOUS REACTIONS

• Duloxetine use may slightly increase the patient's heart rate.

• Colitis, dysphagia, gastritis, and irritable bowel syndrome occur rarely.

INTERACTIONS

Drugs

Duloxetine: Substrate for CYP1A2, CYP2D6; moderate inhibitor of CYP2D6

▣ *Amitriptylline, desipramine, tricyclic antidepressants:* inhibits CYP-2D6-mediated tricyclic agent metabolism, increased bioavailability of tricyclics, increasing risk of adverse events (anticholinergic effects, sedation, confusion, cardiac arrhythmias)

▣ *Class I-C Antiarrhythmic Agents:* inhibits CYP2D6-mediated metabolism of class I-C antiarrhythmic agents (flecainide, propafenone, moricizine); increased risk of cardiotoxicity (QT prolongation, torsades de points, cardiac arrest)

▣ *Fluroquinolone antibiotics (ciprofloxacin, enoxacin):* inhibit CYP1A2-mediated duloxetine metabolism, increased risk of adverse effects

▣ *Fluoxetine:* moderately potent inhibitor of CYP2D6-mediated metabolism of duloxetine; increased serum levels, increased risk of adverse effects

▣ *Fluvoxamine:* inhibits CYYP1A2-mediated duloxetine metabolism, increased risk of adverse effects

▲ *Monamine oxidase inhibitors:* duloxetine inhibitor effects on both norepineperine and serotonin reuptake set up overlapping therapy with monoamine oxidase inhibitor to cause CNS toxicity or serotonin syndrome

▣ *Paroxetine:* moderately potent inhibitor of CYP2D6-mediated metabolism of duloxetine; increased serum levels, increased risk of adverse effects

▣ *Phenothiazines:* duloxetine inhibition of CYP2D6-mediated pheohtiazine metabolism leads to increased phenothiazine concentrations and potential toxicity

❷ *Quinidine:* quinidine inhibition of CYP2D6-mediated duloxetine metabolism; increased adverse effects

SPECIAL CONSIDERATIONS

• Place in therapy: Similar to venlafaxine, with far less experience and comparative data; alternative in major depression in poor responders to other agents; at least as effective as tricyclics, but with lower toxicity; more efficacious than SSRI's

PATIENT/FAMILY EDUCATION

• Therapeutic response may take 4-6 weeks; be alert for emergence of anxiety, agitation, panic, mania, or worsening of depressive state

MONITORING PARAMETERS

• Efficacy: resolution/improvement in symptoms of depression
• Toxicity: blood pressure and pulse in patients prior to initiating treatment and periodically thereafter; Signs of toxicity: somnolence, sleep disturbances, persistent GI symptoms

---

dyphylline

(dye'-fi-lin)

Rx: Dilor, Dylix, Lufyllin, Neothylline

Combinations

Rx: with guaifenesin (Dilex-G, Dilor-G, Lufyllin-GG); with ephedrine, guaifenesin, phenobarbital (Lufyllin-EPG)

Chemical Class: Xanthine derivative

Therapeutic Class: COPD agent; antiasthmatic; bronchodilator

CLINICAL PHARMACOLOGY

Mechanism of Action: A xanthine derivative that acts as a bronchodilator by directly relaxing smooth muscle of the bronchial airway and pulmonary blood vessels similar to theophylline. *Therapeutic Effect:* Relieves bronchospasm, increases vital capacity, produces cardiac, and skeletal muscle stimulation.

Pharmacokinetics

Rapid absorption after PO administration. Excreted in urine. **Half-life:** 2 hrs.

INDICATIONS AND DOSAGES

Chronic bronchospasm, asthma

PO

Adults, Elderly. 15 mg/kg 4 times/day.

IM

Adults, Elderly. 250-500 mg. Maximum: 15 mg/kg q6h.

Children. 4.4-6.6 mg/kg/day in divided doses.

Dosage in renal impairment

Creatinine Clearance	Dosage Percent
50-80 ml/min	Administer 75% of dose
10-50 ml/min	Administer 50% of dose
<10 ml/min	Administer 25% of dose

S AVAILABLE FORMS/COST

• Elixir-Oral: 100 mg/15 ml, 480 ml: **$29.88-$67.10**
• Sol, Inj-IM: 250 mg/ml, 2 ml: **$9.49**
• Tab-Oral: 200 mg, 100's: **$12.81-$176.14**; 400 mg, 100's: **$13.71-$287.88**

CONTRAINDICATIONS: Uncontrolled arrhythmias, hyperthyroidism, history of hypersensitivity to dyphylline, related xanthine derivatives, or any component of the formulation

PREGNANCY AND LACTATION: Pregnancy category C; excreted into breast milk, compatible with breastfeeding

SIDE EFFECTS

Frequent

Tachycardia, nervousness, restlessness

Occasional

Heartburn, vomiting, headache, mild diuresis, insomnia, nausea

SERIOUS REACTIONS

• Ventricular arrhythmias, hypotension, circulatory failure, seizures, hyperglycemia, and syndrome of inappropriate antidiuretic hormone (SIADH) have been reported.

INTERACTIONS

Drugs

▣ *Probenecid:* Increased serum dyphylline concentrations

SPECIAL CONSIDERATIONS

• Though better tolerated, significantly less bronchodilating activity vs theophylline. Serious dosing errors possible if dyphylline monitored with theophylline serum assays

MONITORING PARAMETERS

• Minimal effective serum concentration 12 mcg/ml

---

econazole

(e-kone'a-zole)

Rx: Spectazole

Chemical Class: Imidazole derivative

Therapeutic Class: Antifungal

CLINICAL PHARMACOLOGY

Mechanism of Action: An imidazole derivative that changes the permeability of the fungal cell wall. *Therapeutic Effect:* Inhibits fungal biosynthesis of triglycerides, phospholipids. Fungistatic.

Pharmacokinetics

Low systemic absorption. Protein binding: 98%. Metabolized in liver to more than 20 metabolites. Primarily excreted in urine; minimal excretion in feces. Not removed by hemodialysis.

INDICATIONS AND DOSAGES

Treatment of tinea pedis, tinea cruris, tinea corporis, tinea versicolor

Topical

Adults, Elderly, Children. Apply once daily to affected area for 2-4 wks.

▣ **AVAILABLE FORMS/COST**

• Cre-Top: 1%, 15, 30, 85, 100 g: **$30.92**/30 g

UNLABELED USES: Cutaneous candidiasis, otomycosis

CONTRAINDICATIONS: Hypersensitivity to econazole

PREGNANCY AND LACTATION: Pregnancy category C; excretion into breast milk unknown; limited systemic absorption would minimize possibility of exposure to nursing infant

SIDE EFFECTS

Occasional (10%-1%)

Vulvar/vaginal burning

Rare (less than 1%)

Itching and burning of sexual partner, polyuria, vulvar itching, soreness, edema, discharge

SERIOUS REACTIONS

• None known.

SPECIAL CONSIDERATIONS

PATIENT/FAMILY EDUCATION

• For external use only; avoid contact with eyes; cleanse skin with soap and water and dry thoroughly prior to application

• Use medication for full treatment time outlined by clinician, even though symptoms may have improved

• Notify clinician if no improvement after 2 wk (jock itch, ringworm) or 4 wk (athlete's foot)

edetate calcium disodium (calcium EDTA)

(ed-eh-tate kal-see-um dye-sow-dee-um)

Rx: Calcium Disodium Versenate

Chemical Class: Chelating agent

Therapeutic Class: Antidote, heavy metal

CLINICAL PHARMACOLOGY

Mechanism of Action: A chelating agent that reduces blood concentration of heavy metals, especially lead, forming stable complexes. *Therapeutic Effect:* Allows heavy metal excretion in urine.

Pharmacokinetics

Well absorbed after parenteral administration; poorly absorbed from the gastrointestinal (GI) tract. Penetrates to extracellular fluid and slowly diffuses into cerebrospinal fluid (CSF). No metabolism occurs. Excreted in the urine either unchanged or as the metal chelates. **Half-life:** 20-60 min (IV), 1.5 hrs (IM).

INDICATIONS AND DOSAGES

Diagnosis of lead poisoning

IM/IV

Adults, Elderly. 500 mg/m2. Maximum: 1 g/m2/day divided in equal doses 8-12 hr apart for 5 days, skip 2-4 days and repeat course if needed.

IM

Children. 500 mg/m2 as single dose or 500 mg/m2 each at 12 hr intervals.

IV

Children. 1 g/m2/day IV infusion over 8-12 hr for 5 days, skip 2-4 days and repeat course as needed. Maximum: 75 mg/kg/day

Lead poisoning (without encephalopathy)

IM/IV

Adults, Elderly, Children. 1-1.5 g/m2 daily for 3-5 days (if blood lead concentration >100 mcg/dl, calcium edetate usually given with dimercaprol.) Allow at least 2-4 days, up to 2-3 wks between courses of therapy. Adults should not be given more than 2 courses of therapy.

Lead poisoning (with encephalopathy)

IM

Adults, elderly, children. Initially, dimercaprol 4 mg/kg; then give dimercaprol 4 mg/kg and calcium EDTA 250 mg/m2; then 4 hrs later and q4h for 5 days.

AVAILABLE FORMS/COST

• Sol, Inj-IV: 200 mg/ml, 5 ml: **$42.20**

CONTRAINDICATIONS: Anuria, severe renal disease, hypersensitivity to EDTA or any component of the formulation

PREGNANCY AND LACTATION: Pregnancy category B; excretion into breast milk unknown; use caution in nursing mothers

SIDE EFFECTS

Frequent

Chills, fever, anorexia, headache, histamine-like reaction (sneezing, stuffy nose, watery eyes), decreased blood pressure (BP), nausea, vomiting, thrombophlebitis

Rare

Frequent urination, secondary gout (severe pain in feet, knees, elbows).

SERIOUS REACTIONS

• Drug may produce same signs of renal damage as severe acute lead poisoning (proteinuria, microscopic hematuria). Transient anemia/bone marrow depression, hypercalcemia (constipation, drowsiness, dry mouth, metallic taste) occurs occasionally.

SPECIAL CONSIDERATIONS

PATIENT/FAMILY EDUCATION

• Notify clinician immediately if no urine output in a 12 hr period

MONITORING PARAMETERS

• Urinalysis and urine sediment daily during therapy to detect signs of progressive renal tubular damage

• Renal function tests, liver function tests, and serum electrolytes before and periodically during therapy

• ECG during IV therapy

edetate disodium

(ed-'eh-tate dye-sow-dee-um)

Rx: Disotate, Endrate

Chemical Class: Chelating agent

Therapeutic Class: Antidote, digitalis; antihypercalcemic

CLINICAL PHARMACOLOGY

Mechanism of Action: A chelating agent that forms a soluble chelate with calcium, resulting in rapid decrease in plasma calcium concentrations. *Therapeutic Effect:* Allows calcium to be excreted in urine.

Pharmacokinetics

Distributed in extracellular fluid and does not appear in red blood cells. No metabolism occurs. Rapidly excreted in the urine. **Half-life:** 1.4-3 hrs.

INDICATIONS AND DOSAGES

Digitalis toxicity, hypercalcemia

IV

Adults, Elderly. 500 mg/kg/day over 3 hrs or more, daily for 5 days, skip 2 days, repeat as needed up to 15 doses. Maximum: 3 g/day.

Children. 40 mg/kg/day over 3 hrs or more, daily for 5 days, skip 5 days, repeat as needed. Maximum: 70 mg/kg/day.

$ **AVAILABLE FORMS/COST**

• Sol, Inj-IV: 150 mg/ml, 20 ml: **$3.48-$26.90**

CONTRAINDICATIONS: Anuria, renal impairment, hypersensitivity to EDTA or any component of the formulation

PREGNANCY AND LACTATION: Pregnancy category C; excretion into breast milk unknown; use caution in nursing mothers

SIDE EFFECTS

Frequent

Abdominal cramps or pain, diarrhea, nausea, vomiting, circumoral paresthesia, headache, numbness, postural hypotension

Rare

Exfoliative dermatitis, toxic skin and mucous membrane reactions, thrombophlebitis (at injection site)

SERIOUS REACTIONS

• Nephrotoxicity may occur with excessive dosages.

• Hypomagnesemia may occur with prolonged use.

SPECIAL CONSIDERATIONS

• Have patient remain supine for a short time after INF due to the possibility of orthostatic hypotension

MONITORING PARAMETERS

• ECG, blood pressure during INF

• Renal function before and during therapy

• Serum calcium, magnesium, potassium levels

edrophonium
(ed-roe-foe'nee-um)
Rx: Enlon, Reversol, Tensilon
Combinations
  Rx: with atropine (Enlon-Plus)
Chemical Class: Cholinesterase inhibitor; quaternary ammonium derivative
Therapeutic Class: Antidote, curare; cholinergic

CLINICAL PHARMACOLOGY
Mechanism of Action: A parasympathetic, anticholinesterase agent that inhibits destruction of acetylcholine by acetylcholinesterase, thus causing accumulation of acetylcholine at cholinergic synapses. Results in an increase in cholinergic responses such as miosis, increased tonus of intestinal and skeletal muscles, bronchial and ureteral constriction, bradycardia and increased salivary and sweat gland secretions. *Therapeutic Effect:* Diagnosis of myasthenia gravis.
Pharmacokinetics
Onset of action occurs within 30-60 seconds and has duration of 10 minutes. Rapid absorption after IV administration. Exact method of metabolism is unknown. Rapidly excreted in urine. **Half-life:** 1.8 hrs.

INDICATIONS AND DOSAGES
Diagnosis of myasthenia gravis
IV
Adults, Elderly. 2 mg test dose over 15-30 seconds. If no reaction in 45 seconds, give additional dose of 8 mg. Test dose may be repeated after 30 minutes.
Children more than 34 kg. Initially, 2 mg over 1 minute. If no reaction in 45 seconds, may repeat at a rate of 1 mg every 30-45 seconds. Maximum cumulative dose: 10 mg.
Children less than 34 kg. Initially, 1 mg over 1 minute. If no reaction in 45 seconds, may repeat at a rate of 1 mg every 30-45 seconds. Maximum cumulative dose: 5 mg.
Infants. 0.5 mg infused over 1 minute.
IM/SC
Adults, Elderly, Children. Initially, 10 mg as a single dose. If no cholinergic reaction occurs, give 2 mg 30 minutes later to rule out false-negative reaction.
Children more than 34 kg. 5 mg as a single dose.
Children less than 34 kg. 2 mg as a single dose.
Infants. 0.5-1 mg as a single dose.
Neuromuscular blockade antagonism
IV
Adults, Elderly. 10 mg over 30-45 seconds. May be repeated as needed until a cholinergic response is detected. Maximum: 40 mg.
IM
Children. 233 mcg/kg as a single dose.
Infants. 145 mcg/kg as a single dose.
Dosage in Renal Impairment
Dose may need to be reduced in patients with chronic renal failure.

⒮ AVAILABLE FORMS/COST
• Sol, Inj-IM, IV: 10 mg/ml, 1, 10, 15 ml: **$4.68**/1 ml

CONTRAINDICATIONS: Gastrointestinal (GI) or genitourinary (GU) obstruction, hypersensitivity to edrophonium, sulfites, or any component of the formulation

PREGNANCY AND LACTATION: Pregnancy category C; because it is ionized at physiologic pH, would not be expected to cross placenta in significant amounts; may cause premature labor; because it is ionized at physiologic pH, would not be expected to be excreted into breast milk

SIDE EFFECTS
Frequent

Increase salivation, intestinal secretions, lacrimation, urinary urgency, hyperperistalsis, sweating

Occasional

Bradycardia, hypotension, convulsions, dysphagia, nausea, vomiting, diarrhea

Rare

Bronchoconstriction, cardiac arrest, central respiratory paralysis

SERIOUS REACTIONS
• Overdosage causes symptoms of cholinergic crisis such as muscle weakness, nausea, vomiting, miosis, bronchospasm, and respiratory paralysis.

INTERACTIONS
Drugs

▣ *Procainamide:* Edrophonium tests in patients with myasthenia gravis may be unreliable in procainamide-treated patients

▣ *Tacrine:* Increased cholinergic effects of edrophonium

SPECIAL CONSIDERATIONS
MONITORING PARAMETERS
• Preinjection and postinjection strength
• Heart rate, respiratory rate, blood pressure

---

efalizumab

Rx: Raptiva
Chemical Class: Monoclonal antibody
Therapeutic Class: Antipsoriatic; immunomodulatory agent

CLINICAL PHARMACOLOGY
Mechanism of Action: A monoclonal antibody that interferes with lymphocyte activation by binding to the lymphocyte antigen, inhibiting the adhesion of leukocytes to other cell types. *Therapeutic Effect:* Prevents the release of cytokines and the growth and migration of circulating total lymphocytes, predominant in psoriatic lesions.

Pharmacokinetics

Clearance is affected by body weight, not by gender or race, after subcutaneous injection. Serum concentration reaches steady state at 4 wk. Mean time to elimination: 25 days.

INDICATIONS AND DOSAGES
Psoriasis

Subcutaneous

Adults, Elderly. Initially, 0.7 mg/kg followed by weekly doses of 1 mg/kg. Maximum: 200 mg (single dose).

💲 AVAILABLE FORMS/COST
• Powder, Inj-SC: 125 mg/vial: **$343.00**

CONTRAINDICATIONS: Concurrent use of immunosuppressive agents

PREGNANCY AND LACTATION: Pregnancy category C; breast milk excretion unknown

SIDE EFFECTS
Frequent (32%–10%)

Headache, chills, nausea, injection site pain

Occasional (8%–7%)

Myalgia, flu-like symptoms, fever

Rare (4%)

Back pain, acne

SERIOUS REACTIONS
• Hypersensitivity reaction, malignancies, serious infections (abscess, cellulitis, postoperative wound infection, pneumonia), thrombocytopenia, and worsening of psoriasis occur rarely.

INTERACTIONS
Drugs

⚠ *Immunosuppressives:* Efalizumab should not be given with other immunosuppressive drugs

⚠ *Acellular, live and live-attenuated vaccines:* Administration during efalizumab therapy is not recommended

Labs

• Increased lymphocyte counts related to pharmacologic mechanism of action

SPECIAL CONSIDERATIONS

• Evaluate for latent tuberculosis infection with a tuberculin skin test before initiation of therapy

PATIENT/FAMILY EDUCATION

• Intended for use under the guidance and supervision of clinician; patients may self-inject if appropriate and with medical follow-up, after proper training in injection technique, including proper syringe and needle disposal

MONITORING PARAMETERS

• *Efficacy:* Improvement of clinical signs/symptoms of psoriasis (*e.g.,* itching, redness, scaling, psoriatic body surface area coverage); PASI scores are based on plaque thickness, scaling, and redness, adjusted for percentage of affected body surface area; quality of life assessments

• *Toxicity:* CBC with differential periodically, particularly platelets; vital signs in patients with a history of hypersensitivity to any medication (first injection); temperature periodically (infection)

---

efavirenz
(e-fahv′er-ins)
Rx: Sustiva
Chemical Class: Benzoxazinone, substituted; nonnucleoside reverse transcriptase inhibitor
Therapeutic Class: Antiretroviral

CLINICAL PHARMACOLOGY

Mechanism of Action: A nonnucleoside reverse transcriptase inhibitor that inhibits the activity of HIV reverse transcriptase of HIV-1 and the transcription of HIV-1 RNa to DNA. *Therapeutic Effect:* Interrupts HIV replication, slowing the progression of HIV infection.

Pharmacokinetics

Rapidly absorbed after PO administration. Protein binding: 99%. Metabolized to major isoenzymes in the liver. Eliminated in urine and feces. **Half-life:** 40-55 hr.

INDICATIONS AND DOSAGES

HIV infection (in combination with other antiretrovirals)

PO

Adults, Elderly, Children 3 yr and older weighing 40 kg or more. 600 mg once a day at bedtime.

Children 3 yr and older weighing 32.5 kg-less than 40 kg. 400 mg once a day.

Children 3 yr and older weighing 25 kg-less than 32.5 kg. 350 mg once a day.

Children 3 yr and older weighing 20 kg-less than 25 kg. 300 mg once a day.

Children 3 yr and older weighing 15 kg-less than 20 kg. 250 mg once a day.

Children 3 yr and older weighing 10 kg-less than 15 kg. 200 mg once a day.

🛎 AVAILABLE FORMS/COST
• Cap-Oral: 50 mg, 30's: **$37.08**; 100 mg, 30's: **$74.10**; 200 mg, 90's: **$463.13**
• Tab-Oral: 600 mg, 30's: **$463.13**

CONTRAINDICATIONS: Concurrent use with ergot derivatives, midazolam, or triazolam; efavirenz as monotherapy; hypersensitivity to efavirenz

PREGNANCY AND LACTATION: Pregnancy category C (fetal malformations observed in monkeys); breast-feeding not recommended

SIDE EFFECTS
Frequent (52%)
Mild to severe: Dizziness, vivid dreams, insomnia, confusion, impaired concentration, amnesia, agitation, depersonalization, hallucinations, euphoria, somnolence (mild symptoms don't interfere with daily activities; severe symptoms interrupt daily activities)
Occasional
Mild to moderate: Maculopapular rash (27%); nausea, fatigue, headache, diarrhea, fever, cough (less than 26%) (moderate symptoms may interfere with daily activities)

SERIOUS REACTIONS
• None known.

INTERACTIONS
Drugs
❷ *Amprenavir:* Efavirenz decreases amprenavir plasma level; amprenavir dose adjustment recommended

❸ *Barbiturates:* Barbiturates decrease plasma efavirenz levels; dose adjustment not recommended

❸ *Carbamazepine:* Carbamazepine decreases plasma efavirenz levels; dose adjustment not recommended

❷ *Cisapride:* Efavirenz increases cisapride plasma level; coadministration not recommended

❸ *Clarithromycin:* Efavirenz decreases clarithromycin plasma levels; coadministration not recommended

❷ *Ergotamines:* Efavirenz increases ergotamine plasma level; coadministration not recommended

❸ *Ethinyl estradiol:* Efavirenz increases ethinyl estradiol plasma levels; dose adjustment not recommended

❸ *Indinavir:* Efavirenz reduces indinavir AUC by 31%; increase indinavir dose to 1000 mg q8h

❸ *Lopinavir:* Decreased plasma lopinavir concentrations; consider increase dose of lopinavir/ritonavir combination to 533 mg lopinavir and 133 mg ritonavir

❸ *Lovastatin:* Efavirenz increases lovastatin plasma level; dose adjustment not recommended

❷ *Midazolam:* Efavirenz increases midazolam plasma level; coadministration not recommended

❸ *Nelfinavir:* Efavirenz increases nelfinavir AUC by 20%; dose adjustment not recommended

❸ *Phenobarbital:* Decreased plasma efavirenz concentrations

❸ *Phenytoin:* Phenytoin decreases plasma efavirenz level; dose adjustment not recommended

❸ *Psychoactive drugs:* Potential for additive CNS effects

❷ *Rifabutin:* Efavirenz decreases plasma rifabutin level by 35%; no change in plasma efavirenz level; increase rifabutin dose to 450 mg qday

❸ *Rifampin:* Rifampin decreases plasma efavirenz level by 25%; dose adjustment not recommended

❸ *Ritonavir:* Ritonavir increases efavirenz AUC by 21%; efavirenz increases ritonavir AUC by 18%; dose adjustment not recommended

E

3️⃣ *St. John's Wort (Hypericum perforatum):* Substantial decrease in plasma efavirenz concentrations likely; coadministration not recommended

2️⃣ *Saquinavir:* Saquinavir reduces efavirenz AUC by 12%; efavirenz reduces saquinavir AUC by 62%; coadministration not recommended

3️⃣ *Simvastatin:* Efavirenz increases simvastatin plasma level; dose adjustment not recommended

2️⃣ *Triazolam:* Efavirenz increases triazolam plasma level; coadministration not recommended

3️⃣ *Warfarin:* Efavirenz potentially increases or decreases plasma warfarin concentrations

Labs

• *False positive: Cannabinoid screening test by CEDIA DAU Multi-level THC assay*

SPECIAL CONSIDERATIONS
PATIENT/FAMILY EDUCATION

• May be taken without regard for meals; absorption increased by a high-fat meal, which should be avoided

• Take at bedtime for first 2-4 wk of therapy; may continue at bedtime if desired

• Use caution in driving or other activities requiring alertness

• Avoid alcohol ingestion

MONITORING PARAMETERS

• ALT, AST, CBC, cholesterol, triglycerides

---

eflornithine
(eh-floor-nigh-theen)
Rx: *Injection:* Ornidyl
Rx: *Topical:* Vaniqa
Chemical Class: Ornithine decarboxylase inhibitor
Therapeutic Class: Antiprotozoal

CLINICAL PHARMACOLOGY
Mechanism of Action: A topical antiprotozoal that inhibits ornithine deczarboxylase cell division and synthetic function in the skin. ***Therapeutic Effect:*** Reduces rate of hair growth.

Pharmacokinetics
Absorption is less than 1% from intact skin. Not metabolized. Primarily excreted as unchanged drug in urine. **Half life:** 8 hrs

INDICATIONS AND DOSAGES
For reduction of unwanted facial hair in women
Topical
Adults, Elderly. Apply thin layer to affected area of face and adjacent involved areas under chin; rub in thoroughly. Use twice daily at least 8 hrs apart. Do not wash area for at least 4 hrs.

🆂 **AVAILABLE FORMS/COST**
• Cre-Topical: 13.9%, 30 g: **$48.09**
CONTRAINDICATIONS: Hypersensitivity to eflornithine or any component of the formulation
PREGNANCY AND LACTATION: Pregnancy category C; excretion into breast milk unknown; use caution in nursing mothers
SIDE EFFECTS
Frequent
Acne
Occasional
Headache, stinging/burning skin, dry skin, pruritus, erythema

Rare

Tingling skin, rash, dyspepsia (heartburn, GI distress)

SERIOUS REACTIONS

• Bleeding skin, cheilitis, contact dermatitis, herpes simplex, lip swelling, nausea, numbness, rosacea, and weakness have been reported.

SPECIAL CONSIDERATIONS

• The most frequent, serious, toxic effect of eflornithine is myelosuppression, which may be unavoidable if successful treatment is to be completed; decisions to modify dosage or to interrupt or cease treatment depend on the severity of the observed adverse event(s) and the availability of support facilities

MONITORING PARAMETERS

• Serial audiograms if feasible

• CBC with platelets before and twice weekly during therapy and qwk after completion of therapy until hematologic values return to baseline levels

• Follow-up for at least 24 mo is advised to ensure further therapy should relapses occur

---

eletriptan

Rx: Relpax

Chemical Class: Serotonin derivative

Therapeutic Class: Antimigraine agent

CLINICAL PHARMACOLOGY

Mechanism of Action: A serotonin receptor agonist that binds selectively to vascular receptors, producing a vasoconstrictive effect on cranial blood vessels. *Therapeutic Effect:* Relieves migraine headache.

Pharmacokinetics

Well absorbed after PO administration. Metabolized by the liver to inactive metabolite. Eliminated in urine. **Half-life:** 4.4 hr (increased in hepatic impairment and the elderly (older than 65 yr).

INDICATIONS AND DOSAGES

Acute migraine headache

PO

Adults, Elderly. 20-40 mg. If headache improves but then returns, dose may be repeated after 2 hr. Maximum: 80 mg/day.

S AVAILABLE FORMS/COST

• Tab, Film-Coated-Oral: 20, 40 mg, 12's: **$189.60**

CONTRAINDICATIONS: Arrhythmias associated with conduction disorders, coronary artery disease, ischemic heart disease, severe hepatic impairment, uncontrolled hypertension

PREGNANCY AND LACTATION: Pregnancy category C; excreted in human breast milk-approximately 0.02% of the administered dose; breast milk to plasma ratio 1:4, with great variability; caution should be exercised when eletriptan hydrobromide is administered to nursing women

SIDE EFFECTS

Occasional (6%-5%)

Dizziness, somnolence, asthenia, nausea

Rare (3%-2%)

Paresthesia, headache, dry mouth, warm or hot sensation, dyspepsia, dysphagia

SERIOUS REACTIONS

• Cardiac reactions (including ischemia, coronary artery vasospasm, and MI) and noncardiac vasospasm-related reactions (such as hemorrhage and CVA) occur rarely, particularly in patients with hypertension, diabetes, or a strong family history of coronary artery disease;

obese patients; smokers; males older than 40 years; and postmenopausal women.

INTERACTIONS

Drugs

❷ *Ergot-containing drugs (dihydroergotamine, methysergide):* Additive vasospastic effects; avoid use within 24 hours of each other

❷ *Clarithromycin, Erythromycin, Troleandomycin:* Avoid use within 72 hours of treatment with potent CYP3A4 inhibitors

❸ *Fluconazole:* 1.4-fold increase in C_{max}, 2-fold increase in AUC of eletriptan

❷ *Itraconazole, ketoconazole:* Avoid use within 72 hours of treatment with potent CYP3A4 inhibitors

❷ *Nefazodone:* Avoid use within 72 hours of treatment with potent CYP3A4 inhibitors

❷ *Nelfinavir, ritonavir:* Avoid use within 72 hours of treatment with potent CYP3A4 inhibitors

❸ *Verapamil:* 2-fold increase in C_{max}, 3-fold increase in AUC of eletriptan

SPECIAL CONSIDERATIONS

• First dose should be administered under medical supervision, particularly in patients with risk factors for coronary artery disease

PATIENT/FAMILY EDUCATION

• Use for treatment of migraines, not prophylaxis

MONITORING PARAMETERS

• *Efficacy:* Headache response 1-4 hours after a dose (reduction from moderate or severe pain to minimal or no pain); headache recurrence within 24 hours

• *Toxicity:* Vital signs (pulse blood pressure), electrocardiogram particularly in patient with coronary artery disease risk factors

emtricitabine

Rx: Emtriva
Combinations
  Rx: with tenofovir (Truvada)
Chemical Class: Nucleoside analog
Therapeutic Class: Antiretroviral

CLINICAL PHARMACOLOGY

Mechanism of Action: An antiretroviral that inhibits HIV-1 reverse transcriptase by incorporating itself into viral DNA, resulting in chain termination. *Therapeutic Effect:* Interrupts HIV replication, slowing the progression of HIV infection.

Pharmacokinetics

Rapidly and extensively absorbed from the GI tract. Excreted primarily in urine (86%) and, to a lesser extent, in feces (14%); 30% removed by hemodialysis. Unknown if removed by peritoneal dialysis. **Half-life:** 10 hr.

INDICATIONS AND DOSAGES

HIV infection (in combination with other antiretrovirals)

PO

Adults, Elderly. 200 mg once a day.

Dosage in renal impairment

Dosage and frequency are modified based on creatinine clearance.

Creatinine Clearance	Dosage
30-49 ml/min	200 mg q48h
15-29 ml/min	200 mg q72h
less than 15 ml/min, hemodialysis patients	200 mg q96h

$ **AVAILABLE FORMS/COST**

• Cap-Oral: 200 mg, 30's: **$303.40**

CONTRAINDICATIONS: None known

PREGNANCY AND LACTATION:
Pregnancy category B; breast milk excretion unknown (breast-feeding not advised for HIV infected women)

SIDE EFFECTS

Frequent (23%-13%)

Headache, rhinitis, rash, diarrhea, nausea

Occasional (14%-4%)

Cough, vomiting, abdominal pain, insomnia, depression, paresthesia, dizziness, peripheral neuropathy, dyspepsia, myalgia

Rare (3%-2%)

Arthralgia, abnormal dreams

SERIOUS REACTIONS

• Lactic acidosis and hepatomegaly with steatosis occur rarely and may be severe.

SPECIAL CONSIDERATIONS

• Current treatment guidelines use emtricitabine as an alternative to lamivudine in the nucleoside reverse transcriptase "backbone" that is part of combination antiretroviral therapy; it has no known advantages over lamivudine

• Reduced susceptibility to emtricitabine is associated with HIV reverse transcriptase gene mutation M184V/I

• Always check updated treatment guidelines before initiating or changing antiretroviral therapy (http://AIDSinfo.nih.gov)

PATIENT/FAMILY EDUCATION

• Success of an antiretroviral regimen requires >95% adherence to dosing schedule

MONITORING PARAMETERS

• CBC, renal function, ALT, AST, triglycerides, HIV RNA, CD4 count

enalapril
(en-al'a-pril)
Rx: Vasotec
Combinations
   Rx: with diltiazem (Teczem);
   with felodipine (Lexxel);
   with hydrochlorothiazide
   (Vaseretic)
Chemical Class: Angiotensin-converting enzyme (ACE) inhibitor, nonsulfhydryl
Therapeutic Class: Antihypertensive

CLINICAL PHARMACOLOGY
Mechanism of Action: This angiotensin-converting enzyme (ACE) inhibitor suppresses the renin-angiotensin-aldosterone system, and prevents conversion of angiotensin I to angiotensin II, a potent vasoconstrictor; may inhibit angiotensin II at local vascular, renal sites. Decreases plasma angiotensin II, increases plasma renin activity, decreases aldosterone secretion. *Therapeutic Effect:* In hypertension, reduces peripheral arterial resistance. In congestive heart failure (CHF), increases cardiac output; decreases peripheral vascular resistance, blood pressure (BP), pulmonary capillary wedge pressure, heart size.
Pharmacokinetics

Route	Onset	Peak	Duration
PO	1 hr	4-6 hr	24 hr
IV	15 min	1-4 hr	6 hr

Readily absorbed from the gastrointestinal (GI) tract (not affected by food). Protein binding: 50%–60%. Converted to active metabolite. Primarily excreted in urine. Removed by hemodialysis. **Half-life:** 11 hrs (half-life is increased in those with impaired renal function).

INDICATIONS AND DOSAGES
Hypertension alone or in combination with other antihypertensives
PO
Adults, Elderly. Initially, 2.5-5 mg/day. Range: 10-40 mg/day in 1-2 divided doses.
Children. 0.1 mg/kg/day in 1-2 divided doses. Maximum: 0.5 mg/kg/day.
Neonates. 0.1 mg/kg/day q24h.
IV
Adults, Elderly. 0.625-1.25 mg q6h up to 5 mg q6h.
Children,   Neonates.   5-10 mcg/kg/dose q8–24h.
Adjunctive therapy for CHF
PO
Adults, Elderly. Initially, 2.5-5 mg/day. Range: 5-20 mg/day in 2 divided doses.
Dosage in renal impairment
Dosage is modified based on creatinine clearance.

Creatinine Clearance	% Usual Dose
10-50 ml/min	75-100
less than 10 ml/min	50

Ⓢ AVAILABLE FORMS/COST
• Sol, Inj-IV: 1.25 mg/ml, 1 ml: **$3.84-$15.30**
• Tab-Oral: 2.5 mg, 100's: **$7.54-$80.90**; 5 mg, 100's: **$97.64-$124.55**; 10 mg, 100's: **$10.05-$130.73**; 20 mg, 100's: **$14.30-$178.49**

UNLABELED USES: Treatment of diabetic nephropathy or renal crisis in scleroderma

CONTRAINDICATIONS: History of angioedema from previous treatment with ACE inhibitors

PREGNANCY AND LACTATION: Pregnancy category C (1st trimester), category D (2nd and 3rd trimesters); ACE inhibitors can cause fetal and neonatal morbidity and death when administered to pregnant women; when pregnancy is detected, discontinue ACE inhibitors as soon as possible; detectable in breast milk in trace amounts; effect on nursing infant has not been determined; use with caution in nursing mothers

SIDE EFFECTS
Frequent (7%-5%)
Headache, dizziness
Occasional (3%-2%)
Orthostatic hypotension, fatigue, diarrhea, cough, syncope
Rare (less than 2%)
Angina, abdominal pain, vomiting, nausea, rash, asthenia (loss of strength, energy), syncope

SERIOUS REACTIONS
• Excessive hypotension (first-dose syncope) may occur in patients with CHF and in those who are severely salt or volume depleted.
• Angioedema (swelling of face, lips) and hyperkalemia occur rarely.
• Agranulocytosis and neutropenia may be noted in patients with collagen vascular diseases, including scleroderma and systemic lupus erythematosus, and impaired renal function.
• Nephrotic syndrome may be noted in those with history of renal disease.

INTERACTIONS
Drugs
❷ *Allopurinol:* Predisposition to hypersensitivity reactions to ACE inhibitors
❸ *Aspirin, NSAIDs:* Inhibition of the antihypertensive response to ACE inhibitors
❸ *Azathioprine:* Increased myelosuppression
❸ *Insulin:* Enhanced insulin sensitivity
❸ *Iron:* Increased risk of anaphylaxis with administration of parenteral (IV) iron

3 *Lithium:* Increased risk of serious lithium toxicity

3 *Loop diuretics:* Initiation of ACE inhibitor therapy in the presence of intensive diuretic therapy results in a precipitous fall in blood pressure in some patients; ACE inhibitors may induce renal insufficiency in the presence of diuretic-induced sodium depletion

3 *Potassium:* Increased risk for hyperkalemia

3 *Potassium-sparing diuretics:* Increased risk for hyperkalemia

3 *Prazosin, terazosin, doxazosin:* Exaggerated first-dose hypotensive response to α-blockers

3 *Trimethoprim:* Additive risk of hyperkalemia, especially in patient predisposed to renal insufficiency

Labs

• ACE inhibition can account for approximately 0.5mEq/L rise in serum potassium

SPECIAL CONSIDERATIONS
PATIENT/FAMILY EDUCATION

• Caution with salt substitutes containing potassium chloride

• Rise slowly to sitting/standing position to minimize orthostatic hypotension

• Dizziness, fainting, lightheadedness may occur during first few days of therapy

• May cause altered taste perception or cough; persistent dry cough usually does not subside unless medication is stopped; notify clinician if these symptoms persist

MONITORING PARAMETERS

• BUN, creatinine, potassium within 2 wk after initiation of therapy (increased levels may indicate acute renal failure)

enfuvirtide
Rx: Fuzeon
Chemical Class: Fusion inhibitor, HIV; polypeptide, synthetic
Therapeutic Class: Antiretroviral

CLINICAL PHARMACOLOGY
Mechanism of Action: A fusion inhibitor that interferes with the entry of HIV-1 into CD4+ cells by inhibiting the fusion of viral and cellular membranes. *Therapeutic Effect:* Impairs HIV replication, slowing the progression of HIV infection.

Pharmacokinetics

Comparable absorption when injected into subcutaneous tissue of abdomen, arm, or thigh. Protein binding: 92%. Undergoes catabolism to amino acids. **Half-life:** 3.8 hr.

INDICATIONS AND DOSAGES
HIV infection (in combination with other antiretrovirals)

Subcutaneous

Adults, Elderly. 90 mg (1 ml) twice a day.

Children 6-16 yr. 2 mg/kg twice a day. Maximum 90 mg twice a day.

Pediatric Dosing Guidelines	
Weight: kg (lb)	Dose: mg (ml)
11-15.5 (24-34)	27 (0.3)
15.6-20 (more than 35-44)	36 (0.4)
20.1-24.5 (more than 45-54)	45 (0.5)
24.6-29 (more than 55-64)	54 (0.6)
29.1-33.5 (more than 65-74)	63 (0.7)
33.6-38 (more than 75-84)	72 (0.8)
38.1-42.5 (more than 85-94)	81 (0.9)
greater than 42.5 (greater than 94)	90 (1)

$ AVAILABLE FORMS/COST
• Powder, Inj-SC: 108 mg/vial, 90 mg/ml reconstituted: **$33.32**

CONTRAINDICATIONS: None known.

PREGNANCY AND LACTATION: Pregnancy category B; breast milk excretion unknown (breast-feeding not advised for HIV infected women)

SIDE EFFECTS
Expected (98%)
Local injection site reactions (pain, discomfort, induration, erythema, nodules, cysts, pruritus, ecchymosis)

Frequent (26%-16%)
Diarrhea, nausea, fatigue

Occasional (11%-4%)
Insomnia, peripheral neuropathy, depression, cough, decreased appetite or weight loss, sinusitis, anxiety, asthenia, myalgia, cold sores

Rare (3%-2%)
Constipation, influenza, upper abdominal pain, anorexia, conjunctivitis

SERIOUS REACTIONS
• Enfuvirtide use may potentiate bacterial pneumonia.
• Hypersensitivity (rash, fever, chills, rigors, hypotension), thrombocytopenia, neutropenia, and renal insufficiency or failure may occur rarely.

SPECIAL CONSIDERATIONS
• Not active against HIV-2
• In heavily pretreated patients, randomized to receiving an "optimized" backbone regimen (based on treatment history and resistance testing) versus an optimized backbone regimen plus enfuvirtide, changes in HIV RNA at 24 weeks were -0.73 $\log_{10}$ copies/ml and -1.52 $\log_{10}$ copies/ml, respectively; CD4 cell count changes from baseline were 35 and 71 cells/mm³, respectively; clinical outcomes were not improved by enfuvirtide during this study

PATIENT/FAMILY EDUCATION
• Injection site reactions occur commonly
• Hypersensitivity reactions have included individually and in combination: rash, fever, nausea and vomiting, chills, rigors, hypotension
• Increased rate of bacterial pneumonia was observed in subjects treated with enfuvirtide in clinical trials (4.68 pneumonia events per 100 patient-years in the treatment group versus 0.61 events per 100 patient-years in the control group)
• More information is available for patients at www.FUZEON.com, or 877-438-9366

MONITORING PARAMETERS
• CBC with differential (eosinophilia), ALT, AST, triglycerides

---

enoxaparin
(e-nox-ah-pair'in)
Rx: Lovenox
Chemical Class: Heparin derivative, depolymerized; low-molecular weight heparin
Therapeutic Class: Anticoagulant

CLINICAL PHARMACOLOGY
Mechanism of Action: A low-molecular-weight heparin that potentiates the action of antithrombin III and inactivates coagulation factor Xa. *Therapeutic Effect:* Produces anticoagulation. Does not significantly influence bleeding time, PT, or aPTT.

Pharmacokinetics

Route	Onset	Peak	Duration
Subcutaneous	N/A	3–5 hr	12 hr

Well absorbed after subcutaneous administration. Eliminated primarily in urine. Not removed by hemodialysis. **Half-life:** 4.5 hr.

INDICATIONS AND DOSAGES

Prevention of deep vein thrombosis (DVT) after hip and knee surgery
Subcutaneous
Adults, Elderly. 30 mg twice a day, generally for 7–10 days.

Prevention of DVT after abdominal surgery
Subcutaneous
Adults, Elderly. 40 mg a day for 7–10 days.

Prevention of long-term DVT in nonsurgical acute illness
Subcutaneous
Adults, Elderly. 40 mg once a day for 3 wk.

Prevention of ischemic complications of unstable angina and non-Q-wave MI (with oral aspirin therapy)
Subcutaneous
Adults, Elderly. 1 mg/kg q12h.

Acute DVT
Subcutaneous
Adults, Elderly. 1 mg/kg q12h or 1.5 mg/kg once daily.

Usual pediatric dosage
Subcutaneous
Children. 0.5 mg/kg q12h (prophylaxis); 1 mg/kg q12h (treatment).

Dosage in renal impairment
Clearance of enoxaparin is decreased when creatinine clearance is less than 30 ml/min. Monitor patient and adjust dosage as necessary. When enoxaparin is used in abdomonal, hip, or knee surgery or acute illness, the dosage in renal impairment is 30 mg once a day. When enoxaparin is used to treat DVT, angina, or MI the dosage in renal impairment is 1 mg/kg once a day.

$ AVAILABLE FORMS/COST

• Sol, Inj-SC: 30 mg/0.3 ml: **$18.35**; 40 mg/0.4 ml: **$27.23**; 60 mg/0.6 ml: **$40.89**; 80 mg/0.8 ml: **$54.53**; 100 mg/1 ml: **$68.15**; 120 mg/0.8 ml: **$81.80**; 150 mg/1 ml: **$102.26**

UNLABELED USES: Prevention of DVT following general surgical procedures

CONTRAINDICATIONS: Active major bleeding, concurrent heparin therapy, hypersensitivity to heparin or pork products, thrombocytopenia associated with positive in vitro test for antiplatelet antibodys

PREGNANCY AND LACTATION: Pregnancy category B; reports of congenital anomalies and fetal death, cause and effect relationship has not been determined; excretion into breast milk unknown; use caution in nursing mothers

SIDE EFFECTS

Occasional (4%–1%)
Injection site hematoma, nausea, peripheral edema

SERIOUS REACTIONS

• Overdose may lead to bleeding complications ranging from local ecchymoses to major hemorrhage. Antidote: Protamine sulfate (1% solution) equal to the dose of enoxaparin injected. One mg protamine sulfate neutralizes 1 mg enoxaparin. A second dose of 0.5 mg protamine sulfate per 1 mg enoxaparin may be given if aPTT tested 2–4 hr after first injection remains prolonged.

INTERACTIONS

Drugs
3 *Aspirin:* Increased risk of hemorrhage
3 *Oral anticoagulants:* Additive anticoagulant effects

SPECIAL CONSIDERATIONS

• Cannot be used interchangeably with unfractionated heparin or other low molecular weight heparins

• 1.5 mg/kg qday dosing should not be used in patients with cancer or obese patients

• Recent labeling changes regarding use in patients with mechanical prosthetic heart valves based on study involving a small number of pregnant women with mechanical valves; other evidence exists to substantiate cautious use in non-pregnant patients with mechanical valves

PATIENT/FAMILY EDUCATION

• Administer by deep SC inj into abdominal wall; alternate inj sites

• Report any unusual bruising or bleeding to clinician

MONITORING PARAMETERS

• CBC with platelets, stool occult blood, urinalysis

• Monitoring aPTT is not required

---

entacapone
(en-tak'a-pone)
Rx: Comtan
Chemical Class: Catechol-o-methyl-tranferase (COMT) inhibitor; nitrocatechol
Therapeutic Class: Anti-Parkinson's agent

CLINICAL PHARMACOLOGY
Mechanism of Action: An antiparkinson agent that inhibits the enzyme, catechol-O-methyltransferase (COMT), potentiating dopamine activity and increasing the duration of action of levodopa. *Therapeutic Effect:* Decreases signs and symptoms of Parkinson's disease.

Pharmacokinetics
Rapidly absorbed after PO administration. Protein binding: 98%. Metabolized in the liver. Primarily eliminated by biliary excretion. Not removed by hemodialysis. **Half-life:** 2.4 hr.

INDICATIONS AND DOSAGES
Adjunctive treatment of Parkinson's disease
PO
Adults, Elderly. 200 mg concomitantly with each dose of carbidopa and levodopa up to a maximum of 8 times a day (1,600 mg).

$ **AVAILABLE FORMS/COST**
• Tab-PO: 200 mg, 100's: **$197.60**
CONTRAINDICATIONS: Hypersensitivity, use within 14 days of MAOIs

PREGNANCY AND LACTATION:
Pregnancy category C; use caution in nursing mothers

SIDE EFFECTS
Frequent (greater than 10%)
Dyskinesia, nausea, dark yellow or orange urine and sweat, diarrhea
Occasional (9%-3%)
Abdominal pain, vomiting, constipation, dry mouth, fatigue, back pain
Rare (less than 2%)
Anxiety, somnolence, agitation, dyspepsia, flatulence, diaphoresis, asthenia, dyspnea

SERIOUS REACTIONS
• None known.

INTERACTIONS
Drugs
❷ *Nonselective MAO inhibitors (phenelzine, tranylcypromine):* Inhibition of the majority of the pathways responsible for normal catecholamine metabolism

❸ *Iron:* Decreased absorption of iron via chelation

❸ *Isoproterenol, epinephrine, norepinephrine, dopamine, dobutamine, α-methyldopa, apomorphine, isoetherine, and bitolterol:* Decreased metabolism of these drugs

ephedrine
(eh-fed'-rin)
OTC: Pretz-D, Kondon's
Nasal
Combinations
  Rx: with potassium iodide,
  phenobarbital, theophylline
  (Quadrinal), with hydrox-
  yzine, theophylline
  (Hydrophed DF, Marax-
  DF); with guaifenesin
  (Broncholate, Ephex SR)
Chemical Class: Catechol-
amine
Therapeutic Class: Bronchodi-
lator; decongestant;
vasopressor

CLINICAL PHARMACOLOGY
Mechanism of Action: A adrenergic
agonist that stimulates alpha-adrenergic receptors causing vasoconstriction and pressor effects, beta$_1$-
adrenergic receptors, resulting in
cardiac stimulation, and beta$_2$-ad-
renergic receptors, resulting in bronchial dilation and vasodilation.
Therapeutic Effect: Increases blood
pressure (BP) and pulse rate.
Pharmacokinetics
Well absorbed after nasal and parenteral absorption. Metabolized in
liver. Excreted in urine. **Half-life:**
3-6 hrs.
INDICATIONS AND DOSAGES
Asthma
PO
Adults. 25-50 mg q3-4h as needed.
Children. 3 mg/kg/day in 4 divided
doses.
Hypotension
IM
Adults. 25-50 mg as a single dose.
Maximum 150 mg/day.
Children. 0.2-0.3 mg/kg/dose
q4-6h.

IV
Adults. 5 mg/dose slow IVP as pre-
vention. 10-25 mg/dose slow IVP
repeated q5-10min as treatment.
Maximum: 150 mg/day.
Children. 0.2-0.3 mg/kg/dose slow
IVP q4-6h
SC
Adults. 25-50 q4-6h. Maximum 150
mg/day.
Children. 3 mg/kg/day q4-6h.
Nasal congestion
PO
Adults. 25-50 mg q6h as needed.
Children. 3 mg/kg/day in 4 divided
doses.
Nasal
Adults, Children 12 years and older.
2-3 sprays into each nostril q4h
Children 6-12 yrs. 1-2 sprays into
each nostril q4h
AVAILABLE FORMS/COST
• Cap, Gel-Oral: 25 mg, 100's:
$4.50-$14.00; 50 mg, 100's: **$5.95**
• Sol, Inj-IM, IV, SC: 50 mg/ml, 1
ml: **$0.56-$1.01**
• Spray-Nasal: 0.25%, 50 ml: **$5.00**
UNLABELED USES: Obesity, pro-
pofol-induced pain, radiocontrast
media reactions

CONTRAINDICATIONS: Anesthesia with cyclopropane or halothane,
diabetes (ephedrine injection), hypersensitivity to ephedrine or other
sympathomimetic amines, hypertension or other cardiovascular disorders, pregnancy with maternal
blood pressure above 130/80, thyrotoxicosis

PREGNANCY AND LACTATION:
Pregnancy category C; routinely
used to treat or prevent maternal hypotension following spinal anesthesia; may cause fetal heart rate
changes; excretion into breast milk
unknown; one case report of adverse
effects (excessive crying, irritability, and disturbed sleeping patterns)

E

in a 3-month-old nursing infant whose mother consumed disoephedrine

SIDE EFFECTS
Frequent
Hypertension, anxiety
Occasional
Nausea, vomiting, palpitations, tremor
Nasal: Burning, stinging, runny nose
Rare
Psychosis, decreased urination, necrosis at injection site from repeated injections

SERIOUS REACTIONS
• Excessive doses may cause hypertension, intracranial hemorrhage, anginal pain, and fatal arrhythmias.
• Prolonged or excessive use may result in metabolic acidosis due to increased serum lactic acid concentrations.
• Observe for disorientation, weakness, hyperventilation, headache, nausea, vomiting, and diarrhea.

INTERACTIONS
Drugs
3 *Antacids:* Increased ephedrine serum concentrations
3 *Furazolidone:* Hypertensive response possible
3 *Guanadrel:* Inhibits antihypertensive response
3 *Guanethidine:* Inhibits antihypertensive response
2 *MAOIs:* Substantially enhanced pressor response to ephedrine, severe hypertension
3 *Sodium bicarbonate:* Increased ephedrine serum concentrations
Labs
• *False increase:* Urine amino acids, urine 5-HIAA

SPECIAL CONSIDERATIONS
• Found in many OTC weight-loss products containing MaHuang; use should be avoided

PATIENT/FAMILY EDUCATION
• May cause wakefulness or nervousness; take last dose 4-6 hr prior to bedtime
• Do not use nasal products for >3-5 days

MONITORING PARAMETERS
• Heart rate, ECG, blood pressure (when using for vasopressor effect)

---

epinephrine
(ep-i-nef′rin)
Rx: Adrenalin, Sus-Phrine, Adrenaline, Ana-Guard, Epifrin, Glaucon, Ana-Kit, EpiPen, EpiPen Jr.
OTC: Adrenalin, AsthmaHaler Mist, Asthma-Nefrin, microNefrin, Nephron, Primatene Mist, S-2
Combinations
   Rx: with etidocaine (Duranest with Epinephrine); with prilocaine (Citanest Forte); with lidocaine (Xylocaine with Epinephrine); with pilocarpine (E-Pilo Ophthalmic)
Chemical Class: Catecholamine
Therapeutic Class: Antiglaucoma agent; bronchodilator; decongestant; vasopressor

---

CLINICAL PHARMACOLOGY
Mechanism of Action: A sympathomimetic, adrenergic agonist that stimulates alpha-adrenergic receptors causing vasoconstriction and pressor effects, $beta_1$-adrenergic receptors, resulting in cardiac stimulation, and $beta_2$-adrenergic receptors, resulting in bronchial dilation and vasodilation. With ophthalmic form, increases outflow of aqueous humor from anterior eye chamber. *Therapeutic Effect:* Relaxes

smooth muscle of the bronchial tree, produces cardiac stimulation, and dilates skeletal muscle vasculature. The ophthalmic form dilates pupils and constricts conjunctival blood vessels.

Pharmacokinetics

Route	Onset	Peak	Duration
IM	5–10 min	20 min	1–4 hr
Subcutaneous	5–10 min	20 min	1–4 hr
Inhalation	3–5 min	20 min	1–3 hr
Ophthalmic	1 hr	4–8 hr	12–24 hr

Well absorbed after parenteral administration; minimally absorbed after inhalation. Metabolized in the liver, other tissues, and sympathetic nerve endings. Excreted in urine. The ophthalmic form may be systemically absorbed as a result of drainage into nasal pharyngeal passages. Mydriasis occurs within several min and persists several hr; vasoconstriction occurs within 5 min, and lasts less than 1 hr.

INDICATIONS AND DOSAGES

Asystole

IV

Adults, Elderly. 1 mg q3–5min up to 0.1 mg/kg q3–5min.

Children. 0.01 mg/kg (0.1 ml/kg of 1:10,000 solution). May repeat q3–5min. Subsequent doses of 0.1 mg/kg (0.1 ml/kg) of a 1:1000 solution q3–5min.

Bradycardia

IV infusion

Adults, Elderly. 1–10 mcg/min titrated to desired effect.

IV

Children. 0.01 mg/kg (0.1 ml/kg of 1:10,000 solution) q3–5min. Maximum: 1 mg/10 ml.

Bronchodilation

IM, Subcutaneous

Adults, Elderly. 0.1–0.5 mg (1:1000) q10–15min to 4 hrs.

Subcutaneous

Children. 10 mcg/kg (0.01 ml/kg of 1:1,000) Maximum: 0.5 mg or suspension (1:200) 0.005 ml/kg/dose (0.025 mg/kg/dose) to a maximum of 0.15 ml (0.75 mg for single dose) q8–12h.

Hypersensitivity reaction

IM, Subcutaneous

Adults, Elderly. 0.3–0.5 mg q15–20min.

Subcutaneous

Children. 0.01 mg/kg q15min for 2 doses, then q4h. Maximum single dose: 0.5 mg.

Inhalation

Adults, Elderly, Children 4 yr and older. 1 inhalation, may repeat in at least 1 min. Give subsequent doses no sooner than 3 hr.

Nebulizer

Adults, Elderly, Children 4 yr and older. 1–3 deep inhalations. Give subsequent doses no sooner than 3 hr.

Glaucoma

Ophthalmic

Adults, Elderly. 1–2 drops 1–2 times a day.

$ AVAILABLE FORMS/COST

• Aer—INH: 0.3 mg/INH, 15 g: **$6.58-$11.86**
• Sol, Inj, Pen—IM: 0.15 mg, 0.3 mg; all: **$52.38**
• Sol, Inj—IM, IV, SC: 0.1 mg/ml, 10 ml: **$2.60-$13.92**; 1 mg/ml, 1 ml: **$2.34-$2.51**
• Susp, Inj—SC: 5 mg/ml, 5 ml: **$38.50**
• Sol—Ophth: 0.5%, 7.5 ml: **$17.13**; 1%, 7.5 ml: **$12.38**; 2%, 7.5 ml: **$13.02**

UNLABELED USES: Systemic: Treatment of gingival or pulpal hemorrhage, priapism

Ophthalmic: Treatment of conjunctival congestion during surgery, secondary glaucoma

CONTRAINDICATIONS: Cardiac arrhythmias, cerebrovascular insufficiency, hypertension, hyperthyroidism, ischemic heart disease, narrow-angle glaucoma, shock

PREGNANCY AND LACTATION: Pregnancy category C; excreted into breast milk; use caution in nursing mothers

SIDE EFFECTS

Frequent

Systemic: Tachycardia, palpitations, nervousness

Ophthalmic: Headache, eye irritation, watering of eyes

Occasional

Systemic: Dizziness, lightheadedness, facial flushing, headache, diaphoresis, increased BP, nausea, trembling, insomnia, vomiting, fatigue

Ophthalmic: Blurred or decreased vision, eye pain

Rare

Systemic: Chest discomfort or pain, arrhythmias, bronchospasm, dry mouth or throat

SERIOUS REACTIONS

• Excessive doses may cause acute hypertension or arrhythmias.

• Prolonged or excessive use may result in metabolic acidosis due to increased serum lactic acid concentrations. Metabolic acidosis may cause disorientation, fatigue, hyperventilation, headache, nausea, vomiting, and diarrhea.

INTERACTIONS

Drugs

3 *Antihistamines:* Effects of epinephrine may be potentiated by certain antihistamines; diphenhydramine, tripelennamine, d-chlorpheniramine

3 *β-blockers:* Noncardioselective β-blockers enhance pressor response to epinephrine resulting in hypertension and bradycardia

3 *Chlorpromazine, clozaril, thioridazine:* Reversal of epinephrine pressor response

2 *Cyclic antidepressants:* Pressor response to IV epinephrine markedly enhanced

3 *Levothyroxine:* Effects of epinephrine may be potentiated

SPECIAL CONSIDERATIONS

PATIENT/FAMILY EDUCATION

• Do not exceed recommended doses

• Wait at least 3-5 min between inhalations with MDI

• Notify clinician of dizziness or chest pain

• Do not use nasal preparations for >3-5 days to prevent rebound congestion

• To avoid contamination of ophth preparations, do not touch tip of container to any surface

• Do not use ophth preparations while wearing soft contact lenses

• Transitory stinging may occur on instillation of ophth preparations

• Report any decrease in visual acuity immediately

• Use of OTC asthma preparations containing epinephrine should be discouraged

MONITORING PARAMETERS

• Blood pressure, heart rate

• Intraocular pressure

eplerenone

(e-plear'a-nown)

Rx: Inspra

Chemical Class: Pregnene methyl ester

Therapeutic Class: Selective aldosterone receptor antagonist

CLINICAL PHARMACOLOGY

Mechanism of Action: An aldosterone receptor antagonist that binds to the mineralocorticoid receptors in the kidney, heart, blood vessels, and brain, blocking the binding of aldosterone. *Therapeutic Effect:* Reduces BP.

Pharmacokinetics

Absorption unaffected by food. Protein binding: 50%. No active metabolites. Excreted in the urine with a lesser amount eliminated in the feces. Not removed by hemodialysis. **Half-life:** 4–6 hr.

INDICATIONS AND DOSAGES

Hypertension

PO

Adults, Elderly. 50 mg once a day. If 50 mg once a day produces an inadequate BP response, may increase dosage to 50 mg twice a day. If patient is concurrently receiving erythromycin, saquinavir, verapamil, or fluconazole, reduce initial dose to 25 mg once a day.

CHF following MI

PO

Adults, Elderly. Initially, 25 mg once a day. If tolerated, titrate up to 50 mg once a day within 4 wk.

AVAILABLE FORMS/COST

• Tab—Oral: 25 mg, 50 mg, 90's; all: **$337.50**

CONTRAINDICATIONS: Concurrent use of potassium supplements or potassium-sparing diuretics (such as amiloride, spironolactone, and triamterene), or strong inhibitors of the cytochrome P450 3A4 enzyme system (including ketoconazole and itraconazole), creatinine clearance less than 50 ml/min, serum creatinine level greater than 2 mg/dl in males or 1.8 mg/dl in females, serum potassium level greater than 5.5 mEq/L, type 2 diabetes mellitus with microalbuminuria

PREGNANCY AND LACTATION: Pregnancy category B; excreted into breast milk of lactating rabbits; human information unknown

SIDE EFFECTS

Rare (3%–1%)

Dizziness, diarrhea, cough, fatigue, flu-like symptoms, abdominal pain

SERIOUS REACTIONS

• Hyperkalemia may occur, particularly in patients with type 2 diabetes mellitus and microalbuminuria.

INTERACTIONS

Drugs

② *Angiotensin-converting enzyme inhibitors, and Angiotensin II receptor antagonists:* Increased risk of hyperkalemia

② *Azole antifungal agents (fluconazole [less significant], itraconazole, ketoconazole, miconazole, voriconazole):* Inhibition of hepatic metabolism (CYP3A4) leads to increased eplerenone levels (2-6 times)

③ *Lithium:* Increased risk of lithium toxicity

③ *Macrolide antibiotics (erythromycin, clarithromycin):* Caution, up to two-fold increases in eplerenone levels due to inhibition of hepatic metabolism (CYP3A4)

③ *Nonsteroidal Antiinflammatory Drugs:* Reduction in antihypertensive effect of eplerenone

③ *Saquinavir:* Caution, up to two-fold increases in eplerenone levels due to inhibition of hepatic metabolism (CYP3A4)

3 *Verapamil:* Caution, up to two-fold increases in eplerenone levels due to inhibition of hepatic metabolism (CYP3A4)

SPECIAL CONSIDERATIONS
• Primary advantage of eplerenone over spironolactone is a potentially decreased incidence of endocrine-related adverse effects, such as gynecomastia or sexual dysfunction

MONITORING PARAMETERS
• *Efficacy:* Blood pressure, heart rate, ECG, urine output, cardiac output, improvement in symptoms of heart failure
• *Toxicity:* Serum electrolytes (especially potassium), renal function tests, BP, ECG (hyperkalemia), signs and symptoms of toxicity

---

epoetin alfa
(erythropoietin)
(eh-poh´-ee-tin al´-fa)
Rx: Epogen, Procrit
Chemical Class: Amino acid glycoprotein
Therapeutic Class: Hematopoietic agent

CLINICAL PHARMACOLOGY
Mechanism of Action: A glycoprotein that stimulates division and differentiation of erythroid progenitor cells in bone marrow. *Therapeutic Effect:* Induces erythropoiesis and releases reticulocytes from bone marrow.

Pharmacokinetics
Well absorbed after subcutaneous administration. Following administration, an increase in reticulocyte count occurs within 10 days, and increases in Hgb, Hct, and RBC count are seen within 2–6 wk. **Half-life:** 4–13 hr.

INDICATIONS AND DOSAGES
Treatment of anemia in chemotherapy patients
IV, Subcutaneous
Adults, Elderly, Children. 150 units/kg/dose 3 times a wk. Maximum: 1,200 units/kg/wk.

Reduction of allogenic blood transfusions in elective surgery
Subcutaneous
Adults, Elderly. 300 units/kg/day 10 days before day of, and 4 days after surgery.

Chronic renal failure
IV bolus, Subcutaneous
Adults, Elderly. Initially, 50–100 units/kg 3 times a wk. Target Hct range: 30%–36%. Adjust dosage no earlier than 1-mo intervals unless prescribed. Decrease dosage if Hct is increasing and approaching 36%. Plan to temporarily withhold doses if Hct continues to rise and to reinstate lower dosage when Hct begins to decrease. If Hct increases by more than 4 points in 2 wk, monitor Hct twice a wk for 2–6 wk. Increase dose if Hct does not increase 5–6 points after 8 wk (with adequate iron stores) and if Hct is below target range. Maintenance: *For patients on dialysis:* 75 units/kg 3 times a wk. Range: 12.5–525 units/kg. *For patients not on dialysis:* 75–150 units/kg/wk.

HIV infection in patients treated with AZT
IV, Subcutaneous
Adults. Initially, 100 units/kg 3 times a wk for 8 wk; may increase by 50–100 units/kg 3 times a wk. Evaluate response q4–8wk thereafter. Adjust dosage by 50–100 units/kg 3 times a wk. If dosages larger than 300 units/kg 3 times a wk are not eliciting response, it is unlikely patient will respond. Maintenance: Titrate to maintain desired Hct.

AVAILABLE FORMS/COST
• Inj, Sol—IV, SC: 2000 U/ml, 1 ml: **$26.71-$28.04**; 3000 U/ml, 1 ml: **$40.07-$42.06**; 4000 U/ml, 1 ml: **$53.42-$56.08**; 10,000 U/ml, 1 ml: **$133.56-$146.94**; 20,000 U/ml, 1 ml: **$267.12-$301.53**; 40,000 U/ml, 1 ml: **$534.24-$591.66**

UNLABELED USES: Prevention of anemia in patients donating blood before elective surgery or autologous transfusion, treatment of anemia associated with neoplastic diseases.

CONTRAINDICATIONS: History of sensitivity to mammalian cell-derived products or human albumin, uncontrolled hypertension

PREGNANCY AND LACTATION: Pregnancy category C; excretion into breast milk unknown; use caution in nursing mothers

SIDE EFFECTS
Patients receiving chemotherapy
Frequent (20%–17%)
Fever, diarrhea, nausea, vomiting, edema
Occasional (13%–11%)
Asthenia, shortness of breath, paresthesia
Rare (5%–3%)
Dizziness, trunk pain
Patients with chronic renal failure
Frequent (24%–11%)
Hypertension, headache, nausea, arthralgia
Occasional (9%–7%)
Fatigue, edema, diarrhea, vomiting, chest pain, skin reactions at administration site, asthenia, dizziness
Patients with HIV infection treated with AZT
Frequent (38%–15%)
Fever, fatigue, headache, cough, diarrhea, rash, nausea
Occasional (14%–9%)
Shortness of breath, asthenia, skin reaction at injection site, dizziness

SERIOUS REACTIONS
• Hypertensive encephalopathy, thrombosis, cerebrovascular accident, MI, and seizures have occurred rarely.
• Hyperkalemia occurs occasionally in patients with chronic renal failure, usually in those who do not conform to medication regimen, dietary guidelines, and frequency of dialysis regimen.

SPECIAL CONSIDERATIONS
• Iron supplementation should be given during therapy to provide for increased requirements during expansion of red cell mass secondary to marrow stimulation by erythropoietin
• Use prior to elective surgery should be limited to patients with presurgery hemoglobin of >10 but ≤13 g/dl undergoing noncardiac, nonvascular procedures

PATIENT/FAMILY EDUCATION
• Do not shake vials as this may denature the glycoprotein rendering the drug inactive
• Notify clinician if severe headache develops
• Frequent blood tests required to determine optimal dose

MONITORING PARAMETERS
• Hct (target range 30%-33%, max 36%), serum iron, ferritin (keep >100 ng/dl)
• Baseline erythropoietin level (treatment of patients with erythropoietin levels >200 mU/ml is not recommended)
• Blood pressure
• BUN, uric acid, creatinine, phosphorus, potassium on a regular basis

epoprostenol (prostacyclin)

(e-poe-pros'ten-ol)

Rx: Flolan

Chemical Class: Prostaglandin I_2

Therapeutic Class: Vasodilator

CLINICAL PHARMACOLOGY

Mechanism of Action: An antihypertensive that directly dilates pulmonary and systemic arterial vascular beds and inhibits platelet aggregation. *Therapeutic Effect:* Reduces right and left ventricular afterload; increases cardiac output and stroke volume.

INDICATIONS AND DOSAGES

Long-term treatment of New York Heart Association Class III and IV primary pulmonary hypertension

IV infusion

Adults, Elderly. Procedure to determine dose range: Initially, 2 ng/kg/min, increased in increments of 2 ng/kg/min q15min until dose-limiting adverse effects occur. Chronic infusion: Start at 4 ng/kg/min less than the maximum dose rate tolerated during acute dose ranging (or one half of the maximum rate if rate was less than 5 ng/kg/min).

S AVAILABLE FORMS/COST

• Powder, Inj—IV: 0.5 mg/vial: **$19.01**; 1.5 mg/vial: **$39.91**

UNLABELED USES: Cardiopulmonary bypass surgery; hemodialysis; pulmonary hypertension associated with acute respiratory distress syndrome, systemic lupus erythematosus, or congenital heart disease; neonatal pulmonary hypertension, refractory CHF; severe community-acquired pneumonia

CONTRAINDICATIONS: Long-term use in patients with CHF (severe ventricular systolic dysfunction)

PREGNANCY AND LACTATION: Pregnancy category B; women with pulmonary hypertension should avoid pregnancy; unknown if excreted in breast milk

SIDE EFFECTS

Frequent

Acute phase: Flushing (58%), headache (49%), nausea (32%), vomiting (32%), hypotension (16%), anxiety (11%), chest pain (11%), dizziness (8%)

Chronic phase (greater than 20%): Dyspnea, asthenia, dizziness, headache, chest pain, nausea, vomiting, palpitations, edema, jaw pain, tachycardia, flushing, myalgia, nonspecific muscle pain, paresthesia, diarrhea, anxiety, chills, fever, or flu-like symptoms

Occasional

Acute phase (5%–2%): Bradycardia, abdominal pain, muscle pain, dyspnea, back pain

Chronic phase (20%–10%): Rash, depression, hypotension, pallor, syncope, bradycardia, ascites

Rare

Acute phase: Paresthesia

Chronic phase (less than 2%): Diaphoresis, dyspepsia, tachycardia

SERIOUS REACTIONS

• Overdose may cause hyperglycemia or ketoacidosis manifested as increased urination, thirst, and fruit-like breath odor.

• Angina, MI, and thrombocytopenia occur rarely.

• Abrupt withdrawal, including a large reduction in dosage or interruption in drug delivery, may produce rebound pulmonary hypertension as evidenced by dyspnea, dizziness, and asthenia.

INTERACTIONS
Drugs
3 *Antihypertensives, diuretics, vasodilators:* Additive effects on blood pressure

3 *Digoxin:* Possible elevations of plasma digoxin concentrations

SPECIAL CONSIDERATIONS
• Clinically shown to improve exercise capacity, dyspnea, and fatigue as early as 1st week of therapy

• Drug is administered chronically on an ambulatory basis with a portable infusion pump through a permanent central venous cathether; peripheral IV infusions may be used temporarily until central venous access obtained

• Patients must be taught sterile technique, drug reconstitution, and care of catheter

• Do not interrupt infusion or decrease rate abruptly, may cause rebound symptoms (dyspnea, dizziness, asthenia, death)

• Unless contraindicated, patients should be anticoagulated to reduce risk of pulmonary thromboembolism or systemic embolism through a patent foramen ovale

MONITORING PARAMETERS
• Postural BP and heart rate for several hr following dosage adjustments

---

eprosartan
(eh-pro-sar'tan)
Rx: Teveten
Chemical Class: Angiotensin II receptor antagonist
Therapeutic Class: Antihypertensive

CLINICAL PHARMACOLOGY
Mechanism of Action: An angiotensin II receptor antagonist that blocks the vasoconstrictor and aldosterone-secreting effects of angiotensin II, inhibiting the binding of angiotensin II to the AT_1 receptors. *Therapeutic Effect:* Causes vasodilation, decreases peripheral resistance, and decreases BP.

Pharmacokinetics
Rapidly absorbed after PO administration. Protein binding: 98%. Undergoes first-pass metabolism in the liver to active metabolites. Excreted in urine and biliary system. Minimally removed by hemodialysis. **Half-life:** 5–9 hr.

INDICATIONS AND DOSAGES
Hypertension
PO
Adults, Elderly. Initially, 600 mg/day. Range: 400–800 mg/day.

S **AVAILABLE FORMS/COST**
• Tab—Oral: 400 mg, 100's: **$108.28**; 600 mg, 100's: **$144.00**

CONTRAINDICATIONS: Bilateral renal artery stenosis, hyperaldosteronism

PREGNANCY AND LACTATION: Pregnancy category C, first trimester—category D, second and third trimesters; drugs acting directly on the renin-angiotensin-aldosterone system are documented to cause fetal harm (hypotension, oligohydramnios, neonatal anemia, hyperkalemia, neonatal skull hypoplasia, anuria, and renal failure; neonatal limb contractures, craniofacial deformities, and hypoplastic lung development)

SIDE EFFECTS
Occasional (5%–2%)
Headache, cough, dizziness
Rare (less than 2%)
Muscle pain, fatigue, diarrhea, upper respiratory tract infection, dyspepsia

SERIOUS REACTIONS
• Overdosage may manifest as hypotension and tachycardia. Bradycardia occurs less often.

SPECIAL CONSIDERATIONS

SPECIAL CONSIDERATIONS
• Potentially as or more effective than angiotensin-converting enzyme inhibitors, without cough; no evidence for reduction in morbidity and mortality as first line agents in hypertension, yet; whether they provide the same cardiac and renal protection also still tentative; like ACE inhibitors, less effective in black patients

PATIENT/FAMILY EDUCATION
• Call your clinician immediately if note following side effects: wheezing, lip, throat, or face swelling; hives or rash

MONITORING PARAMETERS
• Baseline electrolytes, urinalysis, blood urea nitrogen and creatinine with recheck at 2-4 wk after initiation (sooner in volume-depleted patients); monitor sitting blood pressure; watch for symptomatic hypotension, particulary in volume-depleted patients

---

eptifibatide
(ep-tih-fib′ah-tide)
Rx: Integrilin
Chemical Class: Glycoprotein (GP) IIb/IIIa inhibitor
Therapeutic Class: Antiplatelet agent

CLINICAL PHARMACOLOGY
Mechanism of Action: A glycoprotein IIb/IIIa inhibitor that rapidly inhibits platelet aggregation by preventing binding of fibrinogen to receptor sites on platelets. *Therapeutic Effect:* Prevents closure of treated coronary arteries. Also prevents acute cardiac ischemic complications.

INDICATIONS AND DOSAGES
Adjunct to percutaneous coronary intervention
IV bolus, IV infusion
Adults, Elderly. 180 mcg/kg before PCI initiation; then continuous drip of 2 mcg/kg/min and a second 180 mcg/kg bolus 10 min after the first. Maximum: 15 mg/h. Continue until hospital discharge or for up to 18-24 hours. Minimum 12 hours is recommended. Concurrent aspirin and heparin therapy is recommended.

Acute coronary syndrome
IV bolus, IV infusion
Adults, Elderly. 180 mcg/kg bolus then 2 mcg/kg/min until discharge or coronary artery bypass graft, up to 72 hr. Maximum: 15 mg/h. Concurrent aspirin and heparin therapy is recommended.

Dosage in renal impairment
Serum creatinine 2-4 mg/dl. Use 180 mcg/kg bolus (maximum 22.6 mg) and 1 mcg/kg/min infusion (maximum: 7.5 mg/h).

§ AVAILABLE FORMS/COST
• Inj, Sol—IV: 0.75 mg/ml, 100 ml: **$211.25**; 2 mg/ml, 10 ml: **$613.13**

CONTRAINDICATIONS: Active internal bleeding, AV malformation or aneurysm, history of cerebrovascular accident (CVA) within 2 years or CVA with residual neurologic defect, history of vasculitis, intracranial neoplasm, oral anticoagulant use within last 7 days unless PT is less than 1.22 times the control, recent (6 wk or less) GI or GU bleeding, recent (6 wk or less) surgery or trauma, prior IV dextran use before or during PTCA, severe uncontrolled hypertension, thrombocytopenia (less than 100,000 cells/mcl)

PREGNANCY AND LACTATION: Pregnancy category B; use caution in nursing mothers

SIDE EFFECTS

Occasional (7%)

Hypotension

SERIOUS REACTIONS

• Minor to major bleeding complications may occur, most commonly at arterial access site for cardiac catheterization.

INTERACTIONS

Drugs

▣ Anticoagulants *(heparin, warfarin)*, Antiplatelet agents *(ticlopidine, clopidogrel, dipyridamole)*, Thrombolytics *(alteplase, streptokinase)*, NSAIDs, aspirin: Increased risk of bleeding

SPECIAL CONSIDERATIONS

• When bleeding cannot be controlled with pressure, discontinue INF

• Most major bleeding occurs at arterial access site for cardiac catheterization; prior to pulling femoral artery sheath, discontinue heparin for 3-4 hr and document activated clotting time (ACT) <150 sec or aPTT <45 sec; achieve sheath hemostasis 2-4 hr before discharge

• In patients who undergo CABG, discontinue eptifibatide INF prior to surgery

• Eptifibatide, tirofiban, and abciximab can all decrease the incidence of cardiac events associated with acute coronary syndromes; direct comparisons are needed to establish which, if any, is superior; for angioplasty, until more data become available, abciximab appears to be the drug of choice

MONITORING PARAMETERS

• Platelet count, hemoglobin, hematocrit, PT/aPTT (baseline, within 6 hr following bolus dose, then daily thereafter)

• In patients undergoing PCI, also measure ACT; maintain aPTT between 50 and 70 sec unless PCI is to be performed; during PCI, maintain ACT between 300 and 350 sec

---

ergoloid mesylates

(ur-go-loyd mess-ah-lates)

Rx: Gerimal, Hydergine

Chemical Class: Ergot alkaloid

Therapeutic Class: Cerebral metabolic enhancer

CLINICAL PHARMACOLOGY

Mechanism of Action: An ergot alkaloid that centrally acts and decreases vascular tone, slows heart rate. Peripheral action blocks alpha adrenergic receptors. *Therapeutic Effect:* Improved O_2 uptake and improves cerebral metabolism.

Pharmacokinetics

Rapidly, incompletely absorbed from GI tract. Metabolized in liver. Eliminated primarily in feces. **Half-life:** 2-5 hrs.

INDICATIONS AND DOSAGES

Age-related decline in mental capacity

PO

Adults, Elderly. Initially, 1 mg 3 times/day. Range: 1.5-12 mg/day.

Ⓢ **AVAILABLE FORMS/COST**

• Tab—Oral: 0.5 mg, 100's: **$15.75**; 1 mg, 100's: **$16.45-$105.50**

• Tab—SL: 0.5 mg, 100's: **$8.85**; 1 mg, 100's: **$10.58**

CONTRAINDICATIONS: Acute or chronic psychosis (regardless or etiology), hypersensitivity to ergoloid mesylates or any component of the formulation

SIDE EFFECTS

Occasional

GI distress, transient nausea, sublingual irritation

SERIOUS REACTIONS

- Overdose may produce blurred vision, dizziness, syncope, headache, flushed face, nausea, vomiting, decreased appetite, stomach cramps, and stuffy nose.

SPECIAL CONSIDERATIONS

PATIENT/FAMILY EDUCATION

- Results may not be observed for 3-4 wk
- May cause transient GI disturbances; allow sublingual tablets to completely dissolve under tongue; do not chew or crush sublingual tablets

MONITORING PARAMETERS

- Before prescribing, exclude the possibility that the patient's signs and symptoms arise from a potentially reversible and treatable condition
- Periodically reassess the diagnosis and the benefit of current therapy to the patient; discontinue if no benefit

ergonovine

(er-goe-noe-veen)

Rx: Ergotrate Maleate

Chemical Class: Ergot alkaloid

Therapeutic Class: Oxytocic

CLINICAL PHARMACOLOGY

Mechanism of Action: An oxytoxic agent that directly stimulates uterine muscle. (Stimulates alpha adrenergic, serotonin receptors producing arterial vasoconstriction. Causes vasospasm of coronary arteries. *Therapeutic Effect:* Increases force and frequency of contractions. Induces cervical contractions.

Pharmacokinetics

None reported.

INDICATIONS AND DOSAGES

Oxytocic

IM/IV

Adults. Initially, 0.2 mg. May repeat no more than q2-4h for no more than 5 doses total.

[$] **AVAILABLE FORMS/COST**

- Tab—Oral: 0.2 mg, 100's: **$45.80**

UNLABELED USES: Treatment of incomplete abortion, diagnosis of angina pectoris

CONTRAINDICATIONS: Induction of labor, threatened spontaneous abortions, hypersensitivity to ergonovine maleate or any component of the formulation

PREGNANCY AND LACTATION: Not recommended for routine use prior to delivery of the placenta; may lower prolactin levels, which may decrease lactation

SIDE EFFECTS

Frequent

Uterine cramping

Occasional

Diarrhea, dizziness, nasal congestion, sweating, ringing in ears

Rare

Headache, nausea, vomiting, allergic reaction

SERIOUS REACTIONS

- Severe hypertensive episodes may result in cerebrovascular accident, serious arrhythmias, seizures; hypertensive effects more frequent with rapid IV administration, concurrent regional anesthesia or vasoconstrictors.
- Peripheral ischemia may lead to gangrene.
- Overdose includes symptoms of angina, bradycardia, confusion, drowsiness, fast, weak pulse; miosis, severe peripheral vasoconstriction (numbness in arms or legs, blue skin color), seizures, tachycardia, thirst, and severe uterine cramping.

INTERACTIONS
Drugs
3 *Dopamine:* Excessive vasoconstriction
SPECIAL CONSIDERATIONS
• Symptoms of ergotism occur with overdosage (nausea, vomiting, diarrhea, seizure, hallucinations delirium, numb/gangrenous extremities)
MONITORING PARAMETERS
• Blood pressure, pulse, and uterine response

---

ergotamine
(er-got′a-meen)
Rx: Ergomar
Combinations
   Rx: with caffeine (Cafergot, Ercaf, Wigraine); with belladonna alkaloids, phenobarbital (Bellergal-S)
Chemical Class: Ergot alkaloid
Therapeutic Class: Antimigraine agent

CLINICAL PHARMACOLOGY
Mechanism of Action: An ergotamine derivative and alpha-adrenergic blocker that directly stimulates vascular smooth muscle, resulting in peripheral and cerebral vasoconstriction. May also have antagonist effects on serotonin. *Therapeutic Effect:* Suppresses vascular headaches.
Pharmacokinetics
Slowly and incompletely absorbed from the GI tract; rapidly and extensively absorbed after rectal administration. Protein binding: greater than 90%. Undergoes extensive first-pass metabolism in the liver to active metabolite. Eliminated in feces by the biliary system. **Half-life:** 21 hr.

INDICATIONS AND DOSAGES
Vascular headaches
PO (Cafergot [fixed-combination of ergotamine and caffeine])
Adults, Elderly. 2 mg at onset of headache, then 1–2 mg q30min. Maximum: 6 mg/episode; 10 mg/wk.
Sublingual
Adults, Elderly. 1 tablet at onset of headache, then 1 tablet q30min. Maximum: 3 tablets/24 hr; 5 tablets/wk.
PO, Sublingual
Children. 1 mg at onset of headache, then 1 mg q30min. Maximum: 3 mg/episode.
IV
Adults, Elderly. 1 mg at onset of headache; may repeat hourly. Maximum: 2 mg/day; 6 mg/wk.
IM, Subcutaneous (dihydroergotamine)
Adults, Elderly. 1 mg at onset of headache; may repeat hourly. Maximum: 3 mg/day; 6 mg/wk.
Intranasal
Adults, Elderly. 1 spray (0.5 mg) into each nostril; may repeat in 15 min. Maximum: 4 sprays/day; 8 sprays/wk.
Rectal
Adults, Elderly. 1 suppository at onset of headache; may repeat dose in 1 hr. Maximum: 2 suppositories/episode; 5 suppositories/wk.
AVAILABLE FORMS/COST
• Supp—Rectal (caffeine/ergotamine): 100 mg-2 mg, 12's: **$89.25**
• Tab—Oral (caffeine/ ergotamine): 100 mg-1 mg, 100's: **$77.39-$124.41**
CONTRAINDICATIONS: Coronary artery disease, hypertension, impaired hepatic or renal function, malnutrition, peripheral vascular diseases (such as thromboangiitis obliterans, syphilitic arteritis, se-

vere arteriosclerosis, thrombophlebitis, and Raynaud's disease), sepsis, severe pruritus

PREGNANCY AND LACTATION: Pregnancy category X; excreted into breast milk; has caused symptoms of ergotism (e.g., vomiting, diarrhea) in the infant; excessive dosage or prolonged administration may inhibit lactation

SIDE EFFECTS
Occasional (5%-2%)
Cough, dizziness
Rare (less than 2%)
Myalgia, fatigue, diarrhea, upper respiratory tract infection, dyspepsia

SERIOUS REACTIONS
• Prolonged administration or excessive dosage may produce ergotamine poisoning, manifested as nausea and vomiting; paresthesia, muscle pain or weakness; precordial pain; tachycardia or bradycardia; and hypertension or hypotension. Vasoconstriction of peripheral arteries and arterioles may result in localized edema and pruritus. Muscle pain will occur when walking and later, even at rest. Other rare effects include confusion, depression, drowsiness, seizures, and gangrene.

INTERACTIONS
Drugs
❷ *Azithromycin, dirithromycin, erythromycin:* Coadministration may result in ergotism
❷ *Nitroglycerin:* Decreased antianginal effects of nitroglycerin

SPECIAL CONSIDERATIONS

PATIENT/FAMILY EDUCATION
• Initiate therapy at first sign of attack
• DO NOT exceed recommended dosage
• Notify clinician of irregular heart beat, nausea, vomiting, numbness or tingling of fingers or toes, pain or weakness of extremities

• Regular use may lead to withdrawal headaches

---

ertapenem
(er-ta-pen'em)
Rx: Invanz
Chemical Class: Carbapenem
Therapeutic Class: Antibiotic

CLINICAL PHARMACOLOGY
Mechanism of Action: A carbapenem that penetrates the bacterial cell wall of microorganisms and binds to penicillin-binding proteins, inhibiting cell wall synthesis. *Therapeutic Effect:* Produces bacterial cell death.

Pharmacokinetics
Almost completely absorbed after IM administration. Protein binding: 85%-95%. Widely distributed. Primarily excreted in urine with smaller amount eliminated in feces. Removed by hemodialysis. **Half-life:** 4 hr.

INDICATIONS AND DOSAGES
Intraabdominal infection
IM, IV
Adults, Elderly. 1 g/day for 5-14 days.
Skin and skin structure infection
IM, IV
Adults, Elderly. 1 g/day for 7-14 days.
Pneumonia, urinary tract infection (UTI)
IM, IV
Adults, Elderly. 1 g/day for 10-14 days.
Pelvic infection
IM, IV
Adults, Elderly. 1 g/day for 3-10 days.
Dosage in renal impairment
For adults and elderly patients with creatinine clearance less than 30 ml/min dosage is 500 mg once a day.

AVAILABLE FORMS/COST
• Powder, Inj—IM, IV: 1 g/vial: **$51.48**

CONTRAINDICATIONS: History of hypersensitivity to beta-lactams (imipenem and cilastin, meropenem), hypersensitivity to amide-type local anesthetics (IM)

PREGNANCY AND LACTATION: Pregnancy category B; excreted into breast milk, bottle feeding recommended during and for 5 days after therapy

SIDE EFFECTS
Frequent (10%-6%)
Diarrhea, nausea, headache
Occasional (5%-2%)
Altered mental status, insomnia, rash, abdominal pain, constipation, vomiting, edema, fever
Rare (less than 2%)
Dizziness, cough, oral candidiasis, anxiety, tachycardia, phlebitis at IV site

SERIOUS REACTIONS
• Antibiotic-associated colitis and other superinfections may occur.
• Anaphylactic reactions have been reported.
• Seizures may occur in those with CNS disorders (including patients with brain lesions or a history of seizures), bacterial meningitis, or severe renal impairment.

INTERACTIONS
Drugs
▪ *Probenecid:* Increased ertapenem half-life

SPECIAL CONSIDERATIONS
• Daily dosing is advantage over imipenem or meropenem

---

erythromycin
(er-ith-roe-mye'sin)
Rx: *Systemic:* E-Mycin, Eryc, Ery-Tab, PCE Dispertab, Ilosone, E.E.S., Eryped, Ilotycin
Rx: *Topical:* A/T/S, Akne-Mycin, C-Solve 2, Emgel, Erycette, Eryderm, Erygel, Erymax, E-Solve 2, ETS-2%, Staticin, Theramycin Z, T-Stat
Rx: *Ophth:* AK-Mycin, Ilotycin
Combinations
  Rx: with sulfisoxazole (Pediazole); with benzoyl peroxide (Benzamycin)
Chemical Class: Macrolide derivative
Therapeutic Class: Antibiotic

CLINICAL PHARMACOLOGY
Mechanism of Action: A macrolide that reversibly binds to bacterial ribosomes, inhibiting bacterial protein synthesis. *Therapeutic Effect:* Bacteriostatic.
Pharmacokinetics
Variably absorbed from the GI tract (depending on dosage form used). Protein binding: 70%–90%. Widely distributed. Metabolized in the liver. Primarily eliminated in feces by bile. Not removed by hemodialysis.
Half-life: 1.4-2 hr (increased in impaired renal function).

INDICATIONS AND DOSAGES
Mild to moderate infections of the upper and lower respiratory tract, pharyngitis, skin infections
PO
Adults, Elderly. 250 mg q6h, 500 mg q12h, or 333 mg q8h. Maximum: 4 g/day.

Children. 30-50 mg/kg/day in divided doses up to 60-100 mg/kg/day for severe infections.

Neonates. 20-40 mg/kg/day in divided doses q6-12h.

IV

Adults, Elderly, Children. 15-20 mg/kg/day in divided doses. Maximum: 4 g/day.

Preoperative intestinal antisepsis

PO

Adults, Elderly. 1 g at 1 pm, 2 pm, and 11 pm on day before surgery (with neomycin).

Children. 20 mg/kg at 1pm, 2pm, and 11 pm on day before surgery (with neomycin).

Acne vulgaris

Topical

Adults. Apply thin layer to affected area twice a day.

Gonococcal ophthalmia neonatorum

Ophthalmic

Neonates. 0.5-2 cm no later than 1 hr after delivery.

S **AVAILABLE FORMS/COST**

Erythromycin Base

• Gel—Top: 2%, 30, 50, 60 g: **$14.75-$43.61**/30 g

• Oint—Ophth: 0.5%, 3.5 g: **$2.75-$8.49**

• Oint—Top: 2%, 25 g: **$42.95**

• Sol—Top: 1.5%, 60 ml: **$5.25-$28.36**; 2%, 60, 120 ml: **$2.90-$31.42**/60 ml

• Swab, Medicated—Top: 2%, 60's: **$25.34-$30.70**

• Tab—Oral: 250 mg, 100's: **$14.78**; 500 mg, 100's: **$27.15**

• Tab, Sus Action—Oral: 250 mg, 100's: **$25.25-$59.28**; 333 mg, 100's: **$20.56-$50.85**; 500 mg, 100's: **$42.52**

Erythromycin Estolate

• Cap, Gel—Oral: 250 mg, 100's: **$31.80-$48.70**

• Susp—Oral: 125 mg/5 ml, 100, 120, 200, 480 ml: **$31.50-$39.50**/480 ml; 250 mg/5 ml, 100, 120, 200, 480 ml: **$56.85-$66.75**/480 ml

Erythromycin Ethyl Succinate

• Granules Reconst—Oral: 200 mg/5 ml, 100, 200, 480 ml: **$14.02-$19.25**/200 ml; 400 mg/5 ml, 100, 200 ml: **$21.62-$30.54**/200 ml

• Granules Reconst, Drops—Oral: 100 mg/2.5 ml, 50 ml: **$6.85**

• Susp—Oral: 200 mg/5 ml, 100, 200, 480 ml: **$20.76-$23.50**/480 ml; 400 mg/5 ml, 100, 200, 480 ml: **$38.67-$42.48**/480 ml

• Tab—Oral: 400 mg, 100's: **$20.75-$31.20**

• Tab, Chewable—Oral: 200 mg, 40's: **$25.46**

Erythromycin Gluceptate

• Inj, Dry Sol—IV: 1 g/ampule, 50 ml: **$25.07**

Erythromycin Lactobionate

• Powder, Inj—IV: 500 mg/vial, 1's: **$3.70-$4.09**; 1 g/vial, 1's: **$7.65-$12.58**

Erythromycin Stearate

• Tab, Plain Coated—Oral: 250 mg, 100's: **$9.00-$21.28**; 500 mg, 100's: **$24.67-$56.00**

UNLABELED USES: Systemic: Treatment of acne vulgaris, chancroid, *Campylobacter* enteritis, gastroparesis, Lyme disease

Topical: Treatment of minor bacterial skin infections

Ophthalmic: Treatment of blepharitis, conjunctivitis, keratitis, chlamydial trachoma

CONTRAINDICATIONS: Administration of fixed-combination product, Pediazole, to infants younger than 2 months; history of hepatitis due to macrolides; hypersensitivity to macrolides; pre-existing hepatic disease.

PREGNANCY AND LACTATION:
Pregnancy category B; excreted into breast milk; compatible with breast-feeding

SIDE EFFECTS

Frequent
IV: Abdominal cramping or discomfort, phlebitis or thrombophlebitis
Topical: Dry skin (50%)

Occasional
Nausea, vomiting, diarrhea, rash, urticaria

Rare
Ophthalmic: Sensitivity reaction with increased irritation, burning, itching, and inflammation
Topical: Urticaria

SERIOUS REACTIONS
• Antibiotic-associated colitis and other superinfections may occur.
• High dosages in patients with renal impairment may lead to reversible hearing loss.
• Anaphylaxis and hepatotoxicity occur rarely.
• Ventricular arrhythmias and prolonged QT interval occur rarely with the IV drug form.

INTERACTIONS

Drugs

▨ *Alfentanil:* Prolonged anesthesia and respiratory depression

▨ *Alprazolam:* Increased plasma alprazolam concentration

▨ *Amprenavir:* Plasma concentrations of erythromycin may be increased by amprenavir; plasma concentrations of amprenavir may be increased by erythromycin

▨ *Atorvastatin:* Increased plasma atorvastatin concentration with risk of rhabdomyolysis

▨ *Bromocriptine:* Increased bromocriptine concentration with toxicity

▨ *Buspirone:* Increased plasma buspirone concentration

▨ *Carbamazepine:* Markedly increased plasma carbamazepine concentrations

❷ *Cisapride:* QT prolongation and dysrhythmia

❷ *Clozapine:* Increased plasma clozapine concentrations

▨ *Colchicine:* Potential colchicine toxicity

▨ *Cyclosporine:* Increased plasma cyclosporine concentrations

▨ *Diazepam:* Increased plasma concentration of diazepam

▨ *Digoxin:* Reduced bacterial flora may increase plasma digoxin concentrations

▨ *Disopyramide:* Increased plasma disopyramide concentrations

❷ *Ergotamine:* Potential for ergotism

▨ *Ethanol:* Ethanol reduces plasma erythromycin concentration

▨ *Felodipine:* Increased plasma felodipine concentrations

▨ *Food:* Food may increase or decrease the bioavailability of erythromycin

▨ *Indinavir:* Plasma concentrations of erythromycin may be increased by indinavir; plasma concentrations of indinavir may be increased by erythromycin

▨ *Itraconazole:* Increased plasma itraconazole concentration

▨ *Lovastatin:* Increased plasma lovastatin concentration with risk of rhabdomyolysis

▨ *Methylprednisolone:* Increased plasma methylprednisolone concentrations

▨ *Midazolam:* Increased plasma concentration of midazolam

▨ *Nelfinavir:* Plasma concentrations of erythromycin may be increased by nelfinavir; plasma concentrations of nelfinavir may be increased by erythromycin

3 *Penicillin:* Decreased activity of penicillin

3 *Quinidine:* Increased plasma concentration of quinidine

3 *Ritonavir:* Plasma concentrations of erythromycin may be increased by ritonavir; plasma concentrations of ritonavir may be increased by erythromycin

3 *Saquinavir:* Plasma concentrations of erythromycin may be increased by saquinavir; plasma concentrations of saquinavir may be increased by erythromycin

3 *Sildenafil:* Increased plasma sildenafil concentration

2 *Simvastatin:* Increased plasma simvastatin concentration with risk of rhabdomyolysis

3 *Tacrolimus:* Increased plasma tacrolimus concentration

3 *Theophylline:* Increased plasma theophylline concentration

3 *Triazolam:* Increased plasma triazolam concentration

3 *Valproic acid:* Increased plasma valproic acid concentration

3 *Warfarin:* Markedly increased hypoprothrombinemic response to warfarin

3 *Zafirlukast:* Reduced plasma zafirlukast concentration probably by reducing bioavailability

3 *Zopiclone:* Increased plasma zopiclone concentration

Labs

• *False decrease:* Folate assay
• *False increase:* Urine 17-ketosteroids, AST, urine amino acids

SPECIAL CONSIDERATIONS

PATIENT/FAMILY EDUCATION

• Take with food to minimize GI discomfort
• Take each dose with 180-240 ml of water
• Wash, rinse, and dry affected area prior to top application
• Keep top preparations away from eyes, nose, and mouth

• Ophth ointments may cause temporary blurring of vision following administration

MONITORING PARAMETERS

• LFTs if hepatotoxicity suspected
• Check daily for vein irritation and phlebitis in patients receiving IV forms

---

escitalopram

(es-sy-tal'oh-pram)
Chemical Class: Bicyclic phthalane derivative
Therapeutic Class: Antidepressant, selective serotonin reuptake inhibitor (SSRI)

CLINICAL PHARMACOLOGY

Mechanism of Action: A selective serotonin reuptake inhibitor that blocks the uptake of the neurotransmitter serotonin at neuronal presynaptic membranes, increasing its availability at postsynaptic receptor sites. *Therapeutic Effect:* Relieves depression.

Pharmacokinetics

Well absorbed after PO administration. Primarily metabolized in the liver. Primarily excreted in feces with a lesser amount eliminated in urine. **Half-life:** 35 hr.

INDICATIONS AND DOSAGES

Depression, general anxiety disorder (GAD)

PO

Adults. Initially, 10 mg once a day in the morning or evening. May increase to 20 mg after a minimum of 1 wk.

Elderly, Patients with hepatic impairment. 10 mg/day.

S **AVAILABLE FORMS/COST**

• Liq—Oral: 5 mg/5 ml, 240 ml: *cost not available*
• Tab—Oral: 10 mg, 100's: **$222.35**; 20 mg, 100's: **$232.04**

CONTRAINDICATIONS: Breast-feeding, use within 14 days of MAOIs

PREGNANCY AND LACTATION: Pregnancy category C; excreted in human breast milk; reports of infants experiencing excessive somnolence, decreased feeding, and weight loss in association with breast-feeding from a citalopram-treated mother

SIDE EFFECTS

Frequent (21%-11%)

Nausea, dry mouth, somnolence, insomnia, diaphoresis

Occasional (8%-4%)

Tremor, diarrhea, abnormal ejaculation, dyspepsia, fatigue, anxiety, vomiting, anorexia

Rare (3%-2%)

Sinusitis, sexual dysfunction, menstrual disorder, abdominal pain, agitation, decreased libido

SERIOUS REACTIONS

• Overdose is manifested as dizziness, drowsiness, tachycardia, somnolence, confusion, and seizures.

INTERACTIONS

Drugs

▨ *Cimetidine:* Increased citalopram levels

▲ *MAOIs:* See Precautions

▨ *Sumatriptan:* Syndrome of weakness, hyperreflexia, and incoordination following combination (rarely)

SPECIAL CONSIDERATIONS

• Patent extension for a useful agent; not different from citalopram

MONITORING PARAMETERS

• Improvement of symptoms of depression or anxiety/depression, suicidal ideation, signs of toxicity (e.g., somnolence, sleep disturbances, persistent GI symptoms)

---

esmolol

(ess'moe-lol)

Rx: Brevibloc

Chemical Class: β_1-adrenergic blocker, cardioselective

Therapeutic Class: Antiarrhythmic, class II

CLINICAL PHARMACOLOGY

Mechanism of Action: An antiarrhythmic that selectively blocks beta$_1$-adrenergic receptors. *Therapeutic Effect:* Slows sinus heart rate, decreases cardiac output, reducing BP.

INDICATIONS AND DOSAGES

Arrythmias

IV

Adults, Elderly. Initially, loading dose of 500 mcg/kg/min for 1 min, followed by 50 mcg/kg/min for 4 min. If optimum response is not attained in 5 min, give second loading dose of 500 mcg/kg/min for 1 min, followed by infusion of 100 mcg/kg/min for 4 min. Additional loading doses can be given and infusion increased by 50 mcg/kg/min, up to 200 mcg/kg/min, for 4 min. Once desired response is attained, cease loading dose and increase infusion by no more than 25 mcg/kg/min. Interval between doses may be increased to 10 min. Infusion usually administered over 24–48 hr in most patients. Range: 50–200 mcg/kg/min, with average dose of 100 mcg/kg/min.

Intra-operative tachycardia or hypertension (immediate control)

IV

Adults, Elderly. Initially, 80 mg over 30 seconds, then 150 mcg/kg/min infusion up to 300 mcg/kg/min.

$ AVAILABLE FORMS/COST
• Sol, Inj—IV: 10 mg/ml, 10: **$22.07-$22.99**; 250 mg/ml, 10 ml: **$108.91**

CONTRAINDICATIONS: Cardiogenic shock, overt cardiac failure, second- and third-degree heart block, sinus bradycardia

PREGNANCY AND LACTATION: Pregnancy category C; potential for hypotension and subsequent decreased uterine blood flow and fetal hypoxia should be considered; excretion into breast milk unknown; use caution in nursing mothers

SIDE EFFECTS
Esmolol is generally well tolerated, with transient and mild side effects.

Frequent

Hypotension (systolic BP less than 90 mm Hg) manifested as dizziness, nausea, diaphoresis, headache, cold extremities, fatigue

Occasional

Anxiety, drowsiness, flushed skin, vomiting, confusion, inflammation at injection site, fever

SERIOUS REACTIONS
• Overdose may produce profound hypotension, bradycardia, dizziness, syncope, drowsiness, breathing difficulty, bluish fingernails or palms of hands, and seizures.

• Esmolol administration may potentiate insulin-induced hypoglycemia in diabetic patients.

INTERACTIONS
Drugs

▪ *α₁-adrenergic blockers:* Potential enhanced first dose response (marked initial drop in blood pressure, particularly on standing (especially prazocin)

▪ *Amiodarone:* Symptomatic bradycardia and sinus arrest; AV node refractory period is prolonged and sinus node automaticity is decreased by amiodarone. The sinus rate can be further slowed or AV block worsened in patients with bradycardia, sick sinus syndrome, or partial AV block

▪ *Dihydropyridine calcium channel blockers:* Severe hypotension or impaired cardiac performance; most prevalent with impaired left ventricular function, cardiac arrhythmias, or aortic stenosis

▪ *Digoxin:* Additive prolongation of atrioventricular (AV) conduction time

▪ *Diltiazem:* Potentiates β-adrenergic effects; hypotension, left ventricular failure, and AV conduction disturbances problematic in elderly, patients with left ventricular dysfunction, aortic stenosis, or with large doses of either drug

▪ *Hypoglycemic agents:* Masked hypoglycemia, hyperglycemia

▪ *Verapamil:* Potentiates β-adrenergic effects; hypotension, left ventricular failure, and AV conduction disturbances problematic in elderly, patients with left ventricular dysfunction, aortic stenosis, or with large doses of either drug

SPECIAL CONSIDERATIONS
• Transfer to alternative agent (e.g., propranolol, digoxin, verapamil): ½ hr after first dose of alternative agent, reduce esmolol INF rate by 50%; following second dose of alternative agent, monitor patient's response and, if satisfactory control is maintained for the first hr, discontinue esmolol INF

• Do not discontinue abruptly; may require taper; rapid withdrawal may produce rebound hypertension or angina

MONITORING PARAMETERS
• Angina: Reduction in nitroglycerin usage; frequency, severity, onset, and duration of angina pain; heart rate

• Arrhythmias: Heart rate

• Hypertension: Blood pressure

• Postmyocardial infarction: Left ventricular function, lower resting heart rate
• Toxicity: Blood glucose, bronchospasm, hypotension, bradycardia, depression, confusion, hallucination, sexual dysfunction

---

esomeprazole
(es-om-eh-pray'zole)
Rx: Nexium
Chemical Class: Benzimidazole derivative
Therapeutic Class: Antiulcer agent; gastrointestinal antisecretory agent

CLINICAL PHARMACOLOGY
Mechanism of Action: A proton pump inhibitor that is converted to active metabolites that irreversibly bind to and inhibit hydrogen-potassium adenosine triphosphates, an enzyme on the surface of gastric parietal cells. Inhibits hydrogen ion transport into gastric lumen. *Therapeutic Effect:* Increases gastric pH, reducing gastric acid production.
Pharmacokinetics
Well absorbed after oral administration. Protein binding: 97%. Extensively metabolized by the liver. Primarily excreted in urine. **Half-life:** 1–1.5 hrs.
INDICATIONS AND DOSAGES
Erosive esophagitis
PO
Adults, Elderly. 20–40 mg once daily for 4–8 wk.
To maintain healing of erosive esophagitis
PO
Adults, Elderly. 20 mg/day.
Gastroesophageal reflux disease
PO
Adults, Elderly. 20 mg once a day for 4 wk.

Duodenal ulcer caused by Helicobacter pylori
PO
Adults, Elderly. 40 mg (esomeprazole) once a day, with amoxicillin 1,000 mg and clarithromycin 500 mg twice a day for 10 days.

$ AVAILABLE FORMS/COST
• Cap, Delayed-Release—Oral: 20 mg, 40 mg, 100's; all: **$399.66**
CONTRAINDICATIONS: None known
PREGNANCY AND LACTATION: Pregnancy category B; likely to be excreted into breast milk, use caution in nursing mothers (suppression of gastric acid secretion is potential effect in nursing infant, clinical significance unknown)
SIDE EFFECTS
Frequent (7%)
Headache
Occasional (3%–2%)
Diarrhea, abdominal pain, nausea
Rare (less than 2%)
Dizziness, asthenia or loss of strength, vomiting, constipation, rash, cough
SERIOUS REACTIONS
• None known.
INTERACTIONS
Drugs
⚠ *Ketoconazole, iron salts, digoxin:* Reduced gastric acidity may result in decreased absorption of these and other drugs where gastric pH is an important determinant of bioavailability
SPECIAL CONSIDERATIONS
• S-isomer of omeprazole (racemate)
• No advantage over other proton-pump inhibitors, cost should govern choice
PATIENT/FAMILY EDUCATION
• Take at least 1 hr before meals

• Capsules may be opened, mixed with cold applesauce and swallowed immediately without chewing for patients who cannot swallow capsules whole

---

estazolam
(es-tay-zoe-lam)
Rx: ProSom
Chemical Class: Benzodiazepine
Therapeutic Class: Sedative/hypnotic
DEA Class: Schedule IV

CLINICAL PHARMACOLOGY
Mechanism of Action: A benzodiazepine that enhances action of gamma aminobutyric acid (GABA) neurotransmission in the central nervous system (CNS). *Therapeutic Effect:* Produces depressant effect at all levels of central nervous system (CNS).

Pharmacokinetics
Rapidly absorbed from gastrointestinal (GI) tract. Protein binding: 93%. Metabolized in liver. Primarily excreted in urine, minimal in feces. **Half-life:** 10-24 hrs.

INDICATIONS AND DOSAGES
Insomnia
PO
Adults (older than 18 yrs). 1-2 mg at bedtime.
Elderly, debilitated, liver disease, low serum albumin. 0.5-1 mg at bedtime.

$ AVAILABLE FORMS/COST
• Tab—Oral: 1 mg, 100's: **$88.70-$134.90**; 2 mg, 100's: **$98.92-$150.29**

CONTRAINDICATIONS: Pregnancy, hypersensitivity to other benzodiazepines

PREGNANCY AND LACTATION:
Pregnancy category X; may cause fetal damage when administered during pregnancy; excreted into breast milk; may accumulate in breast-fed infants and is therefore not recommended

SIDE EFFECTS
Frequent
Drowsiness, sedation, rebound insomnia (may occur for 1-2 nights after drug is discontinued), dizziness, confusion, euphoria
Occasional
Weakness, anorexia, diarrhea
Rare
Paradoxical CNS excitement, restlessness (particularly noted in elderly/debilitated)

SERIOUS REACTIONS
• Overdosage results in somnolence, confusion, diminished reflexes, and coma.

INTERACTIONS
Drugs
▣ *Cimetidine:* Increased serum benzodiazepine concentrations
▣ *Disulfiram:* May increase benzodiazepine serum concentrations
▣ *Erythromycin:* Increased estazolam sedative effects
▣ *Ethanol:* Enhanced adverse psychomotor effects of benzodiazepines
▣ *Rifampin:* Reduced serum benzodiazepine concentrations

SPECIAL CONSIDERATIONS
PATIENT/FAMILY EDUCATION
• Do not discontinue abruptly after prolonged therapy
• May experience disturbed sleep for the first or second night after discontinuing the drug

estradiol

(ess-tra-dye′ole)

Rx: *Oral:* Estrace, Vagifem
Rx: *Estradiol Cypionate Inj:* Depo-Estradiol, DepoGen, Estro-Cyp
Rx: *Estradiol Valerate Inj:* Delestrogen, Valergen
Rx: *Transdermal:* Alora, Climara, E$_2$ III, Esclim, Estraderm, Menostar, Vivelle, Vivelle-Dot
Rx: *Vaginal Insert:* Estring
Combinations
  Rx: with medroxyprogesterone (Lunelle)
  Rx: with norgestimate (Ortho-Prefest)
  Rx: with testosterone cypionate (Depo-Testadiol)
  Rx: with testosterone enanthate (Deladumone)
  Rx: Transdermal with levonorgestrel (Climara Pro); Transdermal with norethindrone (Combi-Patch)
Chemical Class: Estrogen derivative
Therapeutic Class: Antineoplastic; antiosteoporotic; estrogen

CLINICAL PHARMACOLOGY

Mechanism of Action: An estrogen that increases synthesis of DNA, RNA, and proteins in target tissues; reduces release of gonadotropin-releasing hormone from the hypothalamus; and reduces follicle-stimulating hormone and luteinizing hormone (LH) release from the pituitary. *Therapeutic Effect:* Promotes normal growth, promotes development of female sex organs, and maintains GU function and vasomotor stability. Prevents accelerated bone loss by inhibiting bone resorption, restoring balance of bone resorption and formation. Inhibits LH and decreases serum testosterone concentration.

Pharmacokinetics

Well absorbed from the GI tract. Widely distributed. Protein binding: 50%–80%. Metabolized in the liver. Primarily excreted in urine. **Half-life:** Unknown.

INDICATIONS AND DOSAGES

Prostate cancer

IM (valerate)
Adults, Elderly. 30 mg or more q1-2 wk.
PO
Adults, Elderly. 10 mg 3 times a day for at least 3 mo.

Breast cancer

PO
Adults, Elderly. 10 mg 3 times a day for at least 3 mo.

Osteoporosis prophylaxis in postmenopausal females

PO
Adults, Elderly. 0.5 mg/day cyclically (3 weeks on, 1 week off).
Transdermal (Climara)
Adults, Elderly. Initially, 0.025 mg weekly, adjust dose as needed.
Transdermal (Alora, Vivelle, Vivelle-Dot):
Adults, Elderly. Initially, 0.025 mg patch twice weekly, adjust dose as needed.
Transdermal (Estraderm)
Adults, Elderly. 0.05 mg twice weekly.
Transdermal (Menostar)
Adults, Elderly.: 1 mg weekly.

Female hypoestrogenism

PO
Adults, Elderly. 1-2 mg/day, adjust dose as needed.
IM (cypionate)
Adults, Elderly. 1.5-2 mg monthly.
IM (valerate)
Adults, Elderly. 10-20 mg q4wk.

Vasomotor symptoms associated with menopause
PO
Adults, Elderly. 1-2 mg/day cyclically (3 weeks on, 1 week off), adjust dose as needed.
IM (cypionate)
Adults, Elderly. 1-5 mg q3-4wk.
IM (valerate)
Adults, Elderly. 10-20 mg q4wk.
Topical emulsion (Estrasorb)
Adults, Elderly. 3.84 g once a day in the morning.
Topical Gel (Estrogel)
Adults, Elderly. 1.25 g/day.
Transdermal (Climara)
Adults, Elderly. 0.025 mg weekly. Adjust dose as needed.
Transderamal (Alora, Esclim, Estrader, Vivelle-Dot)
Adults, Elderly. 0.05 mg twice a week.
Transdermal (Vivelle)
Adults, Elderly. 0.0375 mg twice a week.
Vaginal ring (Femring)
Adults, Elderly. 0.05 mg. May increase to 0.1 mg if needed.
Vaginal atrophy
Vaginal Ring (Estring)
Adults, Elderly. 2 mg.
Atrophic vaginitis
Vaginal tablet (Vagifem)
Adults, Elderly. Initially, 1 tablet/day for 2 weeks. Maintenance: 1 tablet twice a week.

[$] **AVAILABLE FORMS/COST**
• Cre—Vag: 0.01%, 42.5 g: **$39.49-$67.75**
• Film, Cont Rel—Transdermal: 0.025 mg/24 hr 8's: **$30.49-$34.63**; 0.0375 mg/24 hr, 8's: **$25.68-$34.89**; 0.05 mg/24 hr, 8's: **$24.60** (Vivelle); 0.05 mg/24 hr, 8's: **$18.38-$35.55**; 0.075 mg/24 hr, 8's: **$30.38-$36.30**; 0.1 mg/24 hr, 8's: **$20.04-$37.06**; 0.05 mg/0.14 mg norethindrone/24 hr, 8's: **$33.60**; 0.05 mg/0.25 mg norethindrone/24 hr, 8's: **$34.44**
• Sol, Inj—IM (Cypionate): 5 mg/ml, 5, 10 ml: **$5.50-$15.52**/10 ml
• Sol, Inj (Valerate)—IM: 10 mg/ml, 5, 10 ml: **$6.95-$7.45**/10 ml; 20 mg/ml, 1, 5, 10 ml: **$8.95-$45.68**/10 ml; 40 mg/ml, 5, 10 ml: **$12.60-$75.79**/10 ml
• Ring, Cont Rel—Vag: 2 mg (0.0075 mg/24 hr), 1's: **$108.61**
• Ring, Cont Rel-Vag (acetate): 0.05 mg/24 hr, 1's: **$95.63**; 0.1 mg/24 hr, 1's: **$101.88**
• Tab—Oral: 0.5 mg, 100's: **$22.81-$61.30**; 1 mg, 100's: **$30.39-$81.68**; 1.5 mg, 100's: **$50.83**; 2 mg, 100's: **$44.38-$119.28**; 1 mg/0.5 mg norethindrone, 28's: **$26.09** (Activella)

UNLABELED USES: Treatment of Turner's syndrome

CONTRAINDICATIONS: Abnormal vaginal bleeding, active arterial thrombosis, blood dyscrasias, estrogen-dependent cancer, known or suspected breast cancer, pregnancy, thrombophlebitis or thromboembolic disorders, thyroid dysfunction

PREGNANCY AND LACTATION: Pregnancy category X; may reduce quantity and quality of breast milk

SIDE EFFECTS
Frequent
Anorexia, nausea, swelling of breasts, peripheral edema marked by swollen ankles and feet
Transdermal: Skin irritation, redness
Occasional
Vomiting, especially with high doses; headache that may be severe; intolerance to contact lenses; hypertension; glucose intolerance; brown spots on exposed skin

Vaginal: Local irritation, vaginal discharge, changes in vaginal bleeding, including spotting, and breakthrough or prolonged bleeding

Rare

Chorea or involuntary movements, hirsutism or abnormal hairiness, loss of scalp hair, depression

SERIOUS REACTIONS

• Prolonged administration increases the risk of gallbladder disease, thromboembolic disease, and breast, cervical, vaginal, endometrial, and hepatic carcinoma.

• Cholestatic jaundice occurs rarely.

INTERACTIONS

Drugs

3 *P450 inducers (e.g., rifampin, barbiturates):* Decreased estrogen levels

3 *Corticosteroids:* Increased steroid effect

3 *Phenytoin:* Loss of seizure control, decreased estrogen levels

3 *Warfarin:* Theoretical increased risk thromboembolism

SPECIAL CONSIDERATIONS

• Progestins recommended in non-hysterectomized women. Estring may have minimal systemic absorption

estrogens, conjugated

Rx: Cenestin, Enjuvia, Premarin

Combinations

Rx: with medroxyprogesterone (Prempro [daily product], Premphase [cycled product]); with meprobamate (PMB); with methyltestosterone (Premarin with methyltestosterone)

Chemical Class: Estrogen derivative

Therapeutic Class: Antineoplastic; antiosteoporotic; estrogen

CLINICAL PHARMACOLOGY

Mechanism of Action: An estrogen that increases synthesis of DNA, RNA, and various proteins in target tissues; reduces release of gonadotropin-releasing hormone from the hypothalamus; and reducies follicle-stimulating hormone (FSH) and leuteinizing hormone (LH) release from the pituitary gland. *Therapeutic Effect:* Promotes normal growth, promotes development of femal sex organs, and maintains GU function and vasomotor stability. Prevents accelerated bone loss by inhibiting bone resorption, restoring balance of bone resorption and formation. Inhibits LH and decreases serum concentration of testosterone.

Pharmacokinetics

Well absorbed from the GI tract. Widely distributed. Protein binding: 50%–80%. Metabolized in the liver. Primarily excreted in urine.

INDICATIONS AND DOSAGES

Vasomotor symptoms associated with menopause, atrophic vaginitis, kraurosis vulvae
PO
Adults, Elderly. 0.3–0.625 mg/day cyclically (21 days on, 7 days off) or continuously.
Intravaginal
Adults, Elderly. 0.5–2 g/day cyclically, such as 21 days on and 7 days off.

Female hypogonadism
PO
Adults. 0.3–0.625 mg/day in divided doses for 20 days; then a rest period of 10 days.

Female castration, primary ovarian failure
PO
Adults. Initially, 1.25 mg/day cyclically. Adjust dosage, upward or downward, according to severity of symptoms and patient response. For Maintenance, adjust dosage to lowest level that will provide effective control.

Osteoporosis
PO
Adults, Elderly. 0.3–0.625 mg/day, cyclically, such as 25 days on and 5 days off.

Breast cancer
PO
Adults, Elderly. 10 mg 3 times a day for at least 3 mo.

Prostate cancer
PO
Adults, Elderly. 1.25–2.5 mg 3 times a day.

Abnormal uterine bleeding
PO
Adults. 1.25 mg q4h for 24 hr, then 1.25 mg/day for 7–10 days.
IV, IM
Adults. 25 mg; may repeat once in 6–12 hr.

Ⓢ AVAILABLE FORMS/COST

• Cre, Top—Vag: 0.625 mg/g, 42.5 g: **$68.69**
• Powder, Inj—IM, IV: 25 mg/5 ml: **$58.00**
• Tab—Oral: 0.3 mg, 100's: **$91.38**; 0.45 mg, 100's: **$104.25**; 0.625 mg, 100's: **$39.45-$104.25**; 0.9 mg, 100's: **$69.53-$125.38**; 1.25 mg, 100's: **$88.90-$133.50**; 2.5 mg, 100's: **$179.83**
Combination Products
• Tab—Oral: 0.3 mg/1.5 mg medroxyprogesterone, 28's: **$118.38**; 0.45 mg-1.5 mg medroxyprogesterone, 28's: **$39.46**; 0.625 mg-2.5 mg medroxyprogesterone, 28's: **$17.88-$39.46**; 0.625 mg-5.0 mg medroxyprogesterone, 28's: **$21.60-$39.46**; 0.625 mg/5 mg medroxyprogesterone (Premphase), 28's: **$18.38-$38.50**

UNLABELED USES: Prevention of estrogen deficiency–induced premenopausal osteoporosis
Cream: Prevention of nosebleeds

CONTRAINDICATIONS: Breast cancer with some exceptions, hepatic disease, thrombophlebitis, undiagnosed vaginal bleeding

PREGNANCY AND LACTATION: Pregnancy category X; may decrease quantity and quality of breast milk

SIDE EFFECTS

Frequent
Vaginal bleeding, such as spotting or breakthrough bleeding; breast pain or tenderness; gynecomastia
Occasional
Headache, hypertension, intolerance to contact lenses
High-doses: Anorexia, nausea
Rare
Loss of scalp hair, depression

SERIOUS REACTIONS

• Prolonged administration may increase the risk of gallbladder disease, thromboembolic disease, and breast, cervical, vaginal, endometrial, and hepatic carcinoma.

INTERACTIONS

Drugs

3 *P450 inducers (e.g., rifampin, barbiturates):* Decreased estrogen levels

3 *Corticosteroids:* Increased steroid effect

3 *Phenytoin:* Loss of seizure control, decreased estrogen levels

3 *Warfarin:* Theoretical increased risk thromboembolism

SPECIAL CONSIDERATIONS

• Progestins recommended in non-hysterectomized women

• Premarin is derived from pregnant mare's urine; Cenestin from yams and soy. Although probably therapeutically equivalent, they are not substitutable by the pharmacist

• Consider topical products if treatment is solely for vulvar or vaginal atrophy

• Currently recommended that use of hormone replacement therapy be limited to treating symptomatic women, preferrably for ≤5 yrs. Risk felt to outweigh benefit in asymptomatic women using only for prophylaxis of other conditions

---

estrogens, esterified

Rx: Estratab, Menest
Combinations
   Rx: with methyltestosterone
   (Estratest, Menogen)
Chemical Class: Estrogen derivative
Therapeutic Class: Antineoplastic; antiosteoporotic; estrogen

E

CLINICAL PHARMACOLOGY

Mechanism of Action: A combination of sodium salts of sulfate esters of estrogenic substances (principle component is estrone) that increases synthesis of DNA, RNA, and various proteins in responsive tissues. Reduces release of gonadotropin-releasing hormone, reducing follicle-stimulating hormone (FSH) and leuteinizing hormone (LH). *Therapeutic Effect:* Promotes vasomotor stability, maintains genitourinary (GU) function, normal growth, development of female sex organs. Prevents accelerated bone loss by inhibiting bone resorption, restoring balance of bone resorption and formation.

Pharmacokinetics

Readily absorbed from the gastrointestinal (GI) tract. Widely distributed. Protein binding: 50%-80%. Rapidly metabolized in liver and GI tract to estrone sulfate and conjugated and unconjugated metabolites. Excreted in urine and bile. **Half-life:** Unknown.

INDICATIONS AND DOSAGES

Vasomotor symptoms associated with menopause, atrophic vaginitis, kraurosis vulvae

PO

Adults, Elderly. 0.3-1.25 mg/day.

Female hypogonadism
PO
Adults. 2.5-7.5 mg/day in divided doses for 20 days; rest 10 days.
Female castration, primary ovarian failure
PO
Adults. Initially, 1. 25 mg/day cyclically.
Breast cancer
PO
Adults, Elderly. 10 mg 3 times/day for at least 3 mos.
Prostate cancer
PO
Adults, Elderly. 1.25-2. 5 mg 3 times/day.

$ AVAILABLE FORMS/COST
• Tab—Oral: 0.3 mg, 100's: **$14.53-$41.18**; 0.625 mg, 100's: **$51.37-$61.72**; 1.25 mg, 100's: **$81.63**; 2.5 mg, 50's: **$76.00**; 0.625 mg/1.25 mg methyltestosterone, 100's: **$63.25-$162.16**; 1.25 mg/2.5 mg methyltestosterone, 100's: **$79.00-$198.54**

CONTRAINDICATIONS: Breast cancer with some exceptions, liver disease, thrombophlebitis, undiagnosed vaginal bleeding

PREGNANCY AND LACTATION: Pregnancy category X; may decrease quantity and quality of breast milk

SIDE EFFECTS
Frequent
Change in vaginal bleeding, such as spotting or breakthrough bleeding, breast pain or tenderness, gynecomastia
Occasional
Headache, increased blood pressure (BP), intolerance to contact lenses, nausea
Rare
Loss of scalp hair, clinical depression

SERIOUS REACTIONS
• Prolonged administration may increase risk of gallbladder, thromboembolic disease, breast, cervical, vaginal, endometrial, and liver carcinoma.

INTERACTIONS
Drugs
▣ *P450 inducers (e.g., rifampin, barbiturates):* Decreased estrogen levels
▣ *Corticosteroids:* Increased steroid effect
▣ *Phenytoin:* Loss of seizure control, decreased estrogen levels
▣ *Warfarin:* Theoretical increased risk thromboembolism

SPECIAL CONSIDERATIONS
• Progestins recommended in non-hysterectomized women

---

estrone
(ess'trone)
Rx: Estragyn-5, Estro-A, Kestrone-5, Primestrin
Chemical Class: Estrogen derivative
Therapeutic Class: Antineoplastic; estrogen

CLINICAL PHARMACOLOGY
Mechanism of Action: An estrogen that increases synthesis of DNA, RNA, proteins in target tissues; reduces release of gonadotropin-releasing hormone from hypothalamus; reduces follicle-stimulating hormone (FSH) and luteinizing hormone (LH) release from the pituitary. *Therapeutic Effect:* Promotes normal growth, development of female sex organs, maintaining genitourinary (GU) function, vasomotor stability. Prevents accelerated bone loss by inhibiting bone resorption, restoring balance of bone resorption

and formation. Inhibits LH, decreases serum concentration of testosterone.

Pharmacokinetics

Well absorbed from the gastrointestinal (GI) tract. Widely distributed. Protein binding: 50%-80%. Metabolized in liver as well as a certain proportion excreted into the bile and reabsorbed from the intestine. Primarily excreted in urine. **Half-life:** Unknown.

INDICATIONS AND DOSAGES

Atrophic vaginitis, female castration, female hypogonadism, Kraurosis vulvae, menopausal symptoms, primary ovarian failure, prostatic carcinoma

IM

Adults. Initially, 0.1 or 0.5 mg 2-3 times weekly cyclically (21 days on; 7 days off or continuously). When progestin is given concomitantly, begin progestin after 10-13 days of each estrogen cycle.

§ AVAILABLE FORMS/COST

• Susp, Inj—IM: 2 mg/ml, 10, 30 ml: **$5.00-$9.98**/10 ml; 5 mg/ml, 10, 30 ml: **$10.00-$18.50**/10 ml

CONTRAINDICATIONS: Abnormal vaginal bleeding, active arterial thrombosis, blood dyscrasias, estrogen-dependent cancer, known or suspected breast cancer, pregnancy, thrombophlebitis or thromboembolic disorders, hypersensitivity to estrone or any of its components.

PREGNANCY AND LACTATION: Pregnancy category X; may reduce quantity and quality of breast milk

SIDE EFFECTS

Frequent

Transient menstrual abnormalities including spotting, change in menstrual flow or cervical secretions, and amenorrhea at initiation of therapy

Occasional

Edema, weight change, breast tenderness, nervousness, insomnia, fatigue, dizziness

Rare

Alopecia, mental depression, dermatologic changes, headache, fever, nausea

SERIOUS REACTIONS

• Thrombophlebitis, pulmonary or cerebral embolism, and retinal thrombosis occur rarely.

INTERACTIONS

Drugs

3 *P450 inducers (e.g., rifampin, barbiturates):* Decreased estrogen levels

3 *Corticosteroids:* Increased steroid effect

3 *Phenytoin:* Loss of seizure control, decreased estrogen levels

3 *Warfarin:* Theoretical increased risk thromboembolism

SPECIAL CONSIDERATIONS

• Progestins recommended in non-hysterectomized women

• Consider topical products if treatment is solely for vulvar or vaginal atrophy

• Currently recommended that use of hormone replacement therapy be limited to treating symptomatic women, preferably for ≤5 yrs. Risk felt to outweigh benefit in asymptomatic women using only for prophylaxis of other conditions

estropipate
(es-tro-pip'ate)
Rx: Ogen, Ortho-Est
Chemical Class: Estrogen derivative
Therapeutic Class: Antiosteoporotic; estrogen

CLINICAL PHARMACOLOGY
Mechanism of Action: An estrogen that increases synthesis of DNA, RNA, abd proteins in target tissues; reduces release of gonadotropin-releasing hormone from the hypothalamus; and reduces follicle-stimulating hormone (FSH) and luteinizing hormone (LH) from the pituitary. *Therapeutic Effect:* Promotes normal growth, promotes development of female sex organs, and maintains GU function and vasomotor stability. Prevents accelerated bone loss by inhibiting bone resorption, restoring balance of bone resorption and formation. Inhibits LH and decreases serum testosterone concentration.

INDICATIONS AND DOSAGES
Vasomotor symptoms, atrophic vaginitis, kraurosis vulvae
PO
Adults, Elderly. 0.625–5 mg/day cyclically.
Atrophic vaginitis, kraurosis vulvae
Intravaginal
Adults, Elderly. 2–4 g/day cyclically.
Female hypogonadism, castration, primary ovarian failure
PO
Adults, Elderly. 1.25–7.5 mg/day for 21 days; then off for 8–10 days. Repeat if bleeding does not occur by end of off cycle.
Prevention of osteoporosis
PO
Adults, Elderly. 0.625 mg/day (25 days of 31-day cycle/mo).

$ **AVAILABLE FORMS/COST**
• Tab—Oral: 0.75 mg, 100's: **$21.40-$90.69**; 1.5 mg, 100's: **$29.43-$126.68**; 3 mg, 100's: **$100.35-$220.49**

CONTRAINDICATIONS: Abnormal vaginal bleeding, active arterial thrombosis, blood dyscrasias, estrogen-dependent cancer, known or suspected breast cancer, pregnancy, thrombophlebitis or thromboembolic disorders, thyroid dysfunction

PREGNANCY AND LACTATION: Pregnancy category X; may reduce quantity and quality of breast milk

SIDE EFFECTS
Frequent
Anorexia, nausea, swelling of breasts, peripheral edema marked by swollen ankles and feet
Occasional
Vomiting, especially with high doses; headache that may be severe; intolerance to contact lenses; hypertension; glucose intolerance; brown spots on exposed skin
Vaginal: Local irritation, vaginal discharge, changes in vaginal bleeding, including spotting, and breakthrough or prolonged bleeding
Rare
Chorea or involuntary movements, hirsutism or abnormal hairiness, loss of scalp hair, depression

SERIOUS REACTIONS
• Prolonged administration increases the risk of gallbladder disease, thromboembolic disease and breast, cervical, vaginal, endometrial, and hepatic carcinoma.
• Cholestatic jaundice occurs rarely.

INTERACTIONS
Drugs
3 *P450 inducers (e.g., rifampin, barbiturates):* Decreased estrogen levels

3 *Corticosteroids:* Increased steroid effect

3 *Phenytoin:* Loss of seizure control, decreased estrogen levels

3 *Warfarin:* Theoretical increased risk thromboembolism

SPECIAL CONSIDERATIONS

• Unopposed estrogen increases risk of endometrial cancer; recommended administration of concurrent progestational agents for non-hysterectomized women

---

etanercept

(e-tan′er-cept)

Rx: Enbrel

Chemical Class: Recombinant human fusion protein

Therapeutic Class: Disease-modifying antirheumatic drug (DMARD); immunomodulatory agent

---

CLINICAL PHARMACOLOGY

Mechanism of Action: A protein that binds to tumor necrosis factor (TNF), blocking its interaction with cell surface receptors. Elevated levels of TNF, which is involved in inflammatory and immune responses, are found in the synovial fluid of rheumatoid arthritis patients. *Therapeutic Effect:* Relieves symptoms of rheumatoid arthritis.

Pharmacokinetics

Well absorbed after subcutaneous administration. **Half-life:** 115 hr.

INDICATIONS AND DOSAGES

Rheumatoid arthritis, psoriatic arthritis, ankylosing spondylitis

Subcutaneous

Adults, Elderly. 25 mg twice weekly given 72–96 hr apart. Alternative weekly dosing: 0.8 mg/kg/dose once a week. Maximum: 50 mg/week. Maximum: 25 mg/dose.

Juvenile rheumatoid arthritis

Children 4–17 yr. 0.4 mg/kg (Maximum: 25 mg dose) twice weekly given 72–96 hr apart. Alternative weekly dosing: 50 mg once weekly. Maximum: 25 mg/dose.

Plaque psoriasis

Subcutaneous

Adults, Elderly. 50 mg twice a week (give 3-4 days apart) for 3 mo. Maintenance: 50 mg once a week.

$ **AVAILABLE FORMS/COST**

• Powder, Inj—SQ: 25 mg; 1's: **$155.70**

UNLABELED USES: Treatment of Crohn's disease

CONTRAINDICATIONS: Serious active infection or sepsis

PREGNANCY AND LACTATION: Pregnancy category B; information on breast milk excretion is unknown; breast-feeding not advised

SIDE EFFECTS

Frequent (37%)

Injection site erythema, pruritus, pain, and swelling; abdominal pain, vomiting (more common in children than adults)

Occasional (16%–4%)

Headache, rhinitis, dizziness, pharyngitis, cough, asthenia, abdominal pain, dyspepsia

Rare (less than 3%)

Sinusitis, allergic reaction

SERIOUS REACTIONS

• Infections (such as pyelonephritis, cellulitis, osteomyelitis, wound infection, leg ulcer, septic arthritis, diarrhea, bronchitis, and pneumonia), occur in 38%–29% of patients.

• Rare adverse effects include heart failure, hypertension, hypotension, pancreatitis, GI hemorrhage, and dyspnea. The patient also may develop autoimmune antibodies.

SPECIAL CONSIDERATIONS

• Immunizations should be up to date, especially in children prior to starting therapy

PATIENT/FAMILY EDUCATION
• Review injection techniques to ensure safe self-administration
MONITORING PARAMETERS
• Efficacy: ESR, C-reactive protein, rheumatoid factor, improvement in tender/painful swollen joints, quality of life

---

ethambutol
(e-tham′byoo-tole)
Rx: Myambutol
Chemical Class: Diisopropyl-ethylene diamide derivative
Therapeutic Class: Antituberculosis agent

CLINICAL PHARMACOLOGY
Mechanism of Action: An isonicotinic acid derivative that interferes with RNA synthesis. *Therapeutic Effect:* Suppresses the multiplication of mycobacteria.
Pharmacokinetics
Rapidly and well absorbed from the GI tract. Protein binding: 20%-30%. Widely distributed. Metabolized in the liver. Primarily excreted in urine. Removed by hemodialysis. **Half-life:** 3-4 hr (increased in impaired renal function).

INDICATIONS AND DOSAGES
Tuberculosis
PO
Adults, Elderly, Children. 15-25 mg/kg/day as a single dose or 50 mg/kg 2 times/wk. Maximum: 2.5 g/dose.
Atypical mycobacterial infections
PO
Adults, Elderly, Children. 15 mg/kg/day. Maximum: 1 g/day.
Dosage in renal impairment
Dosage interval is modified based on creatinine clearance.

Creatinine Clearance	Dosage Interval
10-50 ml/min	q24-36h
less than 10 ml/min	q48h

S AVAILABLE FORMS/COST
• Tab—Oral: 100 mg, 100's: **$59.21-$67.69**; 400 mg, 100's: **$177.92-$226.29**
UNLABELED USES: Treatment of atypical mycobacterial infections
CONTRAINDICATIONS: Optic neuritis
PREGNANCY AND LACTATION: Pregnancy category B; compatible with breast-feeding
SIDE EFFECTS
Occasional
Acute gouty arthritis (chills, pain, swelling of joints with hot skin), confusion, abdominal pain, nausea, vomiting, anorexia, headache
Rare
Rash, fever, blurred vision, eye pain, red-green color blindness
SERIOUS REACTIONS
• Optic neuritis (more common with high-dosage or long-term ethambutol therapy), peripheral neuritis, thrombocytopenia, and an anaphylactoid reaction occur rarely.
SPECIAL CONSIDERATIONS
• Initial therapy in tuberculosis should include 4 drugs: isoniazid, rifampin, pyrazinamide, and ethambutol, until drug susceptibility results available
PATIENT/FAMILY EDUCATION
• Administer with meals to decrease GI symptoms
MONITORING PARAMETERS
• Perform visual acuity testing before beginning therapy and periodically during drug administration (qmo if dose >15 mg/kg/day)

ethinyl estradiol
(ess-tra-dye-ole)
Rx: Estinyl
Combinations
See oral contraceptives monograph for combined oral contraceptives containing ethinyl estradiol
Chemical Class: Estrogen derivative
Therapeutic Class: Contraceptive; estrogen

CLINICAL PHARMACOLOGY
Mechanism of Action: A synthetic derivative of estradiol that increases synthesis of DNA, RNA, proteins in target tissues; reduces release of gonadotropin-releasing hormone from hypothalamus; reduces follicle-stimulating hormone (FSH) and luteinizing hormone (LH) release from the pituitary. *Therapeutic Effect:* Promotes normal growth, development of female sex organs, maintaining genitourinary (GU) function, vasomotor stability. Prevents accelerated bone loss by inhibiting bone resorption, restoring balance of bone resorption and formation. Inhibits LH, decreases serum concentration of testosterone.
Pharmacokinetics
Well absorbed from the gastrointestinal (GI) tract. Widely distributed. Protein binding: 50%-80%. Rapidly metabolized in liver to estrone and estriol. Excreted in urine and feces. **Half-life:** 8-25 hrs.

INDICATIONS AND DOSAGES
Female hypogonadism
PO
Adults. 0.05 mg 1-3 times/day during the first 2 wks of menstrual cycle, followed by progesterone during the last half of cycle for 3-6 mos.

Menopausal symptoms
PO
Adults. 0.02- 0.05 mg/day cyclically (3 wks on, 1 wk off).
Breast cancer
PO
Adults. 1 mg 3 times/day for at least 3 mos.
Prostate cancer
PO
Adults. 0.15- 2 mg/day.

$ AVAILABLE FORMS/COST
• Tab, Coated—Oral: 0.02 mg, 100's: **$40.96**; 0.05 mg, 100's: **$68.98**

CONTRAINDICATIONS: Abnormal vaginal bleeding, active arterial thrombosis, blood dyscrasias, estrogen-dependent cancer, known or suspected breast cancer, pregnancy, thrombophlebitis or thromboembolic disorders, thyroid dysfunction, hypersensitivity to estrogens

PREGNANCY AND LACTATION: Pregnancy category X; may reduce quantity and quality of breast milk

SIDE EFFECTS
Frequent
Anorexia, nausea, swelling of breasts, peripheral edema, evidenced by swollen ankles, feet
Occasional
Vomiting, especially with high dosages, headache that may be severe, intolerance to contact lenses, increased blood pressure (BP), glucose intolerance, brown spots on exposed skin
Rare
Chorea or involuntary movements, hirsutism or abnormal hairiness, loss of scalp hair, depression

SERIOUS REACTIONS
• Prolonged administration increases risk of gallbladder disease, thromboembolic disease, and breast, cervical, vaginal, endometrial, and liver carcinoma.

• Cholestatic jaundice occurs rarely.

INTERACTIONS

Drugs

☒ *P450 inducers (e.g., rifampin, barbiturates):* Decreased estrogen levels

☒ *Corticosteroids:* Increased steroid effect

☒ *Phenytoin:* Loss of seizure control, decreased estrogen levels

☒ *Warfarin:* Theoretical increased risk of thromboembolism

SPECIAL CONSIDERATIONS

• Unopposed estrogen increases risk of endometrial cancer; recommended administration of concurrent progestational agents for non-hysterectomized women

---

ethionamide
(e-thye-on'am-ide)
Rx: Trecator-SC
Chemical Class: Thiomine derivative
Therapeutic Class: Antituberculosis agent

CLINICAL PHARMACOLOGY
Mechanism of Action: An antitubercular agent that inhibits peptide synthesis. *Therapeutic Effect:* Suppresses mycobacterial multiplication. Bactericidal.

Pharmacokinetics
Rapidly absorbed from the gastrointestinal (GI) tract. Widely distributed. Protein binding: 10%. Metabolized in liver. Primarily excreted in urine. Removed by hemodialysis. **Half-life:** 2-3 hrs (half-life is increased with impaired renal function).

INDICATIONS AND DOSAGES
Tuberculosis
PO
Adults, Elderly. 500-1000 mg/day as a single to 3 divided doses.

Children. 15-20 mg/kg/day. Maximum 1 g/day.

Dosage in renal impairment
Creatinine clearance less than 50 ml/min, reduce dose by 50%.

§ **AVAILABLE FORMS/COST**
• Tab—Oral: 250 mg, 100's: **$309.00**

UNLABELED USES: Treatment of atypical mycobacterial infections

CONTRAINDICATIONS: Severe hepatic impairment, hypersensitivity to ethionamide

PREGNANCY AND LACTATION: Pregnancy category D

SIDE EFFECTS
Occasional
Abdominal pain, nausea, vomiting, weakness, postural hypotension, psychiatric disturbances, drowsiness, dizziness, headache, confusion, anorexia, headache, metallic taste, anorexia, diarrhea, stomatitis, peripheral neuritis

Rare
Rash, fever, blurred vision, optic neuritis, seizures, hypothyroidism, hypoglycemia, gynecomastia, thrombocytopenia, jaundice

SERIOUS REACTIONS
• Peripheral neuropathy, anorexia, and joint pain rarely occur.

INTERACTIONS
Labs
• *False decrease:* Urine alkaline phosphatase, urine lactate dehydrogenase

SPECIAL CONSIDERATIONS
• Use only with at least 1 other effective antituberculous agent

MONITORING PARAMETERS
• Serum transaminases (AST, ALT) biweekly during therapy

ethosuximide
(eth-oh-sux'i-mide)
Rx: Zarontin
Chemical Class: Succinimide
derivative
Therapeutic Class: Anticonvulsant

CLINICAL PHARMACOLOGY
Mechanism of Action: An anticonvulsant that increases the seizure threshold and suppresses paroxysmal spike-and-wave pattern in absence seizures; depresses nerve transmission in the motor cortex. *Therapeutic Effect:* Produces anticonvulsant activity.

Pharmacokinetics
Well absorbed from the gastrointestinal (GI) tract. Metabolized in liver. Excreted in urine. Removed by hemodialysis. **Half-life:** 50-60 hrs (in adults); 30 hrs (in children).

INDICATIONS AND DOSAGES
Absence seizures
PO
Adults, Elderly, Children older than 6 yrs. Initially, 250 mg/day or 15 mg/kg/day in 2 divided doses. Maintenance: 15-40 mg/kg/day in 2 divided doses.
Children 3-6 yrs. Initially, 250 mg in 2 divided doses, increased by 250 mg as needed every 4-7 days. Maintenance: 20-40 mg/kg/day in 2 divided doses.
Use with caution in patients with renal impairment.

🅢 AVAILABLE FORMS/COST
• Cap, Gel—Oral: 250 mg, 100's: **$90.70-$108.14**
• Syr—Oral: 250 mg/5 ml, 480 ml: **$79.95-$113.75**
UNLABELED USES: Treatment of learning problems
CONTRAINDICATIONS: Hypersensitivity to succinimides

PREGNANCY AND LACTATION:
Pregnancy category C; freely enters breast milk; no adverse effects on infants reported; compatible with breast-feeding

SIDE EFFECTS
Occasional
Dizziness, drowsiness, double vision, headache, ataxia, nausea, diarrhea, vomiting, somnolence, urticaria
Rare
Arganulocytosis, gum hypertrophy, leucopenia, myopia, swelling of the tongue, systemic lupus erythematosus, vaginal bleeding

SERIOUS REACTIONS
• Abrupt withdrawal may increase seizure frequency.
• Overdosage results in nausea, vomiting, and CNS depression including coma with respiratory depression.

SPECIAL CONSIDERATIONS
PATIENT/FAMILY EDUCATION
• Take doses at regularly spaced intervals
• OK with food or milk
MONITORING PARAMETERS
• Blood counts, renal function tests, liver function tests, urinalysis periodically
• Therapeutic serum concentrations 40-100 mcg/ml

etidronate

(ee-tid'roe-nate)
Rx: Didronel
Chemical Class: Pyrophosphate analog
Therapeutic Class: Bisphosphonate; bone resorption inhibitor

CLINICAL PHARMACOLOGY

Mechanism of Action: A bisphosphonate that decreases mineral release and matrix in bone and inhibits osteocytic osteolysis. *Therapeutic Effect:* Decreases bone resorption.

INDICATIONS AND DOSAGES

Paget's disease
PO
Adults, Elderly. Initially, 5–10 mg/kg/day not to exceed 6 mo, or 11–20 mg/kg/day not to exceed 3 mo. Repeat only after drug-free period of at least 90 days.

Heterotopic ossification caused by spinal cord injury
PO
Adult, Elderly. 20 mg/kg/day for 2 wk; then 10 mg/kg/day for 10 wks.

Heterotopic ossification complicating total hip replacement
PO
Adults, Elderly. 20 mg/kg/day for 1 mo before surgery; then 20 mg/kg/day for 3 mo after surgery.

Hypercalcemia associated with malignancy
IV
Adults, Elderly. 7.5 mg/kg/day for 3 days. For retreatment, allow 7 days between treatment courses. Follow with oral therapy on day after last infusion. Begin with 20 mg/kg/day for 30 days; may extend up to 90 days.

$ **AVAILABLE FORMS/COST**
• Sol, Inj—IV: 300 mg/6 ml, 6 ml: **$67.00**

• Tab—Oral: 200 mg, 60's: **$201.53**; 400 mg, 60's: **$402.96**

CONTRAINDICATIONS: Clinically overt osteomalacia

PREGNANCY AND LACTATION: Pregnancy category B; breast milk excretion not known; problems in humans have not been documented

SIDE EFFECTS

Frequent
Nausea; diarrhea; continuing or more frequent bone pain in patients with Paget's disease
Occasional
Bone fractures, especially of the femur
Parenteral: Metallic, altered taste
Rare
Hypersensitivity reaction

SERIOUS REACTIONS
• Nephrotoxicity, including hematuria, dysuria, and proteinuria, has occurred with parenteral route.

SPECIAL CONSIDERATIONS

PATIENT/FAMILY EDUCATION
• Administer on empty stomach with H_2O, 2 hr ac
• Exceeding the 2 wk treatment periods for osteoporosis may lead to bone demineralization and osteomalacia

etodolac

(e-toe-doe'lak)
Rx: Lodine
Chemical Class: Acetic acid derivative
Therapeutic Class: NSAID; antipyretic; nonnarcotic analgesic

CLINICAL PHARMACOLOGY

Mechanism of Action: An NSAID that produces analgesic and anti-inflammatory effects by inhibiting prostaglandin synthesis. *Therapeutic Effect:* Reduces the inflammatory response and intensity of pain.

Pharmacokinetics

Route	Onset	Peak	Duration
PO (analgesic)	30 min	N/A	4–12 hr

Completely absorbed from the GI tract. Protein binding: greater than 99%. Widely distributed. Metabolized in the liver. Primarily excreted in urine. Not removed by hemodialysis. **Half-life:** 6–7 hr.

INDICATIONS AND DOSAGES

Osteoarthritis

PO

Adults, Elderly. Initially, 800–1,200 mg/day in 2–4 divided doses. Maintenance: 600–1,200 mg/day.

Rheumatoid arthritis

PO

Adults, Elderly. Initially, 300 mg 2–3 times a day or 400–500 mg twice a day. Maintenance: 600–1,200 mg/day.

Analgesia

PO

Adults, Elderly. 200–400 mg q6–8h as needed. Maximum: 1,200 mg/day.

S AVAILABLE FORMS/COST

• Cap, Gel—Oral: 200 mg, 100's: **$40.00-$155.24**; 300 mg, 100's: **$125.23-$175.80**
• Tab—Oral: 400 mg, 100's: **$117.76-$185.86**; 500 mg, 100's: **$43.75-$187.05**
• Tab, Sus Action—Oral: 400 mg, 100's: **$140.17-$170.53**; 500 mg 100's: **$146.48-$178.20**; 600 mg, 100's: **$265.21-$322.63**

UNLABELED USES: Treatment of acute gouty arthritis, vascular headache

CONTRAINDICATIONS: Active peptic ulcer disease, chronic inflammation of GI tract, GI bleeding or ulceration, history of hypersensitivity to aspirin or NSAIDs

PREGNANCY AND LACTATION: Pregnancy category C (category D if used near term); breast milk excretion unknown; problems in humans have not been documented

SIDE EFFECTS

Occasional (9%–4%)

Dizziness, headache, abdominal pain or cramps, bloated feeling, diarrhea, nausea, indigestion

Rare (3%–1%)

Constipation, rash, pruritus, visual disturbances, tinnitus

SERIOUS REACTIONS

• Overdose may result in acute renal failure.
• Rare reactions with long-term use include peptic ulcer disease, GI bleeding, gastritis, severe hepatic reactions (jaundice), nephrotoxicity (hematuria, dysuria, proteinuria), and a severe hypersensitivity reaction (bronchospasm, angioedema).

INTERACTIONS

Drugs

3 *Aminoglycosides:* Reduced clearance with elevated aminoglycoside levels and potential for toxicity (especially indomethacin in premature infants; other NSAIDs probably)

3 *Antihypertensives (α-blockers, angiotensin-converting enzyme inhibitors, angiotensin II receptor blockers, β-blockers, diuretics):* Inhibition of antihypertensive and other favorable hemodynamic effects

3 *Corticosteroids:* Increased risk of GI ulceration

3 *Anticoagulants:* Excessive hypoprothrombinemia, decreased platelet aggregation with increased risk of GI bleeding; may be less

likely to increase bleeding risk than other NSAIDs due to preferential effects on COX-2

③ *Cyclosporine:* Increased nephrotoxicity risk

③ *Lithium:* Decreased clearance of lithium (mediated via prostaglandins) resulting in elevated serum lithium levels and risk of toxicity

③ *Methotrexate:* Decreased renal secretion of methotrexate resulting in elevated methotrexate levels and risk of toxicity

③ *Phenylpropanolamine:* Possible acute hypertensive reaction

③ *Potassium-sparing diuretics:* Additive hyperkalemia potential

③ *Triamterene:* Acute renal failure reported with addition of indomethacin; caution with other NSAIDs

SPECIAL CONSIDERATIONS
MONITORING PARAMETERS

• Initial hemogram and fecal occult blood test within 3 mo of starting regular chronic therapy; repeat every 6-12 mo (more frequently in high-risk patients [>65 years, peptic ulcer disease, concurrent steroids or anticoagulants]); electrolytes, creatinine, and BUN within 3 mo of starting regular chronic therapy; repeat every 6-12 mo

ezetimibe
(eh-zet′eh-mibe)
Rx: Zetia
Combinations
　Rx: with simvastatin (Vytorin)
Chemical Class: Substituted azetidinone
Therapeutic Class: Selective cholesterol absorption inhibitor

CLINICAL PHARMACOLOGY
Mechanism of Action: An antihyperlipidemic that inhibits cholesterol absorption in the small intestine, leading to a decrease in the delivery of intestinal cholesterol to the liver. *Therapeutic Effect:* Reduces total serum cholesterol, LDL cholesterol, and triglyceride levels; and increases HDL cholesterol concentration.

Pharmacokinetics **.**
Well absorbed following oral administration. Protein binding: greater than 90%. Metabolized in the small intestine and liver. Excreted by the kidneys and bile. **Half-life:** 22 hr.

INDICATIONS AND DOSAGES
Hypercholesterolemia
PO
Adults, Elderly. Initially, 10 mg once a day, given with or without food. If the patient is also receiving a bile acid sequestrant, give ezetimibe at least 2 hr before or at least 4 hr after the bile acid sequestrant.

🛡 **AVAILABLE FORMS/COST**
• Tab—Oral: 10 mg, 90's: **$229.50**

CONTRAINDICATIONS: Concurrent use of an HMG-CoA reductase inhibitor (atorvastatin, cerivastatin, fluvastatin, lovastatin, pravastatin, or simvastatin) in patients with active hepatic disease or unexplained persistent elevations in serum transaminase levels, moderate or severe hepatic insufficiency

PREGNANCY AND LACTATION: Pregnancy category C; human breast milk exposure unknown; up to half of exposure of maternal plasma in animal pups

SIDE EFFECTS

Occasional (4%–3%)

Back pain, diarrhea, arthralgia, sinusitis, abdominal pain

Rare (2%)

Cough, pharyngitis, fatigue

SERIOUS REACTIONS

• None known.

INTERACTIONS

Drugs

❷ *Cholestyramine:* Decreased ezetimibe plasma levels 55-80%

SPECIAL CONSIDERATIONS

• Modest cholesterol reductions as monotherapy (15%); primary use in combination with statins to achieve and sustain LDL goals

MONITORING PARAMETERS

• Lipid profile, LFT's, serum CPK, electrolytes, blood glucose, signs and symptoms of toxicity (GI symptoms, headache, rash)

---

famciclovir

(fam-si'klo-veer)

Rx: Famvir

Chemical Class: Acyclic purine nucleoside analog

Therapeutic Class: Antiviral

CLINICAL PHARMACOLOGY

Mechanism of Action: A synthetic nucleoside that inhibits viral DNA synthesis. *Therapeutic Effect:* Suppresses replication of herpes simplex virus and varicella-zoster virus.

Pharmacokinetics

Rapidly and extensively absorbed after PO administration. Protein binding: 20%-25%. Rapidly metabolized to penciclovir by enzymes in the gastrointestinal (GI) wall, liver, and plasma. Eliminated unchanged in urine. Removed by hemodialysis.

Half-life: 2 hr.

INDICATIONS AND DOSAGES

Herpes zoster

PO

Adults. 500 mg q8h for 7 days.

Recurrent genital herpes

PO

Adults. 125 mg twice a day for 5 days.

Suppression of recurrent genital herpes

PO

Adults. 250 mg twice a day for up to 1 yr.

Recurrent herpes simplex

PO

Adults. 500 mg twice a day for 7 days.

Dosage in renal impairment

Dosage and frequency are modified based on creatinine clearance.

Creatinine Clearance	Herpes Zoster	Genital Herpes
40-59 ml/min	500 mg q12h	125 mg q12h
20-39 ml/min	500 mg q24h	125 mg q24h
less than 20 ml/min	250 mg q24h	125 mg q24h

Dosage in hemodialysis patients

For adults with herpes zoster, give 250 mg after each dialysis treatment; for adults with genital herpes, give 125 mg after each dialysis treatment.

§ AVAILABLE FORMS/COST

• Tab—Oral: 125 mg, 30's: **$111.70**; 250 mg, 30's: **$121.45**; 500 mg, 30's: **$221.30**

CONTRAINDICATIONS: None known

PREGNANCY AND LACTATION: Pregnancy category B; excreted in breast milk

SIDE EFFECTS
Frequent
Headache (23%), nausea (12%)
Occasional (10%-2%)
Dizziness, somnolence, numbness of feet, diarrhea, vomiting, constipation, decreased appetite, fatigue, fever, pharyngitis, sinusitis, pruritus
Rare (less than 2%)
Insomnia, abdominal pain, dyspepsia, flatulence, back pain, arthralgia

SERIOUS REACTIONS
• None known.

SPECIAL CONSIDERATIONS
• Reserve chronic suppressive therapy for patients without prodromal symptoms who have frequent recurrences

---

famotidine
(fam-o'tah-deen)
Rx: Pepcid, Pepcid RPD
OTC: Mylanta AR, Pepcid AC
Combinations
   OTC: with calcium carbonate and magnesium hydroxide (Pepcid Complete)
Chemical Class: Thiazole derivative
Therapeutic Class: Antiulcer agent

CLINICAL PHARMACOLOGY
Mechanism of Action: An antiulcer agent and gastric acid secretion inhibitor that inhibits histamine action at histamine 2 receptors of parietal cells. *Therapeutic Effect:* Inhibits gastric acid secretion when fasting, at night, or when stimulated by food, caffeine, or insulin.

Pharmacokinetics

Route	Onset	Peak	Duration
PO	1 hr	1–4 hr	10–12 hr
IV	1 hr	0.5–3 hr	10–12 hr

Rapidly, incompletely absorbed from the GI tract. Protein binding: 15%–20%. Partially metabolized in the liver. Primarily excreted in urine. Not removed by hemodialysis. **Half-life:** 2.5–3.5 hr (increased with impaired renal function).

INDICATIONS AND DOSAGES
Acute treatment of duodenal and gastric ulcers
PO
Adults, Elderly, Children 12 yr and older. 40 mg/day at bedtime.
Children 1–11 yr. 0.5 mg/kg/day at bedtime. Maximum: 40 mg/day.
Duodenal ulcer maintenance
PO
Adults, Elderly. 20 mg/day at bedtime.
Gastroesophageal reflux disease
PO
Adults, Elderly, Children 12 yr and older. 20 mg twice a day.
Children 1–11 yr. 1 mg/kg/day in 2 divided doses.
Children 3 mos to younger than 1 yr. 0.5 mg/kg/dose twice a day.
Children younger than 3 mos. 0.5 mg/kg/dose once a day.
Esophagitis
PO
Adults, Elderly, Children 12 yr and older. 2-40 mg twice a day.
Hypersecretory conditions
PO
Adults, Elderly, Children 12 yr and older. Initially, 20 mg q6h. May increase up to 160 mg q6h.
Acid indigestion, heartburn (over-the-counter)
PO
Adults, Elderly, Children 12 yr and older. 10-20 mg 15–60 min before eating. Maximum: 2 doses per day.
Usual Parenteral Dosage
IV
Adults, Elderly, Children 12 yr and older. 20 mg q12h.

Dosage in renal impairment
Dosing frequency is modified based on creatinine clearance.

Creatinine Clearance	Dosing Frequency
10–50 ml/min	q24h
less than 10 ml/min	q36–48h

$ AVAILABLE FORMS/COST
• Powder, Reconst—Oral: 40 mg/5 ml, 50 ml: **$107.71**
• Sol, Inj—IV: 10 mg/ml, 2, 4 ml: **$1.11-$4.73/2 ml**
• Tab, Chewable—Oral: 10 mg, 30's (OTC): **$9.36**
• Tab, Oral Disintegrating—Oral: 40 mg, 100's: **$362.50**
• Tab—Oral: 10 mg, 18's (OTC): **$3.59-$6.99**; 20 mg, 100's: **$170.00-$202.79**; 40 mg, 100's: **$297.78-$391.95**

UNLABELED USES: Autism, prevention of aspiration pneumonitis
CONTRAINDICATIONS: None known

PREGNANCY AND LACTATION: Pregnancy category B; concentrated in breast milk (less than cimetidine or ranitidine); no problems reported with other H$_2$-histamine receptor antagonists; compatible with breast-feeding

SIDE EFFECTS
Occasional (5%)
Headache
Rare (2% or less)
Constipation, diarrhea, dizziness
SERIOUS REACTIONS
• None known.
INTERACTIONS
Drugs
 Cefpodoxime, cefuroxime, enoxacin, ketoconazole: Reduction in gastric acidity reduces absorption, decreased plasma levels, potential for therapeutic failure
 Glipizide; glyburide; tolbutamide: Increased absorption of these drugs, potential for hypoglycemia

 Nifedipine; nitrendipine; nisoldipine: Increased concentrations of these drugs
SPECIAL CONSIDERATIONS
• No advantage over other agents in this class, base selection on cost
PATIENT/FAMILY EDUCATION
• Stagger doses of famotidine and antacids

---

felodipine
(fell-o'da-peen)
Rx: Plendil
Combinations
   Rx: with enalapril (Lexxel)
Chemical Class: Dihydropyridine
Therapeutic Class: Antianginal; antihypertensive; calcium channel blocker

CLINICAL PHARMACOLOGY
Mechanism of Action: An antihypertensive and antianginal agent that inhibits calcium movement across cardiac and vascular smooth-muscle cell membranes. Potent peripheral vasodilator (does not depress SA or AV nodes). *Therapeutic Effect:* Increases myocardial contractility, heart rate, and cardiac output; decreases peripheral vascular resistance and BP.
Pharmacokinetics

Route	Onset	Peak	Duration
PO	2–5 hr	N/A	N/A

Rapidly, completely absorbed from the GI tract. Protein binding: greater than 99%. Undergoes first-pass metabolism in the liver. Primarily excreted in urine. Not removed by hemodialysis. **Half-life:** 11–16 hr.
INDICATIONS AND DOSAGES
Hypertension
PO
Adults. Initially, 5 mg/day as single dose.

Elderly, patients with impaired hepatic function. Initially, 2.5 mg/day. Adjust dosage at no less than 2-wk intervals. Maintenance: 2.5–10 mg/day.

$ AVAILABLE FORMS/COST

• Tab, Sus Action—Oral: 2.5, 5 mg, 100's: **$123.97**; 10 mg, 100's: **$222.77**

UNLABELED USES: Treatment of CHF, chronic angina pectoris, Raynaud's phenomenon

CONTRAINDICATIONS: None known

PREGNANCY AND LACTATION: Pregnancy category C

SIDE EFFECTS

Frequent (22%–18%)
Headache, peripheral edema
Occasional (6%–4%)
Flushing, respiratory infection, dizziness, light-headedness, asthenia (loss of strength, weakness)
Rare (less than 3%)
Paresthesia, abdominal discomfort, nervousness, muscle cramping, cough, diarrhea, constipation

SERIOUS REACTIONS

• Overdose produces nausea, somnolence, confusion, slurred speech, hypotension, and bradycardia.

INTERACTIONS

Drugs
▣ *Barbiturates:* Decreased felodipine bioavailability
▣ *Digitalis glycosides:* Increased digitalis levels; increased risk of toxicity
▣ *Erythromycin:* Increased felodipine concentrations
▣ *Fentanyl:* Severe hypotension or increased fluid volume requirements
▣ *Grapefruit juice:* Inhibits felodipine metabolism, 200% increase in AUC
▣ *Histamine H_2 antagonists:* Increased bioavailability of felodipine

▣ *Hydantoins:* Serum felodipine level may be decreased
▣ *Propranolol:* Enhanced hypotension, increased propranolol concentrations

SPECIAL CONSIDERATIONS

• Results of V-HeFT III indicate felodipine may be used safely in patients with left ventricular dysfunction

PATIENT/FAMILY EDUCATION

• Administer as whole tablet (do not crush or chew)
• Avoid grapefruit juice (see drug interactions)

---

fenofibrate
(fee-no-fye′brate)
Rx: Tricor
Chemical Class: Fibric acid derivative
Therapeutic Class: Antilipemic

CLINICAL PHARMACOLOGY

Mechanism of Action: An antihyperlipidemic that enhances synthesis of lipoprotein lipase and reduces triglyceride-rich lipoproteins and VLDLs. *Therapeutic Effect:* Increases VLDL catabolism and reduces total plasma triglyceride levels.

Pharmacokinetics
Well absorbed from the GI tract. Absorption increased when given with food. Protein binding: 99%. Rapidly metabolized in the liver to active metabolite. Excreted primarily in urine; lesser amount in feces. Not removed by hemodialysis. **Half-life:** 20 hr.

INDICATIONS AND DOSAGES

Reduction of very high serum triglyceride levels in patients at risk for pancreatitis

PO

Adults, Elderly. Initially, 67 mg/day(capsule); may increase to 200 mg/day. Or initially, 54 mg/day(tablet); may increase to 160 mg/day.

Hypercholesterolemia

PO

Adults, Elderly. 200 mg/day (capsule) with meals. Or 160 mg/day-(tablet) with meals.

$ **AVAILABLE FORMS/COST**

• Cap—Oral: 67 mg 100's: **$81.65**; 134 mg 100's: **$155.07-$157.28**; 200 mg 100's: **$232.60-$244.96**

• Tab—Oral: 54 mg 90's: **$95.85**; 160 mg 90's: **$287.51**

CONTRAINDICATIONS: Gallbladder disease, hypersensitivity to fenofibrate, severe renal or hepatic dysfunction (including primary biliary cirrhosis, unexplained persistent liver function abnormality)

PREGNANCY AND LACTATION: Pregnancy category C; embryocidal and teratogenic in rats; no adequate and well-controlled studies in pregnant women; tumorigenicity seen in animal studies; avoid breast-feeding

SIDE EFFECTS

Frequent (8%–4%)

Pain, rash, headache, asthenia or fatigue, flu syndrome, dyspepsia, nausea or vomiting, rhinitis

Occasional (3%–2%)

Diarrhea, abdominal pain, constipation, flatulence, arthralgia, decreased libido, dizziness, pruritus

Rare (less than 2%)

Increased appetite, insomnia, polyuria, cough, blurred vision, eye floaters, earache

SERIOUS REACTIONS

• Fenofibrate may increase excretion of cholesterol into bile, leading to cholelithiasis.

• Pancreatitis, hepatitis, thrombocytopenia, and agranulocytosis occur rarely.

INTERACTIONS

Drugs

[3] *β-Blockers:* Antagonistic effects; exacerbate hypertriglyceridemia

[3] *Estrogens:* Antagonistic effects; exacerbate hypertriglyderidemia

[2] *HMG-CoA reductase inhibitors (statins):* Increased risk of markedly elevated creatine kinase (CK), rhabdomyolysis, myoglobinuria, acute renal failure

[3] *Resins (bile acid sequestrants):* Decreased absorption if taken concomitantly; separate by 1 hr before or 4 hr after to avoid interaction

[3] *Thiazide diuretics:* Antagonistic effects; exacerbate hypertriglyceridemia

[3] *Warfarin:* Potentiation leading to prolonged PT/INR; all oral coumarin-type anticoagulants

Labs

• *Uric acid:* Decreased

SPECIAL CONSIDERATIONS

• Plasma concentrations of fenofibric acid after administration of 54 mg and 160 mg tablets are equivalent to 67 and 200 mg capsules

PATIENT/FAMILY EDUCATION

• Signs, symptoms, and resources for management of myositis

MONITORING PARAMETERS

• Serum cholesterol, triglycerides, LDL-cholesterol, HDL-cholesterol, LFTs (serum transaminases), periodic CBC

F

fenoldopam

(fhe-knowl'doh-pam)
Rx: Corlopam
Chemical Class: Benzazepine derivative
Therapeutic Class: Vasodilator

CLINICAL PHARMACOLOGY

Mechanism of Action: A rapid-acting vasodilator. An agonist for D_1-like dopamine receptors; also produces vasodilation in coronary, renal, mesenteric, and peripheral arteries. *Therapeutic Effect:* Reduces systolic and diastolic BP and increases heart rate.

Pharmacokinetics

After IV administration, metabolized in the liver. Primarily excreted in urine. Unknown if removed by hemodialysis. **Half-life:** Approximately 5 min.

INDICATIONS AND DOSAGES

Short-term management of severe hypertension when rapid, but quickly reversible emergency reduction of BP is clinically indicated, including malignant hypertension with deteriorating end-organ function

IV infusion (continuous)

Adults. Initially, 0.1 mcg/kg/min. May increase in increments of 0.05-0.2 mcg/kg/min until target blood pressure is achieved. Usual length of treatment is 1-6 hours with tapering of dose q15-30min. Average rate: 0.25-0.5 mcg/kg/min.

$ AVAILABLE FORMS/COST

• Sol, Inj—IV: 10 mg/ml, 1 ml: **$238.00-$275.60**

CONTRAINDICATIONS: None known

PREGNANCY AND LACTATION: Pregnancy category B; animal studies show no evidence of impaired fertility or fetal harm; no human data available; excreted into breast milk of rats; human information unknown

SIDE EFFECTS

Expected

Beta blockers may cause unforeseen hypotension.

Occasional

Headache (7%), flushing (3%), nausea (4%), hypotension (2%)

Rare (2% or less)

Nervousness or anxiety, vomiting, constipation, nasal congestion, diaphoresis, back pain

SERIOUS REACTIONS

• Excessive hypotension occurs occasionally.

• Substantial tachycardia may lead to ischemic cardiac events or worsened heart failure.

• Allergic-type reactions, including anaphylaxis and life-threatening asthmatic exacerbation, may occur in patients with sulfite sensitivity.

INTERACTIONS

Drugs

🖪 *Acetaminophen:* May increase fenoldopam serum concentrations due to competition for sulfation (especially with oral fenoldopam)

Labs

• Hypokalemia, increased blood urea nitrogen and serum creatinine, elevated liver transaminases, elevated LDH

SPECIAL CONSIDERATIONS

• *Preparation of infusion solution:* Contents of ampules must be diluted prior to infusion: 1 ml of 10 mg/ml solution in 250 ml 0.9% sodium chloride or 5% dextrose yields a final concentration of 40 mcg/ml

• *Potential advantage over sodium nitroprusside in hypertensive crisis:* Induction of natriuresis, diuresis; ability to increase creatinine clearance, preserve renal function

MONITORING PARAMETERS

• Blood pressure, pulse, serum electrolytes, urine volume, urinary sodium, serum creatinine, blood urea nitrogen, electrocardiogram, hepatic function tests

---

fenoprofen

(fen-oh-proe'fen)
Rx: Nalfon
Chemical Class: Propionic acid derivative
Therapeutic Class: NSAID; antipyretic; nonnarcotic analgesic

CLINICAL PHARMACOLOGY
Mechanism of Action: An NSAID that produces analgesic and anti-inflammatory effects by inhibiting prostaglandin synthesis. *Therapeutic Effect:* Reduces the inflammatory response and intensity of pain.

INDICATIONS AND DOSAGES
Mild to moderate pain
PO
Adults, Elderly. 200 mg q4–6h as needed.
Rheumatoid arthritis, osteoarthritis
PO
Adults, Elderly. 300–600 mg 3–4 times a day.

$ AVAILABLE FORMS/COST
• Cap, Gel—Oral: 200 mg, 100's: **$23.60-$68.69**; 300 mg, 100's: **$27.37-$53.79**
• Tab—Oral: 600 mg, 100's: **$37.80-$70.66**

UNLABELED USES: Treatment of ankylosing spondylitis, psoriatic arthritis, vascular headaches

CONTRAINDICATIONS: Active peptic ulcer disease, chronic inflammation of GI tract, GI bleeding or ulceration, history of hypersensitivity to aspirin or NSAIDs, significant renal impairment

PREGNANCY AND LACTATION: Pregnancy category B (category D, 3rd trimester); excreted in breast milk

SIDE EFFECTS
Frequent (9%–3%)
Headache, somnolence, dyspepsia, nausea, vomiting, constipation
Occasional (2%–1%)
Dizziness, pruritus, nervousness, asthenia, diarrhea, abdominal cramps, flatulence, tinnitus, blurred vision, peripheral edema and fluid retention

SERIOUS REACTIONS
• Overdose may result in acute hypotension and tachycardia.
• Rare reactions with long-term use include peptic ulcer disease, GI bleeding, gastritis, severe hepatic reaction (jaundice), nephrotoxicity (hematuria, dysuria, proteinuria), and a severe hypersensitivity reaction (bronchospasm, angioedema).

INTERACTIONS
Drugs
▣ *Aminoglycosides:* Reduced clearance with elevated aminoglycoside levels and potential for toxicity (especially indomethacin in premature infants; other NSAIDs probably)
▣ *Antihypertensives (α-blockers, angiotensin-converting enzyme inhibitors, angiotensin II receptor blockers, β-blockers, diuretics):* Inhibition of antihypertensive and other favorable hemodynamic effects
▣ *Corticosteroids:* Increased risk of GI ulceration
▣ *Anticoagulants:* Excessive hypoprothrombinemia, decreased platelet aggregation with increased risk of GI bleeding

3 *Cyclosporine:* Increased nephrotoxicity risk

3 *Lithium:* Decreased clearance of lithium (mediated via prostaglandins) resulting in elevated serum lithium levels and risk of toxicity

3 *Methotrexate:* Decreased renal secretion of methotrexate resulting in elevated methotrexate levels and risk of toxicity

3 *Phenylpropranolamine:* Possible acute hypertensive reaction

3 *Potassium-sparing diuretics:* Additive hyperkalemia potential

3 *Triamterene:* Acute renal failure reported with addition of indomethacin; caution with other NSAIDs

Labs

• *False increase:* Free and total triiodothyronine levels, plasma cortisol

• *False positive:* Urine barbiturate, urine benzodiazepine

SPECIAL CONSIDERATIONS

• No significant advantage over other NSAIDs; cost should govern use

MONITORING PARAMETERS

• Initial hemogram and fecal occult blood test within 3 mo of starting regular chronic therapy; repeat every 6-12 mo (more frequently in high-risk patients [>65 years, peptic ulcer disease, concurrent steroids or anticoagulants]); electrolytes, creatinine, and BUN within 3 mo of starting regular chronic therapy; repeat every 6-12 mo

---

fentanyl

(fen'ta-nill)

Rx: *Injection:* Sublimaze
Rx: *Transdermal:* Duragesic
Rx: *Lozenge:* Fentanyl Oralet, Actiq
Combinations
  Rx: with droperidol (Innovar)
Chemical Class: Opiate derivative; phenylpiperidine derivative
Therapeutic Class: Narcotic analgesic
DEA Class: Schedule II

CLINICAL PHARMACOLOGY

Mechanism of Action: An opioid agonist that binds to opioid receptors in the CNS, reducing stimuli from sensory nerve endings and inhibiting ascending pain pathways. *Therapeutic Effect:* Alters pain reception and increases the pain threshold.

Pharmacokinetics

Route	Onset	Peak	Duration
IV	1–2 min	3–5 min	0.5–1 hr
IM	7–15 min	20–30 min	1–2 hrs
Transdermal	6–8 hr	24 hr	72 hr
Transmucosal	5–15 min	20–30 min	1–2 hr

Well absorbed after IM or topical administration. Transmucosal form absorbed through the buccal mucosa and GI tract. Protein binding: 80%–85%. Metabolized in the liver. Primarily eliminated by biliary system. **Half-life:** 2–4 hr IV; 17 hr transdermal; 6.6 hr transmucosal.

INDICATIONS AND DOSAGES
Sedation in minor procedures, analgesia
IM/IV

Adults, Elderly, Children 12 yr and older. 0.5–1 mcg/kg/dose; may repeat in 30–60 min.
Children 1–11 yr. 1–2 mcg/kg/dose.
Children younger than 1 yr. 1–4 mcg/kg/dose.

Preoperative sedation, postoperative pain, adjunct to regional anesthesia
IV, IM

Adults, Elderly, Children 12 yr and older. 50–100 mcg/dose.

Adjunct to general anesthesia
IV

Adults, Elderly, Children 12 yr and older. 2–50 mcg/kg.
Usual transdermal dose
Adults, Elderly, Children 12 yr and older. Initially, 25 mcg/hr. May increase after 3 days.
Usual transmucosal dose
Adults, Children. 200–400 mcg for breakthrough cancer pain.
Usual epidural dose
Adults, Elderly. Bolus dose of 100 mcg, followed by continuous infusion of 10 mcg/ml concentration at 4–12 ml/hr.

Continuous analgesia
IV

Adults, Elderly, Children 1–12 yr. Bolus dose of 1–2 mcg/kg, followed by continuous infusion of 1 mcg/kg/hr. Range: 1–5 mcg/kg/hr.
Children younger than 1 yr. Bolus dose of 1–2 mcg/kg, followed by continuous infusion of 0.5–1 mcg/kg/hr.

Dosage in renal impairment
Dosage is modified based on creatinine clearance.

Creatinine Clearance	Dosage
10–50 ml/min	75% of usual dose
less than 10 ml/min	50% of usual dose

$\boxed{\text{S}}$ AVAILABLE FORMS/COST
• Film, Cont Rel—Transdermal: 25 mcg/hr, 5's: **$75.73**; 50 mcg/hr, 5's: **$133.38**; 75 mcg/hr, 5's: **$203.45**; 100 mcg/hr, 5's: **$270.01**
• Sol, Inj—IM, IV: 0.05 mg/ml, 2, 5, 10, 20, 30, 50 ml: **$0.64-$2.25**/2 ml
• Loz—Top Device: 0.2 mg, 1's: **$8.30**; 0.4 mg, 1's: **$10.60**; 0.6 mg, 1's: **$12.93**; 0.8 mg, 1's: **$15.33**; 1.2 mg, 1's: **$19.97**; 1.6 mg, 1's: **$24.67**
• Loz, Top—Oral: 100, 200, 300, 400 mcg, 1's: **$28.81-$30.86**

CONTRAINDICATIONS: Increased intracranial pressure, severe hepatic or renal impairment, severe respiratory depression

PREGNANCY AND LACTATION: Pregnancy category C; excreted in breast milk

SIDE EFFECTS
Frequent
IV: Postoperative drowsiness, nausea, vomiting
Transdermal (10%–3%): Headache, pruritus, nausea, vomiting, diaphoresis, dyspnea, confusion, dizziness, somnolence, diarrhea, constipation, decreased appetite
Occasional
IV: Postoperative confusion, blurred vision, chills, orthostatic hypotension, constipation, difficulty urinating
Transdermal (3%–1%): Chest pain, arrhythmias, erythema, pruritus, swelling of skin, syncope, agitation, tingling or burning of skin

SERIOUS REACTIONS
• Overdose or too rapid IV administration may produce severe respiratory depression and skeletal and thoracic muscle rigidity (which may

lead to apnea), laryngospasm, bronchospasm, cold and clammy skin, cyanosis, and coma.

• The patient who uses fentanyl repeatedly may develop a tolerance to the drug's analgesic effect.

INTERACTIONS

Drugs

3 *Antihistamines, chloral hydrate, glutethimide, methocarbamol:* Enhanced depressant effects

3 *Barbiturates:* Additive respiratory and CNS-depressant effects

3 *Cimetidine:* Increased respiratory and CNS depression

3 *Diazepam:* Cardiovascular depression

3 *Ethanol:* Additive CNS effects

3 *Nitrous oxide:* Cardiovascular depression

Labs

• False elevations of serum amylase and lipase

SPECIAL CONSIDERATIONS

• Increased skin temperature increases absorption rate of transdermal preparation

• Lozenge should be used only in a monitored anesthesia care setting

• Following removal of transdermal system, 17 hr are required for 50% decrease in serum fentanyl concentrations

• Do not administer agonist/antagonist analgesics (i.e., pentazocine, nalbuphine, butorphanol, dezocine, buprenorphine) to patient who has received a prolonged course of fentanyl (a pure agonist). In opioid-dependent patients, mixed agonist/antagonist analgesics may precipitate withdrawal symptoms

ferrous salts
(fer-rous)

OTC: *Sulfate:* Feosol, Feratab, Fer-in-sol, Fer-Iron, Fero-Gradumet, Mol-Iron

OTC: *Sulfate exsiccated:* Feosol, Fer-in-Sol, Ferra-TD, Slow Fe

OTC: *Gluconate:* Fergon, Simron

OTC: *Fumarate:* Femiron, Feostat, Hemocyte, Ircon, Nephro-Fer

OTC: *Polysaccharide-Iron complex:* Hytinic, Niferex, Nu-Iron

Combinations

OTC: with magnesium and aluminum hydroxide (Fermalox); with docusate (Ferocyl, Ferro-Sequels, Ferro-Docusate, Ferro-dok TR, Ferro-DSS SR); with vitamin C (Mol-Iron with Vitamin C, Ferancee-HP, Vitron-C Plus, Cevi-Fer, Irospan, Fero-Grad, Hemaspan); with folate (Palafer CF); with multivitamins (Flintstones Plus Iron, Stresstabs with Iron)

Chemical Class: Iron preparation

Therapeutic Class: Hematinic

CLINICAL PHARMACOLOGY

Mechanism of Action: An enzymatic mineral that is as an essential component in the formation of Hgb, myoglobin, and enzymes. Promotes effective erythropoiesis and transport and utilization of oxygen (O_2). *Therapeutic Effect:* Prevents iron deficiency.

Pharmacokinetics

Absorbed in the duodenum and upper jejunum. Ten percent absorbed in patients with normal iron stores; increased to 20%–30% in those with inadequate iron stores. Primarily bound to serum transferrin. Excreted in urine, sweat, and sloughing of intestinal mucosa and by menses.
Half-life: 6 hr.

INDICATIONS AND DOSAGES
Iron deficiency anemia

Dosage is expressed in terms of milligrams of elemental iron, degree of anemia, patient weight, and presence of any bleeding. Expect to use periodic hematologic determinations as guide to therapy.
PO (ferrous fumarate)

Adults, Elderly. (ferrous fumarate): 60–100 mg twice a day; (ferrous gluconate): 60 mg 2-4 times a day; (ferrous sulfate): 325 mg 2-4 times a day.

Children. (ferrous fumarate, ferrous gluconate, ferrous sulfate) 3-6 mg/kg/day in 2–3 divided doses.

Prevention of iron deficiency
PO

Adults, Elderly. (ferrous fumarate): 60–100 mg/day; (ferrous gluconate): 60 mg/day; (ferrous sulfate): 325 mg/day.

Children. (ferrous fumarate, ferrous gluconate, ferrous sulfate) 1–2 mg/kg/day.

Ⓢ **AVAILABLE FORMS/COST**
Ferrous Fumarate
• Liq-Oral: 45 mg/0.6 ml, 60 ml: **$18.20**
• Susp-Oral: 100 mg/5 ml, 240 ml: **$23.16**
• Tab, Chewable-Oral: 100 mg, 100's: **$18.73**
• Tab-Oral: 63 mg, 40's: **$4.93-$5.87**; 200 mg, 100's: **$16.25**; 300 mg, 100's: **$3.00-$5.95**; 325 mg, 100's: **$0.77-$3.25**

Ferrous Gluconate
• Cap-Oral: 86 mg, 100's: **$35.65**
• Tab-Oral: 240 mg, 100's: **$3.79-$6.52**; 300 mg, 100's: **$2.81-$5.10**; 325 mg, 100s: **$0.78-$4.43**

Ferrous Sulfate
• Cap, Sus Action-Oral: 250 mg, 100's: **$4.15-$5.29**
• Elixir-Oral: 220 mg/5 ml, 120, 480 ml: **$3.74-$9.98/480 ml**
• Liq-Oral: 75 mg/0.6 ml, 50 ml: **$2.50-$9.69**; 300 mg/5 ml, 100 ml: **$41.00**
• Syr-Oral: 90 mg/5 ml, 480 ml: **$14.75**
• Tab-Oral: 195 mg, 100's: **$5.42**; 200 mg, 100's: **$7.76**; 300 mg, 100's: **$6.02**; 325 mg, 100's: **$0.65-$20.25**
• Tab, Enteric Coated-Oral: 325 mg, 100's: **$4.68**
• Tab, Sus Action-Oral: 160 mg, 90's: **$18.92**; 525 mg, 100's: **$27.65**

CONTRAINDICATIONS: Hemochromatosis, hemosiderosis, hemolytic anemias, peptic ulcer disease, regional enteritis, ulcerative colitis

PREGNANCY AND LACTATION: Pregnancy category A; excreted in breast milk

SIDE EFFECTS
Occasional
Mild, transient nausea
Rare
Heartburn, anorexia, constipation, diarrhea

SERIOUS REACTIONS
• Large doses may aggravate existing GI tract disease, such as peptic ulcer disease, regional enteritis, and ulcerative colitis.
• Severe iron poisoning occurs most often in children and is manifested as vomiting, severe abdominal pain, diarrhea, and dehydration, followed by hyperventilation, pallor or cyanosis, and cardiovascular collapse.

INTERACTIONS
Drugs
☒ *Antacids:* Reduce iron absorption

☒ *Ciprofloxacin, levodopa, levofloxacin, methyldopa, norfloxacin, penicillamine, tetracyclines, vitamin E:* Absorption reduced by iron

☒ *Enalapril:* Three patients on enalapril developed systemic reactions following IV iron; causal relationship not established

Labs
• Urine discoloration black, brown, or dark color

• *Glucose:* Decreased with clinistix, diastix; no effect observed with te-stape

• *Occult blood:* 25-65% false positives

SPECIAL CONSIDERATIONS
PATIENT/FAMILY EDUCATION
• Best absorbed on empty stomach, may take with food if GI upset occurs

• Drink liquid iron preparations in water or juice and through a straw to prevent tooth stains

• 4-6 mo of therapy generally required

• Iron changes stools black or dark green

MONITORING PARAMETERS
• Hemoglobin, hematocrit

---

fexofenadine
(fex-oh-fen'eh-deen)

Rx: Allegra
Combinations
   Rx: with pseudoephedrine
   (Allegra-D)
Chemical Class: Piperidine derivative
Therapeutic Class: Antihistamine

CLINICAL PHARMACOLOGY
Mechanism of Action: A piperidine that competes with histamine for H_1-receptor sites on effector cells.
Therapeutic Effect: Relieves allergic rhinitis symptoms.

Pharmacokinetics
Rapidly absorbed after PO administration. Protein binding: 60%–70%. Does not cross the blood-brain barrier. Minimally metabolized. Eliminated in feces and urine. Not removed by hemodialysis. **Half-life:** 14.4 hr (increased in renal impairment).

INDICATIONS AND DOSAGES
Allergic rhinitis, urticaria
PO

Adults, Elderly, Children 12 yr and older. 60 mg twice a day or 180 mg once a day.

Children 6–11 yr. 30 mg twice a day.

Dosage in renal impairment
For adults, elderly, and children 12 years and older, dosage is reduced to 60 mg once a day. For children 6-11 years, dosage is reduced to 30 mg once a day.

Ⓢ AVAILABLE FORMS/COST
• Cap—Oral: 60 mg, 100's: **$107.67**
• Tab—Oral: 30 mg, 100's: **$70.58**; 60 mg, 100's: **$141.04**; 180 mg, 100's: **$244.55**

• Tab, Sus Action—Oral (with pseudoephedrine): 60 mg-120 mg, 100's: **$143.39**

CONTRAINDICATIONS: None known.

PREGNANCY AND LACTATION: Pregnancy category C; breast milk excretion unknown

SIDE EFFECTS

Rare (less than 2%)

Somnolence, headache, fatigue, nausea, vomiting, abdominal distress, dysmenorrhea

SERIOUS REACTIONS

• None known.

INTERACTIONS

Drugs

▪ *Antacids:* Decreased plasma fexofenadine concentrations; avoid taking aluminum and magnesium containing antacids with fexofenadine

▪ *Erythromycin:* Increased plasma fexofenadine concentrations

▪ *Ketoconazole:* Increased plasma fexofenadine concentrations

SPECIAL CONSIDERATIONS

• Essentially the same as terfenadine without the potential for QT prolongation; relatively weak antihistamine with minimal sedation

• Consider alternating q hs chlorpeniramine with qam fexofenadine 60 mg to minimize cost

---

finasteride

(feen-as′ter-ide)

Rx: Proscar, Propecia

Chemical Class: 5α-reductase inhibitor

Therapeutic Class: Antiandrogen; hair growth stimulant

CLINICAL PHARMACOLOGY

Mechanism of Action: An androgen hormone inhibitor that inhibits 5-alpha reductase, an intracellular enzyme that converts testosterone into dihydrotestosterone (DHT) in the prostate gland, resulting in a decreased serum DHT level. *Therapeutic Effect:* Reduces size of the prostate gland.

Pharmacokinetics

Route	Onset	Peak	Duration
PO	24 hr	1–2 days	5–7 days

Rapidly absorbed from the GI tract. Protein binding: 90%. Widely distributed. Metabolized in the liver. **Half-life:** 6–8 hr. Onset of clinical effect: 3–6 mo of continued therapy.

INDICATIONS AND DOSAGES

Benign prostatic hyperplasia (BPH)

PO

Adults, Elderly. 5 mg once a day (for a minimum of 6 mo).

Hair loss

PO

Adults. 1 mg/day.

Ⓢ **AVAILABLE FORMS/COST**

• Tab, Plain Coated—Oral: 1 mg, 30's: **$54.69**; 5 mg, 100's: **$287.50**

UNLABELED USES: Adjuvant monotherapy after radical prostatectomy in treatment of prostate cancer

CONTRAINDICATIONS: Exposure to the patient's semen or handling of finasteride tablets by those who are or may be pregnant

PREGNANCY AND LACTATION: Pregnancy category X; not indicated for use in women; pregnant women should not handle crushed tablets

SIDE EFFECTS

Rare (4%–2%)

Gynecomastia, sexual dysfunction (impotence, decreased libido, decreased volume of ejaculate)

SERIOUS REACTIONS

• None known.

SPECIAL CONSIDERATIONS
• Minimal benefit for benign prostatic hypertrophy if the prostate is not very large; response is not immediate
• Combination therapy with α-blocker may be optimal
• Whether long-term treatment can reduce prostate cancer risk is unknown; decreases prostate specific antigen (PSA)

PATIENT/FAMILY EDUCATION
• Condoms should be used if the female partner is at risk of pregnancy
• Withdrawal of drug for hair loss leads to reversal within 12 mo

MONITORING PARAMETERS
• 6-12 mo of therapy may be necessary in some patients to assess effectiveness (BPH), 3 or more mo for hair loss

---

flavoxate
(fla-vox'ate)
Rx: Urispas
Chemical Class: Flavone derivative
Therapeutic Class: Genitourinary muscle relaxant

CLINICAL PHARMACOLOGY
Mechanism of Action: An anticholinergic that relaxes detrusor and other smooth muscle by cholinergic blockade, counteracting muscle spasm in the urinary tract. *Therapeutic Effect:* Produces anticholinergic, local anesthetic, and analgesic effects, relieving urinary symptoms.

INDICATIONS AND DOSAGES
To relieve symptoms of cystitis, prostatitis, urethritis, urethrocystitis, or urethrotrigonitis
PO
Adults, Elderly, Adolescents. 100–200 mg 3–4 times a day.

$ AVAILABLE FORMS/COST
• Tab, Plain Coated—Oral: 100 mg, 100's: **$146.32**

CONTRAINDICATIONS: Duodenal or pyloric obstruction, GI hemorrhage or obstruction, ileus, lower urinary tract obstruction

PREGNANCY AND LACTATION: Pregnancy category B; excretion into breast milk unknown; use caution in nursing mothers

SIDE EFFECTS
Frequent
Somnolence, dry mouth and throat
Occasional
Constipation, difficult urination, blurred vision, dizziness, headache, increased light sensitivity, nausea, vomiting, abdominal pain
Rare
Confusion (primarily in elderly), hypersensitivity, increased IOP, leukopenia

SERIOUS REACTIONS
• Overdose may produce anticholinergic effects, including unsteadiness, severe dizziness, somnolence, fever, facial flushing, dyspnea, nervousness, and irritability.

SPECIAL CONSIDERATIONS
• Urinary antispasmodic that is no more effective than propantheline or other similar agents

---

flecainide
(fle'kah-nide)
Rx: Tambocor
Chemical Class: Benzamide derivative
Therapeutic Class: Antiarrhythmic, class IC

CLINICAL PHARMACOLOGY
Mechanism of Action: An antiarrhythmic that slows atrial, AV, His-Purkinje, and intraventricular conduction. Decreases excitability,

conduction velocity, and automaticity. *Therapeutic Effect:* Controls atrial, supraventricular, and ventricular arrhythmias.

INDICATIONS AND DOSAGES

Life-threatening ventricular arrhythmias, sustained ventricular tachycardia

PO

Adults, Elderly. Initially, 100 mg q12h, increased by 100 mg (50 mg twice a day) every 4 days until effective dose or maximum of 400 mg/day is attained.

Paroxysmal supraventricular tachycardias (PSVT), paroxysmal atrial fibrillation (PAF)

PO

Adults, Elderly. Initially, 50 mg q12h, increased by 100 mg (50 mg twice a day) every 4 days until effective dose or maximum of 300 mg/day is attained.

[$] **AVAILABLE FORMS/COST**

- Tab—Oral: 50 mg, 100's: **$173.95-$208.92**; 100 mg, 100's: **$272.80-$327.72**; 150 mg, 100's: **$375.45-$451.02**

CONTRAINDICATIONS: Cardiogenic shock, pre-existing second- or third-degree AV block, right bundle-branch block (without presence of a pacemaker)

PREGNANCY AND LACTATION: Pregnancy category C; excreted into breast milk with milk-plasma ratios 1.6:3.7, but considered compatible with breast-feeding

SIDE EFFECTS

Frequent (19%-10%)

Dizziness, dyspnea, headache

Occasional (9%-4%)

Nausea, fatigue, palpitations, chest pain, asthenia (loss of strength, energy), tremor, constipation

SERIOUS REACTIONS

- Flecainide may worsen existing arrhythmias or produce new ones.
- CHF may occur or existing CHF may worsen.
- Overdose may increase QRS duration, prolong QT interval, cause conduction disturbances, reduce myocardial contractility, and cause hypotension.

INTERACTIONS

Drugs

[3] *Acetazolamide, ammonium chloride, antacids, sodium bicarbonate:* Increases in urine pH decreases flecanide urinary clearance

[3] *Amiodarone:* Reduced flecainide dosage requirements

[3] *Cimetidine:* Inhibits metabolism of flecainide

[3] *Propranolol:* Inhibitors of each other's metabolism; additive negative inotropic effects

[3] *Sotolol:* Additive myocardial conduction depression; cardiac arrest reported

SPECIAL CONSIDERATIONS

- Not first line therapy
- Reserve for resistant arrhythmias due to proarrhythmic effects
- Initiate therapy in facilities capable of providing continuous ECG monitoring and managing life-threatening dysrhythmias

MONITORING PARAMETERS

- Monitor trough plasma levels periodically, especially in patients with moderate to severe chronic renal failure or severe hepatic disease and CHF; therapeutic range 0.2-1 mcg/ml

fluconazole
(floo-con'a-zole)
Rx: Diflucan
Chemical Class: Triazole derivative
Therapeutic Class: Antifungal

CLINICAL PHARMACOLOGY

Mechanism of Action: A fungistatic antifungal that interferes with cytochrome P-450, an enzyme necessary for ergosterol formation. *Therapeutic Effect:* Directly damages fungal membrane, altering its function.

Pharmacokinetics

Well absorbed from GI tract. Widely distributed, including to CSF. Protein binding: 11%. Partially metabolized in liver. Excreted unchanged primarily in urine. Partially removed by hemodialysis. **Half-life:** 20-30 hr (increased in impaired renal function).

INDICATIONS AND DOSAGES

Oropharyngeal candidiasis

PO, IV

Adults, Elderly. 200 mg once, then 100 mg/day for at least 14 days.
Children. 6 mg/kg/day once, then 3 mg/kg/day.

Esophageal candidiasis

PO, IV

Adults, Elderly. 200 mg once, then 100 mg/day (up to 400 mg/day) for 21 days and at least 14 days following resolution of symptoms.
Children. 6 mg/kg/day once, then 3 mg/kg/day (up to 12 mg/kg/day) for 21 days at at least 14 days following resolution of symptoms.

Vaginal candidiasis

PO

Adults. 150 mg once.

Prevention of candidiasis in patients undergoing bone marrow transplantation

PO

Adults. 400 mg/day.

Systemic candidiasis

PO, IV

Adults, Elderly. 400 mg once, then 200 mg/day (up to 400 mg/day) for at least 28 days and at least 14 days following resolution of symptoms.
Children. 6-12 mg/kg/day.

Cryptococcal meningitis

PO, IV

Adults, Elderly. 400 mg once, then 200 mg/day (up to 800 mg/day) for 10-12 wk after CSF becomes negative (200 mg/day for suppression of relapse in patients with AIDS).
Children. 12 mg/kg/day once, then 6-12 mg/kg/day (6 mg/kg/day for suppression of relapse in patients with AIDS).

Onychomycosis

PO

Adults. 150 mg/wk.

Dosage in Renal Impairment

After a loading dose of 400 mg, the daily dosage is based on creatinine clearance:

Creatinine Clearance	% of Recommended Dose
greater than 50 ml/min	100
21-50 ml/min	50
11-20 ml/min	25
Dialysis	Dose after dialysis

AVAILABLE FORMS/COST

• Sol, Inj—IV: 2 mg/ml, 100 ml: **$107.04**
• Powder, Reconst—Oral: 10 mg/ml 35 ml: **$37.04**; 40 mg/ml 35 ml: **$134.53**
• Tab, Plain Coated—Oral: 50 mg, 30's: **$172.90**; 100 mg, 30's: **$271.69**; 150 mg, 12's: **$172.92**; 200 mg, 30's: **$444.60**

UNLABELED USES: Treatment of coccidioidomycosis, cryptococcosis, fungal pneumonia, onychomycosis, ringworm of the hand, septicemia

CONTRAINDICATIONS: None known.

PREGNANCY AND LACTATION: Pregnancy category C; excreted into breast milk in concentrations similar to plasma; not recommended in nursing mothers

SIDE EFFECTS

Occasional (4%-1%)

Hypersensitivity reaction (including chills, fever, pruritus, and rash), dizziness, drowsiness, headache, constipation, diarrhea, nausea, vomiting, abdominal pain

SERIOUS REACTIONS

• Exfoliative skin disorders, serious hepatic effects, and blood dyscrasias (such as eosinophilia, thrombocytopenia, anemia, and leukopenia) have been reported rarely.

INTERACTIONS

Drugs

3 *Alprazolam:* Increased plasma alprazolam concentration

3 *Atevirdine:* Increased plasma atevirdine concentration

3 *Atorvastatin:* Increased plasma atorvastatin concentration with risk of rhabdomyolysis

3 *Buspirone:* Increased plasma buspirone concentration

3 *Caffeine:* Increased plasma caffeine concentration

3 *Chlordiazepoxide:* Increased plasma chlordiazepoxide concentration

2 *Cisapride:* QT prolongation and dysrhythmia

3 *Cyclosporine:* Increased plasma cyclosporine concentration

3 *Diazepam:* Increased plasma diazepam concentration

3 *Felodipine:* Increased plasma felodipine concentration

3 *Fluvastatin:* Increased plasma fluvastatin concentration with risk of rhabdomyolysis

3 *Losartan:* Reduced concentration of losartan's active metabolite may reduce efficacy of losartan

2 *Lovastatin:* Increased plasma lovastatin concentration with risk of rhabdomyolysis

3 *Methadone:* Increased plasma methadone concentration

3 *Midazolam:* Increased plasma midazolam concentration

2 *Phenytoin:* Markedly reduced plasma fluconazole concentration

3 *Pravastatin:* Increased plasma pravastatin concentration with risk of rhabdomyolysis

3 *Quinidine:* Increased plasma quinidine concentration

3 *Rifampin:* Decreased plasma fluconazole concentration; decreased plasma rifampin concentration

2 *Simvastatin:* Increased plasma simvastatin concentration with risk of rhabdomyolysis

3 *Tacrolimus:* Increased plasma tacrolimus concentration

2 *Triazolam:* Increased plasma triazolam concentration

3 *Tolbutamide:* Increased plasma tolbutamide concentration

3 *Warfarin:* Increased hypoprothrombinemic response

Labs

• *Benzoylecgonine:* False negative urine results

SPECIAL CONSIDERATIONS

MONITORING PARAMETERS

• Periodic liver function tests with prolonged therapy

flucytosine

(floo-sye'-toe-seen)
Rx: Ancobon
Chemical Class: Pyrimidine derivative, fluorinated
Therapeutic Class: Antifungal

CLINICAL PHARMACOLOGY

Mechanism of Action: An antifungal that penetrates fungal cells and is converted to fluorouracil which competes with uracil interfering with fungal RNA and protein synthesis. *Therapeutic Effect:* Damages fungal membrane.

Pharmacokinetics

Well absorbed from gastrointestinal (GI) tract. Widely distributed, including cerebrospinal fluid (CSF). Protein binding: 2-4%. Metabolized in liver. Partially removed by hemodialysis. **Half-life:** 3-8 hrs (half-life is increased with impaired renal function).

INDICATIONS AND DOSAGES

Fungal infections, candidiasis, cryptococcosis

PO

Adults, Elderly, Children. 50 to 150 mg/kg/day in 4 equally divided doses.

Dosage in renal function impairment

Based on creatinine clearance:

Creatinine Clearance	Dosage Interval
20-40 ml/min	q12h
10-20 ml/min	q24h
0-10 ml/min	q24-48h

$ AVAILABLE FORMS/COST

• Cap, Gel—Oral: 250 mg, 100's: **$431.95**; 500 mg, 100's: **$859.26**
CONTRAINDICATIONS: Hypersensitivity to flucytosine.

PREGNANCY AND LACTATION:

Pregnancy category C; 4% of drug metabolized to 5-fluorouracil, an antineoplastic suspected of producing congenital defects in humans; excretion into breast milk unknown; use caution in nursing mothers

SIDE EFFECTS

Occasional

Pruritus, rash, photosensitivity, dizziness, drowsiness, headache, diarrhea, nausea, vomiting, abdominal pain, increased liver enzymes, jaundice, increased BUN and creatinine, weakness, hearing loss

SERIOUS REACTIONS

• Hepatic dysfunction and severe bone marrow suppression occur rarely.

INTERACTIONS

Drugs

▨ *Cytosine arabinoside:* Inactivates antifungal activity by competitive inhibition

Labs

• *False increase:* Serum creatinine (when Ektachem analyzer is used)

SPECIAL CONSIDERATIONS

• Rarely used as monotherapy; generally used in combination with amphotericin B

PATIENT/FAMILY EDUCATION

• Reduce or avoid GI upset by taking caps a few at a time over a 15 min period

MONITORING PARAMETERS

• Creatinine, BUN, alk phosphatase, AST, ALT, CBC
• Serum flucytosine concentrations (therapeutic range 25-100 mcg/ml)

fludrocortisone

(floo-droe-kor'ti-sone)

Rx: Florinef

Chemical Class: Mineralocorticoid, synthetic

Therapeutic Class: Mineralocorticoid

CLINICAL PHARMACOLOGY

Mechanism of Action: A mineralocorticoid that acts at distal tubules. *Therapeutic Effect:* Increases potassium and hydrogen ion excretion. Replaces sodium loss and raises blood pressure (with low dosages). Inhibits endogenous adrenal cortical secretion, thymic activity, and secretion of corticotropin by pituitary gland (with higher dosages).

Pharmacokinetics

Well absorbed from the GI tract. Protein binding: 42%. Widely distributed. Metabolized in the liver and kidney. Primarily excreted in urine. **Half-life:** 3.5 hr.

INDICATIONS AND DOSAGES

Addison's disease

PO

Adults, Elderly. 0.05–0.1 mg/day. Range: 0.1 mg 3 times a wk to 0.2 mg/day. Administration with cortisone or hydrocortisone preferred.

Salt-losing adrenogenital syndrome

PO

Adults, Elderly. 0.1–0.2 mg/day.

Usual pediatric dosage

Children. 0.05–0.1 mg/day.

🆂 AVAILABLE FORMS/COST

• Tab—Oral: 0.1 mg, 100's: **$74.77-$88.26**

UNLABELED USES: Treatment of acidosis in renal tubular disorders, idiopathic orthostatic hypotension

CONTRAINDICATIONS: CHF, systemic fungal infection

PREGNANCY AND LACTATION: Pregnancy category C; observe newborn for signs and symptoms of adrenocortical insufficiency; corticosteroids are found in breast milk; use caution in nursing mothers

SIDE EFFECTS

Frequent

Increased appetite, exaggerated sense of well-being, abdominal distention, weight gain, insomnia, mood swings

High dosages, prolonged therapy, too rapid withdrawal: Increased susceptibility to infection with masked signs and symptoms, delayed wound healing, hypokalemia, hypocalcemia, GI distress, diarrhea or constipation, hypertension

Occasional

Headache, dizziness, menstrual difficulty or amenorrhea, gastric ulcer development

Rare

Hypersensitivity reaction

SERIOUS REACTIONS

• Long-term therapy may cause muscle wasting (especially in the arms and legs), osteoporosis, spontaneous fractures, amenorrhea, cataracts, glaucoma, peptic ulcer disease, and CHF.

• Abruptly withdrawing the drug after long-term therapy may cause anorexia, nausea, fever, headache, joint pain, rebound inflammation, fatigue, weakness, lethargy, dizziness, and orthostatic hypotension.

INTERACTIONS

Drugs

🇼 *Amphotericin:* Excessive potassium depletion

🇼 *Diuretics, loop:* Opposite therapeutic effect; excessive potassium loss

🇼 *Diuretics, thiazide:* Opposite therapeutic effect; excessive potassium loss

3 *Digitalis:* Increased potential for digitalis toxicity associated with hypokalemia

SPECIAL CONSIDERATIONS
PATIENT/FAMILY EDUCATION
• Notify clinician of dizziness, severe headache, swelling of feet or lower legs, unusual weight gain
• Do not discontinue abruptly
MONITORING PARAMETERS
• Serum electrolytes, blood pressure, serum renin

---

flumazenil
(flew-maz-ah-nil)

Rx: Romazicon
Chemical Class: Imidazobenzodiazepine derivative
Therapeutic Class: Benzodiazepine antagonist

CLINICAL PHARMACOLOGY
Mechanism of Action: An antidote that antagonizes the effect of benzodiazepines on the gamma-aminobutyric acid receptor complex in the CNS. *Therapeutic Effect:* Reverses sedative effect of benzodiazepines.

Pharmacokinetics

Route	Onset	Peak	Duration
IV	1–2 min	6–10 min	less than 1 hr

Duration and degree of benzodiazepine reversal depend on dosage and plasma concentration. Protein binding: 50%. Metabolized by the liver; excreted in urine.

INDICATIONS AND DOSAGES
Reversal of conscious sedation or general anesthesia
IV

Adults, Elderly. Initially, 0.2 mg (2 ml) over 15 sec; may repeat dose in 45 sec; then at 60-sec intervals. Maximum: 1 mg (10-ml) total dose.

Children, Neonates. Initially, 0.01 mg/kg; may repeat in 45 sec, then at 60-sec intervals. Maximum: 0.2 mg single dose; 0.05 mg/kg or 1 mg cumulative dose.

Benzodiazepine overdose
IV

Adults, Elderly. Initially, 0.2 mg (2 ml) over 30 sec; if desired LOC is not achieved after 30 sec, 0.3 mg (3 ml) may be given over 30 sec. Further doses of 0.5 mg (5 ml) may be administered over 30 sec at 60-sec intervals. Maximum: 3 mg (30 ml) total dose.

Children, Neonates. Initially, 0.01 mg/kg; may repeat in 45 sec, then at 60-sec intervals. Maximum: 0.2 mg single dose; 1 mg cumulative dose.

S   **AVAILABLE FORMS/COST**
• Sol, Inj—IV: 0.1 mg/ml, 5, 10 ml: **$75.88**/5 ml

CONTRAINDICATIONS: Anticholinergic signs (such as mydriasis, dry mucosa, and hypoperistalsis), arrhythmias, cardiovascular collapse, history of hypersensitivity to benzodiazepines, patients with signs of serious cyclic antidepressant overdose (such as motor abnormalities), patients who have been given a benzodiazepine for control of a potentially life-threatening condition (such as control of status epilepticus or increased intracranial pressure)

PREGNANCY AND LACTATION: Pregnancy category C; excretion into breast milk unknown; use caution in nursing mothers

SIDE EFFECTS
Frequent (11%–4%)
Agitation, anxiety, dry mouth, dyspnea, insomnia, palpitations, tremors, headache, blurred vision, dizziness, ataxia, nausea, vomiting, pain at injection site, diaphoresis
Occasional (3%–1%)

Fatigue, flushing, auditory disturbances, thrombophlebitis, rash
Rare (less than 1%)
Urticaria, pruritus, hallucinations
SERIOUS REACTIONS
• Toxic effects, such as seizures and arrhythmias, of other drugs taken in overdose, especially tricyclic antidepressants, may emerge with reversal of sedative effect of benzodiazepines.
• Flumazenil may provoke a panic attack in those with a history of panic disorder.

SPECIAL CONSIDERATIONS
PATIENT/FAMILY EDUCATION
• Resedation may occur; do not engage in any activities requiring complete alertness or operate hazardous machinery or a motor vehicle until at least 18 to 24 hr after discharge
• Do not use any alcohol or non-prescription drugs for 18 to 24 hr after flumazenil administration

MONITORING PARAMETERS
• Monitor for seizures, sedation, respiratory depression, or other residual benzodiazepine effects for an appropriate period (up to 120 min) based on dose and duration of effect of the benzodiazepine employed; pharmacokinetics of benzodiazepines are not altered in the presence of flumazenil

flunisolide
(floo-niss'oh-lide)
Rx: *Aerosol INH:* AeroBid
Rx: *Nasal:* Nasalide, Nasarel
Chemical Class: Glucocorticoid, synthetic
Therapeutic Class: Antiasthmatic; corticoseroid, antiinflammatory; corticosteroid, nasal

F

CLINICAL PHARMACOLOGY
Mechanism of Action: An adrenocorticosteroid that controls the rate of protein synthesis, depresses migration of polymorphonuclear leukocytes, reverses capillary permeability, and stabilizes lysosomal membranes. *Therapeutic Effect:* Prevents or controls inflammation.
INDICATIONS AND DOSAGES
Long-term control of bronchial asthma, assists in reducing or discontinuing oral corticosteroid therapy
Inhalation
Adults, Elderly. 2 inhalations twice a day, morning and evening. Maximum: 4 inhalations twice a day.
Children 6–15 yr. 2 inhalations twice a day.
Relief of symptoms of perennial and seasonal rhinitis
Intranasal
Adults, Elderly. Initially, 2 sprays each nostril twice a day, may increase at 4-7 day intervals to 2 sprays 3 times a day. Maximum: 8 sprays in each nostril daily.
Children 6–14 yr. Initially, 1 spray 3 times a day or 2 sprays twice a day. Maximum: 4 sprays in each nostril daily. Maintenance: 1 spray into each nostril each day.
$ AVAILABLE FORMS/COST
• Aer—Inhaler: 250 mcg/inh, 100 doses, 7 g: **$76.95**

• Spray—Nasal: 25 mcg/inh, 200 doses, 25 ml: **$46.49-$56.55**

UNLABELED USES: To prevent recurrence of nasal polyps after surgery

CONTRAINDICATIONS: Hypersensitivity to any corticosteroid, persistently positive sputum cultures for *Candida albicans,* primary treatment of status asthmaticus, systemic fungal infections

PREGNANCY AND LACTATION: Pregnancy category C; excretion into breast milk unknown; use caution in nursing mothers

SIDE EFFECTS
Frequent
Inhalation (25%–10%): Unpleasant taste, nausea, vomiting, sore throat, diarrhea, upset stomach, cold symptoms, nasal congestion
Occasional
Inhalation (9%–3%): Dizziness, irritability, nervousness, tremors, abdominal pain, heartburn, oropharynx candidiasis, edema
Nasal: Mild nasopharyngeal irritation or dryness, rebound congestion, bronchial asthma, rhinorrhea, altered taste

SERIOUS REACTIONS
• An acute hypersensitivity reaction, marked by urticaria, angioedema, and severe bronchospasm, occurs rarely.
• A transfer from systemic to local steroid therapy may unmask previously suppressed bronchial asthma condition.

SPECIAL CONSIDERATIONS
PATIENT/FAMILY EDUCATION
• To be used on a regular basis, not for acute symptoms
• Use bronchodilators before oral inhaler (for patients using both)
• Nasal sol may cause drying and irritation of nasal mucosa
• Clear nasal passages prior to use of nasal sol

MONITORING PARAMETERS
• Monitor children for growth as well as for effects on the HPA axis during chronic therapy
• Monitor patients switched from chronic systemic corticosteroids to avoid acute adrenal insufficiency in response to stress

---

fluocinolone acetonide
(floo-oh-sin′-oh-lone a-seat′-oh-nide)
Rx: Derma-Smoothe/FS, FS Shampoo, Synalar, Synemol Combinations
   Rx: with hydroquinone/tretinoin (Tri-Luma)
Chemical Class: Corticosteroid, synthetic
Therapeutic Class: Corticosteroid, topical

CLINICAL PHARMACOLOGY
Mechanism of Action: A fluorinated topical corticosteroid that controls the rate of protein synthesis; depresses migration of polymorphonuclear leukocytes and fibroblasts; reduces capillary permeability; prevents or controls inflammation. *Therapeutic Effect:* Decreases tissue response to inflammatory process.
Pharmacokinetics
Use of occlusive dressings may increase percutaneous absorption. Protein binding: more than 90%. Excreted in urine. **Half-life:** Unknown.

INDICATIONS AND DOSAGES
Atopic dermatitis
Topical
Adults, Elderly. Apply 3 times/day.
Children 2 yrs and older. Apply 2 times/day.

Scalp psoriasis
Topical

Adults, Elderly. Apply to damp or wet hair and leave on overnight or for at least 4 hrs. Remove by washing hair with shampoo.

Seborrheic dermatitis, scalp
Shampoo

Adults, Elderly. Apply once daily allowi to remain on scalp for at least 5 min.

S AVAILABLE FORMS/COST
• Cre—Top: 0.01%, 15, 60, 100, 425 g: **$3.20-$4.73**/60 g; 0.025%, 15, 60, 100, 425 g: **$4.20-$66.43**/60 g
• Oil—Top: 0.01%, 120 ml: **$33.53**
• Oint—Top: 0.025%, 15, 30, 60 g: **$9.95-$61.42**/60 g
• Shampoo—Top: 0.01%, 120 ml: **$41.19**
• Sol—Top: 0.01%, 20, 60 ml: **$4.81-$70.06**/60 ml

UNLABELED USES: Vitiligo
CONTRAINDICATIONS: Hypersensitivity to fluocinolone or other corticosteroids

PREGNANCY AND LACTATION: Pregnancy category C; unknown whether topical application could result in sufficient systemic absorption to produce detectable amounts in breast milk (systemic corticosteroids are secreted into breast milk in quantities not likely to have detrimental effects on infant)

SIDE EFFECTS
Occasional
Burning, dryness, itching, stinging
Rare
Allergic contact dermatitis, purpura or blood-containing blisters, thinning of skin with easy bruising, telangiectasis or raised dark red spots on skin

SERIOUS REACTIONS
• When taken in excessive quantities, systemic hypercorticism and adrenal suppression may occur.

SPECIAL CONSIDERATIONS
• Topical oil contains refined peanut oil

PATIENT/FAMILY EDUCATION
• Apply sparingly only to affected area
• Avoid contact with eyes
• Do not put bandages or dressings over treated area unless directed by clinician
• Do not use on weeping, denuded, or infected areas
• Discontinue drug, notify clinician if local irritation or fever develops

---

fluocinonide
(floo-oh-sin'oh-nide)
Rx: Lidex, Lidex-E
Chemical Class: Corticosteroid, synthetic
Therapeutic Class: Corticosteroid, topical

CLINICAL PHARMACOLOGY
Mechanism of Action: A topical corticosteroid that has anti-inflammatory, antipruritic, and vasoconstrictive properties. The exact mechanism of the anti-inflammatory process is unclear. *Therapeutic Effect:* Reduces or prevents tissue response to the inflammatory process.

Pharmacokinetics
Well absorbed systemically. Large variation in absorption among sites. Protein binding: varies. Metabolized in liver. Primarily excreted in urine.

INDICATIONS AND DOSAGES
Dermatoses
Topical

Adults, Elderly. Apply sparingly 2- 4 times/day.

S AVAILABLE FORMS/COST
• Cre—Top: 0.05%, 15, 30, 60, 120 g: **$3.39-$46.96**/30 g

• Gel—Top: 0.05%, 15, 30, 60, 120 g: **$46.01-$78.78**/60 g
• Oint—Top: 0.05%, 15, 30, 60, 120 g: **$18.01-$46.96**/30 g
• Sol—Top: 0.05%, 20, 60 ml: **$18.75-$76.35**/60 ml

CONTRAINDICATIONS: History of hypersensitivity to fluocinonide or other corticosteroids

PREGNANCY AND LACTATION: Pregnancy category C; unknown whether topical application could result in sufficient systemic absorption to produce detectable amounts in breast milk (systemic corticosteroids are secreted into breast milk in quantities not likely to have detrimental effects on infant)

SIDE EFFECTS

Occasional

Itching, redness, irritation, burning at site of application, dryness, folliculitis, acneiform eruptions, hypopigmentation

Rare

Allergic contact dermatitis, maceration of the skin, secondary infection, skin atrophy

SERIOUS REACTIONS

• The serious reactions of long-term therapy and the addition of occlusive dressings are reversible hypothalamic-pituitary-adrenal (HPA) axis suppression, manifestations of Cushing's syndrome, hyperglycemia, and glucosuria.

SPECIAL CONSIDERATIONS

PATIENT/FAMILY EDUCATION

• Apply sparingly only to affected area
• Avoid contact with eyes
• Do not put bandages or dressings over treated area unless directed by clinician
• Do not use on weeping, denuded, or infected areas

• Discontinue drug, notify clinician if local irritation or fever develops

---

fluorescein
(flure'-e-seen sow-dee-um)

Rx: AK-Fluor, Angioscein, Fluorescite, Fluorets, Fluor-I-Strip, Fluor-I-Strip-A.T., Ful-Glo, Ocu-Flur 10
Combinations
   Rx: with proparacaine (Fluoracaine)
Chemical Class: Xanthine dye
Therapeutic Class: Ophthalmic diagnostic agent

CLINICAL PHARMACOLOGY

Mechanism of Action: An indicator dye used as a diagnostic agent with a low molecular weight, high water solubility, and fluorescence that penetrates any break in epithelial barrier to permit rapid penetration. Emits light at a wavelength of 520 to 530 nanometers (green-yellow) when exposed to light in the blue wavelength (465 to 490 nanometers). *Therapeutic Effect:* Diagnosis of corneal and conjunctival abnormalities.

Pharmacokinetics

Rapidly absorbed. Protein binding: 85%. Widely distributed. Metabolized in liver to an active metabolite, fluorescein monoglucuronide. Primarily excreted in urine. **Half-life:** 24 min (parent compound), 4 hrs (metabolite).

INDICATIONS AND DOSAGES

Retinal angiography

Injection

Adults, Elderly. Inject contents of ampule or vial of 10% or 25% solution rapidly into the antecubital vein

Applanation tonometry
Ophthlalmic strips
Adults, Elderly. Place strip, which has been moistened with a drop of sterile water, at the fornix in the lower cul-de-sac close to the punctum. Patient should close lid tightly over strip until desired amount of staining is observed or retract upper lid and touch tip of strip to the bulbar conjunctiva on the temporal side until adequate staining is achieved

AVAILABLE FORMS/COST
• Sol, Inj—Intraocular: 10% 5 ml: **$3.90-$22.19**
• Sol, Inj—IV: 25%, 2 ml: **$3.90-$23.88**
• Sol—Ophth: 2%, 1 ml: **$2.08**; 10%, 5 ml: **$0.25**
• Strip—Ophth: 0.6 mg, 300's: **$36.87**; 1 mg, 9 mg, 300's: **$67.20-$77.80**

CONTRAINDICATIONS: Concomitant soft contact lens use (ophthalmic strips), hypersensitivity to fluorescein or any component of the formulation

PREGNANCY AND LACTATION: Pregnancy category C; avoid parenteral use, especially in 1st trimester; excreted into breast milk; use caution in nursing mothers

SIDE EFFECTS
Occasional
Ophthalmic: Burning sensation in the eye
Injection: Stinging, bronchospasm, generalized hives and itching, hypersensitivity, headache gastrointestinal distress, nausea, strong taste, vomiting, hypotension, syncope
Rare
Injection: anaphylaxis, basilar artery ischemia, cardiac arrest, severe shock, convulsions, thrombophlebitis at injection site

SERIOUS REACTIONS
• Anaphylactic reactions have occurred leading to laryngeal edema, bronchospasm, shock and even death.

SPECIAL CONSIDERATIONS
PATIENT/FAMILY EDUCATION
• May cause temporary yellowish discoloration of skin (fades in 6-12 hr)
• Urine will appear bright yellow (fades in 24-36 hr)
• Soft contact lenses may become stained, wait at least 1 hr after thorough rinsing of eye before replacing lenses

MONITORING PARAMETERS
• Luminescence appears in the retina and choroidal vessels 9-15 min following IV inj; can be observed by standard viewing equipment

---

fluoride, sodium
Rx: Fluorinse, Fluoritab, Flura, Gel-Kam, Karidium, Karigel, Listermint with Fluoride, Luride, Minute-Gel, Pediaflor, Pharmaflur, Phos-Flur, Prevident, Stop, Thera-Flur
OTC: Fluorigard, Gel-Tin
Chemical Class: Fluoride ion
Therapeutic Class: Anti-dental caries agent; antiosteoporotic

---

CLINICAL PHARMACOLOGY
Mechanism of Action: A trace element that increases tooth resistance to acid dissolution. *Therapeutic Effect:* Promotes remineralization of decalcified enamel, inhibits dental plaque bacteria, increases resistance to development of caries, maintains bone strength.

INDICATIONS AND DOSAGES
Dietary supplement for prevention of dental caries in children

Fluoride Level in Water	Age	Dosage
less than 0.3 ppm*	younger than 2 yr	0.25 mg/day
	2–3 yr	0.5 mg/day
	older than 3–13 yr	1 mg/day
0.3–0.7 ppm*	younger than 2 yr	None
	2–3 yr	0.25 mg/day
	older than 3–13 yr	0.5 mg/day
greater than 0.7 ppm*	None	None

* ppm = parts per million

§ AVAILABLE FORMS/COST
• Liq—Oral: 0.25 mg/0.6 ml, 60 ml: **$3.13**
• Lozenge—Oral: 1 mg, 60's: **$7.25**
• Solution—Oral: 0.2%, 480 ml: **$7.49**; 0.5 mg/ml, 50 ml: **$7.00-$15.46**; 1 mg/ml, 30, 60 ml: **$4.25-$6.30**/30 ml
• Tab—Oral: 1 mg, 100's: **$0.59-$2.50**
• Tab, Chewable—Oral: 0.25 mg, 100's: **$2.16**; 0.5 mg, 100's: **$1.98-$5.54**; 1 mg, 100's: **$1.50-$5.54**

CONTRAINDICATIONS: Arthralgia, GI ulceration, severe renal insufficiency

PREGNANCY AND LACTATION: Administration from 3rd-9th mo of gestation safe (no information on teratogenicity); small amounts excreted into breast milk, inadequate therapeutically due to small amount of excretion and complexation with calcium

SIDE EFFECTS
Rare
Oral mucous membrane ulceration

SERIOUS REACTIONS
• Hypocalcemia, tetany, bone pain (especially in ankles and feet), electrolyte disturbances, and arrhythmias occur rarely.
• Fluoride use may cause skeletal fluorosis, osteomalacia, and osteosclerosis.

SPECIAL CONSIDERATIONS
• Therapy begun prenatally and continued through age 16 is effective in reducing the number of decayed, missing, or filled surfaces and teeth; especially beneficial in areas where fluoride content of drinking water is below 0.7 ppm
• Treatment of osteoporosis, combined with 1 or more of the following—calcium, estrogen, or vitamin D—increases bone density, reduces rate of new vertebral fractures, if correct dose and in slow-release preparation; role in steroid-induced osteoporosis being investigated, reports to date indicate a poor response rate

PATIENT/FAMILY EDUCATION
• Avoid use with dairy products

---

fluoxetine
(floo-ox'e-teen)
Rx: Prozac, Prozac Weekly, Sarafem
Combinations
  Rx: with olanzapine (Symbyax)
Chemical Class: Aryloxypropylamine
Therapeutic Class: Antidepressant, selective serotonin reuptake inhibitor (SSRI)

CLINICAL PHARMACOLOGY
Mechanism of Action: A psychotherapeutic agent that selectively inhibits serotonin uptake in the CNS, enhancing serotonergic function.

Therapeutic Effect: Relieves depression; reduces obsessive-compulsive and bulimic behavior.

Pharmacokinetics

Well absorbed from the GI tract. Crosses the blood-brain barrier. Protein binding: 94%. Metabolized in the liver to active metabolite. Primarily excreted in urine. Not removed by hemodialysis. **Half-life:** 2-3 days; metabolite 7-9 days.

INDICATIONS AND DOSAGES

Depression, obsessive-compulsive disorder

PO

Adults. Initially, 20 mg each morning. If therapeutic improvement does not occur after 2 wk, gradually increase to maximum of 80 mg/day in 2 equally divided doses in morning and at noon. Prozac Weekly: 90 mg/wk, begin 7 days after last dose of 20 mg.

Elderly. Initially, 10 mg/day. May increase by 10-20 mg q2wk.

Children 7-17 yr. Initially, 5-10 mg/day. Titrate upward as needed. Usual dosage is 20 mg/day.

Panic disorder

PO

Adults, Elderly. Initially, 10 mg/day. May increase to 20 mg/day after 1 week. Maximum: 60 mg/day.

Bulimia nervosa

PO

Adults. 60 mg each morning.

Premenstrual dysphoric disorder

PO

Adults. 20 mg/day.

$ AVAILABLE FORMS/COST

• Cap—Oral: 10 mg, 100's: **$27.62-$361.91**; 20 mg, 100's: **$23.92-$371.24**; 40 mg, 100's: **$550.00**
• Cap—Oral (Sarafem): 10 mg, 28's: **$94.72**; 20 mg, 28's: **$97.16**
• Cap, Sus Action—Oral: 90 mg, 4's: **$90.88**
• Sol—Oral: 20 mg/5 ml, 120 ml: **$118.00-$164.86**
• Tab—Oral: 10 mg, 100's: **$361.91**; 20 mg, 100's: **$280.06-$311.21**

UNLABELED USES: Treatment of hot flashes

CONTRAINDICATIONS: Use within 14 days of MAOIs

PREGNANCY AND LACTATION: Pregnancy category B; excreted into breast milk; use caution in nursing mothers

SIDE EFFECTS

Frequent (more than 10%)

Headache, asthenia, insomnia, anxiety, nervousness, somnolence, nausea, diarrhea, decreased appetite

Occasional (9%-2%)

Dizziness, tremor, fatigue, vomiting, constipation, dry mouth, abdominal pain, nasal congestion, diaphoresis, rash

Rare (less than 2%)

Flushed skin, light-headedness, impaired concentration

SERIOUS REACTIONS

• Overdose may produce seizures, nausea, vomiting, agitation, and restlessness.

INTERACTIONS

Drugs

③ *Benzodiazepines (alprazolam, diazepam):* Probable inhibition of metabolism (CYP3A4) leading to accumulation of diazepam and alprazolam

③ *β-blockers (metroprolol, propranolol, sotalol):* Inhibition of metabolism (CYP2D6) leads to increased plasma concentrations of selective β-blockers and potential cardiac toxicity; atenolol may be safer choice

③ *Buspirone:* Reduced therapeutic effect of both drugs; possible seizures

③ *Carbamazepine:* Inhibition of hepatic metabolism of carbamazepine, but the formation of carbamazepine epoxide is not inhibited, contributing to increased toxicity

🔞 *Clozapine:* Increased serum clozapine concentrations

🔞 *Cyproheptadine:* Serotonin antagonist may partially reverse antidepressant and other effects

🔞 *Dextromethorphan:* Inhibition of dextromethorphan's metabolism (CYP2D6) by fluoxetine and additive serotonergic effects

🔞 *Diuretics, loop (bumetanide, furosemide, torsemide):* Possible additive hyponatremia; 2 fatal case reports with furosemide and fluoxetine

②️ *Fenfluramine:* Duplicate effects on inhibition of serotonin reuptake; inhibition of dexfenfluramine metabolism (CYP2D6) exaggerates effect; both mechanisms increase risk of serotonin syndrome

🔞 *Haloperidol:* Inhibition of haloperidol's metabolism (CYP2D6) may increase risks of extrapyramidal symptoms

②️ *HMG-Co A reductase inhibitors (atorvastatin, lovastatin, simvastatin):* Inhibition of statin metabolism (CYP3A4), by fluoxetine, may lead to rhabdomyolysis

🔞 *Lithium:* Neurotoxicity (tremor, confusion, ataxia, dizziness, dysarthria, and absence seizures) reported in patients receiving this combination; mechanism unknown

⚠️ *MAOI's (isocarboxazid, phenelzine, tranylcypromine):* Increased CNS serotonergic effect has been associated with severe or fatal reactions with this combination

🔞 *Phenytoin:* Inhibition of metabolism and phenytoin toxicity

🔞 *Selegiline:* Sporadic cases of mania and hypertension

⚠️ *Thioridazine:* Increased serum thioridazine concentrations resulting in an increased risk of QTc interval prolongation, serious ventricular arrhythmias, and death

🔞 *Tricyclic antidepressants (clomipramine, desipramine, doxepin, imipramine, nortriptylline, trazodone):* Marked increases in tricyclic antidepressant levels due to inhibition of metabolism (CYP2D6)

②️ *Tryptophan:* Additive serotonergic effects

🔞 *Warfarin:* Altered anti-coagulant effects, including increased bleeding

SPECIAL CONSIDERATIONS
PATIENT/FAMILY EDUCATION

• Therapeutic response may take 4-6 wk

• May cause insomnia, administer in am; sedating antidepressants, in small doses (i.e. trazodone 50 mg), frequently administered H.S., concurrently

---

fluoxymesterone
(floo-ex-ih-mes-the-rone)

Rx: Halotestin

Chemical Class: Testosterone derivative

Therapeutic Class: Androgen; antineoplastic

DEA Class: Schedule III

CLINICAL PHARMACOLOGY

Mechanism of Action: An androgen that suppresses gonadotropin-releasing hormone, LH, and FSH. *Therapeutic Effect:* Stimulates spermatogenesis, development of male secondary sex characteristics, and sexual maturation at puberty. Stimulates production of red blood cells (RBCs).

Pharmacokinetics

Rapidly absorbed from the gastrointestinal (GI) tract. Protein binding: 98%. Metabolized in liver. Excreted in urine. **Half-life:** 9.2 hrs.

INDICATIONS AND DOSAGES

Males (hypogonadism)

PO

Adults. 5-20 mg/day.

Males (delayed puberty)

PO

Adults. 2.5-20 mg/day for 4-6 mos.

Females (inoperable breast cancer)

PO

Adults. 10-40 mg/day in divided doses for 1-3 mos.

Females (prevent postpartum breast pain/engorgement)

PO

Adults. Initially, 2.5 mg shortly after delivery, then 5-10 mg/day in divided doses for 4-5 days.

$ **AVAILABLE FORMS/COST**

- Tab—Oral: 2 mg, 100's: **$99.05**; 5 mg, 100's: **$223.11**; 10 mg, 100's: **$236.21-$301.12**

CONTRAINDICATIONS: Serious cardiac, renal, or hepatic dysfunction, men with carcinomas of the breast or prostate, hypersensitivity to fluoxymesterone or any component of the formulation including tartrazine

PREGNANCY AND LACTATION: Pregnancy category X; causes virilization of external genitalia of female fetus; excretion into breast milk unknown; use extreme caution in nursing mothers

SIDE EFFECTS

Frequent

Females: Amenorrhea, virilism (e.g., acne, decreased breast size, enlarged clitoris, male pattern baldness), deepening voice

Males: UTI, breast soreness, gynecomastia, priapism, virilism (e.g., acne, early pubic hair growth)

Occasional

Edema, nausea, vomiting, mild acne, diarrhea, stomach pain

Males: Impotence, testicular atrophy

SERIOUS REACTIONS

- Peliosis hepatitis (liver, spleen replaced with blood-filled cysts), hepatic neoplasms, and hepatocellular carcinoma have been associated with prolonged high dosage.

INTERACTIONS

Drugs

❷ *Cyclosporine, tacrolimus:* Increased cyclosporine and tacrolimus levels with potential toxicity

❷ *Oral anticoagulants:* Enhanced hypoprothrombinemic response to oral anticoagulants

SPECIAL CONSIDERATIONS

MONITORING PARAMETERS

- Frequent urine and serum calcium determinations (breast cancer)
- Periodic LFTs, Hct
- X-ray examinations of bone age q6mo during treatment of prepubertal males

---

fluphenazine

(floo-fen'a-zeen)

Rx: Permitil, Prolixin

Chemical Class: Piperazine phenothiazine derivative

Therapeutic Class: Antipsychotic

CLINICAL PHARMACOLOGY

Mechanism of Action: A phenothiazine that antagonizes dopamine neurotransmission at synapses by blocking postsynaptic dopaminergic receptors in the brain. *Therapeutic Effect:* Decreases psychotic behavior. Also produces weak anticholinergic, sedative, and antiemetic effects and strong extrapyramidal effects.

INDICATIONS AND DOSAGES

Psychosis

PO

Adults, Elderly. 0.5-10 mg/day in divided doses q6-8h.

IM

Adults, Elderly. 1.5-10 mg/day in divided doses q6-8h or 12.5 mg (decanoate) q2wk.

[$] **AVAILABLE FORMS/COST**

• Conc—Oral: 5 mg/ml, 120 ml: **$106.94-$160.44**

• Elixir—Oral: 2.5 mg/5 ml, 60 ml: **$16.10-$25.50**

• Sol, Inj—IM, SC: 2.5 mg/ml, 10 ml: **$65.13**

• Tab, Plain Coated—Oral: 1 mg, 100's: **$14.73-$125.24**; 2.5 mg, 100's: **$21.70-$155.40**; 5 mg, 100's: **$27.55-$229.06**; 10 mg 100's: **$33.05-$278.90**

• Sol, Inj (decanoate)—IM, SC: 25 mg/ml, 5 ml: **$14.29-$125.45**

• Sol, Inj (enanthate)—SC: 25 mg/ml, 5 ml: **$128.50**

UNLABELED USES: Treatment of neurogenic pain (adjunct to tricyclic antidepressants)

CONTRAINDICATIONS: Angle-closure glaucoma, myelosuppression, severe cardiac or hepatic disease, severe hypertension or hypotension, subcortical brain damage

PREGNANCY AND LACTATION: Pregnancy category C; EPS in the newborn have been attributed to *in utero* exposure; other reports have indicated that phenothiazines are relatively safe during pregnancy; excretion into breast milk unknown; use caution in nursing mothers

SIDE EFFECTS

Frequent

Hypotension, dizziness, and syncope (occur frequently after first injection, occasionally after subsequent injections, and rarely with oral doses)

Occasional

Somnolence (during early therapy), dry mouth, blurred vision, lethargy, constipation or diarrhea, nasal congestion, peripheral edema, urine retention

Rare

Ocular changes, altered skin pigmentation (with prolonged use of high doses)

SERIOUS REACTIONS

• Extrapyramidal symptoms appear to be related to high dosages and are divided into 3 categories: akathisia (inability to sit still, tapping of feet), parkinsonian symptoms (such as hypersalivation, masklike facial expression, shuffling gait, and tremors), and acute dystonias (such as torticollis, opisthotonos, and oculogyric crisis).

• Tardive dyskinesia, manifested as tongue protrusion, puffing of the cheeks, and chewing or puckering of the mouthoccurs rarely but may be irreversible.

• Abrupt withdrawal after long-term therapy may precipitate dizziness, gastritis, nausea and vomiting, and tremors.

• Blood dyscrasias, particularly agranulocytosis and mild leukopenia, may occur.

• Fluphenzine use may lower the seizure threshold.

INTERACTIONS

Drugs

[3] *Anticholinergics:* Inhibition of therapeutic response to neuroleptics, additive anticholinergic effects

[3] *Antimalarials (amodiaquine, chloroquine, sulfadoxine-pyrimethamine):* Increased neuroleptic concentrations

[3] *Barbiturates:* Reduced serum neuroleptic concentrations

[3] *β-blockers:* Potential increases in serum concentrations of both drugs

[3] *Bromocriptine:* Reduced effects of both drugs

[3] *Clonidine:* Acute organic brain syndrome

3 *Cyclic antidepressants:* Increased serum concentrations of both drugs

3 *Epinephrine:* Reversal of pressor response to epinephrine

3 *Guanadrel:* Inhibits antihypertensive response

2 *Levodopa:* Inhibition of the antiparkinsonian effect of levodopa

3 *Lithium:* Rare cases of severe neurotoxicity have been reported in acute manic patients

3 *Meperidine:* Hypotension, excessive CNS depression

3 *Orphenadrine:* Reduced serum neuroleptic concentrations

Labs

• Urine pregnancy test: false positive

SPECIAL CONSIDERATIONS

• Concentrate must be diluted prior to administration; use only the following diluents: water, saline, 7-Up, homogenized milk, carbonated orange beverage, and pineapple, apricot, prune, orange, V-8, tomato, and grapefruit juices; do not mix with beverages containing caffeine, tannics (tea), or pectinates (apple juice), as physical incompatibility may result

PATIENT/FAMILY EDUCATION

• May cause drowsiness; use caution while driving or performing other tasks requiring alertness

• Avoid contact with skin when using concentrates

• Avoid prolonged exposure to sunlight

• May discolor urine pink or reddish-brown

• Use caution in hot weather, heatstroke may result

• Arise slowly from a reclining position

MONITORING PARAMETERS

• Monitor closely for the appearance of tardive dyskinesia

---

flurandrenolide
(flure-an-dren'oh-lide)
Rx: Cordran, Cordran SP,
Cordran Tape
Chemical Class: Corticosteroid, synthetic
Therapeutic Class: Corticosteroid, topical

F

CLINICAL PHARMACOLOGY
Mechanism of Action: A fluorinated orticosteroid that decreases inflammation by suppression the migration of polymorphonuclear leukocytes and reversal of increased capillary permeability. *Therapeutic Effect:* Decreases tissue response to inflammatory process.

Pharmacokinetics
Repeated applications may lead to percutaneous absorption. Absorption is about 36% from scrotal area, 7% from the forehead, 4% from scalp, and 1% from forearm. Metabolized in liver. Excreted in urine.
Half-life: Unknown.

INDICATIONS AND DOSAGES
Anti-inflammatory, immunosuppressant, corticosteroid replacement therapy
Topical
Adults, Elderly. Apply 2-3 times/day.
Children. Apply 1-2 times/day.

$ **AVAILABLE FORMS/COST**
• Cre—Top: 0.025%, 30, 60 g: **$22.33**/30 g; 0.05%, 15, 30, 60 g: **$28.50**/30 g
• Lotion—Top: 0.05%, 15, 60 ml: **$41.33**/60 ml
• Oint—Top: 0.025%, 30, 60 g: **$31.54**/60 g; 0.05%, 15, 30, 60 g: **$47.65**/60 g
• Tape, Medicated—Top: 4 mcg/cm^2: **$22.03-$47.31**

CONTRAINDICATIONS: Hypersensitivity to flurandrenolide or any componenet of the formulation, viral, fungal, or tubercular skin lesions

PREGNANCY AND LACTATION: Pregnancy category C; unknown whether topical application could result in sufficient systemic absorption to produce detectable amounts in breast milk (systemic corticosteroids are secreted into breast milk in quantities not likely to have detrimental effects on infant)

SIDE EFFECTS
Occasional
Itching, dry skin, folliculitis
Rare
Intracranial hemorrhage, acne, striae, miliaria, allergic contact dermatitis, telangiectasis or raised dark red spots on skin

SERIOUS REACTIONS
• When taken in excessive quantities, systemic hypercorticism and adrenal suppression may occur.

SPECIAL CONSIDERATIONS
PATIENT/FAMILY EDUCATION
• Apply sparingly only to affected area
• Avoid contact with the eyes
• Do not put bandages or dressings over treated area unless directed by clinician
• Do not use on weeping, denuded, or infected areas
• Discontinue drug, notify clinician if local irritation or fever develops

---

flurazepam
(flure-az'e-pam)
Rx: Dalmane
Chemical Class: Benzodiazepine
Therapeutic Class: Sedative/hypnotic
DEA Class: Schedule IV

CLINICAL PHARMACOLOGY
Mechanism of Action: A benzodiazepine that enhances action of inhibitory neurotransmitter gamma-aminobutyric acid (GABA). *Therapeutic Effect:* Produces hypnotic effect due to central nervous system (CNS) depression.

Pharmacokinetics

Route	Onset	Peak	Duration
PO	15-20 min	3-6 hr	7-8 hr

Well absorbed from the gastrointestinal (GI) tract. Protein binding: 97%. Crosses blood-brain barrier. Widely distributed. Metabolized in liver to active metabolite. Primarily excreted in urine. Not removed by hemodialysis. **Half-life:** 2.3 hrs; metabolite: 40–114 hrs.

INDICATIONS AND DOSAGES
Insomnia
PO
Adults. 15–30 mg at bedtime.
Elderly, debilitated, liver disease, low serum albumin, Children 15 yr and older. 15 mg at bedtime.

S AVAILABLE FORMS/COST
• Cap, Gel—Oral: 15 mg, 100's: **$23.50-$152.13**; 30 mg, 100's: **$9.98-$165.48**

CONTRAINDICATIONS: Acute alcohol intoxication, acute angle-closure glaucoma, pregnancy or breastfeeding

PREGNANCY AND LACTATION:
Pregnancy category X; administration to nursing mothers is not recommended

SIDE EFFECTS

Frequent

Drowsiness, dizziness, ataxia, sedation

Morning drowsiness may occur initially.

Occasional

GI disturbances, nervousness, blurred vision, dry mouth, headache, confusion, skin rash, irritability, slurred speech

Rare

Paradoxical CNS excitement or restlessness, particularly noted in elderly or debilitated

SERIOUS REACTIONS

• Abrupt or too-rapid withdrawal after long-term use may result in pronounced restlessness and irritability, insomnia, hand tremors, abdominal or muscle cramps, vomiting, diaphoresis, and seizures.

• Overdose results in somnolence, confusion, diminished reflexes, and coma.

INTERACTIONS

Drugs

❷ *Azole antifungals (fulconazole, itraconazole, ketoconazole):* Increased serum concentrations of flurazepam via inhibition of oxidative metabolism (CYP3A4)

❸ *β-blockers (labetaolol, metoprolol, propranolol):* Reduces the metabolism of benzodiazepines and may increase the pharmacodynamic effects

❸ *Cimetidine:* Increased plasma levels of flurazepam and metabolites via inhibition of hepatic oxidative metabolism

❸ *Clozapine:* Isolated cases of cardiorespiratory collapse, but a causal relationship not established

❸ *Disulfiram:* May increase serum concentrations of flurazepam via inhibition of oxidative metabolism (CYP3A4)

❸ *Isoniazid:* May increase flurazepam serum concentrations via inhibition of metabolism

❸ *Loxapine:* Isolated cases of respiratory depression, stupor, and hypotension reported; role of drug interaction not established

❸ *Macrolide antibiotics (clarithromycin, erythromycin, troleandomycin):* Macrolides increase flurazepam plasma concentrations via inhibition of metabolism (CYP3A4)

❸ *Omeprazole:* Increases plasma concentrations of flurazepam via inhibition of hepatic metabolism

❸ *Rifampin:* Reduced serum concentrations of flurazepam via enhanced hepatic metabolism (CYP3A4)

❸ *Serotonin reuptake inhibitors (fluoxetine, fluvoxamine):* May increase serum concentrations of flurazepam via inhibition of oxidative metabolism (CYP3A4)

SPECIAL CONSIDERATIONS

• Poor choice for elderly patients

PATIENT/FAMILY EDUCATION

• Avoid alcohol and other CNS depressants

• Do not discontinue abruptly after prolonged therapy

• May experience disturbed sleep for the first or second night after discontinuing the drug

• May cause drowsiness or dizziness; use caution while driving or performing other tasks requiring alertness; hangover daytime drowsiness possible secondary to long duration of action

• Inform clinician if you are planning to become pregnant, you are pregnant, or if you become pregnant while taking this medicine

flurbiprofen
(flure-bi' proe-fen)
Rx: Ansaid, Ocufen
(ophthalmic)
Chemical Class: Propionic acid
derivative
Therapeutic Class: NSAID;
antipyretic; nonnarcotic analgesic

CLINICAL PHARMACOLOGY
Mechanism of Action: A phenylalkanoic acid that produces analgesic and anti-inflammatory effect by inhibiting prostaglandin synthesis. Also relaxes the iris sphincter. *Therapeutic Effect:* Reduces the inflammatory response and intensity of pain. Prevents or decreases miosis during cataract surgery.

Pharmacokinetics
Well absorbed from the GI tract; ophthalmic solution penetrates cornea after administration, and may be systemically absorbed. Protein binding: 99%. Widely distributed. Metabolized in the liver. Primarily excreted in urine. **Half-life:** 3–4 hr.

INDICATIONS AND DOSAGES
Rheumatoid arthritis, osteoarthritis
PO
Adults, Elderly. 200–300 mg/day in 2–4 divided doses. Maximum: 100 mg/dose or 300 mg/day.

Dysmenorrhea, pain
PO
Adults. 50 mg 4 times a day
Usual opthalmic dosage
Adults, Elderly, Children. Apply 1 drop q30min starting 2 hr before surgery for total of 4 doses.

ⓢ AVAILABLE FORMS/COST
• Sol—Ophth: 0.03%, 2.5 ml:
$8.73-$20.48

• Tab, Coated—Oral: 50 mg, 100's:
$68.02-$82.50; 100 mg, 100's:
$106.38-$238.04
CONTRAINDICATIONS: Active peptic ulcer, chronic inflammation of GI tract, GI bleeding or ulceration, history of hypersensitivity to aspirin or NSAIDs
PREGNANCY AND LACTATION: Pregnancy category C; excreted into breast milk; use caution in nursing mothers
SIDE EFFECTS
Occasional
PO (9%–3%): Headache, abdominal pain, diarrhea, indigestion, nausea, fluid retention
Ophthalmic: Burning or stinging on instillation, keratitis, elevated intraocular pressure
Rare (less than 3%)
PO: Blurred vision, flushed skin, dizziness, somnolence, nervousness, insomnia, unusual fatigue, constipation, decreased appetite, vomiting, confusion
SERIOUS REACTIONS
• Overdose may result in acute renal failure.
• Rare reactions with long-term use include peptic ulcer disease, GI bleeding, gastritis, severe hepatic reaction (jaundice), nephrotoxicity (hematuria, dysuria, proteinuria), a severe hypersensitivity reaction (angioedema, bronchospasm) and cardiac arrhythmias.
INTERACTIONS
Drugs
▣ *Aminoglycosides:* Reduced clearance with elevated aminoglycoside levels and potential for toxicity (especially indomethacin in premature infants; other NSAIDs probably)
▣ *Antihypertensives (α-blockers, angiotensin-converting enzyme inhibitors, angiotensin II receptor blockers, β-blockers, diuretics):* In-

hibition of antihypertensive and other favorable hemodynamic effects

▣ *Aspirin:* 50% decrease in plasma flurbiprofen concentrations, concurrent use not recommended

▣ *Corticosteroids:* Increased risk of GI ulceration

▣ *Anticoagulants:* Excessive hypoprothrombinemia, decreased platelet aggregation with increased risk of GI bleeding

▣ *Cyclosporine:* Increased nephrotoxicity risk

▣ *Lithium:* Decreased clearance of lithium (mediated via prostaglandins) resulting in elevated serum lithium levels and risk of toxicity

▣ *Methotrexate:* Decreased renal secretion of methotrexate resulting in elevated methotrexate levels and risk of toxicity

▣ *Phenylpropanolamine:* Possible acute hypertensive reaction

▣ *Potassium-sparing diuretics:* Additive hyperkalemia potential

▣ *Triamterene:* Acute renal failure reported with addition of indomethacin; caution with other NSAIDs

Labs

• *Cortisol:* Increased at high flurbiprofen levels

SPECIAL CONSIDERATIONS
PATIENT/FAMILY EDUCATION

• Avoid aspirin and alcoholic beverages

• Take with food, milk, or antacids to decrease GI upset

• Notify clinician if edema, black stools, or persistent headache occurs

MONITORING PARAMETERS

• Initial hemogram and fecal occult blood test within 3 mo of starting regular chronic therapy; repeat every 6-12 mo (more frequently in high-risk patients (>65 years, peptic ulcer disease, concurrent steroids or anticoagulants); elecrolytes, creatinine, and BUN within 3 mo of starting regular chronic therapy; repeat every 6-12 mo

---

flutamide
(floo′ta-mide)

Rx: Eulexin
Chemical Class: Acetanilid derivative
Therapeutic Class: Anitandrogen; antineoplastic

CLINICAL PHARMACOLOGY

Mechanism of Action: An antiandrogen hormone that inhibits androgen uptake and prevents androgen from binding to androgen receptors in target tissue. Used in conjuction with leuprolide to inhibit the stimulant effects of flutamide on serum testosterone levels. *Therapeutic Effect:* Suppresses testicular androgen production and decreases growth of prostate carcinoma.

Pharmacokinetics

Completely absorbed from the GI tract. Protein binding: 94%-96%. Metabolized in the liver to active metabolite. Primarily excreted in urine. Not removed by hemodialysis. **Half-life:** 6 hr (increased in elderly).

INDICATIONS AND DOSAGES
Prostatic carcinoma (in combination with leuprolide)
PO
Adults, Elderly. 250 mg q8h.

Ⓢ **AVAILABLE FORMS/COST**
• Cap, Gel—Oral: 125 mg, 100's: **$209.22-$272.35**

CONTRAINDICATIONS: Severe hepatic impairment

PREGNANCY AND LACTATION: Pregnancy category D

SIDE EFFECTS
Frequent

Hot flashes (50%); decreased libido, diarrhea (24%); generalized pain (23%); asthenia (17%); constipation (12%); nausea, nocturia (11%)

Occasional (8%-6%)

Dizziness, paresthesia, insomnia, impotence, peripheral edema, gynecomastia

Rare (5%-4%)

Rash, diaphoresis, hypertension, hematuria, vomiting, urinary incontinence, headache, flu-like syndromes, photosensitivity

SERIOUS REACTIONS

• Hepatoxicity, including hepatic encephalopathy, and hemolytic anemia may be noted.

INTERACTIONS
Drugs

3 *Warfarin:* Increased hypoprothrombinemic effect

SPECIAL CONSIDERATIONS

• Begin 8 wks before radiation therapy in Stage B_2-C carcinoma, continue during radiation
• In metastatic carcinoma continue until progression noted

PATIENT/FAMILY EDUCATION

• Feminization may occur during therapy
• Do not discontinue therapy without discussion with clinician

MONITORING PARAMETERS

• Periodic LFTs during long-term treatment

fluticasone

(flu-tic′a-zone)

Rx: Cutivate, Flonase, Flovent, Flovent Rotadisk

Combinations

Rx: with salmeterol (Advair Diskus)

Chemical Class: Corticosteroid, synthetic

Therapeutic Class: Corticosteroid, inhaled; corticosteroid, systemic; corticosteroid, topical

CLINICAL PHARMACOLOGY

Mechanism of Action: A corticosteroid that controls the rate of protein synthesis, depresses migration of polymorphonuclear leukocytes, reverses capillary permeability, and stabilizes lysosomal membranes. *Therapeutic Effect:* Prevents or controls inflammation.

Pharmacokinetics

Inhalation/intranasal: Protein binding: 91%. Undergoes extensive first-pass metabolism in liver. Excreted in urine. **Half-life:** 3–7.8 hrs. Topical: Amount absorbed depends on affected area and skin condition (absorption increased with fever, hydration, inflamed or denuded skin).

INDICATIONS AND DOSAGES
Allergic Rhinitis

Intranasal

Adults, Elderly. Initially, 200 mcg (2 sprays in each nostril once daily or 1 spray in each nostril q12h). Maintenance: 1 spray in each nostril once daily. Maximum: 200 mcg/day.

Children older than 4 yr. Initially, 100 mcg (1 spray in each nostril once daily). Maximum: 200 mcg/day.

F

Relief of inflammation and pruritus associated with steroid-responsive disorders, such as contact dermatitis and eczema

Topical

Adults, Elderly, Children older than 3 mo. Apply sparingly to affected area once or twice a day.

Maintenance treatment for asthma for those previously treated with bronchodilators

Inhalation Powder (Flovent Diskus)

Adults, Elderly, Children 12 yr and older. Initially, 100 mcg q12h. Maximum: 500 mcg/day.

Inhalation (Oral, Flovent)

Adults, Elderly, Children 12 yr and older. 88 mcg twice a day. Maximum: 440 mcg twice a day.

Maintenance treatment for asthma for those previously treated with inhaled steroids

Inhalation Powder (Flovent Diskus)

Adults, Elderly, Children 12 yr and older. Initially, 100–250 mcg q12h. Maximum: 500 mcg q12h.

Inhalation, Oral (Flovent)

Adults, Elderly, Children 12 yr and older. 88-220 mcg twice a day. Maximum: 440 mcg twice a day.

Maintenance treatment for asthma for those previously treated with oral steroids

Inhalation Powder (Flovent Diskus)

Adults, Elderly, Children 12 yr and older. 500–1,000 mcg twice a day.

Inhalation, (Oral, Flovent)

Adults, Elderly, Children 12 yrs and older. 880 mcg twice a day.

§ **AVAILABLE FORMS/COST**

• Aer, metered—Inh: 44 mcg/inh, 13 g (120 puffs): **$58.31**; 110 mcg/inh, 13 g (120 puffs): **$81.06**; 220 mcg/inh, 13 g (120 puffs): **$125.91**

• Spray—Nasal: 0.05 mg/inh, 16 g: **$68.26**

• Cre—Top: 0.05%, 15, 30, 60 g: **$35.36/30 g**

• Disk—Inh: 50 mcg/inh, 60's: **$43.54**; 100 mcg/inh, 60's: **$61.21**; 250 mcg/inh, 60's: **$85.14**

• Oint—Top: 0.005%, 15, 30, 60 g: **$35.36/30 g**

CONTRAINDICATIONS: Primary treatment of status asthmaticus or other acute asthma episodes (inhalation); untreated localized infection of nasal mucosa

PREGNANCY AND LACTATION: Pregnancy category C; no information on excretion into human breast milk

SIDE EFFECTS

Frequent

Inhalation: Throat irritation, hoarseness, dry mouth, cough, temporary wheezing, oropharyngeal candidiasis (particularly if mouth is not rinsed with water after each administration)

Intranasal: Mild nasopharyngeal irritation; nasal burning, stinging, or dryness; rebound congestion; rhinorrhea; loss of taste

Occasional

Inhalation: Oral candidiasis

Intranasal: Nasal and pharyngeal candidiasis, headache

Topical: Skin burning, pruritus

SERIOUS REACTIONS

• None known.

INTERACTIONS

Drugs

③ *Ketoconazole:* Possible increased plasma fluticasone concentrations

Labs

• Cholesterol: Increased

SPECIAL CONSIDERATIONS

• Improvement following inhalation, 24 hr to 1-2 wk

• Systemic corticosteroid effects from inhaled and nasal steroids inadequate to prevent adrenal insufficiency in most patients withdrawn abruptly from corticosteroids

• Observe for evidence of inadequate adrenal response following periods of stress; use caution with extended use in children and adolescents as reduction in growth velocity may occur

PATIENT/FAMILY EDUCATION

• Rinsing the mouth following INH and using a spacer device reduces common EENT adverse effects

• Review proper MDI administration technique regularly

---

fluvastatin

(floo'va-sta-tin)
Rx: Lescol, Lescol XL
Chemical Class: Substituted hexahydronaphthalene
Therapeutic Class: HMG-CoA reductase inhibitor; antilipemic

CLINICAL PHARMACOLOGY

Mechanism of Action: An antihyperlipidemic that inhibits HMG-CoA reductase, the enzyme that catalyzes the early step in cholesterol synthesis. *Therapeutic Effect:* Decreases LDL cholesterol, VLDL, and plasma triglyceride levels. Slightly increases HDL cholesterol concentration.

Pharmacokinetics

Well absorbed from the GI tract and is unaffected by food. Does not cross the blood-brain barrier. Protein binding: greater than 98%. Primarily eliminated in feces. **Half-life:** 1.2 hr.

INDICATIONS AND DOSAGES

Hyperlipoproteinemia

PO

Adults, Elderly. Initially, 20 mg/day (capsule) in the evening. May increase up to 40 mg/day. Maintenance: 20–40 mg/day in a single dose or divided doses.

Patients requiring more than a 25% decrease in LDL cholesterol. 40 mg (capsule) 1–2 times a day. Or 80 mg tablet once a day.

AVAILABLE FORMS/COST

• Cap—Oral: 20 mg, 40 mg, 100's: **$185.19**

• Tab, Coated, Sus Action—Oral: 80 mg, 100's: **$237.58**

CONTRAINDICATIONS: Active hepatic disease, unexplained increased serum transaminase levels

PREGNANCY AND LACTATION: Pregnancy category X; contraindicated in breast-feeding—present in breast milk (2:1 milk: plasma ratio)

SIDE EFFECTS

Frequent (8%–5%)

Headache, dyspepsia, back pain, myalgia, arthralgia, diarrhea, abdominal cramping, rhinitis

Occasional (4%–2%)

Nausea, vomiting, insomnia, constipation, flatulence, rash, pruritus, fatigue, cough, dizziness

SERIOUS REACTIONS

• Myositis (inflammation of voluntary muscle) with or without increased CK, and muscle weakness, occur rarely. These conditions may progress to frank rhabdomyolysis and renal impairment.

INTERACTIONS

Drugs

Alcohol: 20 g of alcohol within 1 hr of dosing, increased fluvastatin AUC by 30%

Azole antifungals (fluconazole, itraconazole, ketoconazole, miconazole): Increased fluvastatin levels via inhibition of metabolism with increased risk of rhabdomyolysis

Cholestyramine, colestipol: Reduced bioavailability of fluvastatin

Cimetidine, ranitidine, omeprazole: Coadministration increases fluvastatin Cmax 43%-70% with 18%-23% decrease in plasma clearance

3 *Cyclosporine:* Concomitant administration increases risk of severe myopathy or rhabdomyolysis

3 *Danazol:* Inhibition of metabolism (CYP3A4) thought to yield increased fluvastatin levels with increased risk of rhabdomyolysis

3 *Diclofenac:* Increased plasma diclofenac concentrations

3 *Fluoxetine:* Less likely to inhibit CYP3A4 hepatic metabolism (vs lovastatin) with less risk of rhabdomyolysis

2 *Gemfibrozil:* Small increased risk of myopathy with combination, especially at high doses of statin

3 *Glyburide:* Increased plasma concentrations of glyburide and fluvastatin

3 *Isradipine:* Isradipine probably decreases fluvastatin plasma concentrations minimally

3 *Macrolide antibiotics (clarithromycin, erythromycin, troleandomycin):* Increased fluvastatin levels via inhibition of metabolism with increased risk of rhabdomyolysis

3 *Niacin:* Concomitant administration increases risk of severe hepatotoxicity

3 *Nefazadone:* Less likely to inhibit CYP3A4 hepatic metabolism (vs lovastatin) with less risk of rhabdomyolysis

3 *Phenytoin:* Increased plasma concentrations of phenytoin and fluvastatin

3 *Rifampin:* Coadministration decreases fluvastatin Cmax and AUC

3 *Terbinafine:* Minimal effect on the metabolism of fluvastatin

3 *Warfarin:* Addition of fluvastatin may increase hypoprothrombinemic response to warfarin via inhibition of metabolism (CYP2C9)

SPECIAL CONSIDERATIONS

• Statin selection based on lipid-lowering prowess, cost, and availability

PATIENT/FAMILY EDUCATION

• Report symptoms of myalgia, muscle tenderness, or weakness

• Take daily doses in the evening for increased effect

• May take without regard to food

MONITORING PARAMETERS

• Cholesterol (max therapeutic response 4-6 wk)

• LFT's (AST, ALT) at baseline and at 12 wk of therapy; if no change, nor further monitoring necessary (discontinue if elevations persists at >3 times upper limit of normal)

• CPK in patients complaining of diffuse myalgia, muscle tenderness, or weakness

---

fluvoxamine

(floo-vox'a-meen)

Rx: Luvox

Chemical Class: Aralkylketone derivative

Therapeutic Class: Antidepressant, selective serotonin reuptake inhibitor (SSRI)

CLINICAL PHARMACOLOGY

Mechanism of Action: An antidepressant and antiobsessive agent that selectively inhibits neuronal reuptake of serotonin. *Therapeutic Effect:* Relieves depression and symptoms of obsessive-compulsive disorder.

INDICATIONS AND DOSAGES

Obsessive-compulsive disorder

PO

Adults. 50 mg at bedtime; may increase by 50 mg every 4–7 days. Dosages greater than 100 mg/day given in 2 divided doses. Maximum: 300 mg/day.

Children 8–17 yrs. 25 mg at bedtime; may increase by 25 mg every 4–7 days. Dosages greater than 50 mg/day given in 2 divided doses. Maximum: 200 mg/day.

💲 **AVAILABLE FORMS/COST**
• Tab, Uncoated—Oral: 25 mg, 100's: **$229.18-$294.48**; 50 mg, 100's: **$257.35-$329.06**; 100 mg, 100's: **$262.67-$337.51**

UNLABELED USES: Treatment of depression, panic disorder, anxiety disorders in children

CONTRAINDICATIONS: Use within 14 days of MAOIs

PREGNANCY AND LACTATION: Pregnancy category C; excreted into breast milk; use caution in nursing mothers

SIDE EFFECTS
Frequent
Nausea (40%), headache, somnolence, insomnia (21%–22%)
Occasional (14%–8%)
Nervousness, dizziness, diarrhea, dry mouth, asthenia, weakness, dyspepsia, constipation, abnormal ejaculation
Rare (6%–3%)
Anorexia, anxiety, tremor, vomiting, flatulence, urinary frequency, sexual dysfunction, altered taste

SERIOUS REACTIONS
• Overdose may produce seizures, nausea, vomiting, and extreme agitation and restlessness.

INTERACTIONS
Drugs
⚠ *Antihistamines, nonsedating (astemizole, terfenadine):* Fluvoxamine inhibits metabolism (CYP3A4) for detoxifying these antihistamines; cardiac rhythm disturbances

▣ *Benzodiazepines (alprazolam, midazolam, triazolam, diazepam):* Probable inhibition of metabolism (CYP3A4) leading to accumulation of benzodiazepines, avoid combination

▣ *β-blockers (metoprolol, propranolol, sotalol):* Inhibition of metabolism (CYP2D6) leads to increased plasma concentrations of selective β-blockers and potential cardiac toxicity; atenolol may be safer choice

▣ *Buspirone:* Reduced therapeutic effect of both drugs; possible seizures

▣ *Carbamazepine:* Inhibition of hepatic metabolism of carbamazepine, but the formation of carbamazepine epoxide is not inhibited, contributing to increased toxicity

❷ *Clozapine:* Fluvoxamine markedly increases clozapine concentrations as a potent inhibitor of CYP1A2

▣ *Cyclic antidepressants (clomipramine, desipramine, doxepin, imipramine, nortriptylline, trazadone):* Inhibition of metabolism (CYP1A2 and CYP3A4) leading to accumulation of cyclic antidepressants; dosage adjustments necessary

▣ *Cyproheptadine:* Serotonin antagonist may partially reverse antidepressant and other effects

❷ *Dexfenfluramine:* Duplicate effects on inhibition of serotonin reuptake; inhibition of dexfenfluramine metabolism (CYP2D6) exaggerates effect; both mechanisms increase risk of serotonin syndrome

❷ *Fenfluramine:* Duplicate effects on inhibition of serotonin reuptake; inhibition of dexfenfluramine metabolism (CYP2D6) exaggerates effect; both mechanisms increase risk of serotonin syndrome

❷ *HMG-Co A reductase inhibitors (atorvastatin, lovastatin, simvastatin):* Inhibition of statin metabolism (CYP3A4), by fluoxetine, may lead to rhabdomyolysis

3 *Lithium:* Neurotoxicity (tremor, confusion, ataxia, dizziness, dysarthria, and abscence seizures) reported in patients receiving this combination; mechanism unknown

⚠ *MAOIs (isocarboxazid, phenelzine, tranylcypromine):* Increased CNS serotonergic effects have been associated with severe or fatal reactions with this combination

3 *Mexiletine:* Reduced clearance of mexiletine, monitor serum mexiletine levels if co-administered

3 *Methadone:* Significantly increased plasma methadone concentrations

3 *Phenytoin:* Inhibition of metabolism and phenytoin toxicity

❷ *Selegiline:* Sporadic cases of mania and hypertension

3 *Sumatriptan:* Reports of weakness, hyperreflexia and incoordination with SSRI and sumatriptan use, caution is advised

3 *Tacrine:* Increased plasma tacrine concentrations, cholinergic side effects possible

❷ *Theophylline:* Theophylline toxicity increased via accumulation due to inhibition of metabolism (CYP1A2) by fluvoxamine

⚠ *Thioridazine:* Dose related prolongation of the QTc interval, do not co-administer thioridazine and fluvoxamine

❷ *Tryptophan:* Additive serotonergic effects

3 *Warfarin:* Increased hypothrombinemic response

SPECIAL CONSIDERATIONS
PATIENT/FAMILY EDUCATION
• May cause dizziness or drowsiness; use caution driving or performing tasks requiring alertness

folic acid
(foe'lik)
OTC: Folicin, FA-8
Chemical Class: Vitamin B complex
Therapeutic Class: Hematinic; vitamin

CLINICAL PHARMACOLOGY
Mechanism of Action: A coenzyme that stimulates production of platelets, RBCs, and WBCs. *Therapeutic Effect:* Essential for nucleoprotein synthesis and maintenance of normal erythropoiesis.

Pharmacokinetics
PO form almost completely absorbed from the GI tract (upper duodenum). Protein binding: High. Metabolized in the liver and plasma to active form. Excreted in urine. Removed by hemodialysis.

INDICATIONS AND DOSAGES
Vitamin B$_9$ deficiency
PO, IV, IM, Subcutaneous
Adults, Elderly, Children 12 yr and older. Initially, 1 mg/day. Maintenance: 0.5 mg/day.
Children 1–11 yr. Initially 1 mg/day. Maintenance: 0.1–0.4 mg/day.
Infants. 50 mcg/day.

Dietary supplement
PO, IV, IM, Subcutaneous
Adults, Elderly, Children 4 yr and older. 0.4 mg/day.
Children 1–younger than 4 yr. 0.3 mg/day.
Children younger than 1 yr. 0.1 mg/day.
Pregnant women. 0.8 mg/day.

💲 AVAILABLE FORMS/COST
• Sol, Inj—IM, IV, SC: 5 mg/ml, 10 ml: **$12.50-$14.33**
• Tab—Oral: 1 mg, 100's: **$0.66-$34.50**; 0.4 mg, 100's (OTC): **$1.17-$2.15**; 0.8 mg, 100's (OTC): **$2.40-$3.94**

UNLABELED USES: To decrease the risk of colon cancer

CONTRAINDICATIONS: Anemias (aplastic, normocytic, pernicious, refractory)

PREGNANCY AND LACTATION: Pregnancy category A; folic acid deficiency during pregnancy is a common problem in undernourished women and in women not receiving supplements; evidence has accumulated that folic acid deficiency, or abnormal folate metabolism, may be related to the occurrence of neural tube defects; actively excreted in human breast milk; compatible with breast-feeding; recommended daily allowance during lactation is 0.5 mg/day

SIDE EFFECTS
None known.

SERIOUS REACTIONS
• Allergic hypersensitivity occurs rarely with parenteral form. Oral folic acid is nontoxic.

INTERACTIONS
Drugs
🔢 *Phenytoin:* Decreased serum phenytoin concentrations; long-term phenytoin frequently leads to subnormal folate levels
❷ *Pyrimethamine:* Inhibition of antimicrobial effect of pyrimethamine

SPECIAL CONSIDERATIONS
• Recent evidence supports the premise that lowering elevated plasma homocysteine levels may reduce the risk of coronary heart disease

PATIENT/FAMILY EDUCATION
• Take only under medical supervision

MONITORING PARAMETERS
• CBC; serum folate concentrations <0.005 mcg/ml indicate folic acid deficiency and concentrations <0.002 mcg/ml usually result in megaloblastic anemia

fomepizole
(foe-mep′i-zoll)
Rx: Antizol
Chemical Class: Pyrazole derivative
Therapeutic Class: Antidote, ethylene glycol (antifreeze)

CLINICAL PHARMACOLOGY
Mechanism of Action: An alcohol dehydrogenase inhibitor that inhibits the enzyme that catalyzes the metabolism of ethanol, ethylene glycol, and methanol to their toxic metabolites. *Therapeutic Effect:* Inhibits conversion of ethylene glycol and methanol into toxic metabolites.

Pharmacokinetics
Protein binding: low. Rapidly distributes to total body water after IV infusion. Extensively metabolized by the liver. Minimal excretion in the urine. Removed by hemodialysis. **Half-life:** 5 hrs.

INDICATIONS AND DOSAGES
Ethylene glycol or methanol intoxication
IV infusion
Adults, Elderly. 15 mg/kg as loading dose, followed by 10 mg/kg q12h for 4 doses, then 15 mg/kg q12h until ethylene glycol or methanol concentrations are below 20 mg/dL. All doses should be administered as a slow IV infusion over 30 minutes.

Dosage in renal impairment
During hemodialysis. 15 mg/kg as a loading dose, followed by 10 mg/kg q4h for 4 doses, then 15 mg/kg q4h until ethylene glycol or methanol concentrations are below 20 mg/dL. *After hemodialysis.* If the time between the last dose and end of hemodialysis is less than 1 hour, do not give dose. If the time between is 1-3

hours, give 50% of next scheduled dose. If time is greater than 3 hours give next scheduled dose.

§ **AVAILABLE FORMS/COST**
• Conc—IV: 1 g/ml, 1.5 ml: **$1,270.75**

UNLABELED USES: Butoxyethanol intoxication, diethylene glycol intoxication, ethanol sensitivity

CONTRAINDICATIONS: Hypersensitivity to fomepizole or other pyrazoles

PREGNANCY AND LACTATION: Pregnancy category C; use caution in nursing mothers

SIDE EFFECTS
Frequent
Hypertriglyceridemia, headache, nausea, dizziness
Occasional
Abnormal sense of smell, nystagmus, visual disturbances, ringing in ears, agitation, seizures, anorexia, heartburn, anxiety, vertigo, lightheadedness, altered sense of awareness
Rare
Anuria, disseminated intravascular coagulopathy

SERIOUS REACTIONS
• Mild allergic reactions including rash and eosinophilia occur rarely.
• Overdose may cause nausea, dizziness, and vertigo.

INTERACTIONS
Drugs
③ *Ethanol:* Reduced elimination rate of ethanol; reduced elimination rate of fomepizole

SPECIAL CONSIDERATIONS
MONITORING PARAMETERS
• Frequently monitor both ethylene glycol levels and acid-base balance, as determined by serum electrolyte (anion gap) or arterial blood gas analysis
• In patients with high ethylene glycol levels ($\geq$50 mg/dl), significant metabolic acidosis or renal failure, consider hemodialysis to remove ethylene glycol and its toxic metabolites
• Treatment with fomepizole may be discontinued when ethylene glycol levels have been reduced to <20 mg/dl

---

fomivirsen
(foh-mih-ver´-sen)
Rx: Vitravene
Chemical Class: Antisense oligonucleotide
Therapeutic Class: Antiviral

CLINICAL PHARMACOLOGY
Mechanism of Action: An antiviral that binds to messenger RNA, inhibiting the synthesis of viral proteins.
Therapeutic Effect: Blocks replication of cytomegalovirus (CMV).

INDICATIONS AND DOSAGES
CMV retinitis
Intravitreal injection
Adults. 330 mcg (0.05 ml) every other week for 2 doses, then 330 mcg every 4 weeks.

§ **AVAILABLE FORMS/COST**
• Sol, Inj—Intravitreal: 330 mcg/0.25 ml: **$1,000.00**

CONTRAINDICATIONS: None significant.

PREGNANCY AND LACTATION: Pregnancy category C; breast milk excretion unlikely

SIDE EFFECTS
Frequent (10%-5%)
Fever, headache, nausea, diarrhea, vomiting, abdominal pain, anemia, uveitis, abnormal vision
Occasional (5%-2%)
Chest pain, confusion, dizziness, depression, neuropathy, anorexia, weight loss, pancreatitis, dyspnea, cough

SERIOUS REACTIONS
• Thrombocytopenia may occur.

SPECIAL CONSIDERATIONS

PATIENT/FAMILY EDUCATION

- Does not treat systemic aspects of CMV infection

MONITORING PARAMETERS

- Ophthalmologic examination

fondaparinux

(fawn-da-pear'ih-nux)

Rx: Arixtra

Chemical Class: Pentasaccharide

Therapeutic Class: Anticoagulant

CLINICAL PHARMACOLOGY

Mechanism of Action: A factor Xa inhibitor and pentasaccharide that selectively binds to antithrombin, and increases its affinity for factor Xa, thereby inhibiting factor Xa and stopping the blood coagulation cascade. *Therapeutic Effect:* Indirectly prevents formation of thrombin and subsequently the fibrin clot.

Pharmacokinetics

Well absorbed after subcutaneous administration. Undergoes minimal, if any, metabolism. Highly bound to antithrombin III. Distributed mainly in blood and to a minor extent in extravascular fluid. Excreted unchanged in urine. Removed by hemodialysis. **Half-life:** 17–21 hr (prolonged in patients with impaired renal function).

INDICATIONS AND DOSAGES

Prevention of venous thromboembolism

Subcutaneous

Adults. 2.5 mg once a day for 5–9 days after surgery. Initial dose should be given 6–8 hr after surgery. Dosage should be adjusted in the elderly and in those with renal impairment.

[$] **AVAILABLE FORMS/COST**

- Sol, Inj—SC: 2.5 mg/0.5 ml: **$43.50**

CONTRAINDICATIONS: Active major bleeding, bacterial endocarditis, severe renal impairment (with creatinine clearance less than 30 ml/min), thrombocytopenia associated with antiplatelet antibody formation in the presence of fondaparinux, body weight less than 50 kg

PREGNANCY AND LACTATION: Pregnancy category B; excreted in milk of lactating rats but human studies lacking; use caution in nursing mothers

SIDE EFFECTS

Occasional (14%)

Fever

Rare (4%–1%)

Injection site hematoma, nausea, peripheral edema

SERIOUS REACTIONS

- Accidental overdose may lead to bleeding complications ranging from local ecchymoses to major hemorrhage.
- Thrombocytopenia occurs rarely.

INTERACTIONS

Drugs

[3] *Antithrombotic agents (aspirin, clopidogrel, ticlopidine, warfarin):* Increased risk of bleeding, close monitoring required

SPECIAL CONSIDERATIONS

- Slightly better at preventing DVT than enoxaparin; caused more bleeding than enoxaparin after knee replacement surgery; therapeutic niche not well defined

MONITORING PARAMETERS

- Periodic CBC, serum Cr, stool occult blood

formoterol
(for-moe′ter-ol)
Rx: Foradil Aerolizer
Chemical Class: Sympathomimetic amine; β_2-adrenergic agonist
Therapeutic Class: Antiasthmatic; bronchodilator

CLINICAL PHARMACOLOGY
Mechanism of Action: A long-acting bronchodilator that stimulates beta$_2$-adrenergic receptors in the lungs, resulting in relaxation of bronchial smooth muscle. Also inhibits release of mediators from various cells in the lungs, including mast cells, with little effect on heart rate. *Therapeutic Effect:* Relieves bronchospasm, reduces airway resistance. Improves bronchodilation, nighttime asthma control, and peak flow rates.

Pharmacokinetics

Route	Onset	Peak	Duration
Inhalation	1–3 min	0.5–1 hr	12 hr

Absorbed from bronchi after inhalation. Metabolized in the liver. Primarily excreted in urine. Unknown if removed by hemodialysis. **Half-life:** 10 hr.

INDICATIONS AND DOSAGES
Asthma, chronic obstructive pulmonary disease (COPD)
Inhalation
Adults, Elderly, Children 5 yrs and older. 12 mcg capsule q12h.

Exercise-induced bronchospasm
Inhalation
Adults, Elderly, Children 5 yr and older. 12 mcg capsule at least 15 min before exercise. Do not repeat for another 12 hours.

§ AVAILABLE FORMS/COST
• Cap, Gelatin—Inh: 12 mcg, 60's: **$79.58**
CONTRAINDICATIONS: None known.
PREGNANCY AND LACTATION: Pregnancy category C; β-agonists may potentially interfere with uterine contractility during labor; excretion into breast milk unknown; use caution in nursing mothers

SIDE EFFECTS
Occasional
Tremor, muscle cramps, tachycardia, insomnia, headache, irritability, irritation of mouth or throat

SERIOUS REACTIONS
• Excessive sympathomimetic stimulation may produce palpitations, extrasystole, and chest pain.

INTERACTIONS
Drugs
3 *Non-potassium sparing diuretics, xanthine derivatives, steroids:* Theoretical increase in the potential for hypokalemia
2 *β-blockers:* Decreased action of formoterol, cardioselective β-blockers preferable if concurrent use necessary (e.g., following myocardial infarction)
3 *MAO-inhibitors, tricyclic antidepressants:* Theoretical increase in the potential for prolongation of QTc interval

SPECIAL CONSIDERATIONS
• Not indicated for patients whose asthma can be managed by occasional use of inhaled, short-acting, β_2-agonists
• Can be used concomitantly with short-acting β_2-agonists, inhaled or systemic corticosteroids, and theophylline
• Does not eliminate the need for treatment with an inhaled anti-inflammatory agent

• Do not initiate therapy in patients with significantly worsening or acutely deteriorating asthma

• For use only with the Aerolizer Inhaler

PATIENT/FAMILY EDUCATION

• Should never be used more frequently than twice daily (morning and evening) at the recommended dose; do not use to treat acute symptoms

• Discontinue the regular use of short-acting β_2-agonists and use them only for symptomatic relief of acute asthma symptoms

• Seek medical advice immediately if a previously effective asthma medication regimen fails to provide the usual response

• For inhalation only, do not take orally

• Store in blister packaging, only remove immediately before use; handle capsules with dry hands

• Use the new Aerolizer Inhaler provided with each new prescription

MONITORING PARAMETERS

• Pulmonary function tests

• Serum potassium

---

fosamprenavir
(fos'-am-pren-a-veer)
Rx: Lexiva
Chemical Class: HIV protease inhibitor
Therapeutic Class: Antiretroviral

CLINICAL PHARMACOLOGY
Mechanism of Action: An antiretroviral that is rapidly converted to amprenavir, which inhibits HIV-1 protease by binding to the enzyme's active site, thus preventing the processing of viral precursors and resulting in the formation of immature, noninfectious viral particles. *Therapeutic Effect:* Impairs HIV replication and proliferation.

Pharmacokinetics
Rapidly absorbed after PO administration. Protein binding: 90%. Metabolized in the liver. Excreted in urine and feces. **Half-life:** 7.7 hr.

INDICATIONS AND DOSAGES
HIV infection in patients who have not had previous protease inhibitor therapy
PO
Adults, Elderly. 1,400 mg twice daily without ritonavir; or 1,400 mg twice daily plus ritonavir 200 mg once daily; or 700 mg twice daily plus ritonavir 100 mg twice daily.

HIV infection in patients who have had previous protease inhibitor therapy
PO
Adults, Elderly. 700 mg twice daily plus ritonavir 100 mg twice daily.

Concurrent therapy with efavirenz
PO
Adults, Elderly. In patients receiving fosamprenavir plus once-daily ritonavir in combination with efavirenz, an additional 100 mg/day ritonavir (300 mg total/day) should be given.

CONTRAINDICATIONS: Concurrent use of amprenavir, dihydroergotamine, ergonovine, ergotamine, methylergonovine, pimozide, midazolam, or triazolam. If fosamprenavir is given concurrently with ritonavir, flecainide and propafenone are also contraindicated.

PREGNANCY AND LACTATION: Pregnancy category C; breast-feeding unsafe

SIDE EFFECTS
Frequent (39%-35%)
Nausea, rash, diarrhea
Occasional (19%-8%)
Headache, vomiting, fatigue, depression

Rare (7%-2%)
Pruritus, abdominal pain, perioral paresthesia

SERIOUS REACTIONS
• Severe and possibly life-threatening dermatologic reactions occur rarely.

INTERACTIONS

Drugs

▣ *Abacavir:* Mild increase in fosamprenavir plasma level when given with abacavir

② *Alfuzosin:* Decreased clearance of alfuzosin

② *Alprazolam:* Decreased clearance of alprazolam

② *Amiodarone:* Decreased clearance of amiodarone

② *Amlodipine:* Decreased clearance of amlodipine

▣ *Atorvastatin:* Decreased clearance of atorvastatin

▣ *Barbiturates:* Increased clearance of fosamprenavir; reduced clearance of barbiturates

⚠ *Bepredil:* Decreased clearance of bepredil

② *Carbamazepine:* Increased clearance of fosamprenavir; reduced clearance of carbamazepine

⚠ *Cisapride:* Increased plasma levels of cisapride

▣ *Cyclosporine:* Decreased clearance of cyclosporine

▣ *Delavirdine:* Reduced clearance of fosamprenavir; fosamprenavir reduces clearance of erythromycin

② *Dexamethasone:* Decreased concentration of fosamprenavir

② *Efavirenz:* Efavirenz increases clearance of fosamprenavir

② *Eletriptan:* Decreased clearance of eletriptan; do not use within 72 hours of fosamprenavir

⚠ *Ergot alkaloids:* Increased plasma levels of ergot alkaloids

▣ *Erythromycin:* Reduced clearance of fosamprenavir; fosamprenavir reduces clearance of erythromycin

② *Felodipine:* Decreased clearance of felodipine

② *Garlic:* Decreased concentrations of fosamprenavir

② *Isradipine:* Decreased clearance of isradipine

② *Lidocaine:* Decreased clearance of lidocaine

⚠ *Lovastatin:* Fosamprenavir reduces clearance of lovastatin

▣ *Methadone:* Decreased fosamprenavir concentrations

⚠ *Midazolam:* Increased plasma levels of midazolam and prolonged effect

▣ *Nevirapine:* Reduces plasma fosamprenavir levels

▣ *Oral contraceptives:* Fosamprenavir may reduce efficacy

▣ *Phenytoin:* Increased clearance of fosamprenavir; reduced clearance of phenytoin

② *Quinidine:* Decreased clearance of quinidine

② *Rifabutin:* Increased clearance of fosamprenavir; reduced clearance of rifabutin

⚠ *Rifampin:* Increased clearance of fosamprenavir

⚠ *Rifapentine:* Increased clearance of fosamprenavir

▣ *Ritonavir:* Decreased clearance of fosamprenavir

▣ *Saquinavir:* Decreased clearance of saquinavir; reduce dose of Fortovase (saquinavir soft gel capsule) to 800 mg tid

▣ *Sildenafil:* Decreased clearance of sildenafil

⚠ *Simvastatin:* Decreased clearance of simvastatin

⚠ *St. John's wort:* Increased clearance of fosamprenavir

3 *Tacrolimus:* Decreased clearance of tacrolimus

2 *Tadalafil:* Decreased clearance of tadalafil

⚠ *Triazolam:* Increased plasma levels of triazolam and prolonged effect

2 *Tricyclic antidepressants:* Decreased clearance of tricyclic antidepressants

2 *Vardenafil:* Decreased clearance of vardenafil

2 *Verapamil:* Decreased clearance of verapamil

SPECIAL CONSIDERATIONS

• Fosamprenavir is a prodrug for amprenavir, and allows fewer capsules to be administered per day, due to improved absorption

MONITORING PARAMETERS

• HIV RNA level, CD4 count, CBC, metabolic panel, liver function tests, triglyceride and cholesterol levels

---

foscarnet
(foss-car′net)
Rx: Foscavir
Chemical Class: Pyrophosphate analog
Therapeutic Class: Antiviral

CLINICAL PHARMACOLOGY
Mechanism of Action: An antiviral that selectively inhibits binding sites on virus-specific DNA polymerase and reverse transcriptase. *Therapeutic Effect:* Inhibits replication of herpes virus.
Pharmacokinetics
Sequestered into bone and cartilage. Protein binding: 14%-17%. Primarily excreted unchanged in urine. Removed by hemodialysis. **Half-life:** 3.3-6.8 hr (increased in impaired renal function).

INDICATIONS AND DOSAGES
Cytomegalovirus (CMV) retinitis
IV
Adults, Elderly. Initially, 60 mg/kg q8h or 100 mg/kg q12h for 2-3 wk. Maintenance: 90-120 mg/kg/day as a single IV infusion.
Herpes infection
IV
Adults. 40 mg/kg q8-12h for 2-3 wk or until healed.
Dosage in renal impairment
Dosages are individualized based on creatinine clearance. Refer to the dosing guide provided by the manufacturer.

§ **AVAILABLE FORMS/COST**
• Sol—IV: 24 mg/ml, 250 ml: **$85.01**; 24 mg/ml, 500 ml: **$169.30**
CONTRAINDICATIONS: None known.
PREGNANCY AND LACTATION: Pregnancy category C; excretion into breast milk unknown; use caution in nursing mothers
SIDE EFFECTS
Frequent
Fever (65%); nausea (47%); vomiting, diarrhea (30%)
Occasional (5% or greater)
Anorexia, pain and inflammation at injection site, fever, rigors, malaise, headache, paresthesia, dizziness, rash, diaphoresis, abdominal pain
Rare (5%-1%)
Back or chest pain, edema, flushing, pruritus, constipation, dry mouth
SERIOUS REACTIONS
• Nephrotoxicity occurs to some extent in most patients.
• Seizures and serum mineral or electrolyte imbalances may be life-threatening.
INTERACTIONS
Drugs
3 *Quinolones: Increased seizure risk (rare)*

SPECIAL CONSIDERATIONS

• Hydration to establish diuresis both prior to and during administration is recommended to minimize renal toxicity; the standard 24 mg/ml sol may be used undiluted via a central venous catheter, dilute to 12 mg/ml with D_5W or NS when a peripheral vein catheter is used

PATIENT/FAMILY EDUCATION

• Foscarnet is not a cure for CMV retinitis

• Notify clinician of perioral tingling, numbness in the extremities, or paresthesias (could signify electrolyte imbalances)

MONITORING PARAMETERS

• Serum creatinine, calcium, phosphorus, potassium, magnesium at baseline and 2-3 times/wk during induction and at least every 1-2 wk during maintenance

• Hemoglobin

• Regular ophthalmologic examinations

---

fosfomycin

(foss-fo-mye'sin)

Rx: Monurol
Chemical Class: Phosphoric acid derivative
Therapeutic Class: Antibiotic

CLINICAL PHARMACOLOGY

Mechanism of Action: An antibiotic that prevents bacterial cell wall formation by inhibiting the synthesis of peptidoglycan. *Therapeutic Effect:* Bactericidal.

INDICATIONS AND DOSAGES

Uncomplicated UTIs in females
PO
Females. 3 g mixed in 4 oz water as a single dose.

Uncomplicated UTIs in males
Males. 3 g/day for 2-3 days.

$ AVAILABLE FORMS/COST

• Powder, Reconst—Oral: 3 g/packet, 3's: **$114.04**

CONTRAINDICATIONS: None known

PREGNANCY AND LACTATION: Pregnancy category B; excretion into breast milk unknown

SIDE EFFECTS

Occasional (9%-3%)
Diarrhea, nausea, headache, back pain
Rare (less than 2%)
Dysmenorrhea, pharyngitis, abdominal pain, rash

SERIOUS REACTIONS

• None known.

INTERACTIONS

Drugs

❸ *Metoclopramide:* Decreased serum concentration and urinary excretion of fosfomycin

SPECIAL CONSIDERATIONS

• Inferior 5-11 day posttherapy microbiologic eradication rates compared to ciprofloxacin and co-trimoxazole for acute cystitis; eradication rates comparable to nitrofurantoin

• Reserve for women unable to tolerate or unlikely to comply with 3-day courses of co-trimoxazole or trimethoprim

PATIENT/FAMILY EDUCATION

• Always mix with water before ingesting

fosinopril
(fo-sin'o-pril)
Rx: Monopril
Chemical Class: Angiotensin-converting enzyme (ACE) inhibitor, nonsulfhydryl
Therapeutic Class: Antihypertensive

CLINICAL PHARMACOLOGY
Mechanism of Action: An ACE inhibitor that suppresses the renin-angiotensin-aldosterone system and prevents conversion of angiotensin I to angiotensin II, a potent vasoconstrictor; may also inhibit angiotensin II at local vascular and renal sites. Decreases plasma angiotensin II, increases plasma renin activity, and decreases aldosterone secretion. *Therapeutic Effect:* Reduces peripheral arterial resistance, pulmonary capillary wedge pressure; improves cardiac output, and exercise tolerance.

Pharmacokinetics

Route	Onset	Peak	Duration
PO	1 hr	2–6 hr	24 hr

Slowly absorbed from the GI tract. Protein binding: 97%–98%. Metabolized in the liver and GI mucosa to active metabolite. Primarily excreted in urine. Minimal removal by hemodialysis. **Half-life:** 11.5 hr.

INDICATIONS AND DOSAGES
Hypertension (monotherapy)
PO
Adults, Elderly. Initially, 10 mg/day. Maintenance: 20–40 mg/day. Maximum: 80 mg/day.
Hypertension (with diuretic)
PO
Adults, Elderly. Initially, 10 mg/day titrated to patient's needs.

Heart failure
PO
Adults, Elderly. Initially, 5–10 mg. Maintenance: 20–40 mg/day.

Ⓢ AVAILABLE FORMS/COST
• Tab—Oral: 10 mg, 90's: **$65.69-$118.98**; 20 mg, 90's: **$107.08-$118.98**; 40 mg, 90's: **$107.08-$118.98**

UNLABELED USES: Treatment of diabetic and nondiabetic nephropathy, post-myocardial infarction left ventricular dysfunction, renal crisis in scleroderma

CONTRAINDICATIONS: History of angioedema from previous treatment with ACE inhibitors

PREGNANCY AND LACTATION: Pregnancy category C (1st trimester), category D (2nd and 3rd trimesters); ACE inhibitors can cause fetal and neonatal morbidity and death when administered to pregnant women; when pregnancy is detected, discontinue ACE inhibitors as soon as possible; detectable in breast milk in trace amounts, a newborn would receive <0.1% of the mg/kg maternal dose; effect on nursing infant has not been determined; use with caution in nursing mothers

SIDE EFFECTS
Frequent (12%–9%)
Dizziness, cough
Occasional (4%–2%)
Hypotension, nausea, vomiting, upper respiratory tract infection

SERIOUS REACTIONS
• Excessive hypotension (first-dose syncope) may occur in patients with CHF and in those who are severely salt and volume depleted.
• Angioedema (swelling of face and lips) and hyperkalemia occur rarely.
• Agranulocytosis and neutropenia may be noted in those with collagen vascular disease, including sclero-

derma and systemic lupus erythematosus, and impaired renal function.

• Nephrotic syndrome may be noted in those with history of renal disease.

INTERACTIONS
Drugs
❷ *Allopurinol:* Combination may predispose to hypersensitivity reactions

❸ *α-adrenergic blockers:* Exaggerated first dose hypotensive response when added to fosinopril

❸ *Aspirin:* May reduce hemodynamic effects of fosinopril; less likely at doses under 236 mg; less likely with nonacetylated salicylates

❸ *Azathioprine:* Increased myelosuppression

❸ *Cyclosporine:* Combination may cause renal insufficiency

❸ *Insulin:* Fosinopril may enhance insulin sensitivity

❸ *Iron:* Fosinopril may increase chance of systemic reaction to IV iron

❸ *Lithium:* Reduced lithium clearance

❸ *Loop diuretics:* Initiation of fosinopril may cause hypotension and renal insufficiency in patients taking loop diuretics

❸ *NSAIDs:* May reduce hemodynamic effects of fosinopril

❸ *Potassium-sparing diuretics:* Increased risk of hyperkalemia

❸ *Trimethoprim:* Additive risk of hyperkalemia, especially in patient predisposed to renal insufficiency

Labs
• ACE inhibition can account for approximately 0.5 mEq/L rise in serum potassium

SPECIAL CONSIDERATIONS
PATIENT/FAMILY EDUCATION
• Caution with salt substitutes containing potassium chloride

• Rise slowly to sitting/standing position to minimize orthostatic hypotension

• Dizziness, fainting, lightheadedness may occur during 1st few days of therapy

• May cause altered taste perception or cough; persistent dry cough usually does not subside unless medication is stopped; notify clinician if these symptoms persist

MONITORING PARAMETERS
• BUN, creatinine, potassium within 2 wk after initiation of therapy (increased levels may indicate acute renal failure)

---

frovatriptan
(fro-va-trip′tan)
Rx: Frova
Chemical Class: Serotonin derivative
Therapeutic Class: Antimigraine agent

CLINICAL PHARMACOLOGY
Mechanism of Action: A serotonin receptor agonist that binds selectively to vascular receptors, producing a vasoconstrictive effect on cranial blood vessels. *Therapeutic Effect:* Relieves migraine headache.

Pharmacokinetics
Well absorbed after PO administration. Metabolized by the liver to inactive metabolite. Eliminated in urine. **Half-life:** 26 hr (increased in hepatic impairment).

INDICATIONS AND DOSAGES
Acute migraine attack
PO
Adults, Elderly. Initially 2.5 mg. If headache improves but then returns, dose may be repeated after 2 hr. Maximum: 7.5 mg/day.

Ⓢ **AVAILABLE FORMS/COST**
• Tab—Oral: 2.5 mg, 9's: **$147.04**

CONTRAINDICATIONS: Basilar or hemiplegic migraine, cerebrovascular or peripheral vascular disease, coronary artery disease, ischemic heart disease (including angina pectoris, history of MI, silent ischemia, and Prinzmetal's angina), severe hepatic impairment (Child-Pugh grade C), uncontrolled hypertension, use within 24 hours of ergotamine-containing preparations or another serotonin receptor agonist, use within 14 days of MAOIs

PREGNANCY AND LACTATION: Pregnancy category C; excretion into breast milk unknown; use caution in nursing mothers

SIDE EFFECTS
Occasional (8%-4%)
Dizziness, paresthesia, fatigue, flushing
Rare (3%-2%)
Hot or cold sensation, dry mouth, dyspepsia

SERIOUS REACTIONS
• Cardiac reactions (including ischemia, coronary artery vasospasm, and MI), and noncardiac vasospasm-related reactions (such as hemorrhage and CVA), occur rarely, particularly in patients with hypertension, diabetes, or a strong family history of coronary artery disease; obese patients; smokers; males older than 40 years; and postmenopausal women.

INTERACTIONS
Drugs
⚠ *Ergot containing drugs:* Prolonged vasospastic reactions
❷ *SSRIs:* Weakness, hyperreflexia, incoordination when coadministered

SPECIAL CONSIDERATIONS
• Triptans and dihydroergotamine are drugs of choice for moderate to severe migraine attacks; nasal sumatriptan is usually considered the triptan of choice due to its rapid onset; there are a number of oral triptans, including frovatriptan with more favorable biopharmaceutic profiles and high costs; comparisons not available
• There is no evidence that a second dose of frovatriptan is effective in patients who do not respond to a first dose of the drug for the same headache

PATIENT/FAMILY EDUCATION
• Useful medication for treatment of acute migraine attacks, not prevention

MONITORING PARAMETERS
• Headache response 1-4 hr after a dose (reduction from moderate or severe pain to minimal or no pain), functional disability, need for a second dose, headache recurrence, pulse, blood pressure

---

fulvestrant
(full'veh-strant)
Rx: Faslodex
Chemical Class: Estrogen derivative
Therapeutic Class: Antineoplastic

CLINICAL PHARMACOLOGY
Mechanism of Action: An estrogen antagonist that competes with endogenous estrogen at estrogen receptor binding sites. *Therapeutic Effect:* Inhibits tumor growth.
Pharmacokinetics
Extensively and rapidly distributed after IM administration. Protein binding: 99%. Metabolized in the liver. Eliminated by hepatobiliary route; excreted in feces. **Half-life:** 40 days in postmenopausal women. Peak serum levels occur in 7-9 days.

INDICATIONS AND DOSAGES
Breast cancer
IM

Adults, Elderly. 250 mg given once monthly.

AVAILABLE FORMS/COST
• Sol, Inj—IM: 50 mg/ml, 2.5, 5 ml: **$944.32**/5 ml

CONTRAINDICATIONS: Known or suspected pregnancy

PREGNANCY AND LACTATION: Pregnancy category D; found in rat milk at levels significantly higher (approximately 12-fold) than plasma; excretion in human milk unknown; use with extreme caution in nursing mothers because of the potential for serious adverse reactions from fulvestrant in nursing infants

SIDE EFFECTS
Frequent (26%-13%)

Nausea, hot flashes, pharyngitis, asthenia, vomiting, vasodilatation, headache

Occasional (12%-5%)

Injection site pain, constipation, diarrhea, abdominal pain, anorexia, dizziness, insomnia, paresthesia, bone or back pain, depression, anxiety, peripheral edema, rash, diaphoresis, fever

Rare (2%-1%)

Vertigo, weight gain

SERIOUS REACTIONS
• UTIs, vaginitis, anemia, thromboembolic phenomena, and leukopenia occur rarely.

SPECIAL CONSIDERATIONS
• Store in refrigerator

---

furosemide
(fur-oh'se-mide)
Rx: Furocot, Fumide, Lasix, Lo-Aqua, Myrosemide, Terbolan
Chemical Class: Anthranilic acid derivative
Therapeutic Class: Antihypertensive; diuretic, loop

F

CLINICAL PHARMACOLOGY
Mechanism of Action: A loop diuretic that enhances excretion of sodium, chloride, and potassium by direct action at the ascending limb of the loop of Henle. *Therapeutic Effect:* Produces diuresis and lower BP.

Pharmacokinetics

Route	Onset	Peak	Dura-tion
PO	30–60 min	1–2 hr	6–8 hr
IV	5 min	20–60 min	2 hr
IM	30 min	N/A	N/A

Well absorbed from the GI tract. Protein binding: 91%–97%. Partially metabolized in the liver. Primarily excreted in urine (nonrenal clearance increases in severe renal impairment). Not removed by hemodialysis. **Half-life:** 30–90 min (increased in renal or hepatic impairment, and in neonates).

INDICATIONS AND DOSAGES
Edema, hypertension
PO

Adults, Elderly. Initially, 20–80 mg/dose; may increase by 20–40 mg/dose q6-8h. May titrate up to 600 mg/day in severe edematous states.

Children. 1–6 mg/kg/day in divided doses q6–12h.

IV, IM

Adults, Elderly. 20–40 mg/dose; may increase by 20 mg/dose q1–2h.

Children. 1–2 mg/kg/dose q6–12h.

Neonates. 1–2 mg/kg/dose q12–24h.

IV infusion

Adults, Elderly. Bolus of 0.1 mg/kg, followed by infusion of 0.1 mg/kg/hr; may double q2h. Maximum: 0.4 mg/kg/hr.

Children. 0.05 mg/kg/hr; titrate to desired effect.

AVAILABLE FORMS/COST
• Sol, Inj—IM, IV: 10 mg/ml, 2, 4, 8, 10 ml: **$4.58-$14.96**/10 ml
• Sol—Oral: 10 mg/ml, 60, 120 ml: **$13.96-$20.10**/120 ml; 40 mg/5 ml, 500 ml: **$39.66**
• Tab—Oral: 20 mg, 100's: **$2.00-$22.66**; 40 mg, 100's: **$2.50-$36.24**; 80 mg, 100's: **$12.04-$43.70**

UNLABELED USES: Hypercalcemia

CONTRAINDICATIONS: Anuria, hepatic coma, severe electrolyte depletion

PREGNANCY AND LACTATION: Pregnancy category C; cardiovascular disorders such as pulmonary edema, severe hypertension, or CHF are probably the only valid indications for this drug during pregnancy; furosemide has been used after the first trimester without causing fetal or newborn adverse effects; does not appear to significantly alter amniotic fluid volume; maternal use during pregnancy has not been associated with toxic or teratogenic effects, although metabolic complications have been observed (hyponatremia, hyperuricemia); reduces placental and/or maternal hepatic perfusion; excreted into breast milk; no reports of adverse effects in nursing infants

SIDE EFFECTS

Expected

Increased urinary frequency and urine volume

Frequent

Nausea, dyspepsia, abdominal cramps, diarrhea or constipation, electrolyte disturbances

Occasional

Dizziness, light-headedness, headache, blurred vision, paresthesia, photosensitivity, rash, fatigue, bladder spasm, restlessness, diaphoresis

Rare

Flank pain

SERIOUS REACTIONS
• Vigorous diuresis may lead to profound water loss and electrolyte depletion, resulting in hypokalemia, hyponatremia, and dehydration.
• Sudden volume depletion may result in increased risk of thrombosis, circulatory collapse, and sudden death.
• Acute hypotensive episodes may occur, sometimes several days after beginning therapy.
• Ototoxicity - manifested as deafness, vertigo, or tinnitus - may occur, especially in patients with severe renal impairment.
• Furosemide use can exacerbate diabetes mellitus, systemic lupus erythematosus, gout, and pancreatitis.
• Blood dyscrasias have been reported.

INTERACTIONS

Drugs

❷ *Aminoglycosides (gentamicin, kanamycin, neomycin, streptomycin):* Additive ototoxicity (ethacrynic acid > furosemide, torsemide, bumetanide)

❸ *Angiotensin converting enzyme inhibitors:* Initiation of ACEI with intensive diuretic therapy may result in precipitous fall in blood pressure; ACEIs may induce renal insufficiency in the presence of diuretic-induced sodium depletion

❸ *Barbiturates (phenobarbital):* Reduced diuretic response

3 *Bile acid-binding resins (cholestyramine, colestipol):* Resins markedly reduce the bioavailability and diuretic response of furosemide

3 *Carbenoxolone:* Severe hypokalemia from coadministration

3 *Cephalosporins (cephaloridine, cephalothin):* Enhanced nephrotoxicity with coadministration

2 *Cisplatin:* Additive ototoxicity (ethacrynic acid > furosemide, torsemide, bumetanide)

3 *Clofibrate:* Enhanced effects of both drugs, especially in hypoalbuminemic patients

3 *Corticosteroids:* Concomitant loop diuretic and corticosteroid therapy can result in excessive potassium loss

3 *Digitalis glycosides (digoxin, digitoxin):* Diuretic-induced hypokalemia may increase risk of digitalis toxicity

3 *Nonsteroidal antiinflammatory drugs (flurbiprofen, ibuprofen, indomethacin, naproxen, piroxicam, aspirin, sulindac):* Reduced diuretic and antihypertensive effects

3 *Phenytoin:* Reduced diuretic response

3 *Serotonin-reuptake inhibitors (fluoxetine, paroxetine, sertraline):* Case reports of sudden death; enhanced hyponatremia proposed; causal relationships not established

3 *Terbutaline:* Additive hypokalemia

3 *Tubocurarine:* Prolonged neuromuscular blockade

Labs

• *Cortisol:* False increases

• *Glucose:* Falsely low urine tests with clinistix and diastix

• *Thyroxine:* Increased serum concentration

• *T_3 uptake:* Interference causes increased serum values

SPECIAL CONSIDERATIONS
PATIENT/FAMILY EDUCATION

• May cause GI upset, take with food or milk

• Take early in the day

• Avoid prolonged exposure to sunlight

MONITORING PARAMETERS

• Urine volume, creatinine clearance, BUN electrolytes, reduction in edema, increased diuresis, decrease in body weight, reduction in blood pressure, glucose, uric acid, serum calcium (tetany), tinnitus, vertigo, hearing loss (especially in those at risk for ototoxicity—IV doses >120 mg; concomitant ototoxic drugs; renal disease)

gabapentin
(ga'ba-pen-tin)
Rx: Neurontin
Chemical Class: Cyclohexanacetic acid derivative
Therapeutic Class: Anticonvulsant

CLINICAL PHARMACOLOGY
Mechanism of Action: An anticonvulsant and antineuralgic agent whose exact mechanism unknown. May increase the synthesis or accumulation of gamma-aminobutyric acid by binding to as-yet-undefined receptor sites in brain tissue. *Therapeutic Effect:* Reduces seizure activity and neuropathic pain.

Pharmacokinetics

Well absorbed from the GI tract (not affected by food). Protein binding: less than 5%. Widely distributed. Crosses the blood-brain barrier. Primarily excreted unchanged in urine. Removed by hemodialysis. **Half-life:** 5-7 hr (increased in impaired renal function and the elderly).

INDICATIONS AND DOSAGES
Adjunctive therapy for seizure control
PO

Adults, Elderly, Children 12 yr and older. Initially, 300 mg 3 times a day. May titrate dosage. Range: 900-1800 mg/day in 3 divided doses. Maximum: 3,600 mg/day.

Children 3-12 yr. Initially, 10-15 mg/kg/day in 3 divided doses. May titrate up to 25-35 mg/kg/day (for children 5-12 yr) and 40 mg/kg/day (for children 3-4 yr) Maximum: 50 mg/kg/day.

Adjunctive therapy for neuropathic pain
PO

Adults, Elderly. Initially, 100 mg 3 times a day; may increase by 300 mg/day at weekly intervals. Maximum: 3,600 mg/day in 3 divided doses.

Children. Initially, 5 mg/kg/dose at bedtime, followed by 5 mg/kg/dose for 2 doses on day 2, then 5 mg/kg/dose for 3 doses on day 3. Range: 8-35 mg/kg/day in 3 divided doses.

Postherpetic neuralgia
PO

Adults, Elderly. 300 mg on day 1, 300 mg twice a day on day 2, and 300 mg 3 times a day on day 3. Titrate up to 1,800 mg/day.

Dosage in renal impairment
Dosage and frequency are modified based on creatinine clearance:

Creatinine Clearance	Dosage
60 ml/min or higher	400 mg q8h
30-59 ml/min	300 mg q12h
16-29 ml/min	300 mg daily
less than 16 ml/min	300 mg every other day
Hemodialysis	200-300 mg after each 4-hr hemodialysis session

🟦 AVAILABLE FORMS/COST
- Cap, Gel—Oral: 100 mg, 100's: **$55.60**; 300 mg, 100's: **$139.00**; 400 mg, 100's: **$166.78**
- Sol—Oral: 250 mg/5 ml, 480 ml: **$103.71**
- Tab—Oral: 600 mg, 100's: **$239.03**; 800 mg, 100's: **$286.83**

UNLABELED USES: Treatment of essential tremor, hot flashes, hyperhidrosis, migraines, psychiatric disorders

CONTRAINDICATIONS: None known

PREGNANCY AND LACTATION: Pregnancy category C; excretion into breast milk unknown

SIDE EFFECTS
Frequent (19%-10%)

Fatigue, somnolence, dizziness, ataxia

Occasional (8%-3%)

Nystagmus, tremor, diplopia, rhinitis, weight gain

Rare (less than 2%)

Nervousness, dysarthria, memory loss, dyspepsia, pharyngitis, myalgia

SERIOUS REACTIONS
- Abrupt withdrawal may increase seizure frequency.
- Overdosage may result in diplopia, slurred speech, drowsiness, lethargy, and diarrhea.

INTERACTIONS
Drugs
🟦 *Antacids:* Reduce bioavailability of gabapentin by 20%

SPECIAL CONSIDERATIONS
PATIENT/FAMILY EDUCATION
- Do not stop abruptly; taper over 1 wk

MONITORING PARAMETERS
- Drug level monitoring not necessary

galantamine
(ga-lan'ta-mene)

Rx: Reminyl

Chemical Class: Benzazepine derivative; cholinesterase inhibitor

Therapeutic Class: Acetylcholinesterase inhibitor

CLINICAL PHARMACOLOGY

Mechanism of Action: A cholinesterase inhibitor that inhibits the enzyme acetylcholinesterase, thus increasing the concentration of acetylcholine at cholinergic synapses and enhancing cholinergic function in the CNS. *Therapeutic Effect:* Slows the progression of Alzheimer's disease.

Pharmacokinetics

Rapidly absorbed from the GI tract. Protein binding: 18%. Distributed to blood cells; binds to plasma proteins, mainly albumin. Metabolized in the liver. Excreted in urine. **Half-life:** 7 hr.

INDICATIONS AND DOSAGES
Alzheimer's disease

PO

Adults, Elderly. Initially, 4 mg twice a day (8 mg/day). After a minimum of 4 wk (if well tolerated), may increase to 8 mg twice a day (16 mg/day). After another 4 wk, may increase to 12 mg twice daily (24 mg/day). Range: 16-24 mg/day in 2 divided doses.

Dosage in renal impairment

For moderate impairment, maximum dosage is 16 mg/day. Drug is not recommended for patients with severe impairment.

$ AVAILABLE FORMS/COST
• Sol—Oral: 4 mg/ml, 100 ml: **$157.35**
• Tab, Coated—Oral: 4 mg, 8 mg, 12 mg, 60's; all: **$157.31**

CONTRAINDICATIONS: Severe hepatic or renal impairment

PREGNANCY AND LACTATION: Pregnancy category B; breast milk excretion information not known

SIDE EFFECTS
Frequent (17%-5%)

Nausea, vomiting, diarrhea, anorexia, weight loss

Occasional (9%-4%)

Abdominal pain, insomnia, depression, headache, dizziness, fatigue, rhinitis

Rare (less than 3%)

Tremors, constipation, confusion, cough, anxiety, urinary incontinence

SERIOUS REACTIONS
• Overdose may cause cholinergic crisis, characterized by increased salivation, lacrimation, severe nausea and vomiting, bradycardia, respiratory depression, hypotension, and increased muscle weakness. Treatment usually consists of supportive measures and an anticholinergic such as atropine.

INTERACTIONS
Drugs

3 *Anesthetics (inhaled):* Decreases neuromuscular blocking effects

3 *Anesthetics (local, esters):* Increases effects (possible toxicity) of local anesthetic (pseudocholinesterase competition)

3 *Anticholinergics:* Antagonistic effects; use to counteract undesirable muscarinic effects of cholinesterase inhibitors

2 *Bethanechol, pilocarpine, dexpanthanol, echothiophate:* Galantamine potentiates cholinergic agonists

3 *Cimetidine:* Increased bioavailability of galantamine (16%)

◨ *Ketoconazole:* Strong inhibitor of CYP3A4; increases AUC of galantamine by 30%

◨ *Erythromycin:* Moderate inhibitor of CYP3A4; increases AUC of galantamine 10%

◨ *Fluoxetine:* Inhibition of CYP2D6 may increase levels of galantamine

◨ *Fluvoxamine:* Inhibition of CYP2D6 may increase levels of galantamine

◨ *Paroxetine:* Strong inhibitor of CYP2D6; increases AUC of galantamine 40%

② *Succinylcholine:* Potentiates neuromuscular blockade

SPECIAL CONSIDERATIONS

• Extracted from the bulbs of the daffodil, *Narcissus pseudonarcissus*

PATIENT/FAMILY EDUCATION

• Patient and caregiver should be advised of high incidence of gastrointestinal effects and directions for resource and resolution

MONITORING PARAMETERS

• Cognitive function (e.g., ADAS, Mini-Mental Status Exam [MMSE]), activities of daily living, global functioning, blood chemistry, complete blood counts, heart rate, blood pressure

---

ganciclovir
(gan-sy'clo-ver)
Rx: Cytovene
Chemical Class: Acyclic purine nucleoside analog
Therapeutic Class: Antiviral

CLINICAL PHARMACOLOGY

Mechanism of Action: This synthetic nucleoside competes with viral DNA polymerase and is incorporated into growing viral DNa chains.

Therapeutic Effect: Interferes with synthesis and replication of viral DNA.

Pharmacokinetics

Widely distributed. Protein binding: 1%-2%. Undergoes minimal metabolism. Excreted unchanged primarily in urine. Removed by hemodialysis. **Half-life:** 2.5-3.6 hr (increased in impaired renal function).

INDICATIONS AND DOSAGES

Cytomegalovirus (CMV) retinitis

IV

Adults, Children 3 mo and older. 10 mg/kg/day in divided doses q12h for 14-21 days, then 5 mg/kg/day as a single daily dose.

Prevention of CMV disease in transplant patients

IV

Adults, Children. 10 mg/kg/day in divided doses q12h for 7-14 days, then 5 mg/kg/day as a single daily dose.

Other CMV infections

IV

Adults. Initially, 10 mg/kg/day in divided doses q12h for 14-21 days, then 5 mg/kg/day as a single daily dose. Maintenance: 1,000 mg 3 times a day or 500 mg q3h (6 times a day).

Children. Initially, 10 mg/kg/day in divided doses q12h for 14-21 days, then 5 mg/kg/day as a single daily dose. Maintenance: 30 mg/kg/dose q8h.

Intravitreal implant

Adults. 1 implant q6-9mo plus oral ganciclovir.

Children 9 yr and older. 1 implant q6-9mo plus oral ganciclovir (30 mg/dose q8h).

Adult dosage in renal impairment

Dosage and frequency are modified based on CrCl.

CrCl	*Induction Dosage*	*Maintenance Dosage*	*Oral*
50-69 ml/ min	2.5 mg/kg q12h	2.5 mg/kg q24h	1,500 mg/ day
25-49 ml/ min	2.5 mg/kg q24h	1.25 mg/ kg q24h	1,000 mg/ day
10-24 ml/ min	1.25 mg/kg q24h	0.625 mg/ kg q24h	500 mg/ day
less than 10 ml/ min	1.25 mg/kg 3 times/ wk	0.625 mg/kg 3 times/ wk	500 mg 3 times/ wk

CrCl = creatinine clearance

$ **AVAILABLE FORMS/COST**

• Cap, Gel—Oral: 250 mg, 180's: **$780.90-$901.84**; 500 mg, 180's: **$1,614.28-$1,734.29**

• Implant—Ophth: 4.5 mg: **$5,000.00**

• Powder, Inj—IV: 500 mg/vial: **$38.64**

UNLABELED USES: Treatment of other CMV infections, such as gastroenteritis, hepatitis, and pneumonitis

CONTRAINDICATIONS: Absolute neutrophil count less than 500/mm^3, platelet count less than 25,000/mm^3, hypersensitivity to acyclovir or ganciclovir, immunocompetent patients, patients with congenital or neonatal CMV disease.

PREGNANCY AND LACTATION: Pregnancy category C; excretion into breast milk unknown, not recommended in nursing mothers due to potential for serious adverse reactions in the nursing infant; do not resume nursing for at least 72 hr after last dose of ganciclovir

SIDE EFFECTS

Frequent

Diarrhea (41%), fever (40%), nausea (25%), abdominal pain (17%), vomiting (13%)

Occasional (11%-6%)

Diaphoresis, infection, paresthesia, flatulence, pruritus

Rare (4%-2%)

Headache, stomatitis, dyspepsia, phlebitis

SERIOUS REACTIONS

• Hematologic toxicity occurs commonly: leukopenia in 41%-29% of patients and anemia in 25%-19%.

• Intraocular insertion occasionally results in visual acuity loss, vitreous hemorrhage, and retinal detachment.

• GI hemorrhage occurs rarely.

INTERACTIONS

Drugs

[3] *Didanosine:* Increased hematological toxicity

⚠ *Zidovudine:* Increased hematological toxicity

SPECIAL CONSIDERATIONS

PATIENT/FAMILY EDUCATION

• Compliance with laboratory monitoring is essential

MONITORING PARAMETERS

• CBC with differential and platelets q2 days during induction and weekly thereafter

• Serum creatinine q2 wk

gatifloxacin

(gah-tee-floks'a-sin)

Rx: Tequin

Chemical Class: Fluoroquinolone derivative

Therapeutic Class: Antibiotic

CLINICAL PHARMACOLOGY

Mechanism of Action: A fluoroquinolone that inhibits two enzymes, topoisomerase II and IV, in susceptible microorganisms. *Therapeutic*

Effect: Interferes with bacterial DNA replication. Prevents or delays resistance emergence. Bactericidal.

Pharmacokinetics

Well absorbed from the gastrointestinal (GI) tract after PO administration. Protein binding: 20%. Widely distributed. Metabolized in liver. Primarily excreted in urine. **Half-life:** 7–14 hrs.

INDICATIONS AND DOSAGES

Chronic bronchitis, complicated urinary tract infections, pyelonephritis, skin infections
PO/IV
Adults, Elderly. 400 mg/day for 7–10 days (5 days for chronic bronchitis).

Sinusitis
PO/IV
Adults, Elderly. 400 mg/day for 10 days.

Pneumonia
PO/IV
Adults, Elderly. 400 mg/day for 7–14 days.

Cystitis
PO/IV
Adults, Elderly. 400 mg as a single dose or 200 mg/day for 3 days.

Urethral gonorrhea in men and women, endocervical and rectal gonorrhea in women
PO/IV
Adults, Elderly. 400 mg as a single dose.

Topical treatment of bacterial conjunctivitis due to susceptible strains of bacteria
Ophthalmic
Adults, Elderly, Children 1 yr and older. 1 drop q2h while awake for 2 days, then 1 drop up to 4 times/day for days 3–7.

Dosage in renal impairment

Creatinine Clearance	Dosage
40 ml/min	400 mg/day
less than 40 ml/min	Initially, 400 mg/day then 200 mg/day
Hemodialysis	Initially, 400 mg/day then 200 mg/day
Peritoneal dialysis	Initially, 400 mg/day then 200 mg/day

$ AVAILABLE FORMS/COST

• Sol—Ophth: 0.3%, 5 ml: **$49.30**
• Sol, Inj—IV: 10 mg/ml, 40 ml: **$38.05**
• Tab—Oral: 200 mg 30's: **$282.08**; 400 mg 7's: **$48.97**; 400 mg 100's: **$940.25**

CONTRAINDICATIONS: Hypersensitivity to quinolones

PREGNANCY AND LACTATION: Pregnancy category C; breast milk excretion unknown

SIDE EFFECTS

Occasional (8%–3%)
Nausea, vaginitis, diarrhea, headache, dizziness
Ophthalmic: conjunctival irritation, increased tearing, corneal inflammation

Rare (3%–0.1%)
Abdominal pain, constipation, dyspepsia, stomatitis, edema, insomnia, abnormal dreams, diaphoresis, altered taste, rash
Ophthalmic: corneal swelling, dry eye, eye pain, eyelid swelling, headache, red eye, reduced visual acuity, altered taste

SERIOUS REACTIONS

• Pseudomembranous colitis as evidenced by severe abdominal pain and cramps, severe watery diarrhea, and fever, may occur.
• Superinfection manifested as genital or anal pruritus, ulceration or changes in oral mucosa, and moderate to severe diarrhea, may occur.

INTERACTIONS
Drugs
3 *Aluminum:* Reduced absorption of gatifloxacin; do not take within 4 hr of dose

2 *Amiodarone:* Additive cardiac toxicity

3 *Antacids (containing aluminum or magnesium):* Reduced absorption of gatifloxacin; do not take within 4 hr of dose

2 *Antipsychotics:* Additive cardiac toxicity

3 *Didanosine (buffered formulation):* Markedly reduced absorption of gatifloxacin; take gatifloxacin 2 hr before didanosine

2 *Erythromycin:* Coadministration may increase risk of cardiac toxicity due to gatifloxacin

3 *Foscarnet:* Coadministration increase seizure risk

3 *Iron:* Reduced absorption of gatifloxacin; do not take within 4 hr of dose

3 *Magnesium:* Reduced absorption of gatifloxacin; do not take within 4 hr of dose

3 *Probenecid:* Inhibits excretion of gatifloxacin

2 *Procainamide:* Additive cardiac toxicity

2 *Quinidine:* Additive cardiac toxicity

3 *Sodium bicarbonate:* Reduced absorption of gatifloxacin; do not take within 4 hr of dose

2 *Sotalol:* Additive cardiac toxicity

3 *Sucralfate:* Reduced absorption of gatifloxacin; do not take within 4 hr of dose

2 *Tricyclic antidepressants:* Additive cardiac toxicity

3 *Zinc:* Reduced absorption of gatifloxacin; do not take within 4 hr of dose

SPECIAL CONSIDERATIONS
PATIENT/FAMILY EDUCATION
• May be taken with or without meals

• Should be taken at least 4 hr before or 8 hr after multivitamins (containing iron or zinc), antacids (containing magnesium, calcium, or aluminum), sucralfate, or didanosine chewable/buffered tablets

• Discontinue treatment, rest and refrain from exercise, and inform prescriber if pain, inflammation, or rupture of a tendon occur

• Test reaction to this drug before operating an automobile or machinery or engaging in activities requiring mental alertness or coordination

G

---

gemfibrozil
(gem-fi'broe-zil)
Rx: Lopid
Chemical Class: Fibric acid derivative
Therapeutic Class: Antilipemic

CLINICAL PHARMACOLOGY
Mechanism of Action: A fibric acid derivative that inhibits lipolysis of fat in adipose tissue; decreases liver uptake of free fatty acids and reduces hepatic triglyceride production. Inhibits synthesis of VLDL carrier apolipoprotein B. *Therapeutic Effect:* Lowers serum cholesterol and triglycerides (decreases VLDL, LDL; increases HDL).

Pharmacokinetics
Well absorbed from the gastrointestinal (GI) tract. Protein binding: 99%. Metabolized in liver. Primarily excreted in urine. Not removed by hemodialysis. **Half-life:** 1.5 hrs.

INDICATIONS AND DOSAGES
Hyperlipidemia
PO

Adults, Elderly. 1200 mg/day in 2 divided doses 30 min before breakfast and dinner.

⑧ AVAILABLE FORMS/COST
• Tab, Plain Coated-Oral: 600 mg, 100's: **$89.50-$138.66**

CONTRAINDICATIONS: Liver dysfunction (including primary biliary cirrhosis), preexisting gallbladder disease, severe renal dysfunction

PREGNANCY AND LACTATION: Pregnancy category C; excretion into breast milk unknown; use caution in nursing mothers

SIDE EFFECTS
Frequent (20%)
Dyspepsia
Occasional (10%-2%)
Abdominal pain, diarrhea, nausea, vomiting, fatigue
Rare (less than 2%)
Constipation, acute appendicitis, vertigo, headache, rash, pruritus, altered taste

SERIOUS REACTIONS
• Cholelithiasis, cholecystitis, acute appendicitis, pancreatitis, and malignancy occur rarely.

INTERACTIONS
Drugs
❸ *Binding resins:* Reduced bioavailability of gemfibrozil, separate doses by >2 hr
❸ *Glyburide:* Increased risk of hypoglycemia
❷ *HMG CoA reductase inhibitors (atorvastatin, fluvastatin, lovastatin, pravastatin, simvastatin):* Increased likelihood of drug-induced myopathy
❷ *Warfarin:* Increased hypoprothrombinemic, response to warfarin

SPECIAL CONSIDERATIONS
PATIENT/FAMILY EDUCATION
• May cause dizziness or blurred vision; use caution while driving or performing other tasks requiring alertness
• Notify clinician if GI side effects become pronounced

MONITORING PARAMETERS
• Serum CK level in patients complaining of muscle pain, tenderness, or weakness
• Periodic CBC during first 12 mo of therapy
• Periodic LFTs; discontinue therapy if abnormalities persist
• Blood glucose

---

gemifloxacin
Rx: Factive
Chemical Class: Fluoroquinolone derivative
Therapeutic Class: Antibiotic

CLINICAL PHARMACOLOGY
Mechanism of Action: A fluoroquinolone that inhibits the enzyme DNA gyrase in susceptible microorganisms, interfering with bacterial cell replication and repair. *Therapeutic Effect:* Bactericidal.
Pharmacokinetics
Rapidly and well absorbed from the GI tract. Protein binding: 70%. Widely distributed. Penetrates well into lung tissue and fluid. Undergoes limited metabolism in the liver. Primarily excreted in feces; lesser amount eliminated in urine. Partially removed by hemodialysis. **Half-life:** 4-12 hr.

INDICATIONS AND DOSAGES
Acute bacterial exacerbation of chronic bronchitis
PO

Adults, Elderly. 320 mg once a day for 5 days.

Community-acquired pneumonia
PO

Adults, Elderly. 320 mg once a day for 7 days.

Dosage in renal impairment
Dosage and frequency are modified based on creatinine clearance.

Creatinine Clearance	Dosage
greater than 40 ml/min	320 mg once a day
40 ml/min or less	160 mg once a day

$ AVAILABLE FORMS/COST
• Tab-Oral: 320 mg, 5's and 7's: *Cost not available*

CONTRAINDICATIONS: Concurrent use of amiodarone, quinidine, procainamide, or sotalol; history of prolonged QTc interval; hypersensitivity fo fluoroquinolones; uncorrected electrolyte disorders (such as hypokalemia and hypomagnesemia)

PREGNANCY AND LACTATION: Pregnancy category C; breast milk excretion in humans unknown

SIDE EFFECTS
Occasional (4%-2%)
Diarrhea, rash, nausea
Rare (1% or less)
Headache, abdominal pain, dizziness

SERIOUS REACTIONS
• Antibiotic-associated colitis may result from altered bacterial balance. Hypersensitivity reactions, including photosensitivity (as evidenced by rash, pruritus, blisters, edema, and burning skin), have occurred in patients receiving fluoroquinolones.

INTERACTIONS
Drugs
▣ *Antacids containing aluminum, magnesium or calcium:* Reduced absorption of gemifloxacin; do not take within 3 hrs of dose of gemifloxacin

⚠ *Amiodarone:* Additive QT interval prolongation

▣ *Didanosine, buffered form:* Markedly reduced absorption of gemifloxacin; do not take within 3 hrs of dose of gemifloxacin

⚠ *Erythromycin:* Additive QT interval prolongation

▣ *Iron:* Reduced absorption of gemifloxacin; do not take within 3 hrs of dose of gemifloxacin

⚠ *Procainamide:* Additive QT interval prolongation

▣ *Propranolol:* Inhibits metabolism of propranolol; increased plasma propranolol level

⚠ *Quinidine:* Additive QT interval prolongation

⚠ *Sotalol:* Additive QT interval prolongation

▣ *Sucralfate:* Reduced absorption of gemifloxacin; do not take within 2 hrs of dose of gemifloxacin

▣ *Zinc:* Reduced absorption of gemifloxacin; do not take within 3 hrs of dose of gemifloxacin

SPECIAL CONSIDERATIONS
• Use with caution in pneumonia due to *Klebsiella pneumoniae*. In clinical trials, 2 treatment failures occurred out of 13 cases

PATIENT/FAMILY EDUCATION
• May be taken with or without meals
• Do not chew pills
• Should not be taken within 3 hours of multivitamins (containing iron or zinc), antacids (containing magnesium, calcium, or aluminum), sucralfate, or didanosine chewable/buffered tablets
• Discontinue treatment, rest and refrain from exercise, and inform prescriber if pain, inflammation, or rupture of a tendon occurs
• Test reaction to this drug before operating an automobile or machinery or engaging in activities requiring mental alertness or coordination

G

gentamicin

(jen-ta-mye'sin)

Rx: *Cre/oint:* Ed-Mycin, G-Myticin, Garamycin

Rx: *Ophth:* Ed-Mycin, Garamycin, Genoptic, Gent-AK, Gentrasul, Infa-Gen, Spectro Genta

Rx: *Systemic:* G Mycin, Garamycin

Combinations

Rx: with prednisolone (Pred-G)

Chemical Class: Aminoglycoside

Therapeutic Class: Antibiotic

CLINICAL PHARMACOLOGY

Mechanism of Action: An aminoglycoside antibiotic that irreversibly binds to the protein of bacterial ribosomes. *Therapeutic Effect:* Interferes with protein synthesis of susceptible microorganisms. Bactericidal.

Pharmacokinetics

Rapid, complete absorption after IM administration. Protein binding: less than 30%. Widely distributed (doesn't cross the blood-brain barrier, low concentrations in CSF). Excreted unchanged in urine. Removed by hemodialysis. **Half-life:** 2-4 hr (increased in impaired renal function and neonates; decreased in cystic fibrosis and burn or febrile patients).

INDICATIONS AND DOSAGES

Acute pelvic, bone, intraabdominal, joint, respiratory tract, burn wound, postoperative, and skin or skin-structure infections; complicated UTIs; septicemia; meningitis

IV, IM

Adults, Elderly. Usual dosage, 3-6 mg/kg/day in divided doses q8h or 4-6.6 mg/kg once a day.

Children 5-12 yr. Usual dosage 2-2.5 mg/kg/dose q8h.

Children younger than 5 yr. Usual dosage, 2.5 mg/kg/dose q8h.

Neonates. Usual dosage 2.5-3.5 mg/kg/dose q8-12h.

Hemodialysis

IV, IM

Adults, Elderly. 0.5-0.7 mg/kg/dose after dialysis.

Children. 1.25-1.75 mg/kg/dose after dialysis.

Intrathecal

Adults. 4-8 mg/day.

Children 3 mo-12 yr. 1-2 mg/day.

Neonates. 1 mg/day.

Superficial eye infections

Ophthalmic Ointment

Adults, Elderly. Usual dosage, apply thin strip to conjunctiva 2-3 times a day.

Ophthalmic Solution

Adults, Elderly, Children. Usual dosage, 1-2 drops q2-4h up to 2 drops/hr.

Superficial skin infections

Topical

Adults, Elderly. Usual dosage, apply 3-4 times/day.

Dosage in renal impairment

Creatinine clearance greater than 40-60 ml/min. dosage interval q12h.

Creatinine clearance 20-40 ml/min. dosage interval q24h.

Creatinine clearance less than 20 ml/min. monitor levels to determine dosage interval.

$ AVAILABLE FORMS/COST

- Cre—Top: 0.1%, 15, 30 g: **$3.00-$24.13**/15 g
- Sol, Inj-IM; IV: 10 mg/ml, 2 ml: **$0.78-$1.24**; 40 mg/ml, 2 ml: **$0.84-$6.31**
- Oint—Ophth: 0.3%, 3.5 g: **$4.10-$24.95**
- Oint—Top: 0.1%, 15, 30, 45 g: **$3.00-$18.60**/15 g
- Sol—Ophth: 0.3%, 5, 15 ml: **$2.75-$28.94**/5 ml

UNLABELED USES: Topical: Prophylaxis of minor bacterial skin infections, treatment of dermal ulcer

CONTRAINDICATIONS: Hypersensitivity to gentamicin, other aminoglycosides (cross-sensitivity), or their components. Sulfite sensitivity may result in anaphylaxis, especially in asthmatic patients.

PREGNANCY AND LACTATION: Pregnancy category C; ototoxicity has not been reported as an effect of *in utero* exposure; 8th cranial nerve toxicity in the fetus is well known following exposure to other aminoglycosides and could potentially occur with gentamicin; potentiation of magnesium sulfate-induced neuromuscular weakness in neonates has been reported, use caution during the last 32 hr of pregnancy; data on excretion into breast milk are lacking

SIDE EFFECTS

Occasional

IM: Pain, induration

IV: Phlebitis, thrombophlebitis, hypersensitivity reactions (fever, pruritus, rash, urticaria)

Ophthalmic: Burning, tearing, itching, blurred vision

Topical: Redness, itching

Rare

Alopecia, hypertension, weakness

SERIOUS REACTIONS

• Nephrotoxicity (as evidenced by increased BUN and serum creatinine levels and decreased creatinine clearance) may be reversible if the drug is stopped at the first sign of symptoms.

• Irreversible ototoxicity (manifested as tinnitus, dizziness, ringing or roaring in the ears, and diminished hearing), and neurotoxicity (as evidenced by headache, dizziness, lethargy, tremor, and visual disturbances) occur occasionally. The risk of these effects increases with higher dosages or prolonged therapy and when the solution is applied directly to the mucosa.

• Superinfections, particularly with fungal infections, may result from bacterial imbalance no matter which administration route is used.

• Ophthalmic application may cause paresthesia of conjunctiva or mydriasis.

INTERACTIONS

Drugs

🔳 *Amphotericin B:* Synergistic nephrotoxicity

❷ *Atracurium:* Gentamicin potentiates respiratory depression by atracurium

🔳 *Carbenicillin:* Potential for inactivation of gentamicin in patients with renal failure

🔳 *Carboplatin:* Additive nephrotoxicity or ototoxicity

🔳 *Cephalosporins:* Increased potential for nephrotoxicity in patients with preexisting renal disease

🔳 *Cisplatin:* Additive nephrotoxicity or ototoxicity

🔳 *Cyclosporine:* Additive nephrotoxicity

❷ *Ethacrynic acid:* Additive ototoxicity

🔳 *Indomethacin:* Reduced renal clearance of gentamicin in premature infants

🔳 *Methoxyflurane:* Additive nephrotoxicity

❷ *Neuromuscular blocking agents:* Gentamicin potentiates respiratory depression by neuromuscular blocking agents

🔳 *NSAIDs:* May reduce renal clearance of gentamicin

🔳 *Penicillins (extended spectrum):* Potential for inactivation of gentamicin in patients with renal failure

🔳 *Piperacillin:* Potential for inactivation of gentamicin in patients with renal failure

[2] *Succinylcholine:* Gentamicin potentiates respiratory depression by succinylcholine
[3] *Ticarcillin:* Potential for inactivation of gentamicin in patients with renal failure
[3] *Vancomycin:* Additive nephrotoxicity or ototoxicity
[2] *Vecuronium:* Gentamicin potentiates respiratory depression by vecuronium

Labs

- *Amino acids:* Increase in urine amino acids
- *AST:* False elevations
- *Protein:* False urine elevations

SPECIAL CONSIDERATIONS

PATIENT/FAMILY EDUCATION

- Report headache, dizziness, loss of hearing, ringing, roaring in ears, or feeling of fullness in head
- Tilt head back, place medication in conjunctival sac, and close eyes
- Apply light finger pressure on lacrimal sac for 1 min following instillation (gtt)
- May cause temporary blurring of vision following administration (ophth)
- Notify clinician if stinging, burning, or itching becomes pronounced or if redness, irritation, swelling, decreasing vision, or pain persists or worsens (ophth)
- Do not touch tip of container to any surface (ophth)
- For external use only (ophth)
- Cleanse affected area of skin prior to application (top)
- Notify clinician if condition worsens or if rash or irritation develops (top)

MONITORING PARAMETERS

- Urinalysis for proteinuria, cells, casts
- Urine output
- Serum peak, drawn at 30-60 min after IV INF or 60 min after IM inj, trough level drawn just before next dose; adjust dosage per levels (usual therapeutic plasma levels, peak 4-8 mcg/ml, trough ≤2 mcg/ml)
- Serum creatinine for CrCl calculation
- Serum calcium, magnesium, sodium
- Audiometric testing, assess hearing before, during, after treatment

---

glatiramer

(gla-teer'a-mer)

Rx: Copaxone

Chemical Class: Polypeptide, synthetic

Therapeutic Class: Multiple sclerosis agent

CLINICAL PHARMACOLOGY

Mechanism of Action: An immunosuppressive whose exact mechanism is unknown. May act by modifying immune processes thought to be responsible for the pathogenesis of multiple sclerosis (MS). *Therapeutic Effect:* Slows progression of MS.

Pharmacokinetics

Substantial fraction of glatiramer is hydrolyzed locally. Some fraction of injected material enters lymphatic circulation, reaching regional lymph nodes; some may enter systemic circulation intact.

INDICATIONS AND DOSAGES

MS

Subcutaneous

Adults, Elderly. 20 mg once a day.

[$] **AVAILABLE FORMS/COST**

- Sol, Inj-SC: 20 mg/vial, 30's: **$1,211.81**

CONTRAINDICATIONS: Hypersensitivity to glatiramer or mannitol

PREGNANCY AND LACTATION: Pregnancy category B; excretion into breast milk unknown, use caution in nursing mothers

SIDE EFFECTS
Expected (73%–40%)
Pain, erythema, inflammation, or pruritus at injection site; asthenia
Frequent (27%–18%)
Arthralgia, vasodilation, anxiety, hypertonia, nausea, transient chest pain, dyspnea, flu-like symptoms, rash, pruritus
Occasional (17%–10%)
Palpitations, back pain, diaphoresis, rhinitis, diarrhea, urinary urgency
Rare (8%–6%)
Anorexia, fever, neck pain, peripheral edema, ear pain, facial edema, vertigo, vomiting

SERIOUS REACTIONS
• Infection is a common effect.
• Lymphadenopathy occurs occasionally.

SPECIAL CONSIDERATIONS
• May be useful for relapsing-remitting multiple sclerosis in patients who are not benefiting from, or are intolerant of, interferon β-1 a/b; less effective in patients with advanced disease or chronic-progressive multiple sclerosis; not a cure for multiple sclerosis and benefits achieved are relatively modest
• Sites for injection include arms, abdomen, hips, and thighs

---

glimepiride
(gly-mep′er-ide)
Rx: Amaryl
Chemical Class: Sulfonylurea (2nd generation)
Therapeutic Class: Antidiabetic; hypoglycemic

CLINICAL PHARMACOLOGY
Mechanism of Action: A second-generation sulfonylurea that promotes release of insulin from beta cells of the pancreas and increases insulin sensitivity at peripheral sites. *Therapeutic Effect:* Lowers blood glucose concentration.

Pharmacokinetics

Route	Onset	Peak	Dura-tion
PO	N/A	2–3 hr	24 hr

Completely absorbed from the GI tract. Protein binding: greater than 99%. Metabolized in the liver. Excreted in urine and eliminated in feces. **Half-life:** 5–9.2 hr.

INDICATIONS AND DOSAGES
Diabetes mellitus
PO
Adults, Elderly. Initially, 1–2 mg once a day, with breakfast or first main meal. Maintenance: 1–4 mg once a day. After dose of 2 mg is reached, dosage should be increased in increments of up to 2 mg q1–2wk, based on blood glucose response. Maximum: 8 mg/day.

Dosage in renal impairment
PO
Adults. 1 mg once/day.

AVAILABLE FORMS/COST
• Tab—Oral: 1 mg, 100's: **$36.49**; 2 mg, 100's: **$59.15**; 4 mg, 100's: **$111.55**

CONTRAINDICATIONS: Diabetic complications, such as ketosis, acidosis, and diabetic coma; severe hepatic or renal impairment; monotherapy for type 1 diabetes mellitus; stress situations, including severe infection, trauma, and surgery

PREGNANCY AND LACTATION: Pregnancy category C; inappropriate for use during pregnancy due to inadequacy for blood glucose control, potential for prolonged neonatal hypoglycemia, and risk of congenital abnormalities; insulin is the drug of choice for control of blood sugars during pregnancy; breast milk secretion, unknown; the potential for neonatal hypoglycemia dictates caution in nursing mothers

SIDE EFFECTS

Frequent

Altered taste sensation, dizziness, somnolence, weight gain, constipation, diarrhea, heartburn, nausea, vomiting, stomach fullness, headache

Occasional

Increased sensitivity of skin to sunlight, peeling of skin, itching, rash

SERIOUS REACTIONS

• Overdose or insufficient food intake may produce hypoglycemia, especially with increased glucose demands.

• GI hemorrhage, cholestatic hepatic jaundice, leukopenia, thrombocytopenia, pancytopenia, agranulocytosis, and aplastic or hemolytic anemia occur rarely.

INTERACTIONS

Drugs

▣ *Anabolic steroids:* Enhanced hypoglycemic response

▣ *Angiotensin converting enzyme inhibitors:* Increased risk of hypolycemia

▣ *Antacids:* Enhanced rate of absorption

▣ *Aspirin:* Enhanced hypoglycemic effect

▣ β-*Adrenergic blockers:* Altered response to hypoglycemia; prolonged recovery of normoglycemia, hypertension, blockade of tachycardia; may increase blood glucose concentration

▣ *Clofibrate:* Enhanced effects of oral hypoglycemic drugs

▣ *Corticosteroids:* Increased blood glucose in diabetic patients

▣ *Cyclosporine:* Increased cyclosporine levels

⚠ *Ethanol:* Excessive intake may lead to altered glycemic control; "Antabuse"-like reaction may occur

▣ *Gemfibrozil:* Increased risk of hypoglycemia

▣ *H$_2$-receptor antagonists:* Enhanced rate of absorption

▣ *MAOIs:* Excessive hypoglycemia may occur in patients with diabetes

❷ *Phenylbutazole:* Increases serum concentrations of oral hypoglycemic drugs

▣ *Proton pump blockers:* Enhanced rate of absorption

▣ *Rifampin:* Reduced sulfonylurea concentrations

▣ *Sulfonamides:* Enhanced hypoglycemic effects of sulfonylureas

▣ *Thiazide diuretics:* Potential increased dosage requirement of antidiabetic drugs

SPECIAL CONSIDERATIONS

• No demonstrated advantage over existing second generation sulfonylureas

PATIENT/FAMILY EDUCATION

• Multiple drug interactions, including alcohol and salicylates

• Symptoms of hypoglycemia: tingling lips/tongue, nausea, confusion, fatigue, sweating, hunger, visual changes (spots)

MONITORING PARAMETERS

• Self-monitored blood glucoses; glycosolated hemoglobin q 3-6 mo

glipizide
(glip'i-zide)

Rx: Glucotrol, Glucotrol XL
Combinations
　Rx: with metformin (Meta-glip)
Chemical Class: Sulfonylurea
(2nd generation)
Therapeutic Class: Antidia-betic; hypoglycemic

CLINICAL PHARMACOLOGY
Mechanism of Action: A second-generation sulfonylurea that pro-motes the release of insulin from beta cells of the pancreas and in-creases insulin sensitivity at periph-eral sites. *Therapeutic Effect:* Low-ers blood glucose concentration.

Pharmacokinetics

Route	Onset	Peak	Dura-tion
PO	15–30 min	2–3 hr	12–24 hr
Ex-tended-release	2–3 hr	6–12 hr	24 hr

Well absorbed from the GI tract. Protein binding: 99%. Metabolized in the liver. Excreted in urine. **Half-life:** 2–4 hr.

INDICATIONS AND DOSAGES
Diabetes mellitus
PO
Adults. Initially, 5 mg/day or 2.5 mg in the elderly or those with hepatic disease. Adjust dosage in 2.5- to 5-mg increments at intervals of sev-eral days. Maximum single dose: 15 mg. Maximum dose/day: 40 mg. Maintenance (extended-release tab-let): 20 mg/day.
Elderly. Initially, 2.5–5 mg/day. May increase by 2.5–5 mg/day q1–2wk.

AVAILABLE FORMS/COST
• Tab-Oral: 5 mg, 100's: **$8.55-$46.58**; 10 mg, 100's: **$18.18-$85.50**
• Tab, Coated, Sus Action—Oral: 2.5 mg, 30's: **$12.20-$13.56**; 5 mg, 100's: **$40.66-$45.23**; 10 mg, 100's: **$80.53-$89.58**
• Tab, Film Coated—Oral (with metformin): 2.5 mg-250 mg, 100's: **$89.51**; 2.5 mg-500 mg, 100's: **$106.78**; 5 mg-500 mg, 100's: **$106.78**

CONTRAINDICATIONS: Diabetic ketoacidosis with or without coma, type 1 diabetes mellitus

PREGNANCY AND LACTATION: Pregnancy category C; inappropri-ate for use during pregnancy due to inadequate for blood glucose con-trol, potential for prolonged neona-tal hypoglycemia, and risk of con-genital abnormalities; insulin is the drug of choice for control of blood sugars during pregnancy; breast milk secretion unknown; the poten-tial for neonatal hypoglycemia dic-tates caution in nursing mothers

SIDE EFFECTS
Frequent
Altered taste sensation, dizziness, somnolence, weight gain, constipa-tion, diarrhea, heartburn, nausea, vomiting, stomach fullness, head-ache
Occasional
Increased sensitivity of skin to sun-light, peeling of skin, itching, rash

SERIOUS REACTIONS
• Overdose or insufficiet food intake may produce hypoglycemia, espe-cially with increased glucose de-mands.
• GI hemorrhage, cholestatic he-patic jaundice, leukopenia, thrombo-cytopenia, pancytopenia, agranu-locytosis, and aplastic or hemolytic anemia occurs rarely.

INTERACTIONS
Drugs
▣ *Anabolic steroids:* Enhanced hypoglycemic response

▣ *Angiotensin converting enzyme inhibitor:* Increased risk of hypoglycemia

▣ *Antacids:* Enhanced rate of absorption

▣ *Aspirin:* Enhanced hypoglycemic effects

▣ *β-Adrenergic blockers:* Altered response to hypoglycemia; prolonged recovery of normoglycemia, hypertension, blockade of tachycardia; may increase blood glucose concentration

▣ *Clofibrate:* Enhanced effects of oral hypoglycemic drugs

▣ *Corticosteroids:* Increased blood glucose in diabetic patients

⚠ *Ethanol:* Excessive intake may lead to altered glycemic control; Antabuse-like reaction may occur

▣ *Gemfibrozil:* Increased risk of hypoglycemia

▣ *H_2-receptor antagonists (cimetidine, ranitidine, etc.):* Enhanced rate of absorption

▣ *MAOIs:* Excessive hypoglycemia may occur in patient with diabetes

▣ *Phenylbutazone:* Increases serum concentrations of oral hypoglycemics

▣ *Rifampin:* Reduced sulfonylurea concentrations

▣ *Sulfonamides:* Enhanced hypoglycemic effects of sulfonylureas

▣ *Thiazide diuretics:* Potential increased dosage requirement of antidiabetic drugs

SPECIAL CONSIDERATIONS
PATIENT/FAMILY EDUCATION
• Administer 30 min ac

• Notify clinician of fever, sore throat, rash, unusual bruising, or bleeding

• Multiple drug interactions, including alcohol and salicylates

• Symptoms of hypoglycemia: tingling lips/tongue, nausea, confusion, fatigue, sweating, hunger, visual changes (spots)

• Notify clinician of fever, sore throat, rash, unusual bruising, or bleeding

MONITORING PARAMETERS
• Self-monitored blood glucose; glycosylated hemoglobin q 3-6 mo

---

glucagon hydrochloride
(gloo′-ka-gon)
Rx: Glucagon
Chemical Class: Polypeptide hormone
Therapeutic Class: Antihypoglycemic

CLINICAL PHARMACOLOGY
Mechanism of Action: A glucose elevating agent that promotes hepatic glycogenolysis, gluconeogenesis. Stimulates production of cyclic adenosine monophosphate (cAMP), which results in increased plasma glucose concentration, smooth muscle relaxation, and an inotropic myocardial effect. *Therapeutic Effect:* Increases plasma glucose level.

INDICATIONS AND DOSAGES
Hypoglycemia
IV, IM, Subcutaneous

Adults, Elderly, Children weighing more than 20 kg. 0.5–1 mg. May give 1 or 2 additional doses if response is delayed.

Children weighing 20 kg or less. 0.5 mg.

Diagnostic aid
IV, IM

Adults, Elderly. 0.25–2 mg 10 min prior to procedure.

AVAILABLE FORMS/COST
• Powder, Inj-IM, IV, SC: 1 mg: **$48.00**; 1 mg/vial (Glucagon emergency kit): **$71.39-$78.13**

UNLABELED USES: Treatment of esophageal obstruction due to foreign bodies, toxicity associated with beta blockers or calcium channel blockers

CONTRAINDICATIONS: Hypersensitivity to glucagon or beef or pork proteins, known pheochromocytoma

PREGNANCY AND LACTATION: Pregnancy category B; excretion into breast milk unknown; use caution in nursing mothers

SIDE EFFECTS
Occasional
Nausea, vomiting
Rare
Allergic reaction, such as urticaria, respiratory distress, and hypotension

SERIOUS REACTIONS
• Overdose may produce persistent nausea and vomiting and hypokalemia, marked by severe weakness, decreased appetite, irregular heartbeat, and muscle cramps.

INTERACTIONS
Drugs
3 *Oral anticoagulants:* Enhanced hypoprothrombinemic response to warfarin and possibly other oral anticoagulants

SPECIAL CONSIDERATIONS

PATIENT/FAMILY EDUCATION
• Notify clinician when hypoglycemic reactions occur so that antidiabetic therapy can be adjusted

MONITORING PARAMETERS
• Blood sugar, level of consciousness

---

glyburide
(glye′byoor-ide)
Rx: DiaBeta, Glynase
Prestab, Micronase
Combinations
  Rx: with metformin (Glucovance)
Chemical Class: Sulfonylurea (2nd generation)
Therapeutic Class: Antidiabetic; hypoglycemic

CLINICAL PHARMACOLOGY
Mechanism of Action: A second-generation sulfonylurea that promotes release of insulin from beta cells of the pancreas and increases insulin sensitivity at peripheral sites. *Therapeutic Effect:* Lowers blood glucose concentration.
Pharmacokinetics

Route	Onset	Peak	Duration
PO	0.25–1 hr	1–2 hr	12–24 hr

Well absorbed from the GI tract. Protein binding: 99%. Metabolized in the liver to weakly active metabolite. Primarily excreted in urine. Not removed by hemodialysis. **Half-life:** 1.4–1.8 hr.

INDICATIONS AND DOSAGES
Diabetes mellitus
PO
Adults. Initially 2.5–5 mg. May increase by 2.5 mg/day at weekly intervals. Maintenance: 1.25–20 mg/day. Maximum: 20 mg/day.
Elderly. Initially, 1.25–2.5 mg/day. May increase by 1.25–2.5 mg/day at 1- to 3-wk intervals.
PO (micronized tablets [Glynase])
Adults, Elderly. Initially 0.75–3 mg/day. May increase by 1.5 mg/day at weekly intervals. Maintenance: 0.75–12 mg/day as a single dose or in divided doses.

Dosage in renal impairment

Glyburide is not recommended in patients with creatinine clearance less than 50 ml/min.

$ **AVAILABLE FORMS/COST**

• Tab-Oral: 1.25 mg, 100's: **$9.75-$39.03**; 2.5 mg, 100's: **$17.35-$65.01**; 5 mg, 100's: **$24.77-$109.90**
• Tab, Micronized-Oral: 1.5 mg, 100's: **$37.40-$58.16**; 3 mg, 100's: **$60.20-$98.33**; 4.5 mg, 100's: **$98.50**; 6 mg, 100's: **$84.09-$155.05**
• Tab-Oral (with metformin): 2.5 mg-500 mg, 100's: **$106.78**; 5 mg-500 mg, 100's: **$106.78**

CONTRAINDICATIONS: Diabetic ketoacidosis with or without coma, monotherapy for type 1 diabetes mellitus

PREGNANCY AND LACTATION: Pregnancy category B; inappropriate for use during pregnancy due to inadequacy for blood glucose control, potential for prolonged neonatal hypoglycemia, and risk of congenital abnormalities; insulin is the drug of choice for control of blood sugars during pregnancy; breast milk secretion unknown; the potential for neonatal hypoglycemia dictates caution in nursing mothers

SIDE EFFECTS

Frequent

Altered taste sensation, dizziness, somnolence, weight gain, constipation, diarrhea, heartburn, nausea, vomiting, stomach fullness, headache

Occasional

Increased sensitivity of skin to sunlight, peeling of skin, itching, rash

SERIOUS REACTIONS

• Overdose or insufficient food intake may produce hypoglycemia, especially in patients with increased glucose demands.

• Cholestatic jaundice, leukopenia, thrombocytopenia, pancytopenia, agranulocytosis, and aplastic or hemolytic anemia occur rarely.

INTERACTIONS

Drugs

3 *Anabolic steroids:* Enhanced hypoglycemic response
3 *Angiotensin converting enzyme inhibitor:* Increased risk of hypoglycemia
3 *Antacids:* Enhanced rate of absorption
3 *Aspirin:* Enhanced hypoglycemic effects
3 *β-Adrenergic blockers:* Altered response to hypoglycemia; prolonged recovery of normoglycemia, hypertension, blockade of tachycardia; may increase blood glucose concentration
3 *Clofibrate:* Enhanced effects of oral hypoglycemic drugs
3 *Corticosteroids:* Increased blood glucose in diabetic patients
⚠ *Ethanol:* Excessive intake may lead to altered glycemic control; Antabuse-like reaction may occur
3 *Gemfibrozil:* Increased risk of hypoglycemia
3 *H$_2$-receptor antagonists (cimetidine, ranitidine, etc.):* Enhanced rate of absorption
3 *MAOIs:* Excessive hypoglycemia may occur in patient with diabetes
3 *Phenylbutazone:* Increases serum concentrations of oral hypoglycemics
3 *Rifampin:* Reduced sulfonylurea concentrations
3 *Sulfonamides:* Enhanced hypoglycemic effects of sulfonylureas
3 *Thiazide diuretics:* Potential increased dosage requirement of antidiabetic drugs

Labs

• *Protein:* False-urine increases with Ponceaus dye method

SPECIAL CONSIDERATIONS
• Micronized formulations do not provide bioequivalent serum concentrations to non-micronized formulations; retitrate patients when transferring from any hypoglycemic to micronized glyburide

PATIENT/FAMILY EDUCATION
• Multiple drug interactions including alcohol and salicylates
• Notify clinician of fever, sore throat, rash, unusual bruising, or bleeding

MONITORING PARAMETERS
• Self-monitored blood glucose; glycosylated Hgb q3-6 mo

---

glycerin
(gli'ser-in)
OTC: *Laxative:* Fleets Babylax, Glycerol, Sani-Supp
Rx: *Ophth:* Ophthalgan
Rx: *Oral:* Osmoglyn
Chemical Class: Trihydric alcohol
Therapeutic Class: Antiglaucoma agent; diuretic, osmotic; laxative

---

CLINICAL PHARMACOLOGY
Mechanism of Action: A osmotic dehydrating agent that increases osmotic pressure and draws fluid into colon and stimulates evaulcation of inspissated feces. Lowers both intraocular and intracranial pressure by osmotic dehydrating effects. Increases blood flow to ischemic areas, decreases serum free fatty acids, and increases synthesis of glycerides in the brain. *Therapeutic Effect:* Aids in fecal evacuation.

Pharmacokinetics
Well absorbed after PO administration but poorly absorbed after rectal administration. Widely distributed to extracellular space. Rapidly me-

tabolized in liver. Primarily excreted in urine. **Half-life:** 30- 45 min.

INDICATIONS AND DOSAGES
Constipation
Rectal
Adults, Elderly, Children 6 yrs and older. 3 g/day.
Children younger than 6 yrs. 1-1.5 g/day.
Ophthalmologic procedures
Ophthalmic
Adults, Elderly Children. 1 or 2 drops prior to examination q3-4h.
Reduction of intracranial pressure
PO
Adults, Elderly, Children. 1.5 g/kg/day q4h or 1 g/kg/dose q6h.
Reduction of intraocular pressure
PO
Adults, Elderly, Children. 1-1.8 g/kg 1-1.5 hrs preoperatively.

S AVAILABLE FORMS/COST
• Sol—Oral: 50%, 220 ml: **$2.69**
• Supp—Rect: Adult 12's: **$0.75-$4.82**; Pediatric 12's: **$0.78-$4.82**

UNLABELED USES: Viral meningoencephalitis

CONTRAINDICATIONS: Hypersensitivity to any component in the preparation, well-established anuria, severe dehydration, frank or impending acute pulmonary edema, severe cardiac decompensation

PREGNANCY AND LACTATION: Pregnancy category C; data regarding use in breast-feeding are unavailable

SIDE EFFECTS
Frequent
Oral: Nausea, headache, vomiting
Rectal: Some degree of abdominal discomfort, nausea, mild cramps, headache, vomiting
Occasional
Oral: Diarrhea, dizziness, dry mouth or increased thirst

Ophthalmic: pain and irritation may occur upon instillation

Rectal: faintness, weakness, abdominal pain, bloating

SERIOUS REACTIONS

• Laxative abuse includes symptoms of abdominal pain, weakness, fatigue, thirst, vomiting, edema, bone pain, fluid and electrolyte imbalance, hypoalbuminemia, and syndromes that mimic colitis.

INTERACTIONS

Labs

• *Increase:* Amniotic fluid phosphatidylglycerol, serum triglycerides

• *Decrease:* Serum ionized calcium

SPECIAL CONSIDERATIONS

PATIENT/FAMILY EDUCATION

• Do not use laxative in the presence of abdominal pain, nausea, or vomiting

• Do not use longer than 1 wk

• Prolonged or frequent use may result in dependency or electrolyte imbalance

• Notify clinician if unrelieved constipation, rectal bleeding, muscle cramps, weakness, or dizziness occurs

MONITORING PARAMETERS

• Blood glucose, intraocular pressure

---

glycopyrrolate

(glye-koe-pye′roe-late)

Rx: Robinul, Robinul Forte

Chemical Class: Quaternary ammonium derivative

Therapeutic Class: Anticholinergic; antiulcer agent (adjunct); gastrointestinal

---

CLINICAL PHARMACOLOGY

Mechanism of Action: A quaternary anticholinergic that inhibits action of acetylcholine at postgangli-onic parasympathetic sites in smooth muscle, secretory glands, and CNS. *Therapeutic Effect:* Reduces salivation and excessive secretions of respiratory tract; reduces gastric secretions and acidity.

INDICATIONS AND DOSAGES

Preoperative inhibition of salivation and excessive respiratory tract secretions

IM

Adults, Elderly. 4.4 mcg/kg 30–60 min before procedure.

Children 2 yr and older. 4.4 mcg/kg.

Children younger than 2 yr. 4.4–8.8 mcg/kg.

To block effects of anticholinesterase agents

IV

Adults, Elderly. 0.2 mg for each 1 mg neostigmine or 5 mg pyridostigmine.

$ **AVAILABLE FORMS/COST**

• Sol, Inj-IM, IV: 0.2 mg/ml, 1, 2, 5, 20 ml: **$1.07-$1.44**/2 ml

• Tab-Oral: 1 mg, 100's: **$75.91**; 2 mg, 100's: **$127.17**

CONTRAINDICATIONS: Acute hemorrhage, myasthenia gravis, narrow-angle glaucoma, obstructive uropathy, paralytic ileus, tachycardia, ulcerative colitis

PREGNANCY AND LACTATION: Pregnancy category B; has been used prior to cesarean section to decrease gastric secretions; quaternary structure results in limited placental transfer; excretion into breast milk is unknown, but should be minimal due to quaternary structure

SIDE EFFECTS

Frequent

Dry mouth, decreased sweating, constipation

Occasional

Blurred vision, gastric bloating, urinary hesitancy, somnolence (with high dosage), headache, intolerance to light, loss of taste, nervousness, flushing, insomnia, impotence, mental confusion or excitement (particularly in the elderly and children), temporary light-headedness (with parenteral form), local irritation (with parenteral form)

Rare

Dizziness, faintness

SERIOUS REACTIONS

• Overdose may produce temporary paralysis of ciliary muscle; pupillary dilation; tachycardia; palpitations; hot, dry, or flushed skin; absence of bowel sounds; hyperthermia; increased respiratory rate; EKG abnormalities; nausea; vomiting; rash over face or upper trunk; CNS stimulation; and psychosis (marked by agitation, restlessness, rambling speech, visual hallucinations, paranoid behavior, and delusions, followed by depression).

---

gonadorelin hydrochloride

(goe-nad-oh-rell'in)

Rx: Factrel

Chemical Class: Gonadotropin-releasing hormone, synthetic
Therapeutic Class: Diagnostic agent; ovulation stimulant

CLINICAL PHARMACOLOGY

Mechanism of Action: A synthetic luteinzing hormone that binds to specific transmembrane glycoprotein receptors on gonadotrophic cells of the anterior pituitary which then stimulates synthesis and secretion of gonadotropins through mobilization of intracellular calcium, activation of protein kinase C, and gene transcription. *Therapeutic Effect:* Stimulates synthesis, release of luteinizing hormone (LH), follicle-stimulating hormone (FSH) from anterior pituitary. Stimulates release of gonadotropin-releasing hormone from hypothalamus.

Pharmacokinetics

Maximal LH release occurs within 20 minutes. Metabolized in plasma. Excreted in urine as inactive metabolites. **Half-life:** 4 minutes.

INDICATIONS AND DOSAGES

Gonadotropin function evaluation

IV/Subcutaneous

Adults. 100 mcg. In females, perform test in early follicular phase of menstrual cycle.

S **AVAILABLE FORMS/COST**

• Sol, Inj-IV, SC: 100 mcg/vial: **$212.61**

UNLABELED USES: Hypothalmic anovulation, hypogonadotropic hypogonadism

CONTRAINDICATIONS: Any condition exacerbated by pregnancy, patients with ovarian cysts or causes of anovulation other than hypothalamic origin, the presence of a hormonally-dependent tumor, any conditions worsened by an increase of reproductive hormones, hypersensitivity to gonadorelin acetate or hydrochloride

PREGNANCY AND LACTATION: Pregnancy category B; possibility of fetal harm appears remote if used during pregnancy

SIDE EFFECTS

Occasional

Swelling, pain, or itching at injection site with subcutaneous administration, local or generalized skin rash with chronic subcutaneous administration

Rare

Headache, nausea, lightheadedness, abdominal discomfort, hypersensitivity reactions (bronchospasm, tachycardia, flushing, urticaria), induration at injection site

SERIOUS REACTIONS

• Anaphylactic reaction occurs rarely.

INTERACTIONS

Drugs

3 *Androgen, Estrogen, Glucocorticoid, Progestin-containing preparations:* May reduce LH release from anterior pituitary

Labs

• Do not conduct diagnostic tests during administration of these agents

---

goserelin

(go'seh-rel-in)

Rx: Zoladex

Chemical Class: Gonadotropin-releasing hormone analog

Therapeutic Class: Antiendometriosis agent; antineoplastic

CLINICAL PHARMACOLOGY

Mechanism of Action: A gonadotropin-releasing hormone analogue and antineoplastic agent that stimulates the release of luteinizing hormone (LH) and follicle-stimulating hormone (FSH) from the anterior pituitary gland. In males, increases testosterone concentrations initially, then suppresses secretion of LH and FSH, resuting in decreased testosterone levels. *Therapeutic Effect:* In females, causes a reduction in ovarian size and function, reduction in uterine and mammary gland size, and regression of sex-hormone-responsive tumors. In males, produces pharmacologic castration and decreases the growth of abnormal prostate tissue.

INDICATIONS AND DOSAGES

Prostatic carcinoma

Implant

Adults older than 18 yr, Elderly. 3.6 mg every 28 days or 10.8 mg q12wk subcutaneously into upper abdominal wall.

Breast carcinoma, endometriosis

Implant

Adults. 3.6 mg every 28 days subcutaneously into upper abdominal wall.

Endometrial thinning

Implant

Adults. 3.6 mg subcutaneously into upper abdominal wall as a single dose or in 2 doses 4 wk apart.

§ **AVAILABLE FORMS/COST**

• Implant, Cont Rel—SC: 3.6 mg: **$469.99**; 10.8 mg: **$1,409.98**

CONTRAINDICATIONS: Pregnancy

PREGNANCY AND LACTATION: Pregnancy category X; excretion into breast milk unknown; use caution in nursing mothers

SIDE EFFECTS

Frequent

Headache (60%), hot flashes (55%), depression (54%), diaphoresis (45%), sexual dysfunction (21%), decreased erection (18%), lower urinary tract symptoms (13%)

Occasional (10%-5%)

Pain, lethargy, dizziness, insomnia, anorexia, nausea, rash, upper respiratory tract infection, hirsutism, abdominal pain

Rare

Pruritus

SERIOUS REACTIONS

• Arrhythmias, CHF, and hypertension occur rarely.

• Ureteral obstruction and spinal cord compression have been observed. An immediate orchiectomy may be necessary if these conditions occur.

INTERACTIONS

• *Increase:* Alk phosphatase, estradiol, FSH, LH, testosterone levels (first week)

• *Decrease:* Testosterone levels (after first week), progesterone

SPECIAL CONSIDERATIONS

PATIENT/FAMILY EDUCATION

• Notify clinician if regular menstruation persists (females)

• An initial flare in bone pain may occur (prostate cancer therapy)

MONITORING PARAMETERS

• Prostate-specific antigen, acid phosphatase, alk phosphatase

• Testosterone level (<25 ng/dl)

• Bone density if therapy prolonged

---

granisetron
(gra-ni′se-tron)

Rx: Kytril

Chemical Class: Carbazole derivative

Therapeutic Class: Antiemetic

CLINICAL PHARMACOLOGY

Mechanism of Action: A 5-HT$_3$ receptor antagonist that acts centrally in the chemoreceptor trigger zone or peripherally at the vagal nerve terminals. *Therapeutic Effect:* Prevents nausea and vomiting.

Pharmacokinetics

Route	Onset	Peak	Dura-tion
IV	1–3 min	N/A	24 hr

Rapidly and widely distributed to tissues. Protein binding: 65%. Metabolized in the liver to active metabolite. Eliminated in urine and feces. **Half-life:** 10–12 hr (increased in the elderly).

INDICATIONS AND DOSAGES

Prevention of chemotherapy-induced nausea and vomiting

PO

Adults, Elderly. 1 mg once a day up to 1 hr before chemotherapy or 1 mg twice a day.

IV

Adults, Elderly, Children 2 yr and older. 10 mcg/kg/dose (or 1 mg/dose) within 30 min of chemotherapy.

Prevention of radiation-induced nausea and vomiting

PO

Adults, Elderly. 2 mg once a day given 1 hr before radiation therapy.

Postoperative nausea or vomiting

PO

Adults, Elderly, Children 4 yr and older. 20-40 mcg/kg as a single postoperative dose.

IV

Adults, Elderly. 1 mg as a single postoperative dose.

Children older than 4 yr. 20-40 mcg/kg. Maximum: 1 mg.

Ⓢ AVAILABLE FORMS/COST

• Sol, Inj-IV: 1 mg/ml, 1, 4 ml: **$195.20**/1 ml

• Sol—Oral: 2 mg/10 ml, 30 ml: **$282.30**

• Tab-Oral: 1 mg, 2's: **$94.10**

UNLABELED USES: PO: Prophylaxis of nausea or vomiting associated with radiation therapy

CONTRAINDICATIONS: None known.

PREGNANCY AND LACTATION: Pregnancy category B; breast milk excretion unknown

SIDE EFFECTS

Frequent (21%-14%)

Headache, constipation, asthenia

Occasional (8%-6%)

Diarrhea, abdominal pain

Rare (less than 2%)

Altered taste, hypersensitivity reaction

SERIOUS REACTIONS

• None known.

griseofulvin

Rx: Fulvicin P/G, Fulvicin-U/F, Grifulvin V, Grisactin, Grisactin 500, Grisactin-Ultra, Gris-PEG

Chemical Class: Penicillium griseofulvum derivative

Therapeutic Class: Antifungal

CLINICAL PHARMACOLOGY

Mechanism of Action: An antifungal that inhibits fungal cell mitosis by disrupting mitotic spindle structure. *Therapeutic Effect:* Fungistatic.

INDICATIONS AND DOSAGES

Tinea capitis, tinea corporis, tinea cruris, tinea pedis, tinea unguium

Microsize Tablets, Oral Suspension

Adults. Usual dosage, 500-1,000 mg as a single dose or in divided doses.

Children 2 yr and older. Usual dosage, 10-20 mg/kg/day.

Ultramicrosize Tablets

Adults. Usual dosage, 330-750 mg/day as a single dose or in divided doses.

Children 2 yr and older. 5-10 mg/kg/day.

[$] **AVAILABLE FORMS/COST**

Microsize

• Cap, Gel—Oral: 250 mg, 100's: **$87.68**

• Susp—Oral: 125 mg/5 ml, 120 ml: **$41.20**

• Tab-Oral: 250 mg, 60's: **$60.40**; 500 mg, 60's: **$103.50**

Ultramicrosize

• Tab-Oral: 125 mg, 100's: **$33.11-$69.00**; 165 mg, 100's: **$47.65-$85.19**; 250 mg, 100's: **$64.96-$138.00**; 330 mg, 100's: **$82.25-$151.42**

CONTRAINDICATIONS: Hepatocellular failure, porphyria

PREGNANCY AND LACTATION: Pregnancy category C; since the use of an antifungal is seldom essential during pregnancy, avoid use during this time; excretion into breast milk unknown; use caution in nursing mothers

SIDE EFFECTS

Occasional

Hypersensitivity reaction (including pruritus, rash, and urticaria), headache, nausea, diarrhea, excessive thirst, flatulence, oral thrush, dizziness, insomnia

Rare

Paresthesia of hands or feet, proteinuria, photosensitivity reaction

SERIOUS REACTIONS

• Granulocytopenia occurs rarely.

INTERACTIONS

Drugs

[3] *Aspirin:* Reduces plasma salicylate level

[3] *Cyclosporine:* Reduces plasma cyclosporine level

[3] *Oral contraceptives:* Menstrual irregularities, increased risk of pregnancy possible

[3] *Phenobarbital:* Reduces plasma griseofulvin level

[3] *Tacrolimus:* Reduces plasma tacrolimus level

[3] *Warfarin:* Reduces anticoagulant response

SPECIAL CONSIDERATIONS

• Prior to therapy, the type of fungus responsible for the infection should be identified

PATIENT/FAMILY EDUCATION

• Response to therapy may not be apparent for some time; complete entire course of therapy

• Avoid prolonged exposure to sunlight or sunlamps

• Notify clinician if sore throat or skin rash occurs

• Store oral suspensions at room temp in light-resistant container

MONITORING PARAMETERS

• Periodic assessments of renal, hepatic, and hematopoietic function during prolonged therapy

guaifenesin

(gwye-fen'e-sin)

Rx: Allfen, Amibid LA, Aquamist, Bidex, Duratuss G, Fenesin, GG-200 NR, Ganidin NR, Gua-SR, Guaibid-LA, Guaifenesin Expectorant, Guaifenesin LA, Guaifenesin-SR, Guaifenex G, Guaifenex LA, Humavent LA, Humibid LA, Humibid Pediatric, Iofen-NR, Iophen-NR, Liquibid, Monafed, Muco-Fen 800, Muco-Fen 1200, Muco-Fen LA, Orgadin, Organ-1 NEF, Organidin NR, Pneumomist, Q-Bid LA, Respa-GF, Simumist-SR, Touro EX

OTC: Anti-Tuss, Breonesin, Genatuss, Glytuss, Guiatuss, Hytuss, Hytuss 2X, Mytussin, Naldecon Senior EX, Robitussin

Combinations

Rx: with codeine (Guiatussin AC); with dextromethorphan (Guaibid-DM); with hydrocodone (Hycotuss); with phenylpropanolamine (Entex LA)

Chemical Class: Glyceryl derivative

Therapeutic Class: Expectorant; mucolytic

CLINICAL PHARMACOLOGY

Mechanism of Action: An expectorant that stimulates respiratory tract secretions by decreasing adhesiveness and viscosity of phlegm. *Therapeutic Effect:* Promotes removal of viscous mucus.

Pharmacokinetics

Well absorbed from the GI tract. Metabolized in the liver. Excreted in urine.

INDICATIONS AND DOSAGES

Expectorant

PO

Adults, Elderly, Children older than 12 yr. 200–400 mg q4h.

Children 6–12 yr. 100–200 mg q4h. Maximum: 1.2 g/day.

Children 2–5 yr. 50–100 mg q4h.

Children younger than 2 yr. 12 mg/kg/day in 6 divided doses.

PO (Extended-Release)

Adults, Elderly, Children older than 12 yr. 600-1200 mg q12h. Maximum: 2.4 g/day.

Children 2-5 yr. 600 mg q12h. Maximum: 600 mg/day.

[$] **AVAILABLE FORMS/COST**

• Cap—Oral: 200 mg, 100's: **$14.91-$18.79**

• Cap, Sus Action—Oral: 300 mg, 100's: **$55.73**

• Liq—Oral: 100 mg/5 ml, 120, 240, 480 ml: **$3.26-$149.08**; 200 mg/5 ml, 118 ml: **$5.72**

• Tab—Oral: 100 mg, 100's: **$9.21**; 200 mg, 100's: **$7.07-$56.98**

• Tab, Sus Action—Oral: 575 mg, 100's: **$49.98**; 600 mg 100's: **$4.54-$49.00**; 800 mg, 100's: **$26.29-$35.38**; 1000 mg, 100's: **$29.99-$80.74**; 1200 mg, 100's: **$33.75-$73.70**

CONTRAINDICATIONS: None known.

PREGNANCY AND LACTATION: Pregnancy category C; excretion into breast milk unknown

SIDE EFFECTS

Rare

Dizziness, headache, rash, diarrhea, nausea, vomiting, abdominal pain

G

SERIOUS REACTIONS
• Overdose may produce nausea and vomiting.

INTERACTIONS
Labs
• *Interference:* Urine 5-HIAA, VMA

SPECIAL CONSIDERATIONS

PATIENT/FAMILY EDUCATION
• Drink a full glass of water with each dose to help further loosen mucus
• Notify clinician if cough persists after medication has been used for 7 days or cough is associated with headache, high fever, skin rash, or sore throat

---

guanabenz
(gwan'a-benz)
Rx: Wytensin
Chemical Class: Dichlorobenzene derivative
Therapeutic Class: Antihypertensive; centrally acting sympathoplegic

---

CLINICAL PHARMACOLOGY
Mechanism of Action: An alpha-adrenergic agonist that stimulates alpha2-adrenergic receptors. Inhibits sympathetic cardioaccelerator and vasoconstrictor center to heart, kidneys, peripheral vasculature. *Therapeutic Effect:* Decreases systolic, diastolic blood pressure (BP). Chronic use decreases peripheral vascular resistance.

Pharmacokinetics
Well absorbed from gastrointestinal (GI) tract. Widely distributed. Protein binding: 90%. Metabolized in liver. Excreted in urine and feces. Not removed by hemodialysis. **Half-life:** 6 hrs.

INDICATIONS AND DOSAGES
Hypertension
PO
Adults. Initially, 4 mg 2 times/day. Increase by 4-8 mg at 1-2 wk intervals. Elderly. Initially, 4 mg/day. May increase q1-2 wks. Maintenance: 8-16 mg/day. Maximum: 32 mg/day.

Ⓢ **AVAILABLE FORMS/COST**
• Tab-Oral: 4 mg, 100's: **$66.20-$97.99**; 8 mg, 100's: **$99.40-$190.57**

CONTRAINDICATIONS: History of hypersensitivity to guanabenz or any component of the formulation

PREGNANCY AND LACTATION: Pregnancy category C; excretion into breast milk unknown; use caution in nursing mothers

SIDE EFFECTS
Frequent
Drowsiness, dry mouth, dizziness
Occasional
Weakness, headache, nausea, decreased sexual ability
Rare
Ataxia, sleep disturbances, rash, itching, diarrhea, constipation, altered taste, muscle aches

SERIOUS REACTIONS
• Abrupt withdrawal may result in rebound hypertension manifested as nervousness, agitation, anxiety, insomnia, hand tingling, tremor, flushing, and sweating.
• Overdosage produces hypotension, somnolence, lethargy, irritability, bradycardia, and miosis (pupillary constriction).

INTERACTIONS
Drugs
Ⓑ *β-blockers:* Rebound hypertension from guanabenz withdrawal exacerbated by noncardioselective β-blockers
Ⓑ *Tricyclic antidepressants:* Inhibit the antihypertensive response

SPECIAL CONSIDERATIONS
PATIENT/FAMILY EDUCATION
• Avoid hazardous activities, since drug may cause drowsiness
• Do not discontinue drug abruptly, or withdrawal symptoms may occur (anxiety, increased BP, headache, insomnia, increased pulse, tremors, nausea, sweating)
• Do not use OTC (cough, cold, or allergy) products unless directed by clinician
• Rise slowly to sitting or standing position to minimize orthostatic hypotension, especially elderly
• May cause dizziness, fainting, lightheadedness during first few days of therapy
• May cause dry mouth; use hard candy, saliva product, or frequent rinsing of mouth

MONITORING PARAMETERS
• Blood pressure (posturally), mental depression

---

guanfacine
(gwan'fa-seen)
Rx: Tenex
Chemical Class: Phenylacyl guanidine
Therapeutic Class: Antihypertensive, centrally acting sympathoplegic

---

CLINICAL PHARMACOLOGY
Mechanism of Action: An alpha-adrenergic agonist that stimulates alpha2-adrenergic receptors and inhibits sympathetic cardioaccelerator and vasoconstrictor center to heart, kidneys, peripheral vasculature. *Therapeutic Effect:* Decreases systolic, diastolic blood pressure (BP). Chronic use decreases peripheral vascular resistance.

Pharmacokinetics
Well absorbed from gastrointestinal (GI) tract. Widely distributed. Protein binding: 71%. Metabolized in liver. Excreted in urine and feces. Not removed by hemodialysis. **Half-life:** 17 hrs.

INDICATIONS AND DOSAGES
Hypertension
PO
Adults, Elderly. Initially, 1 mg/day. Increase by 1 mg/day at intervals of 3-4 wks up to 3 mg/day in single or divided doses.

$ AVAILABLE FORMS/COST
• Tab-Oral: 1 mg, 100's: **$12.33-$87.20**; 2 mg, 100's: **$96.75-$138.25**

UNLABELED USES: Attention deficit hyperactivity disorder (ADHD), tic disorders

CONTRAINDICATIONS: History of hypersensitivity to guanfacine or any component of the formulation

PREGNANCY AND LACTATION: Pregnancy category B; excretion into human breast milk unknown

SIDE EFFECTS
Frequent
Dry mouth, somnolence
Occasional
Fatigue, headache, asthenia (loss of strength, energy), dizziness

SERIOUS REACTIONS
• Overdosage may produce difficult breathing, dizziness, faintness, severe drowsiness, bradycardia.

INTERACTIONS
Drugs
▨ *β-blockers:* Rebound hypertension from guanfacine withdrawal exacerbated by noncardioselective β-blockers
▨ *Cyclosporine, tacrolimus:* Increased immunosuppressant plasma levels
▨ *Insulin, sulfonylureas hypoglycemics:* Diminished symptoms of hypoglycemia

3 *Neuroleptics, nitroprusside:* Severe hypotension possible

3 *Tricyclic antidepressants:* Inhibit the antihypertensive response

SPECIAL CONSIDERATIONS
PATIENT/FAMILY EDUCATION
• Avoid hazardous activities, since drug may cause drowsiness
• Do not discontinue oral drug abruptly, or withdrawal symptoms may occur after 3-4 days (anxiety, increased BP, headache, insomnia, increased pulse, tremors, nausea, sweating)
• Do not use OTC (cough, cold, or allergy) products unless directed by clinician
• Rise slowly to sitting or standing position to minimize orthostatic hypotension, especially elderly
• Dizziness, fainting, lightheadedness may occur during 1st few days of therapy
• May cause dry mouth; use hard candy, saliva product, or frequent rinsing of mouth

MONITORING PARAMETERS
• Blood pressure (posturally), blood glucose in patients with diabetes mellitus; confusion, mental depression

---

halcinonide
(hal-sin'o-nide)
Rx: Halog, Halog-E
Chemical Class: Corticosteroid, synthetic
Therapeutic Class: Corticosteroid, topical

CLINICAL PHARMACOLOGY
Mechanism of Action: A topical corticosteroid that has anti-inflammatory, antipruritic, and vasoconstrictive properties. The exact mechanism of the anti-inflammatory process is unclear. *Therapeutic Effect:* Reduces or prevents tissue response to the inflammatory process.

Pharmacokinetics
Well absorbed systemically. Large variation in absorption among sites. Protein binding: varies. Metabolized in liver. Primarily excreted in urine.

INDICATIONS AND DOSAGES
Dermatoses
Topical
Adults, Elderly. Apply sparingly 1-3 times/day.

$ AVAILABLE FORMS/COST
• Cre—Top: 0.1%, 15, 30, 60, 240 g: **$38.60**/30 g
• Oint—Top: 0.1%, 15, 30, 60, 240 g: **$38.60**/30 g
• Sol—Top: 0.1%, 20, 60 ml: **$28.44**/20 ml

CONTRAINDICATIONS: History of hypersensitivity to halcinonide or other corticosteroids

PREGNANCY AND LACTATION: Pregnancy category C; unknown whether top application could result in sufficient systemic absorption to produce detectable amounts in breast milk (systemic corticosteroids are secreted into breast milk in quantities not likely to have detrimental effects on infant)

SIDE EFFECTS
Occasional
Itching, redness, irritation, burning at site of application, dryness, folliculitis, acneiform eruptions, hypopigmentation
Rare
Allergic contact dermatitis, maceration of the skin, secondary infection, skin atrophy

SERIOUS REACTIONS
• The serious reactions of long-term therapy and the addition of occlusive dressings are reversible hypothalamic-pituitary-adrenal (HPA)

axis suppression, manifestations of Cushing's syndrome, hyperglycemia, and glucosuria.

SPECIAL CONSIDERATIONS
PATIENT/FAMILY EDUCATION
• Apply sparingly only to affected area
• Avoid contact with the eyes
• Do not put bandages or dressings over treated area unless directed by clinician
• Do not use on weeping, denuded, or infected areas
• Discontinue drug, notify clinician if local irritation or fever develops

---

halobetasol
(hal-oh-be′ta-sol)
Rx: Ultravate
Chemical Class: Corticosteroid, synthetic
Therapeutic Class: Corticosteroid, topical

CLINICAL PHARMACOLOGY
Mechanism of Action: A corticosteroid that inhibits accumulation of inflammatory cells at inflammation sites, phagocytosis, lysosomal enzyme release and synthesis or release of mediators of inflammation. *Therapeutic Effect:* Decreases or prevents tissue response to inflammatory process.

Pharmacokinetics
Variation in absorption among individuals and sites: scrotum 36%, forehead 7%, scalp 4%, forearm 1%.

INDICATIONS AND DOSAGES
Dermatoses, corticosteroid-unresponsive
Topical
Adults, Elderly, Children more than 12 yrs and older. Apply 1-2 times/day. Maximum: 50 g for 2 weeks.

AVAILABLE FORMS/COST
• Cre—Top: 0.05%, 15, 50 g: **$33.50**/15 g
• Oint—Top: 0.05%, 15, 50 g: **$33.50**/15 g

CONTRAINDICATIONS: Hypersensitivity to halobetasol or other corticosteroids.

PREGNANCY AND LACTATION: Pregnancy category C; unknown whether top application could result in sufficient systemic absorption to produce detectable amounts in breast milk (systemic corticosteroids are secreted into breast milk in quantities not likely to have detrimental effects on infant)

SIDE EFFECTS
Frequent
Burning, stinging, pruritus
Rare
Cushing's syndrome, hyperglycemia, glucosuria, hypothalamic-pituitary-adrenal axis suppression

SERIOUS REACTIONS
• Overdosage can occur from topically applied halobetasol absorbed in sufficient amounts to produce systemic effects producing reversible adrenal suppression, manifestations of Cushing's syndrome, hyperglycemia, and glucosuria in some patients.

SPECIAL CONSIDERATIONS
PATIENT/FAMILY EDUCATION
• Apply sparingly only to affected area
• Avoid contact with the eyes
• Do not put bandages or dressings over treated area
• Do not use on weeping, denuded, or infected areas
• Discontinue drug, notify clinician if local irritation or fever develops
• Treatment should be limited to 2 wk, and amounts greater than 50 g/wk should not be used

haloperidol
(ha-loe-per'idole)
Rx: Haldol
Chemical Class: Butyrophenone derivative
Therapeutic Class: Antipsychotic

CLINICAL PHARMACOLOGY
Mechanism of Action: An antipsychotic, antiemetic, and antidyskinetic agent that competitively blocks postsynaptic dopamine receptors, interrupts nerve impulse movement, and increases turnover of dopamine in the brain. Has strong extrapyramidal and antiemetic effects; weak anticholinergic and sedative effects. *Therapeutic Effect:* Produces tranquilizing effect.

Pharmacokinetics
Readily absorbed from the GI tract. Protein binding: 92%. Extensively metabolized in the liver. Primarily excreted in urine. Not removed by hemodialysis. **Half-life:** 12-37 hr PO; 10-19 hr IV; 17-25 hr IM.

INDICATIONS AND DOSAGES
Treatment of psychotic disorders
PO
Adults, Children 12 yr and older. Initially, 0.5-5 mg 2-3 times/day. Dosage gradually adjusted as needed.
Elderly. 0.5-2 mg 2-3 times/day. Dosage gradually adjusted as needed.
Children 3-12 yr or weighing 15-40 kg. Initially, 0.05 mg/kg/day in 2-3 divided doses. May increase by 0.5 mg increments at 5-7 day intervals. Maximum: 0.15 mg/kg/day in divided doses.
IM
Adults, Elderly, Children 12 yr and older. Initially, 2-5. May repeat at 1 hour intervals as needed. Maximum: 100 mg/day.
IM (Decanoate)
Adults, Elderly, Children 12 yr and older. Initially, 10-15 times previous daily oral dose up to maximum initial dose of 100 mg. Maximum: 300 mg/month.

Treatment of non-psychotic disorders, Tourette's syndrome
PO
Children 3-12 yr or weighing 15-40 kg. Initially, 0.05 mg/kg/day in 2-3 divided doses. May increase by 0.5 mg at 5-7 day intervals. Maximum: 0.075 mg/kg/day.

Ⓢ **AVAILABLE FORMS/COST**
• Conc-Oral (lactate): 2 mg/ml, 15, 120 ml: **$13.69-$54.32**/120 ml
• Sol, Inj-IM (lactate): 5 mg/ml, 1, 10 ml: **$1.78-$10.48**/1 ml
• Sol, Inj-IM (decanoate): 50 mg/ml, 1, 5 ml: **$14.40-$44.20**; 100 mg/ml, 1, 5 ml: **$30.00-$57.60**/1 ml
• Tab-Oral: 0.5 mg, 100's: **$4.09-$24.80**; 1 mg, 100's: **$6.18-$61.04**; 2 mg, 100's: **$10.95-$48.15**; 5 mg, 100's: **$6.68-$137.60**; 10 mg, 100's: **$11.18-$131.00**; 20 mg, 100's: **$63.52-$251.78**

UNLABELED USES: Treatment of Huntington's chorea, infantile autism, nausea or vomiting associated with cancer chemotherapy

CONTRAINDICATIONS: Angle-closure glaucoma, CNS depression, myelosuppression, Parkinson's disease, severe cardiac or hepatic disease

PREGNANCY AND LACTATION: Pregnancy category C; has been used for hyperemesis gravidarum, chorea gravidarum, and manic-depressive illness during pregnancy; excreted into breast milk; effect on nursing infant unknown, but may be of concern

SIDE EFFECTS
Frequent

Blurred vision, constipation, orthostatic hypotension, dry mouth, swelling or soreness of female breasts, peripheral edema

Occasional

Allergic reaction, difficulty urinating, decreased thirst, dizziness, decreased sexual function, drowsiness, nausea, vomiting, photosensitivity, lethargy

SERIOUS REACTIONS

• Extrapyramidal symptoms appear to be dose-related and typically occur in the first few days of therapy. Marked drowsiness and lethargy, excessive salivation, and fixed stare occur frequently. Less common reactions include severe akathisia (motor restlessness) and acute dystonias (such as torticollis, opisthotonos, and oculogyric crisis).

• Tardive dyskinesia (tongue protrusion, puffing of the cheeks, chewing or puckering of the mouth) may occur during long-term therapy or after discontinuing the drug and may be irreversible. Elderly female patients have a greater risk of developing this reaction.

INTERACTIONS
Drugs

▨ *Anticholinergics:* Inhibition of therapeutic effect of neuroleptics

▨ *Barbiturates:* Potential reduction of serum neuroleptic concentrations

▨ *Bromocriptine:* Inhibition of bromocriptine's ability to lower serum prolactin concentrations in patients with pituitary adenoma; theoretical inhibition of antipsychotic effects of neuroleptics

▨ *Carbamazepine:* Decreased serum haloperidol concentrations

▨ *Guanethidine:* Inhibition of antihypertensive effect of guanethidine

❷ *Levodopa:* Inhibition of antiparkinsonian effects of levodopa

▨ *Lithium:* Rare reports of severe neurotoxicity in patients receiving lithium and neuroleptics

▨ *Quinidine:* Increases haldol concentrations; increased risk of toxicity

SPECIAL CONSIDERATIONS
PATIENT/FAMILY EDUCATION

• Do not mix liquid formulation with coffee or tea
• Use calibrated dropper
• Take with food or milk
• Arise slowly from reclining position
• Do not discontinue abruptly
• Use a sunscreen during sun exposure to prevent burns
• Take special precautions to stay cool in hot weather

MONITORING PARAMETERS

• Observe closely for signs of tardive dyskinesia

---

heparin
(hep'a-rin)

Rx: Heparin
Chemical Class: Glycosaminoglycan, sulfated
Therapeutic Class: Anticoagulant

CLINICAL PHARMACOLOGY
Mechanism of Action: A blood modifier that interferes with blood coagulation by blocking conversion of prothrombin to thrombin and fibrinogen to fibrin. *Therapeutic Effect:* Prevents further extension of existing thrombi or new clot formation. Has no effect on existing clots.

Pharmacokinetics

Well absorbed following subcutaneous administration. Protein binding: Very high. Metabolized in the liver. Removed from the circulation via uptake by the reticuloendothelial system. Primarily excreted in urine. Not removed by hemodialysis. **Half-life:** 1–6 hr.

INDICATIONS AND DOSAGES

Line flushing

IV

Adults, Elderly, Children. 100 units q6–8h.

Infants weighing less than 10 kg. 10 units q6–8h.

Treatment of venous thrombosis, pulmonary embolism, peripheral arterial embolism, atrial fibrillation with embolism

Intermittent IV

Adults, Elderly. Initially, 10,000 units, then 50–70 units/kg (5,000–10,000 units) q4–6h.

Children 1 yr and older. Initially, 50–100 units/kg, then 50–100 units q4h.

IV infusion

Adults, Elderly. Loading dose: 80 units/kg, then 18 units/kg/hr, with adjustments based on aPTT. Range: 10–30 units/kg/hr.

Children 1 yr and older. Loading dose: 75 units/kg, then 20 units/kg/hr with adjustments based on aPTT.

Children younger than 1 yr. Loading dose: 75 units/kg, then 28 units/kg/hr.

Prevention of venous thrombosis, pulmonary embolism, peripheral arterial embolism, atrial fibrillation with embolism

Subcutaneous

Adult, Elderly. 5,000 units q8–12h.

[$] **AVAILABLE FORMS/COST**

• Sol, Inj-IV, SC: 1000 U/ml, 1, 2, 10, 30 ml: **$0.80-$1.08**/ml; 5000 U/ml, 0.5, 1, 10, 20 ml: **$1.00-$1.29**; 7500 U/ml, 1 ml: **$1.21**; 10,000 U/ml, 0.5, 1, 2, 4, 5, 10 ml: **$1.61-$1.94**/ml; 20,000 U/ml, 1, 2, 5 ml: **$2.39-$4.81**/ml

CONTRAINDICATIONS: Intracranial hemorrhage, severe hypotension, severe thrombocytopenia, subacute bacterial endocarditis, uncontrolled bleeding

PREGNANCY AND LACTATION: Pregnancy category C; does not cross the placenta, has major advantages over oral anticoagulants as the treatment of choice during pregnancy; is not excreted into breast milk due to its high molecular weight

SIDE EFFECTS

Occasional

Itching, burning (particularly on soles of feet) caused by vasospastic reaction

Rare

Pain, cyanosis of extremity 6–10 days after initial therapy lasting 4–6 hours; hypersensitivity reaction, including chills, fever, pruritus, urticaria, asthma, rhinitis, lacrimation, and headache

SERIOUS REACTIONS

• Bleeding complications ranging from local ecchymoses to major hemorrhage occur more frequently in high-dose therapy, intermittent IV infusion, and in women 60 years of age and older.

• Antidote: Protamine sulfate 1–1.5 mg, IV, for every 100 units heparin subcutaneous within 30 minutes of overdose, 0.5–0.75 mg for every 100 units heparin subcutaneous if within 30–60 minutes of overdose, 0.25–0.375 mg for every 100 units heparin subcutaneous if 2 hours have elapsed since overdose, 25–50 mg if heparin was given by IV infusion.

INTERACTIONS

Drugs

[3] *Aspirin:* Increased risk of hemorrhage

3 *Warfarin:* Warfarin may prolong the aPTT in patients receiving heparin; heparin may prolong the PT in patients receiving warfarin

SPECIAL CONSIDERATIONS

PATIENT/FAMILY EDUCATION
• Report any signs of bleeding: gums, under skin, urine, stools

MONITORING PARAMETERS
• aPTT (usual goal is to prolong aPTT to a value that corresponds to a plasma heparin level of 0.2 to 0.4 U/ml by protamine titration or to an antifactor Xa level of about 0.3 to 0.6 U/ml; this range must be determined for each individual laboratory), usually measure 6-8 hr after initiation of IV and 6-8 hr after INF rate changes; increase or decrease INF by 2-4 U/kg/hr dependent on aPTT
• For intermittent inj, measure aPTT 3.5-4 hr after IV inj; at midinterval after SC inj
• Platelet counts, signs of bleeding, Hgb, hct

---

hydralazine
(hye-dral'a-zeen)
Rx: Apresoline
Combinations
  Rx: with hydrochlorothiazide (Apresazide); with hydrochlorothiazide, reserpine (Ser-Ap-Es)
Chemical Class: Phthalazine derivative
Therapeutic Class: Antihypertensive; direct vasodilator

CLINICAL PHARMACOLOGY
Mechanism of Action: An antihypertensive with direct vasodilating effects on arterioles. *Therapeutic Effect:* Decreases BP and systemic resistance.

Pharmacokinetics

Route	Onset	Peak	Duration
PO	20–30 min	N/A	2–4 hr
IV	5–20 min	N/A	2–6 hr

Well absorbed from the GI tract. Widely distributed. Protein binding: 85%–90%. Metabolized in the liver to active metabolite. Primarily excreted in urine. Not removed by hemodialysis. **Half-life:** 3–7 hr (increased with impaired renal function).

INDICATIONS AND DOSAGES
Moderate to severe hypertension
PO
Adults. Initially, 10 mg 4 times a day. May increase by 10–25 mg/dose q2–5 days. Maximum: 300 mg/day.
Children. Initially, 0.75–1 mg/kg/day in 2–4 divided doses, not to exceed 25 mg/dose. May increase over 3–4 wk. Maximum: 7.5 mg/kg/day (5 mg/kg/day in infants).
IV, IM
Adults, Elderly. Initially, 10–20 mg/dose q4–6h. May increase to 40 mg/ dose.
Children. Initially, 0.1–0.2 mg/kg/dose (maximum: 20 mg) q4–6h, as needed, up to 1.7–3.5 mg/kg/day in divided doses q4–6h.
Dosage in renal impairment
Dosage interval is based on creatinine clearance.

Creatinine Clearance	Dosage Interval
10–50 ml/min	q8h
less than 10 ml/min	q8–24h

S AVAILABLE FORMS/COST
• Sol, Inj-IM, IV: 20 mg/ml, 1 ml: **$15.00-$18.75**
• Tab-Oral: 10 mg, 100's: **$2.75-$20.60**; 25 mg, 100's: **$1.02-$43.50**; 50 mg, 100's: **$1.48-$63.30**; 100 mg, 100's: **$6.90-$11.97**

UNLABELED USES: Treatment of CHF, hypertension secondary to eclampsia and preeclampsia, primary pulmonary hypertension.

CONTRAINDICATIONS: Coronary artery disease, lupus erythematosus, rheumatic heart disease

PREGNANCY AND LACTATION: Pregnancy category C; commonly used in pregnant women; excreted into breast milk; compatible with breast-feeding

SIDE EFFECTS

Frequent

Headache, palpitations, tachycardia (generally disappears in 7–10 days)

Occasional

GI disturbance (nausea, vomiting, diarrhea), paresthesia, fluid retention, peripheral edema, dizziness, flushed face, nasal congestion

SERIOUS REACTIONS

• High dosage may produce lupus erythematosus–like reaction, including fever, facial rash, muscle and joint aches, and splenomegaly.

• Severe orthostatic hypotension, skin flushing, severe headache, myocardial ischemia, and cardiac arrhythmias may develop.

• Profound shock may occur with severe overdosage.

INTERACTIONS

Drugs

3 *Diazoxide:* Severe hypotension

3 *NSAIDs:* Inhibited antihypertensive response to hydralazine

Labs

• *False increase:* Ca^{++} (slight); urine 17-ketogenic steroids; glucose, uric acid

• *False decrease:* Glucose, uric acid

SPECIAL CONSIDERATIONS

• Lupus-like syndrome more common in "slow acetylators" and following higher doses for prolonged periods

PATIENT/FAMILY EDUCATION

• Take with meals

• Notify clinician of any unexplained prolonged general tiredness or fever, muscle or joint aching, or chest pain

• Stools may turn black

MONITORING PARAMETERS

• CBC and ANA titer before and during prolonged therapy

hydrochlorothiazide
(hye-droe-klor-oh-thye′a-zide)
Rx: Aquazide-H, Diaqua, Esidrix, Ezide, HydroDiuril, Hydro-Par, Lexor, Microzide, Oretic, Zide
Combinations
Rx: with angiotensin-converting inhibitors: quinapril (Accuretic); captopril (Acediur, Capozide); lisinopril (Prinzide, Zestoretic); benazepril (Lotensin HCT); moexipril (Uniretic); enalapril (Vaseretic); with spironolactone (Aldactazide, Spirozide) with methyldopa (Aldoril), with hydralazine (Apresazide) with reserpine (Aqwesine, Hydropres, Hydroserpine, Hydrotensin, Mallopres, Marpres, Unipres) with angiotensin II receptor blockers: irbesartan (Avalide), valsartan (Diovan HCT), losartan (Hyzaar), with hydralazine and reserpine (Cam-ap-es, H.H.R., Hyserp, Lo-Ten, Ser-A-Gen, Seralazide, Ser-Ap-Es, Serpex, Uni-Serp), with triamterene: (Dyazide, Maxzide) with potassium (Esidrix-K) with guanethidine (Esimil), with β-blockers: propranolol: (Inderide); metoprolol: (Lopressor HCT); labetolol (Normazide, Trandate-HCT); timolol: (Timolide); bisoprolol (Ziac) with amiloride (Moduretic)
Chemical Class: Sulfonamide derivative
Therapeutic Class: Antihypertensive; diuretic, thiazide

CLINICAL PHARMACOLOGY
Mechanism of Action: A sulfonamide derivative that acts as a thiazide diuretic and antihypertensive. As a diuretic blocks reabsorption of water, sodium, and potassium at the cortical diluting segment of the distal tubule. As an antihypertensive reduces plasma, extracellular fluid volume, and peripheral vascular resistance by direct effect on blood vessels. *Therapeutic Effect:* Promotes diuresis; reduces BP.

Pharmacokinetics

Route	Onset	Peak	Duration
PO (diuretic)	2 hr	4–6 hr	6–12 hr

Variably absorbed from the GI tract. Primarily excreted unchanged in urine. Not removed by hemodialysis. **Half-life:** 5.6–14.8 hr.

INDICATIONS AND DOSAGES
Edema, hypertension
PO
Adults. 12.5–100 mg/day. Maximum: 200 mg/day.
Usual pediatric dosage
PO
Children 6 mo - 12 yr. 2 mg/kg/day in 2 divided doses. Maximum: 200 mg/day.
Children younger than 6 mo. 2-4 mg/kg/day in 2 divided doses. Maximum: 37.5 mg/day.

S **AVAILABLE FORMS/COST**
• Cap-Oral: 12.5 mg, 100's: **$42.45-$68.89**
• Sol—Oral: 50 mg/5 ml, 500 ml: **$16.91**
• Tab-Oral: 25 mg, 100's: **$0.69-$15.12**; 50 mg, 100's: **$0.74-$25.45**; 100 mg, 100's: **$1.04-$5.25**
UNLABELED USES: Treatment of diabetes insipidus, prevention of calcium-containing renal calculi

CONTRAINDICATIONS: Anuria, history of hypersensitivity to sulfonamides or thiazide diuretics, renal decompensation

PREGNANCY AND LACTATION: Pregnancy category B; 1st trimester use may increase risk of congenital defects, use in later trimesters does not seem to carry this risk; therapy for preexisting hypertension can be continued throughout pregnancy with minimal risk; initiating for simple edema not recommended; few unequivocal indications for diuretic therapy in pregnancy except for pulmonary edema or congestive heart failure, excreted into breast milk in small amounts; considered compatible with breast-feeding

SIDE EFFECTS

Expected
Increase in urinary frequency and urine volume

Frequent
Potassium depletion

Occasional
Orthostatic hypotension, headache, GI disturbances, photosensitivity

SERIOUS REACTIONS
• Vigorous diuresis may lead to profound water and electrolyte depletion, resulting in hypokalemia, hyponatremia, and dehydration.
• Acute hypotensive episodes may occur.
• Hyperglycemia may occur during prolonged therapy.
• Pancreatitis, blood dyscrasias, pulmonary edema, allergic pneumonitis, and dermatologic reactions occur rarely.
• Overdose can lead to lethargy and coma without changes in electrolytes or hydration.

INTERACTIONS

Drugs
❷ *Angiotensin-converting enzyme inhibitors:* Risk of postural hypotension when added to ongoing diuretic therapy; more common with loop diuretics; first dose hypotension possible in patients with sodium depletion or hypovolemia due to diuretics or sodium restriction; hypotensive response is usually transient; hold diuretic day of first dose

▣ *Calcium (high doses):* Risk of milk-alkali syndrome; monitor for hypercalcemia

▣ *Carbenoxolone:* Additive potassium wasting; severe hypokalemia

▣ *Cholestyramine/colestipol:* Reduced serum concentrations of thiazide diuretics

▣ *Corticosteroids:* Concomitant therapy may result in excessive potassium loss

▣ *Diazoxide:* Hyperglycemia

▣ *Digitalis glycosides:* Diuretic-induced hypokalemia may increase the risk of digitalis toxicity

▣ *Hypoglycemic agents:* Thiazide diuretics tend to increase blood glucose, may increase dosage requirements of antidiabetic drugs

▣ *Lithium:* Increased serum lithium concentrations, toxicity may occur

▣ *Methotrexate:* Increased bone marrow suppression

▣ *Nonsteroidal antiinflammatory drugs:* Concurrent use may reduce diuretic and antihypertensive effects

Labs
• *False decrease:* Urine estriol

SPECIAL CONSIDERATIONS
• May protect against osteoporotic hip fractures
• Loop diuretics or metolazone more effective if CrCl <40-50 ml/min
• Combinations with triamterene, lisinopril have potassium sparing effect

• Doses above 25 mg provide no further blood pressure reduction, but are more likely to induce metabolic disturbance (i.e., hypokalemia, hyperuricemia, etc.)

PATIENT/FAMILY EDUCATION
• Will increase urination temporarily (for about 3 wk); take early in the day
• May cause sensitivity to sunlight; avoid prolonged exposure to the sun and other ultraviolet light
• May cause gout attacks; notify clinician if sudden joint pain occurs

MONITORING PARAMETERS
• Weight, urine output, serum electrolytes, BUN, creatinine, CBC, uric acid, glucose, lipids

hydrocodone
(hye-droe-koe-done)
Rx: Hycodan
Combinations
  Rx: with acetaminophen (Anexsia, Bancap-HC, Cetaplus, Co-gesic, Duocet, Hydrocet, Hydrogesic, Hy-Phen, Lorcet, Lortab, Margesic-H, Norco, Panacet, Stagesic, T-Gesic, Vicodin, Zydone); with aspirin (Alor, Azdone, Damason-P, Lortab); with ibuprofen (Vicoprofen); with pseudoephedrine, guaifenesin (Duratuss, Pizotuss-D, Deconamine CX, Entuss-D, Cophene XP, SRC Liquid, Tussafin), with pseudoephedrine, chlorpheniramine, guaifenesin (Ztuss); with phenylpropanolamine, pyrilamine, guaifenesin (Triaminic Expectorant DH, S-T Forte, Vetuss HC, Statuss); with phenindamine, guaifenesin (P-V-Tussin); with phenylpropanolamine, guaifenesin (Tussanil); with phenylephrine, chlorpheniramine (Atuss-HD); with phenylephrine, guaifenesin (Donatussin DC, Tussafed HC, Atuss-G)
Chemical Class: Opiate derivative; phenanthrene derivative
Therapeutic Class: Antitussive; narcotic analgesic
DEA Class: Schedule III

CLINICAL PHARMACOLOGY
Mechanism of Action: Hydrocodone blocks pain perception in the cerebral cortex by binding to specific opiate receptors (mu and

kappa) neuronal membranes of synapses. This binding results in a decreased synaptic chemical transmission throughout the CNS thus inhibiting the flow of pain sensations into the higher centers and cause analgesia. *Therapeutic Effect:* Alters perception of pain and produces analgesic effect.

Pharmacokinetics

Well absorbed. Metabolized in liver. Excreted in urine. **Half-life:** 3.3-3.4 hrs.

INDICATIONS AND DOSAGES

Hydrocodone & acetaminophen

Analgesia: PO: *Adults, Children older than 13 yrs or more than 50 kg.* 2.5-10 mg q4-6h. Maximum: 60 mg/day hydrocodone. Maximum dose of acetaminophen: 4 g/day. *Elderly.* 2.5-5 mg hydrocodone q4-6h. Titrate dose to appropriate analgesic effect. Maximum: 4 g/day acetaminophen.: *Children 2-13 yrs or less than 50 kg.* 0.135 mg/kg/dose hydrocodone q4-6h. Maximum: 6 doses/day of hydrocodone or maximum recommended dose of acetaminophen.

Hydrocodone & aspirin

PO

Adults. 2.5-10 mg q4-6h. Maximum: 60 mg/day hydrocodone.

Elderly. 2.5-5 mg hydrocodone q4-6h. Titrate dose to appropriate analgesic effect.

Children 2-13 yrs or less than 50 kg. 0.135 mg/kg/dose hydrocodone q4-6h.

Hydrocodone & chlorpheniramine

Adults, Elderly, Children 12 yrs and older. 5 ml q12h. Maximum: 10 ml/24h.

Children 6-12yrs. 2.5 ml q12h. Maximum: 5 ml/24h.

Hydrocodone & guaifenesin

Adults, Elderly, Children 12 yrs and older. 5 ml q4h. Maximum: 30 ml/24h.

Children 2-12yrs. 2.5 ml q4h.

Children less than 2 yrs. 0.3 mg/kg/day (hydrocodone) in 4 divided doses.

Hydrocodone & homatropine

Adults, Elderly. 10 mg (hydrocodone) q4-6h. A single dose should not exceed 15 mg and not more frequently than q4h.

Children. 0.6mg/kg/day (hydrocodone) in 3-4 divided doses. Do not administer more frequently than q4h.

Hydrocodone & ibuprofen

Adults. 7.5-15 mg (hydrocodone) q4-6h as needed for pain. Maximum: 5 tablets/day.

Hydrocodone & pseudoephedrine

Adults, Elderly. 5 ml 4 times/day.

Hydrocodone, chlorpheniramine, phenylephrine, acetaminophen, & caffeine

Adults, Elderly. 1 tablet q4h up to 4 times/day.

Ⓢ AVAILABLE FORMS/COST

• Cap, Gel—Oral: 500 mg (acetaminophen)/5 mg, 100's: **$15.24-$112.22**

• Elixir—Oral: 500 mg (acetaminophen)/7.5 mg/15 ml, 480 ml: **$25.31-$99.34**; 100 mg (guiafenisen)/5 mg/15 ml, 480 ml: **$7.76-$98.56**

• Tab-Oral: 500 mg (acetaminophen)/2.5 mg, 100's: **$29.95-$90.15**; 500 mg (acetaminophen)/5 mg, 100's: **$8.27-$90.15**; 500 mg (acetaminophen)/7.5 mg, 100's: **$39.75-$99.85**; 500 mg (acetaminophen)/10 mg, 100's: **$53.27-$253.03**; 650 mg (acetaminophen)/7.5, 100's: **$38.35-$99.25**; 650 mg (acetaminophen)/10 mg, 100's: **$50.78-$145.45**; 750 mg (acetaminophen)/7.5 mg, 100's: **$12.90-$70.25**; 200 mg (ibuprofen)/7.5 mg, 100's: **$93.00-$127.39**

CONTRAINDICATIONS: CNS depression, severe respiratory depression, hypersensitivity to hydrocodone, or any component of the formulation

PREGNANCY AND LACTATION: Pregnancy category B (category D if used for prolonged periods or in high doses at term); withdrawal could theoretically occur in infants exposed *in utero* to prolonged maternal ingestion; excretion into breast milk unknown; use caution in nursing mothers

SIDE EFFECTS

Frequent

Dizziness, sedation, drowsiness, bradycardia

Occasional

Anxiety, dysphoria, euphoria, fear, lethargy, lightheadedness, malaise, mental clouding, mental impairment, mood changes, physiological dependence, sedation, somnolence, constipation, bradycardia, heartburn, nausea, vomiting

Rare

Hypersensitivity reaction, rash

SERIOUS REACTIONS

• Cardiac arrest, circulatory collapse, coma, hypotension, hypoglycemic coma, ureteral spasm, urinary retention, vesical sphincter spasm, agranulocytosis, bleeding time prolonged, hemolytic anemia, iron deficiency anemia, occult blood loss, thrombocytopenia, hepatic necrosis, hepatits, skeletal muscle rigidity, renal toxicity, renal tubular necrosis have been reported.

• Hearing impairment or loss have been reported with chronic overdose.

• Acute airway obstruction, apnea, dyspnea, and respiratory depression occur rarely and are usually dose related.

INTERACTIONS

Drugs

3 *Antihistamines, chloral hydrate, glutethimide, methocarbamol:* Enhanced depressant effects

3 *Barbiturates:* Additive respiratory and CNS depressant effects

3 *Cimetidine:* Increased respiratory and CNS depression

3 *Ethanol:* Additive CNS effects

3 *Protease inhibitors:* Enhanced CNS and respiratory depression

Labs

• False elevations of amylase and lipase

SPECIAL CONSIDERATIONS

PATIENT/FAMILY EDUCATION

• Report any symptoms of CNS changes, allergic reactions

• Physical dependency may result when used for extended periods

• Change position slowly, orthostatic hypotension may occur

• Avoid hazardous activities if drowsiness or dizziness occurs

• Avoid alcohol, other CNS depressants

• Minimize nausea by administering with food and remain lying down following dose

• Do not administer agonist/antagonist analgesics (i.e., pentazocine, nalbuphine, butorphanol, dezocine, buprenorphine) to patient who has received a prolonged course of hydrocodone (a pure agonist). In opioid-dependent patients, mixed agonist/antagonist analgesics may precipitate withdrawal symptoms

H

hydrocortisone
(hye-dro-kor'ti-sone)

Rx: *Ano-Rectals:* Proctocort, Anusol-HC, Proctofoam-HC, Anucort-HC, Cortenema

Rx: *Systemic:* Cortef, Hydrocortone, Hydrocortone Phosphate, Hydrocortone Acetate, Solu-Cortef

Rx: *Topical:* Cetacort, Cort-Dome, Dermacort, Hytone, Locoid, Synacort, Westcort

OTC: Cortizone, Cortaid, Lanacort-5, Gynecort Female Creme, Dermolate, Tegrin-HC

Combinations

    Rx: with choloramphenicol (Chloromycetin/HC suspension—ophthalmic); with neomycin and polymyxin B (Cortisporin Otic, Drotic, Otocort—otic); with neomycin, polymyxin B, and bacitracin (Cortisporin Ointment, Neotricin HC—ophthalmic); with oxytetracycline (Terra-Cortril—ophthalmic); with urea (Carmol HC)

Chemical Class: Glucocorticoid

Therapeutic Class: Corticosteroid, systemic; corticosteroid, topical

---

CLINICAL PHARMACOLOGY
Mechanism of Action: An adrenocortical steroid that inhibits accumulation of inflammatory cells at inflammation sites, phagocytosis, lysosomal enzyme release and synthesis and release of mediators of inflammation. *Therapeutic Effect:* Prevents or suppresses cell-mediated immune reactions. Decreases or prevents tissue response to inflammatory process.

Pharmacokinetics

Route	Onset	Peak	Duration
IV	N/A	4–6 hr	8–12 hr

Well absorbed after IM administration. Widely distributed. Metabolized in the liver. **Half-life:** Plasma, 1.5–2 hr; biologic, 8–12 hr.

INDICATIONS AND DOSAGES
Acute adrenal insufficiency
IV

Adults, Elderly. 100 mg IV bolus; then 300 mg/day in divided doses q8h.
Children. 1–2 mg/kg IV bolus; then 150–250 mg/day in divided doses q6–8h.
Infants. 1–2 mg/kg/dose IV bolus; then 25–150 mg/day in divided doses q6–8h.

Anti-inflammation, immunosuppression
IV, IM

Adults, Elderly. 15–240 mg q12h.
Children. 1–5 mg/kg/day in divided doses q12h.

Physiologic replacement
PO

Children. 0.5–0.75 mg/kg/day in divided doses q8h.
IM
Children. 0.25–0.35 mg/kg/day as a single dose.

Status asthmaticus
IV

Adults, Elderly. 100–500 mg q6h.
Children. 2 mg/kg/dose q6h.

Shock
IV

Adults, Elderly, Children 12 yr and older. 100–500 mg q6h.
Children younger than 12 yr. 50 mg/kg. May repeat in 4 hr, then q24h as needed.

Adjunctive treatment of ulcerative colitis

Rectal

Adults, Elderly. 100 mg at bedtime for 21 nights or until clinical and proctologic remission occurs (may require 2–3 mo of therapy).

Rectal (Cortifoam)

Adults, Elderly. 1 applicator 1–2 times a day for 2–3 wk, then every second day until therapy ends.

Topical

Adults, Elderly. Apply sparingly 2–4 times a day.

Ⓢ AVAILABLE FORMS/COST

• Cre, Oint (butyrate)—Top: 0.1%, 15, 45 g: **$23.35-$29.46**/15 g
• Cre—Rect: 1%, 30 g: **$3.73-$46.54**; 2.5%, 30 g: **$5.25-$39.35**
• Cre—Top: 0.5%, 15, 30, 45, 60, 120, 454 g: **$0.80-$9.13**/30 g; 2.5%, 20, 30, 120, 454 g: **$4.55-$44.21**/30 g
• Foam-Rect: 10%, 15 g: **$88.73**
• Gel-Top: 1%, 15, 30g: **$4.01**/30 g
• Susp, Inj (acetate)-IA, IM: 25 mg/ml, 5, 10 ml: **$3.60**/10 ml
• Powder, Inj (sodium succinate)-IM, IV: 100 mg/vial: **$2.00-$3.75**; 250 mg/vial: **$3.51-$9.50**; 500 mg/vial: **$8.95-$15.00**; 1000 mg/vial: **$29.00**
• Sol, Inj (sodium phosphate)-IM, IV, SC: 50 mg/ml, 2 ml: **$11.71**
• Lotion—Top: 0.5%, 60, 120 ml: **$16.25**/60 ml; 2.5%, 60, 120 ml: **$29.67-$54.10**/60 ml
• Oint—Top: 0.5%, 30, 60, 120, 240 g: **$1.44-$1.89**/30 g; 1%, 20, 30, 60, 120, 454 g: **$1.63-$10.24**/30 g; 2.5%, 20, 30, 454 g: **$11.00-$20.66**/30 g
• Sol (butyrate)—Top: 0.1%, 20, 60 ml: **$31.43**/20 ml
• Sol—Top: 1%, 30, 60 ml: **$9.92-$11.22**/30 ml; 2.5%, 30 ml: **$21.61**
• Supp-Rect: 30 mg, 12's: **$45.63-$51.75**
• Supp (acetate)—Rect: 25 mg, 12's: **$1.98-$43.79**
• Susp (cypionate)—Oral: 10 mg/5 ml, 120 ml: **$28.26**
• Susp-Rect: 100 mg/60 ml: **$11.17-$12.40**
• Tab-Oral: 5 mg, 50's: **$11.16**; 10 mg, 100's: **$23.93-$39.53**; 20 mg, 100's: **$11.25-$74.94**

CONTRAINDICATIONS: Fungal, tuberculosis, or viral skin lesions; serious infections

PREGNANCY AND LACTATION: Pregnancy category C; excreted in breast milk, could interfere with infant's growth and endogenous corticosteroid production

SIDE EFFECTS

Frequent

Insomnia, heartburn, nervousness, abdominal distention, diaphoresis, acne, mood swings, increased appetite, facial flushing, delayed wound healing, increased susceptibility to infection, diarrhea or constipation

Occasional

Headache, edema, change in skin color, frequent urination

Topical: Itching, redness, irritation

Rare

Tachycardia, allergic reaction (such as rash and hives), psychological changes, hallucinations, depression

Topical: Allergic contact dermatitis, purpura

Systemic: Absorption more likely with use of occlusive dressings or extensive application in young children

SERIOUS REACTIONS

• Long-term therapy may cause hypocalcemia, hypokalemia, muscle wasting (especially in arms and legs), osteoporosis, spontaneous fractures, amenorrhea, cataracts, glaucoma, peptic ulcer disease, and CHF.

• Abruptly withdrawing the drug after long-term therapy may cause anorexia, nausea, fever, headache, sudden severe joint pain, rebound inflammation, fatigue, weakness, lethargy, dizziness, and orthostatic hypotension.

INTERACTIONS
Drugs
▣ *Aminoglutethamide:* Enhanced elimination of hydrocortisone; reduction in corticosteroid response

▣ *Antidiabetics:* Increased blood glucose in patients with diabetes

▣ *Barbiturates:* Reduction in the serum concentrations of corticosteroids

▣ *Cholestyramine, colestipol:* Possible reduced absorption of corticosteroids

▣ *Cyclosporine:* Increased levels of both drugs increases the risk of seizures

▣ *Estrogens:* Enhanced effects of corticosteroids

▣ *Isoniazid (INH):* Reduced INH levels, enhanced corticosteroid effect

▣ *IUDs:* Inhibition of inflammation may decrease contraceptive effect

▣ *NSAIDs:* Increased risk GI ulceration

▣ *Phenytoin:* Reduced therapeutic effect of corticosteroids

▣ *Rifampin:* Reduced therapeutic effect of corticosteroids

▣ *Salicylates:* Enhanced elimination of salicylates; subtherapeutic salicylate concentrations possible

Labs
• *False negative:* Skin allergy tests

SPECIAL CONSIDERATIONS
PATIENT/FAMILY EDUCATION
• May cause GI upset; take with meals or snacks
• Take single daily doses in am

• Increased dose of rapidly acting corticosteroids may be necessary in patients subjected to unusual stress
• Signs of adrenal insufficiency include fatigue, anorexia, nausea, vomiting, diarrhea, weight loss, weakness, dizziness, and low blood sugar
• Avoid abrupt withdrawal of therapy following high-dose or long-term therapy
• May mask infections
• Do not give live virus vaccines to patients on prolonged therapy
• Patients on chronic steroid therapy should wear medical alert bracelet

MONITORING PARAMETERS
• Serum K and glucose
• Edema, blood pressure, CHF, mental status, weight
• Growth in children on prolonged therapy

---

hydroflumethiazide
(high-drow-floo-meth-eye-'ah-zide)
Rx: Diucardin, Saluron
Combinations
  Rx: reserpine (Salutensin, Salutensin-Demi)
Chemical Class: Sulfonamide derivative
Therapeutic Class: Antihypertensive; diuretic, thiazide

CLINICAL PHARMACOLOGY
Mechanism of Action: A diuretic that blocks reabsorption of water, the electrolytes sodium and potassium at cortical diluting segment of distal tubule. As an antihypertensive it reduces plasma and extracellular fluid volume and decreases peripheral vascular resistance (PVR) by direct effect on blood vessels. *Therapeutic Effect:* Promotes diuresis, reduces blood pressure (BP).

Pharmacokinetics
Rapidly but incompletely absorbed from the gastrointestinal (GI) tract. Metabolized to metabolite that is extensively bound to red blood cells and has a longer half-life than parent compound. Primarily excreted in urine. Not removed by hemodialysis. **Half-life:** 2-17 hrs.

INDICATIONS AND DOSAGES
Edema
PO
Adults, Elderly. Initially, 50 mg 2 times/day. Maintenance: 25-200 mg/day.

Hypertension
Adults, Elderly. Children. 1 mg/kg/day.
Initially, 50 mg 2 times/day. Maintenance: 50-100 mg/day.

S AVAILABLE FORMS/COST
• Tab-Oral: 50 mg, 100's: **$59.05-$72.94**

UNLABELED USES: Treatment of diabetes insipidus
CONTRAINDICATIONS: Anuria, history of hypersensitivity to sulfonamides or thiazide diuretics, renal decompensation, pregnancy
PREGNANCY AND LACTATION: Pregnancy category C; therapy for preexisting hypertension can be continued throughout pregnancy with minimal risk; initiating for simple edema not recommended; few unequivocal indications for diuretic therapy in pregnancy except for pulmonary edema or congestive heart failure, excreted into breast milk in small amounts; considered compatible with breast-feeding

SIDE EFFECTS
Expected
Increase in urine frequency and volume
Frequent
Potassium depletion
Occasional

Postural hypotension, headache, gastrointestinal (GI) disturbances, photosensitivity reaction

SERIOUS REACTIONS
• Vigorous diuresis may lead to profound water loss and electrolyte depletion, resulting in hypokalemia, hyponatremia, and dehydration.
• Acute hypotensive episodes may occur.
• Hyperglycemia may be noted during prolonged therapy.
• GI upset, pancreatitis, dizziness, paresthesias, headache, blood dyscrasias, pulmonary edema, allergic pneumonitis, and dermatologic reactions occur rarely.
• Overdosage can lead to lethargy and coma without changes in electrolytes or hydration.

INTERACTIONS
Drugs
❷ *Angiotensin-converting enzyme inhibitors:* Risk of postural hypotension when added to ongoing diuretic therapy; more common with loop diuretics; first dose hypotension possible in patients with sodium depletion or hypovolemia due to diuretics or sodium restriction; hypotensive response is usually transient; hold diuretic day of first dose
❸ *Calcium (high dose):* Risk of milk-alkali syndrome. Monitor for hypoglycemia
❸ *Cholestyramine, Colestipol:* Reduced serum concentrations of thiazide diuretics
❸ *Corticosteroids:* Concomitant therapy may result in excessive potassium loss
❸ *Diazoxide:* Hyperglycemia
❸ *Digitalis glycosides:* Diuretic-induced hypokalemia may increase the risk of digitalis toxicity

3 *Hypoglycemic agents:* Thiazide diuretics tend to increase blood glucose; may increase dosage requirements of hypoglycemic agents

3 *Lithium:* Increased serum lithium concentrations, toxicity may occur

3 *Methotrexate:* Increased bone marrow suppression

3 *Nonsteroidal antiinflammatory drugs:* Concurrent may reduce diuretic and antihypertensive effects

Labs

• *False decrease:* Urine estriol

SPECIAL CONSIDERATIONS

• May protect against osteoporotic hip fractures

• Loop diuretics or metolazone more effective if CrCl <40-50 ml/min

PATIENT/FAMILY EDUCATION

• Will increase urination temporarily (approximately 3 wk); take early in the day to prevent sleep disturbance

• May cause sensitivity to sunlight; avoid prolonged exposure to the sun and other ultraviolet light

• May cause gout attacks; notify clinician if sudden joint pain occurs

MONITORING PARAMETERS

• Weight, urine output, serum electrolytes, BUN, creatinine, CBC, uric acid, glucose, lipids

hydromorphone

(hye-droe-mor'fone)

Rx: Dilaudid, Palladone
Chemical Class: Opiate derivative; phenanthrene derivative
Therapeutic Class: Antitussive; narcotic analgesic
DEA Class: Schedule II

CLINICAL PHARMACOLOGY

Mechanism of Action: An opioid agonist that binds to opioid receptors in the CNS, reducing the intensity of pain stimuli from sensory nerve endings. *Therapeutic Effect:* Alters the perception of and emotional response to pain; suppresses cough reflex.

Pharmacokinetics

Route	Onset	Peak	Duration
PO	30 min	90–120 min	4 hr
IV	10–15 min	15–30 min	2–3 hr
IM	15 min	30–60 min	4–5 hr
Subcutaneous	15 min	30–90 min	4 hr
Rectal	15–30 min	N/A	N/A

Well absorbed from the GI tract after IM administration. Widely distributed. Metabolized in the liver. Excreted in urine. **Half-life:** 1–3 hr.

INDICATIONS AND DOSAGES

Analgesia

PO

Adults, Elderly, Children weighing 50 kg and more. 2-4 mg q3-4h. Range: 2-8 mg/dose.

Children older than 6 mo and weighing less than 50 kg. 0.03-0.08 mg/kg/dose q3-4h.

PO (Extended-Release)

Adults, Elderly. 12-32 mg once a day.

IV

Adults, Elderly, Children weighing more than 50 kg. 0.2-0.6 mg q2-3h. *Children weighing 50 kg or less.* 0.015 mg/kg/dose q3-6h as needed.

Rectal

Adults, Elderly. 3 mg q4-8h.

Patient-controlled analgesia (PCA)

IV

Adults, Elderly. 0.05-0.5 mg at 5-15 min lockout. Maximum (4-hr): 4-6 mg.

Epidural

Adults, Elderly. Bolus dose of 1-1.5 mg at rate of 0.04-0.4 mg/hr. Demand dose of 0.15 mg at 30 min lockout.

Cough

PO

Adults, Elderly, Children older than 12 yr. 1 mg q3–4h.

Children 6-12 yr. 0.5 mg q3–4h.

S AVAILABLE FORMS/COST

• Sol, Inj-IM, IV, SC: 1 mg/ml, 1, 10 ml: **$1.26**/1 ml; 2 mg/ml, 1, 10, 20 ml: **$1.05-$1.40**/1 ml; 4 mg/ml, 1, 10, 20 ml: **$1.00-$1.70**/1 ml; 10 mg/ml, 1, 5, 10 ml: **$3.54**/1 ml
• Sol—Oral: 1 mg/ml, 120, 480 ml: **$108.18**/480 ml
• Supp—Rect: 3 mg, 6's: **$23.97**
• Tab-Oral: 2 mg, 100's: **$18.00-$49.34**; 4 mg, 100's: **$30.00-$80.54**; 8 mg, 100's: **$131.93-$146.59**

CONTRAINDICATIONS: None known.

PREGNANCY AND LACTATION: Pregnancy category C (category D if used for prolonged periods or in high doses at term); use during labor produces neonatal respiratory depression; excretion into breast milk unknown; use caution in nursing mothers

SIDE EFFECTS

Frequent

Somnolence, dizziness, hypotension (including orthostatic hypotension), decreased appetite

Occasional

Confusion, diaphoresis, facial flushing, urine retention, constipation, dry mouth, nausea, vomiting, headache, pain at injection site

Rare

Allergic reaction, depression

SERIOUS REACTIONS

• Overdose results in respiratory depression, skeletal muscle flaccidity, cold or clammy skin, cyanosis, and extreme somnolence progressing to seizures, stupor, and coma.

• The patient who uses hydromorphone repeatedly may develop a tolerance to the drug's analgesic effect as well as physical dependence.

• This drug may have a prolonged duration of action and cumulative effect in patients with hepatic or renal impairment.

INTERACTIONS

Drugs

▣ *Antihistamines, chloral hydrate, glutethimide, methocarbamol:* Enhanced depressant effects

▣ *Barbiturates:* Additive respiratory and CNS depressant effects

▣ *Cimetidine:* Increased respiratory and CNS depression

▣ *Ethanol:* Additive CNS effects

Labs

• *False increase:* Amylase and lipase

SPECIAL CONSIDERATIONS

• Do not administer agonist/antagonist analgesics (i.e., pentazocine, nalbuphine, butorphanol, dezocine, buprenorphine) to patient who has received a prolonged course of hydromorphone (a pure agonist). In opioid-dependent patients, mixed agonist/antagonist analgesics may precipitate withdrawal symptoms.

H

PATIENT/FAMILY EDUCATION
• Physical dependency may result when used for extended periods
• Avoid hazardous activities if drowsiness or dizziness occurs
• Avoid alcohol, other CNS depressants unless directed by clinician
• Minimize nausea by administering with food and remain lying down following dose

---

hydroquinone
(hye-droe-kwin′-one)
Rx: Alphaquin HP, Eldopaque-Forte, Eldoquin-Forte, Lustra, Solaquin Forte, Melpaque HP, Melquin HP, Melquin 3, NuQuin HP, Melanex, Viquin Forte
Combinations
   Rx: with fluocinolone/tretinoin (Tri-Luma)
Chemical Class: Monobenzone derivative
Therapeutic Class: Depigmenting agent

CLINICAL PHARMACOLOGY
Mechanism of Action: A depigmenting agent that suppresses melanocyte metabolic processes of the skin. Inhibits the enzymatic oxidation of tyrosine to DOPA (3, 4-dihydroxyphenylalanine). Sun exposure reverses this effect and causes repigmentation. Therapeutic Effect: Lighten hyperpigmented areas.
Pharmacokinetics
Onset and duration of depigmentation vary among individuals. About 35% is absorbed.

INDICATIONS AND DOSAGES
Hyperpigmentation, melanin
Topical
Adults, Elderly, Children 12 yrs and older. Apply twice daily.

$ AVAILABLE FORMS/COST
• Cre—Top: 2%, 15, 28, 90, 120 g: **$6.27**/90 g; 4%, 15, 30, 45, 60, 120 g: **$19.75-$81.25**/30 g
• Gel—Top: 4%, 15, 30, 60 g: **$35.50-$51.40**/30 g
• Sol—Top: 3%, 30 ml: **$8.70-$13.13**
UNLABELED USES: *None known.*
CONTRAINDICATIONS: Hypersensitivity to hydroquinone, sulfites, or any other component of its formulation
PREGNANCY AND LACTATION: Pregnancy category C; degree of systemic absorption unknown; excretion into breast milk unknown
SIDE EFFECTS
Occasional
Burning, itching, stinging, erythema such as localized contact dermatitis
Rare
Conjunctival changes, fingernail staining
SERIOUS REACTIONS
• Gradual blue-black darkening of skin has been reported.
• Occasional cutaneous hypersensitivity (localized contact dermatitis) may occur.
INTERACTIONS
Labs
• *False decrease:* Urine glucose
SPECIAL CONSIDERATIONS
PATIENT/FAMILY EDUCATION
• Apply small amount to an unbroken patch of skin and check in 24 hr; if vesicle formation, itching, or excessive inflammation occurs, further treatment not advised
• Positive response may require 3 wk to 6 mo
• Protect the treated area from UV light by using a sunscreen, sun block, or protective clothing
• Avoid application to lips or near eyes

hydroxocobalamin (vitamin B_{12})

(hye-drox'oh-co-bal'a-min)

Rx: Hydroxy-Cobal, LA-12

Chemical Class: Vitamin B complex

Therapeutic Class: Antidote, nitroprusside; hematinic; vitamin

CLINICAL PHARMACOLOGY

Mechanism of Action: A coenzyme for metabolic functions, including fat and carbohydrate metabolism and protein synthesis. *Therapeutic Effect:* Necessary for growth, cell replication, hematopoiesis, and myelin synthesis.

Pharmacokinetics

Rapidly absorbed after IM administration. Protein binding: High. Primarily excreted in urine. Metabolized in liver. **Half-life:** 6 days.

INDICATIONS AND DOSAGES

Vitamin B_{12} deficiency

IM

Adults, Elderly. 30 mcg/day for 5-10 days then 100- 200 mcg monthly. Children. 1-5 mg in single doses of 100 mcg over 2 or more weeks then 30-50 mcg monthly.

[$] **AVAILABLE FORMS/COST**

• Sol, Inj-IM: 1000 mcg/ml, 10, 30 ml: **$9.75**/30 ml

CONTRAINDICATIONS: Folate deficient anemia, hereditary optic nerve atrophy, hypersensitivity to cobalt, hypersensitivity to hydroxocobalamin or any component of the formulatioin

PREGNANCY AND LACTATION: Pregnancy category A (C if dose exceeds recommended daily allowance); vitamin B_{12} is an essential vitamin and needs are increased during pregnancy; excreted into breast milk; 2.6 mcg/day should be consumed during pregnancy and lactation

SIDE EFFECTS

Occasional

Diarrhea, itching, pain at injection site

SERIOUS REACTIONS

• Rare allergic reaction generally due to impurities in preparation, may occur.

• May produce peripheral vascular thrombosis, pulmonary edema, hypokalemia, and congestive heart failure (CHF).

INTERACTIONS

Labs

• *False positive:* Intrinsic factor

• *Interference:* Methotrexate, pyrimethamine and most antibiotics interfere with vitamin B_{12} assay

SPECIAL CONSIDERATIONS

PATIENT/FAMILY EDUCATION

• Therapy may require life-long monthly injections

MONITORING PARAMETERS

• Serum potassium for 1st 48 hr during treatment of severe megaloblastic anemia

• Reticulocyte counts, Hct, vitamin B_{12}, iron, and folic acid plasma levels prior to treatment, between days 5 and 7 of treatment, then frequently until Hct is normal

hydroxychloroquine
(hye-drox-ee-klor'oh-kwin)
Rx: Plaquenil, Quineprox
Chemical Class: 4-amino-
quinoline derivative
Therapeutic Class: Antimalarial; disease-modifying
antirheumatic drug (DMARD)

CLINICAL PHARMACOLOGY
Mechanism of Action: An antimalarial and antirheumatic that concentrates in parasite acid vesicles,
increasing the pH of the vesicles and
interfering with parasite protein
synthesis. Antirheumatic action
may involve suppressing formation
of antigens responsible for hypersensitivity reactions. *Therapeutic
Effect:* Inhibits parasite growth.

INDICATIONS AND DOSAGES
*Treatment of acute attack of ma-
laria (dosage in mg base)*
PO

Dose	Times	Adults	Children
Initial	Day 1	620 mg	10 mg/kg
Second	6 hr later	310 mg	5 mg/kg
Third	Day 2	310 mg	5 mg/kg
Fourth	Day 3	310 mg	5 mg/kg

Suppression of malaria
PO
Adults. 310 mg base weekly on same
day each week, beginning 2 wk before entering an endemic area and
continuing for 4-6 wk after leaving
the area.
Children. 5 mg base/kg/wk, beginning 2 wk before entering an endemic area and continuing for 4-6
wk after leaving the area. If therapy
is not begun before exposure, administer a loading dose of 10 mg
base/kg in 2 equally divided doses 6
hr apart, followed by the ususal dosage regimen.

Rheumatoid arthritis
PO
Adults. Initially, 400-600 mg
(310-465 mg base) daily for 5-10
days, gradually increased to optimum response level. Maintenance
(usually within 4-12 wk): Dosage
decreased by 50% and then continued at maintenance dose of 200-400
mg/day. Maximum effect may not
be seen for several months.

Lupus erythematosus
PO
Adults. Initially, 400 mg once or
twice a day for several weeks or
months. Maintenance: 200-400
mg/day.

$ AVAILABLE FORMS/COST
• Tab-Oral: 200 mg, 100's: **$23.53-
$189.20**

UNLABELED USES: Treatment of
juvenile arthritis, sarcoid-associated hypercalcemia

CONTRAINDICATIONS: Long-
term therapy for children, porphyria, psoriasis, retinal or visual field
changes

PREGNANCY AND LACTATION:
Pregnancy category C; excreted in
breast milk; safe use during nursing
has not been established

SIDE EFFECTS
Frequent
Mild, transient headache; anorexia;
nausea; vomiting
Occasional
Visual disturbances, nervousness,
fatigue, pruritus (especially of
palms, soles, and scalp), irritability,
personality changes, diarrhea
Rare
Stomatitis, dermatitis, impaired
hearing

SERIOUS REACTIONS
• Ocular toxicity, especially retinopathy, may occur and may progress
even after drug is discontinued.

• Prolonged therapy may result in peripheral neuritis, neuromyopathy, hypotension, EKG changes, agranulocytosis, aplastic anemia, thrombocytopenia, seizures, and psychosis.

• Overdosage may result in headache, vomiting, visual disturbances, drowsiness, seizures, and hypokalemia followed by cardiovascular collapse and death.

INTERACTIONS
Drugs
▣ *Digitalis glycosides:* Increased serum digoxin concentrations
▣ *Praziquantel:* Reduced praziquantel concentration

SPECIAL CONSIDERATIONS
PATIENT/FAMILY EDUCATION
• Report any muscle weakness, visual disturbances, difficulty hearing, or ringing in ears to clinician

MONITORING PARAMETERS
• Baseline and periodic ophthalmologic examinations (visual acuity, slit lamp, funduscopic, and visual field tests); periodic tests of knee and ankle reflexes to detect muscular weakness

• Periodic CBCs during prolonged therapy

---

hydroxyprogesterone
Rx: Hylutin, Prodrox
Chemical Class: Progestin derivative
Therapeutic Class: Antineoplastic; progestin

CLINICAL PHARMACOLOGY
Mechanism of Action: A hormone that influences proliferative endometrium and transforms into secretory endometrium. Secretion of pituitary gonadotropins is inhibited which prevents follicular maturation and ovulation. *Therapeutic*

Effect: Facilitates ureteral dilatation associated with hydronephrosis of pregnancy.

INDICATIONS AND DOSAGES
Amenorrhea
IM

Adults. 375 mg given at any point in the menstrual cycle.

Endogenous estrogen production
IM

Adults. 125 to 250 mg beginning on the tenth day of cycle and repeated every 7 days until suppression is no longer desired.

Endometrial carcinoma
IM

Adults. 1000 mg 1 or more times weekly.

Abnormal uterine bleeding
IM

Adults. 5-10 mg for 6 days. When estrogen is given concomitantly, begin progesterone after 2 wks of estrogen therapy; discontinue when menstrual flow begins.

Prevention of endometrial hyperplasia
IM

Adults. 200 mg in evening for 12 days per 28-day cycle in combination with daily conjugated estrogen.

Premature labor
IM

Adults. 250 to 500 mg once weekly.

▣ AVAILABLE FORMS/COST
• Sol, Inj-IM: 250 mg/ml, 5 ml: **$13.15-$29.95**

UNLABELED USES: Alopecia, stress incontinence, menopausal symptoms, preterm delivery, treatment of prostatic hyperplasia, seborrhea, ureteral stones

CONTRAINDICATIONS: Breast cancer, cerebral apoplexy or history of these conditions, missed abortion, severe liver dysfunction, thromboembolic disorders, throm-

H

bophlebitis, undiagnosed vaginal bleeding, genital malignancy, use as a diagnostic test for pregnancy

PREGNANCY AND LACTATION: Pregnancy category D; an increased risk of hypospadias in the male fetus and mild virilization of the female fetus have been reported with progestin use; progestins compatible with breast-feeding

SIDE EFFECTS

Frequent

Breakthrough bleeding or spotting at beginning of therapy, amenorrhea, change in menstrual flow, breast tenderness

Occasional

Edema, weight gain or loss, rash, pruritus, photosensitivity, skin pigmentation

Rare

Pain or swelling at injection site, acne, mental depression, alopecia, hirsutism

SERIOUS REACTIONS

• Thrombophlebitis, cerebrovascular disorders, retinal thrombosis, and pulmonary embolism rarely occur.

INTERACTIONS

Drugs

3 *Aminoglutethimide:* Decreases progestin concentration

SPECIAL CONSIDERATIONS

PATIENT/FAMILY EDUCATION

• Take protective measures against exposure to UV light or sunlight

---

hydroxyzine
(hye-drox′i-zeen)
Rx: Atarax, Vistaril, Vistazine
Chemical Class: Piperidine derivative
Therapeutic Class: Antiemetic (parenteral); antihistamine; anxiolytic; sedative/hypnotic

CLINICAL PHARMACOLOGY
Mechanism of Action: A piperazine derivative that competes with histamine for receptor sites in the GI tract, blood vessels, and respiratory tract. May exert CNS depressant activity in subcortical areas. Diminishes vestibular stimulation and depresses labyrinthine function. *Therapeutic Effect:* Produces anxiolytic, anticholinergic, antihistaminic, and analgesic effects; relaxes skeletal muscle; controls nausea and vomiting.

Pharmacokinetics

Route	Onset	Peak	Duration
PO	15-30 min	N/A	4-6 hr

Well absorbed from the GI tract and after parenteral administration. Metabolized in the liver. Primarily excreted in urine. Not removed by hemodialysis. **Half-life:** 20-25 hr (increased in the elderly).

INDICATIONS AND DOSAGES
Anxiety
PO
Adults, Elderly. 25-100 mg 4 times a day. Maximum: 600 mg/day.
Nausea and vomiting
IM
Adults, Elderly. 25-100 mg/dose q4-6h.
Pruritus
PO
Adults, Elderly. 25 mg 3-4 times a day.

Preoperative sedation
PO
Adults, Elderly. 50-100 mg.
IM
Adults, Elderly. 25-100 mg.
Usual pediatric dosage
PO
Children. 2 mg/kg/day in divided doses q6-8h.
IM
Children. 0.5-1 mg/kg/dose q4-6h.

⛊ AVAILABLE FORMS/COST

• Cap—Oral: 25 mg, 100's: **$7.95-$112.40**; 50 mg, 100's: **$8.44-$132.94**; 100 mg, 100's: **$18.95-$163.35**

• Sol, Inj-IM: 25 mg/ml, 10 ml: **$3.00-$6.38**; 50 mg/ml, 10 ml: **$3.50-$20.53**

• Sus—Oral: 25 mg/5 ml, 120, 480 ml: **$28.00-$41.60**/120 ml

• Syr—Oral: 10 mg/5 ml, 120, 480 ml: **$7.17-$12.70**/120 ml

• Tab—Oral: 10 mg, 100's: **$5.25-$69.68**; 25 mg, 100's: **$6.95-$102.19**; 50 mg, 100's: **$8.75-$124.58**; 100 mg, 100's: **$22.50-$153.08**

CONTRAINDICATIONS: None known.

PREGNANCY AND LACTATION: Pregnancy category C (but no excess in birth defects documented); safe during labor for relief of anxiety; no data on breast-feeding

SIDE EFFECTS
Side effects are generally mild and transient.
Frequent
Somnolence, dry mouth, marked discomfort with IM injection
Occasional
Dizziness, ataxia, asthenia, slurred speech, headache, agitation, increased anxiety
Rare
Paradoxical CNS reactions, such as hyperactivity or nervousness in children and excitement or restlessness in elderly or debilitated patients (generally noted during first 2 weeks of therapy, particularly in presence of uncontrolled pain)

SERIOUS REACTIONS
• A hypersensitivity reaction, including wheezing, dyspnea, and chest tightness, may occur.

INTERACTIONS
Labs
• *False increase:* Urine 17-hydroxycorticosteroids and 17-ketogenic steroids

---

hyoscyamine
(hye-oh-sye'a-meen)
Rx: A-Spas S/L, Anaspaz, Cystospaz, Cystospaz-M, Donnamar, ED-SPAZ, Gastrosed, Hyco Drops, Hyosol/SL, Hyospaz, Levbid, Levsin, Levsin/SL, Levsinex, Liqui-Sooth, Medispaz, Spacol, Spasdel, Symax-SL, Symax-SR
Combinations
  Rx: with phenobarbital (Levsin PB)
Chemical Class: Belladonna alkaloid
Therapeutic Class: Anticholinergic; gastrointestinal

CLINICAL PHARMACOLOGY
Mechanism of Action: A GI antispasmodic and anticholinergic agent that inhibits the action of acetylcholine at post-ganglionic (muscarinic) receptor sites. *Therapeutic Effect:* Decreases secretions (bronchial, salivary, sweat gland) and gastric juices and reduces motility of GI and urinary tract.

INDICATIONS AND DOSAGES
GI tract disorders
PO

Adults, Elderly, Children 12 yr and older. 0.125–0.25 mg q4h as needed. Extended-release: 0.375–0.75 mg q12h. Maximum: 1.5 mg/day.

Children 2-11 yr. 0.0625–0.125 mg q4h as needed. Extended-release: 0.375 mg q12h. Maximum: 0.75 mg/day.

IM, IV

Adults, Elderly, Children 12 yr and older. 0.25–0.5 mg q4h for 1–4 doses.

Hypermotility of lower urinary tract
PO, Sublingual

Adults, Elderly. 0.15–0.3 mg 4 times a day; or extended-release 0.375 mg q12h.

Infant colic
PO

Infants. Individualized drops dosed q4h as needed.

$ AVAILABLE FORMS/COST
• Cap, Gel, Sus Action—Oral: 0.375 mg, 100's: **$13.11-$133.50**

• Elixir—Oral: 0.125 mg/5 ml, 480 ml: **$11.45-$38.10**

• Sol, Inj-IM, IV, SC: 0.5 mg/ml, 1 ml: **$18.01**

• Tab-SL: 0.125 mg, 100's: **$4.37-$70.18**

• Tab-Oral: 0.125 mg, 100's: **$4.37-$72.80**; 0.15 mg, 100's: **$21.25-$47.81**

• Tab, Sus Action—Oral: 0.375 mg, 100's: **$13.88-$118.69**

CONTRAINDICATIONS: GI or GU obstruction, myasthenia gravis, narrow-angle glaucoma, paralytic ileus, severe ulcerative colitis

PREGNANCY AND LACTATION: Pregnancy category C; excreted in breast milk; infants sensitive to anticholinergics

SIDE EFFECTS
Frequent

Dry mouth (sometimes severe), decreased sweating, constipation

Occasional

Blurred vision; bloated feeling; urinary hesitancy; somnolence (with high dosage); headache; intolerance to light; loss of taste; nervousness; flushing; insomnia; impotence; mental confusion or excitement (particularly in the elderly and children); temporary light-headedness (with parenteral form); local irritation (with parenteral form)

Rare

Dizziness, faintness

SERIOUS REACTIONS
• Overdose may produce temporary paralysis of ciliary muscle; pupillary dilation; tachycardia; palpitations; hot, dry, or flushed skin; absence of bowel sounds; hyperthermia; increased respiratory rate; EKG abnormalities; nausea; vomiting; rash over face or upper trunk; CNS stimulation; and psychosis (marked by agitation, restlessness, rambling speech, visual hallucinations, paranoid behavior, and delusions, followed by depression).

---

ibandronate
Rx: Boniva
Chemical Class: Pyrophosphate analog
Therapeutic Class: Antiosteoporotic; bisphosphonate

CLINICAL PHARMACOLOGY
Mechanism of Action: A bisphosphonate that binds to bone hydroxyapatite (part of the mineral matrix of bone) and inhibits osteoclast activity. *Therapeutic Effect:*

Reduces rate of bone turnover and bone resorption, resulting in a net gain in bone mass.

Pharmacokinetics

Absorbed in the upper GI tract. Extent of absorption impaired by food or beverages (other than plain water). Rapidly binds to bone. Unabsorbed portion is eliminated in urine. Protein binding: 90%. **Half-life:** 10–60 hr.

INDICATIONS AND DOSAGES

Osteoporosis

PO

Adults, Elderly. 2.5 mg daily.

[$] **AVAILABLE FORMS/COST**

- Tab, Film-Coated—Oral: 2.5 mg, 90's: *Cost not available*

CONTRAINDICATIONS: Hypersensitivity to other bisphosphonates, including alendronate, etidronate, pamidronate, risedronate, and tiludronate; inability to stand or sit upright for at least 60 minutes; severe renal impairment with creatinine clearance less than 30 ml/min; uncorrected hypocalcemia

PREGNANCY AND LACTATION: Pregnancy category C; breast milk excretion unknown

SIDE EFFECTS

Frequent (13%–6%)

Back pain; dyspepsia, including epigastric distress and heartburn; peripheral discomfort; diarrhea; headache; myalgia

Occasional (4%–3%)

Dizziness, arthralgia, asthenia

Rare (2% or less)

Vomiting, hypersensitivity reaction

SERIOUS REACTIONS

- Upper respiratory tract infection occurs occasionally.
- Overdose causes hypocalcemia, hypophosphatemia, and significant GI disturbances

INTERACTIONS

Drugs

[3] *Antacids: calcium and other multivalent cations (aluminum, magnesium, iron):* Reduced absorption

[3] *Food (including coffee and juice):* Decreases bioavailability drastically (see pharmacokinetics)

[3] *Aspirin, nonsteroidal anti-inflammatory drugs:* Theoretical increased risk of gastropathy

Labs

- Decreases in alkaline phosphatase levels
- Bisphosphonate class effect — interference with the use of bone-imaging agents

SPECIAL CONSIDERATIONS

- Clinicians should remain alert to signs or symptoms signaling possible esophageal irritation reaction (dysphagia, retrosternal pain, or heartburn)

PATIENT/FAMILY EDUCATION

- To maximize absorption and clinical benefit, patients should be instructed to take drug at least 60 minutes before first food or drink of the day or other oral medications (particularly calcium, antacids or vitamins)
- To reduce potential for esophageal irritation, patients should be instructed to swallow tablets intact (not chew or suck) with a full glass of plain water (not mineral water) while remaining in the standing or sitting upright position for 60 minutes
- Patients should receive supplemental calcium and vitamin D if dietary intake is inadequate

MONITORING PARAMETERS

- Bone mass density (T-score, hip, spine), N-telopeptide; serum calcium (adjusted for hypoalbuminemia), phosphorus, magnesium, renal function, liver function, serum electrolytes, signs and symptoms of toxicity (*i.e.,* esophageal irritation)

---

ibuprofen
(eye-byoo′pro-fen)
Rx: Motrin, Ibuprohm, IBU, Rufen, Saleto
OTC: Arthritis Foundation Pain Reliever, Advil, Ibuprin, Motrin IB, Nuprin
Combinations
> **Rx:** with Hydrocodone (Vicoprofen); with oxycodone (Combunox)
> **OTC:** With pseudoephedrine (Sine-Aid IB, Motrin IB Sinus)

Chemical Class: Propionic acid derivative
Therapeutic Class: NSAID; antipyretic; nonnarcotic analgesic

CLINICAL PHARMACOLOGY
Mechanism of Action: An NSAID that inhibits prostaglandin synthesis. Also produces vasodilation by acting centrally on the heat-regulating center of the hypothalamus. *Therapeutic Effect:* Produces analgesic and anti-inflammatory effects and decreases fever.
Pharmacokinetics

Route	Onset	Peak	Duration
PO (analgesic)	0.5 hr	N/A	4–6 hr
PO (antirheumatic)	2 days	1–2 wk	N/A

Rapidly absorbed from the GI tract. Protein binding: greater than 90%. Metabolized in the liver. Primarily excreted in urine. Not removed by hemodialysis. **Half-life:** 2–4 hr.

INDICATIONS AND DOSAGES
Acute or chronic rheumatoid arthritis, osteoarthritis, migraine pain, gouty arthritis
PO
Adults, Elderly. 400–800 mg 3–4 times a day. Maximum: 3.2 g/day.
Mild to moderate pain, primary dysmenorrhea
PO
Adults, Elderly. 200–400 mg q4–6h as needed. Maximum: 1.6 g/day.
Fever, minor aches or pain
PO
Adults, Elderly. 200–400 mg q4–6h. Maximum: 1.6 g/day.
Children. 5–10 mg/kg/dose q6–8h. Maximum: 40 mg/kg/day. OTC: 7.5 mg/kg/dose q6–8h. Maximum: 30 mg/kg/day.
Juvenile arthritis
PO
Children. 30–70 mg/kg/day in 3–4 divided doses. Maximum: 400 mg/day in children weighing less than 20 kg, 600 mg/day in children weighing 20–30 kg, 800 mg/day in children weighing greater than 30–40 kg.

S AVAILABLE FORMS/COST
• Cap—Oral: 200 mg, 40's: **$6.12**
• Susp—Oral: 40 mg/5 ml, 15 ml: **$4.44-$4.97**; 100 mg/5 ml, 60, 120 ml: **$2.94-$13.85**
• Tab, Chewable—Oral: 50 mg, 24's: **$2.76-$3.29**; 100 mg, 100's: **$2.95-$4.58**
• Tab—Oral: 200 mg, 100's: **$1.75-$23.42**; 400 mg, 100's: **$3.95-$41.00**; 600 mg, 100's: **$4.35-$45.90**; 800 mg, 100's: **$6.25-$49.89**

UNLABELED USES: Treatment of psoriatic arthritis, vascular headaches

CONTRAINDICATIONS: Active peptic ulcer, chronic inflammation of GI tract, GI bleeding disorders or ulceration, history of hypersensitivity to aspirin or NSAIDs

PREGNANCY AND LACTATION: Pregnancy category B; reduces amniotic fluid volume, constriction of the ductus arteriosus in 3rd trimester; compatible with breast-feeding

SIDE EFFECTS

Occasional (9%–3%)

Nausea with or without vomiting, dyspepsia, dizziness, rash

Rare (less than 3%)

Diarrhea or constipation, flatulence, abdominal cramps or pain, pruritus

SERIOUS REACTIONS

• Acute overdose may result in metabolic acidosis.

• Rare reactions with long-term use include peptic ulcer disease, GI bleeding, gastritis, a severe hepatic reaction (cholestasis, jaundice), nephrotoxicity (dysuria, hematuria, proteinuria, nephrotic syndrome), and a severe hypersensitivity reaction (particularly in patients with systemic lupus erythematosus or other collagen diseases).

INTERACTIONS

Drugs

3 *Aminoglycosides:* Reduced clearance with elevated aminoglycoside levels and potential for toxicity (especially indomethacin in premature infants; other NSAIDs probably)

3 *Anticoagulants:* Excessive hypoprothrombinemia, decreased platelet aggregation with increased risk of GI bleeding

3 *Antihypertensives (α-blockers, angiotensin-converting enzyme inhibitors, angiotensin II receptor blockers, β-blockers, diuretics):* Inhibition of antihypertensive and other favorable hemodynamic effects

3 *Corticosteroids:* Increased risk of GI ulceration

3 *Cyclosporine:* Increased nephrotoxicity risk

3 *Lithium:* Decreased clearance of lithium (mediated via prostaglandins) resulting in elevated serum lithium levels and risk of toxicity

3 *Methotrexate:* Decreased renal secretion of methotrexate resulting in elevated methotrexate levels and risk of toxicity

3 *Phenylpropanolamine:* Possible acute hypertensive reaction

3 *Potassium-sparing diuretics:* Additive hyperkalemia potential

3 *Triamterene:* Acute renal failure reported with addition of indomethacin; caution with other NSAIDs

Labs

• *False decrease:* ALT, AST

SPECIAL CONSIDERATIONS

• Administer with food or antacids if GI symptoms occur

MONITORING PARAMETERS

• Initial hemogram and fecal occult blood test within 3 mo of starting regular chronic therapy; repeat every 6-12 mo (more frequently in high-risk patients, >65 years, peptic ulcer disease, concurrent steroids or anticoagulants); electrolytes, creatinine, and BUN within 3 mo of starting regular chronic therapy; repeat every 6-12 mo

ibutilide

(eye-byoo'ti-lide)

Rx: Corvert

Chemical Class: Methane-sulfonamide derivative

Therapeutic Class: Antiar-rhythmic, class III

CLINICAL PHARMACOLOGY

Mechanism of Action: An antiar-rhythmic that prolongs both atrial and ventricular action potential duration and increases the atrial and ventricular refractory period. Activates slow, inward current (mostly of sodium), produces mild slowing of sinus node rate and AV conduction, and causes dose-related prolongation of QT interval. *Therapeutic Effect:* Converts arrhythmias to sinus rhythm.

Pharmacokinetics

After IV administration, highly distributed, rapidly cleared. Protein binding: 40%. Primarily excreted in urine as metabolite. **Half-life:** 2–12 hr (average: 6 hrs).

INDICATIONS AND DOSAGES

Rapid conversion of atrial fibrillation or flutter of recent onset to normal sinus rhythm

IV infusion

Adults, Elderly weighing 60 kg or more. One vial (1 mg) given over 10 min. If arrhythmia does not stop within 10 min after end of initial infusion, a second 1 mg/10-min infusion may be given.

Adults, Elderly weighing less than 60 kg. 0.01 mg/kg given over 10 min. If arrhythmia does not stop within 10 min after end of initial infusion, a second 0.01 mg/kg, 10-min infusion may be given.

Ⓢ AVAILABLE FORMS/COST

• Sol—IV: 0.1 mg/ml, 10 ml: **$275.60**

CONTRAINDICATIONS: None known

PREGNANCY AND LACTATION: Pregnancy category C; excretion into breast milk unknown, breast-feeding not recommended

SIDE EFFECTS

Ibutilide is generally well tolerated.

Occasional

Ventricular extrasystoles (5.1%), ventricular tachycardia (4.9%), headache (3.6%), hypotension, orthostatic hypotension (2%)

Rare

Bundle-branch block, AV block, bradycardia, hypertension

SERIOUS REACTIONS

• Sustained polymorphic ventricular tachycardia, occasionally with QT prolongation (torsades de pointes) occurs rarely.

• Overdose results in CNS toxicity, including CNS depression, rapid gasping breathing, and seizures.

• Expect prolongation of repolarization may be exaggerated.

• Existing arrhythmias may worsen or new arrhythmias may develop.

INTERACTIONS

Drugs

❸ *Disopyramide, quinidine, procainamide, amiodarone, sotalol:* Potential to prolong refractoriness

❷ *Phenothiazines, tricyclic antidepressants, terfenadine, astemizole:* Increased potential for prodysrhythmia due to prolongation of QT interval

SPECIAL CONSIDERATIONS

MONITORING PARAMETERS

• Continuous ECG monitoring for at least 4 hr following infusion or until QTc returns to baseline (longer monitoring if dysrhythmic activity noted). Defibrillator must be available

imatinib
(im'a-tin-ib)
Rx: Gleevec
Chemical Class: Phenylaminopyrimidine derivative
Therapeutic Class: Antineoplastic

CLINICAL PHARMACOLOGY
Mechanism of Action: Inhibits Bcr-Abl tyrosine kinase, an enzyme created by the Philadelphia chromosome abnormality found in patients with chronic myeloid leukemia (CML). *Therapeutic Effect:* Suppresses tumor growth during the three stages of CML; blast crisis, accelerated phase, and chronic phase.

Pharmacokinetics
Well absorbed after PO administration. Binds to plasma proteins, particularly albumin. Metabolized in the liver. Eliminated mainly in the feces as metabolites. **Half-life:** 18 hr.

INDICATIONS AND DOSAGES
CML
PO
Adults, Elderly. 400 mg/day for patients in chronic-phase CML; 600 mg/day for patients in accelerated phase or blast crisis. May increase dosage from 400 to 600 mg/day for patients in chronic phase or from 600 to 800 mg (given as 300-400 mg twice a day) for patients in accelerated phase or blast crisis in the absence of a severe drug reaction or severe neutropenia or thrombocytopenia in the following circumstances: progression of the disease, failure to achieve a satisfactory hematologic response after 3 months or more of treatment, or loss of a previously achieved hematologic response.

Children. 260 mg/m^2 a day as a single daily dose or in 2 divided doses.

Ⓢ **AVAILABLE FORMS/COST**
• Cap—Oral: 100 mg, 120's: **$2,555.94**
• Tab—Oral: 100 mg, 100's: **$2,208.75**; 400 mg, 30's: **$2,650.51**
CONTRAINDICATIONS: Known hypersensitivity to imatinib
PREGNANCY AND LACTATION: Pregnancy category D, breast-feeding not recommended

SIDE EFFECTS
Frequent (68%-24%)
Nausea, diarrhea, vomiting, headache, fluid retention (periorbital, lower extremities), rash, musculoskeletal pain, muscle cramps, arthralgia
Occasional (23%-10%)
Abdominal pain, cough, myalgia, fatigue, fever, anorexia, dyspepsia, constipation, night sweats, pruritus
Rare (less than 10%)
Nasopharyngitis, petechiae, asthenia, epistaxis

SERIOUS REACTIONS
• Severe fluid retention (manifested as pleural effusion, pericardial effusion, pulmonary edema, and ascites) and hepatotoxicity occur rarely.
• Neutropenia and thrombocytopenia are expected responses to the drug.
• Respiratory toxicity, manifested as dyspnea and pneumonia, may occur.

INTERACTIONS
Drugs
③ *Ketoconazole, itraconazole, erythromycin, clarithromycin (CYP3A4 inhibitors):* Increased imatinib concentrations
③ *Simvastatin, cyclosporin, dihydropyridine calcium channel blockers, triazolo-benzodiazepines, pi-*

mozide (inhibition of CYP3A4 by imatinib): Increased concentrations of these drugs

3 *Phenytoin, dexamethasone, carbamezepine, rifampicin, phenobarbital, St. John's wort (CYP3A4 inducers):* Decreased imatinib concentrations

2 *Warfarin:* Altered metabolism of warfarin, use standard or low molecular weight heparin

2 *Acetaminophen:* Possible increased hepatotoxicity (single report of patient death)

SPECIAL CONSIDERATIONS
• Median time to hematologic response 1 month
• Manage fluid retention with interruption of therapy, diuretics, dose reduction
• If bilirubin increases >3 × upper limits normal (ULN) or transaminases >5 × ULN, withhold until bilirubin <1.5 × ULN and transaminases <2.5 × ULN; reduce dose and continue treatment
• If in chronic phase and ANC <1 × 10^9/L and/or platelets <50 × 10^9/L stop therapy until ANC = 1.5 × 10^9/L and platelets = 75 × 10^9/L, resume at reduced dose; if patient in accelerated phase or blast crisis, check if cytopenia related to leukemia
• There are no controlled trials in pediatric patients demonstrating a clinical benefit, such as improvement in disease related symptoms or increased survival

PATIENT/FAMILY EDUCATION
• Take with food and large glass of water to minimize GI side effects
• Avoid acetaminophen (hepatotoxicity)
• Numerous drugs may interact with imatinib, discuss with prescriber

MONITORING PARAMETERS
• Follow weights and monitor for fluid retention

• LFTs before treatment and q month, CBC, serum chemistry, bone marrow assessment (including cytogenic analysis)

---

imipenem-cilastatin
(i-me-pen'em sye-la-stat'in)
Rx: Primaxin
Chemical Class: Carbapenem; renal dipeptidase inhibitor (cilastatin); thienamycin derivative
Therapeutic Class: Antibiotic

CLINICAL PHARMACOLOGY
Mechanism of Action: A fixed-combination carbapenem. Imipenem penetrates the bacterial cell membrane and binds to penicillin-binding proteins, inhibiting cell wall synthesis. Cilastatin competitively inhibits the enzyme dehydropeptidase, preventing renal metabolism of imipenem. *Therapeutic Effect:* Produces bacterial cell death.

Pharmacokinetics
Readily absorbed after IM administration. Protein binding: 13%-21%. Widely distributed. Metabolized in the kidneys. Primarily excreted in urine. Removed by hemodialysis. **Half-life:** 1 hr (increased in impaired renal function).

INDICATIONS AND DOSAGES
Serious respiratory tract, skin and skin-structure, gynecologic, bone, joint, intraabdominal, nosocomial, and polymicrobic infections; UTIs; endocarditis; septicemia
IV
Adults, Elderly. 2-4 g/day in divided doses q6h.

Mild to moderate respiratory tract, skin and skin-structure, gynecologic, bone, joint, intraabdominal, and polymicrobic infections; UTIs; endocarditis; septicemia

IV

Adults, Elderly. 1-2 g/day in divided doses q6–8h.

Children older than 3 mo-12 yr. 60-100 mg/kg/day in divided doses q6h. Maximum: 4 g/day.

Children 1-3 mo. 100 mg/kg/day in divided doses q6h.

Children younger than 1 mo. 20-25 mg/kg/dose q8–24h.

IM

Adults, Elderly. 500-750 mg q12h.

Dosage in renal impairment

Dosage and frequency are modified based on creatinine clearance and the severity of the infection.

Creatinine Clearance	Dosage (IV)
31-70 ml/min	500 mg q8h
21-30 ml/min	500 mg q12h
5-20 ml/min	250 mg q12h

$ AVAILABLE FORMS/COST

• Powder, Inj-IM: 750 mg-750 mg/vial: **$43.20**
• Powder, Inj-IV: 250 mg-250 mg/vial: **$17.37**
• Powder, Inj-IV, IM: 500-500 mg/vial: **$32.69**

CONTRAINDICATIONS: None known.

PREGNANCY AND LACTATION: Pregnancy category C; unknown if excreted in breast milk

SIDE EFFECTS

Occasional (3%-2%)

Diarrhea, nausea, vomiting

Rare (2%-1%)

Rash

SERIOUS REACTIONS

• Antibiotic-associated colitis and other superinfections may occur.
• Anaphylactic reactions have been reported.

INTERACTIONS

Drugs

▨ *Cyclosporine, tacrolimus:* Risk of CNS toxicity

▨ *Theophylline:* Increased seizure risk without elevated theophylline levels

Labs

• *Interference:* Clindamycin, erythromycin, metronidazole, polymyxin, tetracycline, trimethoprim colistin levels

---

imipramine

Rx: Tofranil, Tofranil PM

Chemical Class: Dibenzazepine derivative; tertiary amine

Therapeutic Class: Antidepressant, tricyclic; antiincontinence agent

---

CLINICAL PHARMACOLOGY

Mechanism of Action: A tricyclic antidepressant, antibulimic, anticataplectic, antinarcoleptic, antineuralgic, antineuritic, and antipanic agent that blocks the reuptake of neurotransmitters, such as norepinephrine and serotonin, at presynaptic membranes, increasing their concentration at postsynaptic receptor sites. *Therapeutic Effect:* Relieves depression and controls nocturnal enuresis.

INDICATIONS AND DOSAGES

Depression

PO

Adults. Initially, 75-100 mg/day. May gradually increase to 300 mg/day for hospitalized patients, or 200 mg/day for outpatients; then reduce dosage to effective maintenance level, 50-150 mg/day.

Elderly. Initially, 10-25 mg/day at bedtime. May increase by 10-25 mg every 3-7 days. Range: 50-150 mg/day.

Children. 1.5 mg/kg/day. May increase by 1 mg/kg every 3-4 days. Maximum: 5 mg/kg/day.

Enuresis
PO
Children older than 6 yr.: Initially, 10-25 mg at bedtime. May increase by 25 mg/day. Maximum: 50 mg for children older than 12 yr.

$ AVAILABLE FORMS/COST
• Cap, Gel—Oral (pamoate): 75 mg, 100's: **$563.71**; 100 mg, 100's: **$563.71**; 125 mg, 100's: **$426.34**; 150 mg, 100's: **$563.71**
• Tab-Oral: 10 mg, 100's: **$3.25-$119.86**; 25 mg, 100's: **$4.50-$200.24**; 50 mg, 100's: **$5.75-$340.06**

UNLABELED USES: Treatment of attention-deficit hyperactivity disorder, cataplexy associated with narcolepsy, neurogenic pain, panic disorder

CONTRAINDICATIONS: Acute recovery period after MI, use within 14 days of MAOIs

PREGNANCY AND LACTATION: Pregnancy category C

SIDE EFFECTS
Frequent
Somnolence, fatigue, dry mouth, blurred vision, constipation, delayed micturition, orthostatic hypotension, diaphoresis, impaired concentration, increased appetite, urine retention, photosensitivity.
Occasional
GI disturbances (nausea, metallic taste).
Rare
Paradoxical reactions, (agitation, restlessness, nightmares, insomnia), extrapyramidal symptoms (particularly fine hand tremor).

SERIOUS REACTIONS
• Overdose may produce seizures; cardiovascular effects, such as severe orthostatic hypotension, dizziness, tachycardia, palpitations, and arrhythmias; and altered temperature regulation, including hyperpyrexia or hypothermia.

• Abrupt discontinuation after prolonged therapy may produce headache, malaise, nausea, vomiting, and vivid dreams.

INTERACTIONS
Drugs
▣ *Altretamine:* Orthostatic hypotension
▣ *Amphetamines:* Theoretical increase in amphetamine effect
▣ *Antidiabetics:* Possible enhanced hypoglycemic effects
❷ *Bethanidine, clonidine:* Inhibition of antihypertensive effect, possible hypertensive crisis
▣ *Carbamazepine, cholestyramine, colestipol, barbiturates:* Reduces imipramine levels
❷ *Epinephrine, norepinephrine:* Hypertension and dysrhythmias
▣ *Ethanol:* Enhanced motor skill impairment
▣ *Guanethidine, guanfacine:* Inhibition of antihypertensive effect
▣ *Isoproterenol and possibly other β-agonists:* Increased risk of arrhythmias
▣ *Lithium:* Possible increased CNS toxicity, especially in elderly
⚠ *MAOIs:* Serotonin syndrome, some fatal
❷ *Moclobemide:* Risk serotonin syndrome
▣ *Phenothiazines, cimetidine (not with other H_2 blockers), calcium channel blockers, selective serotonin reuptake inhibitors, quinidine, ritonavir, indinavir:* Increased imipramine levels
▣ *Phenylephrine:* Enhanced pressor response
▣ *Propantheline:* Excessive anticholinergic effects
Labs
• *False increase:* Carbamazepine levels
• *False decrease:* Urine 5-HIAA, VMA

SPECIAL CONSIDERATIONS
PATIENT/FAMILY EDUCATION
• Withdrawal symptoms (headache, nausea, vomiting, muscle pain, weakness) may occur if drug discontinued abruptly
• At doses of 20 mg/kg ventricular arrhythmias occur

---

imiquimod
(im-ick'wih-mod)
Rx: Aldara
Chemical Class: Imidazoquinoline amine
Therapeutic Class: Antiviral

CLINICAL PHARMACOLOGY
Mechanism of Action: An immune response modifier whose mechanism of action is uknown. *Therapeutic Effect:* Reduces genital and perianal warts.
Pharmacokinetics
Minimal absorption after topical administration. Minimal excretion in urine and feces.

INDICATIONS AND DOSAGES
Warts/condyloma acuminata
Topical
Adults, Elderly, Children 12 yrs and older. Apply 3 times/wk before normal sleeping hours; leave on skin 6-10 hrs. Remove following treatment period. Continue therapy for maximum of 16 weeks.

AVAILABLE FORMS/COST
• Cre—Topical: 5%, 250 mg/single-use packet, 12's: **$148.50**
CONTRAINDICATIONS: History of hypersensitivity to imiquimod
PREGNANCY AND LACTATION: Pregnancy category B; excretion into breast milk unknown but would be expected to be small given minimal systemic absorption

SIDE EFFECTS
Frequent
Local skin reactions: erythema, itching, burning, erosion, excoriation /flaking, fungal infections (women)
Occasional
Pain, induration, ulceration, scabbing, soreness, headache, flulike symptoms
SERIOUS REACTIONS
• None reported.
SPECIAL CONSIDERATIONS
• New option for treatment of genital and perianal warts which can be applied by patient at home and appears to have low toxicity compared to podofilox
• Response rates approximately 50% and relapses are common
PATIENT/FAMILY EDUCATION
• Apply thin layer to wart(s) and rub in until cream is no longer visible
• Do not occlude application site
• Should severe local reaction occur, remove cream by washing with soap and water; treatment may be resumed once skin reaction has subsided

---

inamrinone lactate
(in-am'-ri-nohn)
Chemical Class: Bipyridine derivative
Therapeutic Class: Cardiac inotropic agent

CLINICAL PHARMACOLOGY
Mechanism of Action: A positive inotropic agent that inhibits myocardial myocardial cyclic adenosine monophosphate (cAMP) phosphodiesterase activity and directly stimulates cardiac contractility. Peripheral vasodilation reduces both

preload and afterload. *Therapeutic Effect:* Reduces preload and afterload; increases cardiac output.

Pharmacokinetics

After IV administration, rapidly absorbed from the gastrointestinal (GI) tract. Protein binding: 10-49%. Partially metabolized in liver. Excreted in urine as both inamrinone and its metabolites. **Half-life:** 3-6 hrs (half-life increased with congestive heart failure).

INDICATIONS AND DOSAGES

Short-term management of intractable heart failure

IV infusion (continuous)

Adults. Initially, 0.75 mg/kg loading dose over 2-3 minutes followed by a maintenance infusion of 5 and 10 mcg/kg/min. A bolus dose of 0.75 mg/kg may be given 30 minutes after the initiation of therapy. Use within 24 hours and do not dilute with solutions that contain dextrose. Maximum: 10 mg/kg/day.

§   AVAILABLE FORMS/COST

• Sol, Inj-IV: 5 mg/ml, 20 ml vial: **$61.75-$88.75**

CONTRAINDICATIONS: Severe aortic or pulmonic valvular disease; hypersensitivity to inamrinone or bisulfites.

PREGNANCY AND LACTATION: Pregnancy category C

SIDE EFFECTS

Occasional

Arrhythmia, nausea, hypotension, thrombocytopenia

Rare

Fever, vomiting, abdominal pain, anorexia, chest pain, decreased tear production hepatotoxicity, and burning at the site of injection, hypersensitivity to inamrinone

SERIOUS REACTIONS

• Overdose may cause severe hypotension.

INTERACTIONS

Drugs

• *Furosemide:* Precipitates when furosemide is injected into an IV line infusing inamrinone

Labs

• *Increase:* Serum digoxin (Abbott TdX method)

MONITORING PARAMETERS

• BP and pulse q5 min during infusion; if BP drops 30 mm Hg, stop infusion

• Cardiac output and pulmonary capillary wedge pressure

• Monitor platelet count and serum K, Na, Cl, Ca, BUN, creatinine, ALT, AST, and bilirubin daily

---

indapamide

(in-dap′a-mide)

Rx: Lozol

Chemical Class: Indoline derivative

Therapeutic Class: Antihypertensive; diuretic, thiazide-like

CLINICAL PHARMACOLOGY

Mechanism of Action: A thiazide-like diuretic that blocks reabsorption of water, sodium, and potassium at the cortical diluting segment of the distal tubule; also reduces plasma and extracellular fluid volume and peripheral vascular resistance by direct effect on blood vessels. *Therapeutic Effect:* Promotes diuresis and reduces BP.

INDICATIONS AND DOSAGES

Edema

PO

Adults. Initially, 2.5 mg/day, may increase to 5 mg/day after 1 wk.

Hypertension

PO

Adults, Elderly. Initially, 1.25 mg, may increase to 2.5 mg/day after 4

wk or 5 mg/day after additional 4 wk.

$ AVAILABLE FORMS/COST

• Tab-Oral: 1.25 mg, 100's: **$61.40-$99.16**; 2.5 mg, 100's: **$73.12-$101.84**

CONTRAINDICATIONS: None known.

PREGNANCY AND LACTATION: Pregnancy category B; therapy for preexisting hypertension can be continued throughout pregnancy with minimal risk; initiating for edema not recommended; few unequivocal indications for diuretic therapy in pregnancy except for pulmonary edema or congestive heart failure; not known if excreted in breast milk

SIDE EFFECTS

Frequent (5% and greater)
Fatigue, numbness of extremities, tension, irritability, agitation, headache, dizziness, light-headedness, insomnia, muscle cramps
Occasional (less than 5%)
Tingling of extremities, urinary frequency, urticaria, rhinorrhea, flushing, weight loss, orthostatic hypotension, depression, blurred vision, nausea, vomiting, diarrhea or constipation, dry mouth, impotence, rash, pruritus

SERIOUS REACTIONS

• Vigorous diuresis may lead to profound water and electrolyte depletion, resulting in hypokalemia, hyponatremia, and dehydration.
• Acute hypotensive episodes may occur.
• Hyperglycemia may occur during prolonged therapy.
• Pancreatitis, blood dyscrasias, pulmonary edema, allergic pneumonitis, and dermatologic reactions occur rarely.
• Overdose can lead to lethargy and coma without changes in electrolytes or hydration.

INTERACTIONS

Drugs

❷ *Angiotensin-converting enzyme inhibitors:* Risk of postural hypotension when added to ongoing diuretic therapy; more common with loop diuretics; first dose hypotension possible in patients with sodium depletion or hypovolemia due to diuretics or sodium restriction; hypotensive response is usually transient; hold diuretic day of first dose

❸ *Corticosteroids:* Concomitant therapy may result in excessive potassium loss

❸ *Diazoxide:* Blunt insulin secretion; results in hyperglycemia

❸ *Lithium:* Concurrent use may result in elevated serum levels of lithium; monitor carefully

❸ *Nonsteroidal antiinflammatory drugs:* Concurrent may reduce diuretic and antihypertensive effects

SPECIAL CONSIDERATIONS

PATIENT/FAMILY EDUCATION

• May cause sensitivity to sunlight; avoid prolonged exposure to the sun and other ultraviolet light
• May cause gout attacks; notify clinician if sudden joint pain occurs
• May worsen control or increase requirements of hypoglycemic agents

MONITORING PARAMETERS

• Weight, urine output, serum electrolytes, BUN, creatinine, CBC, uric acid, glucose, lipids

indinavir

(in-din'ah-veer)

Rx: Crixivan

Chemical Class: Protease inhibitor, HIV

Therapeutic Class: Antiretroviral

CLINICAL PHARMACOLOGY

Mechanism of Action: A protease inhibitor that suppresses HIV protease, an enzyme necessary for splitting viral polyprotein precursors into mature and infectious viral particles. *Therapeutic Effect:* Interrupts HIV replication, slowing the progression of HIV infection.

Pharmacokinetics

Rapidly absorbed after PO administration. Protein binding: 60%. Metabolized in the liver. Primarily excreted in urine. Unknown if removed by hemodialysis. **Half-life:** 1.8 hr (increased in impaired hepatic function).

INDICATIONS AND DOSAGES

HIV infection (in combination with other antiretrovirals)

PO

Adults. 800 mg (two 400-mg capsules) q8h.

HIV infection in patients with hepatic insufficiency

PO

Adults. 600 mg q8h.

$ **AVAILABLE FORMS/COST**

• Cap—Oral: 200 mg, 270's: **$375.98**; 333 mg, 135's: **$341.14**; 400 mg, 180's: **$546.37**

UNLABELED USES: Prophylaxis following occupational exposure to HIV

CONTRAINDICATIONS: Hypersensitivity to indinavir; nephrolithiasis

PREGNANCY AND LACTATION: Pregnancy category C; not recommended for breast-feeding mothers

SIDE EFFECTS

Frequent

Nausea (12%), abdominal pain (9%), headache (6%), diarrhea (5%)

Occasional

Vomiting, asthenia, fatigue (4%); insomnia; accumulation of fat in waist, abdomen, or back of neck

Rare

Abnormal taste sensation, heartburn, symptomatic urinary tract disease, transient renal dysfunction

SERIOUS REACTIONS

• Nephrolithiasis (flank pain with or without hematuria) occurs in 4% of patients.

INTERACTIONS

Drugs

[3] *Barbiturates:* Increased clearance of indinavir; reduced clearance of barbiturates

[2] *Carbamazepine:* Increased clearance of indinavir; reduced clearance of carbamazepine

⚠ *Cisapride:* Increased plasma levels of cisapride

[3] *Clarithromycin:* Indinavir reduces clearance of clarithromycin

[3] *Delavirdine:* Decreased clearance of indinavir; reduce dose of indinavir to 600 mg q8h

[2] *Efavirenz:* Reduced indinavir level; increase indinavir dose to 1000 mg q8h

⚠ *Ergot alkaloids:* Increased plasma levels of ergot alkaloids

[3] *Erythromycin:* Reduced clearance of indinavir; indinavir reduces clearance of erythromycin

[3] *Ketoconazole:* Decreased clearance of indinavir; decrease indinavir dose to 600 mg tid

⚠ *Lovastatin:* Indinavir reduces clearance of lovastatin

⚠ *Midazolam:* Increased plasma levels of midazolam and prolonged effect

🔳 *Nelfinavir:* Decreased clearance of indinavir; reduce dose of indinavir to 1200 mg bid

🔳 *Nevirapine:* Reduces plasma indinavir levels; no dose adjustment needed

🔳 *Oral contraceptives:* Indinavir may reduce efficacy

🔳 *Phenytoin:* Increased clearance of indinavir; reduced clearance of phenytoin

❷ *Rifabutin:* Increased clearance of indinavir; reduced clearance of rifabutin—reduce rifabutin dose to 150 mg qday and increase indinavir dose to 1000 mg tid

⚠ *Rifampin:* Increased clearance of indinavir

🔳 *Ritonavir:* Decreased clearance of indinavir; decrease indinavir dose to 400 mg bid

🔳 *Saquinavir:* Decreased clearance of saquinavir; reduce dose of Fortovase (saquinavir soft gel capsule) to 800 mg tid

⚠ *Simvastatin:* Indinavir reduces clearance of simvastatin

⚠ *Terfenadine:* Increased plasma levels of terfenadine

⚠ *Triazolam:* Increased plasma levels of triazolam and prolonged effect

🔳 *Troleandomycin:* Reduced clearance of indinavir; indinavir reduces clearance of troleandomycin

SPECIAL CONSIDERATIONS

• Antiretroviral activity of indinavir may be increased when used in combination with reverse transcriptase inhibitors

PATIENT/FAMILY EDUCATION

• Drink plenty of water, at least 48 oz/day

• Take with water or light, low-fat meals (dry toast, apple juice, corn flakes, skim milk). High fat meals and grapefruit juice reduce absorption

• Capsules sensitive to moisture. Keep dessicant in bottle

• If dose is missed take next dose on schedule; do not double this dose

• Separate dosing with didanosine by 1 hour

• Take 1 hr before or 2 hr after meals; may take with skim milk or low-fat meal

indomethacin
(in-doe-meth′a-sin)

Rx: Indocin, Indocin IV, Indocin SR, Indochron, Indo-Lemmon
Chemical Class: Indole acetic acid derivative
Therapeutic Class: NSAID; antipyretic; nonnarcotic analgesic

CLINICAL PHARMACOLOGY
Mechanism of Action: An NSAID that produces analgesic and anti-inflammatory effects by inhibiting prostaglandin synthesis. Also increases the sensitivity of the premature ductus to the dilating effects of prostaglandins. *Therapeutic Effect:* Reduces the inflammatory response and intensity of pain. Closure of the patent ductus arteriosus.

INDICATIONS AND DOSAGES
Moderate to severe rheumatoid arthritis, osteoarthritis, ankylosing spondylitis
PO
Adults, Elderly. Initially, 25 mg 2–3 times a day; increased by 25–50 mg/wk up to 150–200 mg/day. Or 75 mg/day (extended-release) up to 75 mg twice a day.

Children. 1–2 mg/kg/day. Maximum: 150–200 mg/day.

Acute gouty arthritis
PO
Adults, Elderly. Initially, 100 mg, then 50 mg 3 times a day.

Acute shoulder pain
PO
Adults, Elderly. 75–150 mg/day in 3–4 divided doses.

Usual rectal dosage
Adults, Elderly. 50 mg 4 times a day.
Children. Initially, 1.5–2.5 mg/kg/day, increased up to 4 mg/kg/day. Maximum: 150–200 mg/day.

Patent ductus arteriosus
IV
Neonates. Initially, 0.2 mg/kg. Subsquent doses are based on age, as follows:
Neonates older than 7 days. 0.25 mg/kg for 2nd and 3rd doses.
Neonates 2–7 days. 0.2 mg/kg for 2nd and 3rd doses.
Neonates less than 48 hr. 0.1 mg/kg for 2nd and 3rd doses.

$ AVAILABLE FORMS/COST
• Cap, Gel—Oral: 25 mg, 100's: **$6.50-$67.46**; 50 mg, 100's: **$7.50-$110.14**
• Cap, Gel, Sus Action—Oral: 75 mg, 100's: **$64.13-$193.00**
• Powder, Inj-IV: 1 mg/vial: **$32.40**
• Supp—Rect: 50 mg, 30's: **$46.20-$49.90**
• Susp—Oral: 25 mg/5 ml, 237, 500 ml: **$50.65**/237 ml

UNLABELED USES: Treatment of fever due to malignancy, pericarditis, psoriatic arthritis, rheumatic complications associated with Paget's disease of bone, vascular headache

CONTRAINDICATIONS: Active GI bleeding or ulcerations; hypersensitivity to aspirin, indomethacin, or other NSAIDs; renal impairment, thrombocytopenia

PREGNANCY AND LACTATION: Pregnancy category B; crosses placenta; excreted in breast milk

SIDE EFFECTS
Frequent (11%–3%)
Headache, nausea, vomiting, dyspepsia, dizziness
Occasional (less than 3%)
Depression, tinnitus, diaphoresis, somnolence, constipation, diarrhea, bleeding disturbances in patent ductus arteriosus
Rare
Hypertension, confusion, urticaria, pruritus, rash, blurred vision

SERIOUS REACTIONS
• Paralytic ileus and ulceration of the esophagus, stomach, duodenum, or small intestine may occur.
• Patients with impaired renal function may develop hyperkalemia and worsening of renal impairment.
• Indomethacin use may aggravate epilepsy, parkinsonism, and depression or other psychiatric disturbances.
• Nephrotoxicity, including dysuria, hematuria, proteinuria, and nephrotic syndrome, occurs rarely.
• Metabolic acidosis or alkalosis, apnea, and bradycardia occur rarely in patients with patent ductus arteriosus.

INTERACTIONS
Drugs
3 *Aminoglycosides:* Reduced clearance with elevated aminoglycoside levels and potential for toxicity (especially indomethacin in premature infants; other NSAIDs probably)
3 *Anticoagulants:* Excessive hypoprothrombinemia, decreased platelet aggregation with increased risk of GI bleeding
3 *Antihypertensives (α-blockers, angiotensin-converting enzyme inhibitors, angiotensin II receptor blockers, β-blockers, diuretics:* In-

hibition of antihypertensive and other favorable hemodynamic effects

[3] *Corticosteroids:* Increased risk of GI ulceration

[3] *Cyclosporine:* Increased nephrotoxicity risk

[3] *Lithium:* Decreased clearance of lithium (mediated via prostaglandins) resulting in elevated serum lithium levels and risk of toxicity

[3] *Methotrexate:* Decreased renal secretion of methotrexate resulting in elevated methotrexate levels and risk of toxicity

[3] *Phenylpropanolamine:* Possible acute hypertensive reaction

[3] *Potassium-sparing diuretics:* Additive hyperkalemia potential

[3] *Triamterene:* Acute renal failure reported with addition of indomethacin; caution with other NSAIDs

SPECIAL CONSIDERATIONS
PATIENT/FAMILY EDUCATION
• Take with food
• No significant advantage over other oral NSAIDs; cost and clinical situation should govern use

MONITORING PARAMETERS
• Renal and hepatic function with prolonged use: check after 3 months, then q6-12 months
• Initial CBC and fecal occult blood test within 3 months of starting regular chronic therapy; repeat q6-12 months (more frequently in high-risk patients)

infliximab
(in-flicks'ih-mab)

Rx: Remicade
Chemical Class: Monoclonal antibody
Therapeutic Class: Tumor necrosis factor α (TNF-α) antibody

CLINICAL PHARMACOLOGY
Mechanism of Action: A monoclonal antibody that binds to tumor necrosis factor (TNF), inhibiting functional activity of TNF. Reduces infiltration of inflammatory cells. *Therapeutic Effect:* Decreases inflamed areas of the intestine.

Pharmacokinetics

Route	Onset	Peak	Duration
IV (Crohn's disease)	1–2 wk	N/A	8–48 wk
IV (Rheumatoid arthritis [RA])	3–7 days	N/A	6–12 wk

Absorbed into the GI tissue; primarily distributed in the vascular compartment. **Half-life:** 9.5 days.

INDICATIONS AND DOSAGES
Moderate to severe Crohn's disease
IV infusion
Adults, Elderly. 5 mg/kg as a single IV infusion.

Fistulizing Crohn's disease
IV infusion
Adults, Elderly. Initially, 5 mg/kg followed by additional 5-mg/kg doses at 2 and 6 wk after first infusion.

RA
IV infusion
Adults, Elderly. 3 mg/kg; followed by additional doses at 2 and 6 wk after first infusion: Then q8wk.

$ AVAILABLE FORMS/COST
• Sol, Inj-IV: 100 mg/20 ml vial: **$691.61**

UNLABELED USES: Ankylosing spondylitis, sciatica

CONTRAINDICATIONS: Sensitivity to infliximab or murine proteins, sepsis, serious active infection

PREGNANCY AND LACTATION: Pregnancy category B; breast milk excretion unknown; nursing not recommended

SIDE EFFECTS
Frequent (22%–10%)
Headache, nausea, fatigue, fever
Occasional (9%–5%)
Fever or chills during infusion, pharyngitis, vomiting, pain, dizziness, bronchitis, rash, rhinitis, cough, pruritus, sinusitis, myalgia, back pain
Rare (4%–1%)
Hypotension or hypertension, paresthesia, anxiety, depression, insomnia, diarrhea, urinary tract infection

SERIOUS REACTIONS
• Hypersensitivity reaction and lupus-like syndrome may occur.

INTERACTIONS
Drugs
• *Live virus vaccines:* No information on vaccine response or secondary transmission of infection

SPECIAL CONSIDERATIONS
• Evaluate for risk of TB (TB skin test) prior to initiating therapy

PATIENT/FAMILY EDUCATION
• More susceptible to infections; avoid crowds, people with URI, flu, etc.

MONITORING PARAMETERS
• Decreased levels of serum IL-6, C-reactive protein, ESR, rheumatoid factor, signs and symptoms of disease, urinalysis, blood chemistry, human anti-cA2 titers, blood pressure (during and after infusion), temperature, body weight, signs and symptoms of infection (including TB)

---

insulin

Rx: *RAPID-ACTING: Insulin Analogs:* Apidra (Glulisine), Humalog (Lispro), NovoLog (Aspart)

Rx: *LONG-ACTING: Insulin Analog:* Lantus (Glargine)

Rx: *REGULAR CONCENTRATED INSULIN:* Humulin RU-500, Regular Iletin II U-500 (Pork)

OTC: *RAPID-ACTING: Regular Insulin* Humulin R, Regular Iletin II (Pork), Novolin R, Velosulin

OTC: *INTERMEDIATE ACTING: Insulin-Zinc Suspension:* Humulin L, Iletin II Lente (Pork)

OTC: *INTERMEDIATE ACTING: Isophane-Insulin Suspension (NPH):* Humulin N, Iletin II NPH (Pork), Novolin N

OTC: *LONG-ACTING: Extended Insulin-Zinc Suspension:* Humulin-U

Rx: *INSULIN MIXTURES: Isophane and Regular:* Humalog Mix 50/50, Humalog Mix 75/25, NovoLog Mix 70/30

OTC: *INSULIN MIXTURES: Isophane and Regular:* Humulin 50/50, Humulin 70/30, Novolin 70/30

Chemical Class: Exogenous insulin

Therapeutic Class: Antidiabetic; hypoglycemic

CLINICAL PHARMACOLOGY
Mechanism of Action: An exogenous insulin that facilitates passage

of glucose, potassium, and magnesium across the cellular membranes of skeletal and cardiac muscle and adipose tissue. Controls storage and metabolism of carbohydrates, protein, and fats. Promotes conversion of glucose to glycogen in the liver. *Therapeutic Effect:* Controls glucose levels in diabetic patients.

Pharmacokinetics

Drug Form	Onset (hr)	Peak (hr)	Duration (hr)
Lispro	0.25	0.5-1.5	4-5
Insulin aspart	1/6	1-3	3-5
Regular	0.5-1	2-4	5-7
NPH	1-2	6-14	24+
Lente	1-3	6-14	24+
Insulin glargine	N/A	N/A	24

INDICATIONS AND DOSAGES

Treatment of insulin-dependent type 1 diabetes mellitus and non-insulin-dependent type 2 diabetes mellitus when diet or weight control has failed to maintain satisfactory blood glucose levels or in event of fever, infection, pregnancy, surgery, or trauma, or severe endocrine, hepatic or renal dysfunction; emergency treatment of ketoacidosis (regular insulin); to promote passage of glucose across cell membrane in hyperalimentation (regular insulin): to facilitate intracellular shift of potassium in hyperkalemia (regular insulin)

Subcutaneous

Adults, Elderly, Children. 0.5-1 unit/kg/day.

Adolescents (during growth spurt). 0.8-1.2 unit/kg/day.

S **AVAILABLE FORMS/COST**

Rapid-Acting Insulin Analog

• Sol, Inj—SC: 100 U/ml, 10 ml (Lispro): **$66.95**; 100 U/ml, 10 ml (Aspart): **$66.95**

Long-Acting Insulin Analog

• Sol, Inj—SC: 100 U/ml, 10 ml (Glargine): **$55.83**

Rapid-Acting Regular Insulin

• Sol, Inj—IM, IV, SC: 100 U/ml 10 ml, (human): **$24.10-$30.50**; (pork): **$46.13-$49.98**

Intermediate-Acting Insulin-Zinc Suspension

• Susp, Inj—SC: 100 U/ml, 10 ml (human): **$30.50**; 100 U/ml, 10 ml (pork): **$47.98**

Isophane Insulin Suspension (NPH)

• Susp, Inj—SC: 100 U/ml, 10 ml: **$24.10-$30.50**

Long-Acting Insulin-Zinc Suspension

• Susp, Inj—SC: 100 U/ml, 10 ml: **$30.50**

Mixed Insulin 70/30 (NPH/Regular)

• Sol, Inj—SC: 100 U/ml, 10 ml: **$24.10-$30.50**

Mixed Insulin 50/50 (NPH/Regular)

• Susp, Inj—SC: 50 U/ml, 10 ml: **$30.50**

Mixed Insulin 70/30 (Aspart Protamine/Aspart)

• Susp, Inj—SC: 100 U/ml, 10 ml: **$66.95**

Mixed Insulin 75/25 (Lispro Protamine/Lispro)

• Susp, Inj—SC: 100 U/ml, 10 ml: **$66.95**

Mixed Insulin 50/50 (Lispro Protamine/Lispro)

• Susp, Inj—SC: 100 U/ml, 3 ml: **$17.53**

Concentrated Regular Insulin

• Sol, Inj—SC: 500 U/ml, 20 ml: **$219.46**

CONTRAINDICATIONS: Hypersensitivity or insulin resistance may require change of type or species source of insulin

PREGNANCY AND LACTATION:
Pregnancy category B; insulin requirements of pregnant diabetic patients often decreased in first half and increased in the latter half of pregnancy; elevated blood glucose levels associated with congenital abnormalities; does not pass into breast milk

SIDE EFFECTS

Occasional

Localized redness, swelling, and itching caused by improper injection technique or allergy to cleansing solution or insulin

Infrequent

Somogyi effect, including rebound hyperglycemia with chronically excessive insulin dosages: systemic allergic reaction, marked by rash, angioedema, and anaphylaxis; lipodystrophy or depression at injection site due to breakdown of adipose tissue; lipohypertrophy or accumulation of subcutaneous tissue at injection site due to inadequate site rotation

Rare

Insulin resistance

SERIOUS REACTIONS

• Severe hypoglycemia caused by hyperinsulinism may occur with insulin overdose, decrease or delay of food intake, or excessive exercise and in those with brittle diabetes.

• Diabetic ketoacidosis may result from stress, illness, omission of insulin dose, or long-term poor insulin control.

INTERACTIONS

Drugs

▣ β-*blockers:* Increased glucose levels, hypoglycemia symptoms masked (except sweating)

▣ *Cigarette smoking, marijuana, corticosteroids, thiazides:* Increased glucose levels

▣ *Clonidine, Guanfacine, Guanabenz:* Hypoglycemia symptoms masked

⚠ *Ethanol (excessive):* Hypoglycemia

▣ *Salicylates, ACE inhibitors, anabolic steroids, MAO inhibitors:* Enhanced hypoglycemic response

SPECIAL CONSIDERATIONS

PATIENT/FAMILY EDUCATION

• Symptoms of hypoglycemia include: fatigue, weakness, confusion, headache, convulsions, hunger, nausea, pallor, sweating, rapid breathing

• For hypoglycemia, give 1 mg glucagon, glucose 25 g IV (via dextrose 50% sol, 50 ml) or oral glucose if tolerated

• When mixing insulins, draw up short-acting first

• Dosage adjustment may be necessary when changing insulin products

• Human insulin considered insulin of choice secondary to antigenicity of animal insulins

---

interferon alfa-2a/2b

Rx: Roferon-A (alfa-2a), Intron-A (alfa-2b)
Combinations
   Rx: Interferon alfa 2b with ribavirin (Rebetron Combination Therapy)
Chemical Class: Recombinant interferon
Therapeutic Class: Antineoplastic; antiviral

CLINICAL PHARMACOLOGY

Mechanism of Action: A biologic response modifier that inhibits viral replication in virus-infected cells.

Therapeutic Effect: Suppresses cell proliferation; increases phagocytic action of macrophages; augments specific lymphocytic cell toxicity.

Pharmacokinetics

Interferon alfa-2a

Well absorbed after IM, subcutaneous administration. Undergoes proteolytic degradation during reabsorption in kidney. **Half-life:** IM: 2 hrs; Subcutaneous: 3 hrs.

Interferon alfa-2b

Well absorbed after IM, subcutaneous administration. Undergoes proteolytic degradation during reabsorption in kidney. **Half-life:** 2-3 hrs.

INDICATIONS AND DOSAGES

Hairy cell leukemia

Interferon alfa-2a

Subcutaneous/IM

Adults. Initially, 3 million units/day for 16- 24 wks. Maintenance: 3 million units 3 times/wk. Do not use 36-million-unit vial.

Interferon alfa-2b

Subcutaneous/IM

Adults. 2 million units/m2 3 times/wk. If severe adverse reactions occur, modify dose or temporarily discontinue.

Chronic myelocytic leukemia (CML)

Interferon alfa-2a

Subcutaneous/IM

Adults. 9 million units daily.

Condylomata acuminate

Interferon alfa-2b

Intralesional

Adults. 1 million units/lesion 3 times/wk for 3 wks. Use only 10-million-units vial, reconstitute with no more than 1 ml diluent. Use tuberculin (TB) syringe with 25- or 26-gauge needle. Give in evening with acetaminophen, which alleviates side effects.

Melanoma

Interferon alfa-2a

Subcutaneous/IM

Adults, Elderly. 12 million units/m2 3 times/wk for 3 mos.

Interferon alfa-2b

IV

Adults. Initially, 20 million units/m2 5 times/wk for 4 wks. Maintenance: 10 million units IM/Subcutaneous for 48 wks.

AIDS-related Kaposi's sarcoma

Interferon alfa-2a

Subcutaneous/IM

Adults. Initially, 36 million units/day for 10- 12 wks, may give 3 million units on day 1; 9 million units on day 2; 18 million units on day 3; then begin 36 million units/day for remainder of 10- 12 wks. Maintenance: 36 million units/day 3 times/wk.

Interferon alfa-2b

Subcutaneous/IM

Adults. 30 million units/m2 3 times/wk. Use only 50 million units vials. If severe adverse reactions occur, modify dose or temporarily discontinue.

Chronic hepatitis B

Interferon alfa-2b

Subcutaneous/IM

Adults. 30- 35 million units/wk, 5 million units/day or 10 million units 3 times/wk.

Chronic hepatitis C

Interferon alfa-2a

Subcutaneous/IM

Adults. Initially, 6 million units once a day for 3 wks, then 3 million units 3 times/wk for 6 mos.

Interferon alfa-2b Subcutaneous/IM

Adults. 3 million units 3 times/wk for up to 6 mos, for up to 18-24 mos for chronic hepatitis C.

AVAILABLE FORMS/COST

Interferon alfa-2a

• Sol, Inj-IM, SC: 3 million IU/vial: **$38.25**; 6 million IU/vial: **$76.48**; 9 million IU/vial: **$107.68**; 36 million IU/vial: **$419.26**

Interferon alfa-2b

• Powder, Inj-IM, SC, IV: 3 million IU/vial: **$35.63**; 5 million IU/vial: **$71.04**; 10 million IU/vial: **$163.10**; 18 million IU/vial: **$293.61**; 25 million IU/vial: **$355.25**; 50 million IU/vial: **$815.64**; 60 million IU/vial: **$293.61**

UNLABELED USES: Interferon alfa-2a

Treatment of active, chronic hepatitis, bladder or renal carcinoma, malignant melanoma, multiple myeloma, mycosis fungoides, non-Hodgkin's lymphoma

Interferon alfa-2b

Treatment of bladder, cervical, renal carcinoma, chronic myelocytic leukemia, laryngeal papillomatosis, multiple myeloma, mycosis fungoides

CONTRAINDICATIONS: Hypersensitivity to any component of the formulations

PREGNANCY AND LACTATION: Pregnancy category C; abortifacient in animal models; avoid breastfeeding

SIDE EFFECTS

Frequent

Interferon alfa-2a

Flu-like symptoms, including fever, fatigue, headache, aches, pains, anorexia, and chills, nausea, vomiting, coughing, dyspnea, hypotension, edema, chest pain, dizziness, diarrhea, weight loss, taste change, abdominal discomfort, confusion, paresthesia, depression, visual and sleep disturbances, diaphoresis, lethargy

Interferon alfa-2b

Flu-like symptoms, including fever, fatigue, headache, aches, pains, anorexia, and chills, rash with hairy cell leukemia (Kaposi's sarcoma only)

Kaposi's sarcoma: All previously mentioned side effects plus depression, dyspepsia, dry mouth or thirst, alopecia, rigors

Occasional

Interferon alfa-2a

Partial alopecia, rash, dry throat or skin, pruritus, flatulence, constipation, hypertension, palpitations, sinusitis

Interferon alfa-2b

Dizziness, pruritus, dry skin, dermatitis, alteration in taste

Rare

Interferon alfa-2a

Hot flashes, hypermotility, Raynaud's syndrome, bronchospasm, earache, ecchymosis

Interferon alfa-2b

Confusion, leg cramps, back pain, gingivitis, flushing, tremor, nervousness, eye pain

SERIOUS REACTIONS

• Arrhythmias, stroke, transient ischemic attacks, congestive heart failure (CHF), pulmonary edema, and myocardial infarction (MI) occur rarely with interferon alfa-2a.

• Hypersensitivity reaction occurs rarely with interferon alfa-2b.

• Severe adverse reactions of flu-like symptoms appear dose related with interferon alfa-2b.

INTERACTIONS

Drugs

▣ *Theophylline:* Increased theophylline levels

SPECIAL CONSIDERATIONS

• Rebetron Combination Therapy (kit containing interferon alfa-2b inj plus ribavirin capsules) more effective than interferon alfa-2b monotherapy for chronic hepatitis C infection

PATIENT/FAMILY EDUCATION

• Drink plenty of fluids

• Flu-like symptoms decrease during treatment. Acetaminophen (do not exceed recommended dose) may alleviate fever and headache

interferon alfacon-1

(in-ter-feer′on)

Rx: Infergen

Chemical Class: Recombinant interferon

Therapeutic Class: Antiviral

CLINICAL PHARMACOLOGY

Mechanism of Action: A biological response modifier that stimulates the immune system. *Therapeutic Effect:* Inhibits hepatitis C virus.

INDICATIONS AND DOSAGES

Chronic hepatitis C

Subcutaneous

Adults. 9 mcg 3 times a week for 24 wk. May increase to 15 mcg 3 times a week in patients who tolerate but fail to respond to 9-mcg dose.

[$] **AVAILABLE FORMS/COST**

• Sol, Inj-SC: 9 mcg/0.3 ml vial: **$42.00**; 15 mcg/0.5 ml vial: **$70.04**

CONTRAINDICATIONS: History of autoimmune hepatitis or severe psychiatric disorders

PREGNANCY AND LACTATION: Pregnancy category C; unknown if excreted in breast milk

SIDE EFFECTS

Frequent (greater than 50%)

Headache, fatigue, fever, depression

INTERACTIONS

Drugs

[3] *Theophylline:* Increased theophylline levels

SPECIAL CONSIDERATIONS

• Response rates (normal ALT, HCV RNA negative) of 9 mcg dose approx 35%, about half those have sustained response 24 wk after treatment

• Withold dosage temporarily if severe adverse reaction occurs, consider decreasing dose to 7.5 mcg

PATIENT/FAMILY EDUCATION

• Needs to be refrigerated (36-46° F), may allow to reach room temp before injection; call manufacturer for advice if left out

MONITORING PARAMETERS

• CBC, plts, TSH, triglycerides, LFTs initially, repeat after 2 wk treatment and periodically thereafter

• Withold for ANC $<0.5 \times 10^9$/L or platelets $<50 \times 10^9$/L

interferon alfa-n3

(in-ter-feer′on)

Rx: Alferon N

Chemical Class: Human leukocyte interferon

Therapeutic Class: Antiviral

CLINICAL PHARMACOLOGY

Mechanism of Action: A biological response modifier that inhibits viral replication in virus-infected cells, suppresses cell proliferation, increases phagocytic action of macrophages, and augments specific cytotoxicity of lymphocytes for target cells. *Therapeutic Effect:* Inhibits viral growth in condylomata acuminatum.

INDICATIONS AND DOSAGES

Condyloma acuminatum

Intralesional

Adults, Children 18 yr and older. 0.05 ml (250,000 international units) per wart twice a week up to 8 wk. Maximum dose/treatment session: 0.5 ml (2.5 million international units). Do not repeat for 3 mo after initial 8 wk course unless warts enlarge or new warts appear.

$ AVAILABLE FORMS/COST

• Sol, Inj-Intralesional: 5 million U/ml: **$172.03**

UNLABELED USES: Treatment of active chronic hepatitis, bladder carcinoma, chronic myelocytic leukemia, laryngeal papillomatosis, malignant melanoma, multiple myeloma, mycosis fungoides, non-Hodgkin's lymphoma

CONTRAINDICATIONS: Previous history of anaphylactic reaction to egg protein, mouse immunoglobulin, or neomycin

PREGNANCY AND LACTATION: Pregnancy category C: Abortifacient in animal models; unknown if excreted into breast milk

SIDE EFFECTS

Frequent

Flu-like symptoms

Occasional

Dizziness, pruritus, dry skin, dermatitis, altered taste

Rare

Confusion, leg cramps, back pain, gingivitis, flushing, tremor, nervousness, eye pain

SERIOUS REACTIONS

• Hypersensitivity reaction occurs rarely.

• Severe flu-like symptoms may occur at higher doses.

INTERACTIONS

Drugs

3 *Theophylline:* Increased theophylline levels

---

interferon beta-1a/b

Rx: Avonex (beta-1a), Betaseron (beta-1b)
Chemical Class: Recombinant interferon
Therapeutic Class: Multiple sclerosis agent

CLINICAL PHARMACOLOGY

Mechanism of Action: A biologic response modifier that interacts with specific cell receptors found on surface of human cells. *Therapeutic Effect:* Possesses antiviral and immunoregulatory activities.

Pharmacokinetics

Interferon beta-1a

After IM administration, peak serum levels attained in 3-15 hrs. Biologic markers increase within 12 hrs and remain elevated for 4 days. **Half-life:** 10 hrs (IM).

Interferon beta-1b

Half-life: 8 min-4.3 hrs.

INDICATIONS AND DOSAGES

Relapsing-remitting multiple sclerosis

Interferon beta-1a

IM

Adults. 30 mcg Avonex once weekly.

Subcutaneous

Adults. Initially 8. 8 mcg Rebif 3 times/wk, may increase over 4- 6 wks to 44 mcg Rebif 3 times/wk.

Interferon beta-1b

Subcutaneous

Adults. 0. 25 mg (8 million units) every other day.

$ AVAILABLE FORMS/COST

• Powder, Inj-SC (beta-1a): 30 mcg/vial: **$269.06**

• Sol, Inj-SC (beta-1a): 22 mcg, 44 mcg/0.5 ml; all: **$117.11**

• Inj-SC (beta-1b): 0.3 mg/vial: **$87.37**

UNLABELED USES: Treatment of acquired immune deficiency syndrome (AIDS), AIDS-related Kaposi's sarcoma, malignant melanoma, renal cell carcinoma

CONTRAINDICATIONS: Hypersensitivity to albumin, interferon

PREGNANCY AND LACTATION: Pregnancy category C; possible abortifacient; not known if excreted into breast milk; avoid in nursing mothers

SIDE EFFECTS

Frequent

Interferon beta-1a: Headache (67%), flu-like symptoms (61%), myalgia (34%), upper respiratory infection (31%), pain (24%), asthenia, chills (21%), sinusitis (18%), infection (11%)

Interferon beta-1a: Injection site reaction (85%), headache (84%), flu-like symptoms (76%), fever (59%), pain (52%), asthenia (49%), myalgia (44%), sinusitis (36%), diarrhea, dizziness (35%), mental status changes (29%), constipation (24%), diaphoresis (23%), vomiting (21%)

Occasional

Interferon beta-1a: Abdominal pain, arthralgia (9%), chest pain, dyspnea (6%), malaise, syncope (4%)

Interferon beta-1b: Malaise (15%), somnolence (6%), alopecia (4%)

Rare

Interferon beta-1a: Injection site reaction, hypersensitivity reaction (3%)

SERIOUS REACTIONS

• Anemia occurs in 8% of patients taking interferon beta-1a.

• Seizures occur rarely in patients taking interferon beta-1b.

INTERACTIONS

Drugs

3 *Zidovudine, theophylline:* Increased levels of these drugs

SPECIAL CONSIDERATIONS

PATIENT/FAMILY EDUCATION

• Use acetaminophen for relief of flu-like symptoms

• Avoid prolonged sun exposure (photosensitivity)

• Benefit in chronic progressive multiple sclerosis has not been evaluated

• Patients treated × 2 yr had significantly longer time to progression of disability compared with placebo group

MONITORING PARAMETERS

• CBC, platelets, liver function tests, and blood chemistries q3 mo

• DC for ANC <750/m^3, ALT/AST >10 × upper normal limits; when labs return to these levels, restart at 50% of dose

---

interferon gamma-1b

(in-ter-feer'on)

Rx: Actimmune

Chemical Class: Recombinant interferon

Therapeutic Class: Biologic response modifier

CLINICAL PHARMACOLOGY

Mechanism of Action: A biological response modifier that induces activation of macrophages in blood monocytes to phagocytes, which is necessary in the body's cellular immune response to intracellular and extracellular pathogens. Enhances phagocytic function and antimicrobial activity of monocytes. *Therapeutic Effect:* Decreases signs and symptoms of serious infections in chronic granulomatous disease.

Pharmacokinetics

Slowly absorbed after subcutaneous administration.

INDICATIONS AND DOSAGES
Chronic granulomatous disease; severe, malignant osteopetrosis
Subcutaneous

Adults, Children older than 1 yr. 50 mcg/m^2 (1.5 million units/m^2) in patients with body surface area (BSA) greater than 0.5 m^2; 1.5 mcg/kg/dose in patients with BSA 0.5 m^2 or less. Give 3 times a week.

$ **AVAILABLE FORMS/COST**
• Sol, Inj-SC: 2 million IU/0.5 ml: **$242.93**

CONTRAINDICATIONS: Hypersensitivity to *Escherichia coli*-derived products

PREGNANCY AND LACTATION: Pregnancy category C; possible abortifacient; not known if excreted in breast milk; not recommended in breast-feeding

SIDE EFFECTS
Frequent

Fever (52%); headache (33%); rash (17%); chills, fatigue, diarrhea (14%)

Occasional (13%–10%)

Vomiting, nausea

Rare (6%–3%)

Weight loss, myalgia, anorexia

SERIOUS REACTIONS
• Interferon gamma-1b may exacerbate pre-existing CNS disturbances, including decreased mental status, gait disturbance, and dizziness, as well as cardiac disorders.

INTERACTIONS
Drugs

3 *Theophylline, zidovudine:* Increased levels of these drugs

SPECIAL CONSIDERATIONS
• Optimal sites for inj are the right and left deltoid and anterior thigh

PATIENT/FAMILY EDUCATION
• Use acetaminophen to relieve fever, headache

---

iodoquinol
(eye-oh-do-kwin′ole)
Rx: Yodoxin
Chemical Class: Hydroxyquinoline derivative
Therapeutic Class: Amebicide

CLINICAL PHARMACOLOGY
Mechanism of Action: An antibacterial, antifungal, and antitrichomonal agent that works in the intestinal lumen by an unknown mechanism. *Therapeutic Effect:* Amebicidal.

Pharmacokinetics

Partially and irregularly absorbed from the gastrointestinal (GI) tract. Metabolized in liver. Primarily excreted in feces.

INDICATIONS AND DOSAGES
Intestinal amebiasis
PO

Adults, Elderly. 630-650 mg 3 times a day for 20 days.

Children. 40 mg/kg in 3 divided doses for up to 20 days. Maximum: 650 mg/day.

$ **AVAILABLE FORMS/COST**
• Tab-Oral: 210 mg, 100's: **$69.27**; 650 mg, 100's: **$19.50-$89.09**

CONTRAINDICATIONS: Hepatic impairment, renal impairment, chronic diarrhea (especially in children), hypersensitivity to iodine and 8-hydroxyquinolones

PREGNANCY AND LACTATION: Pregnancy category C; excretion into breast milk unknown

SIDE EFFECTS
Occasional

Fever, chills, headache, nausea, vomiting, diarrhea, cramps, urticaria, pruritus

SERIOUS REACTIONS

• Optic neuritis, atrophy, and peripheral neuropathy have been reported with high dosages and long-term use.

ipecac

(ip'e-kak)

OTC: Ipecac

Chemical Class: Cephaelis ipecacuanha derivative

Therapeutic Class: Emetic

CLINICAL PHARMACOLOGY

Mechanism of Action: An antidote that acts centrally by stimulating medullary chemoreceptor trigger zone and locally by irritating gastric mucosa. *Therapeutic Effect:* Produces emesis.

Pharmacokinetics

Onset of action occurs within 20-30 minutes. Eliminated very slowly in urine.

INDICATIONS AND DOSAGES

Poisoning, acute

PO

Adults, Elderly, Children 12 yrs and older. 15-30 ml followed by 200-300 ml of water

Children 6-12 yrs. 5-10 ml followed by 10-20 ml/kg.

Children 1-12 yrs. 15 ml followed by 10-20 ml/kg.

Children 6 mos-1 yr. 5-10 ml, followed by 10-20 ml/kg.

[$] **AVAILABLE FORMS/COST**

• Syr-Oral: 7%, 30 ml: **$1.18-$23.11**

CONTRAINDICATIONS: Ingestion of petroleum distillate, ingestion of strong acids or bases, ingestion of strychnine, unconsciousness or absence of gag reflex, hypersensitivity to ipecac or any component of the formulation

PREGNANCY AND LACTATION: Pregnancy category C; not known if excreted in breast milk

SIDE EFFECTS

Expected response

Nausea, vomiting, drowsiness and mild CNS depression after vomiting

Occasional

Diarrhea, lethargy, muscle aching, stomach cramps

SERIOUS REACTIONS

• Cardiotoxicity may occur if ipecac syrup is not vomited (noted as hypotension, tachycardia, precordial chest pain, pulmonary congestion, dyspnea, ventricular tachycardia and fibrillation, cardiac arrest).

• Overdose may produce diarrhea, fast/irregular heartbeat, nausea continuing >30 min, stomach pain, respiratory difficulty, unusually tired, and aching/stiff muscles.

INTERACTIONS

Drugs

[3] *Activated charcoal:* Decreased effect of ipecac; if both drugs used, give activated charcoal after emesis induced

SPECIAL CONSIDERATIONS

• May not work on empty stomach

• Do not confuse with ipecac fluid extract (14 times stronger)

ipratropium
(eye-pra-troep'ee-um)
Rx: Atrovent
Combinations
 Rx: with albuterol (Combivent)
Chemical Class: Quaternary ammonium compound
Therapeutic Class: COPD agent; bronchodilator

CLINICAL PHARMACOLOGY
Mechanism of Action: An anticholinergic that blocks the action of acetylcholine at parasympathetic sites in bronchial smooth muscle. *Therapeutic Effect:* Causes bronchodilation and inhibits nasal secretions.

Pharmacokinetics

Route	Onset	Peak	Duration
Inhalation	1–3 min	1–2 hr	4–6 hr

Minimal systemic absorption after inhalation. Metabolized in the liver (systemic absorption). Primarily eliminated in feces. **Half-life:** 1.5–4 hr.

INDICATIONS AND DOSAGES
Bronchospasm, acute treatment
Inhalation
Adults, Elderly, Children. 4-8 puffs as needed.
Nebulization
Adults, Elderly, Children 12 yr and older. 500 mcg q30min for 3 doses, then q2-4h as needed.
Children younger than 12 yr. 250 mcg q20min for 3 doses, then q2-4h as needed.
Bronchospasm, maintenance treatment
Inhalation
Adults, Elderly, Children 12 yr and older. 2-3 puffs q6h.
Children younger than 12 yr. 1-2 puffs q6h.

Nebulization
Adults, Elderly, Children 12 yr and older. 500 mcg q6h.
Children younger than 12 yr. 250-500 mcg q6h.
Rhinorrhea
Intranasal
Adults, Children older than 12 yr. 2 sprays of 0.06% solution 3–4 times a day.
Adults, Children 6–12 yr. 2 sprays of (0.03%) solution 2–3 times a day.

$ **AVAILABLE FORMS/COST**
• Aer—INH: 18 mcg/inh, 14 g (200 puffs): **$57.20**
• Sol—INH: 0.2 mg/ml, 2.5 ml: **$0.70-$3.50**
• Sol—Nasal: 21 mcg/inh, 30 ml: **$37.50-$57.56**; 42 mcg/inh 15 ml: **$32.19-$49.35**
• MDI—INH (with albuterol): 90 mcg-18 mcg/puff, 14.7 g (200 puffs): **$59.91**

CONTRAINDICATIONS: History of hypersensitivity to atropine
PREGNANCY AND LACTATION: Pregnancy category B; not known if excreted in breast milk, but little systemic absorption when administered by INH

SIDE EFFECTS
Frequent
Inhalation (6%–3%): Cough, dry mouth, headache, nausea
Nasal: Dry nose and mouth, headache, nasal irritation
Occasional
Inhalation (2%): Dizziness, transient increased bronchospasm
Rare (less than 1%)
Inhalation: Hypotension, insomnia, metallic or unpleasant taste, palpitations, urine retention
Nasal: Diarrhea or constipation, dry throat, abdominal pain, stuffy nose
SERIOUS REACTIONS
• Worsening of angle-closure glaucoma, acute eye pain, and hypotension occur rarely.

SPECIAL CONSIDERATIONS
• Bronchodilator of choice for COPD

---

irbesartan
(erb'ba-sar-tan)

Rx: Avapro
Combinations
  Rx: with hydrochlorothiazide
  (Avalide)
Chemical Class: Angiotensin II receptor antagonist
Therapeutic Class: Antihypertensive

CLINICAL PHARMACOLOGY
Mechanism of Action: An angiotensin II receptor, type AT_1, antagonist that blocks the vasoconstrictor and aldosterone-secreting effects of angiotensin II, inhibiting the binding of angiotensin II to the AT_1 receptors. *Therapeutic Effect:* Causes vasodilation, decreases peripheral resistance, and decreases BP.

Pharmacokinetics
Rapidly and completely absorbed after PO administration. Protein binding: 90%. Undergoes hepatic metabolism to inactive metabolite. Recovered primarily in feces and, to a lesser extent, in urine. Not removed by hemodialysis. **Half-life:** 11–15 hr.

INDICATIONS AND DOSAGES
Hypertension alone or in combination with other antihypertensives
PO

Adults, Elderly, Children 13 yr and older. Initially, 75–150 mg/day. May increase to 300 mg/day.

Children 6–12 yr. Initially, 75 mg/day. May increase to 150 mg/day.

Nephropathy
PO

Adults, Elderly. Target dose of 300 mg/day.

$\boxed{\text{S}}$ AVAILABLE FORMS/COST
• Cap—Oral: 75 mg, 90's: **$142.20**; 150 mg, 100's: **$166.33**; 300 mg, 100's: **$210.88**

UNLABELED USES: Treatment of heart failure

CONTRAINDICATIONS: Bilateral renal artery stenosis, biliary cirrhosis or obstruction, primary hyperaldosteronism, severe hepatic insufficiency

PREGNANCY AND LACTATION: Pregnancy category C (first trimester—category D, second and third trimesters); drugs acting directly on the renin-angiotensin-aldosterone system are documented to cause fetal harm (hypotension, oligohydramnios, neonatal anemia, hyperkalemia, neonatal skull hypoplasia, anuria, and renal failure; neonatal limb contractures, craniofacial deformities, and hypoplastic lung development; breast milk excretion unknown

SIDE EFFECTS
Occasional (9%–3%)
Upper respiratory tract infection, fatigue, diarrhea, cough
Rare (2%–1%)
Heartburn, dizziness, headache, nausea, rash

SERIOUS REACTIONS
• Overdosage may manifest as hypotension and tachycardia. Bradycardia occurs less often.

SPECIAL CONSIDERATIONS
• Potentially as or more effective than angiotensin-converting enzyme inhibitors, without cough; no evidence for reduction in morbidity and mortality as first line agents in hypertension, yet; whether they provide the same cardiac and renal protection also still tentative; Like ACE inhibitors, less effective in black patients

PATIENT/FAMILY EDUCATION
• Call your clinician immediately if note following side effects: wheezing; lip, throat or face swelling; hives or rash

MONITORING PARAMETERS
• Baseline electrolytes, urinalysis, blood urea nitrogen and creatinine with recheck at 2-4 weeks after initiation (sooner in volume depleted patients); monitor sitting blood pressure; watch for symptomatic hypotension, particularly in volume depleted patients

---

iron dextran

Rx: InFeD, Dexferrum
Chemical Class: Ferric hydroxide complexed with dextran
Therapeutic Class: Hematinic

CLINICAL PHARMACOLOGY
Mechanism of Action: A trace element and essential component in the formation of Hgb. Necessary for effective erythropoiesis and transport and utilization of oxygen. Serves as cofactor of several essential enzymes. *Therapeutic Effect:* Replenishes Hgb and depleted iron stores.

Pharmacokinetics
Readily absorbed after IM administration. Most absorption occurs within 72 hr; remainder within 3–4 wk. Bound to protein to form hemosiderin, ferritin, or transferrin. No physiologic system of elimination. Small amounts lost daily in shedding of skin, hair, and nails and in feces, urine, and perspiration. **Half-life:** 5–20 hr.

INDICATIONS AND DOSAGES
Iron deficiency anemia (no blood loss)
Dosage is expressed in terms of milligrams of elemental iron, degree of anemia, patient weight, and pres-

ence of any bleeding. Expect to use periodic hematologic determinations as guide to therapy.
IV, IM
Adults, Elderly. Mg iron = 0.66 × weight (kg) × (100 − Hgb [g/dl]/14.8

Iron replacement secondary to blood loss
IM, IV
Adults, Elderly. Replacement iron (mg) = blood loss (ml) times Hct.

Maximum daily dosage
Adults weighing more than 50 kg. 100 mg.
Children weighing 10-50 kg. 100 mg.
Children weighing 5-less than 10 kg. 50 mg.
Infants weighing less than 5 kg. 25 mg.

☒ AVAILABLE FORMS/COST
• Sol, Inj-IM, IV: 50 mg/ml, 2 ml: **$37.70**

CONTRAINDICATIONS: All anemias except iron deficiency anemia, including pernicious, aplastic, normocytic, and refractory

PREGNANCY AND LACTATION: Pregnancy category C; excreted in breast milk

SIDE EFFECTS
Frequent
Allergic reaction (such as rash and itching), backache, myalgia, chills, dizziness, headache, fever, nausea, vomiting, flushed skin, pain or redness at injection site, brown discoloration of skin, metallic taste

SERIOUS REACTIONS
• Anaphylaxis has occurred during the first few minutes after injection, causing death rarely.
• Leukocytosis and lymphadenopathy occur rarely.

INTERACTIONS
Drugs
🔳 *Enalapril:* Three patients on enalapril receiving IV iron developed systemic reactions (GI symptoms, hypotension); causality not established

🔳 *Vitamin E:* Decreased reticulocyte response in anemic children
Labs
• *False increase:* Serum calcium, serum glucose, serum iron
• *False positive:* Stool guaiac
SPECIAL CONSIDERATIONS
• Discontinue oral iron before giving
• Delayed reaction (fever, myalgias, arthralgias, nausea) may occur 1-2 days after administration
• When giving IM, give only in gluteal muscle

---

isocarboxazid
(eye-soe-kar-box′a-zid)
Rx: Marplan
Chemical Class: Hydrazine derivative
Therapeutic Class: Antidepressant, monoamine oxidase inhibitor (MAOI)

CLINICAL PHARMACOLOGY
Mechanism of Action: An antidepressant that inhibits the MAO enzyme system at central nervous system (CNS) storage sites. The reduced MAO activity causes an increased concentration in epinephrine, norepinephrine, serotonin, and dopamine at neuron receptor sites. *Therapeutic Effect:* Produces antidepressant effect.

INDICATIONS AND DOSAGES
Depression refractory to other antidepressants or electroconvulsive therapy
PO

Adults, Elderly. Initially, 10 mg 3 times/day. May increase to 60 mg/day.

🆂 **AVAILABLE FORMS/COST**
• Tab-Oral: 10 mg, 100's: **$74.32**
UNLABELED USES: Treatment of panic disorder, vascular or tension headaches
CONTRAINDICATIONS: Cardiovascular disease (CVD), cerebrovascular disease, liver impairment, pheochromocytoma, liver impairment
PREGNANCY AND LACTATION: Pregnancy category C; breastfeeding data not available
SIDE EFFECTS
Frequent (more than 10%)
Postural hypotension, drowsiness, decreased sexual ability, weakness, trembling, visual disturbances
Occasional (10%-1%)
Tachycardia, peripheral edema, nervousness, chills, diarrhea, anorexia, constipation, xerostomia
Rare (less than 1%)
Hepatitis, leukopenia, parkinsonian syndrome
SERIOUS REACTIONS
• Hypertensive crisis, marked by severe hypertension, occipital headache radiating frontally, neck stiffness or soreness, nausea, vomiting, sweating, fever or chilliness, clammy skin, dilated pupils, palpitations, tachycardia or bradycardia, and constricting chest pain.
INTERACTIONS
Drugs
🔳 *Barbiturates:* Prolonged action of barbiturate

⚠ *Dextromethorphan:* Agitation, seizure, increased BP, hyperpyrexia

⚠ *Ephedrine, amphetamines, phenylephrine, phenylpropanolamine, pseudoephedrine:* Hypertension, severe

⚠ *Ethanol:* Alcoholic beverages containing tyramine may cause severe hypertensive reaction

▣ *Guanethidine:* Decreased antihypertensive response to guanethidine

▣ *Levodopa:* Hypertension, severe

② *Lithium:* Hyperpyrexia possible

⚠ *Meperidine:* Sweating, rigidity, hypertension

⚠ *Methotrimeprazine:* Case report of fatality in patient taking these drugs, causality not established

▣ *Norepinephrine:* Increased pressor response to norepinephrine

⚠ *Reserpine:* Potential for hypertensive reaction, clinical evidence lacking

⚠ *Sertraline, fluoxetine, fluvoxamine, paroxetine, venlafaxine:* Increased CNS effects (serotonergic)

⚠ *Tricyclic antidepressants:* Excessive sympathetic response, mania, hyperpyrexia

SPECIAL CONSIDERATIONS
• Phentolamine for severe hypertension

PATIENT/FAMILY EDUCATION
• Avoid high-tyramine foods: cheese (aged), sour cream, beer, wine, pickled products, liver, raisins, bananas, figs, avocados, meat tenderizers, chocolate, yogurt; soy sauce, caffeine
• Do not discontinue medication quickly after long-term use

isoetharine hydrochloride / isoetharine mesylate
(eye-soe-eth'a-reen)
Rx: Isoetharine
Chemical Class: Sympathomimetic amine; β_2-adrenergic agonist
Therapeutic Class: Antiasthmatic; bronchodilator

CLINICAL PHARMACOLOGY
Mechanism of Action: A sympathomimetic (adrenergic agonist) that stimulates beta2-adrenergic receptors in the lungs, resulting in relaxation of bronchial smooth muscle. *Therapeutic Effect:* Relieves bronchospasm, reduces airway resistance.
Pharmacokinetics
Rapidly, well absorbed from the gastrointestinal (GI) tract. Extensive metabolism in GI tract. Unknown extent metabolized in liver and lungs. Excreted in urine. **Half-life:** 4 hrs.

INDICATIONS AND DOSAGES
Bronchospasm
Hand-bulb Nebulizer
Adults, Elderly. 4 inhalations (range: 3-7 inhalations) undiluted. May be repeated up to 5 times/day.
Metered Dose Inhalation
Adults, Elderly. 1-2 inhalations q4h. Wait 1 min before administering 2nd inhalation.
IPPB, Oxygen Aerolization
Adults, Elderly. 0.5-1 ml of a 0.5% or 0.5 ml of a 1% solution diluted 1:3.

Ⓢ **AVAILABLE FORMS/COST**
• Sol—INH: 1%, 30 ml: **$120.14**
CONTRAINDICATIONS: History of hypersensitivity to sympathomimetics

PREGNANCY AND LACTATION:
Pregnancy category C; no breast-feeding data available

SIDE EFFECTS

Occasional

Tremor, nausea, nervousness, palpitations, tachycardia, peripheral vasodilation, dryness of mouth, throat, dizziness, vomiting, headache, increased BP, insomnia.

SERIOUS REACTIONS

• Excessive sympathomimetic stimulation may produce palpitations, extrasystoles, tachycardia, chest pain, slight increase in BP followed by a substantial decrease, chills, sweating, and blanching of skin.

• Too frequent or excessive use may lead to loss of bronchodilating effectiveness and severe and paradoxical bronchoconstriction.

INTERACTIONS

Drugs

❷ *β-blockers:* Decreased action of isoetharine, cardioselective β-blockers preferable if concurrent use necessary

❸ *Furosemide:* Potential for additive hypokalemia

SPECIAL CONSIDERATIONS

• Inhalation technique critical
• Re-educate routinely

isometheptene

(eye-soe-me-thep´teen)

Rx: Amidrine Duradin, I.D.A., Iso-Acetazone, Midchlor, Midrin, Migrapap, Migratine, Migrazone, Migquin, Migrex, VA-Zone

Chemical Class: Sympathomimetic amine

Therapeutic Class: Vasoconstrictor (in combination with analgesic and sedative)

CLINICAL PHARMACOLOGY

Mechanism of Action: Acetaminophen: A central analgesic whose exact mechanism is unknown, but appears to inhibit prostaglandin synthesis in the central nervous system (CNS) and, to a lesser extent, block pain impulses through peripheral action. Acetaminophen acts centrally on hypothalamic heat-regulating center, producing peripheral vasodilation (heat loss, skin erythema, sweating). Isometheptene: An indirect-acting sympathomimetic agent with vasoconstricting activity whose exact mechanism is unknown, but appears to constrict cerebral blood vessels and reduce pulsation in cerebral arteries that may be responsible for the pain of migraine headaches. Dichloralphenazone: A complex of chloral hydrate and antipyrine that acts as a mild sedative and relaxant. *Therapeutic Effect:* Relieves migraine headaches.

Pharmacokinetics

Rapidly, completely absorbed from gastrointestinal (GI) tract; rectal absorption variable. Widely distributed to most body tissues. Acetaminophen is metabolized in liver; excreted in urine. Dichloralphenazone is hydrolyzed to active compounds chloral hydrate and antipyrine. Chloral hydrate is metabolized in the liver and erythrocytes to the active metabolite trichloroethanol, which may be further metabolized to inactive metabolite. It is also metabolized in the liver and kidneys to inactive metabolites. The pharmacokinetics of isometheptene is not reported. Removed by hemodialysis. **Half-life:** Acetaminophen: 1- 4 hrs (half-life is increased in those with liver disease, elderly, neonates; decreased in children).

INDICATIONS AND DOSAGES
Migraine headache
PO
Adults, Elderly. Initially, 2 capsules, followed by 1 capsule every hour until relief is obtained. Maximum: 5 capsules/12 hrs.
Tension headache
PO
Adults, Elderly. 1-2 capsules q4h. Maximum: 8 capsules/24 hrs.

S AVAILABLE FORMS/COST
• Cap, Gel—Oral: acetaminophen 325 mg/dichloralphenazone 100 mg/isometheptene 65 mg, 100's: **$17.95-$62.92**

CONTRAINDICATIONS: Glaucoma, hypersensitivity to acetaminophen, isometheptene, dichloralphenazone, or any component of the formulation, hepatic disease, hypertension, organic heart disease, MAO inhibitor therapy, severe renal disease

PREGNANCY AND LACTATION: Pregnancy category C; excretion into breast milk unknown

SIDE EFFECTS
Occasional
Transient dizziness
Rare
Hypersensitivity reaction

SERIOUS REACTIONS
• Acetaminophen toxicity is the primary serious reaction.

• Early signs and symptoms of acetaminophen toxicity include anorexia, nausea, diaphoresis, and generalized weakness within the first 12 to 24 hrs.
• Later signs of acetaminophen toxicity include vomiting, right upper quadrant tenderness, and elevated liver function tests within 48 to 72 hrs after ingestion.
• The antidote to acetaminophen toxicity is acetylcysteine.

INTERACTIONS
Drugs
▲ *Bromocriptine:* Potential for hypertension and ventricular tachycardia
Labs
• *False positive:* Urine amphetamine

---

isoniazid (INH)
(eye-soe-nye'a-zid)
Rx: *INH:* Nydrazid
Combinations
  Rx: with rifampin (Rifamate); with rifampin, pyrazinamide (Rifater)
Chemical Class: Isonicotinic acid derivative
Therapeutic Class: Antituberculosis agent

CLINICAL PHARMACOLOGY
Mechanism of Action: An isonicotinic acid derivative that inhibits mycolic acid synthesis and causes disruption of the bacterial cell wall and loss of acid-fast properties in susceptible mycobacteria. Active only during bacterial cell division. *Therapeutic Effect:* Bactericidal against actively growing intracelluar and extracellular susceptible mycobacteria.

Pharmacokinetics
Readily absorbed from the GI tract. Protein binding: 10%-15%. Widely distributed (including to CSF). Metabolized in the liver. Primarily excreted in urine. Removed by hemodialysis. **Half-life:** 0.5-5 hr.

INDICATIONS AND DOSAGES
Tuberculosis (in combination with one or more antituberculars)
PO, IM

Adults, Elderly. 5 mg/kg/day as a single dose. Maximum 300 mg/day.
Children. 10-15 mg/kg/day as a single dose. Maximum 300 mg/day.

Prevention of tuberculosis
PO, IM

Adults, Elderly. 300 mg/day as a single dose.
Children. 10 mg/kg/day as a single dose. Maximum 300 mg/day.

AVAILABLE FORMS/COST
• Sol, Inj-IM: 100 mg/ml, 10 ml: **$20.26**
• Syr—Oral: 50 mg/5ml, 480 ml: **$20.00-$22.50**
• Tab-Oral: 100 mg, 100's: **$0.68-$15.45**; 300 mg, 100's: **$6.95-$20.75**

CONTRAINDICATIONS: Acute hepatic disease, history of hypersensitivity reactions or hepatic injury with previous isoniazid therapy

PREGNANCY AND LACTATION: Pregnancy category C; the American Thoracic Society recommends use of isoniazid for tuberculosis during pregnancy; excreted in breast milk; women can safely breast-feed their infants while taking isoniazid if the infant is periodically examined for signs and symptoms of peripheral neuritis or hepatitis

SIDE EFFECTS
Frequent
Nausea, vomiting, diarrhea, abdominal pain

Rare
Pain at injection site, hypersensitivity reaction

SERIOUS REACTIONS
• Rare reactions include neurotoxicity (as evidenced by ataxia and paraesthesia), optic neuritis, and hepatotoxicity.

INTERACTIONS
Drugs
3 *Acetaminophen:* Increased acetaminophen concentrations, potential for hepatotoxicity
3 *Antacids:* Reduced plasma isoniazid concentrations
3 *Carbamazepine:* Increased serum carbamazepine concentrations, toxicity may occur
3 *Corticosteroids:* Reduced plasma concentrations of isoniazid
3 *Cycloserine:* Increased potential for CNS toxicity
3 *Diazepam, triazolam:* Increased concentrations of these drugs
2 *Disulfiram:* Adverse mental changes and coordination problems
3 *Ethanol:* Higher incidence of isoniazid-induced hepatitis in alcoholics
3 *Phenytoin:* Predictable increases in serum phenytoin concentrations, toxicity possible
3 *Rifampin:* Increased hepatotoxicity of isoniazid in some patients; more common with slow acetylators of isoniazid, and/or pre-existing liver disease
3 *Theophylline:* Increased theophylline concentrations, toxicity possible
3 *Valproic acid:* Increased valproic acid concentration possible
3 *Warfarin:* Potential for enhanced hypoprothrombinemic response to warfarin

Labs
• *False increase:* Serum AST, serum uric acid

- *False decrease:* Serum glucose
- *False positive:* Urine sugar

SPECIAL CONSIDERATIONS
PATIENT/FAMILY EDUCATION
- Take on empty stomach if possible; however, may be taken with food to decrease GI upset
- Minimize daily alcohol consumption to lessen the risk of hepatitis
- Notify clinician of weakness, fatigue, loss of appetite, nausea and vomiting, yellowing of skin or eyes, darkening of urine, numbness or tingling of hands and feet

MONITORING PARAMETERS
- Periodic ophthalmologic examinations even when visual symptoms do not occur
- Periodic liver function tests

---

isoproterenol
(eye-soe-proe-ter'e-nole)

Rx: Isuprel, Medihaler-Iso
Combinations
   Rx: with phenylephrine
      (Duo-Medihaler)
Chemical Class: Catecholamine, synthetic
Therapeutic Class: Antiasthmatic; bronchodilator; sympathomimetic; vasopressor; ß-adrenergic agonist

---

CLINICAL PHARMACOLOGY
Mechanism of Action: A sympathomimetic (adrenergic agonist) that stimulates beta1-adrenergic receptors. *Therapeutic Effect:* Increases myocardial contractility, stroke volume, cardiac output.

Pharmacokinetics
Readily absorbed. Metabolized in liver. Primarily excreted in urine. **Half-life:** 2.5-5 min.

INDICATIONS AND DOSAGES
Arrhythmias
IV Bolus
Adults, Elderly. Initially, 0.02-0.06 mg (1-3 ml of diluted solution). Subsequent dose range: 0.01-0.2 mg (0.5-10 ml of diluted solution).
IV Infusion
Adults, Elderly. Initially, 5 mcg/min (1.25 ml/min of diluted solution). Subsequent dose range: 2-20 mcg/min.
Children. 2.5 mcg/min or 0.1 mcg/kg per min.

Complete heart block following closure of ventricular septal defects
IV
Adults, Elderly. 0.04-0.06 mg (2-3 ml of diluted solution).
Infants. 0.01-0.03 (0.5-1.5 ml of diluted solution).

Shock
IV Infusion
Adults, Elderly. Rate of 0.5-5 mcg/min (0.25-2.5 ml of 1:500,000 dilution); rate of infusion based on clinical response (heart rate, central venous pressure, systemic BP, urine flow measurements).

AVAILABLE FORMS/COST
- Sol, Inj-IV: 0.02 mg/ml, 10 ml: **$7.99**; 0.2 mg/ml, 1, 5, 10 ml: **$5.70-$15.78**/5 ml
- Sol—INH: 0.5%, 10ml: **$24.80**

CONTRAINDICATIONS: Tachycardia due to digitalis toxicity, preexisting arrhythmias, angina, precordial distress, hypersensitivity to isoproterenol or any component of the formulation

PREGNANCY AND LACTATION: Pregnancy category C; no reports linking isoproterenol with congenital defects have been located; excretion into breast milk unknown; use caution in nursing mothers

SIDE EFFECTS
Frequent

Palpitations, tachycardia, restlessness, nervousness, tremor, insomnia, anxiety

Occasional

Increased sweating, headache, nausea, flushed skin, dizziness, coughing

SERIOUS REACTIONS

• Excessive sympathomimetic stimulation may cause palpitations, extrasystoles, tachycardia, chest pain, slight increase in BP followed by a substantial decrease, chills, sweating, and blanching of skin.

• Ventricular arrhythmias may occur if heart rate is above 130 beats/min.

• Parotid gland swelling may occur with prolonged use.

INTERACTIONS
Drugs

▨ *Amitriptyline:* Combined use may result in predisposition to cardiac arrhythmias

▨ *β-blockers:* Reduced effectiveness of isoproterenol in the treatment of asthma

Labs

• *False increase:* Serum AST, serum bilirubin, serum glucose

---

isosorbide dinitrate/mononitrate

Rx: *Dinitrate (sublingual chewable):* Isordil, Sorbitrate, Dilatrate-SR

Rx: *Mononitrate (oral):* Monoket, ISMO, Imdur, Isotrate ER

Chemical Class: Nitrate, organic

Therapeutic Class: Antianginal

CLINICAL PHARMACOLOGY

Mechanism of Action: A nitrate that stimulates intracellular cyclic guanosine monophosphate. *Therapeutic Effect:* Relaxes vascular smooth muscle of both arterial and venous vasculature. Decreases preload and afterload.

Pharmacokinetics

Route	Onset	Peak	Duration
Dinitrate			
Sublingual	2–5 min	N/A	1–2 hr
PO (Chewable)	2–5 min	N/A	1–2 hr
PO	15–40 min	N/A	4–6 hr
PO (Sustained Release)	30 min	N/A	12 hr
Mononitrate			
Oral	60 min	N/A	N/A

Dinitrate poorly absorbed and metabolized in the liver to its activate metabolite isosorbide mononitrate. Mononitrate well absorbed after PO administration. Excreted in urine and feces. **Half-life:** Dinitrate, 1–4 hr; mononitrate. 4 hr.

INDICATIONS AND DOSAGES
Angina

PO (isosorbide dinitrate)

Adults, Elderly. 5-40 mg 4 times a day. Sustained-release: 40 mg q8-12h.

PO (isosorbide mononitrate)

Adults, Elderly. 5-10 mg twice a day given 7 hours apart. Sustained-release: Initially, 30-60 mg/day in morning as a single dose. May increase dose at 3 day intervals. Maximum: 240 mg/day.

🔢 AVAILABLE FORMS/COST

Dinitrate

• Cap, Gel, Sus Action—Oral: 40 mg, 100's: **$59.48-$86.64**
• Tab, Chewable—Oral: 5 mg, 100's: **$22.45**
• Tab, Coated, Sus Action—Oral: 40 mg, 100's: **$6.00-$76.18**
• Tab, SL—Oral: 2.5 mg, 100's: **$4.35-$20.65**; 5 mg, 100's: **$2.50-$20.65**; 10 mg, 100's: **$39.95**
• Tab-Oral: 5 mg, 100's: **$2.50-$34.35**; 10 mg, 100's: **$2.34-$40.43**; 20 mg, 100's: **$4.25-$62.00**; 30 mg, 100's: **$9.05-$132.15**; 40 mg, 100's: **$4.95-$75.61**

Mononitrate

• Tab-Oral: 10 mg, 100's: **$102.40**; 20 mg, 100's: **$38.82-$112.96**
• Tab, Coated, Sus Action—Oral: 30 mg, 100's: **$111.56-$192.60**; 60 mg, 100's: **$36.69-$202.70**; 120 mg, 100's: **$195.70-$283.75**

UNLABELED USES: CHF, dysphagia, pain relief, relief of esophageal spasm with gastroesophageal reflux

CONTRAINDICATIONS: Closed-angle glaucoma, GI hypermotility or malabsorption (extended-release tablets), head trauma, hypersensitivity to nitrates, increased intracranial pressure, orthostatic hypotension, severe anemia (extended-release tablets)

PREGNANCY AND LACTATION: Pregnancy category C; excretion into breast milk unknown; use caution in nursing mothers

SIDE EFFECTS

Frequent

Burning and tingling at oral point of dissolution (sublingual), headache (possibly severe) occurs mostly in early therapy, diminishes rapidly in intensity, and usually disappears during continued treatment, transient flushing of face and neck, dizziness (especially if patient is standing immobile or is in a warm environment), weakness, orthostatic hypotension, nausea, vomiting, restlessness

Occasional

GI upset, blurred vision, dry mouth

SERIOUS REACTIONS

• Blurred vision or dry mouth may occur (drug should be discontinued).
• Isosorbide administration may cause severe orthostatic hypotension manifested by fainting, pulselessness, cold or clammy skin, and diaphoresis.
• Tolerance may occur with repeated, prolonged therapy, but may not occur with the extended-release form. Minor tolerance may be seen with intermittent use of sublingual tablets.
• High dosage tends to produce severe headache.

INTERACTIONS

Drugs

▨ *Alcohol:* Exaggerated hypotension and cardiac collapse

▨ *Calcium channel blockers:* Exaggerated symptomatic orthostatic hypotension

▨ *Dihydroergotamine:* Increases the bioavailability of dihydroergotamine with resultant increase in mean standing systolic blood pressure; functional antagonism, decreasing effects

▨ *Sildenafil:* Excessive hypotensive effects

SPECIAL CONSIDERATIONS

PATIENT/FAMILY EDUCATION

- Headache may be a marker for drug activity; do not try to avoid by altering treatment schedule; contact clinician if severe or persistent; aspirin or acetaminophen may be used for relief
- Dissolve SL tablets under tongue; do not crush, chew, or swallow
- Do not crush chewable tablets before administering
- Avoid alcohol
- Make changes in position slowly to prevent fainting

---

isotretinoin

(eye-soe-tret′i-noyn)

Rx: Accutane

Chemical Class: Retinoid; vitamin A derivative

Therapeutic Class: Antiacne agent

CLINICAL PHARMACOLOGY

Mechanism of Action: Reduces the size of sebaceous glands and inhibits their activity. *Therapeutic Effect:* Decreases sebum production; produces antikeratinizing and anti-inflammatory effects.

Pharmacokinetics

Metabolized in the liver; major metabolite active. Eliminated in urine and feces. **Half-life:** 21 hr; metabolite, 21-24 hr.

INDICATIONS AND DOSAGES

Recalcitrant cystic acne that is unresponsive to conventional acne therapies

PO

Adults. Initially, 0.5-2 mg/kg/day divided into 2 doses for 15-20 wk. May repeat after at least 2 mo off therapy.

[$] **AVAILABLE FORMS/COST**

- Cap, Elastic—Oral: 10 mg, 100's: **$703.31-$944.66**; 20 mg, 100's: **$834.01-$1,120.21**; 30 mg, 100's: **$901.48**; 40 mg, 100's: **$968.95-$1,301.48**

UNLABELED USES: Treatment of gram-negative folliculitis, severe keratinization disorders, severe rosacea

CONTRAINDICATIONS: Hypersensitivity to isotretinoin or parabens (component of capsules)

PREGNANCY AND LACTATION: Pregnancy category X; isotretinoin is a potent human teratogen; excretion into breast milk unknown, but based on the close relationship to vitamin A, the presence of isotretinoin in breast milk should be expected; avoid use in nursing mothers

SIDE EFFECTS

Frequent (90%-20%)

Cheilitis (inflammation of lips), dry skin and mucous membranes, skin fragility, pruritus, epistaxis, dry nose and mouth, conjunctivitis, hypertriglyceridemia, nausea, vomiting, abdominal pain

Occasional (16%-5%)

Musculoskeletal symptoms (including bone pain, arthralgia, generalized myalgia), photosensitivity

Rare

Decreased night vision, depression

SERIOUS REACTIONS

- Inflammatory bowel disease and pseudotumor cerebri (benign intracranial hypertension) have been associated with isotretinoin therapy.

INTERACTIONS

Drugs

[3] *Carbamazepine:* Decreased concentrations of carbamazepine in one patient

[3] *Vitamin A supplements:* Possible additive toxic effects

❷ *Tetracyclines:* Concomitant use of isotretinoin and tetracyclines associated with pseudotumor cerebri

SPECIAL CONSIDERATIONS

• Have patient complete consent form included with package insert prior to initiating therapy

PATIENT/FAMILY EDUCATION

• Administer with meals
• Avoid alcohol
• Do not take vitamin supplements containing vitamin A
• **Women of childbearing potential should practice contraception during therapy and for 1 mo before and after therapy**
• Notify clinician immediately if pregnancy is suspected
• A transient exacerbation of acne may occur during the initiation of therapy
• Avoid prolonged exposure to sunlight or sunlamps
• Do not donate blood during and for 30 days after stopping therapy
• Use caution driving or operating any vehicle at night
• Discontinue drug if visual difficulties occur and have an ophthalmologic exam

MONITORING PARAMETERS

• Pregnancy test initially, during first 5 days of menstrual period then monthly
• CBC with differential, platelet count, baseline sedimentation rate, serum triglycerides (baseline and biweekly for 4 wk), liver enzymes

---

isradipine
(is-rad′i-peen)
Rx: DynaCirc
Chemical Class: Dihydropyridine
Therapeutic Class: Antianginal; antihypertensive; calcium channel blocker

---

CLINICAL PHARMACOLOGY
Mechanism of Action: An antihypertensive that inhibits calcium movement across cardiac and vascular smooth-muscle cell membranes. Potent peripheral vasodilator that does not depress SA or AV nodes. *Therapeutic Effect:* Produces relaxation of coronary vascular smooth muscle and coronary vasodilation. Increases myocardial oxygen delivery to those with vasospastic angina.
Pharmacokinetics

Route	Onset	Peak	Duration
PO	2–3 hr	2–4 wks (with multiple doses) 8-16 hr (with single dose)	N/A
PO (Controlled-release)	2 hr	8-10 hr	N/A

Well absorbed from the GI tract. Protein binding: 95%. Metabolized in the liver (undergoes first-pass effect). Primarily excreted in urine. Not removed by hemodialysis. **Half-life:** 8 hr.

INDICATIONS AND DOSAGES
Hypertension
PO
Adults, Elderly. Initially 2.5 mg twice a day. May increase by 2.5 mg at 2- to 4-wk intervals. Range: 5–20 mg/day

$ AVAILABLE FORMS/COST
• Cap, Gel—Oral: 2.5 mg, 100's: **$142.88**; 5 mg, 100's: **$207.94**
• Tab, Sus Action—Oral: 5 mg, 100's: **$182.94**; 10 mg, 100's: **$223.44**

UNLABELED USES: Treatment of chronic angina pectoris, Raynaud's phenomenon

CONTRAINDICATIONS: Cardiogenic shock, CHF, heart block, hypotension, sinus bradycardia, ventricular tachycardia

PREGNANCY AND LACTATION: Pregnancy category C; excretion into breast milk unknown; use caution in nursing mothers

SIDE EFFECTS
Frequent (7%–4%)
Peripheral edema, palpitations (higher frequency in females)
Occasional (3%)
Facial flushing, cough
Rare (2%–1%)
Angina, tachycardia, rash, pruritus

SERIOUS REACTIONS
• Overdose produces nausea, drowsiness, confusion, and slurred speech.
• CHF occurs rarely.

INTERACTIONS
Drugs
3 *Cimetidine:* Increased blood levels of isradipine with cimetidine
3 *Digitalis glycosides:* Increased digitalis levels; increased risk of toxicity
3 *Fentanyl:* Severe hypotension or increased fluid volume requirements
3 *Lovastatin:* Decreased lovastatin concentrations

itraconazole
(it-ra-con′a-zol)
Rx: Sporanox
Chemical Class: Triazole derivative
Therapeutic Class: Antifungal

CLINICAL PHARMACOLOGY
Mechanism of Action: A fungistatic antifungal that inhibits the synthesis of ergosterol, a vital component of fungal cell formation *Therapeutic Effect:* Damages the fungal cell membrane, altering its function.
Pharmacokinetics
Moderately absorbed from the GI tract. Absorption is increased if the drug is taken with food. Protein binding: 99%. Widely distributed, primarily in the fatty tissue, liver, and kidneys. Metabolized in the liver to active metabolite. Primarily excreted in urine. Not removed by hemodialysis. **Half-life:** 21 hr; metabolite, 12 hr.

INDICATIONS AND DOSAGES
Blastomycosis, histoplasmosis
PO
Adults, Elderly. Initially, 200 mg once a day. Maximum: 400 mg/day in 2 divided doses.
IV
Adults, Elderly. 200 mg twice a day for 4 doses, then 200 mg once a day.
Aspergillosis
PO
Adults, Elderly. 600 mg/day in 3 divided doses for 3-4 days, then 200-400 mg/day in 2 divided doses.
IV
Adults, Elderly. 200 mg twice a day for 4 doses, then 200 mg once a day.
Esophageal candidiasis
PO
Adults, Elderly. Swish 10 ml in mouth for several seconds, then swallow. Maximum: 200 mg/day.

Oropharyngeal candidiasis
PO

Adults, Elderly. Vigorously swish 10 ml in mouth for several seconds (20 ml total daily dose) once a day.

§ AVAILABLE FORMS/COST
• Cap, Gel—Oral: 100 mg, 30's: **$280.86**
• Sol-Oral: 10 mg/ml, 150 ml: **$140.18**

UNLABELED USES: Suppression of histoplasmosis; treatment of disseminated sporotrichosis, fungal pneumonia and septicemia, or ringworm of the hand

CONTRAINDICATIONS: Hypersensitivity to itraconazole, fluconazole, ketoconazole, or miconazole

PREGNANCY AND LACTATION: Pregnancy category C; excreted into breast milk; do not administer to nursing mothers

SIDE EFFECTS
Frequent (11%-9%)

Nausea, rash

Occasional (5%-3%)

Vomiting, headache, diarrhea, hypertension, peripheral edema, fatigue, fever

Rare (2% or less)

Abdominal pain, dizziness, anorexia, pruritus

SERIOUS REACTIONS
• Hepatitis (as evidenced by anorexia, abdominal pain, unusual fatigue or weakness, jaundice skin or sclera, and dark urine) occurs rarely.

INTERACTIONS
Drugs

▪ *Alprazolam:* Increased plasma alprazolam concentration

▪ *Aluminum:* Reduced itraconazole absorption

▪ *Amprenavir:* Increased plasma amprenavir concentration

▪ *Antacids:* Reduced itraconazole absorption

▲ *Astemizole:* QT prolongation and life-threatening dysrhythmia

▪ *Atevirdine:* Increased plasma atevirdine concentration

▪ *Atorvastatin:* Increased plasma atorvastatin concentration with risk of rhabdomyolysis

▪ *Buspirone:* Increased plasma buspirone concentration

▪ *Calcium:* Reduced itraconazole absorption

▪ *Cerivastatin:* Increased plasma cerivastatin concentration with risk of rhabdomyolysis

▪ *Chlordiazepoxide:* Increased plasma chlordiazepoxide concentration

▪ *Cimetidine:* Reduced itraconazole absorption

▲ *Cisapride:* QT prolongation and life-threatening dysrhythmia

▪ *Clarithromycin:* Increased plasma itraconazole concentration

▪ *Cyclosporine:* Increased plasma cyclosporine concentration

▪ *Diazepam:* Increased plasma diazepam concentration

▪ *Digoxin:* Increased plasma digoxin concentration

▪ *Didanosine:* Reduced itraconazole absorption

▪ *Erythromycin:* Increased plasma itraconazole concentration

▪ *Ethanol:* Disulfiram-like reaction possible

▪ *Famotidine:* Reduced itraconazole absorption

▪ *Felodipine:* Increased plasma felodipine concentration

▪ *Fluvastatin:* Increased plasma fluvastatin concentration with risk of rhabdomyolysis

▪ *Food:* Increased intraconazole absorption

▪ *Indinavir:* Increased plasma indinavir concentration

▪ *Lansoprazole:* Reduced itraconazole absorption

❷ *Lovastatin:* Increased plasma lovastatin concentration with risk of rhabdomyolysis

3 *Magnesium:* Reduced itraconazole absorption

3 *Methadone:* Increased plasma methadone concentration

3 *Methylprednisolone:* Increased plasma methylprednisolone concentration

3 *Midazolam:* Increased plasma midazolam concentration

3 *Nelfinavir:* Increased plasma nelfinavir concentration

3 *Nizatidine:* Reduced itraconazole absorption

3 *Omeprazole:* Reduced itraconazole absorption

3 *Oral anticoagulants:* Increased hypoprothrombinemic response

2 *Phenytoin:* Markedly reduced plasma itraconazole concentration

⚠ *Pimozide:* Increased plasma pimozide concentration, QT prolongation and life-threatening dysrhythmia

3 *Pravastatin:* Increased plasma pravastatin concentration with risk of rhabdomyolysis

⚠ *Quinidine:* Increased plasma quinidine concentration, QT prolongation and life-threatening dysrhythmia

3 *Rifampin:* Decreased plasma itraconazole concentration; decreased plasma rifampin concentration

3 *Ritonavir:* Increased plasma ritonavir concentration

3 *Saquinavir:* Increased plasma saquinavir concentration

2 *Simvastatin:* Increased plasma simvastatin concentration with risk of rhabdomyolysis

3 *Sodium bicarbonate:* Reduced itraconazole absorption

3 *Sucralfate:* Reduced itraconazole absorption

3 *Tacrolimus:* Increased plasma tacrolimus concentration

⚠ *Terfenadine:* QT prolongation and life-threatening dysrhythmia

3 *Tolbutamide:* Increased plasma tolbutamide concentration

2 *Triazolam:* Increased plasma triazolam concentration

3 *Warfarin:* Increased hypoprothrombinemic response

SPECIAL CONSIDERATIONS
PATIENT/FAMILY EDUCATION
• Take with food to ensure maximal absorption
• Avoid antacids within 2 hr of itraconazole administration
MONITORING PARAMETERS
• Liver function tests in patients with pre-existing abnormalities

ivermectin
(eye-ver-mek'-tin)
Rx: Mectizan, Stromectol
Chemical Class: Avermectin derivative
Therapeutic Class: Antihelmintic

CLINICAL PHARMACOLOGY
Mechanism of Action: Selectively binds to chloride ion channels in invertebrate nerve/muscle cells, increasing permeability to chloride ions. In general the following organisms are susceptible to ivermectin: *Onchocerca volvulus, Pediculosis capitis, Strongyloides stercoralis, Sarcoptes scabiei,* and *Wuchereria bancrofti. Therapeutic effects:* Causes paralysis/death of parasites.
Pharmacokinetics
Does not readily cross the blood-brain barrier. Metabolized in the liver. Excreted in the feces. **Half-life:** 4 hours. Well absorbed with plasma concentrations proportional to the dose.

INDICATIONS AND DOSAGES
Strongyloidiasis
PO

Adults, Elderly, Children >33 pounds: 200 mcg/kg as a single dose.

Onchoceriasis
PO

Adults, Elderly, Children >33 pounds: 150 mcg/kg as a single dose at 3-12 month intervals.

Scabies
PO

Adults. 200 mcg/kg as a single dose and repeat 2 weeks later

Norwegian Scabies (crusted scabies infection), superinfected scabies, or resistant scabies
PO

Adults. 200 mcg/kg with repeated treatments or combined with a topical scabicide

Pediculosis
PO

Adults. A regimen of 2 doses of 200mcg/kg with each dose separated by 10 days

Bancroft's filariasis
PO

Adults, Children >15 kg. 150 mcg/kg as a single dose. May repeat 1 or 2 more times (each dose a week apart) if larva continues to migrate 1 week after the previous dose.

§ **AVAILABLE FORMS/COST**
• Tab-Oral: 3 mg, 20's: **$108.80**; 6 mg, 10's: **$99.74**

UNLABELED USES: Cutaneous larva migrans, filariasis, pediculosis, scabies, *Wuchereria bancrofti*
CONTRAINDICATIONS: Hypersensitivity to ivermectin or to any one of its components. Should not be used in women who are pregnant or infants.
PREGNANCY AND LACTATION: Pregnancy category C; excreted in breast milk in low concentrations

SIDE EFFECTS
Occasional
Abdominal pain, anorexia, arthralgia, constipation, diarrhea, dizziness, drowsiness, edema, fatigue, fever, lymphadenopathy, maculopapular or unspecified rash, nausea, vomiting, orthostatic hypotension, pruritis, Stevens-Johnson syndrome, toxic epidermal necrolysis, tremor, urticaria, vertigo, visual impairment, weakness

SPECIAL CONSIDERATIONS
PATIENT/FAMILY EDUCATION
• Rapid killing of microfilariae may induce systemic or ocular inflammatory response (Mazzotti reaction, manifest by pruritus, rash, lymphadenopathy, and fever)
MONITORING PARAMETERS
• Stool for parasites; blood for microfilaria and eosinophils

---

kanamycin
(kan-a-mye'sin)
Rx: Kantrex
Chemical Class: Aminoglycoside
Therapeutic Class: Antibiotic

CLINICAL PHARMACOLOGY
Mechanism of Action: An aminoglycoside antibiotic that irreversibly binds to protein on bacterial ribosomes. *Therapeutic Effect:* Interferes with protein synthesis of susceptible microorganisms.

INDICATIONS AND DOSAGES
Wound and surgical site irrigation
Adults, Elderly. 0.25% solution to irrigate pleural space, ventricular or abscess cavities, wounds, or surgical sites.

§ **AVAILABLE FORMS/COST**
• Sol, Inj-IM, IV: 1 g/3 ml, 3 ml: **$6.93-$9.61**

CONTRAINDICATIONS: Hypersensitivity to kanamycin, other aminoglycosides (cross-sensitivity), or their components.

PREGNANCY AND LACTATION: Pregnancy category D; 8th cranial nerve toxicity in the fetus has been reported; excreted into breast milk in low concentrations; poor oral availability reduces potential for ototoxicity for the infant; compatible with breast-feeding

SIDE EFFECTS

Occasional

Hypersensitivity reactions (fever, pruritus, rash, urticaria)

Rare

Headache

SERIOUS REACTIONS

• None known.

INTERACTIONS

Drugs

③ *Amphotericin B:* Synergistic nephrotoxicity

② *Atracurium:* Kanamycin potentiates respiratory depression by atracurium

③ *Carbenicillin:* Potential for inactivation of kanamycin in patients with renal failure

③ *Carboplatin:* Additive nephrotoxicity or ototoxicity

③ *Cephalosporins:* Increased potential for nephrotoxicity in patients with preexisting renal disease

③ *Cisplatin:* Additive nephrotoxicity or ototoxicity

③ *Cyclosporine:* Additive nephrotoxicity

② *Ethacrynic acid:* Additive ototoxicity

③ *Indomethacin:* Reduced renal clearance of kanamycin in premature infants

③ *Methoxyflurane:* Additive nephrotoxicity

② *Neuromuscular blocking agents:* Kanamycin potentiates respiratory depression by neuromuscular blocking agents

③ *NSAIDs:* May reduce renal clearance of kanamycin

③ *Penicillins (extended spectrum):* Potential for inactivation of kanamycin in patients with renal failure

③ *Piperacillin:* Potential for inactivation of kanamycin in patients with renal failure

② *Succinylcholine:* Kanamycin potentiates respiratory depression by succinylcholine

③ *Ticarcillin:* Potential for inactivation of kanamycin in patients with renal failure

③ *Vancomycin:* Additive nephrotoxicity or ototoxicity

② *Vecuronium:* Kanamycin potentiates respiratory depression by vecuronium

Labs

• *False increase:* Urine amino acids

SPECIAL CONSIDERATIONS

PATIENT/FAMILY EDUCATION

• Report headache, dizziness, loss of hearing, ringing, roaring in ears, or feeling of fullness in head

MONITORING PARAMETERS

• Urinalysis

• Urine output

• Serum peak drawn at 30-60 min after IV INF or 60 min after IM inj, trough level drawn just before next dose; adjust dosage per levels, especially in renal function impairment (usual therapeutic plasma levels; peak 15-30 mg/L, trough ≤10 mg/L)

• Serum creatinine for CrCl calculation

• Serum calcium, magnesium, sodium

• Audiometric testing; assess hearing before, during, after treatment

K

kaolin-pectin

OTC: Kao-Spen, Kapectolin, Kaolinpec
Combinations
  OTC: with bismuth subcarbonate (K-C); with bismuth subsalicylate (Kaodene nonnarcotic)
Chemical Class: Kaolin: hydrous magnesium aluminum silicate; pectin: purified carbohydrate product
Therapeutic Class: Antidiarrheal

CLINICAL PHARMACOLOGY
Mechanism of Action: An antidiarrheal agent that acts as an adsorbent and protectant. *Therapeutic Effect:* Absorbs bacteria, toxins, and reduces water loss.

Pharmacokinetics
Not absorbed orally. Up to 90% of pectin decomposed in gastrointestinal (GI) tract.

INDICATIONS AND DOSAGES
Antidiarrheal
PO
Adults, Elderly. 60-120 ml after each loose bowel movement (LBM).
Children 12 yrs and older. 60 ml after each LBM.
Children 6-12 yrs. 30-60 ml after each LBM.
Children 3-6 yrs. 15-30 ml after each LBM.

$ AVAILABLE FORMS/COST
• Susp—Oral: 5.8 g (kaolin)/130 mg (pectin)/30 ml, 180 ml: **$1.87**; 5.2 g (kaolin)/260 mg (pectin)/30 ml, 480 ml: **$4.68**
CONTRAINDICATIONS: Diarrhea secondary to pseudomembranous enterocolitis or toxigenic bacteria, hypersensitivity to kaolin/pectin products

PREGNANCY AND LACTATION:
Pregnancy category C; neither agent is systemically absorbed; should have no effect on lactation or nursing infant
SIDE EFFECTS
Rare
Constipation
SERIOUS REACTIONS
• Dehydration may occur.
INTERACTIONS
Drugs
❷ *Clindamycin, lincomycin:* Reduced antibacterial efficacy of these drugs
❸ *Digoxin:* Reduced bioavailability of digoxin tablets, capsules not affected
❸ *Lovastatin:* Pectin inhibits cholesterol lowering effects of lovastatin
❸ *Quinidine:* Reduced plasma quinidine concentrations
SPECIAL CONSIDERATIONS
PATIENT/FAMILY EDUCATION
• Do not self-medicate diarrhea for >48 hr without consulting a provider

ketoconazole
(kee-toe-koe′na-zole)
Rx: Nizoral
Chemical Class: Imidazole derivative
Therapeutic Class: Antifungal

CLINICAL PHARMACOLOGY
Mechanism of Action: A fungistatic antifungal that inhibits the synthesis of ergosterol, a vital component of fungal cell formation. *Therapeutic Effect:* Damages the fungal cell membrane, altering its function.

INDICATIONS AND DOSAGES

Histoplasmosis, blastomycosis, systemic candidiasis, chronic mucocutaneous candidiasis, coccidioidomycosis, paracoccidioidomycosis, chromomycosis, seborrheic dermatitis, tinea corporis, tinea capitis, tinea manus, tinea cruris, tinea pedis, tinea unguium (onychomycosis), oral thrush, candiduria

PO

Adults, Elderly. 200-400 mg/day.
Children. 3.3-6.6 mg/kg/day. Maximum: 800 mg/day in 2 divided doses.

Topical

Adults, Elderly. Apply to affected area 1-2 times a day for 2-4 wk.

Shampoo

Adults, Elderly. Use twice weekly for 4 wk, allowing at least 3 days between shampooing. Use intermittently to maintain control.

§ AVAILABLE FORMS/COST

• Cre—Top: 2%, 15, 30, 60 g: **$27.70-$35.29**/30 g
• Shampoo—Top: 2%, 120 ml: **$23.84-$33.22**
• Tab-Oral: 200 mg, 100's: **$231.25-$474.38**

UNLABELED USES: Systemic: Treatment of fungal pneumonia, prostate cancer, septicemia

CONTRAINDICATIONS: None known.

PREGNANCY AND LACTATION: Pregnancy category C; has been used, apparently without harm, for the treatment of vaginal candidiasis during pregnancy; not detected in plasma with chronic shampoo use; unknown if cream absorbed; oral ketoconazole probably excreted in breast milk; use in breast-feeding not recommended

SIDE EFFECTS

Occasional (10%-3%)
Nausea, vomiting

Rare (less than 2%)
Abdominal pain, diarrhea, headache, dizziness, photophobia, pruritus
Topical: itching, burning, irritation

SERIOUS REACTIONS

• Hematologic toxicity (as evidenced by thrombocytopenia, hemolytic anemia, and leukopenia) occurs occasionally.
• Hepatotoxicity may occur within 1 week to several months after starting therapy.
• Anaphylaxis occurs rarely.

INTERACTIONS

Drugs

▣ *Alprazolam:* Increased plasma alprazolam concentration

▣ *Aluminum:* Reduced ketoconazole absorption

▣ *Amprenavir:* Increased plasma amprenavir concentration

▣ *Antacids:* Reduced ketoconazole absorption

⚠ *Astemizole:* QT prolongation and life-threatening dysrhythmia

▣ *Atevirdine:* Increased plasma atevirdine concentration

▣ *Atorvastatin:* Increased plasma atorvastatin concentration with risk of rhabdomyolysis

▣ *Buspirone:* Increased plasma buspirone concentration

▣ *Calcium:* Reduced ketoconazole absorption

▣ *Chlordiazepoxide:* Increased plasma chlordiazepoxide concentration

▣ *Cimetidine:* Reduced ketoconazole absorption

② *Cisapride:* QT prolongation and dysrhythmia

▣ *Cyclosporine:* Increased plasma cyclosporine concentration

▣ *Diazepam:* Increased plasma diazepam concentration

▣ *Didanosine:* Reduced ketoconazole absorption

K

▪ *Ethanol:* Disulfiram-like reaction possible

▪ *Famotidine:* Reduced ketoconazole absorption

▪ *Felodipine:* Increased plasma felodipine concentration

▪ *Fluvastatin:* Increased plasma fluvastatin concentration with risk of rhabdomyolysis

▪ *Indinavir:* Increased plasma indinavir concentration

▪ *Lansoprazole:* Reduced ketoconazole absorption

❷ *Lovastatin:* Increased plasma lovastatin concentration with risk of rhabdomyolysis

▪ *Magnesium:* Reduced ketoconazole absorption

▪ *Methadone:* Increased plasma methadone concentration

▪ *Methylprednisolone:* Increased plasma methylprednisolone concentration

▪ *Midazolam:* Increased plasma midazolam concentration

▪ *Nelfinavir:* Increased plasma nelfinavir concentration

▪ *Nizatidine:* Reduced ketoconazole absorption

▪ *Omeprazole:* Reduced ketoconazole absorption

▪ *Oral anticoagulants:* Increased hypoprothrombinemic response

▪ *Pravastatin:* Increased plasma pravastatin concentration with risk of rhabdomyolysis

▪ *Quinidine:* Increased plasma quinidine concentration

▪ *Rifampin:* Decreased plasma ketoconazole concentration; decreased plasma rifampin concentration

▪ *Ritonavir:* Increased plasma ritonavir concentration

▪ *Saquinavir:* Increased plasma saquinavir concentration

❷ *Simvastatin:* Increased plasma simvastatin concentration with risk of rhabdomyolysis

▪ *Sodium bicarbonate:* Reduced ketoconazole absorption

▪ *Sucralfate:* Reduced ketoconazole absorption

▪ *Tacrolimus:* Increased plasma tacrolimus concentration

⚠ *Terfenadine:* QT prolongation and life-threatening dysrhythmia

▪ *Tolbutamide:* Increased plasma tolbutamide concentration

▪ *Triazolam:* Increased plasma triazolam concentration

▪ *Warfarin:* Increased hypoprothrombinemic response

SPECIAL CONSIDERATIONS
PATIENT/FAMILY EDUCATION

• For shampoo, moisten hair and scalp, apply shampoo, and gently massage over entire scalp for 1 min; rinse with warm water; repeat, leaving shampoo on scalp for additional 3 min

• Do not take tab with antacids or H_2-receptor antagonists; separate doses by at least 2 hr

• Take tablets with food

MONITORING PARAMETERS

• Liver function tests at baseline and periodically during treatment

---

ketoprofen
(kee-toe-proe′fen)

Rx: Orudis, Oruvail

OTC: Actron, Orudis KT

Chemical Class: Propionic acid derivative

Therapeutic Class: NSAID; antipyretic; nonnarcotic analgesic

CLINICAL PHARMACOLOGY

Mechanism of Action: An NSAID that produces analgesic and anti-inflammatory effects by inhibiting prostaglandin synthesis. *Therapeutic Effect:* Reduces the inflammatory response and intensity of pain.

INDICATIONS AND DOSAGES
Acute or chronic rheumatoid arthritis and osteoarthritis
PO (tablets, capsules)
Adults. Initially, 75 mg 3 times a day or 50 mg 4 times a day.
Elderly. Initially, 25–50 mg 3–4 times a day. Maintenance: 150–300 mg/day in 3–4 divided doses.
PO (Extended-Release)
Adults, Elderly. 100–200 mg once a day.
Mild to moderate pain, dysmenorrhea
PO
Adults, Elderly. 25–50 mg q6–8h. Maximum: 300 mg/day.
Over-the-counter (OTC) dosage
PO
Adults, Elderly. 12.5 mg q4-6h. Maximum: 6 tabs/day.
Dosage in renal impairment
Mild. 150 mg/day maximum.
Severe. 100 mg/day maximum.
ⓈAVAILABLE FORMS/COST
• Cap, Gel—Oral: 25 mg, 100's: **$65.68-$72.15**; 50 mg, 100's: **$80.62-$122.75**; 75 mg, 100's: **$98.90-$124.00**
• Cap, Gel, Sus Action—Oral: 100 mg, 100's: **$225.50-$247.69**; 150 mg, 100's: **$301.05**; 200 mg, 100's: **$249.00-$339.91**
• Tab—Oral: 12.5 mg, 100's (OTC): **$8.93**

UNLABELED USES: Treatment of acute gouty arthritis, psoriatic arthritis, ankylosing spondylitis, vascular headache

CONTRAINDICATIONS: Active peptic ulcer disease, chronic inflammation of the GI tract, GI bleeding or ulceration, history of hypersensitivity to aspirin or NSAIDs

PREGNANCY AND LACTATION: Pregnancy category B (category D if used in 3rd trimester); could cause constriction of the ductus arteriosus *in utero;* persistent pulmonary hypertension of the newborn or prolonged labor; unknown if excreted into human breast milk

SIDE EFFECTS
Frequent (11%)
Dyspepsia
Occasional (more than 3%)
Nausea, diarrhea or constipation, flatulence, abdominal cramps, headache
Rare (less than 2%)
Anorexia, vomiting, visual disturbances, fluid retention

SERIOUS REACTIONS
• Rare reactions with long-term use include peptic ulcer disease, GI bleeding, gastritis, and severe hepatic reactions (cholestasis, jaundice), nephrotoxicity (dysuria, hematuria, proteinuria, nephrotic syndrome), and severe hypersensitivity reaction (bronchospasm, angioedema).

INTERACTIONS
Drugs
▣ *Aminoglycosides:* Reduced clearance with elevated aminoglycoside levels and potential for toxicity (especially indomethacin in premature infants; other NSAIDs probably)

▣ *Anticoagulants:* Excessive hypoprothrombinemia, decreased platelet aggregation with increased risk of GI bleeding

▣ *Antihypertensives (α-blockers, angiotensin-converting enzyme inhibitors, angiotensin II receptor blockers, β-blockers, diuretics):* Inhibition of antihypertensive and other favorable hemodynamic effects

▣ *Corticosteroids:* Increased risk of GI ulceration

▣ *Cyclosporine:* Increased nephrotoxicity risk

K

3 *Lithium:* Decreased clearance of lithium (mediated via prostaglandins) resulting in elevated serum lithium levels and risk of toxicity

3 *Methotrexate:* Decreased renal secretion of methotrexate resulting in elevated methotrexate levels and risk of toxicity

3 *Phenylpropanolamine:* Possible acute hypertensive reaction

3 *Potassium-sparing diuretics:* Additive hyperkalemia potential

3 *Triamterene:* Acute renal failure reported with addition of indomethacin; caution with other NSAIDs

Labs

• *False decrease:* Serum ALT, AST; serum lactate dehydrogenase

SPECIAL CONSIDERATIONS

• No significant advantage over other NSAIDs; cost should govern use

PATIENT/FAMILY EDUCATION

• Avoid aspirin and alcoholic beverages

• Take with food, milk, or antacids to decrease GI upset

MONITORING PARAMETERS

• Initial hemogram and fecal occult blood test within 3 mo of starting regular chronic therapy; repeat every 6-12 mo (more frequently in high-risk patients (>65 years, peptic ulcer disease, concurrent steroids or anticoagulants); electrolytes, creatinine, and BUN within 3 mo of starting regular chronic therapy; repeat every 6-12 mo

---

ketorolac

(kee-toe'role-ak)

Rx: *Systemic:* Toradol

Rx: *Ophthalmic:* Acular, Acular PF

Chemical Class: Acetic acid derivative

Therapeutic Class: NSAID; antipyretic; nonnarcotic analgesic

CLINICAL PHARMACOLOGY

Mechanism of Action: An NSAID that inhibits prostaglandin synthesis and reduces prostaglandin levels in the aqueous humor. *Therapeutic Effect:* Relieves pain stimulus and reduces intraocular inflammation.

Pharmacokinetics

Route	Onset	Peak	Duration
PO	30–60 min	1.5–4 hr	4–6 hr
IV/IM	30 min	1–2 hr	4–6 hr

Readily absorbed from the GI tract, after IM administration. Protein binding: 99%. Largely metabolized in the liver. Primarily excreted in urine. Not removed by hemodialysis. **Half-life:** 3.8–6.3 hr (increased with impaired renal function and in the elderly).

INDICATIONS AND DOSAGES

Short-term relief of mild to moderate pain (multiple doses)

PO

Adults, Elderly. 10 mg q4–6h. Maximum: 40 mg/24 hr.

IV/IM

Adults younger than 65 yr. 30 mg q6h. Maximum: 120 mg/24 hr.

Adults 65 yr and older, those with renal impairment, those weighing less than 50 kg. 15 mg q6h. Maximum: 60 mg/24 hr.

Children 2–16 yr. 0.5 mg/kg q6h.

Short-term relief of mild to moderate pain (single dose)
IV
Adults younger than 65 yr, Children 17 yr and older weighing more than 50 kg. 30 mg.
Adults 65 yr and older, with renal impairment, weighing less than 50 kg. 15 mg.
Children 2-16 yr. 0.5 mg/kg. Maximum: 15 mg.
IM
Adults younger than 65 yr, Children 17 yr and older, weighing more than 50 kg. 60 mg.
Adults 65 yrs and older, with renal impairment, weighing less than 50 kg. 30 mg.
Children 2–16 yr. 1 mg/kg. Maximum: 15 kg.
Allergic conjunctivitis
Ophthalmic
Adults, Elderly, Children 3 yr and older. 1 drop 4 times a day.
Cataract extraction
Ophthalmic
Adults, Elderly. 1 drop 4 times a day. Begin 24 hr after surgery and continue for 2 wk.
Refractive surgery
Ophthalmic
Adults, Elderly. 1 drop 4 times a day for 3 days.

[$] **AVAILABLE FORMS/COST**
• Sol, Inj-IV/IM: 15 mg/ml, 1 ml: **\$3.60-\$9.03**; 30 mg/ml, 1, 2, 10 ml: **\$3.84-\$10.88**/1 ml
• Sol—Ophth: 0.5%, 3, 5, 10 ml: **\$49.90-\$67.08**/5 ml
• Tab-Oral: 10 mg, 100's: **\$56.94-\$150.27**

UNLABELED USES: Prevention or treatment of ocular inflammation (ophthalmic form)

CONTRAINDICATIONS: Active peptic ulcer disease, chronic inflammation of GI tract, GI bleeding or ulceration, history of hypersensitivity to aspirin or NSAIDs

PREGNANCY AND LACTATION: Pregnancy category C; excreted into breast milk; not recommended in lactation

SIDE EFFECTS
Frequent (17%–12%)
Headache, nausea, abdominal cramps or pain, dyspepsia
Occasional (9%–3%)
Diarrhea
Ophthalmic: Transient stinging and burning
Rare (3%–1%)
Constipation, vomiting, flatulence, stomatitis, dizziness
Ophthalmic: Ocular irritation, allergic reactions, superficial ocular infection, keratitis

SERIOUS REACTIONS
• Rare reactions with long-term use include peptic ulcer disease, GI bleeding, gastritis, severe hepatic reactions (cholestasis, jaundice), nephrotoxicity (glomerular nephritis, interstitial nephritis, nephrotic syndrome), and an acute hypersensitivity reaction (including fever, chills, and joint pain).

INTERACTIONS
Drugs
[3] *Aminoglycosides:* Reduced clearance with elevated aminoglycoside levels and potential for toxicity (especially indomethacin in premature infants; other NSAIDs probably)
[3] *Anticoagulants:* Excessive hypoprothrombinemia, decreased platelet aggregation with increased risk of GI bleeding
[3] *Antihypertensives (α-blockers, angiotensin-converting enzyme inhibitors, angiotensin II receptor blockers, β-blockers, diuretics):* Inhibition of antihypertensive and other favorable hemodynamic effects
[3] *Corticosteroids:* Increased risk of GI ulceration

K

3 *Cyclosporine:* Increased nephrotoxicity risk

3 *Lithium:* Decreased clearance of lithium (mediated via prostaglandins) resulting in elevated serum lithium levels and risk of toxicity

3 *Methotrexate:* Decreased renal secretion of methotrexate resulting in elevated methotrexate levels and risk of toxicity

3 *Phenylpropanolamine:* Possible acute hypertensive reaction

3 *Potassium-sparing diuretics:* Additive hyperkalemia potential

3 *Triamterene:* Acute renal failure reported with addition of indomethacin; caution with other NSAIDs

SPECIAL CONSIDERATIONS

PATIENT/FAMILY EDUCATION

• Not for chronic use

• No significant advantage over other oral NSAIDs; cost and clinical situation should govern use; no reason to continue parenteral course of therapy with oral ketorolac (more expensive, more toxic)

• Combined use of ketorolac parenteral and oral should not exceed 5 days

---

labetalol

(la-bet′a-lole)

Rx: Normodyne, Trandate
Combinations
   Rx: with hydrochlorothiazide (Normozide, Trandate HCT)
Chemical Class: α-adrenergic blocker, peripheral; β-adrenergic blocker, nonselective
Therapeutic Class: Antihypertensive

CLINICAL PHARMACOLOGY

Mechanism of Action: An antihypertensive that blocks alpha$_1$-, beta$_1$-, and beta$_2$-(large doses) adrenergic receptor sites. Large doses increase airway resistance. *Therapeutic Effect:* Slows sinus heart rate; decreases peripheral vascular resistance, cardiac output, and BP.

Pharmacokinetics

Route	Onset	Peak	Duration
PO	0.5–2 hr	2–4 hr	8–12 hr
IV	2–5 min	5–15 min	2–4 hr

Completely absorbed from the GI tract. Protein binding: 50%. Undergoes first-pass metabolism. Metabolized in the liver. Primarily excreted in urine. Not removed by hemodialysis. **Half-life:** PO, 6–8 hr; IV, 5.5 hr.

INDICATIONS AND DOSAGES

Hypertension

PO

Adults. Initially, 100 mg twice a day adjusted in increments of 100 mg twice a day q2–3 days. Maintenance: 200–400 mg twice a day. Maximum: 2.4 g/day.

Elderly. Initially, 100 mg 1–2 times a day. May increase as needed.

Severe hypertension, hypertensive emergency

IV

Adults. Initially, 20 mg. Additional doses of 20–80 mg may be given at 10-min intervals, up to total dose of 300 mg.

IV infusion

Adults. Initially, 2 mg/min up to total dose of 300 mg.

PO (after IV therapy)

Adults. Initially, 200 mg; then, 200–400 mg in 6–12 hr. Increase dose at 1-day intervals to desired level.

S AVAILABLE FORMS/COST

• Sol, Inj-IV: 5 mg/ml, 4, 8, 20, 40 ml: **$5.00-$45.35**/20 ml

• Tab, Coated—Oral: 100 mg, 100's: **$36.31-$70.88**; 200 mg, 100's: **$68.10-$100.06**; 300 mg, 100's: **$90.61-$133.10**

UNLABELED USES: Control of hypotension during surgery, treatment of chronic angina pectoris

CONTRAINDICATIONS: Bronchial asthma, cardiogenic shock, second- or third-degree heart block, severe bradycardia, uncontrolled CHF

PREGNANCY AND LACTATION: Pregnancy category C; similar drug, atenolol, frequently used in the third trimester for treatment of hypertension (many studies of efficacy and safety of atenolol in pregnancy-induced hypertension); long-term use has been associated with intrauterine growth retardation; only a small amount of drug appears in milk (0.004% of dose); unlikely to be therapeutically significant

SIDE EFFECTS
Frequent
Drowsiness, difficulty sleeping, unusual fatigue or weakness, diminished sexual ability, transient scalp tingling
Occasional
Dizziness, dyspnea, peripheral edema, depression, anxiety, constipation, diarrhea, nasal congestion, nausea, vomiting, abdominal discomfort
Rare
Altered taste, dry eyes, increased urination, paresthesia

SERIOUS REACTIONS
• Labetolol administration may precipitate or aggravate CHF beacause of decreased myocardial stimulation.
• Abrupt withdrawal may precipitate ischemic heart disease, producing sweating, palpitations, headache, and tremor.

• May mask signs and symptoms of acute hypoglycemia (tachycardia, BP changes) in patients with diabetes.

INTERACTIONS
Drugs
③ *α₁-adrenergic blockers:* Potential enhanced first dose response (marked initial drop in blood pressure, particularly on standing)
③ *Amiodarone:* Symptomatic bradycardia and sinus arrest, especially patients with bradycardia, sick sinus syndrome, or partial AV node block
③ *Cimetidine:* Increased plasma labetolol concentrations
③ *Clonidine:* Withdrawal of clonidine abruptly may exaggerate the hypertension due to unopposed alpha stimulation; safer than other β-blockers, however
③ *Digoxin:* Additive prolongation of AV conduction time
③ *Dihydropyridine calcium channel blockers:* Severe hypotension or impaired cardiac performance; most prevalent with impaired left ventricular function, cardiac arrhythmias, or aortic stenosis
③ *Diltiazem:* Potentiates β-adrenergic effects; hypotension, left ventricular failure, and AV conduction disturbances problematic in elderly, patients with left ventricular dysfunction, aortic stenosis, or with large doses of either drug
③ *Epinephrine:* Increased diastolic pressure and bradycardia during epinephrine infusions
③ *Hypoglycemic agents:* Masked hypoglycemia, hyperglycemia
③ *NSAIDs:* Reduced hypotensive effects of β-blockers
② *Theophylline:* Antagonistic pharmacodynamic effects
③ *Verapamil:* Potentiates β-adrenergic effects; hypotension, left ventricular failure, and AV conduction

disturbances problematic in elderly, patients with ventricular dysfunction, aortic stenosis, or with large doses of either drug

Labs
• *False positive:* Urine amphetamine
• *False increase:* Urinary catecholamines, plasma epinephrine

SPECIAL CONSIDERATIONS

PATIENT/FAMILY EDUCATION
• Do not discontinue abruptly; may require taper; rapid withdrawal may produce rebound hypertension or angina
• Transient scalp tingling may occur, especially when treatment is initiated
• May mask the symptoms of hypoglycemia, except for sweating, in diabetic patients

MONITORING PARAMETERS
• Angina: Reduction in nitroglycerin usage; frequency, severity, onset, and duration of angina pain; heart rate
• Arrhythmias: Heart rate
• Congestive heart failure: Functional status, cough, dyspnea on exertion, paroxysmal nocturnal dyspnea, exercise tolerance, and ventricular function
• Hypertension: Blood pressure
• Postmyocardial infarction: Left ventricular function, lower resting heart rate
• Toxicity: Blood glucose, bronchospasm, hypotension, bradycardia, depression, confusion, hallucination, sexual dysfunction

lactulose
(lak´tyoo-lose)
Rx: Cephulac, Cholac, Chronulac, Constilac, Constulose, Duphalac, Enulose, Generlac, Kristalose
Chemical Class: Disaccharide lactose analog
Therapeutic Class: Ammonia detoxicant; laxative

CLINICAL PHARMACOLOGY
Mechanism of Action: A lactose derivative that retains ammonia in colon and decreases serum ammonia concentration, producing osmotic effect. *Therapeutic Effect:* Promotes increased peristalsis and bowel evacuation, which expels ammonia from the colon.

Pharmacokinetics

Route	Onset	Peak	Duration
PO	24–48 hr	N/A	N/A
Rectal	30–60 min	N/A	N/A

Poorly absorbed from the GI tract. Acts in the colon. Primarily excreted in feces.

INDICATIONS AND DOSAGES
Constipation
PO
Adults, Elderly. 15–30 ml (10-20 g)/day, up to 60 ml (40 g)/day.
Children. 7.5 ml (5 g)/day after breakfast.

Portal-systemic encephalopathy
PO
Adults, Elderly. Initially, 30–45 ml every hr. Then, 30–45 ml (20-30 g) 3–4 times a day. Adjust dose q1–2 days to produce 2–3 soft stools a day.
Children. 40–90 ml/day in divided doses.
Infants. 2.5–10 ml/day in divided doses.
Rectal (as retention enema)

Adults, Elderly, 300 ml with 700 ml water or saline solution; patient should retain 30–60 min. Repeat q4–6h. If evacuation occurs too promptly, repeat immediately.

AVAILABLE FORMS/COST

• Powder, Packet—Oral: 10 g/packet, 30's: **$31.50**; 20 g/packet 30's: **$48.90**

• Syr—Oral: 10 g/15 ml, 480 ml: **$12.43-$34.70**

CONTRAINDICATIONS: Abdominal pain, appendicitis, nausea, patients on a galactose-free diet, vomiting

PREGNANCY AND LACTATION: Pregnancy category B; breastfeeding risk to fetus and the newborn negligible

SIDE EFFECTS

Occasional

Abdominal cramping, flatulence, increased thirst, abdominal discomfort

Rare

Nausea, vomiting

SERIOUS REACTIONS

• Diarrhea indicates overdose.

• Long-term use may result in laxative dependence, chronic constipation, and loss of normal bowel function.

INTERACTIONS

Labs

• *False increase:* Serum creatinine

SPECIAL CONSIDERATIONS

PATIENT/FAMILY EDUCATION

• May be mixed with fruit juice, water, or milk to increase palatability

• Do not take other laxatives while on lactulose therapy

MONITORING PARAMETERS

• Serum electrolytes, carbon dioxide periodically during chronic treatment

lamivudine (3TC)

(la-miv'yoo-deen)

Rx: Epivir, Epivir-HBV
Combinations

Rx: with abacavir (Epzicom); with zidovudine: (Combivir)

Chemical Class: Nucleoside analog

Therapeutic Class: Antiretroviral

CLINICAL PHARMACOLOGY

Mechanism of Action: An antiviral that inhibits HIV reverse transcriptase by viral DNA chain termination. Also inhibits RNA- and DNA-dependent DNA polymerase, an enzyme necessary for HIV replication. *Therapeutic Effect:* Interrupts HIV replication, slowing the progression of HIV infection.

Pharmacokinetics

Rapidly and completely absorbed from the GI tract. Protein binding: 36%. Widely distributed (crosses the blood-brain barrier). Primarily excreted unchanged in urine. Not removed by hemodialysis or peritoneal dialysis. **Half-life:** 11-15 hr (intracellular), 2-11 hr (serum, adults), 1.7-2 hr (serum, children). (increased in impaired renal function).

INDICATIONS AND DOSAGES

HIV infection (in combination with other antiretrovirals)

PO

Adults, Children 12-16 yr, weighing more than 50 kg (100 lb). 150 mg twice a day or 300 mg once a day.

Adults weighing less than 50 kg. 2 mg/kg twice a day.

Children 3 mo-11 yr. 4 mg/kg twice a day (up to 150 mg/dose).

Chronic hepatitis B
PO

Adults, Children 17 yr and older. 100 mg/day.

Children younger than 17 yr. 3 mg/kg/day. Maximum: 100 mg/day.

Dosage in renal impairment

Dosage and frequency are modified based on creatinine clearance.

Creatinine Clearance (ml/min)	Dosage
50 ml/min or higher	150 mg twice a day
30-49 ml/min	150 mg once a day
15-29 ml/min	150 mg first dose, then 100 mg once a day
5-14 ml/min	150 mg first dose, then 50 mg once a day
less than 5 ml/min	50 mg first dose, then 25 mg once a day

$ AVAILABLE FORMS/COST

• Sol—Oral: 5 mg/ml, 240 ml: **$60.67**; 10 mg/ml, 240 ml: **$84.28**
• Tab, Film Coated—Oral: 100 mg, 60's: **$363.16**; 150 mg, 60's: **$316.04**

UNLABELED USES: Prophylaxis in health care workers at risk of acquiring HIV after occupational exposure.

CONTRAINDICATIONS: None known.

PREGNANCY AND LACTATION: Pregnancy category C; not recommended in nursing mothers

SIDE EFFECTS

Frequent

Headache (35%), nausea (33%), malaise and fatigue (27%), nasal disturbances (20%), diarrhea, cough (18%), musculoskeletal pain, neuropathy (12%), insomnia (11%), anorexia, dizziness, fever or chills (10%)

Occasional

Depression (9%); myalgia (8%); abdominal cramps (6%); dyspepsia, arthralgia (5%)

SERIOUS REACTIONS

• Pancreatitis occurs in 13% of pediatric patients.
• Anemia, neutropenia, and thrombocytopenia occur rarely.

---

lamotrigine
(la-moe-trih'jeen)

Rx: Lamictal, Lamictal CD
Chemical Class: Phenyltriazine derivative
Therapeutic Class: Anticonvulsant

CLINICAL PHARMACOLOGY

Mechanism of Action: An anticonvulsant whose exact mechanism is unknown. May block voltage-sensitive sodium channels, thus stabilizing neuronal membranes and regulating presynaptic transmitter release of excitatory amino acids. *Therapeutic Effect:* Reduces seizure activitiy.

INDICATIONS AND DOSAGES

Seizure control in patients receiving enzyme-inducing antiepileptic drug (EIAEDs), but not valproate acid
PO

Adults, Elderly, Children 12 yr and older. Recommended as add-on therapy: 50 mg once a day for 2 wk, followed by 100 mg/day in 2 divided doses for 2 wk. Maintenance: Dosage may be increased by 100 mg/day every week, up to 300-500 mg/day in 2 divided doses.

Children 2-12 yr. 0.6 mg/kg/day in 2 divided doses for 2 wk, then 1.2 mg/kg/day in 2 divided doses for wk 3 and 4. Maintenance: 5-15 mg/kg/day. Maximum: 400 mg/day.

Seizure control in patients receiving combination therapy of EI-AEDs and valproic acid
PO

Adults, Elderly, Children 12 yr and older. 25 mg every other day for 2 wk, followed by 25 mg once a day for 2 wk. Maintenance: Dosage may be increased by 25-50 mg/day q1-2wk, up to 150 mg/day in 2 divided doses.

Children 2-12 yr. 0.15 mg/kg/day in 2 divided doses for 2 wk, then 0.3 mg/kg/day in 2 divided doses for wk 3 and 4. Maintenance: 1-5 mg/kg/day in 2 divided doses. Maximum: 200 mg/day.

Conversion to monotherapy
PO

Adults, Children 12 yr and older. Add lamotrigine 50 mg/day for 2 wk; then 100 mg/day during wk 3 and 4. Increase by 100 mg/day q1-2wk until maintenance dosage (300-500 mg/day in 2 divided doses) is achieved. Gradually discontinue other EIAEDs over 4 wk once maintenance dose is achieved.

Bipolar disorder
PO

Adults, Elderly. Initially, 25 mg/day. May double dose after wk 2, 4, and 5. Target dose: 200 mg/day.

Discontinuation therapy

Adults, Children older than 12 yr. A dosage reduction of approximately 50% per week over at least 2 wk is recommended.

$ AVAILABLE FORMS/COST

• Tab—Oral: 25 mg, 100's: **$312.81**; 100 mg, 100's: **$332.05**; 150 mg, 60's: **$209.36**; 200 mg, 60's: **$219.45**

• Tab, Chewable—Oral: 5 mg, 100's: **$295.59**; 25 mg, 100's: **$309.58**

CONTRAINDICATIONS: None known

PREGNANCY AND LACTATION: Pregnancy category C; passes into breast milk, effects on infants exposed by this route are unknown

SIDE EFFECTS

Frequent

Dizziness (38%), diplopia (28%), headache (29%), ataxia (22%), nausea (19%), blurred vision (16%), somnolence, rhinitis (14%)

Occasional (10%-5%)

Rash, pharyngitis, vomiting, cough, flu-like symptoms, diarrhea, dysmenorrhea, fever, insomnia, dyspepsia

Rare

Constipation, tremor, anxiety, pruritus, vaginitis, hypersensitivity reaction

SERIOUS REACTIONS

• Abrupt withdrawal may increase seizure frequency.

INTERACTIONS

Drugs

🔳 *Carbamazepine:* Increased carbamazepine epoxide levels; decreased lamotrigine levels

🔳 *Phenobarbital, primidone, phenytoin:* Decreased lamotrigine concentrations

🔳 *Valproic acid:* Increased lamotrigine concentration; decreased valproic acid concentration

SPECIAL CONSIDERATIONS

PATIENT/FAMILY EDUCATION

• Notify clinician immediately if a skin rash develops

• Avoid prolonged exposure to direct sunlight

lansoprazole

(lan-soe'pray-zole)

Rx: Prevacid
Combinations
  Rx: with naproxen (Napra-PAC)
Chemical Class: Benzimidazole derivative
Therapeutic Class: Antiulcer agent; gastrointestinal antisecretory agent

CLINICAL PHARMACOLOGY

Mechanism of Action: A proton pump inhibitor that selectively inhibits the parietal cell membrane enzyme system (hydrogen-potassium adenosine triphosphatase) or proton pump. *Therapeutic Effect:* Suppresses gastric acid secretion.

Pharmacokinetics

Route	Onset	Peak	Duration
PO (15 mg)	2–3 hr	N/A	24 hr
PO (30 mg)	1–2 hr	N/A	longer than 24 hr

Rapid and complete absorption (food may decrease absorption) once drug has left stomach. Protein binding: 97%. Distributed primarily to gastric parietal cells and converted to two active metabolites. Extensively metabolized in the liver. Eliminated in bile and urine. Not removed by hemodialysis. **Half-life:** 1.5 hr (increased in the elderly and in those with hepatic impairment).

INDICATIONS AND DOSAGES

Duodenal ulcer

PO

Adults, Elderly. 15 mg/day, before eating, preferably in the morning, for up to 4 wks.

Erosive esophagitis

PO

Adults, Elderly. 30 mg/day, before eating, for up to 8 wks. If healing does not occur within 8 wk (in 5%–10% of cases), may give for additional 8 wk. Maintenance: 15 mg/day.

IV

Adults, Elderly. 30 mg once a day for up to 7 days. Switch to oral lansoprazole therapy as soon as patient can tolerate oral route.

Gastric ulcer

PO

Adults. 30 mg/day for up to 8 wk.

NSAID gastric ulcer

PO

Adults, Elderly. (Healing): 30 mg/day for up to 8 wk. (Prevention): 15 mg/day for up to 12 wk.

Healed duodenal ulcer, gastroesophageal reflux disease

PO

Adults. 15 mg/day.

Usual pediatric dosage

Children 3 mo–14 yr, weighing more than 20 kg. 30 mg once daily.
Children 3 mo–14 yr, weighing 10–20 kg. 15 mg once daily.
Children 3 mo–14 yr, weighing less than 10 kg. 7.5 mg once daily.
Helicobacter pylori infection

PO

Adults. 30 mg twice a day for 10 days (with amoxicillin and clarithromycin).

Pathologic hypersecretory conditions (including Zollinger-Ellison syndrome)

PO

Adults, Elderly. 60 mg/day. Individualize dosage according to patient needs and for as long as clinically indicated. May increase to 120 mg/day in divided doses.

[$] **AVAILABLE FORMS/COST**

• Cap, Gel, Sus Action—Oral: 15 mg, 30's: **$140.36**; 30 mg, 100's: **$476.79**

• Susp—Oral: 15 mg packets, 30's: **$140.36**; 30 mg packets, 30's: **$143.04**

• Tab, Disintegrating—Oral: 15 mg, 30's: **$140.36**; 30 mg, 30's: **$143.04**

CONTRAINDICATIONS: None known

PREGNANCY AND LACTATION: Pregnancy category B; excretion into breast milk unknown

SIDE EFFECTS

Occasional (3%–2%)

Diarrhea, abdominal pain, rash, pruritus, altered appetite

Rare (1%)

Nausea, headache

SERIOUS REACTIONS

• Bilirubinemia, eosinophilia, and hyperlipemia occur rarely.

INTERACTIONS

Drugs

[3] *Cefpodoxime, cefuroxime, ketoconazole, enoxacin:* Reduced concentrations of these drugs

[3] *Digoxin, nifedipine:* Increased serum concentrations of these drugs

[3] *Food:* 50% decrease in absorption if given 30 min after food compared to the fasting condition

[3] *Glipizide, glyburide, tolbutamide:* Increased concentrations of these drugs, potential for hypoglycemia

[3] *Sucralfate:* Delayed absorption of lansoprazole and reduced bioavailability, administer lansoprazole at least 30 min prior to sucralfate

SPECIAL CONSIDERATIONS

• For patients with a nasogastric tube, capsules may be opened and the intact granules mixed with 40 ml of apple juice and injected through tube into stomach

• For patients unable to swallow capsules, capsule can be opened and the intact granules sprinkled on 1 tablespoon of applesauce and swallowed immediately; do not crush or chew granules

• For oral suspension, empty contents of packet into 30 ml of water only, don't use other liquids, do not crush or chew granules, if material remains add more water, stir, and drink immediately

leflunomide

(le-flu′na-mide)

Rx: Arava

Chemical Class: Isoxazole derivative

Therapeutic Class: Disease-modifying antirheumatic drug (DMARD); immunomodulatory agent

CLINICAL PHARMACOLOGY

Mechanism of Action: An immunomodulatory agent that inhibits dihydroorotate dehydrogenase, the enzyme involved in autoimmune process that leads to rheumatoid arthritis. *Therapeutic Effect:* Reduces signs and symptoms of rheumatoid arthritis and slows structural damage.

Pharmacokinetics

Well absorbed after PO administration. Protein binding: greater than 99%. Metabolized to active metabolite in the GI wall and liver. Excreted through both renal and biliary systems. Not removed by hemodialysis. **Half-life:** 16 days.

INDICATIONS AND DOSAGES

Rheumatoid arthritis

PO

Adults, Elderly. Initially, 100 mg/day for 3 days, then 10–20 mg/day.

lepirudin
(leh-peer'u-din)
Rx: Refludan
Chemical Class: Hirudin derivative; thrombin inhibitor
Therapeutic Class: Anticoagulant

AVAILABLE FORMS/COST
• Tab, Coated—Oral: 10 mg, 20 mg, 30's: **$340.02**

CONTRAINDICATIONS: Pregnancy or plans to become pregnant

PREGNANCY AND LACTATION: Pregnancy category X; amount of excretion into breast milk unknown; use of leflunomide by nursing mothers is not recommended since the potential risk to nursing infants is considered serious

SIDE EFFECTS
Frequent (20%–10%)
Diarrhea, respiratory tract infection, alopecia, rash, nausea

SERIOUS REACTIONS
• Transient thrombocytopenia and leukopenia occur rarely.

INTERACTIONS
Drugs
⏹ *Cholestyramine, charcoal:* Coadministration results in rapid and significant decrease in active metabolite
⏹ *Nonsteroidal antiinflammatory drugs:* Inhibition of CYP 2C9, decreases the metabolism of many NSAIDS
⏹ *Rifampin:* Leflunomide levels increased 40%

SPECIAL CONSIDERATIONS
• Discuss potential risks of pregnancy and recommend appropriate contraception

MONITORING PARAMETERS
• *Efficacy:* ESR, C-reactive protein, platelet count, hemoglobin, improvement of RA; *toxicity:* LFTs (baseline, then monthly until stable)

lepirudin
(leh-peer'u-din)
Rx: Refludan
Chemical Class: Hirudin derivative; thrombin inhibitor
Therapeutic Class: Anticoagulant

CLINICAL PHARMACOLOGY
Mechanism of Action: An anticoagulant that inhibits thrombogenic action of thrombin (independent of antithrombin II and not inhibited by platelet factor 4). One molecule of lepirudin binds to one molecule of thrombin. *Therapeutic Effect:* Produces dose-dependent increases aPTT.

Pharmacokinetics
Distributed primarily in extracellular fluid. Primarily eliminated by the kidneys. **Half-life:** 1.3 hr (increased in impaired renal function).

INDICATIONS AND DOSAGES
Heparin-induced thrombocytopenia and associated thromboembolic disease to prevent further thromboembolic complications
IV, IV infusion
Adults, Elderly. 0.2–0.4 mg/kg, IV slowly over 15–20 sec, followed by IV infusion of 0.1–0.15 mg/kg/hr for 2–10 days or longer.

Dosage in renal impairment
Initial dose is decreased to 0.2 mg/kg, with infusion rate adjusted based on creatinine clearance.

Creatinine Clearance (ml/min)	% of Standard Infusion Rate	Infusion Rate (mg/kg/hr)
45–60	50	0.075
30–44	30	0.045
15–29	15	0.0225

AVAILABLE FORMS/COST
• Powder, Inj-IV: 50 mg, 1 vial: **$164.84**

CONTRAINDICATIONS: None known
PREGNANCY AND LACTATION: Pregnancy category B; use caution in nursing mothers
SIDE EFFECTS
Frequent (14%–5%)
Bleeding from gums, puncture sites, or wounds, hematuria, fever, GI and rectal bleeding
Occasional (3%–1%)
Epistaxis; allergic reaction, such as rash and pruritus; vaginal bleeding
SERIOUS REACTIONS
• Overdose is characterized by excessively high aPTT.
• Intracranial bleeding occurs rarely.
• Abnormal hepatic function occurs in 6% of patients.
INTERACTIONS
Drugs
▣ *Thrombolytics:* Increased risk of bleeding complications; enhanced effect of lepirudin on aPTT prolongation
▣ *Antithrombotic agents (warfarin, aspirin, ticlopidine, clopidogrel, dipyridamole):* Inceased risk of bleeding
SPECIAL CONSIDERATIONS
• Untreated, HIT can lead to thrombosis, venous thromboembolism, acute MI, peripheral artery occlusion, and stroke; mortality rate approaches 20% to 30%
• All sources of heparin must be discontinued as soon as HIT is detected
• In clinical trials the cumulative risk of death 35 days after starting treatment was 9% in the lepirudin-treated patients, compared with 18% in historical controls; cumulative risk of new thromboembolic complications was 6% with lepirudin and 22% in historical controls

MONITORING PARAMETERS
• aPTT ratio (patient aPTT over median of laboratory normal range for aPTT); target range 1.5-2.5; do not start in patients with baseline aPTT ratio ≥2.5; determine aPTT ratio 4 hr following start of INF and at least daily thereafter
• CBC with platelet count (to detect bleeding complications and monitor recovery of platelets)

letrozole
(le′tro-zole)
Rx: Femara
Chemical Class: Benzhydryl-triazole derivative
Therapeutic Class: Antineoplastic

CLINICAL PHARMACOLOGY
Mechanism of Action: Decreases the level of circulating estrogen by inhibiting aromatase, an enzyme that catalyzes the final step in estrogen production. *Therapeutic Effect:* Inhibits the growth of breast cancers that are stimulated by estrogens.
Pharmacokinetics
Rapidly and completely absorbed. Metabolized in the liver. Primarily eliminated by the kidneys. Unknown if removed by hemodialysis.
Half-life: Approximately 2 days.
INDICATIONS AND DOSAGES
Breast cancer
PO
Adults, Elderly. 2.5 mg/day. Continue until tumor progression is evident.
▣ **AVAILABLE FORMS/COST**
• Tab—Oral: 2.5 mg, 30's: **$246.70**
CONTRAINDICATIONS: None known.

PREGNANCY AND LACTATION:
Pregnancy category D; excretion into breast milk unknown; use caution in nursing mothers

SIDE EFFECTS
Frequent (21%-9%)
Musculoskeletal pain (back, arm, leg), nausea, headache
Occasional (8%-5%)
Constipation, arthralgia, fatigue, vomiting, hot flashes, diarrhea, abdominal pain, cough, rash, anorexia, hypertension, peripheral edema
Rare (4%-1%)
Asthenia, somnolence, dyspepsia, weight gain, pruritus

SERIOUS REACTIONS
• None known.

INTERACTIONS
Drugs
③ *Tamoxifen:* Decreases letrozole concentrations by 38%

PATIENT/FAMILY EDUCATION
• May take without regard to meals

MONITORING PARAMETERS
• Consider CBC, TFTs, electrolytes, serum transaminases, creatinine until more toxicity information available

---

leucovorin
(loo-koe-vor'in)
Rx: Leucovorin
Chemical Class: Folic acid derivative
Therapeutic Class: Antidote, dihydrofolate reductase inhibitor; hematinic

CLINICAL PHARMACOLOGY
Mechanism of Action: An antidote to folic acid antagonists that may limit methotrexate action on normal cells by competing with methotrexate for the same transport processes into the cells. *Therapeutic Effect:* Reverses toxic effects of folic acid antagonists. Reverses folic acid deficiency.

Pharmacokinetics
Readily absorbed from the GI tract. Widely distributed. Primarily concentrated in the liver. Metabolized in the liver and intestinal mucosa to active metabolite. Primarily excreted in urine. **Half-life:** 15 min; metabolite, 30–35 min.

INDICATIONS AND DOSAGES
Conventional rescue dosage in high-dose methotrexate therapy
PO, IV, IM
Adults, Elderly, Children. 10 mg/m^2 IM or IV one time, then PO q6h until serum methotrexate level is less than 10^{-8} M. If 24-hr serum creatinine level increases by 50% or greater over baseline or methotrexate level exceeds 5×10^{-6} M or 48-hr level exceeds 9×10^{-7} M, increase to 100 mg/m^2 IV q3h until methotrexate level is less than 10^{-8} M.

Folic acid antagonist overdose
PO
Adults, Elderly, Children. 2–15 mg/day for 3 days or 5 mg every 3 days.

Megaloblastic anemia
IM
Adults, Elderly, Children. 3–6 mg/day.

Megaloblastic anemia secondary to folate deficiency
IM
Adults, Elderly, Children. 1 mg/day.

Prevention of hematologic toxicity (for toxoplasmosis), with sulfadiazine
PO, IV
Adults, Elderly, Children. 5–10 mg/day, repeat every 3 days.

Prevention of hematologic toxicity with pyrimethamine, PCP
PO, IV
Adults, Children. 25 mg once weekly.

$ AVAILABLE FORMS/COST
• Powder, Inj-IV/IM: 50 mg/vial: **$3.75**; 100 mg/vial: **$35.00**; 200 mg/vial: **$15.00-$77.90**; 350 mg/vial: **$18.75-$137.95**; 500 mg/vial: **$195.00**
• Tab-Oral: 5 mg, 100's: **$202.68-$551.87**; 10 mg, 24's: **$180.05**; 15 mg, 24's: **$195.62**; 25 mg, 25's: **$600.00-$680.34**

UNLABELED USES: Treatment of Ewing's sarcoma, gestational trophoblastic neoplasms, or non-Hodgkin's lymphoma; treatment adjunct for head and neck carcinoma

CONTRAINDICATIONS: Pernicious anemia, other megaloblastic anemias secondary to vitamin B_{12} deficiency

PREGNANCY AND LACTATION: Pregnancy category C; has been used in the treatment of megaloblastic anemia during pregnancy; compatible with breast-feeding

SIDE EFFECTS
Frequent
When combined with chemotherapeutic agents: Diarrhea, stomatitis, nausea, vomiting, lethargy or malaise or fatigue, alopecia, anorexia
Occasional
Urticaria, dermatitis

SERIOUS REACTIONS
• Excessive dosage may negate chemotherapeutic effects of folic acid antagonists.
• Anaphylaxis occurs rarely.
• Diarrhea may cause rapid clinical deterioration.

SPECIAL CONSIDERATIONS
• Administer as soon as possible following overdoses of dihydrofolate reductase inhibitors

MONITORING PARAMETERS
• CBC with differential and platelets, electrolytes, and liver function tests prior to each treatment with leucovorin/5-fluorouracil combination
• Plasma methotrexate concentrations as a therapeutic guide to high-dose methotrexate therapy with leucovorin rescue; continue leucovorin until plasma methotrexate concentrations are $<5 \times 10^{-8}$M (see dosage)
• Serum creatinine

---

leuprolide
(loo'proe-lide)
Rx: Lupron, Oaklide, Lupron Depot, Lupron Depot-Ped, Viadur
Chemical Class: Gonadotropin-releasing hormone analog
Therapeutic Class: Antiendometriosis agent; antineoplastic

CLINICAL PHARMACOLOGY
Mechanism of Action: A gonadotropin-releasing hormone analogue and antineoplastic agent that stimulates the release of luteinizing hormone (LH) and follicle-stimulating hormone (FSH) from the anterior pituitary gland. *Therapeutic Effect:* Produces pharmacologic castration and decreases the growth of abnormal prostate tissue in males; causes endometrial tissue to become inactive and atrophic in females; and decreases the rate of pubertal development in children with central precocious puberty.
Pharmacokinetics
Rapidly and well absorbed after subcutaneous administration. Absorbed slowly after IM administration. Protein binding: 43%-49%. **Half-life:** 3-4 hr.

INDICATIONS AND DOSAGES
Advanced prostatic carcinoma
IM

Adults, Elderly. (Lupron Depot) 7.5 mg every month or 22.5 mg every 3 months or 30 mg every 4 months.

Subcutaneous

Adults, Elderly. (Eligard) 7.5 mg every month or 22.5 mg every 3 months or 30 mg every 4 months; (Lupron) 1 mg/day; (Viadur) 65 mg implanted every 12 months.

Endometriosis
IM

Adults, Elderly. (Lupron Depot) 3.75 mg/mo for up to 6 months or 11.25 mg every 3 months for up to 2 doses.

Uterine leiomyomata
IM (with iron)

Adults, Elderly. (Lupron Depot) 3.75 mg/mo for up to 3 months or 11.25 mg as a single injection.

Precocious puberty
IM

Children. (Lupron Depot) 0.3 mg/kg/dose every 28 days. Minimum: 7.5 mg. If down regulation is not achieved, titrate upward in 3.75-mg increments q4wk.

Subcutaneous

Children. (Lupron) 20-45 mcg/kg/day. Titrate upward by 10 mcg/kg/day if down regululation is not achieved.

§ AVAILABLE FORMS/COST
• Implant—SC: 65 mg: **$5,683.75**
• Sol, Inj-SC: 5 mg/ml, 2.8 ml: **$369.91-$468.28**
• Inj, Susp (Depot)—IM: 3.75 mg/vial, 1's: **$556.11**; 7.5 mg/vial, 1's: **$643.75**
• Susp, Inj (Depot)-IM: 3.75 mg/vial, 1's: **$518.64**; 7.5 mg/vial, 1's: **$682.38**
• Susp, Inj (Depot-3)-IM: 11.25 mg/vial, 1's: **$1,701.70**; 22.5 mg/vial, 1's: **$2,047.13**
• Susp, Inj (Depot-4)-IM: 30 mg/vial, 1's: **$2,729.50**
• Kit (Depot-Ped)—IM: 7.5 mg/vial, 1's: **$682.38**; 11.25 mg/vial, 1's: **$1,238.85**; 15 mg/vial, 1's: **$1,081.25**

CONTRAINDICATIONS: Pernicious anemia, pregnancy

PREGNANCY AND LACTATION: Pregnancy category X; spontaneous abortions or intrauterine growth retardation are possible; not recommended during lactation

SIDE EFFECTS
Frequent

Hot flashes (ranging from mild flushing to diaphoresis)

Females: Amenorrhea, spotting

Occasional

Arrhythmias; palpitations; blurred vision; dizziness; edema; headache; burning or itching, or swelling at injection site; nausea; insomnia; weight gain

Females: Deepening voice, hirsutism, decreased libido, increased breast tenderness, vaginitis, altered mood

Males: Constipation, decreased testicle size, gynecomastia, impotence, decreased appetite, angina

Rare

Males: Thrombophlebitis

SERIOUS REACTIONS
• Signs and symptoms of metastatic prostatic carcinoma (such as bone pain, dysuria or hematuria, and weakness or paresthesia of the lower extremities) occasionally worsen 1 to 2 weeks after the initial dose but then subside with continued therapy.

• Pulmonary embolism and MI occur rarely.

SPECIAL CONSIDERATIONS
PATIENT/FAMILY EDUCATION
• May cause increase in bone pain and difficulty urinating during first

few weeks of treatment for prostate cancer, may also cause hot flashes
• Gonadotropin and sex steroids rise above baseline initially; side effects greatest in first weeks
• Continuous therapy vital for treatment of central precocious puberty
• Females may experience menses or spotting during first two months of therapy for central precocious puberty; notify provider if continues into second treatment month; nonhormonal contraception should be used

MONITORING PARAMETERS
• Monitor response to therapy for prostate cancer by measuring prostate specific antigen (PSA) levels
• GnRH stimulation test and sex steroid levels 1-2 mo after starting therapy for central precocious puberty, measurement of bone age for advancement q6-12mo

---

levetiracetam

(leva-tir-ass'eh-tam)

Rx: Keppra

Chemical Class: Pyrrolidone derivative

Therapeutic Class: Anticonvulsant

CLINICAL PHARMACOLOGY
Mechanism of Action: An anticonvulsant that inhibits burst firing without affecting normal neuronal excitability. *Therapeutic Effect:* Prevents seizure activity.

INDICATIONS AND DOSAGES
Partial-onset seizures
PO
Adults, Elderly. Initially, 500 mg q12h. May increase by 1,000 mg/day q2wk. Maximum: 3,000 mg/day.

Children 4-16 yr. 10-20 mg/kg/day in 2 divided doses. May increase at weekly intervals by 10-20 mg/kg. Maximum: 60 mg/kg.

Dosage in renal impairment
Dosage is modified based on creatinine clearance.

Creatinine Clearance (ml/min)	Dosage
Higher than 80 ml/min	500-1500 mg q12h
50-80 ml/min	500-1000 mg q12h
30-50 ml/min	250-750 mg q12h
less than 30 ml/min	250-500 mg q12h
End stage renal disease using dialysis	500-1000 mg q12h, after dialysis, a 250- to 500-mg supplemental dose is recommended.

☒ AVAILABLE FORMS/COST
• Tab—Oral: 250 mg, 120's: **$209.87**; 500 mg, 120's: **$256.51**; 750 mg, 120's: **$366.02**

CONTRAINDICATIONS: Hypersensitivity reaction

PREGNANCY AND LACTATION: Pregnancy category C; developmental toxicity in animals; excretion into breast milk unknown

SIDE EFFECTS
Frequent (15%-10%)
Somnolence, asthenia, headache, infection
Occasional (9%-3%)
Dizziness, pharyngitis, pain, depression, nervousness, vertigo, rhinitis, anorexia
Rare (less than 3%)
Amnesia, anxiety, emotional lability, cough, sinusitis, anorexia, diplopia

SERIOUS REACTIONS
• None known.

SPECIAL CONSIDERATIONS
• Reserve as an alternative treatment for patients with partial onset seizures not responding to first-line agents

PATIENT/FAMILY EDUCATION
• Notify clinician if female patients intend to or become pregnant
• Caution about common adverse effects, i.e., dizziness and somnolence

MONITORING PARAMETERS
• Therapeutic plasma concentrations not established; base dosing on therapeutic response (reduction in severity and frequency of seizures)

---

levocabastine
(levo-cab′a-steen)
Rx: Livostin
Chemical Class: Phenyl-isonipecotic acid derivative
Therapeutic Class: Ophthalmic antihistamine

CLINICAL PHARMACOLOGY
Mechanism of Action: An antiallergic agent that selectively antagonizes H1 receptor. *Therapeutic Effect:* Blocks histamine-associated symptoms of seasonal allergic conjunctivitis.

Pharmacokinetics
Duration of action is about 2 hours. Minimal systemic absorbtion.

INDICATIONS AND DOSAGES
Allergic conjunctivitis
Ophthalmic
Adults, Elderly, Children 12 yrs or older. 1 drop 4 times/day, for up to 2 wks.

S AVAILABLE FORMS/COST
• Susp—Ophth: 0.05%, 5, 10 ml: **$53.23**/5 ml

CONTRAINDICATIONS: Wearing of soft contact lenses (product contains benzalkonium chloride), hypersensitivity to levocabastine or any component of the formulation

PREGNANCY AND LACTATION:
Pregnancy category C; excreted in human breast milk at very low concentrations due to minimal systemic absorption following ocular administration

SIDE EFFECTS
Frequent
Transient stinging, burning, discomfort, headache
Occasional
Dry mouth, fatigue, eye dryness, lacrimation/discharge, eyelid edema
Rare
Rash, erythema, nausea, dyspnea

SERIOUS REACTIONS
• None reported.

SPECIAL CONSIDERATIONS
• Shake well before using

---

levodopa
(lev-oh-dope-ah)
Rx: Larodopa
Combinations
   Rx: with Carbidopa (Sinemet, Sinemet CR)
Chemical Class: Catecholamine precursor
Therapeutic Class: Anti-Parkinson's agent; antidyskinetic

CLINICAL PHARMACOLOGY
Mechanism of Action: A dopamine prodrug that is converted to dopamine in basal ganglia. Increases dopamine concentrations in the brain, inhibiting hyperactive cholinergic activity. *Therapeutic Effect:* Decreases signs and symptoms of Parkinson's disease.

Pharmacokinetics
About 30% absorbed. May be reduced with high-protein meal. Protein binding: minimal. Crosses blood-brain barrier. Converted to dopamine. Eliminated primarily in

urine and to a lesser amount in feces and expired air. Not removed by hemodialysis. **Half-life:** 0.75 -1.5 hrs.

INDICATIONS AND DOSAGES
Parkinsonism
PO

Adults, Elderly. Initially, 0.5-1 g 2-4 times/day. May increase in increments not exceeding 0.75 g every 3-7 days, up to a maximum of 8 g/day.

S AVAILABLE FORMS/COST
• (Sinemet) Tab-Oral: 10 mg-100 mg, 100's: **$32.34-$82.69**; 25 mg-100 mg, 100's: **$26.05-$93.36**; 25 mg-250 mg, 100's: **$41.16-$118.96**

• (Sinemet CR) Tab, Sus Action-Oral: 25 mg-100 mg, 100's: **$93.10-$104.59**; 50 mg-200 mg, 100's: **$180.85-$201.16**

CONTRAINDICATIONS: Nonselective MAOI therapy, hypersensitivity to levodopa or any component of its formulation.

PREGNANCY AND LACTATION: Pregnancy category C; do not use in nursing mothers

SIDE EFFECTS
Frequent

Uncontrolled body movements of the face, tongue, arms and upper body, nausea and vomiting, anorexia

Occasional

Depression, anxiety, confusion, nervousness, difficulty urinating, irregular heartbeats, hiccoughs, dizziness, lightheadedness, decreased appetite, blurred vision, constipation, dry mouth, flushed skin, headache, insomnia, diarrhea, unusual tiredness, darkening of urine, discolored sweat

Rare

Hypertension, ulcer, hemolytic anemia, marked by tiredness or weakness.

SERIOUS REACTIONS
• High incidence of involuntary dystonic, and dyskinetic movements may be noted in patients on long-term therapy.

• Mental changes, such as paranoid ideation, psychotic episodes and depression, may be noted.

• Numerous mild to severe central nervous system (CNS) psychiatric disturbances may include reduced attention span, anxiety, nightmares, daytime somnolence, euphoria, fatigue, paranoia, and hallucinations.

INTERACTIONS
Drugs

❸ *Benzodiazepines:* Diazepam and chlordiazepoxide have exacerbated parkinsonism in a few patients receiving levodopa, effect of other benzodiazepines not clinically established

❸ *Food:* High-protein diets may inhibit the efficacy of levodopa

❸ *Iron:* Reduced levodopa bioavailability possible

❸ *Methionine, phenytoin, pyridoxine, spiramycin, tacrine:* Inhibited clinical response to levodopa

❸ *Moclobemide:* Increased risk of adverse effects from levodopa

❸ *MAOIs:* Hypertensive response

❷ *Neuroleptics:* Inhibited clinical response to levodopa

Labs

• *False positive:* Urine ferric chloride test, urine ketones, urine glucose, Coombs test

• *False negative:* Urine glucose (glucose oxidase), urine guaiacols spot test

• *False increase:* Serum acid phosphatase, urine amino acids, serum AST, serum bilirubin, plasma catecholamines, serum cholinesterase, serum creatinine, urine creatinine, creatinine clearance, serum glucose, urine hydroxy-methoxymandelic acid, urine ketones, serum lithium, urine protein, urine sugar, serum uric acid, urine uric acid

• *False decrease:* Serum bilirubin (conjugated and unconjugated), serum glucose, urine glucose, serum triglycerides, serum urea nitrogen, serum uric acid, VMA

SPECIAL CONSIDERATIONS

• Combination with carbidopa is preferred preparation

PATIENT/FAMILY EDUCATION

• Full benefit may require up to 6 mo
• Take with food to minimize GI upset
• Avoid sudden changes in posture
• May cause darkening of the urine or sweat

MONITORING PARAMETERS

• CBC, renal function, liver function, ECG, intraocular pressure

---

levofloxacin

(levo-flox′a-sin)

Rx: *Oral:* Levaquin

Rx: *Ophthalmic:* IQUIX, Quixin

Chemical Class: Fluoroquinolone derivative

Therapeutic Class: Antibiotic

CLINICAL PHARMACOLOGY

Mechanism of Action: A fluoroquinolone that inhibits the enzyme DNA enzyme gyrase in susceptible microorganisms, interfering with bacterial cell replication and repair. *Therapeutic Effect:* Bactericidal.

Pharmacokinetics

Well absorbed after both PO and IV administration. Protein binding: 24%-8%. Penetrates rapidly and extensively into leukocytes, epithelial cells, and macrophages. Lung concentrations are 2-5 times higher than those of plasma. Eliminated unchanged in the urine. Partially removed by hemodialysis. **Half-life:** 8 hr.

INDICATIONS AND DOSAGES

Bronchitis

PO, IV

Adults, Elderly. 500 mg q24h for 7 days.

Community-acquired pneumonia

PO

Adults, Elderly. 750 mg/day for 5 days.

Pneumonia

PO, IV

Adults, Elderly. 500 mg q24h for 7-14 days.

Acute maxillary sinusitis

PO, IV

Adults, Elderly. 500 mg q24h for 10-14 days.

Skin and skin-structure infections

PO, IV

Adults, Elderly. 500 mg q24h for 7-10 days.

UTIs, acute pyelonephritis

PO, IV

Adults, Elderly. 250 mg q24h for 10 days.

Bacterial conjunctivitis

Ophthalmic

Adults, Elderly, Children 1 yr and older. 1-2 drops q2h for 2 days (up to 8 times a day), then 1-2 drops q4h for 5 days.

Corneal ulcer

Ophthalmic

Adults, Elderly, Children older than 5 yr. Days 1-3: Instill 1-2 drops q30min to 2 hours while awake and 4-6 hours after retiring. Days 4 through completion: 1-2 drops q1-4h while awake.

Dosage in renal impairment

For bronchitis, pneumonia, sinusitis, and skin and skin-structure infections, dosage and frequency are modified based on creatinine clearance.

Creatinine Clearance	Dosage
50-80 ml/min	No change
20-49 ml/min	500 mg initially, then 250 mg q24h
10-19 ml/min	500 mg initially, then 250 mg q48h

Dialysis 500 mg initially, then 250 mg q48h

For UTIs and pyelonephritis, dosage and frequency are modified based on creatinine clearance.

Creatinine Clearance	Dosage
20 ml/min	No change
10-19 ml/min	250 mg initially, then 250 mg q48h

S AVAILABLE FORMS/COST
• Sol—IV: 500 mg/20 ml, 1's: **$45.65**
• Sol—Ophth: 0.5%, 5 ml: **$42.85**
• Tab, Film Coated—Oral: 250 mg, 50's: **$461.13**; 500 mg, 50's: **$528.49**; 750 mg, 50's: **$811.35**

CONTRAINDICATIONS: Hypersensitivity to levofloaxcin, other fluoroquinolones, or nalidixic acid

PREGNANCY AND LACTATION: Pregnancy category C; excretion into breast milk unknown; due to the potential for arthropathy and osteochondrosis, use extreme caution in nursing mothers

SIDE EFFECTS
Occasional (3%-1%)
Diarrhea, nausea, abdominal pain, dizziness, drowsiness, headache, light-headedness
Ophthalmic: Local burning or discomfort, margin crusting, crystals or scales, foreign body sensation, ocular itching, altered taste
Rare (less than 1%)
Flatulence; altered taste; pain; inflammation or swelling in calves, hands, or shoulder; chest pain; difficulty breathing; palpitations; edema; tendon pain

Ophthalmic: Corneal staining, keratitis, allergic reaction, eyelid swelling, tearing, reduced visual acuity

SERIOUS REACTIONS
• Antibiotic-associated colitis and other superinfections may occur from altered bacterial balance. Hypersensitivity reactions, incluing photosensitivity (as evidenced by rash, pruritus, blisters, edem, and burning skin), have occurred in patients receiving fluoroquinolones.

INTERACTIONS
Drugs
▨ *Aluminum:* Reduced absorption of levofloxacin; do not take within 4 hr of dose
▨ *Antacids:* Reduced absorption of levofloxacin; do not take within 4 hr of dose
▨ *Calcium:* Reduced absorption of levofloxacin; do not take within 4 hr of dose
▨ *Cimetidine:* Reduced absorption of levofloxacin
▨ *Didanosine:* Markedly reduced absorption of levofloxacin; take levofloxacin 2 hr before didanosine
▨ *Famotidine:* Reduced absorption of levofloxacin
▨ *Iron:* Reduced absorption of levofloxacin; do not take within 4 hr of dose
▨ *Lansoprazole:* Reduced absorption of levofloxacin
▨ *Magnesium:* Reduced absorption of levofloxacin; do not take within 4 hr of dose
▨ *Nizatidine:* Reduced absorption of levofloxacin
▨ *Omeprazole:* Reduced absorption of levofloxacin
▨ *Ranitidine:* Reduced absorption of levofloxacin
▨ *Sodium bicarbonate:* Reduced absorption of levofloxacin; do not take within 4 hr of dose

3 *Sucralfate:* Reduced absorption of levofloxacin; do not take within 4 hr of dose

3 *Warfarin:* May increase hypoprothrombinemic response to warfarin

3 *Zinc:* Reduced absorption of levofloxacin; do not take within 4 hr of dose

SPECIAL CONSIDERATIONS
• L-isomer of the racemate, ofloxacin (a commercially available quinolone antibiotic)

PATIENT/FAMILY EDUCATION
• Avoid direct exposure to sunlight (even when using sunscreen)
• Drink fluids liberally

---

levonorgestrel
(lee-voe-nor-jes'-trel)
Rx: Jadelle, Norplant System, Mirena, Plan B
Combinations
  Rx: Transdermal with estradiol (Climara Pro); See oral contraceptives monograph for combined oral contraceptives containing levonorgestrel
Chemical Class: 19-nortestosterone derivative; progestin derivative
Therapeutic Class: Contraceptive; progestin

CLINICAL PHARMACOLOGY
Mechanism of Action: A contraceptive hormone that causes thickening of cervical mucus, inhibition of ovulation and inhibition of implantation. *Therapeutic Effect:* Prevents ovulation or fertilization.

Pharmacokinetics
Levonorgestrel is rapidly and completely absorbed after oral administration. Maximum serum concentrations of approximately 15 ng/ml occur at an average of 2 hours. Does not appear to be extensively metabolized by the liver. Protein binding: 97.5%. Primarily excreted in the urine, with smaller amounts recovered in the feces.

INDICATIONS AND DOSAGES
Long-term prevention of pregnancy
Intrauterine
Adults, Elderly: Insert 1 system into uterine cavity within 7 days of onset of menstruation or immediately after first trimester abortion. Releases 20mcg levonorgestrol daily over 5 years.

Emergency contraception
PO
Adults, Elderly: One 0.75mg tablet as soon as possible within 72 hours of unprotected sexual intercourse. A second 0.75mg tablet 12 hours after the first dose.

S **AVAILABLE FORMS/COST**
• Device-Intrauteral: 52 mg, 1 device: **$453.75**
• Tab—Oral: 0.75 mg package of 2: **$21.95**
• Tab—Oral: 0.05 mg ethinyl estradiol/0.25 mg levonorgestrel, 4's: **$12.50**

CONTRAINDICATIONS: Active thrombophlebitis or thromboembolic disorders, undiagnosed abnormal genital bleeding, known or suspected pregnancy, acute liver disease; benign or malignant liver tumors, known or suspected carcinoma of the breast, history of idiopathic intracranial hypertension, hypersensitivity to levonorgestrel or any of the components of the levonorgestrel implants.

PREGNANCY AND LACTATION: Pregnancy category X; compatible with breast-feeding

SIDE EFFECTS
Occasional

Hypertension, headache, depression, nervousness, breast pain, dysmenorrheal, decreased libidoabdominal pain, nausea, weight gain, leukorrhea, vaginitis.

Rare

Alopecia, anemia, cervicitis, dyspareunia, eczema, failed insertion, migraine, sepsis, vomiting.

SERIOUS REACTIONS
• None known.

INTERACTIONS
Drugs

3 *Carbamazepine, phenobarbital, phenytoin:* Decreased efficacy of levonorgestrel, pregnancy has occurred

SPECIAL CONSIDERATIONS
PATIENT/FAMILY EDUCATION
• Most women can expect some variation in menstrual bleeding; these irregularities should diminish with continued use

• Capsules can be removed at any time for any reason or at the end of 5 yr. Removal is more difficult than insertion.

• Failure rate 0.2-1.0%, increases to 5% in patients ≥70 kg (Norplant)

• Efficacy of emergency contraception is better as soon as possible after unprotected intercourse. Causes less nausea and vomiting than other products for emergency contraception. Decreases risk of pregnancy from 8% to 19%

• Based on WHO study, levonorgesterel (norgestrel) only pills preferred emergency contraception; equal efficacy and 50% less nausea, vomiting compared to combined regimen

• About 80% of women wishing to become pregnant conceived within 12 mo after removal of intrauterine device

levorphanol
(lee-vor'fa-nole)
Rx: Levo-Dromoran
Chemical Class: Opiate derivative; phenanthrene derivative
Therapeutic Class: Narcotic analgesic
DEA Class: Schedule II

CLINICAL PHARMACOLOGY
Mechanism of Action: An opioid agonist that binds at opiate receptor sites in central nervous system (CNS). *Therapeutic Effect:* Reduced intensity of pain stimuli incoming from sensory nerve endings, altering pain perception and emotional response to pain.

Pharmacokinetics

Rapidly absorbed. Protein binding: 40-50%. Extensively distributed. Metabolized in liver. Excreted in urine. **Half-life:** 11 hrs.

INDICATIONS AND DOSAGES
Pain

PO

Adults, Elderly. 2 mg. May be increased to 3 mg, if needed.

IM/Subcutaneous

Adults, Elderly: 1-2 mg as a single dose. May repeat in 6-8 hrs as needed. Maximum: 3-8 mg/day.

IV

Adults. Up to 1 mg injection in divided doses. May repeat in 3-6 hrs as needed. Maximum: 4-8 mg/day.

Preoperative

IM/Subcutaneous

Adults, Elderly. 1-2 mg as a single dose 60-90 min. before surgery.

AVAILABLE FORMS/COST
• Sol, Inj-SC: 2 mg/ml, 2 ml: **$3.96**
• Tab-Oral: 2 mg, 100's: **$107.25**

CONTRAINDICATIONS: Hypersensitivity to levorphanol or any component of the formulation

PREGNANCY AND LACTATION:
Pregnancy category B (category D if used for prolonged periods or in high doses at term); use during labor produces neonatal depression

SIDE EFFECTS
Effects are dependent on dosage amount, route of administration. Ambulatory patients and those not in severe pain may experience dizziness, nausea, vomiting, hypotension more frequently than those in supine position or having severe pain

Frequent
Dizziness, drowsiness, hypotension, nausea, vomiting

Occasional
Shortness of breath, confusion, decreased urination, stomach cramps, altered vision, constipation, dry mouth, headache, difficult or painful urination

Rare
Allergic reaction (rash, itching), histamine reaction (decreased BP, increased sweating, flushed face, wheezing)

SERIOUS REACTIONS
• Overdosage results in respiratory depression, skeletal muscle flaccidity, cold clammy skin, cyanosis, extreme somnolence progressing to convulsions, stupor, coma.
• Tolerance to analgesic effect, physical dependence may occur with repeated use.
• Paralytic ileus may occur with prolonged use.

INTERACTIONS
Drugs
③ *Antihistamines, chloral hydrate, glutethimide, methocarbamol:* Enhanced depressant effects
③ *Barbiturates:* Additive respiratory and CNS depressant effects
③ *Cimetidine:* Increased respiratory and CNS depression
③ *Ethanol:* Additive CNS effects

Labs
• *False increase:* Amylase and lipase

SPECIAL CONSIDERATIONS
• Do not administer agonist/antagonist analgesics (i.e., pentazocine, nalbuphine, butorphanol, dezocine, buprenorphine) to patient who has received a prolonged course of levorphanol (a pure agonist). In opioid-dependent patients, mixed agonist/antagonist analgesics may precipitate withdrawal symptoms

PATIENT/FAMILY EDUCATION
• Physical dependency may result when used for extended periods
• Change position slowly; orthostatic hypotension may occur
• Minimize nausea by administering with food and remain lying down following dose

---

levothyroxine
(lee-voe-thye-rox'een)
Rx: Levo-T, Levothroid, Levoxine, Synthroid, Levoxyl
Combinations
Rx: with liothyronine (Euthroid, Thyrolar)
Chemical Class: Synthetic levo isomer of thyroxine (T_4)
Therapeutic Class: Thyroid hormone

CLINICAL PHARMACOLOGY
Mechanism of Action: A synthetic isomer of thyroxine involved in normal metabolism, growth, and development, especially of the CNS in infants. Possesses catabolic and anabolic effects. *Therapeutic Effect:* Increases basal metabolic rate, enhances gluconeogenesis and stimulates protein synthesis.

Pharmacokinetics
Variable, incomplete absorption from the GI tract. Protein binding: 99%. Widely distributed. Deiodinated in peripheral tissues, minimal metabolism in the liver. Eliminated by biliary excretion. **Half-life:** 6–7 days.

INDICATIONS AND DOSAGES

Hypothyroidism
PO
Adults, Elderly. Initially, 12.5–50 mcg. May increase by 25–50 mcg/day q2–4wk. Maintenance: 100–200 mcg/day.
Children 13 yr and older. 150 mcg/day.
Children 6–12 yr. 100–125 mcg/day.
Children 1–5 yr. 75–100 mcg/day.
Children 7-11 mo. 50–75 mcg/day.
Children older than 3–6 mo. 25–50 mcg/day.
Children 3 mo and younger. 10–15 mcg/day.

Thyroid suppression therapy
PO
Adults, Elderly. 2–6 mcg/kg/day for 7–10 days.

Thyroid stimulating hormone suppression in thyroid cancer, nodules, euthyroid goiters
PO
Adults, Elderly. 2–6 mcg/kg/day for 7–10 days.
IV
Adults, Elderly, Children. Initial dosage approximately half the previously established oral dosage.

[$] **AVAILABLE FORMS/COST**
• Powder, Inj-IM, IV: 0.2 mg/vial: **$4.38-$62.56**; 0.5 mg/vial: **$4.38-$89.50**
• Tab-Oral: 0.025 mg, 100's: **$4.95-$39.08**; 0.05 mg, 100's: **$5.05-$44.43**; 0.075 mg, 100's: **$4.74-$49.05**; 0.088 mg, 100's: **$14.48-$49.93**; 0.1 mg, 100's: **$3.05-$50.24**; 0.112 mg, 100's: **$14.48-$58.06**; 0.125 mg, 100's: **$5.40-$58.85**; 0.137 mg, 100's: **$14.48-$60.21**; 0.15 mg, 100's: **$3.15-$60.61**; 0.175 mg, 100's: **$14.48-$86.65**; 0.2 mg, 100's: **$3.30-$72.25**; 0.3 mg, 100's: **$6.00-$98.33**

CONTRAINDICATIONS: Hypersensitivity to tablet components, such as tartrazine; allergy to aspirin; lactose intolerance; MI and thyrotoxicosis uncomplicated by hypothyroidism; treatment of obesity

PREGNANCY AND LACTATION: Pregnancy category A; little or no transplacental passage at physiologic serum concentrations; excreted into breast milk in low concentrations (inadequate to protect a hypothyroid infant; too low to interfere with neonatal thyroid screening programs)

SIDE EFFECTS

Occasional
Reversible hair loss at the start of therapy (in children)

Rare
Dry skin, GI intolerance, rash, hives, pseudotumor cerebri or severe headache in children

SERIOUS REACTIONS
• Excessive dosage produces signs and symptoms of hyperthyroidism, including weight loss, palpitations, increased appetite, tremors, nervousness, tachycardia, hypertension, headache, insomnia, and menstrual irregularities.
• Cardiac arrhythmias occur rarely.

INTERACTIONS

Drugs
[3] *Aluminum and magnesium antacids, bile acid sequestrants, calcium carbonate, ferrous sulfate, kayexalate, simethicone, sucralfate:* Reduced serum thyroid concentrations through binding and delaying or preventing absorption of levothyroxine, administer these agents at least 4 hr apart

❸ *Antidepressants (tricyclics, tetracyclics, selective serotonin reuptake inhibitors):* Potential increase in therapeutic and toxic effects of levothyroxine and tri/tetracyclics; increased levothyroxine requirements with sertraline

❸ *Carbamazepine, phenobarbital, phenytoin, rifampin:* Increased elimination of thyroid hormones; possible increased requirement for thyroid hormones in hypothyroid patients

❸ *Digoxin:* Levothyroxin may reduce therapeutic effects of digitalis glycosides

❷ *Ketamine:* Concurrent use with thyroid hormones may cause hypertension and tachycardia

❸ *Oral anticoagulants:* Thyroid hormones increase catabolism of vitamin K-dependent clotting factors; an increase or decrease in clinical thyroid status will increase or decrease the hypoprothrombinemic response to oral anticoagulants

❸ *Sympathomimetics:* Concurrent use may increase the effects of thyroid hormones or sympathomimetics

❸ *Theophylline:* Reduced serum theophylline concentrations with initiation of thyroid therapy

Labs
• *False increase:* Serum triiodothyronine

SPECIAL CONSIDERATIONS
• Bioequivalence problems have been documented in the past for products marketed by different manufacturers; however, studies in patients have shown comparable clinical efficacy between brands based on the results of thyroid function tests; brand interchange should be limited to products with demonstrated therapeutic equivalence

PATIENT/FAMILY EDUCATION
• Transient, partial hair loss may be experienced by children in the first few months of therapy
• Take as a single daily dose, preferably before breakfast

MONITORING PARAMETERS
• TSH

---

lidocaine
(lye'doe-kane)
Rx: Anestacon, Dilocaine, Duo-Trach Kit, Lidoject, Nervocaine, Octocaine, Xylocaine
OTC: DermaFlex, Solarcaine, Zilactin-L
Combinations
   Rx: with epinephrine (LidoSite, Xylocaine with Epinephrine); Prilocaine (EMLA)
Chemical Class: Amide derivative
Therapeutic Class: Anesthetic, local; antiarrhythmic, class IB

CLINICAL PHARMACOLOGY
Mechanism of Action: An amide anesthetic that inhibits conduction of nerve impulses. *Therapeutic Effect:* Causes temporary loss of feeling and sensation. Also an antiarrhythmic that decreases depolarization, automaticity, excitability of the ventricle during diastole by direct action. *Therapeutic Effect:* Inhibits ventricular arrhythmias.
Pharmacokinetics

Route	Onset	Peak	Duration
IV	30-90 sec	N/A	10-20 min
Local anesthetic	2.5 min	N/A	30-60 min

Completely absorbed after IM administration. Protein binding: 60% to 80%. Widely distributed. Metabolized in the liver. Primarily excreted in urine. Minimally removed by hemodialysis. **Half-life:** 1-2 hr.

INDICATIONS AND DOSAGES

Rapid control of acute ventricular arrhythmias after an MI, cardiac catheterization, cardiac surgery, or digitalis-induced ventricular arrhythmias

IM

Adults, Elderly. 300 mg (or 4.3 mg/kg). May repeat in 60–90 min.

IV

Adults, Elderly. Initially, 50–100 mg (1 mg/kg) IV bolus at rate of 25–50 mg/min. May repeat in 5 min. Give no more than 200–300 mg in 1 hr. Maintenance: 20–50 mcg/kg/min (1–4 mg/min) as IV infusion.

Children, Infants. Initially, 0.5–1 mg/kg IV bolus; may repeat but total dose not to exceed 3–5 mg/kg. Maintenance: 10–50 mcg/kg/min as IV infusion.

Dental or surgical procedures, childbirth

Infiltration or nerve block

Adults. Local anesthetic dosage varies with procedure, degree of anesthesia, vascularity, duration. Maximum dose: 4.5 mg/kg. Do not repeat within 2 hrs.

Local skin disorders (minor burns, insect bites, prickly heat, skin manifestations of chickenpox, abrasions), and mucous membrane disorders (local anesthesia of oral, nasal, and laryngeal mucous membranes; local anesthesia of respiratory, urinary tract; relief of discomfort of pruritus ani, hemorrhoids, pruritus vulvae)

Topical

Adults, Elderly. Apply to affected areas as needed.

Treatment of shingles-related skin pain

Topical (Dermal patch)

Adults, Elderly. Apply to intact skin over most painful area (up to 3 applications once for up to 12 hrs in a 24-hr period).

ⓢ AVAILABLE FORMS/COST

Top
• Cream—Top: 0.5%, 120 g: **$3.00**; 5%, 30 g: **$50.16-$52.46**
• Film-Top: 5%, 5's: **$23.68-$26.18**
• Gel—Top: 2%, 5, 10, 15, 20, 30 ml: **$15.50-$23.75**/30 ml; 2.5%, 15 g: **$53.20**
• Oint—Top: 5%, 3, 35, 50, 454 g: **$2.50-$28.80**/35 g
• Liq-Top: 2.5%, 60, 105, 120, 450 ml: **$3.39**/120 ml
• Sol, Visc-Oral: 2%, 5, 20, 60, 100 ml: **$3.42-$21.80**/100 ml

Local
• Sol, Inj: 0.5%, 50 ml: **$4.83-$12.96**; 1%, 50 ml: **$1.95-$25.15**; 1.5%, 20 ml: **$4.52-$13.28**; 2%, 50 ml: **$1.95-$25.19**; 4%, 5 ml: **$6.38-$7.64**

For Direct IV Administration
• Sol, Inj-IV: 1%, 5 ml: **$3.90-$11.55**; 2%, 5 ml: **$2.10-$12.10**

For IV Admixture
• Sol, Inj: 4%, 5 ml: **$2.31**; 10%, 10 ml: **$10.50**; 20%, 10 ml: **$5.78-$9.56**

CONTRAINDICATIONS: Adams-Stokes syndrome, hypersensitivity to amide-type local anesthetics, septicemia (spinal anesthesia), supraventricular arrhythmias, Wolff-Parkinson-White syndrome

PREGNANCY AND LACTATION: Pregnancy category C; has been used as a local anesthetic during labor and delivery; may produce CNS depression and bradycardia in the newborn with high serum levels; compatible with breast-feeding

SIDE EFFECTS

CNS effects are generally dose-related and of short duration.

Occasional

IM: Pain at injection site

Topical: Burning, stinging, tenderness at application site

Rare

Generally with high dose: Drowsiness; dizziness; disorientation; light-headedness; tremors; apprehension; euphoria; sensation of heat, cold, or numbness; blurred or double vision; ringing or roaring in ears (tinnitus); nausea

SERIOUS REACTIONS

• Although serious adverse reactions to lidocaine are uncommon, high dosage by any route may produce cardiovascular depression, bradycardia, hypotension, arrhythmias, heart block, cardiovascular collapse, and cardiac arrest.

• Potential for malignant hyperthermia.

• CNS toxicity may occur, especially with regional anesthesia use, progressing rapidly from mild side effects to tremors, somnolence, seizures, vomiting, and respiratory depression.

• Methemoglobinemia (evidenced by cyanosis) has occurred following topical application of lidocaine for teething discomfort and laryngeal anesthetic spray.

INTERACTIONS

Drugs

▨ *Disopyramide:* Induction of dysrhythmia or heart failure in predisposed patients

▨ *Metoprolol, nadolol, propranolol, cimetidine:* Increased serum lidocaine concentrations

Labs

• *False increase:* Serum creatinine, CSF protein

SPECIAL CONSIDERATIONS

PATIENT/FAMILY EDUCATION

• Do not ingest food for 60 min following oral use (impairs swallowing)

MONITORING PARAMETERS

• Constant ECG monitoring, blood pressure

• Therapeutic serum concentrations are 1.5-6 mcg/ml (concentrations >6-10 mcg/ml are usually associated with toxicity)

---

lindane (gamma benzene hexachloride)

(lin′dane)

Rx: Lindane

Chemical Class: Cyclic chlorinated hydrocarbon

Therapeutic Class: Pediculicide; scabicide

CLINICAL PHARMACOLOGY

Mechanism of Action: A scabicidal agent that is directly absorbed by parasites and ova through the exoskeleton. *Therapeutic Effect:* Stimulates the nervous system resulting in seizures and death of parasitic arthropods.

Pharmacokinetics

May be absorbed systemically. Metabolized in liver. Excreted in the urine and feces. **Half-life:** 17-22 hrs.

INDICATIONS AND DOSAGES

Treatment of scabies

Topical

Adults, Elderly, Children. Apply thin layer. Massage on skin from neck to the toes. Bathe and remove drug after 8-12 hrs.

Head lice, crab lice

Topical

Adults, Elderly, Children. Apply about 30 ml of shampoo to dry hair and massage into hair for 4 min. Add small amounts of water to hair until lather forms, then rinse hair thoroughly and comb with a fine tooth comb to remove nits. Maximum: 60 ml of shampoo.

[$] **AVAILABLE FORMS/COST**

- Liq-Top: 1%, 60 ml: **$6.95**
- Lotion—Top: 1%, 60, 100, 480 ml: **$3.35-$15.18**/60 ml
- Shampoo—Top: 1%, 60, 100, 480 ml: **$2.61-$38.05**/60 ml

CONTRAINDICATIONS: Hypersensitivity to lindane or any component of the formulation, uncontrolled seizure disorders, crusted (Norwegian) scabies, acutely-inflamed skin or raw, weeping surfaces, or other skin conditions which may increase systemic absorption

PREGNANCY AND LACTATION: Pregnancy category B; use no more than twice during a pregnancy; amounts excreted in breast milk probably clinically insignificant

SIDE EFFECTS

Rare (less than 1%)

Burning, stinging, cardiac arrhythmia, ataxia, dizziness, headache, restlessness, seizures, pain, alopecia, contact dermatitis, skin and adipose tissue may act as repositories, eczematous eruptions, pruritus, urticaria, nausea, vomiting, aplastic anemia, hepatitis, paresthesias, hematuria, pulmonary edema

SERIOUS REACTIONS

- Seizures rarely occur.

SPECIAL CONSIDERATIONS

PATIENT/FAMILY EDUCATION

- Do not exceed prescribed dosage
- Do not apply to face
- Avoid getting in eyes
- Wear rubber gloves for application
- Do not use oil-based hair products (e.g., conditioners) after using product
- Treat sexual and household contacts concurrently

linezolid

(li-nee'zoh-lid)

Rx: Zyvox

Chemical Class: Oxazolidinone derivative

Therapeutic Class: Antibiotic

CLINICAL PHARMACOLOGY

Mechanism of Action: An oxalodinone anti-infective that binds to a site on bacterial 23S ribosomal RNA, preventing the formation of a complex that is essential for bacterial translation. *Therapeutic Effect:* Bacteriostatic against enterococci and staphylococci; bactericidal against streptococci.

Pharmacokinetics

Rapidly and extensively absorbed after PO administration. Protein binding: 31%. Metabolized in the liver by oxidation. Excreted in urine. **Half-life:** 4-5.4 hr.

INDICATIONS AND DOSAGES

Vancomycin-resistant infections

PO, IV

Adults, Elderly, Children older than 11 yr. 600 mg q12h for 14-28 days.

Pneumonia, complicated skin and skin structure infections

PO, IV

Adults, Elderly, Children older than 11 yr. 600 mg q12h for 10-14 days.

Uncomplicated skin and skin structure infections

PO

Adults, Elderly. 400 mg q12h for 10-14 days.

Children older than 11 yr. 600 mg q12h for 10-14 days.

Children 5-11 yr. 10 mg/kg/dose q12h for 10-14 days.

Usual neonate dosage

PO, IV

Neonates. 10 mg/kg/dose q8-12h.

💲 AVAILABLE FORMS/COST
• Sol, Inj-IV: 2 mg/ml, 100 ml: **$40.35**
• Powder, Reconst-Oral: 100 mg/5 ml, 150 ml: **$315.76**
• Tab, Coated—Oral: 600 mg, 20's: **$1,263.08**

CONTRAINDICATIONS: None known

PREGNANCY AND LACTATION: Pregnancy category C; breast milk excretion unknown

SIDE EFFECTS
Occasional (5%-2%)
Diarrhea, nausea, headache
Rare (less than 2%)
Altered taste, vaginal candidiasis, fungal infection, dizziness, tongue discoloration

SERIOUS REACTIONS
• Thrombocytopenia and myelosuppression occur rarely.
• Antibiotic-associated colitis and other superinfections may result from altered bacterial balance.

INTERACTIONS
Drugs
❷ *Amphetamines, alcoholic beverages containing tyramine, metaraminol, phenylephrine, phenylpropanolamine, pseudoephedrine, tyramine:* Severe hypertensive reaction
❷ *Antidepressants, cyclic:* Excessive sympathetic response
❷ *Dextromethorphan:* Severe hypertensive reaction
❷ *Dopamine:* Severe hypertensive reaction
❷ *Epinephrine:* Severe hypertensive reaction
❸ *Levodopa:* Hypertension
❷ *Meperidine:* Severe hypertensive reaction
❷ *Selective serotonin reuptake inhibitors (SSRIs):* Serotonin syndrome (hyperpyrexia, cognitive dysfunction)
❷ *Sibutramine:* Serotonin syndrome (hyperpyrexia, cognitive dysfunction)
❷ *Trazodone:* Serotonin syndrome (hyperpyrexia, cognitive dysfunction)
❷ *Venlafaxine:* Serotonin syndrome (hyperpyrexia, cognitive dysfunction)

SPECIAL CONSIDERATIONS
• Most appropriate use is when Vancomycin-resistant *Enterococcus faecium* infection is documented or strongly suspected, or for oral therapy of methicillin resistant *Staphylococcus aureus* infection

PATIENT/FAMILY EDUCATION
• Avoid high tyramine foods (consume less than 100 mg per meal)

MONITORING PARAMETERS
• CBC weekly if treatment longer than 2 weeks, ALT, AST, renal function

---

liothyronine (T3)
(lye-oh-thye'roe-neen)
Rx: Cytomel, Triostat
Combinations
  Rx: with levothyroxine (Euthroid, Thyrolar)
Chemical Class: Synthetic triiodothyronine (T_3)
Therapeutic Class: Thyroid hormone

CLINICAL PHARMACOLOGY
Mechanism of Action: A synthetic form of triiodothyronine (T_3), a thyroid hormone involved in normal metabolism, growth, and development, especially of the CNS in infants. Possesses catabolic and anabolic effects. *Therapeutic Effect:* Increases basal metabolic rate, enhances gluconeogenesis, and stimulates protein synthesis.

INDICATIONS AND DOSAGES
Hypothyroidism
PO

Adults, Elderly. Initially, 25 mcg/day. May increase in increments of 12.5–25 mcg/day q1–2wk. Maximum 100 mcg/day.

Children. Initially, 5 mcg/day. May increase by 5 mcg/day q3–4wk. Maintenance: 100 mcg/day (children older than 3 yr); 50 mcg/day (children 1-3 yr); 20 mcg/day (infants).

Myxedema
PO

Adults, Elderly. Initially, 5 mcg/day. Increase by 5–10 mcg q1–2wk (after 25 mcg/day has been reached, may increase in 12.5-mcg increments). Maintenance: 50–100 mcg/day.

Nontoxic goiter
PO

Adults, Elderly. Initially, 5 mcg/day. Increase by 5–10 mcg/day q1–2wk. When 25 mcg/day has been reached, may increase by 12.5–25 mcg/day q1–2wk. Maintenance: 75 mcg/day. *Children.* 5 mcg/day. May increase by 5 mcg q1–2wk. Maintenance: 15–20 mcg/day.

Congenital hypothyroidism
PO

Children. Initially, 5 mcg/day. Increase by 5 mcg/day q3–4 days. Maintenance: Full adult dosage (children older than 3 yr); 50 mcg/day (children 1-3 yr); 20 mcg/day (infants).

T_3 suppression test
PO

Adults, Elderly. 75–100 mcg/day for 7 days; then repeat I^{131} thyroid uptake test.

Myxedema coma, precoma
IV

Adults, Elderly. Initially, 25–50 mcg (10–20 mcg in patients with cardiovascular disease). Total dose at least 65 mcg/day.

AVAILABLE FORMS/COST
• Inj, Sol—IV: 10 mcg/ml, 1 ml, 1's: **$399.58-$452.99**
• Tab, Uncoated—Oral: 5 mcg, 100's: **$20.18-$52.33**; 25 mcg, 100's: **$24.33-$63.04**; 50 mcg, 100's: **$37.14-$96.29**

CONTRAINDICATIONS: MI and thyrotoxicosis uncomplicated by hypothyroidism; obesity

PREGNANCY AND LACTATION: Pregnancy category A; little or no transplacental passage at physiologic serum concentrations; excreted into breast milk in low concentrations; (inadequate to protect a hypothyroid infant; too low to interfere with neonatal screening programs)

SIDE EFFECTS
Occasional

Reversible hair loss at start of therapy (in children)

Rare

Dry skin, GI intolerance, rash, hives, pseudotumor cerebri or severe headache in children

SERIOUS REACTIONS
• Excessive dosage produces signs and symptoms of hyperthyroidism, including weight loss, palpitations, increased appetite, tremors, nervousness, tachycardia, hypertension, headache, insomnia, and menstrual irregularities.
• Cardiac arrhythmias occur rarely.

INTERACTIONS
Drugs

3 *Bile acid sequestrants:* Reduced serum thyroid hormone concentrations

3 *Carbamazepine, phenytoin, rifampin:* Increased elimination of thyroid hormones; possible increased requirement for thyroid hormones in hypothyroid patients

3 *Oral anticoagulants:* Thyroid hormones increase catabolism of vitamin K-dependent clotting factors;

an increase or decrease in clinical thyroid status will increase or decrease the hypoprothrombinemic response to oral anticoagulants

3 *Theophylline:* Reduced serum theophylline concentrations with initiation of thyroid therapy

SPECIAL CONSIDERATIONS
PATIENT/FAMILY EDUCATION
• Transient, partial hair loss may be experienced by children in the first few months of therapy
• Other thyroid products have longer half-lives. Take this into consideration when switching from them to liothyronine.
• Take as single daily dose, preferably before breakfast
MONITORING PARAMETERS
• TSH

---

lisinopril
(ly-sin'oh-pril)
Rx: Prinivil, Zestril
Combinations
　Rx: with hydrochlorothiazide (Prinzide, Zestoretic)
Chemical Class: Angiotensin-converting enzyme (ACE) inhibitor, nonsulfhydryl
Therapeutic Class: Antihypertensive

CLINICAL PHARMACOLOGY
Mechanism of Action: This angiotensin-converting enzyme (ACE) inhibitor suppresses the renin-angiotensin-aldosterone system and prevents conversion of angiotensin I to angiotensin II, a potent vasoconstrictor; may also inhibit angiotensin II at local vascular and renal sites. Decreases plasma angiotensin II, increases plasma renin activity, and decreases aldosterone secretion.
Therapeutic Effect: Reduces peripheral arterial resistance, blood pressure (BP), afterload, pulmonary capillary wedge pressure (preload), pulmonary vascular resistance. In those with heart failure, also decreases heart size, increases cardiac output, and exercise tolerance time.

Pharmacokinetics

Route	Onset	Peak	Duration
PO	1 hr	6 hrs	24 hrs

Incompletely absorbed from the gastrointestinal (GI) tract. Protein binding: 25%. Primarily excreted unchanged in urine. Removed by hemodialysis. **Half-life:** 12 hrs (half-life is prolonged in those with impaired renal function).

INDICATIONS AND DOSAGES
Hypertension (used alone)
PO
Adults. Initially, 10 mg/day. May increase by 5–10 mcg/day at 1–2 wk intervals. Maximum: 40 mg/day.
Elderly. Initially, 2.5–5 mg/day. May increase by 2.5–5 mg/day at 1- to 2-wk intervals. Maximum: 40 mg/day.

Hypertension (used in combination with other antihypertensives)
PO
Adults. Initially, 2.5–5 mg/day titrated to patient's needs.

Adjunctive therapy for management of heart failure
PO
Adults, Elderly. Initially, 2.5–5 mg/day. May increase by no more than 10 mg/day at intervals of at least 2 wk. Maintenance: 5–40 mg/day.

Improve survival in patients after a myocardial infarction (MI)
PO
Adults, Elderly. Initially, 5 mg, then 5 mg after 24 hr, 10 mg after 48 hr, then 10 mg/day for 6 wk. For pa-

tients with low systolic BP, give 2.5 mg/day for 3 days, then 2.5–5 mg/day.

Dosage in renal impairment

Titrate to patient's needs after giving the following initial dose:

Creatinine Clearance	% Normal Dose
10–50 ml/min	50–75
less than 10 ml/min	25–50

S **AVAILABLE FORMS/COST**

• Tab—Oral: 2.5 mg, 100's: **$63.55-$76.51**; 5 mg, 100's: **$32.11-$114.71**; 10 mg, 100's: **$84.54-$114.84**; 20 mg, 100's: **$90.48-$126.81**; 30 mg, 100's: **$149.10-$179.54**; 40 mg, 100's: **$125.50-$185.45**

UNLABELED USES: Treatment of hypertension or renal crises with scleroderma

CONTRAINDICATIONS: History of angioedema from previous treatment with ACE inhibitors

PREGNANCY AND LACTATION: Pregnancy category C (1st trimester), category D (2nd and 3rd trimesters); ACE inhibitors can cause fetal and neonatal morbidity and death when administered to pregnant women; when pregnancy is detected, discontinue ACE inhibitors as soon as possible; detectable in breast milk in trace amounts; a newborn would receive <0.1% of the mg/kg maternal dose; effect on nursing infant has not been determined

SIDE EFFECTS

Frequent (12%–5%)

Headache, dizziness, postural hypotension

Occasional (4%–2%)

Chest discomfort, fatigue, rash, abdominal pain, nausea, diarrhea, upper respiratory infection

Rare (1% or less)

Palpitations, tachycardia, peripheral edema, insomnia, paresthesia, confusion, constipation, dry mouth, muscle cramps

SERIOUS REACTIONS

• Excessive hypotension ("first-dose syncope") may occur in patients with congestive heart failure (CHF) and severe salt and volume depletion.

• Angioedema (swelling of face and lips) and hyperkalemia occurs rarely.

• Agranulocytosis and neutropenia may be noted in patients with collagen vascular disease, including scleroderma and systemic lupus erythematosus, and impaired renal function.

• Nephrotic syndrome may be noted in patients with history of renal disease.

INTERACTIONS

Drugs

② *Allopurinol:* Predisposition to hypersensitivity reactions to ACE inhibitors

③ *Aspirin, NSAIDs:* Inhibition of the antihypertensive response to ACE inhibitors

③ *Azathioprine:* Increased myelosuppression

③ *Insulin:* Enhanced insulin sensitivity

③ *Lithium:* Increased risk of serious lithium toxicity

③ *Loop diuretics:* Initiation of ACE inhibitor therapy in the presence of intensive diuretic therapy results in a precipitous fall in blood pressure in some patients; ACE inhibitors may induce renal insufficiency in the presence of diuretic-induced sodium depletion

③ *Potassium-sparing diuretics:* Increased risk for hyperkalemia

③ *Prazosin, terazosin, doxazosin:* Exaggerated first-dose hypotensive response to α-blockers

L

3 *Trimethoprim:* Additive risk of hyperkalemia, especially in patient predisposed to renal insufficiency

Labs

• ACE inhibition can account for approximately 0.5mEq/L rise in serum potassium

SPECIAL CONSIDERATIONS

PATIENT/FAMILY EDUCATION

• Caution with salt substitutes containing potassium chloride

• Rise slowly to sitting/standing position to minimize orthostatic hypotension

• Dizziness, fainting, lightheadedness may occur during first few days of therapy

• May cause altered taste perception or cough; persistent dry cough usually does not subside unless medication is stopped; notify clinician if these symptoms persist

MONITORING PARAMETERS

• BUN, creatinine, potassium within 2 wk after initiation of therapy (increased levels may indicate acute renal failure)

---

lithium

Rx: *Tablets:* Eskalith, Lithane, Lithotabs, Lithobid

Rx: *Capsules:* Eskalith, Lithonate

Rx: *Syrup:* Cibalith-S

Chemical Class: Monovalent cation

Therapeutic Class: Antimanic; psychotherapeutic agent

CLINICAL PHARMACOLOGY

Mechanism of Action: A psychotherapeutic agent that affects the storage, release, and reuptake of neurotransmitters. Antimanic effect may result from increased norepinephrine reuptake and serotonin re-

ceptor sensitivity. *Therapeutic Effect:* Produces antimanic and antidepressant effects.

Pharmacokinetics

Rapidly and completely absorbed from the GI tract. Primarily excreted unchanged in urine. Removed by hemodialysis. **Half-life:** 18–24 hr (increased in elderly).

INDICATIONS AND DOSAGES:

Alert: During acute phase, a therapeutic serum lithium concentration of 1–1.4 mEq/L is required. For long-term control, the desired level is 0.5–1.3 mEq/L. Monitor serum drug concentration and clinical response to determine proper dosage.

Prevention or treatment of acute mania, manic phase of bipolar disorder (manic-depressive illness)

PO

Adults. 300 mg 3–4 times a day or 450–900 mg slow-release form twice a day. Maximum: 2.4 g/day.

Elderly. 300 mg twice a day. May increase by 300 mg/day q1wk. Maintenance: 900–1,200 mg/day.

Children 12 yr and older. 600–1,800 mg/day in 3–4 divided doses (2 doses/day for slow-release).

Children younger than 12 yr. 15–60 mg/kg/day in 3–4 divided doses.

S AVAILABLE FORMS/COST

Lithium Carbonate

• Cap, Gel—Oral: 150 mg, 100's: **$13.97**; 300 mg, 100's: **$7.00-$37.19**; 600 mg, 100's: **$39.11**

• Tab-Oral: 300 mg, 100's: **$9.11-$21.52**

• Tab, Coated, Sus Action—Oral: 300 mg, 100's: **$43.32-$46.52**; 450 mg, 100's: **$52.10-$59.66**

Lithium Citrate

• Syr—Oral: 300 mg/5 ml, 480 ml: **$16.22-$19.29**

UNLABELED USES: Prevention of vascular headache; treatment of depression, neutropenia

CONTRAINDICATIONS: Debilitated patients, severe cardiovascular disease, severe dehydration, severe renal disease, severe sodium depletion

PREGNANCY AND LACTATION: Pregnancy category D; avoid use in pregnancy if possible, especially during the 1st trimester; excreted in breast milk; contraindicated in nursing mothers

SIDE EFFECTS

Alert: Side effects are dose related and seldom occur at lithium serum levels less than 1.5 mEq/L.

Occasional

Fine hand tremor, polydipsia, polyuria, mild nausea

Rare

Weight gain, bradycardia or tachycardia, acne, rash, muscle twitching, cold and cyanotic extremities, pseudotumor cerebri (eye pain, headache, tinnitus, vision disturbances)

SERIOUS REACTIONS

• A lithium serum concentration of 1.5–2.0 mEq/L may produce vomiting, diarrhea, drowsiness, confusion, incoordination, coarse hand tremor, muscle twitching, and T-wave depression on EKG.

• A lithium serum concentration of 2.0–2.5 mEq/L may result in ataxia, giddiness, tinnitus, blurred vision, clonic movements, and severe hypotension.

• Acute toxicity may be characterized by seizures, oliguria, circulatory failure, coma, and death.

INTERACTIONS

Drugs

▨ *ACE inhibitors, methyldopa:* Increased risk of lithium toxicity

▨ *Acetazolamide, sodium bicarbonate, urea:* Increased lithium renal clearance, decreased lithium efficacy

▨ *Aminophylline, caffeine, dyphylline, oxtriphylline, theophylline:* Increased lithium renal clearance, decreased lithium efficacy

▨ *Diltiazem, verapamil, amitriptyline, carbamazepine, fluoxetine, fluvoxamine:* Neurotoxicity, including seizures

❷ *MAOIs:* Malignant hyperpyrexia

▨ *Metronidazole:* Increased risk of lithium toxicity

▨ *Neuroleptics:* Reduced neuroleptic response; severe neurotoxicity possible in acute manic patients receiving lithium and neuroleptics

▨ *Neuromuscular blocking agents:* Prolonged effect of neuromuscular blocking agents possible

▨ *NSAIDs (including COX-2 inhibitors):* Increased lithium concentrations

▨ *Phenytoin:* Development of lithium toxicity has been reported

▨ *Potassium iodide:* Increased risk for hypothyroidism

▨ *Sodium bicarbonate:* Decreased plasma lithium concentrations

▨ *Sodium chloride:* High sodium intake may reduce serum lithium concentrations; sodium restriction may increase serum lithium

▨ *Theophylline:* Increased lithium renal clearance, decreased lithium efficacy

▨ *Thiazide diuretics:* Decreased lithium renal clearance, increased lithium concentrations

Labs

• *False increase:* Serum creatinine

SPECIAL CONSIDERATIONS

PATIENT/FAMILY EDUCATION

• Take with meals to avoid stomach upset

• Discontinue medication and contact clinician for diarrhea, vomiting, unsteady walking, coarse hand tremor, severe drowsiness, muscle weakness

• Drink 8-12 glasses of water or other liquid every day
• Do not restrict sodium in diet

MONITORING PARAMETERS

• Serum lithium concentrations drawn immediately prior to next dose (8-12 hr after previous dose), monitor biweekly until stable then q2-3mo; therapeutic range 0.8-1.2 mEq/L (acute), 0.5-1.0 mEq/L (maintenance)
• Serum creatinine, CBC, urinalysis, serum electrolytes, fasting glucose, ECG, TSH

lodoxamide

(loe-dox'a-mide)

Rx: Alomide

Chemical Class: Dioxamic acid derivative; mast cell stabilizer

Therapeutic Class: Ophthalmic antiinflammatory

CLINICAL PHARMACOLOGY

Mechanism of Action: A mast cell stabilizer that prevents increase in cutaneous vascular permeability, antigen-stimulated histamine release and may prevent calcium influx into mast cells. *Therapeutic Effect:* Inhibits sensitivity reaction.

Pharmacokinetics

Non-detectable absorption. **Half-life:** 8.5 hrs.

INDICATIONS AND DOSAGES

Treatment of vernal keratoconjunctivitis, conjunctivitis, and keratitis

Ophthalmic

Adults, Elderly, Children 2 yrs or older. 1-2 drops 4 times/day, for up to 3 mos.

[$] **AVAILABLE FORMS/COST**

• Sol—Ophth: 0.1%, 10 ml: **$72.00**

CONTRAINDICATIONS: Wearing soft contact lenses (product contains benzalkonium chloride), hypersensitivity to lodoxamide tromethamine or any component of the formulation

PREGNANCY AND LACTATION: Pregnancy category B; excretion into breast milk unknown but would be expected to be almost nothing since plasma levels are not measurable following ocular administration of therapeutic doses

SIDE EFFECTS

Frequent

Transient stinging, burning, instillation discomfort

Occasional

Ocular itching, blurred vision, dry eye, tearing/discharge/foreign body sensation, headache

Rare

Scales on lid/lash, ocular swelling, sticky sensation, dizziness, somnolence, nausea, sneezing, dry nose, rash

SERIOUS REACTIONS

• None reported.

lomefloxacin

Rx: Maxaquin

Chemical Class: Fluoroquinolone derivative

Therapeutic Class: Antibiotic

CLINICAL PHARMACOLOGY

Mechanism of Action: A quinolone that inhibits the enzyme DNA gyrase in susceptible microorganisms, interfering with bacterial cell replication and repair. *Therapeutic Effect:* Bactericidal.

Pharmacokinetics

Well absorbed from the GI tract. Protein binding: 10%. Widely distributed. Metabolized in the liver. Primarily excreted in urine. Not removed by hemodialysis. **Half-life:** 4-6 hr (increased with impaired renal function and in the elderly).

INDICATIONS AND DOSAGES
Complicated UTIs
PO

Adults, Elderly. 400 mg/day for 10-14 days.
Uncomplicated UTIs
PO

Adults (females). 400 mg/day for 3 days.
Lower respiratory tract infections
PO

Adults, Elderly. 400 mg/day for 10 days.
Surgical prophylaxis
PO

Adults, Elderly. 400 mg 2-6 hr before surgery.
Dosage in renal impairment
Dosage and frequency are modified based on creatinine clearance.

Creatinine Clearance	Dosage
41 ml/min and higher	No change
10-40 ml/min	400 mg initially, then 200 mg/day for 10–14 days

$ **AVAILABLE FORMS/COST**
• Tab, Coated—Oral: 400 mg, 20's: **$144.46**

CONTRAINDICATIONS: Hypersensitivity to quinolones

PREGNANCY AND LACTATION: Pregnancy category C; excretion into breast milk unknown; due to the potential for arthropathy and osteochondrosis, use extreme caution in nursing mothers

SIDE EFFECTS
Occasional (3%-2%)
Nausea, headache, photosensitivity, dizziness
Rare (1%)
Diarrhea

SERIOUS REACTIONS
• Antibiotic-associated colitis and other superinfections may result from altered bacterial balance.

• Hypersensitivity reactions, including photosensitivity (as evidenced by rash, pruritus, blisters, edema, and burning skin), have occurred in patients receiving fluoroquinolones.

• Arthropathy may occur if the drug is given to children younger than 18 years.

INTERACTIONS
Drugs
3 *Antacids (aluminum and magnesium containing):* Reduced absorption of lomefloxacin; take lomefloxacin 2 hr before or 4 hr after antacids

3 *Calcium, iron, zinc:* Reduced absorption of lomefloxacin; do not take lomefloxacin 2 hr before or after

3 *Cimetidine:* Interference with the elimination of other quinolones

3 *Cyclosporine:* Increased plasma cyclosporine concentrations with other quinolones

3 *Didanosine (buffered formulations):* Markedly reduced absorption of lomefloxacin; take lomefloxacin 2 hr before or 4 hr after didanosine

3 *Probenecid:* Probenecid slows the renal elimination of lomefloxacin possibly resulting in increased plasma lomefloxacin concentrations

3 *Sodium bicarbonate:* Reduced absorption of lomefloxacin; do not take within 4 hr of dose

3 *Sucralfate:* Reduced absorption of lomefloxacin; take lomefloxacin 2 hr before or 4 hr after sucralfate

3 *Warfarin:* May increase hypoprothrombinemic response to warfarin

SPECIAL CONSIDERATIONS
PATIENT/FAMILY EDUCATION
• Avoid direct and indirect exposure to sunlight (even when using sunscreen), discontinue at first signs of

phototoxicity, avoid re-exposure to sunlight until completely recovered from reaction

• Take dose in the evening to reduce risk of phototoxicity
• Take without regard to meals
• Drink fluids liberally
• Do not take antacids containing magnesium or aluminum or products containing iron or zinc within 4 hr before or 2 hr after dosing

loperamide

(loe-per'a-mide)
Rx: Imodium
OTC: Imodium A-D, Maalox Anti-Diarrheal
Combinations
OTC: with simethicone (Imodium Advanced)
Chemical Class: Piperidine derivative
Therapeutic Class: Antidiarrheal

CLINICAL PHARMACOLOGY
Mechanism of Action: An antidiarrheal that directly affects the intestinal wall muscles. *Therapeutic Effect:* Slows intestinal motility and prolongs transit time of intestinal contents by reducing fecal volume, diminishing loss of fluid and electrolytes, and increasing viscosity and bulk of stool.
Pharmacokinetics
Poorly absorbed from the GI tract. Protein binding: 97%. Metabolized in the liver. Eliminated in feces and excreted in urine. Not removed by hemodialysis. **Half-life:** 9.1–14.4 hr.

INDICATIONS AND DOSAGES
Acute diarrhea
PO (capsules)
Adults, Elderly. Initially, 4 mg; then 2 mg after each unformed stool. Maximum: 16 mg/day.
Children 9–12 yr, weighing more than 30 kg. Initially, 2 mg 3 times a day for 24 hr.
Children 6–8 yr, weighing 20–30 kg. Initially, 2 mg twice a day for 24 hr.
Children 2–5 yrs, weighing 13–20 kg. Initially, 1 mg 3 times/day for 24 hrs. Maintenance: 1 mg/10 kg only after loose stool.
Chronic diarrhea
PO
Adults, Elderly. Initially, 4 mg; then 2 mg after each unformed stool until diarrhea is controlled.
Children. 0.08–0.24 mg/kg/day in 2–3 divided doses. Maximum: 2 mg/dose.
Traveler's diarrhea
PO
Adults, Elderly. Initially, 4 mg; then 2 mg after each loose bowel movement (LBM). Maximum: 8 mg/day for 2 days.
Children 9–11 yr. Initially, 2 mg; then 1 mg after each LBM. Maximum: 6 mg/day for 2 days.
Children 6–8 yr. Initially, 1 mg; then 1 mg after each LBM. Maximum: 4 mg/day for 2 days.

[$] **AVAILABLE FORMS/COST**
• Cap, Gel—Oral: 2 mg, 100's: **$11.66-$71.39**
• Liq—Oral: 1 mg/5 ml, 60, 120 ml (OTC): **$2.23-$7.01**/120 ml
• Tab—Oral: 2 mg, 12's (OTC): **$1.50-$17.76**

CONTRAINDICATIONS: Acute ulcerative colitis (may produce toxic megacolon), diarrhea associated with pseudomembranous enterocolitis due to broad-spectrum antibiotics or to organisms that invade intestinal mucosa (such as *Escherichia coli*, shigella, and salmonella), patients who must avoid constipation

PREGNANCY AND LACTATION:
Pregnancy category B; unknown if
excreted in breast milk; compatible
with breast-feeding

SIDE EFFECTS

Rare

Dry mouth, somnolence, abdominal
discomfort, allergic reaction (such
as rash and itching)

SERIOUS REACTIONS

• Toxicity results in constipation, GI
irritation, including nausea and
vomiting, and CNS depression. Activated charcoal is used to treat loperamide toxicity.

SPECIAL CONSIDERATIONS

PATIENT/FAMILY EDUCATION

• Do not self-medicate diarrhea for
>48 hr without consulting provider

---

lopinavir/ritonavir

(lop-in'a-veer/rit-on'a-veer)

Rx: Kaletra

Chemical Class: Protease inhibitor, HIV

Therapeutic Class: Antiviral

CLINICAL PHARMACOLOGY

Mechanism of Action: A protease
inhibitor combination drug in which
lopinavir inhibits the activity of the
enzyme protease late in the HIV replication process and ritonavir increases plasma levels of lopinavir.
Therapeutic Effect: Formation of
immature, noninfectious viral particles.

Pharmacokinetics

Readily absorbed after PO administration (absorption increased when
taken with food). Protein binding:
98%-99%. Metabolized in the liver.
Eliminated primarily in feces. Not
removed by hemodialysis. **Half-
life:** 5-6 hr.

INDICATIONS AND DOSAGES

HIV infection

PO

Adults. 3 capsules (400 mg lopi-
navir/100 mg ritonavir) or 5 ml
twice a day. Increase to 4 capsules
(533 mg lopinavir/133 mg ritonavir)
or 6.5 ml when taken with efavirenz
or nevirapine.

*Children weighing 15-40 kg who are
not taking efavirenz or nevirapine.*
10 mg/kg twice a day.

*Children weighing 7-14 kg who are
not taking Alprenavir, efavirenz,
nelfinavir, nevirapine.* 12 mg/kg
twice a day.

*Children weighing 15-40 kg who are
taking efavirenz or nevirapine.* 11
mg/kg twice a day.

*Children weighing 7-14 kg who are
taking efavirenz or nevirapine.* 13
mg/kg twice a day.

AVAILABLE FORMS/COST

• Cap—Oral: 133.3 mg lopinavir
with 33.3 mg ritonavir, 180's:
$703.50

• Liquid—Oral: 400 mg lopinavir
with 100 mg ritonavir/5 ml, 160 ml:
$351.75

CONTRAINDICATIONS: Concomitant use of ergot derivatives
(causes peripheral ischemia of extremities and vasospasm), flecainide, midazolam, pimozide, propafenone (increases the risk of serious
cardiac arrhythmias), or triazolam
(increases sedation or respiratory
depression); hypersensitivity to
lopinavir or ritonavir

PREGNANCY AND LACTATION:
Pregnancy category C; breast milk
excretion unknown; the CDC recommends that HIV-infected mothers not breast-feed their infants to
avoid risking postnatal transmission
of HIV

SIDE EFFECTS

Frequent (14%)

Mild to moderate diarrhea

Occasional (6%-2%)

Nausea, asthenia, abdominal pain, headache, vomiting

Rare (less than 2%)

Insomnia, rash

SERIOUS REACTIONS

• Anemia, leukopenia, lymphadenopathy, deep vein thrombosis, Cushing's syndrome, pancreatitis, and hemorrhagic colitis occur rarely.

INTERACTIONS

Drags

② *Amiodarone:* Increased plasma levels of amiodarone

③ *Amprenavir:* Increased plasma level of amprenavir; consider dose adjustment of amprenavir to 750 mg bid

⚠ *Astemizole:* Increased plasma levels of astemizole

③ *Atorvastatin:* Increased plasma level of atorvastatin

③ *Atovaquone:* Decreased level of atovaquone

③ *Barbiturates:* Increased clearance of lopinavir/ritonavir; reduced clearance of barbiturates

② *Bepridil:* Increased plasma levels of bepridil

② *Carbamazepine:* Increased clearance of lopinavir/ritonavir; reduced clearance of carbamazepine

③ *Cerivastatin:* Increased plasma level of cerivastatin

⚠ *Cisapride:* Increased plasma levels of cisapride

② *Clarithromycin:* Reduced clearance of lopinavir/ritonavir; lopinavir/ritonavir reduces clearance of clarithromycin; reduce clarithromycin dose for renal insufficiency if coadministered

③ *Cyclosporine:* Increased plasma level of cyclosporine

③ *Dexamethasone:* Decreased plasma level of lopinavir/ritonavir

③ *Didanosine (buffered formulation):* Reduces absorption of lopinavir/ritonavir, take didanosine 1 hr before or 2 hr after dose of lopinavir/ritonavir

③ *Dihydropyridine calcium channel blockers (amlodipine, felodipine, nifedipine, nicardipine):* Increased plasma level of these drugs

③ *Efavirenz:* Increased clearance of lopinavir/ritonavir, increase dose to 533/133 mg bid

② *Encainide:* Increased plasma levels of encainide

⚠ *Ergot alkaloids:* Increased plasma levels of ergot alkaloids

③ *Erythromycin:* Reduced clearance of lopinavir/ritonavir; lopinavir/ritonavir reduces clearance of erythromycin

⚠ *Flecainide:* Increased plasma levels of flecainide

⚠ *Flurazepam:* Increased plasma levels of flurazepam

③ *Indinavir:* Increased plasma level of indinavir; consider dose reduction to 600 mg bid

③ *Itraconazole:* Lopinavir/ritonavir reduces clearance of itraconazole; reduce itraconazole dose

③ *Ketoconazole:* Lopinavir/ritonavir reduces clearance of ketoconazole; reduce ketoconazole dose

② *Lidocaine:* Increased plasma levels of lidocaine

② *Lovastatin:* Lopinavir/ritonavir reduces clearance of lovastatin

② *Meperidine:* Increased plasma levels of meperidine

③ *Methadone:* Lopinavir/ritonavir reduces methadone plasma concentration by 50%

⚠ *Midazolam:* Increased plasma levels of midazolam and prolonged effect

③ *Nevirapine:* Increased clearance of lopinavir/ritonavir, increase dose to 533/133 mg bid

⑧ *Oral contraceptives:* Lopinavir/ritonavir may reduce efficacy

⑧ *Phenytoin:* Increased clearance of lopinavir/ritonavir; reduced clearance of phenytoin

⚠ *Pimozide:* Increased plasma levels of pimozide

⚠ *Propafenone:* Increased plasma levels of propafenone

② *Propoxyphene:* Increased plasma levels of propoxyphene

② *Quinidine:* Increased plasma levels of quinidine

⑧ *Rapamycin:* Increased plasma level of rapamycin

② *Rifabutin:* Increased clearance of lopinavir/ritonavir; reduced clearance of rifabutin; reduce rifabutin dose to 150 mg qod

② *Rifampin:* Increased clearance of lopinavir/ritonavir

⑧ *Saquinavir:* Decreased clearance of saquinavir; reduce dose of Fortovase (saquinavir soft gel capsule) to 800 mg bid

② *Sildenafil:* Increased plasma level of sildenafil, reduce dose to 25 mg q48h

② *Simvastatin:* Lopinavir/ritonavir reduces clearance of simvastatin

② *St. John's Wort (hypericum perforatum):* Increased clearance of lopinavir/ritonavir

⑧ *Tacrolimus:* Increased plasma level of tacrolimus

⚠ *Terfenadine:* Increased plasma levels of terfenadine

⑧ *Tenofovir:* Lopinavir/ritonavir increases tenofovir AUC by 34%; tenofovir decreases AUC of lopinavir/ritonavir by 24% (when co-administered with lopinavir/ritonavir, tenofovir should be administered 2 hours before or one hour after administration of lopinavir/ritonavir)

⚠ *Triazolam:* Increased plasma levels of triazolam and prolonged effect

⑧ *Troleandomycin:* Reduced clearance of lopinavir/ritonavir; lopinavir/ritonavir reduces clearance of troleandomycin

⑧ *Warfarin:* May reduce warfarin effect

② *Zolpidem:* Increased plasma levels of zolpidem

SPECIAL CONSIDERATIONS
PATIENT/FAMILY EDUCATION
• Take with food to improve bioavailability
• Be aware of many potential drug interactions

MONITORING PARAMETERS
• Plasma glucose, lipid levels, hepatic function tests

loracarbef
(lor-a-kar'bef)
Rx: Lorabid
Chemical Class: Carbacephem derivative
Therapeutic Class: Antibiotic

CLINICAL PHARMACOLOGY
Mechanism of Action: A second-generation cephalosporin that binds to bacterial cell membranes and inhibits cell wall synthesis. *Therapeutic Effect:* Bactericidal.

INDICATIONS AND DOSAGES
Bronchitis
PO
Adults, Elderly, Children 12 yr and older. 200-400 mg q12h for 7 days.

Pharyngitis
PO
Adults, Elderly, Children 12 yr and older. 200 mg q12h for 10 days.
Children 6 mo-11 yr. 7.5 mg/kg q12h for 10 days.

Pneumonia
PO
Adults, Elderly, Children 12 yr and older. 400 mg q12h for 14 days.

Sinusitis
PO
Adults, Elderly, Children 12 yr and older. 400 mg q12h for 10 days.
Children 6 mo-11 yr. 15 mg/kg q12h for 10 days.

Skin and soft-tissue infections
PO
Adults, Elderly, Children 12 yr and older. 200 mg q12h for 7 days.
Children 6 mo-11 yr. 7.5 mg/kg q12h for 7 days.

UTIs
PO
Adults, Elderly, Children 6 mo-12 yr. 200-400 mg q12h for 7-14 days.

Otitis media
PO
Children 6 mo-12 yr. 15 mg/kg q12h for 10 days.

S AVAILABLE FORMS/COST
• Cap, Gel—Oral: 200 mg, 100's: **$453.15**; 400 mg, 100's: **$637.88**
• Susp—Oral: 100 mg/5 ml, 100 ml: **$47.53**; 200 mg/5 ml, 100 ml: **$71.85**

CONTRAINDICATIONS: History of anaphylactic reaction to penicillins or hypersensitivity to cephalosporins

PREGNANCY AND LACTATION: Pregnancy category B; unknown if excreted into breast milk

SIDE EFFECTS
Frequent
Abdominal pain, anorexia, nausea, vomiting, diarrhea
Occasional
Rash, pruritus
Rare
Dizziness, headache, vaginitis

SERIOUS REACTIONS
• Antibiotic-associated colitis and other superinfections may result from altered bacterial balance.
• Hypersensitivity reactions (ranging from rash, urticaria, and fever to anaphylaxis) occur in fewer than 5%

of patients—most commonly in patients with a history of drug allergies, especially to penicillins.

SPECIAL CONSIDERATIONS
• Essentially same spectrum and utility as cefaclor
• Take 1 hr before eating or 2 hr after eating

---

loratadine
(loer-at'ah-deen)
Rx: Claritin, Claritin Reditabs
Combinations
  Rx: with pseudoephedrine (Claritin-D)
Chemical Class: Piperidine derivative
Therapeutic Class: Antihistamine

CLINICAL PHARMACOLOGY
Mechanism of Action: A long-acting antihistamine that competes with histamine for H_1 receptor sites on effector cells. *Therapeutic Effect:* Prevents allergic responses mediated by histamine, such as rhinitis, urticaria, and pruritus.

Pharmacokinetics

Route	Onset	Peak	Duration
PO	1–3 hr	8–12 hr	longer than 24 hr

Rapidly and almost completely absorbed from the GI tract. Protein binding: 97%; metabolite, 73%–77%. Distributed mainly to the liver, lungs, GI tract, and bile. Metabolized in the liver to active metabolite; undergoes extensive first-pass metabolism. Eliminated in urine and feces. Not removed by hemodialysis. **Half-life:** 8.4 hr; metabolite, 28 hr (increased in elderly and hepatic impairment).

INDICATIONS AND DOSAGES
Allergic rhinitis, urticaria
PO

Adults, Elderly, Children 6 yr and older. 10 mg once a day.

Children 2–5 yr. 5 mg once a day.

Dosage in hepatic impairment
For adults, elderly, and children 6 years and older dosage is reduced to 10 mg every other day.

$\boxed{\text{S}}$ AVAILABLE FORMS/COST
• Syr—Oral: 5 mg/5 ml, 480 ml: **$122.40**
• Tab-Oral: 10 mg, 100's: **$82.50-$340.12**
• Tab, Disintegrating—Oral: 10 mg, 30's: **$111.71**
• Tab, Sus Action—Oral (with pseudoepedrine): 5 mg-120 mg, 100's: **$181.94**; 10 mg-240 mg, 100's: **$363.84**

UNLABELED USES: Adjunct treatment of bronchial asthma

CONTRAINDICATIONS: Hypersensitivity to loratadine or its ingredients

PREGNANCY AND LACTATION: Pregnancy category B; excreted into breast milk at levels equivalent to serum levels

SIDE EFFECTS
Frequent (12%–8%)
Headache, fatigue, somnolence
Occasional (3%)
Dry mouth, nose, or throat
Rare
Photosensitivity

SERIOUS REACTIONS
• None known.

INTERACTIONS
Drugs
$\boxed{3}$ *Itraconazole, ketoconazole, miconazole:* Increased loratadine levels but no increase in toxicity reported

• Effective, but expensive nonsedating antihistamine; reserve for patients unable to tolerate sedating antihistamines like chlorpheniramine

---

lorazepam
(lor-a′ze-pam)
Rx: Ativan
Chemical Class: Benzodiazepine
Therapeutic Class: Anticonvulsant; anxiolytic; sedative/hypnotic
DEA Class: Schedule IV

CLINICAL PHARMACOLOGY
Mechanism of Action: A benzodiazepine that enhances the action of the inhibitory neurotransmitter gamma-aminobutyric acid in the CNS, affecting memory, as well as motor, sensory, and cognitive function. *Therapeutic Effect:* Produces anxiolytic, anticonvulsant, sedative, muscle relaxant, and antiemetic effects.

Pharmacokinetics

Route	Onset	Peak	Duration
PO	60 min	N/A	8-12 hr
IV	15-30 min	N/A	8-12 hr
IM	30-60 min	N/A	8-12 hr

Well absorbed after PO and IM administration. Protein binding: 85%. Widely distributed. Metabolized in the liver. Primarily excreted in urine. Not removed by hemodialysis. **Half-life:** 10-20 hr.

INDICATIONS AND DOSAGES
Anxiety
PO

Adults. 1-10 mg/day in 2-3 divided doses. Average: 2-6 mg/day.

Elderly. Initially, 0.5-1 mg/day. May increase gradually. Range: 0.5-4 mg.

IV

Adults, Elderly. 0.02-0.06 mg/kg q2-6h.

IV Infusion

Adults, Elderly. 0.01-0.1 mg/kg/h.

PO, IV

Children. 0.05 mg/kg/dose q4-8h. Range: 0.02-0.1 mg/kg. Maximum: 2 mg/dose.

Insomnia due to anxiety

PO

Adults. 2-4 mg at bedtime.

Elderly. 0.5-1 mg at bedtime.

Preoperative sedation

IV

Adults, Elderly. 0.044 mg/kg 15-20 min before surgery. Maximum total dose: 2 mg.

IM

Adults, Elderly. 0.05 mg/kg 2 hr before procedure. Maximum total dose: 4 mg.

Status epilepticus

IV

Adults, Elderly. 4 mg over 2-5 min. May repeat in 10-15 min. Maximum: 8 mg in 12-hr period.

Children. 0.1 mg/kg over 2-5 min. May give second dose of 0.05 mg/kg in 15-20 min. Maximum: 4 mg.

Neonates. 0.05 mg/kg. May repeat in 10-15 min.

$ AVAILABLE FORMS/COST

• Sol, Inj-IM, IV: 2 mg/ml, 0.5, 1, 2, 10 ml: **$2.50-$3.75**/1 ml; 4 mg/ml, 1, 2, 10 ml: **$4.66-$4.74**/1 ml

• Sol—Oral: 2 mg/ml, 30 ml: **$46.63**

• Tab—Oral: 0.5 mg, 100's: **$9.35-$93.50**; 1 mg, 100's: **$10.95-$121.75**; 2 mg, 100's: **$18.70-$177.50**

UNLABELED USES: Treatment of alcohol withdrawal, panic disorders, skeletal muscle spasms, chemotherapy-induced nausea or vomiting, tension headache, tremors; adjunctive treatment before endoscopic procedures (diminishes patient recall)

CONTRAINDICATIONS: Angle-closure glaucoma; pre-existing CNS depression; severe hypotension; severe uncontrolled pain

PREGNANCY AND LACTATION: Pregnancy category D (other benzodiazepines associated with cleft lip, cleft palate, microcephaly, pyloric stenosis); neonatal withdrawal, hypotonia; excreted into breast milk in low quantities; effect on infant unknown

SIDE EFFECTS

Frequent

Somnolence (initially in the morning), ataxia, confusion

Occasional

Blurred vision, slurred speech, hypotension, headache

Rare

Paradoxical CNS restlessness or excitement in elderly or debilitated

SERIOUS REACTIONS

• Abrupt or too-rapid withdrawal may result in pronounced restlessness, irritability, insomnia, hand tremor, abdominal or muscle cramps, diaphoresis, vomiting, and seizures.

• Overdose results in somnolence, confusion, diminished reflexes, and coma.

INTERACTIONS

Drugs

🔳 *Ethanol:* Increased adverse psychomotor effects of lorazepam

② *Fluconazole:* Potential for increased lorazepam concentrations

🔳 *Itraconazole:* Potential for increased lorazepam concentrations

SPECIAL CONSIDERATIONS

• A good choice for elderly or patients with liver dysfunction who need benzodiazepines due to phase II metabolism to inactive metabolites (less likely to accumulate)

PATIENT/FAMILY EDUCATION
• Do not discontinue abruptly after long-term use, withdrawal syndrome (seizures, anxiety, insomnia, nausea, vomiting, flu-like illness, confusion, hallucinations, memory impairment) can occur

---

losartan
(lo-sar′tan)
Rx: Cozaar
Combinations
  Rx: with hydrochlorothiazide (Hyzaar)
Chemical Class: Angiotensin II receptor antagonist
Therapeutic Class: Antihypertensive

CLINICAL PHARMACOLOGY
Mechanism of Action: An angiotensin II receptor, type AT_1, antagonist that blocks vasoconstrictor and aldosterone-secreting effects of angiotensin II, inhibiting the binding of angiotensin II to the AT_1 receptors. *Therapeutic Effect:* Causes vasodilation, decreases peripheral resistance, and decreases BP.

Pharmacokinetics

Route	Onset	Peak	Duration
PO	N/A	6 hr	24 hr

Well absorbed after PO administration. Protein binding: 98%. Undergoes first-pass metabolism in the liver to active metabolites. Excreted in urine and via the biliary system. Not removed by hemodialysis. **Half-life:** 2 hr, metabolite: 6–9 hr.

INDICATIONS AND DOSAGES
Hypertension
PO
Adults, Elderly. Initially, 50 mg once a day. Maximum: May be given once or twice a day, with total daily doses ranging from 25–100 mg.

Nephropathy
PO
Adults, Elderly. Initially, 50 mg/day. May increase to 100 mg/day based on BP response.
Stroke reduction
PO
Adults, Elderly. 50 mg/day. Maximum: 100 mg/day.
Hypertension in patients with impaired hepatic function
PO
Adults, Elderly. Initially, 25 mg/day.
S AVAILABLE FORMS/COST
Cozaar
• Tab—Oral: 25, 50 mg; 100's: **$166.16**; 100 mg, 100's: **$215.99**
Hyzaar
• Tab—Oral: 12.5-50 mg, 100's: **$166.16**; 25-100 mg, 100's: **$226.35**
CONTRAINDICATIONS: None known.
PREGNANCY AND LACTATION: Pregnancy category C, first trimester—Category D, second and third trimesters; drugs acting directly on the renin-angiotensin-aldosterone system are documented to cause fetal harm (hypotension, oligohydramnios, neonatal anemia, hyperkalemia, neonatal skull hypoplasia, anuria, and renal failure; neonatal limb contractures, craniofacial deformities, and hypoplastic lung development); excretion into breast milk unknown
SIDE EFFECTS
Frequent (8%)
Upper respiratory tract infection
Occasional (4%–2%)
Dizziness, diarrhea, cough
Rare (1% or less)
Insomnia, dyspepsia, heartburn, back and leg pain, muscle cramps, myalgia, nasal congestion, sinusitis

SERIOUS REACTIONS

• Overdosage may manifest as hypotension and tachycardia. Bradycardia occurs less often.

INTERACTIONS

Drugs

◙ *Fluconazole:* Decreased conversion to active metabolite (CYP2C9 inhibition), loss of antihypertensive effects

➋ *Lithium:* Increased renal lithium reabsorption at the proximal tubular site due to the natriuresis associated with the inhibition of aldosterone secretion; increased risk of lithium toxicity

◙ *NSAIDs:* May reduce hemodynamic effects of losartan

◙ *Potassium-sparing diuretics:* Increased risk of hyperkalemia

◙ *Rifampin:* Induced metabolism of losartan and metabolite, resulting in a decrease in the area under the concentration-time curve (AUC) and half-life of both compounds and reduced losartan efficacy

SPECIAL CONSIDERATIONS

• Potentially as or more effective than angiotensin-converting enzyme inhibitors, without cough; no evidence for reduction in morbidity and mortality as first line agents in hypertension, yet; whether they provide the same cardiac and renal protection also still tentative; like ACE inhibitors, less effective in black patients

PATIENT/FAMILY EDUCATION

• Call your clinician immediately if note following side effects: wheezing; lip, throat or face swelling; hives or rash

MONITORING PARAMETERS

• Baseline electrolytes, urinalysis, blood urea nitrogen and creatinine with recheck at 2-4 weeks after initiation (sooner in volume depleted patients); monitor sitting blood pressure; watch for symptomatic hypotension, particularly in volume-depleted patients

---

lovastatin

(lo'va-sta-tin)

Rx: Altocor, Mevacor

Combinations

Rx: With niacin extended release (Advicor)

Chemical Class: Substituted hexahydronaphthalene

Therapeutic Class: HMG-CoA reductase inhibitor; antilipemic

CLINICAL PHARMACOLOGY

Mechanism of Action: An antihyperlipidemic that inhibits HMG-CoA reductase, the enzyme that catalyzes the early step in cholesterol synthesis. *Therapeutic Effect:* Decreases LDL cholesterol, VLDL cholesterol, plasma triglycerides; increases HDL cholesterol.

Pharmacokinetics

Route	Onset	Peak	Duration
PO	3 days	4–6 wk	N/A

Incompletely absorbed from the GI tract (increased on empty stomach). Protein binding: 95%. Hydrolyzed in the liver to active metabolite. Primarily eliminated in feces. Not removed by hemodialysis. **Half-life:** 1.1–1.7 hrs.

INDICATIONS AND DOSAGES

Hyperlipoproteinemia, primary prevention of coronary artery disease

PO

Adults, Elderly. Initially, 20–40 mg/day with evening meal. Increase at 4-wk intervals up to maximum of 80 mg/day. Maintenance: 20–80 mg/day in single or divided doses.

PO (extended release)

Adults, Elderly. Initially, 20 mg/day. May increase at 4-wk intervals up to 60 mg/day.

Children 10–17 yr. 10–40 mg/day with evening meal.

Heterozygous familial hypercholesterolemia
PO

Children 10-17 yr. Initially, 10 mg/day. May increase to 20 mg/day after 8 wk and 40 mg/day after 16 wk if needed.

AVAILABLE FORMS/COST

• Tab—Oral: 10 mg, 100's: **$134.55**; 20 mg, 60's: **$142.21–$161.03**; 40 mg, 60's: **$256.00–$286.35**

• Tab, Sus Action—Oral: 20 mg, 30's: **$56.70**; 40 mg, 30's: **$59.06**; 60 mg, 30's: **$67.34**

• Tab—Oral (with Niacin): 20 mg-100 mg, 90's: **$214.18**; 20 mg-500 mg, 90's: **$164.32**; 20 mg-750 mg, 90's: **$200.58**

CONTRAINDICATIONS: Active liver disease, pregnancy, unexplained elevated liver function tests

PREGNANCY AND LACTATION: Pregnancy category X (may produce skeletal malformations); excretion into breast milk unknown, contraindicated in nursing mothers

SIDE EFFECTS

Generally well tolerated. Side effects usually mild and transient.

Frequent (9%–5%)

Headache, flatulence, diarrhea, abdominal pain or cramps, rash and pruritus

Occasional (4%–3%)

Nausea, vomiting, constipation, dyspepsia

Rare (2%–1%)

Dizziness, heartburn, myalgia, blurred vision, eye irritation

SERIOUS REACTIONS

• There is a potential for cataract development.

INTERACTIONS
Drugs

③ *Cholestyramine, colestipol:* Decreased bioavailability of lovastatin possible, potentially reduced benefit overcome by additive lipid-lowering effects of concurrent therapy

② *Clarithromycin, danazol, erythromycin, nefazodone:* Severe myopathy or rhabdomyolysis

② *Clofibrate, fenofibrate, gemfibrozil:* Severe myopathy or rhabdomyolysis with combination possible, especially at high doses; if used concomitantly lovastatin dose should not exceed 20 mg/day

③ *Cyclosporine:* Concomitant administration increases risk of severe myopathy or rhabdomyolysis; if used concomitantly lovastatin dose should not exceed 20 mg/day

③ *Diltiazem, verapamil:* Increased risk of myopathy

② *Fluconazole, itraconazole, ketoconazole:* Large increases in lovastatin concentration, myopathy or rhabdomyolysis possible

③ *Grapefruit juice:* Increased risk of myopathy or rhabdomyolysis with large quantities of grapefruit juice (>1 quart/day)

③ *Imatinib:* Increased risk of myopathy or rhabdomyolysis with combination

③ *Isradipine:* Reduction in lovastatin concentration

③ *Niacin:* Concomitant administration increases risk of severe myopathy or rhabdomyolysis; if used concomitantly lovastatin dose should not exceed 20 mg/day

③ *Pectin:* Reduced cholesterol-lowering effect of lovastatin

② *Protease inhibitors:* Severe myopathy or rhabdomyolysis with combination possible

③ *Warfarin:* Increased prothrombin times and bleeding reported with concomitant use

SPECIAL CONSIDERATIONS
• Less effective in homozygous familial hypercholesterolemia (lack of functional LDL receptors); these patients also more likely to have adverse reaction of elevated transaminases
• Statin selection based on lipid-lowering prowess, cost, and availability

PATIENT/FAMILY EDUCATION
• Report symptoms of myalgia, muscle tenderness, or weakness
• Take daily doses in the evening for increased effect

MONITORING PARAMETERS
• Cholesterol (max therapeutic response 4-6 wk)
• LFTs (AST, ALT) at baseline and at 12 wk of therapy; if no change, no further monitoring necessary (discontinue if elevations persist >3 × upper limit of normal)
• CPK in patients complaining of diffuse myalgia, muscle tenderness, or weakness

---

loxapine
(lox′a-peen)
Rx: Loxitane
Chemical Class: Dibenzoxazepine derivative; tertiary amine
Therapeutic Class: Antipsychotic

CLINICAL PHARMACOLOGY
Mechanism of Action: A dibenzodiazepine derivative that interferes with the binding of dopamine at postsynaptic receptor sites in brain. Strong anticholinergic effects. *Therapeutic Effect:* Suppresses locomotor activity, produces tranquilization.

Pharmacokinetics
Onset of action occurs within 1 hours. Metabolized to active metabolites 8-hydroxyloxapine, 7-hydroxyloxapine, and 8-hydroxyamoxapine. Excreted in urine. **Half-life:** 4 hrs.

INDICATIONS AND DOSAGES
Psychotic disorders
PO
Adults. 10 mg 2 times/day. Increase dosage rapidly during first week to 50 mg, if needed. Usual therapeutic, maintenance range: 60-100 mg daily in 2-4 divided doses. Maximum: 250 mg/day.

S AVAILABLE FORMS/COST
• Cap, Gel—Oral: 5 mg, 100's: **$47.25-$140.66**; 10 mg, 100's: **$69.45-$181.74**; 25 mg, 100's: **$108.90-$274.60**; 50 mg, 100's: **$139.95-$366.40**

CONTRAINDICATIONS: Severe central nervous system (CNS) depression, comatose states, hypersensivitiy to loxapine or any component of the formulation

PREGNANCY AND LACTATION: Pregnancy category C; no data in lactating women

SIDE EFFECTS
Frequent
Blurred vision, confusion, drowsiness, dry mouth, dizziness, lightheadedness
Occasional
Allergic reaction (rash, itching), decreased urination, constipation, decreased sexual ability, enlarged breasts, headache, photosensitivity, nausea, vomiting, insomnia, weight gain

SERIOUS REACTIONS
• Extrapyramidal symptoms frequently noted are akathisia (motor restlessness, anxiety). Less frequently noted are akinesia (rigidity, tremor, salivation, mask-like facial expression, reduced voluntary

movements). Infrequently noted dystonias: torticollis (neck muscle spasm), opisthotonos (rigidity of back muscles), and oculogyric crisis (rolling back of eyes). Tardive dyskinesia (protrusion of tongue, puffing of cheeks, chewing/puckering of mouth) occurs rarely but may be irreversible. Risk is greater in female elderly patients.

INTERACTIONS

Drugs

▪ *Anticholinergics:* Decreased neuroleptic effect

▪ *Bromocriptine:* Decreased lowering of prolactin by bromocriptine in patients with pituitary adenoma

❷ *Epinephrine:* Inhibition of vasopressor effect of epinephrine

▪ *Lithium:* Increased neurotoxicity

▪ *Lorazepam:* Isolated cases of respiratory depression, stupor and hypotension have been observed

SPECIAL CONSIDERATIONS

PATIENT/FAMILY EDUCATION

• Avoid alcohol; caution with activities requiring mental alertness

• Mix oral concentrate in orange or grapefruit juice

---

mafenide

(ma'fe-nide)

Rx: Sulfamylon

Chemical Class: Sulfonamide derivative

Therapeutic Class: Antibiotic, topical

CLINICAL PHARMACOLOGY

Mechanism of Action: A topical anti-infective that decreases number of bacteria avascular tissue of second- and third-degree burns. *Therapeutic Effect:* Bacteriostatic. Promotes spontaneous healing of deep partial-thickness burns.

Pharmacokinetics

Absorbed through devascularzied areas into systemic circulation following topical administration. Excreted in the form of its metabolite rho-carboxybenzenesulfonamide

INDICATIONS AND DOSAGES

Burns

Topical

Adults, Elderly, Children. Apply 1-2 times/day.

Ⓢ   AVAILABLE FORMS/COST

• Cre—Top: 85 mg/g, 60, 120, 454 g: **$24.51**/60 g

• Powder, Reconst-Top: 50 g/packet: **$122.50**

CONTRAINDICATIONS: Hypersensitivity to mafenide or sulfite or any other component of the formulation

PREGNANCY AND LACTATION: Pregnancy category C; compatible with breast-feeding except in G-6-PD deficiency and ill, jaundiced, or premature infants

SIDE EFFECTS

Difficult to distinguish side effects and effects of severe burn

Frequent

Pain, burning upon application

Occasional

Allergic reaction (usually 10-14 days after initiation): itching, rash, facial edema, swelling; unexplained syndrome of marked hyperventilation with respiratory alkalosis

Rare

Delay in eschar separation, excoriation of new skin

SERIOUS REACTIONS

• Hemolytic anemia, porphyria, bone marrow depression, superinfections (especially with fungi), metabolic acidosis occurs rarely.

INTERACTIONS

Labs

• *False increase:* Urine amino acids

M

magaldrate

OTC: Riopan
Combinations
  OTC: with simethicone (Riopan Plus)
Chemical Class: Aluminum and magnesium hydroxide and sulfate mixture
Therapeutic Class: Antacid

CLINICAL PHARMACOLOGY
Mechanism of Action: An antacid that causes less hydrogen ion available for diffusion through the gastrointestinal (GI) mucosa. *Therapeutic Effect:* Reduces and neutralizes gastric acid.

INDICATIONS AND DOSAGES
Hyperacidity and gas
PO
Adults, Elderly. 540 to 1080 mg between meals and at bedtime.

$ AVAILABLE FORMS/COST
• Susp—Oral: 540 mg/5 ml, 360 ml: **$3.45-$5.49**

CONTRAINDICATIONS: Hypersensitivity to magaldrate, colostomy or ileostomy, appendicitis, ulcerative colitis, diverticulits

PREGNANCY AND LACTATION: Pregnancy category C

SIDE EFFECTS
Rare
Constipation, diarrhea, fluid retention, dizziness or lightheadedness, continuing discomfort, irregular heartbeat, loss of appetite, mood or mental changes, muscle weakness, unusual tiredness or weakness, weight loss, chalky taste

SERIOUS REACTIONS
• None known.

INTERACTIONS
Drugs
⬛ *Allopurinol, cefpodoxime, ciprofloxacin, isoniazid, ketoconazole, quinolones, tetracyclines, digoxin, iron salts, indomethacin:* Decreased GI absorption of these drugs
⬛ *Pseudoephedrine, enteric coated aspirin, diazepam:* Increased GI absorption of these drugs
⬛ *Quinidine:* Increased quinidine levels
⬛ *Salicylates:* Increased urinary excretion of salicylates

magnesium

OTC: *Magnesium oxide:* Mag-Ox 400, Maox, Uro-Mag
OTC: *Magnesium hydroxide:* Milk of Magnesia, Phillips' Chewable
OTC: *Magnesium citrate:* Evac-Q-Mag, Citro-Nesia, Citroma
OTC: *Magnesium sulfate:* Epsom Salts
OTC: *Magnesium gluconate:* Almora, Magonate, Magtrate
OTC: *Magnesium chloride:* Slow-Mag
Chemical Class: Divalent cation
Therapeutic Class: Antacid; antiarrhythmic; electrolyte supplement; laxative; uterine relaxant

CLINICAL PHARMACOLOGY
Mechanism of Action: An antacid, laxative, electrolyte, and anticonvulsant. As an antacid acts in the stomach to neutralize gastric acid. *Therapeutic Effect:* Increases pH. As a laxative has an osmotic effect, primarily in the small intestine, and draws water into the intestinal lumen. *Therapeutic Effect:* Produces

distention and promotes peristalsis and bowel evacuation. As a systemic dietary supplement and electrolyte replacement, is found primarily in intracellular fluids and is essential for enzyme activity, nerve conduction, and muscle contraction. As an anticonvulsant, blocks neuromuscular transmission and the amount of acetylcholine released at the motor end plate. *Therapeutic Effect:* Controls seizure. Maintains and restores magnesium levels.

Pharmacokinetics

Antacid, laxative: Minimal absorption through the intestine. Absorbed dose primarily excreted in urine. Systemic: Widely distributed. Primarily excreted in urine.

INDICATIONS AND DOSAGES

Hypomagnesemia (magnesium sulfate)

PO

Adults, Elderly. 3 g q6h for 4 doses as needed.

IV, IM

Adults, Elderly. 1-12 g/day in divided doses.

Children. 25–50 mg/kg/dose q4–6h for 3–4 doses. Maintenance: 30-60 mg/kg/day.

Hypertension, seizures (magnesium sulfate)

IV, IM

Children. 20–100 mg/kg/dose q4–6h as needed.

IV

Adults. Initially, 4 g then 1-4 g/h by continuous infusion.

Arrhythmias (magnesium sulfate)

IV

Adults, Elderly. Initially, 1–2 g then infusion of 1-2 g/h.

Treat constipation (magnesium sulfate)

PO

Adults, Elderly, Children older than 11 yr. 10-30 g/day in divided doses.

Children 6–11 yr. 5-10 g/day in divided doses.

Children 2-5 yr. 2.5-5 g/kg/day in divided doses.

Treat constipation (magnesium hydroxide)

PO

Adults, Elderly, Children older than 11 yr. 6-8 tablets or 30–60 ml/day.

Children 6–11 yr. 3-4 tablets or 7.5-15 ml/day.

Children 2–5 yr. 1-2 tablets or 2.5-7.5 ml/day.

Treatment of hyperacidity (magnesium hydroxide)

PO

Adults, Elderly. 2-4 tablets or 5–15 ml as needed up to 4 times a day.

Children 7-14 yr. 1 tablet or 2.5–5 ml as needed up to 4 times a day.

Magnesium deficiency (magnesium oxide)

PO

Adults, Elderly. 1-2 tablets 2-3 times/day.

Dietary supplement (magnesium chloride)

PO

Adults, Elderly. 54-483 mg/day in 2-4 divided doses.

Cathartic (magnesium citrate)

PO

Adults, Elderly, Children 12 yr and older. 120-300 ml.

Children 6-11 yr. 100-150 ml.

Children younger than 6 yr. 0.5 ml/kg up to maximum of 200 ml.

$ AVAILABLE FORMS/COST

Magnesium Citrate

• Liq—Oral: 8.85%, 300 ml: **$0.75-$4.86**

Magnesium Chloride

• Sol, Inj-IV: 200 mg/ml, 50 ml: **$4.20-$12.50**

Magnesium Gluconate

• Tab—Oral: 500 mg, 100's: **$2.29-$31.53**

M

Magnesium Hydroxide
• Conc, Liq—Oral: 16%, 240 ml: **$4.34**
• Susp-Oral: 8%, 30, 60, 120, 360, 480 ml: **$2.16-$2.27**/120 ml
• Tab, Chewable-Oral: 325 mg, 100's: **$4.30**

Magnesium Oxide
• Cap-Oral: 140 mg, 100's: **$10.83**
• Tab-Oral: 250 mg, 100's: **$1.50-$2.62**; 400 mg, 100's: **$9.99**

Magnesium Sulfate
• Sol, Inj-IV; IM: 10% mg/ml, 50 ml: **$3.40**
• Sol, Inj-IV: 2%, 500 ml: **$11.23**; 4%, 100 ml: **$7.78**; 8%, 50 ml: **$7.79**; 50%, 50 ml: **$5.58**

CONTRAINDICATIONS: Antacid: Appendicitis or symptoms of appendicitis, ileostomy, intestinal obstruction, severe renal impairment
Laxative: Appendicitis, CHF, colostomy, hypersensitivity, ileostomy, intestinal obstruction, undiagnosed rectal bleeding
Systemic: Heart block, myocardial damage, renal failure

PREGNANCY AND LACTATION: Pregnancy category B; compatible with breast-feeding

SIDE EFFECTS
Frequent
Antacid: Chalky taste, diarrhea, laxative effect
Occasional
Antacid: Nausea, vomiting, stomach cramps
Antacid, laxative: With prolonged use or large doses in renal impairment, possible hypermagnesemia, marked by dizziness, irregular heartbeat, mental changes, fatigue, and weakness
Laxative: Cramping, diarrhea, increased thirst, flatulence

Systemic (dietary supplement, electrolyte replacement): Reduced respiratory rate, decreased reflexes, flushing, hypotension, decreased heart rate

SERIOUS REACTIONS
• Magnesium as an antacid or laxative has no known serious reactions.
• Systemic use of magnesium may produce prolonged PR interval and widening of QRS interval.
• Magnesium toxicity may cause loss of deep tendon reflexes, heart block, respiratory paralysis, and cardiac arrest. The antidote for toxicity is 10-20 ml 10% calcium gluconate (5-10 mEq of calcium).

INTERACTIONS
Drugs
▣ *Allopurinol, cefpodoxime, ciprofloxacin, atenolol, tetracyclines, iron salts, isoniazid, ketoconazole, lomefloxacin, norfloxacin, ofloxacin, pefloxacin, penicillamine, trovafloxacin:* Decreased PO effectiveness of these drugs with PO magnesium products
▣ *Aspirin:* Decreased salicylate concentrations due to alkinization of urine with oral magnesium hydroxide
▣ *Glipizide, glyburide:* Increased absorption of these drugs with oral magnesium hydroxide
▣ *Nifedipine:* Decreased effect of nifedipine with parenteral magnesium sulfate
▣ *Quinidine:* Increased quinidine concentrations with oral magnesium products
▣ *Sodium polystyrene sulfonate:* Systemic alkalosis with oral magnesium products
▣ *Succinylcholine:* Increased toxicity of these drugs with parenteral magnesium sulfate
Labs
• *False increase:* Serum alkaline phosphatase

SPECIAL CONSIDERATIONS
MONITORING PARAMETERS
• Parenteral magnesium: knee jerk reflexes prior to each dose (do not administer if absent), respiration rate (do not administer if <16/min), urine output (do not administer if <100 ml during 4 hr preceding each dose), serum magnesium concentrations (normal 1.5-3 mEq/L; therapeutic concentrations for preeclampsia, eclampsia, convulsions 4-7 mEq/L)

---

magnesium salicylate
Rx: Mobidin
OTC: Doan's pills
Chemical Class: Salicylate derivative
Therapeutic Class: NSAID; nonnarcotic analgesic

CLINICAL PHARMACOLOGY
Mechanism of Action: A nonsteroidal anti-inflammatory that inhibits cyclooxygenase and suppresses prostaglandin synthesis. *Therapeutic Effect:* Produces analgesic and anti-inflammatory effect.

Pharmacokinetics
Rapidly absorbed from the gastrointestinal (GI) tract. Widely distributed. Protein binding: 80%-90%. Metabolized in liver. Primarily excreted in urine. Removed by hemodialysis. **Half-life:** 2-3 hrs.

INDICATIONS AND DOSAGES
Arthritis, inflammation, musculoskeletal disorders (backache)
PO
Adults, Elderly. 650 mg times/day or 1090 mg 3 times/day. May increase to 3.6-4.8 g/day in 3-4 divided doses.

▣ **AVAILABLE FORMS/COST**
• Tab—Oral: 325 mg, 24's (OTC): **$4.03-$5.23**; 467 mg, 24's (OTC): **$4.54**; 500 mg, 24's (OTC): **$5.03**; 600 mg, 100's: **$23.22**

CONTRAINDICATIONS: Severe renal impairment, hypersensitivity to magnesium salicylate or any component of the formulation

PREGNANCY AND LACTATION: Pregnancy category C; excreted into breast milk; use caution in nursing mothers due to potential adverse effects in nursing infant

SIDE EFFECTS
Occasional
Gastric mucosal irritation, bleeding

SERIOUS REACTIONS
• Overdosage may cause tinnitus.
• Toxic levels may be reached quickly in dehydrated, febrile children. Marked toxicity is manifested as hyperthermia, restlessness, abnormal breathing patterns, convulsions, respiratory failure, and coma.

INTERACTIONS
Labs
• *False increase:* Serum bicarbonate, CSF protein, serum theophylline
• *False decrease:* Urine cocaine, urine estrogen, serum glucose, urine 17-hydroxycorticosteroids, urine opiates
• *False positive:* Urine ferric chloride test

SPECIAL CONSIDERATIONS
• Consider for patients with GI intolerance to aspirin or patients in whom interference with normal platelet function by aspirin or other NSAIDs is undesirable

MONITORING PARAMETERS
• AST, ALT, bilirubin, creatinine, CBC, if patient is on long-term therapy

M

mannitol
(man'i-tall)

Rx: Osmitrol, Resectisol
Chemical Class: Hexahydric alcohol
Therapeutic Class: Antiglaucoma agent; diuretic, osmotic; genitourinary irrigant

CLINICAL PHARMACOLOGY

Mechanism of Action: An osmotic diuretic, antiglaucoma, and antihemolytic agent that elevates osmotic pressure of the glomerular filtrate, inhibiting tubular reabsorption of water and electrolytes, resulting in increased flow of water into interstitial fluid and plasma. *Therapeutic Effect:* Produces diuresis; reduces IOP; reduces ICP and cerebral edema.

Pharmacokinetics

Route	Onset	Peak	Duration
IV (diuresis)	15-30 min	N/A	2-8 hr
IV (Reduced ICP)	15-30 min	N/A	3-8 hr
IV (Reduced IOP)	N/A	30-60 min	4–8 hrs

Remains in extracellular fluid. Primarily excreted in urine. Removed by hemodialysis. **Half-life:** 100 min.

INDICATIONS AND DOSAGES

Prevention and treatment of oliguric phase of acute renal failure; to promote urinary excretion of toxic substances (such as aspirin, barbiturates, bromides, and imipramine); to reduce increased ICP due to cerebral edema or edema of injured spinal cord; to reduce increased IOP due to acute glaucoma

IV
Adults, Elderly, Children. Initially, 0.5–1 g/kg, then 0.25–0.5 g/kg q4–6h.

S AVAILABLE FORMS/COST
• Sol, Inj-IV: 5%, 1000 ml: **$29.46-$38.59**; 10%, 1000 ml: **$35.05-$55.87**; 15%, 500 ml: **$3.20-$60.09**; 20%, 500 ml: **$18.28-$27.77**; 25%, 50 ml: **$1.85-$3.56**

CONTRAINDICATIONS: Dehydration, intracranial bleeding, severe pulmonary edema and congestion, severe renal disease

PREGNANCY AND LACTATION: Pregnancy category C

SIDE EFFECTS
Frequent
Dry mouth, thirst
Occasional
Blurred vision, increased urinary frequency and urine volume, headache, arm pain, backache, nausea, vomiting, urticaria, dizziness, hypotension or hypertension, tachycardia, fever, angina-like chest pain

SERIOUS REACTIONS
• Fluid and electrolyte imbalance may occur from rapid administration of large doses or inadequate urine output resulting in overexpansion of extracellular fluid.
• Circulatory overload may produce pulmonary edema and CHF.
• Excessive diuresis may produce hypokalemia and hyponatremia.
• Fluid loss in excess of electrolyte excretion may produce hypernatremia and hyperkalemia.

INTERACTIONS
Labs
• *False increase:* Serum osmolality, serum phosphate, CSF protein
• *False decrease:* Serum phosphate

SPECIAL CONSIDERATIONS

MONITORING PARAMETERS
• Serum electrolytes, urine output

maprotiline

(mah-pro-'tih-leen)

Rx: Ludiomil

Chemical Class: Dibenzo-bicy-clo-octadiene derivative

Therapeutic Class: Antidepressant, tetracyclic

CLINICAL PHARMACOLOGY

Mechanism of Action: A tetracyclic compound that blocks reuptake norepinephrine by CNS presynaptic neuronal membranes, increasing availability at postsynaptic neuronal receptor sites, and enhances synaptic activity. *Therapeutic Effect:* Produces antidepressant effect, with prominent sedative effects and low anticholinergic activity.

Pharmacokinetics

Slowly and completely absorbed after PO administration. Protein binding: 88%. Metabolized in liver by hydroxylation and oxidative modification. Excreted in urine. Unknown if removed by hemodialysis. **Half-life:** 27-58 hrs.

INDICATIONS AND DOSAGES
Mild to moderate depression
PO

Adults. 75 mg/day to start, in 1-4 divided doses. Elderly: 50-75 mg/day. In 2 wks, increase dosage gradually in 25 mg increments until therapeutic response is achieved. Reduce to lowest effective maintenance level.

Severe depression
PO

Adults. 100-150 mg/day in 1-4 divided doses. May increase gradually to maximum 225 mg/day.

Usual elderly dosage
PO

Initially, 25 mg at bedtime. May increase by 25 mg q3-7 days. Maintenance: 50-75 mg/day.

$ **AVAILABLE FORMS/COST**
• Tab, Coated—Oral: 25 mg, 100's: **$30.06-$50.00**; 50 mg, 100's: **$39.49-$74.10**; 75 mg, 100's: **$71.43-$93.00**

CONTRAINDICATIONS: Acute recovery period following myocardial infarction (MI), Within 14 days of MAOI ingestion, known or suspected seizure disorder, hypersensitivity to maprotiline or any component of the formulation

PREGNANCY AND LACTATION: Pregnancy category B; excreted into breast milk; milk:plasma ratios of 1.5 and 1.3 have been reported; significance to the nursing infant unknown

SIDE EFFECTS
Frequent

Drowsiness, fatigue, dry mouth, blurred vision, constipation, delayed micturition, postural hypotension, excessive sweating, disturbed concentration, increased appetite, urinary retention

Occasional

GI disturbances (nausea, GI distress, metallic taste sensation), photosensitivity

Rare

Paradoxical reaction (agitation, restlessness, nightmares, insomnia), extrapyramidal symptoms (particularly fine hand tremor)

SERIOUS REACTIONS
• Higher incidence of seizures than with tricyclic antidepressants, especially in those with no previous history of seizures.

• High dosage may produce cardiovascular effects, such as severe postural hypotension, dizziness, tachycardia, palpitations, and arrhythmias.

• May also result in altered temperature regulation (hyperpyrexia or hypothermia).

M

• Abrupt withdrawal from prolonged therapy may produce headache, malaise, nausea, vomiting, and vivid dreams.

INTERACTIONS
Drugs
❸ *Barbiturates:* Reduced serum concentrations of cyclic antidepressants

❷ *Bethanidine:* Reduced antihypertensive effect of bethanidine

❸ *Carbamazepine:* Reduced cyclic antidepressant serum concentrations

❸ *Cimetidine:* Increased maprotiline concentrations

❷ *Clonidine:* Reduced antihypertensive response to clonidine; enhanced hypertensive response with abrupt clonidine withdrawal

❸ *Debrisoquin:* Inhibited antihypertensive response of debrisoquin

❷ *Epinephrine:* Markedly enhanced pressor response to IV epinephrine

❸ *Ethanol:* Additive impairment of motor skills; abstinent alcoholics may eliminate cyclic antidepressants more rapidly than non-alcoholics

❸ *Fluoxetine, fluvoxamine:* Marked increases in cyclic antidepressant plasma concentrations

❸ *Grapefruit juice:* Marked increase in cyclic antidepressant plasma concentrations

❸ *Guanethidine:* Inhibited antihypertensive response to guanethidine

❷ *Moclobemide:* Potential association with fatal or non-fatal serotonin syndrome

⚠ *MAOIs:* Excessive sympathetic response, mania, or hyperpyrexia possible

❸ *Neuroleptics:* Increased therapeutic and toxic effects of both drugs

❷ *Norepinephrine:* Markedly enhanced pressor response to norepinephrine

❷ *Phenylephrine:* Enhanced pressor response to IV phenylephrine

❸ *Propantheline:* Excessive anticholinergic effects

❸ *Propoxyphene:* Enhanced effect of cyclic antidepressants

❸ *Quinidine:* Increased cyclic antidepressant serum concentrations

❸ *Tolazemide:* Enhanced hypoglycemic effects of tolazemide

Labs
• *False negative:* Serum tricyclic antidepressants screen

SPECIAL CONSIDERATIONS
• Not first-line agent due to risk of seizures

PATIENT/FAMILY EDUCATION
• Use caution in driving or other activities requiring alertness
• Do not discontinue abruptly after long-term use

MONITORING PARAMETERS
• CBC
• Weight
• Mental status: mood, sensorium, affect, suicidal tendencies
• Determination of maprotiline plasma concentrations is not routinely recommended, but may be useful in identifying toxicity, drug interactions, or noncompliance (adjustments in dosage should be made according to clinical response not plasma concentrations); therapeutic plasma levels 200-300 ng/ml (including active metabolite)

mazindol
(may-zin-doll)
Rx: Mazanor, Sanorex
Chemical Class: Imidazoline derivative
Therapeutic Class: Anorexiant
DEA Class: Schedule IV

CLINICAL PHARMACOLOGY
Mechanism of Action: An isoindole that stimulates the central nervous system and primarily exerting its effect on the limbic system. *Therapeutic Effect:* Stimulates the hypothalamus to reduce appetite.

Pharmacokinetics
Slow but complete absorption. Protein binding: greater than 99%. Metabolized in liver to metabolites. Primarily excreted in urine as well as feces. Unknown if removed by hemodialysis. **Half-life:** 30- 50 hrs

INDICATIONS AND DOSAGES
Obesity
PO
Adults. 1 mg/day. Maximum: 3 mg/day.

Ⓢ AVAILABLE FORMS/COST
• Tab—Oral: 1 mg, 100's: **$154.25**; 2 mg, 100's: **$244.75**
UNLABELED USES: Narcolepsy
CONTRAINDICATIONS: Agitated states, glaucoma, history of drug abuse, symptomatic cardiovascular disease (arrhythmias), coadministration with or within 14 days of MAOI therapy, hypersensitivity to mazindol
PREGNANCY AND LACTATION: Pregnancy category C
SIDE EFFECTS
Occasional
Insomnia, headache, tachycardia, palpitations, tremors, nervousness, restlessness, dry mouth, constipation

Rare
Blurred vision, impotence, insulin sensitivity, rash, sweating, weakness
SERIOUS REACTIONS
• Overdosage includes symptoms of irritability, agitation, hyperactivity, tachycardia, arrhythmia, tachypnea.
INTERACTIONS
Drugs
🖪 *Furazolidone:* Hypertensive crisis
🖪 *Guanethidine:* Decreased antihypertensive effects
❷ *MAOIs:* Hypertensive crisis
🖪 *Tricyclic antidepressants:* Decreased anorexiant effects
Labs
• *False positive:* Chlordiazepoxide, flurazepam, methadone, methapyrilene, methylphenidate, phendimetrazine
SPECIAL CONSIDERATIONS
PATIENT/FAMILY EDUCATION
• May cause insomnia; avoid taking late in the day
• Use caution while driving or performing other tasks requiring alertness; may cause dizziness or blurred vision
• Take with food if stomach upset occurs
• Do not discontinue abruptly

mebendazole
(meh-ben'-dah-zole)
Rx: Vermox
Chemical Class: Benzimidazole derivative
Therapeutic Class: Antihelmintic

CLINICAL PHARMACOLOGY
Mechanism of Action: A synthetic benzimidazole derivative that degrades parasite cytoplasmic microtubules and irreversibly blocks glu-

M

cose uptake in helminthes and larvae. Vermicidal. *Therapeutic Effect:* depletes glycogen, decreases ATP, causes helminth death.

Pharmacokinetics

Poorly absorbed from GI tract (absorption increases with food). Metabolized in liver. Primarily eliminated in feces. **Half-life:** 2.5-9 hrs (half life increased with impaired renal function.

INDICATIONS AND DOSAGES

Trichuriasis, ascariasis, hookworm

PO

Adults, Elderly, Children older than 2 yrs. 1 tablet in morning and at bedtime for 3 days.

Enterobiasis

PO

Adults, Elderly, Children older than 2 yrs: 1 tablet one time.

[$] **AVAILABLE FORMS/COST**

• Tab, Chewable—Oral: 100 mg, 12's: **$63.85-$85.47**

UNLABELED USES: Ancylostoma duodenale or Necator americanus

CONTRAINDICATIONS: Hypersensitivity to mebendazole or any component of the formulation

PREGNANCY AND LACTATION: Pregnancy category C; consider treatment if the parasite is causing clinical disease or may cause public health problems; it is doubtful that enough mebendazole is absorbed to be excreted into breast milk in significant quantities

SIDE EFFECTS

Occasional

Nausea, vomiting, headache, dizziness, transient abdominal pain, diarrhea with massive infection and expulsion of helminths

Rare

Fever

SERIOUS REACTIONS

• High dosage may produce reversible myelosuppression (granulocytopenia, leukopenia, neutropenia).

INTERACTIONS

Drugs

[3] *Carbamazepine:* Decreased mebendazole concentrations and effect via induction of metabolism

[2] *Phenytoin:* Decreased mebendazole concentrations; possible impairment of therapeutic effect

SPECIAL CONSIDERATIONS

PATIENT/FAMILY EDUCATION

• Chew or crush tablets and administer with food
• Parasite death and removal from digestive tract may take up to 3 days after treatment
• Consult clinician if not cured in 3 wk
• For pinworms, all household contacts of patient should be treated
• Strict hygiene essential to prevent reinfection; disinfect toilet facilities, change and launder undergarments, bed linens, towels, and nightclothes

---

mecamylamine

(mek-a-mil-'a-meen hye-droe-klor-ide)

Rx: Inversine

Chemical Class: Ganglionic blocker

Therapeutic Class: Antihypertensive; ganglionic blocker

CLINICAL PHARMACOLOGY

Mechanism of Action: A ganglionic blocker that inhibits acetylcholine at the autonomic ganglia. Blocks central nicotinic cholinergic receptors, which inhibits effects of nicotine. *Therapeutic Effect:* Reduces blood pressure; decreases desire to smoke.

Pharmacokinetics
Completely absorbed following PO administration. Widely distributed. Excreted in urine. **Half-life:** 24 hrs.

INDICATIONS AND DOSAGES

Hypertension
PO
Adults. Initially, 2.5 mg q12h for 2 days, then increase by 2.5 mg increments at more than 2 day intervals until desired blood pressure is achieved. The average daily dose is 25 mg in 3 divided doses.

Smoking cessation
PO
Adults. Initially, 2.5 mg q12h for 2 days, then increase by 2.5 mg increments during the first week of therapy. Range: 10-20 mg in divided doses.

Ⓢ **AVAILABLE FORMS/COST**
• Tab—Oral: 2.5 mg, 100's: **$255.31**

UNLABELED USES: Tourette's syndrome, hyperreflexia

CONTRAINDICATIONS: Coronary insufficiency, pyloric stenosis, glaucoma, uremia, recent myocardial infarction, unreliable patients

PREGNANCY AND LACTATION: Pregnancy category C; not recommended in nursing mothers

SIDE EFFECTS
Occasional
Nausea, diarrhea, orthostatic hypotension, tachycardia, drowsiness, urinary retention, blurred vision, dilated pupils, confusion, mental depression, decreased sexual ability, loss of appetite
Rare
Pulmonary edema, pulmonary fibrosis, paresthesias

SERIOUS REACTIONS
• Overdosage includes symptoms such as hypotension, nausea, vomiting, urinary retention and constipation.

SPECIAL CONSIDERATIONS
PATIENT/FAMILY EDUCATION
• Take after meals
• Arise slowly from reclining position
• Orthostatic changes are exacerbated by alcohol, exercise, hot weather

MONITORING PARAMETERS
• Maintenance doses should be limited to dose that causes slight faintness or dizziness in the standing position

---

meclizine
(mek'li-zeen)
Rx: Antivert, Medivert, Meclicot
OTC: Bonine
Chemical Class: Piperazine derivative
Therapeutic Class: Antihistamine; antivertigo agent

M

CLINICAL PHARMACOLOGY
Mechanism of Action: An anticholinergic that reduces labyrinthine excitability and diminishes vestibular stimulation of the labyrinth, affecting the chemoreceptor trigger zone. *Therapeutic Effect:* Reduces nausea, vomiting, and vertigo.

Pharmacokinetics

Route	Onset	Peak	Duration
PO	30–60 min	N/A	12–24 hr

Well absorbed from the GI tract. Widely distributed. Metabolized in the liver. Primarily excreted in urine. **Half-life:** 6 hr.

INDICATIONS AND DOSAGES
Motion sickness
PO
Adults, Elderly, Children 12 yr and older. 12.5-25 mg 1 hr before travel. May repeat q12-24h. May require a dose of 50 mg.

Vertigo

PO

Adults, Elderly, Children 12 yr and older. 25-100 mg/day in divided doses, as needed.

§ **AVAILABLE FORMS/COST**
• Tab, Chewable—Oral: 25 mg, 100's: **$1.01-$29.17**
• Tab—Oral: 12.5 mg, 100's: **$0.77-$51.19**; 25 mg, 100's: **$3.25-$74.05**; 50 mg, 100's: **$131.86**

CONTRAINDICATIONS: None known.

PREGNANCY AND LACTATION: Pregnancy category B; used for treatment of nausea and vomiting during pregnancy; excretion into breast milk unknown

SIDE EFFECTS

Frequent

Drowsiness

Occasional

Blurred vision; dry mouth, nose, or throat

SERIOUS REACTIONS
• A hypersensitivity reaction, marked by eczema, pruritus, rash, cardiac disturbances, and photosensitivity, may occur.
• Overdose may produce CNS depression (manifested as sedation, apnea, cardiovascular collapse, or death) or severe paradoxical reactions (such as hallucinations, tremor, and seizures).
• Children may experience paradoxical reactions, including restlessness, insomnia, euphoria, nervousness, and tremors.
• Overdose in children may result in hallucinations, seizures, and death.

---

meclofenamate
(me´-kloe-fen-´a-mate soe-dee-um)
Rx: Meclomen, Meclodium
Chemical Class: Anthranilic acid derivative
Therapeutic Class: NSAID; antipyretic; nonnarcotic analgesic

CLINICAL PHARMACOLOGY
Mechanism of Action: A nonsteroidal anti-inflammatory drug that inhibits prostaglandin synthesis by decreasing activity of the enzyme, cyclooxygenase, which results in decreased formation of prostaglandin precursors. *Therapeutic Effect:* Reduces inflammatory response and intensity of pain stimulus reaching sensory nerve endings.

Pharmacokinetics

PO route, onset 15 minutes, peak 0.5-1.5 hours, duration 2-4 hours. Completely absorbed from the gastrointestinal (GI) tract. Widely distributed. Protein binding: greater than 99%. Metabolized in liver. Primarily excreted in urine and feces as metabolites. Not removed by hemodialysis. **Half-life:** 2-3.3 hrs.

INDICATIONS AND DOSAGES
Mild to moderate pain
PO
Adults, Elderly. 50 mg q4-6h as needed.

Excessive menstrual blood loss and primary dysmenorrhea
PO
Adults, Elderly. 100 mg 3 times/day for 6 days, starting at the onset of menstrual flow.

Rheumatoid arthritis, osteoarthritis
PO
Adults, Elderly. 200-400 mg 3-4 times/day.

$ AVAILABLE FORMS/COST

• Cap, Gel—Oral: 50 mg, 100's: **$34.08-$183.00**; 100 mg, 100's: **$45.40-$339.75**

CONTRAINDICATIONS: Active peptic ulcer disease, chronic inflammation of GI tract, GI bleeding disorders, GI ulceration, history of hypersensitivity to aspirin or NSAIDs

PREGNANCY AND LACTATION: Pregnancy category B (category D if used in 3rd trimester); may inhibit labor and prolong pregnancy, cause constriction of the ductus arteriosus *in utero,* or cause persistent pulmonary hypertension of the newborn

SIDE EFFECTS

Frequent (33%-10%)

Diarrhea, nausea, abdominal cramping/pain, dyspepsia (heartburn, indigestion, epigastric pain)

Occasional (9%-1%)

Flatulence, rash, dizziness

Rare (less than 1%)

Constipation, anorexia, stomatitis, headache, ringing in the ears, rash

SERIOUS REACTIONS

• Overdosage may result in headache, seizure, vomiting, and cerebral edema.

• Peptic ulcer disease, GI bleeding, gastritis, severe hepatic reactions, such as jaundice, nephrotoxicity, marked by hematuria, dysuria, proteinuria, and severe hypersensitivity reaction, including bronchospasm, and facial edema occur rarely.

INTERACTIONS

Drugs

3 *Aminoglycosides:* Reduced clearance with elevated aminoglycoside levels and potential for toxicity (especially indomethacin in premature infants; other NSAIDs probably)

3 *Anticoagulants:* Excessive hypoprothrombinemia, decreased platelet aggregation with increased risk of GI bleeding

3 *Antihypertensives (α-blockers, angiotensin-converting enzyme inhibitors, angiotensin II receptor blockers, β-blockers, diuretics):* Inhibition of antihypertensive and other favorable hemodynamic effects

3 *Corticosteroids:* Increased risk of GI ulceration

3 *Cyclosporine:* Increased nephrotoxicity risk

3 *Lithium:* Decreased clearance of lithium (mediated via prostaglandins) resulting in elevated serum lithium levels and risk of toxicity

3 *Methotrexate:* Decreased renal secretion of methotrexate resulting in elevated methotrexate levels and risk of toxicity

3 *Phenylpropanolamine:* Possible acute hypertensive reaction

3 *Potassium-sparing diuretics:* Additive hyperkalemia potential

3 *Triamterene:* Acute renal failure reported with addition of indomethacin; caution with other NSAIDs

SPECIAL CONSIDERATIONS

• No significant advantage over other NSAIDs; cost should govern use

MONITORING PARAMETERS

• Initial hemogram and fecal occult blood test within 3 mo of starting regular chronic therapy; repeat every 6-12 mo (more frequently in high-risk patients (>65 years, peptic ulcer disease, concurrent steroids or anticoagulants); electrolytes, creatinine, and BUN within 3 mo of starting regular chronic therapy; repeat every 6-12 mo

M

medroxyprogesterone

(me-drox'ee-proe-jess'te-rone)

Rx: Amen, Curretab, Cycrin, Depo-Provera, Provera

Combinations

Rx: with estradiol (Lunelle)

Chemical Class: 17α-hydroxyprogesterone derivative

Therapeutic Class: Antineoplastic; contraceptive; progestin

CLINICAL PHARMACOLOGY

Mechanism of Action: A hormone that transforms endometrium from proliferative to secretory in an estrogen-primed endometrium. Inhibits secretion of pituitary gonadotropins. *Therapeutic Effect:* Prevents follicular maturation and ovulation. Stimulates growth of mammary alveolar tissue and relaxes uterine smooth muscle. Corrects hormonal imbalance.

Pharmacokinetics

Slowly absorbed after IM administration. Protein binding: 90%. Metabolized in the liver. Primarily excreted in urine. **Half-life:** 30 days.

INDICATIONS AND DOSAGES

Endometrial hyperplasia

PO

Adults. 2.5-10 mg/day for 14 days.

Secondary amenorrhea

PO

Adults. 5–10 mg/day for 5–10 days, beginning at any time during menstrual cycle or 2.5 mg/day.

Abnormal uterine bleeding

PO

Adults. 5–10 mg/day for 5–10 days, beginning on calculated day 16 or day 21 of menstrual cycle.

Endometrial, renal carcinoma

IM

Adults, Elderly. Initially, 400–1,000 mg; repeat at 1-wk intervals. If improvement occurs and disease is stabilized, begin maintenance with as little as 400 mg/mo.

Prevention of pregnancy

IM

Adults. 150 mg q3mo.

[$] **AVAILABLE FORMS/COST**

• Susp, Inj-IM: 125 mg/ml, 1 ml: **$41.29**; 150 mg/ml, 1 ml: **$56.11-$60.40**; 400 mg/ml, 2.5, 10 ml: **$110.39**/2.5 ml

• Tab-Oral: 2.5 mg, 100's: **$15.88-$68.55**; 5 mg, 100's: **$16.45-$103.48**; 10 mg, 100's: **$13.94-$128.18**

UNLABELED USES: Hormone replacement therapy in estrogen-treated menopausal women, treatment of endometriosis

CONTRAINDICATIONS: Carcinoma of breast; estrogen-dependent neoplasm; history of or active thrombotic disorders, such as cerebral apoplexy, thrombophlebitis, or thromboembolic disorders; hypersensitivity to progestins; known or suspected pregnancy; missed abortion; severe hepatic dysfunction; undiagnosed abnormal genital bleeding; use as pregnancy test

PREGNANCY AND LACTATION: Pregnancy category X; compatible with breast-feeding

SIDE EFFECTS

Frequent

Transient menstrual abnormalities (including spotting, change in menstrual flow or cervical secretions, and amenorrhea) at initiation of therapy

Occasional

Edema, weight change, breast tenderness, nervousness, insomnia, fatigue, dizziness

Rare

Alopecia, depression, dermatologic changes, headache, fever, nausea

SERIOUS REACTIONS
• Thrombophlebitis, pulmonary or cerebral embolism, and retinal thrombosis occur rarely.

INTERACTIONS

Drugs

▓ *Aminoglutethimide:* Reduced plasma medroxyprogesterone concentrations

Labs

• *Feces:* Green color

SPECIAL CONSIDERATIONS

PATIENT/FAMILY EDUCATION
• Take protective measures against exposure to ultraviolet light
• Diabetic patients must monitor blood glucose carefully during therapy
• Take with food if GI upset occurs
• When used as contraceptive, menstrual cycle may be disrupted and irregular and unpredictable bleeding or spotting results; usually decreases to the point of amenorrhea as treatment continues (55% at 1 yr)
• After stopping injections, 50% of women who become pregnant will do so in about 10 mo after the last injection, 93% within 18 mo; not related to length of time drug used; women with lower body weights conceive sooner
• Failure rate 0.3% in first year of constant use

---

mefenamic acid

(me-fe-nam′ik)

Rx: Ponstel
Chemical Class: Anthranilic acid derivative
Therapeutic Class: NSAID; antipyretic; nonnarcotic analgesic

CLINICAL PHARMACOLOGY

Mechanism of Action: A nonsteroidal anti-inflammatory that produces analgesic and anti-inflammatory effect by inhibiting prostaglandin synthesis. *Therapeutic Effect:* Reduces inflammatory response and intensity of pain stimulus reaching sensory nerve endings.

Pharmacokinetics

Rapidly absorbed from the gastrointestinal (GI) tract. Protein binding: high. Metabolized in liver. Partially excreted in urine and partially in the feces. Not removed by hemodialysis. **Half-life:** 3.5 hrs.

INDICATIONS AND DOSAGES

Mild to moderate pain, lower back pain, dysmenorrhea

PO

Adults, Elderly, Children 14 yrs and older. Initially, 500 mg to start, then 250 mg q4h as needed. Maximum: 1 week of therapy.

Ⓢ **AVAILABLE FORMS/COST**
• Cap, Gel—Oral: 250 mg, 100's: **$150.29**

UNLABELED USES: Cataract prevention, menorrhagia, osteoarthritis, premenstrual syndrome, rheumatoid arthritis

CONTRAINDICATIONS: History of hypersensitivity to aspirin or NSAIDs, pregnancy

PREGNANCY AND LACTATION: Pregnancy category C (category D if used in 3rd trimester)

SIDE EFFECTS
Occasional (10%-1%)
Dyspepsia, including heartburn, indigestion, flatulence, abdominal cramping, constipation, nausea, diarrhea, epigastric pain, vomiting, headache, nervousness, dizziness, bleeding, elevated liver function tests, tinnitus
Rare (less than 1%)
Fluid retention, arrhythmias, tachycardia, confusion, drowsiness, rash, dry eyes, blurred vision, hot flashes

SERIOUS REACTIONS
• Peptic ulcer, GI bleeding, gastritis, and severe hepatic reaction, such as cholestasis and jaundice, occur rarely.
• Nephrotoxicity, including dysuria, hematuria, proteinuria, and nephrotic syndrome and severe hypersensitivity reaction, marked by bronchospasm, and angioedema occur rarely.

INTERACTIONS
Drugs
3 *Aminoglycosides:* Reduced clearance with elevated aminoglycoside levels and potential for toxicity (especially indomethacin in premature infants; other NSAIDs probably)
3 *Anticoagulants:* Excessive hypoprothrombinemia, decreased platelet aggregation with increased risk of GI bleeding
3 *Antihypertensives (α-blockers, angiotensin-converting enzyme inhibitors, angiotensin II receptor blockers, β-blockers, diuretics):* Inhibition of antihypertensive and other favorable hemodynamic effects
3 *Corticosteroids:* Increased risk of GI ulceration
3 *Cyclosporine:* Increased nephrotoxicity risk

3 *Lithium:* Decreased clearance of lithium (mediated via prostaglandins) resulting in elevated serum lithium levels and risk of toxicity
2 *Methotrexate:* Decreased renal secretion of methotrexate resulting in elevated methotrexate levels and risk of toxicity
3 *Phenylpropanolamine:* Possible acute hypertensive reaction
3 *Potassium-sparing diuretics:* Additive hyperkalemia potential
3 *Triamterene:* Acute renal failure reported with addition of indomethacin; caution with other NSAIDs

SPECIAL CONSIDERATIONS
• No significant advantage over other NSAIDs; cost should govern use
• Use beyond 1 wk is not recommended

MONITORING PARAMETERS
• Initial hemogram and fecal occult blood test within 3 mo of starting regular chronic therapy; repeat 6-12 mo (more frequently in high-risk patients (>65 years, peptic ulcer disease, concurrent steroids or anticoagulants); electrolytes, creatinine, and BUN within 3 mo of starting regular chronic therapy; repeat every 6-12 mo

mefloquine
(me′flow-quine)
Rx: Lariam
Chemical Class: Quinolinemethanol derivative
Therapeutic Class: Antimalarial

CLINICAL PHARMACOLOGY
Mechanism of Action: A quinone-methanol compound structurally similar to quinine that destroys the asexual blood forms of malarial pathogens, Plasmodium

falciparum, P.vivax, P.malariae, P.ovale. *Therapeutic Effect:* Inhibits parasite growth.

Pharmacokinetics

Well absorbed from the gastrointestinal (GI) tract. Protein binding: 98%. Widely distributed, including cerebrospinal fluid (CSF). Metabolized in liver. Primarily excreted in urine. **Half-life:** 21-22 days.

INDICATIONS AND DOSAGES

Suppression of malaria

PO

Adults. 250 mg base weekly starting 1 week before travel, continuing weekly during travel and for 4 weeks after leaving endemic area.

Children more than 45 kg. 250 mg weekly starting 1 week before travel, continuing weekly during travel and for 4 weeks after leaving endemic area.

Children 45-31kg. 187.5 mg (3/4 tablet) weekly starting 1 week before travel, continuing weekly during travel and for 4 weeks after leaving endemic area.

Children 30-20 kg. 125 mg (1/2 tablet) weekly starting 1 week before travel, continuing weekly during travel and for 4 weeks after leaving endemic area.

Children 19-15 kg. 62.5 mg (1/4 tablet) weekly starting 1 week before travel, continuing weekly during travel and for 4 weeks after leaving endemic area.

Treatment of malaria

PO

Adults. 1250 mg as a single dose.
Children. 15-25 mg/kg in a single dose. Maximum: 1250 mg.

$ AVAILABLE FORMS/COST

• Tab—Oral: 250 mg, 25's: **$198.98-$294.16**

CONTRAINDICATIONS: Cardiac abnormalities, severe psychiatric disorders, epilepsy, history of hypersensitivity to mefloquine

PREGNANCY AND LACTATION: Pregnancy category C; use caution during the 1st 12-14 wk of pregnancy; excreted in breast milk in amounts not thought to be harmful to the nursing infant and insufficient to provide adequate protection against malaria

SIDE EFFECTS

Occasional

Mild transient headache, difficulty concentrating, insomnia, lightheadedness, vertigo, diarrhea, nausea, vomiting, visual disturbances, tinnitus

Rare

Aggressive behavior, anxiety, bradycardia, depression, hallucinations, hypotension, panic attacks, paranoia, psychosis, syncope, tremor

SERIOUS REACTIONS

• Prolonged therapy may result in peripheral neuritis, neuromyopathy, hypotension, electrocardiogram (EKG) changes, agranulocytosis, aplastic anemia, thrombocytopenia, seizures, and psychosis.

• Overdosage may result in headache, vomiting, visual disturbance, drowsiness, and seizures.

SPECIAL CONSIDERATIONS

PATIENT/FAMILY EDUCATION

• Do not take on an empty stomach
• Take medication with at least 8 oz water
• Caution, initially, when driving, operating machinery, where concentration necessary

MONITORING PARAMETERS

• Liver function tests and ophthalmic examinations during prolonged therapy

M

megestrol
(me-jess'trole)
Rx: Megace
Chemical Class: Progestin derivative
Therapeutic Class: Antineoplastic; appetite stimulant

CLINICAL PHARMACOLOGY
Mechanism of Action: A hormone and antineoplastic agent that suppresses the release of luteinizing hormone from the anterior pituitary gland by inhibiting pituitary function. *Therapeutic Effect:* Shrinks tumors. Also increases appetite by an unknown mechanism.
Pharmacokinetics
Well absorbed from the GI tract. Metabolized in the liver; excreted in urine.

INDICATIONS AND DOSAGES
Palliative treatment of advanced breast cancer
PO
Adults, Elderly. 160 mg/day in 4 equally divided doses.
Palliative treatment of advanced endometrial carcinoma
PO
Adults, Elderly. 40-320 mg/day in divided doses. Maximum: 800 mg/day in 1-4 divided doses.
Anorexia, cachexia, weight loss
PO
Adults, Elderly. 800 mg (20 ml)/day.
☒ AVAILABLE FORMS/COST
• Susp—Oral: 40 mg/ml, 240 ml: **$135.93-$159.95**
• Tab—Oral: 20 mg, 100's: **$29.68-$72.66**; 40 mg, 100's: **$53.12-$129.59**
UNLABELED USES: Appetite stimulant, treatment of hormone-dependent or advanced prostate carcinoma

CONTRAINDICATIONS: None known.
PREGNANCY AND LACTATION: Pregnancy category X; not recommended during the 1st 4 mo of pregnancy
SIDE EFFECTS
Frequent
Weight gain secondary to increased appetite
Occasional
Nausea, breakthrough bleeding, backache, headache, breast tenderness, carpal tunnel syndrome
Rare
Feeling of coldness
SERIOUS REACTIONS
• Thrombophlebitis and pulmonary embolism occur rarely.
SPECIAL CONSIDERATIONS
• Average weight gain in AIDS patients 11 lbs in 12 wk. Begin therapy only after treatable causes of weight loss are sought and addressed

---

meloxicam
(mel-oks'i-kam)
Rx: Mobic
Chemical Class: Oxicam derivative
Therapeutic Class: NSAID; antipyretic; nonnarcotic analgesic

CLINICAL PHARMACOLOGY
Mechanism of Action: An NSAID that produces analgesic and anti-inflammatory effects by inhibiting prostaglandin synthesis. *Therapeutic Effect:* Reduces the inflammatory response and intensity of pain.
Pharmacokinetics

Route	Onset	Peak	Duration
PO (analgesic)	30 min	4–5 hr	N/A

Well absorbed after PO administration. Protein binding: 99%. Metabolized in the liver. Eliminated in urine and feces. Not removed by hemodialysis. **Half-life:** 15–20 hr.

INDICATIONS AND DOSAGES
Osteoarthritis, Rheumatoid arthritis
PO
Adults. Initially, 7.5 mg/day. Maximum: 15 mg/day.

§ AVAILABLE FORMS/COST
• Tab, Coated—Oral: 7.5 mg, 100's: **$275.93**; 15 mg, 100's: **$356.39**

CONTRAINDICATIONS: Aspirin-induced nasal polyps associated with bronchospasm

PREGNANCY AND LACTATION: Pregnancy category C; animal studies document both teratogenic and nonteratongenic (premature PDA closure) in animals; no studies in humans; no human studies on breast milk excretion; in rats, milk concentrations are twice that of plasma

SIDE EFFECTS
Frequent (9%–7%)
Dyspepsia, headache, diarrhea, nausea
Occasional (4%–3%)
Dizziness, insomnia, rash, pruritus, flatulence, constipation, vomiting
Rare (less than 2%)
Somnolence, urticaria, photosensitivity, tinnitus

SERIOUS REACTIONS
• Rare reactions with long-term use include peptic ulcer disease, GI bleeding, gastritis, severe hepatic reaction (jaundice), nephrotoxicity (hematuria, dysuria, proteinuria), and a severe hypersensitivity reaction (bronchospasm, angioedema).

INTERACTIONS
Drugs
❷ *Anticoagulants (heparin, low molecular weight heparin, warfarin, etc.):* Increased risk of hematoma and major and minor bleeding
❷ *Aspirin:* Increased risk of GI ulceration, especially with high dose aspirin; potential negation of protective cardiac effects
❸ *ACE inhibitors, angiotensin II receptor blockers:* Diminished antihypertensive effect
❸ *β-blockers:* Diminished antihypertensive effect
❸ *Cholestyramine:* Increases clearance of meloxicam (50%), with reduction in $t_{1/2}$ and AUC
❸ *Corticosteroids:* Additive effects; increased risk of GI bleeding, sodium/water retention
❸ *Cyclosporine:* Additive nephrotoxicity
❸ *Diuretics:* Reduced natriuretic effects
❷ *Lithium:* Addition of meloxicam may result in increased lithium blood levels (21%)
❷ *Warfarin:* Additive effects on coagulation; prothrombin times as INR have increased with the addition of meloxicam
Labs
• *Guaiac (Hemoccult) assay:* False positives

SPECIAL CONSIDERATIONS
• Partial, not pure, COX-2 selective inhibitor; most studies have compared it with non-selective agents, making final assessment of place in therapy difficult

PATIENT/FAMILY EDUCATION
• Take with food or milk; report gastrointestinal adverse effects

MONITORING PARAMETERS
• Acute phase reactants for efficacy in rheumatoid arthritis; pain, stiffness, number of swollen joints,

M

range of motion, functional capacity, structural damage, fecal occult blood, hemogram, renal and hepatic function

---

memantine

Rx: Namenda
Chemical Class: Adamantane derivative; tricyclic amine
Therapeutic Class: Antidementia agent

CLINICAL PHARMACOLOGY
Mechanism of Action: A neurotransmitter inhibitor that decreases the effects of glutamate, the principle excitatory neurotransmitter in the brain. Persistent CNS excitation by glutamate is thought to cause the symptoms of Alzheimer's disease. *Therapeutic Effect:* May reduce clinical deterioration in moderate to severe Alzheimer's disease.

Pharmacokinetics
Rapidly and completely absorbed after PO administration. Protein binding: 45%. Undergoes little metabolism; most of the dose is excreted unchanged in urine. **Half-life:** 60-80 hr.

INDICATIONS AND DOSAGES
Alzheimer's disease
PO
Adults, Elderly. Initially, 5 mg once a day. May increase dosage at intervals of at least 1 wk in 5-mg increments to 10 mg/day (5 mg twice a day), then 15 mg/day (5 mg and 10 mg as separate doses), and finally 20 mg/day (10 mg twice a day). Target dose: 20 mg/day.

⑧ AVAILABLE FORMS/COST
• Tab, Film-Coated—Oral: 5 mg, 10 mg, 60's; all: **$139.50**

CONTRAINDICATIONS: Severe renal impairment

PREGNANCY AND LACTATION:
Pregnancy category B; breast milk excretion unknown

SIDE EFFECTS
Occasional (7%-4%)
Dizziness, headache, confusion, constipation, hypertension, cough
Rare (3%-2%)
Back pain, nausea, fatigue, anxiety, peripheral edema, arthralgia, insomnia

SERIOUS REACTIONS
• None known.

INTERACTIONS
Drugs
⓷ *Carbonic anhydrase inhibitors (acetazolamide, dichlorphenamide, methazolamide):* Memantine renal clearance reduced by 80% under alkaline urine conditions (pH 8)

SPECIAL CONSIDERATIONS
• Combination memantine-donepezil more likely to show a smaller decline or an improvement

PATIENT/FAMILY EDUCATION
• Twice daily for doses above 5 mg and minimum interval, 1 week dose escalation

MONITORING PARAMETERS
• *Efficacy:* Improvement or maintenance of mental status and functional quality of life scales
• *Toxicity:* Pharmacotoxic psychosis (hallucinations, nervousness, changes in behavior, tremor, akathisia, restlessness, increased motor activity, insomnia, depression

menotropins

(men-oh-troe'-pins)

Rx: Humegon, Pergonal, Repronex

Chemical Class: Human pituitary gonadotropins, purified

Therapeutic Class: Ovulation stimulant

CLINICAL PHARMACOLOGY

Mechanism of Action: A mixture of equal activity of follicle stimulating hormone (FSH) and lutenizing hormone (LH) that are isolated from the urine of postmenopausal women and are necessary for the development, maturation, and release of ova from ovaries and for spermatogenesis in the testes. *Therapeutic Effect:* Promotes ovulation and pregnancy in infertile women.

Pharmacokinetics

Not absorbed from the gastrointestinal (GI) tract. Cleared from circulation by glomular filtration. Degraded in proximal tubule or excreted unchanged in urine. **Half-life:** 2.2-2.9 hrs.

INDICATIONS AND DOSAGES

Follicle maturation, ovulation and pregnancy induction

IM

Adults. Initially, 75 Internation Units (IU) daily for 7-12 days followed by hCG, 5,000-10,000 units one day after the last dose of menotropins. Treat until indices of estrogen activity are equivalent to or greater than those of the normal individual. If signs of ovulation are present but pregnancy does not occur, repeat this dosage regime for at least 2 more courses before increasing the dose of menotropins.

Follicle maturation, Ovulation and pregnancy induction

IM

Adults. After 3 course failures at 75 IU, increase dose to 150 IU daily for 7-12 days followed by 5000-10,000 units of hCG one day after the last dose of menotropins. If signs of ovulation are present but pregnancy does not develop, repeat the same dose for two more courses.

Stimulation of spermatogenesis

IM

Adults. Pretreatment with 5000 units hCG 3 times weekly is required prior to initiating concomitant therapy with menotropins. Continue pretreatment until serum testosterone levels are in the normal range and masculinization is reached (may require 4-6 months); then initiate therapy with menotropins 75 IU 3 times weekly and 2000 units hCG twice weekly for a minimum of 4 months. If the patient has not responded after 4 months, continue treatment with 75 IU menotropins 3 times weekly or increase dose to 150 IU 3 times weekly, keeping the dose for hCG the same

$ **AVAILABLE FORMS/COST**

• Sol, Inj-IM: 75 U, 1's: **$57.00-$66.50**; 150 U, 1's: **$113.12-$129.66**

CONTRAINDICATIONS: Prior hypersensitivity to menotropins

Women: Known or suspected pregnancy, high FSH level indicating primary ovarian failure, abnormal bleeding of undetermined origin, an organic intracranial lesion such as a pituitary tumor, elevated gonadotropin levels indicating primary testicular failure, presence of any cause of infertility other than anovulation, unless they are candidates for in vitro fertilization, ovarian cysts or enlargement not due to polycystic

M

ovary syndrome, uncontrolled thyroid and adrenal dysfunction

Men: infertility disorders other than hypogonadotropic hypogonadism, normal gonadotropin levels indicating normal pituitary function

PREGNANCY AND LACTATION:
Pregnancy category X

SIDE EFFECTS

Occasional

Women: Abdominal pain, bloating, diarrhea, nausea, vomiting, body rash, dizziness, dyspnea, tachypnea, ovarian cysts, ovarian enlargement, pain, rash, swelling at injection site, tachycardia

Men: Gynecomastia

SERIOUS REACTIONS

• Acute respiratory distress syndrome, atelectasis, pulmonary embolism, pulmonary infarction, arterial occlusion, cerebral vascular occlusion, venous thrombophlebitis, congenital abnormalities, ectopic pregnancy, and ovarian hyperstimulation syndrome have been reported.

SPECIAL CONSIDERATIONS

PATIENT/FAMILY EDUCATION

• Multiple births occur in approximately 20% of women treated with menotropins and HCG

• Couple should engage in intercourse daily, beginning on the day prior to HCG administration, until ovulation occurs

• Ovarian enlargement regresses without treatment in 2-3 wk

MONITORING PARAMETERS

• Urinary estrogen; do not administer HCG if >150 mcg/24 hr (increased risk of hyperstimulation of ovaries syndrome)

• Sonographic visualization of ovaries; estradiol levels

---

meperidine

(me-per'i-deen)

Rx: Demerol
Combinations
  Rx: with promethazine (Mepergan)
Chemical Class: Opiate derivative; phenylpiperidine derivative
Therapeutic Class: Narcotic analgesic
DEA Class: Schedule II

CLINICAL PHARMACOLOGY

Mechanism of Action: An opioid agonist that binds to opioid receptors in the CNS. *Therapeutic Effect:* Alters the perception of and emotional response to pain.

Pharmacokinetics

Route	Onset	Peak	Duration
PO	15 min	60 min	2–4 hr
IV	less than 5 min	5–7 min	2–3 hr
IM	10–15 min	30–50 min	2–4 hr
Subcutaneous	10–15 min	30–50 min	2–4 hr

Variably absorbed from the GI tract; well absorbed after IM administration. Protein binding: 60%–80%. Widely distributed. Metabolized in the liver to active metabolite. Primarily excreted in urine. Not removed by hemodialysis. **Half-life:** 2.4–4 hr; metabolite 8-16 hr (increased in hepatic impairment and disease).

INDICATIONS AND DOSAGES

Analgesia

PO, IM, Subcutaneous

Adults, Elderly. 50–150 mg q3–4h.

Children. 1.1–1.5 mg/kg q3–4h. Do not exceed single dose of 100 mg.

Patient-controlled analgesia (PCA)
IV

Adults. Loading dose: 50–100 mg. Intermittent bolus: 5–30 mg. Lockout interval: 10–20 min. Continuous infusion: 5–40 mg/hr. Maximum (4-hr): 200–300 mg.

Dosage in renal impairment
Dosage is based on creatinine clearance.

Creatinine Clearance	Dosage
10–50 ml/min	75% of usual dose
less than 10 ml/min	50% of usual dose

AVAILABLE FORMS/COST
• Sol, Inj-IM, IV, SC: 10 mg/ml, 30 ml: **$118.00**; 25 mg/ml, 1 ml: **$0.95**; 50 mg/ml, 1 ml: **$0.99**; 75 mg/ml, 1 ml: **$0.86-$1.03**; 100 mg/ml, 1 ml: **$1.06**
• Syr—Oral: 50 mg/5 ml, 473 ml: **$105.85**
• Tab-Oral: 50 mg, 100's: **$24.70-$108.31**; 100 mg, 100's: **$38.70-$206.01**

CONTRAINDICATIONS: Delivery of premature infant, diarrhea due to poisoning, use within 14 days of MAOIs

PREGNANCY AND LACTATION: Pregnancy category B (category D if used for prolonged periods or in high doses at term); use during labor may produce neonatal respiratory depression; compatible with breastfeeding

SIDE EFFECTS
Frequent
Sedation, hypotension (including orthostatic hypotension), diaphoresis, facial flushing, dizziness, nausea, vomiting, constipation
Occasional
Confusion, arrhythmias, tremors, urine retention, abdominal pain, dry mouth, headache, irritation at injection site, euphoria, dysphoria

Rare
Allergic reaction (rash, pruritus), insomnia

SERIOUS REACTIONS
• Overdose results in respiratory depression, skeletal muscle flaccidity, cold or clammy skin, cyanosis, and extreme somnolence progressing to seizures, stupor, and coma. The antidote is 0.4 mg naloxone.
• The patient who uses meperidine repeatedly may develop a tolerance to the drug's analgesic effect and physical dependence.

INTERACTIONS
Drugs
▣ *Antihistamines, chloral hydrate, glutethimide, methocarbamol:* Enhanced depressant effects
▣ *Barbiturates:* Additive respiratory and CNS depressant effects
▣ *Cimetidine:* Increased respiratory and CNS depression
▣ *Ethanol:* Additive CNS effects
⚠ *MAOIs:* Accumulation of CNS serotonin leading to agitation, blood pressure changes, hyperpyrexia, seizures
▣ *Neuroleptics:* Hypotension, excessive CNS depression
▣ *Phenytoin:* Enhanced metabolism; reduced meperidine concentrations
❷ *Selegiline:* Though primarily MAO-B inhibitor, residual MAO-A activity; see MAOI description
Labs
• *False increase:* Amylase and lipase

SPECIAL CONSIDERATIONS
PATIENT/FAMILY EDUCATION
• Physical dependency may result when used for extended periods
• Do not administer agonist/antagonist analgesics (i.e., pentazocine, nalbuphine, butorphanol, dezocine, buprenorphine) to patient who has received a prolonged course of meperidine (a pure agonist). In opioid-

M

dependent patients, mixed agonist/antagonist analgesics may precipitate withdrawal symptoms.

• Change position slowly; orthostatic hypotension may occur
• Avoid hazardous activities if drowsiness or dizziness occurs
• Avoid alcohol, other CNS depressants unless directed by clinician
• Minimize nausea by administering with food and remain lying down following dose

---

mephobarbital
(me'foe-bar'bi-tal)
Rx: Mebaral
Chemical Class: Barbituric acid derivative
Therapeutic Class: Anticonvulsant; sedative/hypnotic
DEA Class: Schedule IV

CLINICAL PHARMACOLOGY
Mechanism of Action: A barbiturate that increases seizure threshold in the motor cortex. *Therapeutic Effect:* Depresses monosynaptic and polysynaptic transmission in the central nervous system (CNS).

Pharmacokinetics
PO route onset 20-60 minutes, peak N/A, duration 6-8 hours. Well absorbed after PO administration. Widely distributed. Metabolized in liver to active metabolite, a form of phenobarbital. Minimally excreted in urine. Removed by hemodialysis.
Half-life: 34 hrs.

INDICATIONS AND DOSAGES
Epilepsy
PO
Adults, Elderly. 400-600 mg/day in divided doses or at bedtime.
Children more than 5 yrs. 32-64 mg 3 or 4 times/day.
Children less than 5 yrs. 16-32 mg 3 or 4 times/day.

Sedation
PO
Adults, Elderly. 32-100 mg/day in 3-4 divided doses.
Children. 16-32 mg in 3-4 divided doses.

$ **AVAILABLE FORMS/COST**
• Tab-Oral: 32 mg, 250's: **$95.93**; 50 mg, 250's: **$137.36**; 100 mg, 250's: **$184.10**
CONTRAINDICATIONS: Porphyria, history of hypersensitivity to mephobarbital or other barbituates
PREGNANCY AND LACTATION: Pregnancy category D; has caused major adverse effects in some nursing infants; should be given with caution to nursing women
SIDE EFFECTS
Frequent
Dizziness, lightheadedness, somnolence
Occasional
Confusion, headache, insomnia, mental depression, nervousness, nightmares, unusual excitement
Rare
Rash, paradoxical CNS hyperactivity or nervousness in children, excitement or restlessness in elderly, generally noted during first 2 weeks of therapy, particularly noted in presence of uncontrolled pain
SERIOUS REACTIONS
• Abrupt withdrawal after prolonged therapy may produce effects including markedly increased dreaming, nightmares or insomnia, tremor, sweating, vomiting, to hallucinations, delirium, seizures, and status epilepticus.
• Skin eruptions appear as hypersensitivity reaction.
• Blood dyscrasias, liver disease, and hypocalcemia occur rarely.

• Overdosage produces cold or clammy skin, hypothermia, severe CNS depression, cyanosis, rapid pulse, and Cheyne-Stokes respirations.

• Toxicity may result in severe renal impairment.

INTERACTIONS

Drugs

🔢 *Acetaminophen:* Enhanced hepatotoxic potential of acetaminophen overdoses

🔢 *Antidepressants:* Reduced serum concentration of cyclic antidepressants

🔢 *β-adrenergic blockers:* Reduced serum concentrations of β-blockers which are extensively metabolized

🔢 *Calcium channel blockers:* Reduced serum concentrations of verapamil and dihydropyridines

🔢 *Chloramphenicol:* Increased barbiturate concentrations; reduced serum chloramphenicol concentrations

🔢 *Corticosteroids:* Reduced serum concentrations of corticosteroids; may impair therapeutic effect

🔢 *Cyclosporine:* Reduced serum concentration of cyclosporine

🔢 *Digitoxin:* Reduced serum concentration of digitoxin

🔢 *Disopyramide:* Reduced serum concentration of disopyramide

🔢 *Doxycycline:* Reduced serum doxycycline concentrations

🔢 *Estrogen:* Reduced serum concentration of estrogen

🔢 *Ethanol:* Excessive CNS depression

🔢 *Griseofulvin:* Reduced griseofulvin absorption

🔢 *Methoxyflurane:* Enhanced nephrotoxic effect

🔢 *MAOIs:* Prolonged effect of barbiturates

🔢 *Narcotic analgesics:* Increased toxicity of meperidine; reduced effect of methadone; additive CNS depression

🔢 *Neuroleptics:* Reduced effect of either drug

② *Oral anticoagulants:* Decrease hypoprothrombinemic response to oral anticoagulants

🔢 *Oral contraceptives:* Reduced efficacy of oral contraceptives

🔢 *Phenytoin:* Unpredictable effect on serum phenytoin levels

🔢 *Propafenone:* Reduced serum concentration of propafenone

🔢 *Quinidine:* Reduced quinidine plasma concentrations

🔢 *Tacrolimus:* Reduced serum concentration of tacrolimus

🔢 *Theophylline:* Reduced serum theophylline concentrations

🔢 *Valproic acid:* Increased serum concentrations of amobarbital

② *Warfarin:* See oral anticoagulants

Labs

• *Phenobarbital:* Falsely increased result

SPECIAL CONSIDERATIONS

PATIENT/FAMILY EDUCATION

• Avoid driving or other activities requiring alertness

• Avoid alcohol ingestion or CNS depressants

• Do not discontinue medication abruptly after long-term use

• Notify clinician of fever, sore throat, mouth sores, easy bruising or bleeding, broken blood vessels under skin

MONITORING PARAMETERS

• Periodic CBC, liver and renal function tests, serum folate, vitamin D during prolonged therapy

meprobamate
(me-proe'-ba-mate)
Rx: Equanil, Miltown, Neuramate
Chemical Class: Carbamate derivative
Therapeutic Class: Anxiolytic; sedative/hypnotic
DEA Class: Schedule IV

CLINICAL PHARMACOLOGY
Mechanism of Action: A carbamate derivative that affects the thalamus and limbic system. Appears to inhibit multi-neuronal spinal reflexes. *Therapeutic Effect:* Relieves pain or muscle spasms.

Pharmacokinetics
Slowly absorbed from the gastrointestinal (GI) tract. Protein binding: 0-30%. Metabolized in liver. Excreted in urine and feces. Moderately dialyzable. **Half-life:** 10 hrs.

INDICATIONS AND DOSAGES
Anxiety disorders
PO
Adults, Children 12 yrs and older. 400 mg 3-4 times. Maximum: 2400 mg/day.
Children 6-12 yrs. 100-200 mg 2-3 times/day.
Elderly. Use lowest effective dose. 200 mg 2-3 times/day

Dosage in renal impairment

Creatinine Clearance	Dosage Interval
10-50 ml/min	every 9-12 hrs
less than 10 ml/min	every 12-18 hrs

$ AVAILABLE FORMS/COST
• Tab-Oral: 200 mg, 100's: **$1.08-$105.28**; 400 mg, 100's: **$1.44-$293.56**

UNLABELED USES: Muscle contraction, headache, premenstrual tension, external sphincter spasticity, muscle rigidity, opisthotonos-associated with tetanus

CONTRAINDICATIONS: Acute intermittent porphyria, hypersensitivity to meprobamate or related compounds

PREGNANCY AND LACTATION: Pregnancy category D; excreted into breast milk in concentrations 2-4 times that of maternal plasma; effect on nursing infant unknown

SIDE EFFECTS
Frequent
Drowsiness, dizziness
Occasional
Tachycardia, palpitations, headache, lightheadedness, dermatitis, diarrhea, nausea, vomiting, dyspnea, rash, weakness, blurred vision, wheezing.

SERIOUS REACTIONS
• Agranulocytosis, aplastic anemia, leucopenia, anaphylaxis, cardiac arrhythmias, hypotensive crisis, syncope, Stevens-Johnson syndrome and bullous dermatitis have been reported.

• Overdose may cause CNS depression, ataxia, coma, shock, hypotension and death.

INTERACTIONS
Drugs
3 *Ethanol:* Enhanced CNS depression
Labs
• *17-Hydroxycorticosteroids:* Urine, increased
• *17-Ketogenic Steroids:* Urine, increased

SPECIAL CONSIDERATIONS
PATIENT/FAMILY EDUCATION
• Avoid alcohol
• Do not discontinue abruptly following long-term use
MONITORING PARAMETERS
• Periodic CBC with differential and platelets during prolonged therapy

meropenem
(mear-ro-pen'em)
Rx: Merrem
Chemical Class: Carbapenem
Therapeutic Class: Antibiotic

CLINICAL PHARMACOLOGY
Mechanism of Action: A carbapenem that binds to penicillin-binding proteins and inhibits bacterial cell wall synthesis. *Therapeutic Effect:* Produces bacterial cell death.
Pharmacokinetics
After IV administration, widely distributed into tissues and body fluids, including CSF. Protein binding: 2%. Primarily excreted unchanged in urine. Removed by hemodialysis.
Half-life: 1 hr.

INDICATIONS AND DOSAGES
Mild to moderate infections
IV
Adults, Elderly. 0.5-1 g q8h.
Children 3 mo and older. 20 mg/kg/dose q8h.
Children younger than 3 mo. 20 mg/kg/dose q8-12h.
Meningitis
IV
Adults, Elderly, Children weighing 50 kg or more. 2 g q8h.
Children 3 mo and older weighing less than 50 kg. 40 mg/kg q8h. Maximum: 2 g/dose.
Dosage in renal impairment
Dosage and frequency are modified based on creatinine clearance.

Creatinine Clearance	Dosage	Interval
26-49 ml/min	Recommended dose (1,000 mg)	q12h
10-25 ml/min	1/2 of recommended dose	q12h
less than 10 ml/min	1/2 of recommended dose	q24h

AVAILABLE FORMS/COST
• Powder, Inj-IV: 500 mg, 10ml: **$282.60**; 1 g, 10 ml: **$572.40**
UNLABELED USES: Lower respiratory tract infections, febrile neutropenia, gynecologic and obstetric infections, sepsis
CONTRAINDICATIONS: None known.
PREGNANCY AND LACTATION: Pregnancy category B; unknown if excreted into human milk

SIDE EFFECTS
Frequent (5%-3%)
Diarrhea, nausea, vomiting, headache, inflammation at injection site
Occasional (2%)
Oral candidiasis, rash, pruritus
Rare (less than 2%)
Constipation, glossitis

SERIOUS REACTIONS
• Antibiotic-associated colitis and other superinfections may occur.
• Anaphylactic reactions have been reported.
• Seizures may occur in those with CNS disorders (including brain lesions and a history of seizures), bacterial meningitis, or impaired renal function.

INTERACTIONS
Drugs
▣ *Probenecid:* Inhibits renal excretion of meropenem
▣ *Valproic acid:* Two reports of decreased valproate concentrations

SPECIAL CONSIDERATIONS
• Less likely to induce seizures than imipenem-cilastin

MONITORING PARAMETERS
• Renal, hepatic and hematopoietic function during prolonged therapy

M

mesalamine

(mez-al'a-meen)

Rx: Asacol, Pentasa, Rowasa
Chemical Class: 5-amino derivative of salicylic acid
Therapeutic Class: Gastrointestinal antiinflammatory

CLINICAL PHARMACOLOGY

Mechanism of Action: A salicylic acid derivative that locally inhibits arachidonic acid metabolite production, which is increased in patients with chronic inflammatory bowel disease. *Therapeutic Effect:* Blocks prostaglandin production and diminishes inflammation in the colon.

Pharmacokinetics

Poorly absorbed from the colon. Moderately absorbed from the GI tract. Metabolized in the liver to active metabolite. Unabsorbed portion eliminated in feces; absorbed portion excreted in urine. Unknown if removed by hemodialysis. **Half-life:** 0.5–1.5 hr; metabolite, 5–10 hr.

INDICATIONS AND DOSAGES

Ulcerative colitis, proctosigmoiditis, proctitis

PO (Asacol)

Adults, Elderly. 800 mg 3 times a day for 6 wk.

Children. 50 mg/kg/day q8–12h.

PO (Pentasa)

Adults, Elderly. 1 g 4 times a day for 8 wk.

Children. 50 mg/kg/day q6–12h.

Rectal (retention enema)

Adults, Elderly. 60 ml (4 g) at bedtime; retain overnight (about 8 hr) for 3–6 wk.

Rectal (suppository)

Adults, Elderly. 1 suppository (500 mg) twice a day, retain 1–3 hr for 3–6 wk.

To maintain remission in ulcerative colitis

PO (Asacol)

Adults, Elderly. 1.6 g/day in divided doses.

PO (Pentasa)

Adults, Elderly. 1 g 4 times a day

$ AVAILABLE FORMS/COST

• Cap, Gel, Sus Action—Oral: 250 mg, 240's: **$165.96**
• Enema—Rect: 4 g/60 ml, 60 ml; 7's: **$112.07**
• Supp—Rect: 500 mg, 30's: **$105.00-$132.68**
• Tab, Enteric Coated—Oral: 400 mg, 100's: **$103.85**

CONTRAINDICATIONS: None known

PREGNANCY AND LACTATION: Pregnancy category B; has produced adverse effects in a nursing infant and should be used with caution during breast-feeding; observe nursing infant closely for changes in stool consistency

SIDE EFFECTS

Mesalamine is generally well tolerated, with only mild and transient effects.

Frequent (greater than 6%)

PO: Abdominal cramps or pain, diarrhea, dizziness, headache, nausea, vomiting, rhinitis, unusual fatigue

Rectal: Abdominal or stomach cramps, flatulence, headache, nausea

Occasional (6%–2%)

PO: Hair loss, decreased appetite, back or joint pain, flatulence, acne

Rectal: Hair loss

Rare (less than 2%)

Rectal: Anal irritation

SERIOUS REACTIONS

• Sulfite sensitivity may occur in susceptible patients, manifested by cramping, headache, diarrhea, fever, rash, hives, itching, and wheezing. Discontinue drug immediately.

- Hepatitis, pancreatitis, and pericarditis occur rarely with oral forms.

SPECIAL CONSIDERATIONS
PATIENT/FAMILY EDUCATION
- Swallow tabs whole, do not break the outer coating
- Intact or partially intact tabs may be found in stool; notify clinician if this occurs repeatedly
- Avoid excess handling of suppositories
- Lie on left side during enema administration (to facilitate migration into the sigmoid colon)

---

mesna
(mess'na)

Rx: Mesnex, Mesnex VHA Plus
Chemical Class: Thiol derivative
Therapeutic Class: Antidote, ifosfamide

CLINICAL PHARMACOLOGY
Mechanism of Action: An antineoplastic adjunct and cytoprotective agent that binds with and detoxifies urotoxic metabolites of ifosfamide and cyclophosphamide. *Therapeutic Effect:* Inhibits ifosfamide-and cyclophosphamide-induced hemorrhagic cystitis.

Pharmacokinetics
Rapidly metabolized after IV administration to mesna disulfide, which is reduced to mesna in kidney. Excreted in urine. **Half-life:** 24 min.

INDICATIONS AND DOSAGES
Prevention of hemorrhagic cystitis in patients receiving ifosfamide
IV

Adults, Elderly. 20% of ifosfamide dose at time of ifosfamide administration and 4 and 8 hr after each dose of ifosfamide. Total dose: 60% of ifosfamide dosage. Range: 60%-160% of the daily ifosfamide dose.

Prevention of hemorrhagic cystitis in patients receiving cyclophosphamide
PO

Adults, Elderly. 40% of cyclophosphamide dose q4h for 3 doses.
IV

Adults, Elderly. 20% of cyclophosphamide dose at time of cyclophosphamide administration and q3h for 3–4 doses.

AVAILABLE FORMS/COST
- Sol, Inj-IV: 100 mg/ml, 10 ml: **$177.60-$210.53**
- Tab—Oral: 400 mg, 10's: **$875.00**

CONTRAINDICATIONS: None known.

PREGNANCY AND LACTATION: Pregnancy category B; use caution in nursing mothers

SIDE EFFECTS
Frequent (more than 17%)
Bad taste, soft stools
Large doses: Diarrhea, myalgia, headache, fatigue, nausea, hypotension, allergic reaction

SERIOUS REACTIONS
- Hematuria occurs rarely.

INTERACTIONS
Labs
- *False positive:* Urinary ketones, β-hydroxybutyrate

SPECIAL CONSIDERATIONS
MONITORING PARAMETERS
- Urinalysis each day prior to ifosfamide administration
- Reduction or discontinuation of ifosfamide may be initiated in patients developing hematuria (>50 RBC/hpf)

mesoridazine
(mez-oh-rid'a-zeen)
Rx: Serentil
Chemical Class: Piperidine phenothiazine derivative
Therapeutic Class: Antipsychotic

CLINICAL PHARMACOLOGY
Mechanism of Action: A phenothiazine that blocks dopamine at postsynaptic receptor sites in the brain. *Therapeutic Effect:* Diminishes schizophrenic behavior. Also has anticholinergic and sedative effects.

INDICATIONS AND DOSAGES
Schizophrenia
PO
Adults, Elderly. 25-50 mg 3 times a day. Maximum: 400 mg/day.
IM
Adults, Elderly. Initially, 25 mg. May repeat in 30-60 min. Range: 25-200 mg.
Severe behavioral problems (combativeness or explosive, hyperexcitable behavior) associated with neurologic diseases
PO
Elderly. Initially, 10 mg once or twice a day. May increase at 4-7 day intervals. Maximum: 250 mg.
IM
Adults, Elderly. Initially, 25 mg. May repeat in 30-60 min. Range: 25-200 mg.

Ⓢ AVAILABLE FORMS/COST
• Conc, Liq-Oral: 25 mg/ml, 120 ml: **$78.24**
• Tab-Oral: 25 mg, 100's: **$121.28**; 100 mg, 100's: **$167.54**

CONTRAINDICATIONS: Coma, myelosuppression, severe cardiovascular disease, severe CNS depression, subcortical brain damage

PREGNANCY AND LACTATION: Pregnancy category C; bulk of evidence indicates that phenothiazines are safe for mother and fetus; effect on nursing infant is unknown, but may be of concern

SIDE EFFECTS
Frequent
Orthostatic hypotension, dizziness, syncope (occur frequently after first injection, occasionally after subsequent injections, and rarely with oral form)
Occasional
Somnolence (during early therapy), dry mouth, blurred vision, lethargy, constipation or diarrhea, nasal congestion, peripheral edema, urine retention
Rare
Ocular changes, altered skin pigmentation (in those taking high doses for prolonged periods), darkening of urine

SERIOUS REACTIONS
• Abrupt withdrawal after long-term therapy may precipitate nausea, vomiting, gastritis, dizziness, and tremors.
• Blood dyscrasias, particularly agranulocytosis and mild leukopenia may occur.
• Mesoridazine use may lower the seizure threshold.

INTERACTIONS
Drugs
▣ *Anticholinergics:* Inhibited therapeutic response to antipsychotic; enhanced anticholinergic side effects
▣ *Antidepressants:* Increased serum concentrations of some cyclic antidepressants
▣ *Antimalarials:* Mesoridazine serum levels increased
▣ *Attapulgite:* Reduced mesoridazine via decreased absorption
▣ *Barbiturates:* Reduced effect of antipsychotic

[3] *β-blockers:* Enhanced effects of both drugs
[3] *Bromocriptine, lithium:* Reduced effects of both drugs
[3] *Clonidine:* Hypotension
[3] *Epinephrine:* Reversed pressor response to epinephrine
[3] *Guanadrel:* Mesoridazine inhibits antihypertensive response
[3] *Guanethidine:* Inhibited antihypertensive response to guanethidine
[2] *Levodopa:* Inhibited effect of levodopa on Parkinson's disease
[3] *Narcotic analgesics:* Excessive CNS depression, hypotension, respiratory depression
[3] *Orphenadrine:* Reduced serum neuroleptic concentrations; excessive anticholinergic effects
[3] *Phenylpropanolamine:* Case report of patient death on combination of these two drugs

SPECIAL CONSIDERATIONS

PATIENT/FAMILY EDUCATION

- Do not discontinue abruptly
- Concentrate may be diluted just prior to administration with distilled water, acidified tap water, orange or grape juice

MONITORING PARAMETERS

- Observe closely for signs of tardive dyskinesia
- Periodic CBC with platelets during prolonged therapy

metaproterenol

(met-a-proe-ter'e-nole)
Rx: Alupent
Chemical Class: Sympathomimetic amine; β_2-adrenergic agonist
Therapeutic Class: Antiasthmatic; bronchodilator

CLINICAL PHARMACOLOGY

Mechanism of Action: A sympathomimetic that stimulates beta$_2$-adrenergic receptors, resulting in relaxation of bronchial smooth muscle. *Therapeutic Effect:* Relieves bronchospasm and reduces airway resistance.

INDICATIONS AND DOSAGES

Treatment of bronchospasm

PO

Adults, Children older than 9 yr. 20 mg 3–4 times a day.
Elderly. 10 mg 3–4 times a day. May increase to 20 mg/dose.
Children 6–9 yr. 10 mg 3–4 times a day.
Children 2–5 yr. 1.3–2.6 mg/kg/day in 3–4 divided doses.
Children younger than 2 yr. 0.4 mg/kg 3–4 times a day.

Inhalation

Adults, Elderly, Children 12 yr and older. 2–3 inhalations q3–4h. Maximum: 12 inhalations/24 hr.

Nebulization

Adults, Elderly, Children 12 yr and older. 10–15 mg (0.2–0.3 ml) of 5% q4–6h.
Children younger than 12 yr, Infants. 0.5–1 mg/kg (0.01–0.02 ml/kg) of 5% q4–6h.

[$] **AVAILABLE FORMS/COST**

- MDI—INH: 0.65 mg/inh, 14 g, 200 puffs: **$33.65**
- Sol—INH: 0.4%, 2.5 ml: **$1.23-$1.38**; 0.6%, 2.5 ml: **$0.45-$1.38**; 5%, 30 ml: **$45.83**

- Syr—Oral: 10 mg/5 ml, 120, 480 ml: **$12.30**/480 ml
- Tab-Oral: 10 mg, 100's: **$33.75-$34.20**; 20 mg, 100's: **$46.88-$48.59**

CONTRAINDICATIONS: Angle-closure glaucoma, pre-existing arrhythmias associated with tachycardia

PREGNANCY AND LACTATION: Pregnancy category C; has been used to prevent premature labor; long-term evaluation of infants exposed *in utero* to β-agonists has been reported, but not specifically for metaproterenol, no harmful effects were observed

SIDE EFFECTS
Frequent (over 10%)
Rigors, tremors, anxiety, nausea, dry mouth
Occasional (9%–1%)
Dizziness, vertigo, asthenia, headache, GI distress, vomiting, cough, dry throat
Rare (less than 1%)
Somnolence, diarrhea, altered taste

SERIOUS REACTIONS
- Excessive sympathomimetic stimulation may cause palpitations, extrasystoles, tachycardia, chest pain, a slight increase in BP followed by a substantial decrease, chills, diaphoresis, and blanching of skin.
- Too-frequent or excessive use may lead decreased drug effectiveness and severe, paradoxical bronchoconstriction.

INTERACTIONS
Drugs
▣ *Furosemide:* Potential for additive hypokalemia
② *β-blockers:* Decreased action of metaproterenol, cardio selective β-blockers preferable if concurrent use necessary

Labs
- *Glucose:* Urine, increase via Benedict's reagent

SPECIAL CONSIDERATIONS
PATIENT/FAMILY EDUCATION
- Proper inhalation technique is vital for MDIs
- Excessive use may lead to adverse effects
- Notify clinician if no response to usual doses

---

metaraminol
(met-ar-am'e-nol)
Rx: Aramine
Chemical Class: Catecholamine, synthetic
Therapeutic Class: Vasopressor; α-adrenergic sympathomimetic amine

CLINICAL PHARMACOLOGY
Mechanism of Action: An alpha-adrenergic receptor agonist that causes vasoconstriction, reflex bradycardia, inhibits GI smooth muscle and vascular smooth muscle supplying skeletal muscle and increases heart rate and force of heart muscle contraction. *Therapeutic Effect:* Increases both systolic and diastolic pressure.
Pharmacokinetics

Route	Onset	Peak	Duration
IM (pressor effect)	10 min	N/A	20-60 min
IV	1-2 min	N/A	
SC	5-20 min	N/A	

Metabolized in the liver. Excreted in the urine and the bile.

INDICATIONS AND DOSAGES
Prevention of hypotension
IM/SC
Adults, Elderly. 2-10 mg as a single dose.

Children. 0.01 mg/kg as a single dose.

Adjunctive treatment of hypotension

IV

Adults, Elderly. 15-100 mg IV infusion, administered at a rate to maintain the desired blood pressure.

Severe shock

IV

Adults, Elderly. 0.5-5 mg direct IV injection followed by 15-100 mg IV infusion in 250-500 ml fluid for control of blood pressure.

S AVAILABLE FORMS/COST
• Sol, Inj-IM, IV, SC: 10 mg/ml, 10 ml: **$13.36**

CONTRAINDICATIONS: Cyclopropane or halothane anesthesia, use of MAOIs, pregnancy, hypersensitivity to metaraminol

PREGNANCY AND LACTATION: Pregnancy category D; use could cause reduced uterine blood flow and fetal hypoxia

SIDE EFFECTS

Occasional

Tachycardia, hypertension, cardiac arrhythmias, flushing, palpitations, hypotension, angina, tremors, nervousness, headache, dizziness, weakness, sloughing of skin, nausea, abscess formation, diaphoresis

SERIOUS REACTIONS

• Overdosage produces hypertension, cerebral hemorrhage, cardiac arrest, and seizures.

INTERACTIONS

Drugs

3 *Guanethidine:* Reversed antihypertensive effects

2 *Halogenated hydrocarbon anesthetics:* Sensitized myocardium to the effects of catecholamines, arrhythmias possible

A *MAOIs:* Severe hypertensive response

3 *Oxytocic drugs:* Concomitant use may cause severe persistent hypertension

3 *Tricyclic antidepressant:* Vasopressor response decreased; higher sympathomimetic may be necessary

SPECIAL CONSIDERATIONS

MONITORING PARAMETERS

• Maximum effect is not immediately apparent; allow at least 10 min to elapse before increasing the dose
• BP and pulse

---

metaxalone

(me-tax′a-lone)
Rx: Skelaxin
Chemical Class: Oxazolidinedione derivative
Therapeutic Class: Skeletal muscle relaxant

M

CLINICAL PHARMACOLOGY

Mechanism of Action: A central depressant whose exact mechanism is unknown. Many effects due to its central depressant actions. *Therapeutic Effect:* Relieves pain or muscle spasms.

Pharmacokinetics

PO route onset 1 hour, peak 3 hours, duration 4-6 hours. Well absorbed from the gastrointestinal (GI) tract. Metabolized in liver. Primarily excreted in urine. **Half-life:** 9 hrs.

INDICATIONS AND DOSAGES

Muscle relaxant

PO

Adults, Elderly, Children older than 12 yrs. 800 mg 3-4 times/day.

S AVAILABLE FORMS/COST
• Tab-Oral: 400 mg, 100's: **$49.90-$140.29**

CONTRAINDICATIONS: Impaired renal or hepatic function, history of drug-induced hemolytic anemias or other anemias, history of hypersensitivity to metaxalone

SIDE EFFECTS

Occasional

Drowsiness, headache, lightheadedness, dermatitis, nausea, vomiting, stomach cramps, dyspnea

SERIOUS REACTIONS

• Overdose may cause CNS depression, coma, shock, and respiratory depression.

INTERACTIONS

Labs

• *False positive:* Glucose, urine via Benedict's reagent

---

metformin

(met-for′min)

Rx: Glucophage

Combinations

Rx: with rosiglitazone (Avandamet); with glyburide (Glucovance)

Chemical Class: Biguanide

Therapeutic Class: Antidiabetic; hypoglycemic

CLINICAL PHARMACOLOGY

Mechanism of Action: An antihyperglycemic that decreases hepatic production of glucose. Decreases absorption of glucose and improves insulin sensitivity. *Therapeutic Effect:* Improves glycemic control, stabilizes or decreases body weight, and improves lipid profile.

Pharmacokinetics

Slowly, incompletely absorbed after oral administration. Food delays or decreases the extent of absorption. Protein binding: Negligible. Primarily distributed to intestinal mucosa and salivary glands. Primarily excreted unchanged in urine. Removed by hemodialysis. **Half-life:** 3–6 hr.

INDICATIONS AND DOSAGES

Diabetes mellitus

PO (500-mg, 1,000-mg tablet)

Adults, Elderly. Initially, 500 mg twice a day, with morning and evening meals. May increase in 500-mg increments every week, in divided doses. May give twice a day up to 2,000 mg/day (for example, 1,000 mg twice a day [with morning and evening meals]). If 2,500 mg/day is required, give 3 times a day with meals. Maximum: 2,500 mg/day.

Children 10–16 yr. Initially, 500 mg twice a day. May increase by 500 mg/day at weekly intervals. Maximum: 2,000 mg/day.

PO (850-mg tablet)

Adults, Elderly. Initially, 850-mg/day, with morning meal. May increase dosage in 850-mg increments every other week, in divided doses. Maintenance: 850 mg twice a day, with morning and evening meals. Maximum: 2,550 mg/day (850 mg 3 times a day).

PO (Extended-Release tablets)

Adults, Elderly. Initially, 500 mg once a day. May increase by 500 mg/day at weekly intervals. Maximum: 2,000 mg once a day.

Adjunct to insulin therapy

PO

Adults, Elderly. Initially, 500 mg/day. May increase by 500 mg at 7-day intervals. Maximum: 2,500 mg/day (2,000 mg/day for extended-release form).

S AVAILABLE FORMS/COST

• Tab-Oral: 500 mg, 100's: **$58.70-$81.19**; 850 mg, 100's: **$54.64-$141.50**; 1000 mg, 100's: **$57.53-$167.24**

UNLABELED USES: Treatment of metabolic complications of AIDS, prediabetes, weight reduction

CONTRAINDICATIONS: Acute CHF, MI, cardiovascular collapse, renal disease or dysfunction, respiratory failure, septicemia

PREGNANCY AND LACTATION: Pregnancy category B; breast milk excretion unknown

SIDE EFFECTS

Occasional (greater than 3%)

GI disturbances (including diarrhea, nausea, vomiting, abdominal bloating, flatulence, and anorexia) that are transient and resolve spontaneously during therapy.

Rare (3%–1%)

Unpleasant or metallic taste that resolves spontaneously during therapy

SERIOUS REACTIONS

• Lactic acidosis occurs rarely but is a fatal complication in 50% of cases. Lactic acidosis is characterized by an increase in blood lactate levels (greater than 5 mmol/L), a decrease in blood pH, and electrolyte disturbances. Signs and symptoms of lactic acidosis include unexplained hyperventilation, myalgia, malaise, and somnolence, which may advance to cardiovascular collapse (shock), acute CHF, acute MI, and prerenal azotemia.

INTERACTIONS

Drugs

3 *Cimetidine:* Increased metformin AUC 50%, peak concentrations 81%, and decreased renal clearance 27%, increasing the risk of lactic acidosis

3 *Monoamine oxidase (MAO) inhibitors:* Stimulate insulin secretion via β-adrenergic stimulation; excessive and prolonged hypoglycemia may occur in some individuals

SPECIAL CONSIDERATIONS

• May also lower triglycerides

• May decrease insulin requirement in insulin-requiring diabetics

PATIENT/FAMILY EDUCATION

• Administer with food

• Avoid excessive alcohol

• Notify clinician of diarrhea, severe muscle pain or cramping, shallow and fast breathing, unusual tiredness and weakness, unusual sleepiness (signs of lactic acidosis)

MONITORING PARAMETERS

• Glycosylated hemoglobin q 3-6 mo (<7.0%); self-monitored preprandial blood sugars <150 mg/dL; absence of hyperglycemia (e.g., polyuria, polyphagia, polydipsia, blurred vision)

• Renal and hepatic function tests before and annually during therapy

• Serum vitamin B_{12} annually during chronic therapy

---

methacholine

(meth-a-ko'leen)

Rx: Provocholine

Chemical Class: Choline ester

Therapeutic Class: Diagnostic agent

CLINICAL PHARMACOLOGY

Mechanism of Action: A cholinergic, parasympathomimetic, synthetic analogue of acetylcholine that stimulates muscarinic, postganglionic parasympathetic receptors. *Therapeutic Effect:* Results in smooth muscle contraction of the airways and increased tracheobronchial secretions.

Pharmacokinetics

PO route onset rapid, peak 1-4 minutes, duration 15-75 minues or 5 minutes if methacholine challenge is followed with a beta-agonist agent. Undergoes rapid hydrolysis in the plasma by acetylcholinesterase.

INDICATIONS AND DOSAGES
Asthma diagnosis
Inhalation

Challenge test: Before inhalation challenge, perform baseline pulmonary function tests; the patient must have an FEV1 of at least 70% of the predicted value. The following is a suggested schedule for administration of methacholine challenge. Calculate cumulative units by multiplying number of breaths by concentration given. Total cumulative units are the sum of cumulative units for each concentration given.

Vial E:
- Serial concentration: 0.025 mg/ml
- No. of breaths: 5
- Cumulative units per concentration: 0.125
- Total cumulative units: 0.125

Vial D:
- Serial concentration: 0.25 mg/ml
- No. of breaths: 5
- Cumulative units per concentration: 1.25
- Total cumulative units: 1.375

Vial C:
- Serial concentration: 2.5 mg/ml
- No. of breaths: 5
- Cumulative units per concentration: 12.5
- Total cumulative units: 13.88

Vial B:
- Serial concentration: 10 mg/ml
- No. of breaths: 5
- Cumulative units per concentration: 50
- Total cumulative units: 63.88

Vial A:
- Serial concentration: 25 mg/ml
- No. of breaths: 5
- Cumulative units per concentration: 125
- Total cumulative units: 188.88

Determine FEV1 within 5 minutes of challenge, a positive challenge is a 20% reduction in FEV1.

$ AVAILABLE FORMS/COST
- Powder—INH: 100 mg, 1's: **$39.95**

UNLABELED USES: Adie syndrome diagnosis, familial dysautonomia diagnosis, peripheral ischemia, parotitis

CONTRAINDICATIONS: Asthma, wheezing, or very low baseline pulmonary function tests, concomitant use of beta-blockers, hypersensitivity to the drug; because of the potential for severe bronchoconstriction

PREGNANCY AND LACTATION:
Pregnancy category C

SIDE EFFECTS
Occasional
Headache, lightheadedness, itching, throat irritation, wheezing

SERIOUS REACTIONS
- Severe bronchoconstriction and reduction in respiratory function can result. Patients with severe hyperreactivity of the airways can experience bronchoconstriction at a dosage as low as 0.025 mg/ml (0.125 cumulative units). If severe bronchoconstriction occurs, reverse immediately by administration of a rapid-acting inhaled bronchodilator (beta-agonist).

INTERACTIONS
Drugs
3 β-blockers: Exaggerated response to methacholine challenge, prolonged recovery, poor response to treatment

SPECIAL CONSIDERATIONS
MONITORING PARAMETERS
- FEV_1 3-5 min after administration of each serial concentration; procedure is complete when there is a $\geq 20\%$ reduction in FEV_1 compared to baseline (positive response) or when 5 inhalations have been administered at each concentration and FEV_1 has been reduced by $\leq 14\%$ (negative response)

methadone

(meth'a-done)
Rx: Dolophine
Chemical Class: Diphenylheptane derivative; opiate derivative
Therapeutic Class: Narcotic analgesic
DEA Class: Schedule II

CLINICAL PHARMACOLOGY
Mechanism of Action: An opioid agonist that binds with opioid receptors in the CNS. *Therapeutic Effect:* Alters the perception of and emotional response to pain; reduces withdrawal symptoms from other opioid drugs.

Pharmacokinetics

Route	Onset	Peak	Duration
Oral	0.5–1 hr	1.5–2 hr	6–8 hr
IM	10–20 min	1–2 hr	4–5 hr
IV	N/A	15–30 min	3-4 hr

Well absorbed after IM injection. Protein binding: 80%–85%. Metabolized in the liver. Primarily excreted in urine. Not removed by hemodialysis. **Half-life:** 15–25 hr.

INDICATIONS AND DOSAGES
Analgesia
PO, IV, IM, Subcutaneous
Adults. 2.5–10 mg q3–8h as needed up to 5–20 mg q6–8h.
Elderly. 2.5 mg q8–12h.
Children. Initially, 0.1 mg/kg/dose q4h for 2–3 doses, then q6–12h. Maximum: 10 mg/dose.
Detoxification
PO
Adults, Elderly. 15–40 mg/day.
Temporary maintenance treatment of narcotic abstinence syndrome
PO
Adults, Elderly. 20–120 mg/day.

$ AVAILABLE FORMS/COST
• Conc—Oral: 10 mg/ml, 946 ml: **$79.87-$84.67**
• Sol, Inj-IM, SC: 10 mg/ml, 20 ml: **$15.89**
• Sol—Oral: 1 mg/ml, 500 ml: **$30.85**; 10 mg/5 ml, 500 ml: **$67.05**
• Tab-Oral: 5 mg, 100's: **$8.68-$38.45**; 10 mg, 100's: **$14.10-$43.74**; 40 mg, 100's: **$33.00-$37.26**

CONTRAINDICATIONS: Delivery of premature infant, diarrhea due to poisoning, hypersensitivity to narcotics, labor

PREGNANCY AND LACTATION: Pregnancy category B (category D if used for prolonged periods or in high doses at term); compatible with breast-feeding if mother consumes ≤20 mg/24 hr

SIDE EFFECTS
Frequent
Sedation, decreased BP (including orthostatic hypotension), diaphoresis, facial flushing, constipation, dizziness, nausea, vomiting
Occasional
Confusion, urine retention, palpitations, abdominal cramps, visual changes, dry mouth, headache, decreased appetite, anxiety, insomnia
Rare
Allergic reaction (rash, pruritus)

SERIOUS REACTIONS
• Overdose results in respiratory depression, skeletal muscle flaccidity, cold or clammy skin, cyanosis, and extreme somnolence progressing to seizures, stupor, and coma. The antidote is 0.4 mg naloxone.
• The patient who uses methadone long-term may develop a tolerance to the drug's analgesic effect and physical dependence.

INTERACTIONS
Drugs
3 *Anticoagulants:* Potentiation of warfarin's anticoagulant effect

M

⒊ *Antihistamines, chloral hydrate, glutethimide, methocarbamol:* Enhanced depressant effects

⒊ *Barbiturates:* Additive respiratory and CNS depressant effects

⒊ *Carbamazepine, phenobarbital, primidone, rifampin:* Reduced serum methadone concentrations; increased symptoms associated with narcotic withdrawal

⒊ *Cimetidine:* Increased effect of narcotic analgesics

⒊ *Ethanol:* Additive CNS effects

⒊ *Neuroleptics:* Hypotension and excessive CNS depression

⒉ *Phenytoin:* As with carbamazepine above

⒊ *Protease inhibitors:* Increased respiratory and CNS depression

Labs

• *Morphine:* Urine, increased
• *Pregnancy tests:* Urine, false positive (Gravindex)
• *False increase:* Amylase and lipase

SPECIAL CONSIDERATIONS

• **When used for the treatment of narcotic addiction in detoxification or maintenance programs, can only be dispensed by approved hospital pharmacies, approved community pharmacies, and maintenance programs approved by the Food and Drug Administration and the designated state authority**

• Do not administer agonist/antagonist analgesics (i.e., pentazocine, nalbuphine, butorphanol, dezocine, buprenorphine) to patient who has received a prolonged course of methadone (a pure agonist). In opioid-dependent patients, mixed agonist/antagonist analgesics may precipitate withdrawal symptoms.

PATIENT/FAMILY EDUCATION

• Change position slowly; orthostatic hypotension may occur

• Minimize nausea by administering with food and remain lying down following dose

---

methamphetamine
(meth-am-fet´a-meen)
Rx: Desoxyn
Chemical Class: Amphetamine derivative
Therapeutic Class: Anorexiant; central nervous system stimulant
DEA Class: Schedule II

CLINICAL PHARMACOLOGY
Mechanism of Action: A sympathomimetic amine related to amphetamine and ephedrine that enhances CNS stimulant activity. Peripheral actions include elevation of systolic and diastolic blood pressure and weak bronchodilator and respiratory stimulant action. *Therapeutic Effect:* Increases motor activity, mental alertness; decreases drowsiness, fatigue.

Pharmacokinetics

Rapidly absorbed from the gastrointestinal (GI) tract. Metabolized in liver. Primarily excreted in the urine. Unknown if removed by hemodialysis. **Half-life:** 4-5 hrs.

INDICATIONS AND DOSAGES
Attention deficit/hyperactivity disorder (ADHD)
PO
Adults, Children 6 yrs and older. Initially, 2.5-5 mg 1-2 times/day. Increase by 5 mg/day at weekly intervals until therapeutic response achieved.

Appetite suppressant
PO
Adults, Children 12 yrs and older. 5 mg daily, given 30 min before meals. Extended-release 10-15 mg in the morning.

ⓢ AVAILABLE FORMS/COST
• Tab-Oral: 5 mg, 100's: **$118.66**; 10 mg, 1000's: **$300.00**

UNLABELED USES: Narcolepsy

CONTRAINDICATIONS: Advanced arteriosclerosis, agitated states, glaucoma, history of drug abuse, history of hypersensitivity to sympathomimetic amines, hyperthyroidism, moderate to severe hypertension, symptomatic cardiovascular disease, within 14 days following discontinuation of an MAOI

PREGNANCY AND LACTATION: Pregnancy category C; use of amphetamine for medical indications does not pose a significant risk to the fetus for congenital anomalies; mild withdrawal symptoms may be observed in the newborn; illicit maternal use presents significant risks to the fetus and newborn including intrauterine growth retardation, premature delivery, and the potential for increased maternal, fetal, and neonatal morbidity; concentrated in breast milk; contraindicated during breast-feeding

SIDE EFFECTS
Frequent

Irregular pulse, increased motor activity, talkativeness, nervousness, mild euphoria, insomnia

Occasional

Headache, chills, dry mouth, gastrointestinal (GI) distress, worsening depression in patients who are clinically depressed, tachycardia, palpitations, chest pain

SERIOUS REACTIONS
• Overdose may produce skin pallor, flushing, arrhythmias, and psychosis.

• Abrupt withdrawal following prolonged administration of high dosage may produce lethargy which may last for weeks.

• Prolonged administration to children with ADHD may produce a temporary suppression of normal weight and height patterns.

INTERACTIONS
Drugs

🄱 *Acetazolamide:* Increased serum amphetamine concentrations and prolonged amphetamine effects

🄱 *Antidepressants:* Increased effect of amphetamines, clinical evidence lacking

🄱 *Furazolidone:* Hypertensive reactions

🄱 *Guanadrel, guanethidine:* Inhibition of the antihypertensive response

⚠ *MAOIs:* Severe hypertensive reactions possible

🄱 *Selegiline:* Potential for enhanced pressor effect if used in combination

🄱 *Sodium bicarbonate:* Large doses of sodium bicarbonate inhibit the elimination and increase the effect of amphetamines

Labs

• *Amino acids:* Urine, increased

• *Amphetamine:* Urine, positive at 1.0 mcg/ml

SPECIAL CONSIDERATIONS
PATIENT/FAMILY EDUCATION
• Take early in the day
• Do not discontinue abruptly
• Avoid hazardous activities until stabilized on medication
• Avoid OTC preparations unless approved by clinician

methazolamide

(meth-ah-zole'ah-mide)

Rx: Neptazane
Chemical Class: Carbonic anhydrase inhibitor; sulfonamide derivative
Therapeutic Class: Antiglaucoma agent

CLINICAL PHARMACOLOGY

Mechanism of Action: A noncompetitive inhibitor of carbonic anhydrase that inhibits the enzyme at the luminal border of cells of the proximal tubule. Increases urine volume and changes to an alkaline pH with subsequent decreases in the excretion of titratable acid and ammonia. *Therapeutic Effect:* Produces a diuretic and antiglaucoma effect.

Pharmacokinetics

PO route onset 2-4 hrs, peak 6- 8 hrs, duration10-18 hrs. Well absorbed slowly from the GI tract. Protein binding: 55%. Distributed into the tissues (including CSF). Metabolized slowly from the gastrointestinal (GI) tract. Partially excreted in urine. Not removed by hemodialysis. **Half-life:** 14 hrs.

INDICATIONS AND DOSAGES

Glaucoma

PO

Adults, Elderly. 50- 100 mg/day 2-3 times/day.

Ⓢ AVAILABLE FORMS/COST

• Tab-Oral: 25 mg, 100's: **$45.75-$66.39**; 50 mg, 100's: **$68.20-$99.10**

UNLABELED USES: Motion sickness, essential tremor

CONTRAINDICATIONS: Kidney or liver dysfunction, severe pulmonary obstruction, hypersensitivity to methazolamide or any component of the formulation

PREGNANCY AND LACTATION:
Pregnancy category C

SIDE EFFECTS

Occasional

Paresthesias, hearing dysfunction or tinnitus, fatigue, malaise, loss of appetite, taste alteration, nausea, vomiting, diarrhea, polyuria, drowsiness, confusion, hypokalemia

Rare

Metabolic acidosis, electrolyte imbalance, transient myopia, urticaria, melena, hematuria, glycosuria, hepatic insufficiency, flaccid paralysis, photosensitivity, convulsions, and rarely, crystalluria, renal calculi

SERIOUS REACTIONS

• Malaise and complaints of tiredness and myalgia are signs of excessive dosing and acidosis in the elderly.

• Stevens-Johnson syndrome, toxic epidermal necrolysis, fulminant hepatic necrosis, agranulocytosis, aplastic anemia, and other blood dyscrasias have been reported and have caused fatalities.

INTERACTIONS

Drugs

③ *Amphetamines:* Increased amphetamine serum concentrations and prolonged effects

③ *Antiarrhythmics (flecainide, mexiletine):* Alkalinization of urine increases concentrations of these drugs

③ *Cyclosporine:* Increased trough cyclosporine levels with potential for neurotoxicity and nephropathy

③ *Ephedrine:* Increased ephedrine concentrations

③ *Methenamine compounds:* Interference with antibacterial activity

③ *Phenytoin:* Increased risk of osteomalacia with prolonged use of both agents

3 *Quinidine:* Alkalinization of urine increases quinidine concentrations

2 *Salicylates:* Increased concentrations of methazolamide leading to CNS toxicity; also see furosemide for other general diuretic interactions

Labs

• *Increase:* Blood glucose levels, bilirubin, blood ammonia, calcium, chloride

• *Decrease:* Urine citrate, serum potassium

• *False positive:* Urinary protein

SPECIAL CONSIDERATIONS
PATIENT/FAMILY EDUCATION

• Take with food if GI upset occurs
MONITORING PARAMETERS

• Intraocular pressure, reduction in AMS symptoms, serum electrolytes, creatinine, CO_2

---

methenamine
Rx: *Hippurate:* Hiprex, Urex
Rx: *Mandelate:*
Mandelamine
Chemical Class: Formaldehyde precursors
Therapeutic Class: Urinary anti-infective

CLINICAL PHARMACOLOGY
Mechanism of Action: A hippuric acid salt that hydrolyzes to formaldehyde and ammonia in acidic urine. *Therapeutic Effect:* Formaldehyde has antibacterial action. Bacteriocidal.
Pharmacokinetics
Readily absorbed from the gastrointestinal (GI) tract. Partially metabolized by hydrolysis (unless protected by enteric coating) and partially by the liver. Primarily excreted in urine. **Half-life:** 3-6 hrs.

INDICATIONS AND DOSAGES
Urinary tract infection (UTI)
PO
Adults, Elderly. 1 g 2 times/day (as hippurate). 1 g 4 times/day (as mandelate)
Children 6-12 yrs. 25-50 mg/kg/day q12h (as hippurate). 50-75 mg/kg/day q6h (as mandelate).

$ AVAILABLE FORMS/COST
Methenamine Hippurate
• Tab-Oral: 1 g, 100's: **$136.98-$149.10**
Methenamine Mandelate
• Susp-Oral: 500 mg/5 ml, 480 ml: **$54.70**
• Tab-Oral: 500 mg, 100's: **$1.59-$45.53**; 1 g 100's: **$4.50-$123.28**
UNLABELED USES: Hyperhidrosis
CONTRAINDICATIONS: Moderate to severe renal impairment, hepatic impairment (hippurate salt), tartrazine sensitivity (Hiprex contains tartrazine), hypersensitivity to methenamine or any of its components
PREGNANCY AND LACTATION: Pregnancy category C; excreted into breast milk; no adverse effects on nursing infants have been reported
SIDE EFFECTS
Occasional
Rash, nausea, dyspepsia, difficulty urinating
Rare
Bladder irritation, increased liver enzymes
SERIOUS REACTIONS
• Crystalluria can occur when methenamine is given in large doses.
INTERACTIONS
Drugs
3 *Acetazolamide:* Acetazolamide interferes with the urinary antibacterial activity of methenamine
3 *Antacids (magnesium, aluminum, sodium bicarbonate):* Inter-

M

fere with urinary antibacterial activity of methenamine

■ *Sulfadiazine (sulfamethizole, sulfathiazole):* Combination may yield crystalluria

Labs

• *Catecholamines:* Plasma, increased
• *Estriol:* Urine, decreased
• *Estrogens:* Urine, decreased
• *PSP Excretion:* Urine, increased
• *Sugar:* Urine, increased via Benedict's reagent
• *Urobilinogen:* Urine, increased

SPECIAL CONSIDERATIONS

PATIENT/FAMILY EDUCATION

• Keep urine acidic (pH <5.5) by eating food that acidifies urine (meats, eggs, fish, gelatin products, prunes, plums, cranberries); may need to add ascorbic acid
• Fluids must be increased to 3 L/day to avoid crystallization in kidneys
• Take at evenly spaced intervals around clock for best results

MONITORING PARAMETERS

• Periodic liver function tests (hippurate); urine pH

---

methimazole

(meth-im′a-zole)

Rx: Tapazole
Chemical Class: Thioimidazole derivative
Therapeutic Class: Antithyroid agent

CLINICAL PHARMACOLOGY

Mechanism of Action: A thiomidazole derivative that inhibits synthesis of thyroid hormone by interfering with the incorporation of iodine into tyrosyl residues. *Therapeutic Effect:* Effectively treats hyperthyroidism by decreasing thyroid hormone levels.

INDICATIONS AND DOSAGES

Hyperthyroidism

PO

Adults, Elderly. Initially, 15–60 mg/day in 3 divided doses. Maintenance: 5–15 mg/day.

Children. Initially, 0.4 mg/kg/day in 3 divided doses. Maintenance: One-half the initial dose.

Ⓢ AVAILABLE FORMS/COST

• Tab-Oral: 5 mg, 100's: **$18.38-$53.33**; 10 mg, 100's: **$68.54-$97.65**; 20 mg, 30's: **$54.70**

CONTRAINDICATIONS: None known

PREGNANCY AND LACTATION: Pregnancy category D; use smallest possible dose to control maternal disease (propylthiouracil preferable, less likely to cross the placenta); excreted into breast milk

SIDE EFFECTS

Frequent (5%–4%)

Fever, rash, pruritus

Occasional (3%–1%)

Dizziness, loss of taste, nausea, vomiting, stomach pain, peripheral neuropathy or numbness in fingers, toes, face

Rare (less than 1%)

Swollen lymph nodes or salivary glands

SERIOUS REACTIONS

• Agranulocytosis as long as 4 months after therapy, pancytopenia, and hepatitis have occurred.

INTERACTIONS

Drugs

■ *Oral anticoagulants:* Reduced hypoprothrombinemic response to oral anticoagulants

■ *Theophylline:* Physiologic response to antithyroid drug will increase theophylline concentrations via decreased clearance

Labs

• *False increase:* Glucose

SPECIAL CONSIDERATIONS

• Methimazole is the thioamide of choice based on improved patient adherence and outcomes

PATIENT/FAMILY EDUCATION

• Notify clinician of fever, sore throat, unusual bleeding or bruising, rash, yellowing of skin, vomiting

MONITORING PARAMETERS

• CBC periodically during therapy (especially during initial 3 mo), TSH

---

methocarbamol

(meth-oh-kar-′ba-mole)

Rx: Robaxin, Robaxin-750
Combinations
   Rx: with aspirin (Robaxisal)
Chemical Class: Carbamate derivative
Therapeutic Class: Skeletal muscle relaxant

CLINICAL PHARMACOLOGY

Mechanism of Action: A carbamate derivative of guaifenesin that causes skeletal muscle relaxation by general CNS depression. *Therapeutic Effect:* Relieves muscle spasticity.

Pharmacokinetics

Rapidly and almost completely absorbed from the gastrointestinal (GI) tract. Protein binding: 46-50%. Metabolized in liver by dealkylation and hydroxylation. Primarily excreted in urine as metabolites. **Half-life:** 1-2 hrs.

INDICATIONS AND DOSAGES

Musculoskeletal spasm

IM/IV

Adults, Children 16 yrs and older. 1 g q8h for no more than 3 consecutive days. May repeat course of therapy after a drug-free interval of 48 hrs.

PO

Adults, Children 16 yrs and older. 1.5 g 4 times/day for 2-3 days (up to 8 g/day may be given in severe conditions). Decrease to 4-4.5 g/day in 3-6 divided doses.

Elderly. Initially, 500 mg 4 times a day. May gradually increase dosage.

Tetanus spasm

IV

Adults. 1-3 g q6h until oral dosing is possible. Injection should be used no more than 3 consecutive days.

Children. 15 mg/kg/dose or 500 mg/m^2/dose q6h as needed. Maximum: 1.8 g/m^2/day for 3 days only.

💲 AVAILABLE FORMS/COST

• Sol, Inj-IM, IV: 100 mg/ml, 10 ml: **$2.50-$15.77**
• Tab-Oral: 500 mg, 100's: **$2.64-$81.29**; 750 mg, 100's: **$3.70-$116.18**

CONTRAINDICATIONS: Hypersensitivity to methocarbamol or any component of the formulation, renal impairment (injection formulation)

PREGNANCY AND LACTATION: Pregnancy category C; compatible with breast-feeding

SIDE EFFECTS

Frequent

Transient drowsiness, weakness, dizziness, lightheadedness, nausea, vomiting.

Occasional

Headache, constipation, anorexia, hypotension, confusion, blurred vision, vertigo, facial flushing, rash

Rare

Paradoxical CNS excitement and restlessness, slurred speech, tremor, dry mouth, diarrhea, nocturia, impotence, bradycardia, hypotension, syncope

M

SERIOUS REACTIONS
• Anaphylactoid reactions, leukopenia, and seizures (intravenous form) have been reported.
• Methocarbamol overdosage results in cardiac arrhythmias, nausea, vomiting, drowsiness, and coma.

INTERACTIONS
Labs
• *Color:* Urine brown, green, blue or black on standing
• *5-hydroxyindole acetic acid:* Urine, increased
• *Vanillylmandelic acid (VMA):* Urine, increased

---

methotrexate
(meth-oh-trex′ate)
Rx: Folex, Mexate, Rheumatrex, Trexall
Chemical Class: Dihydrofolate reductase inhibitor
Therapeutic Class: Antineoplastic; antipsoriatic; disease-modifying antirheumatic drug (DMARD)

CLINICAL PHARMACOLOGY
Mechanism of Action: An antimetabolite that competes with enzymes necessary to reduce folic acid to tetrahydrofolic acid, a component essential to DNA, RNA, and protein synthesis. This action inhibits DNA, RNA, and protein synthesis. *Therapeutic Effect:* Causes death of cancer cells.

Pharmacokinetics
Variably absorbed from the GI tract. Completely absorbed after IM administration. Protein binding: 50%-60%. Widely distributed. Metabolized intracellularly in the liver. Primarily excreted in urine. Removed by hemodialysis but not by peritoneal dialysis. **Half-life:** 8-12 hr (large doses, 8-15 hr).

INDICATIONS AND DOSAGES
Trophoblastic neoplasms
PO, IM
Adults, Elderly. 15-30 mg/day for 5 days; repeat in 7 days for 3-5 courses.

Head and neck cancer
PO, IV, IM
Adults, Elderly. 25-50 mg/m^2 once weekly.

Choriocarcinoma, chorioadenoma destruens, hydatidiform mole
PO, IM
Adults, Elderly. 15-30 mg/day for 5 days; repeat 3-5 times with 1-2 wk between courses.

Breast cancer
IV
Adults, Elderly. 30-60 mg/m^2 days 1 and 8 q3-4h.

Acute lymphocytic leukemia
PO, IV, IM
Adults, Elderly. Induction: 3.3 mg/m^2/day in combination with other chemotherapeutic agents. Maintenance: 30 mg/m^2/wk PO or IM in divided doses or 2.5 mg/kg IV every 14 days.

Burkitt's lymphoma
PO
Adults. 10-25 mg/day for 4-8 days; repeat with 7-to 10-day rest between courses.

Lymphosarcoma
PO
Adults, Elderly. 0.625-2.5 mg/kg/day.

Mycosis fungoides
PO
Adults, Elderly. 2.5-10 mg/day.
IM
Adults, Elderly. 50 mg/wk or 25 mg twice a week.

Rheumatoid arthritis
PO
Adults, Elderly. 7.5 mg once weekly or 2.5 mg q12h for 3 doses once weekly. Maximum: 20 mg/wk.

Juvenile rheumatoid arthritis
PO, IM, Subcutaneous

Children. 5-15 mg/m^2/wk as a single dose or in 3 divided doses given q12h.

Psoriasis
PO

Adults, Elderly. 10-25 mg once weekly or 2.5-5 mg q12h for 3 doses once weekly.

IM

Adults, Elderly. 10-25 mg once weekly.

Antineoplastic dosage for children
PO, IM

Children. 7.5-30 mg/m^2/wk or q2wk.

IV

Children. 10-33,000 mg/m^2 bolus or continuous infusion over 6-42 hr.

Dosage in renal impairment
Creatinine clearance 61-80 ml/min.
Reduce dose by 25%.

Creatinine clearance 51-60 ml/min.
Reduce dose by 33%.

Creatinine clearance 10-50 ml/min.
Reduce dose by 50%-70%.

§ AVAILABLE FORMS/COST
• Powder, Inj-Intrathecal: 25 mg/vial, 2 ml: **$5.00**

• Sol, Inj-IM, IV: 25 mg/ml, 2 ml: **$4.56-$5.00**

• Tab-Oral: 2.5 mg, 100's: **$135.24-$363.40**; 5 mg, 30's: **$228.80**; 7.5 mg, 30's: **$343.20**; 10 mg, 30's: **$457.60**; 15 mg, 30's: **$686.40**

UNLABELED USES: Treatment of acute myelocytic leukemia; bladder, cervical, ovarian, prostatic, renal, and testicular carcinomas; psoriatic arthritis; systemic dermatomyositis

CONTRAINDICATIONS: Pre-existing myelosuppression, severe hepatic or renal impairment

PREGNANCY AND LACTATION: Pregnancy category D; contraindicated in breast-feeding

SIDE EFFECTS
Frequent (10%-3%)

Nausea, vomiting, stomatitis; burning and erythema at psoriatic site (in patients with psoriasis)

Occasional (3%-1%)

Diarrhea, rash, dermatitis, pruritus, alopecia, dizziness, anorexia, malaise, headache, drowsiness, blurred vision

SERIOUS REACTIONS
• GI toxicity may produce gingivitis, glossitis, pharyngitis, stomatitis, enteritis, and hematemesis.

• Hepatotoxicity is more likely to occur with frequent small doses than with large intermittent doses.

• Pulmonary toxicity may be characterized by interstitial pneumonitis.

• Hematologic toxicity, which may develop rapidly from marked myelosuppression, may be manifested as leukopenia, thrombocytopenia, anemia, and hemorrhage.

• Dermatologic toxicity may produce a rash, pruritus, urticaria, pigmentation, photosensitivity, petechiae, ecchymosis, and pustules.

• Severe nephrotoxicity may produce azotemia, hematuria, and renal failure.

INTERACTIONS
Drugs

▨ *Aminoglycosides, oral (neomycin, vancomycin):* Reduction of 30-50% in methotrexate absorption in patient receiving concurrent oral aminoglycosides

▨ *Antimalarials (chloroquine, hydroxychloroquine):* Methotrexate concentrations reduced by concurrent antimalarial administration

▨ *Binding resins:* Reduced methotrexate concentrations

▨ *Co-trimoxazole, omeprazole, penicillins:* Increased methotrexate concentrations, possible toxicity

M

3 *Cyclosporine:* Increased toxicity of both agents

3 *Ethanol:* Increased risk of methotrexate-induced liver injury

3 *Etretinate:* Increased risk of hepatotoxicity

2 *NSAIDs, probenecid, salicylates, sulfinpyrazone, trimethoprim/sulfamethoxazole:* Increased methotrexate concentrations, possible toxicity

⚠ *Vaccines:* Increased risk of infection following use of live vaccines; reduced seroconversion rate to vaccine

Labs

• *Alanine aminotransferase:* Serum, decreased

• *Alkaline phosphatase:* Serum, increased

• *Bilirubin:* Serum, increased

• *Cholesterol:* Serum, increased

• *Color:* Feces, black

• *Ethanol:* Serum, increased

• *Lactate dehydrogenase:* Serum, decreased

• *Phosphate:* Serum, increased

• *Protein:* CSF, increased

• *Triglycerides:* Serum, decreased

• *Uric acid:* Serum, decreased

SPECIAL CONSIDERATIONS
PATIENT/FAMILY EDUCATION

• Notify clinician of black, tarry stools, chills, fever, sore throat, bleeding, bruising, cough, shortness of breath, dark or bloody urine

• Hair may be lost during treatment

• Drink 10-12 glasses of fluid/day

• Avoid alcohol, salicylates

MONITORING PARAMETERS

• Tumor response: Objective remissions are usually associated with a 50% decrease in the size of solid tumor as measured by physical measurement or test parameter (e.g., chest X-ray). After intrathecal administration, clearing of malignant cells in the cerebrospinal fluid indicates a positive response

• Rheumatoid arthritis: Tender, swollen joints, visual analogue scale for pain; acute phase reactants (ESR, C-reactive protein), duration of early morning stiffness, preservation of function

• CBC and platelets at 7, 10, and 14 days postdrug administration/injection; due to the possibility of early-onset pancytopenia, a lower initial dose for rheumatoid arthritis treatment along with intensified monitoring during early therapy is recommended—CBC's at 1, 2, and 4 wk of treatment; if stable dose may be increased and subsequent CBC's should be performed at monthly intervals

• BUN, serum uric acid, urine ClCr, electrolytes before, during therapy

• Liver function tests before and during therapy

---

methoxsalen
(meth-ox'a-len)
Rx: 8-Mop, Oxsoralen, Oxsoralen-Ultra
Chemical Class: Psoralen derivative
Therapeutic Class: Antipsoriatic; pigmenting agent

CLINICAL PHARMACOLOGY

Mechanism of Action: A member of the family of psoralens that induces an augmented sunburn reaction followed by hyperpigmentation in the presence of long-wave ultraviolet radiation. Bonds covalently to pyrimidine bases in DNA, inhibits the synthesis of DNA, and suppresses cell division. The augmented sunburn reaction involves excitation of the methoxsalen molecule by radiation in the long-wave ultraviolet light (UVA), resulting in transference of energy to the methoxsalen molecule producing an excited state or "triplet electronic state". The molecule, in this "triplet state", then reacts with cutaneous DNA. *Therapeutic Effect:* Results in symptomatic control of severe, recalcitrant disabling psoriasis, repigmentation of idiopathic vitiligo, palliative treatment of skin manifestations of cutaneous T-cell lymphoma (CTCL), repigmentation of idiopathic vitiligo, and palliative treatment of skin manifestations of CTCL.

Pharmacokinetics

Absorption varies. Food increases peak serum levels. Reversibly bound to albumin. Metabolized in the liver. Excreted in the urine. **Half-life:** 2 hrs.

INDICATIONS AND DOSAGES

Psoriasis

PO

Adults, Elderly. 10-70 mg 1.5 -2 hrs before exposure to UVA light, repeated 2-3 times/week. Give at least 48 hours apart. Dosage is based upon patient's body weight and skin type:

Less than 30 kg: 10 mg, *30-50 kg:* 20 mg, *51-65 kg:* 30 mg, *66-80 kg:* 40 mg, *81-90 kg:* 50 mg, *91-115 kg:* 60 mg, *more than 115 kg:* 70 mg.

Vitiligo

PO

Adults, Elderly, Children older than 12 yrs. 20 mg 2-4 hrs before exposure to UVA light. Give at least 48 hours apart.

Topical

Adults, Elderly, Children older than 12 yrs. Apply 1-2 hrs. before exposure to UVA light, no more than once weekly.

CTCL

Extracorporeal

Adults, Elderly. Inject 200 mcg into the photoactivation bag during collection cycle using the UVAR photopheresis system, 2 consecutive days every 4 weeks for a minimum of 7 treatment cycles.

$ **AVAILABLE FORMS/COST**
• Cap, Gel-Oral: 10 mg, 50's: **$338.58-$389.36**
• Lotion-Top: 1%, 30 ml: **$129.98**
• Sol-Inj: 20 mcg/ml, 10 ml: **$41.50**

UNLABELED USES: Dermographism, eczema, hypereosinophilic syndrome, hypopigmented sarcoidosis, ichthyosis linearis circumflexa, lymphomatoid papulosis, mycosis fungoides, palmoplantar pustulosis, pruritus, scleromyxedema, systemic sclerosis

CONTRAINDICATIONS: Cataract, invasive squamous cell cancer, aphakia, melanoma, pregnancy (Uvadex), diseases associated with photosensitivity, hypersensitivity to methoxsalen (psoralens) or any component of the formulation

PREGNANCY AND LACTATION: Pregnancy category C; excretion into breast milk unknown

SIDE EFFECTS

Occasional

Nausea, pruritus, edema, hypotension, nervousness, vertigo, depression, dizziness, headache, malaise, painful blistering, burning, rash, urticaria, loss of muscle coordination, leg cramps

SERIOUS REACTIONS

• Hypersensitivity reaction, such as nausea and severe burns, may occur.

SPECIAL CONSIDERATIONS

• Hard and soft caps are not equivalent

PATIENT/FAMILY EDUCATION

• Do not sunbathe during 24 hr prior to methoxsalen ingestion and UVA exposure
• Wear UVA-absorbing sunglasses for 24 hr following treatment to prevent cataract
• Avoid sun exposure for at least 8 hr after methoxsalen ingestion

M

• Avoid concurrent photosensitizing drugs
• Avoid furocoumarin-containing foods (e.g., limes, figs, parsley, parsnips, mustard, carrots, celery)
• Repigmentation of vitiligo may require 6-9 mo

methscopolamine

(meth-scoe-pol-a-meen)

Rx: Pamine

Chemical Class: Quaternary ammonium derivative

Therapeutic Class: Antiulcer agent (adjunct)

CLINICAL PHARMACOLOGY

Mechanism of Action: A peripheral anticholinergic agent that has limited ability to cross the blood-brian barrier and provides a peripheral blockade of muscarinic receptors. *Therapeutic Effect:* Reduces the volume and the total acid content of gastric secretions, inhibits salivation, and reduces gastrointestinal motility.

Pharmacokinetics

Poorly and unreliably absorbed from the gastrointestinal (GI) tract. Limited ability to cross the blood brain barrier. Primarily excreted in the urine and the bile. The effects of methscopolamine appear to occur within in 1 hour and last for 4-6 hours. Primarily excreted in urine. **Half-life:** unknown.

INDICATIONS AND DOSAGES

Peptic ulcer

Adults, Elderly. Initially, 2.5 mg 30 minutes before meals and 2.5-5 mg at bedtime. May increase dose to 5 mg every 12 hours

$ **AVAILABLE FORMS/COST**

• Tab-Oral: 2.5 mg, 100's: **$83.95**; 5 mg, 60's: **$63.36**

UNLABELED USES: Gastrointestinal spasm

CONTRAINDICATIONS: Reflux esophagitis; glaucoma, obstructed uropathy, obstructed disease of the GI tract (pyloroduodenal stenosis), paralytic ileus, intestinal atony of elderly or debilitated individuals, unstable cardiovascular status in acute hemorrhage, severe ulcerative colitis, toxic megacolon, complicated ulcerative colitis, myasthenia gravis, hypersensitivity to methscopolamine, any component of the formulation, or related drugs

PREGNANCY AND LACTATION: Pregnancy category C; excretion into breast milk unknown, although would be expected to be minimal due to quaternary structure (see also atropine)

SIDE EFFECTS

Occasional

Dry mouth, throat and nose, urinary hesitancy and/or retention, constipation, tachycardia, palpitations, headache, insomnia, dry skin, urticaria, weakness

SERIOUS REACTIONS

• Overdosage may vary from CNS depression, including sedation, apnea, hypotension, cardiovascular collapse, or death to severe paradoxical reaction (such as hallucinations, tremor, and seizures).

INTERACTIONS

Drugs

[3] *Amantadine, rimantadine:* Methscopolamine potentiates the CNS side effects of antivirals; antivirals potentiate the anticholinergic side effects of other anticholinergics

[3] *Antidepressants (amitriptylline, doxepin, imipramine, maprotiline, nortriptyline, protriptyline, trimipramine):* Excessive anticholinergic effects

3 *Neuroleptics (chlorpromazine, haloperidol):* Methscopolamine may inhibit the therapeutic response to neuroleptics; excessive anticholinergic effects with combination

3 *Tacrine:* Tacrine may inhibit the therapeutic effects of anticholinergic agents; centrally acting anticholinergics may inhibit the therapeutic effects of tacrine

SPECIAL CONSIDERATIONS
• Has not been shown to be effective in contributing to the healing of peptic ulcer, decreasing the rate of recurrence, or preventing complications

---

methsuximide
(meth-sux'i-mide)
Rx: Celontin
Chemical Class: Succinimide derivative
Therapeutic Class: Anticonvulsant

CLINICAL PHARMACOLOGY
Mechanism of Action: An anticonvulsant agent that increases the seizure threshold, suppresses paroxysmal spike-and-wave pattern in absence seizures and depresses nerve transmission in the motor cortex. *Therapeutic Effect:* Controls absence (petit mal) seizures.
Pharmacokinetics
Rapidly metabolized in liver to active metabolite, N-desmethylmethsuximide. Primarily excreted in urine. Unknown if removed by hemodialysis. **Half-life:** 1.4 hrs.
INDICATIONS AND DOSAGES
Absence seizures
PO
Adults, Elderly. Initially, 300 mg/day for the first week. Increase dosage by 300 mg/day at weekly intervals until response is attained.

Maintenance: 1,200 mg/day at 2- 4 times/day. Do not exceed 1,000 mg/day in children 12-15 yrs, 1,200 mg/day in patients older than 15 yrs. *Children.* Initially, 10-15 mg/kg/day 3- 4 times/day. Increase at weekly intervals. Maximum: 30 mg/kg/day.
S AVAILABLE FORMS/COST
• Cap, Gel-Oral: 150 mg, 100's: **$64.75**; 300 mg, 100's: **$106.16**
UNLABELED USES: Partial complex (psychomotor) seizures
CONTRAINDICATIONS: Hypersensitivity to succinimides or any component of the formulation
PREGNANCY AND LACTATION: Pregnancy category C
SIDE EFFECTS
Frequent
Drowsiness, dizziness, nausea, vomiting
Occasional
Visual abnormalities, such as spots before eyes, difficulty focusing, blurred vision, dry mouth or pharynx, tongue irritation, nervousness, insomnia, headache, constipation or diarrhea, rash, weight loss, proteinuria, edema
SERIOUS REACTIONS
• Toxic reactions appear as blood dyscrasias, including aplastic anemia, agranulocytosis, thrombocytopenia, leukopenia, leukocytosis, eosinophilia, cardiovascular disturbances, such as congestive heart failure (CHF), hypotension or hypertension, thrombophlebitis, arrhythmias, and dermatologic effects, such as rash, urticaria, pruritus, photosensitivity.
• Abrupt withdrawal may precipitate status epilepticus.
INTERACTIONS
Labs
• *Ethosuximide:* False positive metabolite cross-reacts

M

SPECIAL CONSIDERATIONS
PATIENT/FAMILY EDUCATION
• Take with food or milk
• Do not discontinue abruptly
MONITORING PARAMETERS
• CBC with differential; liver enzymes
• Serum *N*-desmethylmethsuximide concentrations at trough for efficacy (range 10-40 mcg/ml) and 3 hr post-dose for toxicity (>40 mcg/ml)

---

methyclothiazide
(meth-i-kloe-thye′-ah-zide)
Rx: Aquatensen, Enduron
Combinations
  Rx: with reserpine (Diutensen-R)
Chemical Class: Sulfonamide derivative
Therapeutic Class: Antihypertensive; diuretic, thiazide

CLINICAL PHARMACOLOGY
Mechanism of Action: A sulfonamide derivative that acts as a thiazide diuretic and antihypertensive. As a diuretic it blocks the reabsorption of water, sodium and potassium at cortical diluting segment of distal tubule. As an antihypertensive it reduces plasma and extracellular fluid volume and decreases peripheral vascular resistance (PVR) by direct effect on blood vessels. *Therapeutic Effect:* Promotes diuresis, reduces blood pressure (BP).
Pharmacokinetics
Variably absorbed from the gastrointestinal (GI) tract. Primarily excreted unchanged in urine. Not removed by hemodialysis. **Half-life:** 24 hrs.
INDICATIONS AND DOSAGES
Edema
PO
Adults. 2.5- 10 mg/day.

Hypertension
PO
Adults. 2.5-5 mg/day.
🅢 **AVAILABLE FORMS/COST**
• Tab-Oral: 2.5   mg,   100's: **$6.60-$9.70**; 5 mg, 100's: **$7.95-$52.10**
UNLABELED USES: Treatment of diabetes insipidus, prevention of calcium-containing renal stones
CONTRAINDICATIONS: Anuria, history of hypersensitivity to sulfonamides or thiazide diuretics, renal decompensation
PREGNANCY AND LACTATION: Pregnancy category B; therapy for preexisting hypertension can be continued throughout pregnancy with minimal risk; initiating for simple edema not recommended; few unequivocal indications for diuretic therapy in pregnancy except for pulmonary edema or congestive heart failure; excreted into breast milk in small amounts; considered compatible with breast-feeding
SIDE EFFECTS
Expected
Increase in urinary frequency and volume
Frequent
Potassium depletion
Occasional
Postural hypotension, headache, gastrointestinal (GI) disturbances, photosensitivity reaction, anorexia
SERIOUS REACTIONS
• Vigorous diuresis may lead to profound water loss and electrolyte depletion leading to hypokalemia, hyponatremia, and dehydration.
• Acute hypotensive episodes may occur.
• Hyperglycemia may be noted during prolonged therapy.

• GI upset, pancreatitis, dizziness, paresthesias, headache, blood dyscrasias, pulmonary edema, allergic pneumonitis, and dermatologic reactions occur rarely.

• Overdosage can lead to lethargy and coma without changes in electrolytes or hydration.

INTERACTIONS
Drugs

❷ *Angiotensin converting enzyme inhibitors:* Risk of postural hypotension when added to ongoing diuretic therapy; more common with loop diuretics; first dose hypotension possible in patients with sodium depletion or hypovolemia due to diuretics or sodium restriction; hypotensive response is usually transient; hold diuretic day of first dose

❸ *Calcium:* Large doses can lead to milk-alkali syndrome

❸ *Carbenoxolone:* Severe hypokalemia

❸ *Binding resins (cholestyramine, colestipol):* Reduces thiazide serum levels and lessened diuretic effects

❸ *Corticosteroids:* Concomitant therapy may result in excessive potassium loss

❸ *Diazoxide:* Hyperglycemia

❸ *Digitalis glycosides:* Diuretic-induced hypokalemia may potentiate the risk of digitalis toxicity

❸ *Hypoglycemic agents:* Thiazide diuretics tend to increase blood glucose; may increase dosage requirements of hypoglycemic agents.

❸ *Insulin:* Increased blood glucose, increased dosage requirement of antidiabetic drugs

❸ *Lithium:* Increased lithium concentrations

❸ *Methotrexate:* Increased methotrexate effects; potentiates bone marrow toxicity

❸ *Nonsteroidal antiinflammatory drugs:* Concurrent use may reduce diuretic and antihypertensive effects.

SPECIAL CONSIDERATIONS

• Doses above 2.5 mg provide no further blood pressure reduction, but are more likely to induce metabolic disturbance (i.e., hypokalemia, hyperuricemia, etc.)

• May protect against osteoporotic hip fractures

• Loop diuretics or metolazone more effective if CrCl <40-50 ml/min

PATIENT/FAMILY EDUCATION

• Will increase urination temporarily (approx. 3 weeks); take early in the day to prevent sleep disturbance

• May cause sensitivity to sunlight; avoid prolonged exposure to the sun and other ultraviolet light

• May cause gout attacks; notify clinician if sudden joint pain occurs

MONITORING PARAMETERS

• Weight, urine output, serum electrolytes, BUN, creatinine, CBC, uric acid, glucose, lipids

M

---

methylcellulose
Rx: Citrucel
Chemical Class: Hydrophilic semisynthetic cellulose derivative
Therapeutic Class: Laxative

CLINICAL PHARMACOLOGY
Mechanism of Action: A bulk-forming laxative that dissolves and expands in water. *Therapeutic Effect:* Provides increased bulk and moisture content in stool, increasing peristalsis and bowel motility.

Pharmacokinetics

Route	Onset	Peak	Duration
PO	12–24 hr	N/A	N/A

Acts in small and large intestines. Full effect may not be evident for 2–3 days.

INDICATIONS AND DOSAGES

Constipation

PO

Adults, Elderly. 1 tbsp (15 ml) in 8 oz water 1–3 times a day.

Children 6–12 yr. 1 tsp (5 ml) in 4 oz water 3–4 times a day.

[$] **AVAILABLE FORMS/COST**

• Powder-Oral: 2 g/heaping tablespoon, 454 g: **$7.73**; packet, 20's: **$7.73**

• Tab-Oral: 500 mg, 100's: **$13.05**

CONTRAINDICATIONS: Abdominal pain, dysphagia, nausea, partial bowel obstruction, symptoms of appendicitis, vomiting

PREGNANCY AND LACTATION: Bulk forming laxatives are the laxative of choice during pregnancy; compatible with breast-feeding

SIDE EFFECTS

Rare

Some degree of abdominal discomfort, nausea, mild cramps, griping, faintness

SERIOUS REACTIONS

• Esophageal or bowel obstruction may occur if administered with less than 250 ml or 1 full glass of liquid.

SPECIAL CONSIDERATIONS

PATIENT/FAMILY EDUCATION

• Notify clinician of unrelieved constipation, rectal bleeding

• Ensure adequate fluids, proper dietary fiber intake and regular exercise

methyldopa

(meth-ill-doe′pa)

Rx: Aldomet

Combinations

Rx: with HCTZ (Aldoril); with chlorothiazide (Aldoclor)

Chemical Class: Catecholamine, synthetic

Therapeutic Class: Antihypertensive; centrally acting sympathoplegic

CLINICAL PHARMACOLOGY

Mechanism of Action: An antihypertensive agent that stimulates central inhibitory alpha-adrenergic receptors, lowers arterial pressure, and reduces plasma renin activity. *Therapeutic Effect*: Reduces BP.

INDICATIONS AND DOSAGES

Moderate to severe hypertension

PO

Adults. Initially, 250 mg 2–3 times a day for 2 days. Adjust dosage at intervals of 2 days (minimum).

Elderly. Initially, 125 mg 1–2 times a day. May increase by 125 mg q2–3 days. Maintenance: 500 mg to 2 g/day in 2–4 divided doses.

Children. Initially, 10 mg/kg/day in 2–4 divided doses. Adjust dosage at intervals of 2 days (minimum). Maximum: 65 mg/kg/day or 3 g/day, whichever is less.

IV

Adults. 250–1,000 mg q6-8h. Maximum: 4 g/day.

Children. Initially, 2–4 mg/kg/dose. May increase to 5-10 mg/kg/dose in 4-6h if no response. Maximum: 65 mg/kg/day or 3 g/day, whichever is less.

[$] **AVAILABLE FORMS/COST**

• Sol, Inj-IV: 50 mg/ml, 5, 10 ml: **$12.50**/5 ml (methyldopate)

• Susp-Oral: 250 mg/5 ml, 5 ml: **$7.71**
• Tab-Oral: 125 mg, 100's: **$9.75-$13.95**; 250 mg, 100's: **$12.50-$44.92**; 500 mg, 100's: **$18.40-$68.49**

CONTRAINDICATIONS: Hepatic disease, pheochromocytoma

PREGNANCY AND LACTATION: Pregnancy category B (oral); C (IV); no adverse reactions have been reported despite rather wide use during pregnancy; compatible with breast-feeding

SIDE EFFECTS

Frequent

Peripheral edema, somnolence, headache, dry mouth

Occasional

Mental changes (such as anxiety, depression), decreased sexual function or libido, diarrhea, swelling of breasts, nausea, vomiting, lightheadedness, paraesthesia, rhinitis

SERIOUS REACTIONS

• Hepatotoxicity (abnormal liver function test results, jaundice, hepatitis), hemolytic anemia, unexplained fever and flu-like symptoms may occur. If these conditions appear, discontinue the medication and contact the physician.

INTERACTIONS

Drugs

3 *β-blockers:* Rebound hypertension from methyldopa withdrawal exacerbated by noncardioselective β-blockers

3 *Iron:* Inhibited antihypertensive response to methyldopa

3 *Lithium:* Lithium toxicity not necessarily associated with excessive lithium concentrations

3 *Tricyclic antidepressants:* Inhibit the antihypertensive response

Labs

• *Interference:* Plasma and urine catecholamines, serum creatinine, glucose, serum, urine uric acid, and acetaminophen, AST
• *False increase:* Urine amino acids, serum bilirubin, urine ferric chloride test, urine ketones, metanephrines, VMA
• *False decrease:* Serum cholesterol, triglycerides
• *False positive:* Guaiacols spot test, urine melanogen, urine Thormahlen test

SPECIAL CONSIDERATIONS

• Perform both direct and indirect Coombs test if blood transfusion needed. If indirect Coombs test positive, interference may occur with cross match. Positive direct Coombs test will not interfere

PATIENT/FAMILY EDUCATION

• Urine exposed to air after voiding may darken
• Do not discontinue abruptly
• Initial sedation usually improves

MONITORING PARAMETERS

• CBC, liver function tests periodically during therapy
• Direct Coombs test before therapy and after 6-12 mo. If positive rule out hemolytic anemia

M

---

methylene blue

(meth'-i-leen bloo)

Rx: Urolene Blue

Chemical Class: Thiazine dye

Therapeutic Class: Antidote, cyanide; antidote, drug-induced methemoglobinemia; diagnostic agent

CLINICAL PHARMACOLOGY

Mechanism of Action: A weak germicide which hastens the conversion of methemoglobin to hemoglobin in low concentrations. At high concentrations, it has the opposite effect by converting ferrous ion of reduced hemoglobin to ferric iron to form methemoglobin. In cyanide toxicity, it combines with cyanide to form cyanmethemoglobin preventing interference of cyanide with the cytochrome system. *Therapeutic Effect:* Antidote for drug-induced methemoglobinemia.

Pharmacokinetics

Erratic absorption. Protein binding: unknown. Metabolized in tissues to leucomethylene blue. Excreted unchanged in urine and feces. Unknown if removed by hemodialysis. **Half-life:** Unknown.

INDICATIONS AND DOSAGES

Methemoglobinemia, drug-induced

IV

Adults, Elderly, Children. 1-2 mg/kg (0.1-0.2 ml/kg of 1% solution) injected very slowly over several minutes.

NADPH-methemoglobin reductase deficiency

PO

Children. 1-1.5 mg/kg/day. Maximum: 300 mg/day.

Genitourinary antiseptic

PO

Adults. 65-130 mg 3 times/day. Maximum: 390 mg/day.

Dosage in Renal Impairment

Specific guidelines are unavailable although dosage adjustment should be considered.

🅢 AVAILABLE FORMS/COST

• Sol, Inj-IV: 1%, 1 ml: **$4.70-$7.81**
• Tab-Oral: 65 mg, 100's: **$53.06**

CONTRAINDICATIONS: Hypersensitivity to methylene blue or any component of its formulation, glucose-6-phosphate dehydrogenase (G6PD) deficiency, intraspinal injection, severe renal insufficiency,

treatment of methemoglobinemia in cyanide poisoning

PREGNANCY AND LACTATION: Pregnancy category C (category D if inj intra-amniotically); deep blue staining of the newborn, hemolytic anemia, hyperbilirubinemia, and methemoglobinemia in the newborn may occur after inj into the amniotic fluid

SIDE EFFECTS

Occasional

Dizziness, headache, mental confusion, abdominal pain, diarrhea, nausea, vomiting, hypertension, hypotension, sweating

Rare

Arrhythmias, hemolytic anemia, methemoglobinemia

SERIOUS REACTIONS

• Hemolytic anemia and methemoglobinemia occur rarely.

SPECIAL CONSIDERATIONS

PATIENT/FAMILY EDUCATION

• Photosensitivity may occur

MONITORING PARAMETERS

• Hct

---

methylergonovine

(meth-ill-er-goe-noe'veen)
Rx: Methergine
Chemical Class: Ergot alkaloid
Therapeutic Class: Oxytocic

CLINICAL PHARMACOLOGY

Mechanism of Action: An ergot alkaloid that stimulates alpha-adrenergic and serotonin receptors, producing arterial vasoconstriction. Causes vasospasm of coronary arteries and directly stimulates uterine muscle. *Therapeutic Effect:* Increases strength and frequency of uterine contractions. Decreases uterine bleeding.

Pharmacokinetics

Route	Onset	Peak	Dura-tion
PO	5–10 min	N/A	N/A
IV	Immedi-ate	N/A	3 hr
IM	2–5 min	N/A	N/A

Rapidly absorbed from the GI tract after IM administration. Distributed rapidly to plasma, extracellular fluid, and tissues. Metabolized in the liver and undergoes first-pass effect. Primarily excreted in urine. **Half-life:**IV (alpha phase), 2-3 min or less; IV (beta phase), 20-30 min or longer.

INDICATIONS AND DOSAGES
Prevention and treatment of post-partum and postabortion hemorrhage due to atony or involution
PO
Adults. 0.2 mg 3–4 times a day. Continue for up to 7 days.
IV, IM
Adults. Initially, 0.2 mg. May repeat q2–4h for no more than a total of 5 doses.

§ **AVAILABLE FORMS/COST**
• Sol, Inj-IM, IV: 0.2 mg/ml, 1's: **$3.89-$4.76**
• Tab, Coated-Oral: 0.2 mg, 100's: **$73.91-$86.43**

UNLABELED USES: Treatment of incomplete abortion
CONTRAINDICATIONS: Hypertension, pregnancy, toxemia, untreated hypocalcemia
PREGNANCY AND LACTATION: Pregnancy category C; small quantity appears in breast milk; adverse effects have not been described

SIDE EFFECTS
Frequent
Nausea, uterine cramping, vomiting
Occasional
Abdominal pain, diarrhea, dizziness, diaphoresis, tinnitus, bradycardia, chest pain

Rare
Allergic reaction, such as rash and itching; dyspnea; severe or sudden hypertension

SERIOUS REACTIONS
• Severe hypertensive episodes may result in CVA, serious arrhythmias, and seizures. Hypertensive effects are more frequent with patient susceptibility, rapid IV administration, and concurrent use of regional anesthesia or vasoconstrictors.
• Peripheral ischemia may lead to gangrene.

SPECIAL CONSIDERATIONS
PATIENT/FAMILY EDUCATION
• Report increased blood loss, severe abdominal cramps, increased temperature, or foul-smelling lochia.
• Symptoms of ergotism occur with overdosage (nausea, vomiting, diarrhea, seizure, hallucinations, delirium, numb/gangrenous extremities)

MONITORING PARAMETERS
• Blood pressure, pulse, and uterine response

---

methylphenidate
(meth-ill-fen′i-date)
Rx: Concerta, Ritalin, Ritalin-LA, Ritalin-SR
Chemical Class: Piperidine derivative of amphetamine
Therapeutic Class: Cerebral stimulant
DEA Class: Schedule II

CLINICAL PHARMACOLOGY
Mechanism of Action: A CNS stimulant that blocks the reuptake of norepinephrine and dopamine into presynaptic neurons. *Therapeutic Effect:* Decreases motor restlessness

M

and fatigue; increases motor activity, attention span, and mental alertness; produces mild euphoria.

Pharmacokinetics

Onset	Peak	Duration
Immediate-release	2 hr	3-5 hr
Sustained-release	4-7 hr	3-8 hr
Extended-release	N/A	8-12 hr

Slowly and incompletely absorbed from the GI tract. Protein binding: 15%. Metabolized in the liver. Eliminated in urine and in feces by biliary system. Unknown if removed by hemodialysis. **Half-life:** 2-4 hr.

INDICATIONS AND DOSAGES

Attention deficit hyperactivity disorder (ADHD)

PO

Children 6 yr and older. Immediate release: Initially, 2.5-5 mg before breakfast and lunch. May increase by 5-10 mg/day at weekly intervals. Maximum: 60 mg/day.

PO (Concerta)

Children 6 yr and older. Initially, 18 mg once a day; may increase by 18 mg/day at weekly intervals. Maximum: 54 mg/day.

PO (Metadate CD)

Children 6 yr and older. Initially, 20 mg/day. May increase by 20 mg/day at weekly intervals. Maximum: 60 mg/day.

PO (Ritalin LA)

Children 6 yr and older. Initially, 20 mg/day. May increase by 10 mg/day at weekly intervals. Maximum: 60 mg/day.

Narcolepsy

PO

Adults, Elderly. 10 mg 2-3 times a day. Range: 10-60 mg/day.

AVAILABLE FORMS/COST

• Cap, Sus Action-Oral: 10 mg, 100's: **$212.79**; 20 mg, 100's: **$212.70-$239.04**; 30 mg, 100's: **$212.79-$244.48**; 40 mg, 100's: **$251.26**

• Tab, Plain Coated, Sus Action-Oral: 10 mg, 100's: **$83.59-$101.46**; 20 mg, 100's: **$84.97-$160.34**

• Tab, Sus Action-Oral (Concerta): 18 mg, 100's: **$280.00**; 27 mg, 100's: **$287.50**; 36 mg, 100's: **$295.00**; 54 mg, 100's: **$321.25**

• Tab-Oral: 5 mg, 100's: **$24.97-$51.66**; 10 mg, 100's: **$35.60-$73.66**; 20 mg, 100's: **$54.60-$105.91**

UNLABELED USES: Treatment of secondary mental depression

CONTRAINDICATIONS: Use within 14 days of MAOIs

PREGNANCY AND LACTATION: Pregnancy category C

SIDE EFFECTS

Frequent

Anxiety, insomnia, anorexia

Occasional

Dizziness, drowsiness, headache, nausea, abdominal pain, fever, rash, arthralgia, vomiting

Rare

Blurred vision, Tourette syndrome (marked by uncontrolled vocal outbursts, repetitive body movements, and tics), palpitations

SERIOUS REACTIONS

• Prolonged administration to children with ADHD may delay growth.

• Overdose may produce tachycardia, palpitations, arrhythmias, chest pain, psychotic episode, seizures, and coma.

• Hypersensitivity reactions and blood dyscrasias occur rarely.

INTERACTIONS
Drugs
■ *Guanethidine:* Inhibition of guanethidine antihypertensive effect

❷ *MAOIs:* Hypertensive reactions

■ *Phenytoin:* Increased phenytoin levels with risk of toxicity

■ *Tricyclic antidepressants:* Increased serum concentrations of tricyclic antidepressants

Labs
• *False positive:* Urine amphetamine

SPECIAL CONSIDERATIONS
• Overdosage may cause vomiting, agitation, tremor, muscle twitching, seizures, confusion, tachycardia, hypertension, arrhythmias

PATIENT/FAMILY EDUCATION
• Take last daily dose prior to 6 pm to avoid insomnia

• Do not discontinue abruptly

• Avoid OTC preparations unless approved by clinician

• Do not crush or chew sustained release formulation

MONITORING PARAMETERS
• Periodic CBC with differential and platelet count

---

methylprednisolone
(meth-il-pred-niss′oh-lone)
Rx: *Methylprednisolone:* Medrol
Rx: *Acetate:* Depo-Medrol, depMedalone, Depoject, Depopred, D-Med, Duralone, Medralone, M-Prednisol, Rep-Pred
Rx: *Sodium Succinate:* A-MethaPred, Solu-Medrol
Chemical Class: Glucocorticoid, synthetic
Therapeutic Class: Corticosteroid, systemic

M

CLINICAL PHARMACOLOGY
Mechanism of Action: An adrenocortical steroid that suppresses migration of polymorphonuclear leukocytes and reverses increased capillary permeability. *Therapeutic Effect:* Decreases inflammation.
Pharmacokinetics

Route	Onset	Peak	Duration
PO	N/A	1–2 hr	30–36 hr
IM	N/A	4–8 days	1–4 wk

Well absorbed from the GI tract after IM administration. Widely distributed. Metabolized in the liver. Excreted in urine. Removed by hemodialysis. **Half-life:** 3.5 hr.

INDICATIONS AND DOSAGES
Substitution therapy for deficiency states: acute or chronic adrenal insufficiency, adrenal insufficiency secondary to pituitary insufficiency, and congenital adrenal hyperplasia; nonendocrine disorders: allergic, collagen, hepatic, intestinal tract, ocular, renal, and skin diseases; arthritis; bronchial asthma; cerebral edema; malignancies; and rheumatic carditis

PO

Adults, Elderly. Initially, 4–48 mg/day.

IV (Methylprednisolone Sodium Succinate)

Adults, Elderly. 40–250 mg q4–6h. High dosage: 30 mg/kg over at least 30 min. Repeat q4–6h for 48–72 hr.

Spinal cord injury

IV Bolus

Adults, Elderly. 30 mg/kg over 15 min. Maintenance dose: 5.4 mg/kg/h for 23 hr, to be given within 45 min of bolus dose.

IM (Methylprednisolone Acetate)

Adults, Elderly. 10–80 mg/day.

Intra-articular, intralesional

Adults, Elderly. 4–40 mg, up to 80 mg q1–5wk.

§ **AVAILABLE FORMS/COST**

• Tab-Oral: 2 mg, 100's: **$57.08**; 4 mg, 100's: **$14.29–$107.99**; 4 mg, 21's (dose-pack): **$5.31–$21.96**; 8 mg, 25's: **$37.90**; 16 mg, 50's: **$117.11**; 24 mg, 25's: **$63.16**; 32 mg, 25's: **$87.20**

Methylprednisolone Acetate

• Sol, Inj-IM, intraarticular, intralesional: 20 mg/ml, 10 ml: **$7.50**; 40 mg/ml, 10 ml: **$16.18–$45.31**; 80 mg/ml, 5 ml: **$9.50–$45.31**

Methylprednisolone Sodium Succinate

• Powder, Inj-IM, IV: 40 mg/vial, 1's: **$2.05–$5.53**; 125 mg/vial, 1's: **$3.41–$12.50**; 500 mg/vial, 1's: **$10.21–$37.50**; 1 g/vial, 1's: **$9.71–$65.00**; 2 g/vial, 1's: **$41.21**

CONTRAINDICATIONS: Administration of live virus vaccines, systemic fungal infection

PREGNANCY AND LACTATION: Pregnancy category C; excreted in breast milk, could suppress infant's growth and interfere with endogenous corticosteroid production

SIDE EFFECTS

Frequent

Insomnia, heartburn, anxiety, abdominal distention, diaphoresis, acne, mood swings, increased appetite, facial flushing, GI distress, delayed wound healing, increased susceptibility to infection, diarrhea or constipation

Occasional

Headache, edema, tachycardia, change in skin color, frequent urination, depression

Rare

Psychosis, increased blood coagulability, hallucinations

SERIOUS REACTIONS

• Long-term therapy may cause hypocalcemia, hypokalemia, muscle wasting (especially in arms and legs), osteoporosis, spontaneous fractures, amenorrhea, cataracts, glaucoma, peptic ulcer disease, and CHF.

• Abruptly withdrawing the drug after long-term therapy may cause anorexia, nausea, fever, headache, sudden severe myalgia, rebound inflammation, fatigue, weakness, lethargy, dizziness, and orthostatic hypotension.

INTERACTIONS

Drugs

▣ *Aminoglutethamide:* Enhanced elimination of corticosteroids; marked reduction in corticosteroid response; increased clearance of methylprednisolone; doubling of dose may be necessary

▣ *Antidiabetics:* Increased blood glucose

▣ *Barbiturates, carbamazepine:* Reduced serum concentrations of corticosteroids; increased clearance of methylprednisolone

▣ *Cholestyramine, colestipol:* Possible reduced absorption of corticosteroids

③ *Cyclosporine:* Possible increased concentration of both drugs, seizures

③ *Erythromycin, troleandomycin, clarithromycin, ketoconazole:* Possible enhanced steroid effect

③ *Estrogens, oral contraceptives:* Enhanced effects of corticosteroids

③ *Isoniazid:* Reduced plasma concentrations of isoniazid

③ *IUDs:* Inhibition of inflammation may decrease contraceptive effect

③ *NSAIDs:* Increased risk GI ulceration

③ *Rifampin:* Reduced therapeutic effect of corticosteroids; may reduce hepatic clearance of methylprednisolone

③ *Salicylates:* Subtherapeutic salicylate concentrations possible

Labs
• *False increase:* Cortisol, digoxin, theophylline level
• *False decrease:* Urine glucose (Clinistix, Diastix only, Testape no effect)
• *False negative:* Skin allergy tests

SPECIAL CONSIDERATIONS
PATIENT/FAMILY EDUCATION
• Take single daily doses in am
• May mask infections
• Increased dose of rapidly acting corticosteroids may be necessary in patients subjected to unusual stresses
• Signs of adrenal insufficiency include fatigue, anorexia, nausea, vomiting, diarrhea, weight loss, weakness, dizziness, and low blood sugar
• Avoid abrupt withdrawal of therapy following high dose or long-term therapy. Relative insufficiency may exist for up to 1 yr after discontinuation
• Patients on chronic steroid therapy should wear Medic Alert bracelet
• Do not give live virus vaccines to patients on prolonged therapy

MONITORING PARAMETERS
• Serum K and glucose
• Growth of children on prolonged therapy

methyltestosterone
(meth-il-tes-tos-′te-rone)
Rx: Android, Methitest, Testred, Virilon
Chemical Class: Androgen; testosterone derivative
Therapeutic Class: Androgen; antineoplastic
DEA Class: Schedule III

CLINICAL PHARMACOLOGY
Mechanism of Action: A synthetic testosterone derivative with androgen activity that promotes growth and development of male sex organs and maintains secondary sex characteristics in androgen-deficient males. *Therapeutic Effect:* Treats hypogonadism and delayed puberty in males.

Pharmacokinetics
Well absorbed from the gastrointestinal (GI) tract. Protein binding: 98%. Metabolized in liver. Primarily excreted in urine. Unknown if removed by hemodialysis. **Half-life:** 10- 100 min.

INDICATIONS AND DOSAGES
Breast cancer
PO
Adults, Elderly. 50-200 mg/day.
Delayed puberty
PO
Adults. 10-50 mg/day.
Adults, Elderly. 50-200 mg/day.
Hypogonadism
PO
Adults. 10-50 mg/day.

AVAILABLE FORMS/COST
• Cap, Gel-Oral: 10 mg, 100's: **$43.00-$288.68**
• Tab-Oral: 10 mg, 100's: **$3.52-$171.17**; 25 mg, 100's: **$10.30-$343.32**

UNLABELED USES: Hereditary angiodema

CONTRAINDICATIONS: Pregnancy, prostatic or breast cancer in males, hypersensitivity to methyltestosterone or any other component of its formulation

PREGNANCY AND LACTATION: Pregnancy category X; causes virilization of female fetuses; excretion into breast milk unknown; use extreme caution in nursing mothers

SIDE EFFECTS

Frequent
Gynecomastia, acne, amenorrhea or other menstrual irregularities
Females: Hirsutism, deepening of voice, clitoral enlargement that may not be reversible when drug is discontinued.

Occasional
Edema, nausea, insomnia, oligospermia, priapism, male pattern of baldness, bladder irritability, hypercalcemia in immobilized patients or those with breast cancer, hypercholesterolemia

Rare
Polycythemia

SERIOUS REACTIONS
• Cholestatic jaundice, hepatocellular neoplasms, peliosis hepatitis, edema with or without congestive heart failure and suppression of clotting factors II, V, VII, and X have been reported.

INTERACTIONS

Drugs
■ *Cyclosporine:* Increased cyclosporine concentrations
② *Warfarin:* Enhanced hypoprothrombinemic response to oral anticoagulants

SPECIAL CONSIDERATIONS
PATIENT/FAMILY EDUCATION
• Do not swallow buccal tablets, allow to dissolve between cheek and gum
• Avoid eating, drinking, or smoking while buccal tablet in place

MONITORING PARAMETERS
• LFTs, lipids, Hct
• Growth rate in children (Xrays for bone age q6 mo)

---

metoclopramide
(met'oh-kloe-pra'mide)

Rx: Reglan
Chemical Class: Para-aminobenzoic acid derivative
Therapeutic Class: Antiemetic; gastrointestinal prokinetic agent

---

CLINICAL PHARMACOLOGY
Mechanism of Action: A dopamine receptor antagonist that stimulates motility of the upper GI tract and decreases reflux into the esophagus.. Also raises the threshold of activity in the chemoreceptor trigger zone. *Therapeutic Effect:* Accelerates intestinal transit and gastric emptying; relieves nausea and vomiting.

Pharmacokinetics

Route	Onset	Peak	Duration
PO	30-60 min	N/A	N/A
IV	1-3 min	N/A	N/A
IM	10-15 min	N/A	N/A

Well absorbed from the GI tract. Metabolized in the liver. Protein binding: 30%. Primarily excreted in urine. Not removed by hemodialysis. **Half-life:** 4-6 hr.

INDICATIONS AND DOSAGES
Prevention of chemotherapy-induced nausea and vomiting
IV

Adults, Elderly, Children. 1-2 mg/kg 30 min before chemotherapy; repeat q2h for 2 doses, then q3h as needed.

Postoperative nausea and vomiting
IV

Adults, Elderly, Children 15 yr and older. 10 mg; repeat q6-8h as needed.

Children 14 yr and younger. 0.1-0.2 mg/kg/dose; repeat q6-8h as needed.

Diabetic gastroparesis
PO, IV

Adults. 10 mg 30 min before meals and at bedtime for 2-8 wk.

PO

Elderly. Initially, 5 mg 30 min before meals and at bedtime. May increase to 10 mg.

IV

Elderly. 5 mg over 1-2 min. May increase to 10 mg.

Symptomatic gastroesophageal reflux
PO

Adults. 10-15 mg up to 4 times a day, or single doses up to 20 mg as needed.

Elderly. Initially, 5 mg 4 times a day. May increase to 10 mg.

Children. 0.4-0.8 mg/kg/day in 4 divided doses.

To facilitate small bowel intubation (single dose)
IV

Adults, Elderly. 10 mg as a single dose.

Children 6-14 yr. 2.5-5 mg as a single dose.

Children younger than 6 yr. 0.1 mg/kg as a single dose.

Dosage in renal impairment
Dosage is modified based on creatinine clearance.

Creatinine Clearance	% of normal dose
40-50 ml/min	75%
10-40 ml/min	50%
less than 10 ml/min	25%-50%

ⓢ AVAILABLE FORMS/COST
• Conc—Oral: 10 mg/ml, 30 ml: **$19.49**
• Sol, Inj—IM, IV: 5 mg/ml, 2 ml: **$0.89-$4.04**
• Syr—Oral: 5 mg/5 ml, 480 ml: **$6.44-$19.25**
• Tab—Oral: 5 mg, 100's: **$9.00-$66.15**; 10 mg, 100's: **$7.18-$104.30**

UNLABELED USES: Prevention of aspiration pneumonia; treatment of drug-related postoperative nausea and vomiting, persistent hiccups, slow gastric emptying, vascular headaches

CONTRAINDICATIONS: Concurrent use of medications likely to produce extrapyramidal reactions, GI hemorrhage, GI obstruction or perforation, history of seizure disorders, pheochromocytoma

PREGNANCY AND LACTATION: Pregnancy category B; has been used during pregnancy as an antiemetic and to decrease gastric emptying time; excreted into milk; use during lactation a concern because of the potent CNS effects the drug is capable of producing

SIDE EFFECTS
Frequent (10%)

Somnolence, restlessness, fatigue, lethargy

Occasional (3%)

Dizziness, anxiety, headache, insomnia, breast tenderness, altered menstruation, constipation, rash, dry mouth, galactorrhea, gynecomastia

Rare (less than 3%)

Hypotension or hypertension, tachycardia

M

SERIOUS REACTIONS

• Extrapyramidal reactions occur most commonly in children and young adults (18-30 years) receiving large doses (2 mg/kg) during chemotherapy and are usually limited to akathisia (involuntary limb movement and facial grimacing).

INTERACTIONS

Drugs

▣ *Cyclosporine:* Increased bioavailability and serum concentrations of cyclosporine

▣ *Digitalis glycosides:* Reduced serum digoxin concentration when coadministered with generic formulations

▣ *Ethanol:* Increased sedative effects of ethanol

▣ *MAOIs:* Metoclopramide releases catecholamines, use cautiously with MAOIs

▣ *Insulin:* Dosage and timing of insulin may need to be adjusted

SPECIAL CONSIDERATIONS

• Dystonic reactions can be managed with 50 mg diphenhydramine or 1-2 mg benztropine IM

PATIENT/FAMILY EDUCATION

• Use caution while diving or during other activities requiring alertness; may cause drowsiness

---

metolazone

(met-tole′a-zone)

Rx: Mykrox (rapid acting), Zaroxolyn (slow acting)
Chemical Class: Quinazoline derivative
Therapeutic Class: Antihypertensive; diuretic, thiazide-like

CLINICAL PHARMACOLOGY

Mechanism of Action: A thiazide-like diuretic and antihypertensive. As a diuretic, blocks reabsorption of sodium, potassium, and chloride at the distal convoluted tubule, increasing renal excretion of sodium and water. As an antihypertensive, reduces plasma and extracellular fluid volume and peripheral vascular resistance. *Therapeutic Effect:* Promotes diuresis and reduces BP.

Pharmacokinetics

Route	Onset	Peak	Duration
PO (diuretic)	1 hr	2 hr	12–24 hr

Incompletely absorbed from the GI tract. Protein binding: 95%. Primarily excreted unchanged in urine. Not removed by hemodialysis. **Half-life:** 14 hr.

INDICATIONS AND DOSAGES

Edema

PO

Adults, Elderly. 5-10 mg/day. May increase to 20 mg/day in edema associated with renal disease or heart failure.

Children. 0.2-0.4 mg/kg/day in 1-2 divided doses.

Hypertension

PO (Zaroxolyn)

Adults, Elderly. 2.4-5 mg/day.

PO (Mydrox)

Adults, Elderly. Initially, 0.5 mg/day. May increase up to 1 mg/day.

Usual elderly dosage (Zaroxolyn)

PO

• *Elderly.* Initially, 2.5 mg/day or every other day.

▣ **AVAILABLE FORMS/COST**

• Tab—Oral: 0.5 mg, 100's: **$136.45**; 2.5 mg, 100's: **$42.86-$144.85**; 5 mg, 100's: **$53.21-$164.61**; 10 mg, 100's: **$117.38-$197.09** (Zaroxolyn)

CONTRAINDICATIONS: Anuria, hepatic coma or precoma, history of hypersensitivity to sulfonamides or thiazide diuretics, renal decompensation

PREGNANCY AND LACTATION:
Pregnancy category B; therapy for preexisting hypertension can be continued throughout pregnancy with minimal risk; initiating for simple edema not recommended; few unequivocal indications for diuretic therapy in pregnancy except for pulmonary edema or congestive heart failure; excreted into breast milk in small amounts; considered compatible with breast-feeding

SIDE EFFECTS

Expected
Increase in urinary frequency and urine volume

Frequent (10%–9%)
Dizziness, light-headedness, headache

Occasional (6%–4%)
Muscle cramps and spasm, fatigue, lethargy

Rare (less than 2%)
Asthenia, palpitations, depression, nausea, vomiting, abdominal bloating, constipation, diarrhea, urticaria

SERIOUS REACTIONS
• Vigorous diuresis may lead to profound water and electrolyte depletion, resulting in hypokalemia, hyponatremia, and dehydration.
• Acute hypotensive episodes may occur.
• Hyperglycemia may occur during prolonged therapy.
• Pancreatitis, paresthesia, blood dyscrasias, pulmonary edema, allergic pneumonitis, and dermatologic reactions occur rarely.
• Overdose can lead to lethargy and coma without changes in electrolytes or hydration.

INTERACTIONS

Drugs
② *Angiotensin-converting enzyme inhibitors:* Risk of postural hypotension when added to ongoing diuretic therapy; more common with loop diuretics; first dose hypotension possible in patients with sodium depletion or hypovolemia due to diuretics or sodium restriction; hypotensive response is usually transient; hold diuretic day of first dose

③ *Calcium:* Milk-alkali syndrome
③ *Carbenoxolone:* Enhanced hypokalemia
③ *Cholestyramine, colestipol:* Reduced serum concentrations of metolazone
③ *Corticosteroids:* Concomitant therapy may result in excessive potassium loss
③ *Diazoxide:* Hyperglycemia
③ *Digitalis glycosides:* Diuretic-induced hypokalemia may increase the risk of digitalis toxicity
③ *Hypoglycemic agents:* Metolazone increases blood glucose
③ *Lithium:* Increased serum lithium concentrations, toxicity may occur
③ *Methotrexate:* Enhanced bone marrow suppression
③ *Nonsteroidal antiinflammatory drugs:* Concurrent use may reduce diuretic and antihypertensive effects

SPECIAL CONSIDERATIONS
• More effective than other thiazide-type diuretics in patients with impaired renal function
• Metolazone formulations are not bioequivalent or therapeutically equivalent at the same doses. Mykrox is more rapidly and completely bioavailable; Do not interchange brands.

PATIENT/FAMILY EDUCATION
• Will increase urination; take early in the day to prevent sleep disturbance
• May cause sensitivity to sunlight; avoid prolonged exposure to the sun and other ultraviolet light
• May cause gout attacks; notify clinician if sudden joint pain occurs

M

MONITORING PARAMETERS

• Weight, urine output, serum electrolytes, BUN, creatinine, CBC, uric acid, glucose, lipids

---

metoprolol

(me-toe′pro-lole)
Rx: Lopressor, Toprol XL
Combinations
　Rx: with hydrochlorothiazide (Lopressor Hct)
Chemical Class: β_1-adrenergic blocker, cardioselective
Therapeutic Class: Antianginal; antihypertensive

CLINICAL PHARMACOLOGY

Mechanism of Action: An antianginal, antihypertensive, and MI adjunct that selectively blocks beta$_1$-adrenergic receptors; high dosages may block beta$_2$-adrenergic receptors. Decreases oxygen requirements. Large doses increase airway resistance. *Therapeutic Effect:* Slows sinus node heart rate, decreases cardiac output, and reduces BP. Also decreases myocardial ischemia severity.

Pharmacokinetics

Route	Onset	Peak	Duration
PO	10–15 min	N/A	6 hr
PO (extended release)	N/A	6–12 hr	24 hr
IV	Immediate	20 min	5–8 hr

Well absorbed from the GI tract. Protein binding: 12%. Widely distributed. Metabolized in the liver (undergoes significant first-pass metabolism). Primarily excreted in urine. Removed by hemodialysis. **Half-life:** 3–7 hr.

INDICATIONS AND DOSAGES
Mild to moderate hypertension
PO
Adults. Initially, 100 mg/day as single or divided dose. Increase at weekly (or longer) intervals. Maintenance: 100–450 mg/day.
Elderly. Initially, 25 mg/day. Range: 25–300 mg/day.
PO (extended-release tablets)
Adults. 50–100 mg/day as single dose. May increase at least at weekly intervals until optimum BP attained. Maximum: 200 mg/day.
Chronic, stable angina pectoris
PO
Adults. Initially, 100 mg/day as single or divided dose. Increase at weekly (or longer) intervals. Maintenance: 100–450 mg/day.
PO (extended-release tablets)
Adults. Initially, 100 mg/day as single dose. May increase at least at weekly intervals until optimum clinical response achieved. Maximum: 200 mg/day.
Congestive heart failure
PO (extended-release tablets)
Adults. Initially, 25 mg/day. May double dose q2wk. Maximum: 200 mg/day.
Early treatment of MI
IV
Adults. 5 mg q2min for 3 doses, followed by 50 mg orally q6h for 48 hr. Begin oral dose 15 min after last IV dose. Or, in patients who do not tolerate full IV dose, give 25–50 mg orally q6h, 15 min after last IV dose.
Late treatment and maintenance after an MI
PO
Adults. 100 mg twice a day for at least 3 mo.

▣ AVAILABLE FORMS/COST
• Sol, Inj—IV: 5 mg/5 ml, 1′s: **$3.44-$10.10**

• Tab, Coated—Oral: 50 mg, 100's: **$5.20-$101.41**; 100 mg, 100's: **$9.93-$152.28**
• Tab, Coated, Sus Action—Oral: 25 mg, 100's: **$78.25**; 50 mg, 100's: **$78.25**; 100 mg, 100's: **$117.58**; 200 mg, 100's: **$195.89**
• Tab—Oral (with hydrochlorothiazide): 50 mg-25 mg, 100's: **$116.29**; 100 mg-25 mg, 100's: **$181.73**; 100 mg-50 mg, 100's: **$192.74**

UNLABELED USES: To increase survival rate in diabetic patients with coronary artery disease (CAD); treatment or prevention of anxiety; cardiac arrhythmias; hypertrophic cardiomyopathy; mitral valve prolapse syndrome; pheochromocytoma; tremors; thyrotoxicosis; vascular headache

CONTRAINDICATIONS: Cardiogenic shock, MI with a heart rate less than 45 beats/minute or systolic BP less than 100 mm Hg, overt heart failure, second- or third-degree heart block, sinus bradycardia

PREGNANCY AND LACTATION: Pregnancy category C; similar drug, atenolol, frequently used in the third trimester for treatment of hypertension (many studies of efficacy and safety of atenolol in pregnancy-induced hypertension); long-term use has been associated with intrauterine growth retardation; excreted into breast milk in insignificant concentrations; prudent to monitor infant for signs of β-blockade

SIDE EFFECTS

Metoprolol is generally well tolerated, with transient and mild side effects.

Frequent

Diminished sexual function, drowsiness, insomnia, unusual fatigue or weakness

Occasional

Anxiety, nervousness, diarrhea, constipation, nausea, vomiting, nasal congestion, abdominal discomfort, dizziness, difficulty breathing, cold hands or feet

Rare

Altered taste, dry eyes, nightmares, paraesthesia, allergic reaction (rash, pruritus)

SERIOUS REACTIONS

• Overdose may produce profound bradycardia, hypotension, and bronchospasm.
• Abrupt withdrawal of metoprolol may result in diaphoresis, palpitations, headache, tremulousness, exacerbation of angina, MI, and ventricular arrhythmias.
• Metoprolol administration may precipitate CHF and MI in patients with heart disease; thyroid storm in those with thyrotoxicosis; and peripheral ischemia in those with existing peripheral vascular disease.
• Hypoglycemia may occur in patients with previously controlled diabetes.

INTERACTIONS

Drugs

3 *α-adrenergic blockers:* Potential enhanced first dose response (marked initial drop in blood pressure) particularly on standing (especially prazosin)

3 *Amiodarone:* Bradycardia, cardiac arrest, or ventricular dysrhythmia

3 *Antidiabetics:* Altered response to hypoglycemia, prolonged recovery of normoglycemia, hypertension, blockade of tachycardia; may increase blood glucose and impair peripheral circulation

3 *Antipyrine:* Increased antipyrine concentrations

3 *Barbiturates:* Reduced β-blocker concentrations

M

❷ *β-agonists:* Antagonism of bronchodilating effect

▪ *Bromazepam, diazepam, oxazepam:* Increased benzodiazepine effect (lorazepam and alprazolam unaffected)

▪ *Cimetidine, etintidine, propafenone, propoxyphene, quinidine:* Increased plasma metoprolol concentration

▪ *Clonidine:* Abrupt withdrawal of clonidine while on a β-blocker may exaggerate the rebound hypertension due to unopposed alpha stimulation

▪ *Digoxin:* Additive prolongation of atrioventricular (AV) conduction time

▪ *Dihydropyridines (nicardipine, nifedipine, felodipine, isradipine, nisoldipine):* Increased β-blocker effects

▪ *Diltiazem:* Potentiates β-adrenergic effects; hypotension, left ventricular failure, and AV conduction disturbances problematic in elderly, patients with left ventricular dysfunction, aortic stenosis, or with large doses of either drug

▪ *Dipyridamole, Tacrine:* Bradycardia

▪ *Fluoxetine:* Enhanced effect of β-blocker

▪ *Isoproterenol:* Potential reduction in effectiveness of isoproterenol in the treatment of asthma; less likely with cardioselective agents like metoprolol

▪ *Local anesthetics:* Use of local anesthetics containing epinephrine may result in hypertensive reactions in patients taking β-blockers

▪ *NSAIDs:* Reduced hypotensive effects of β-blockers

▪ *Phenylephrine:* Enhanced pressor response to phenylephrine, particularly when it is administered IV

▪ *Prazosin:* First-dose response to prazosin may be enhanced by β-blockade

▪ *Quinolones:* Inhibition of β-blocker metabolism, increased β-blocker effects

▪ *Rifampin:* Reduced plasma metoprolol concentration

▪ *Theophylline:* Antagonistic pharmacodynamic effects

▪ *Verapamil:* Potentiates β-adrenergic effects; hypotension, left ventricular failure, and AV conduction disturbances problemmatic in elderly, patients with left ventricular dysfunction, aortic stenosis, or with large doses of either drug

SPECIAL CONSIDERATIONS

PATIENT/FAMILY EDUCATION

• Do not discontinue abruptly; may require taper; rapid withdrawal may produce rebound hypertension or angina

• Avoid driving or other activities requiring alertness until response to therapy is determined

• Take with or immediately following meals

• Extended release tablets are scored and can be divided; whole or half tablet should be swallowed whole and not chewed or crushed

MONITORING PARAMETERS

• Angina: Reduction in nitroglycerin usage; frequency, severity, onset, and duration of angina pain; heart rate

• Arrhythmias: heart rate

• Congestive heart failure: Functional status, cough, dyspnea on exertion, paroxysmal nocturnal dyspnea, exercise tolerance, and ventricular function

• Hypertension: Blood pressure

• Migraine headache: Reduction in the frequency, severity, and duration of attacks

• Postmyocardial infarction: Left ventricular function, lower resting heart rate

• Toxicity: Blood glucose, bronchospasm, hypotension, bradycardia, depression, confusion, hallucination, sexual dysfunction

---

metronidazole
(me-troe-ni'da-zole)
Rx: Flagyl, Flagyl ER, Metro IV, MetroCream, MetroGel, Metrolotion, Noritate, Protostat
Rx: Kit: Helidac (metronidazole, bismuth subsalicylate, tetracycline)
Chemical Class: Nitroimidazole derivative
Therapeutic Class: Antibiotic; antihelmintic; antiprotozoal

CLINICAL PHARMACOLOGY
Mechanism of Action: A nitroimidazole derivative that disrupts bacterial and protozoal DNA, inhibiting nucleic acid synthesis. *Therapeutic Effect:* Produces bactericidal, antiprotozoal, amebicidal, and trichomonacidal effects. Produces anti-inflammatory and immunosuppressive effects when applied topically.

Pharmacokinetics

Well absorbed from the GI tract; minimally absorbed after topical application. Protein binding: less than 20%. Widely distributed; crosses blood-brain barrier. Metabolized in the liver to active metabolite. Primarily excreted in urine; partially eliminated in feces. Removed by hemodialysis. **Half-life:** 8 hr (increased in alcoholic hepatic disease and in neonates).

INDICATIONS AND DOSAGES
Amebiasis
PO
Adults, Elderly. 500-750 mg q8h.
Children. 35-50 mg/kg/day in divided doses q8h.
Trichomoniasis
PO
Adults, Elderly. 250 mg q8h or 2 g as a single dose.
Children. 15-30 mg/kg/day in divided doses q8h.
Anaerobic skin and skin-structure, CNS, lower respiratory tract, bone, joint, intraabdominal, and gynecologic infections; endocarditis; septicemia
PO, IV
Adults, Elderly, Children. 30 mg/kg/day in divided doses q6h. Maximum: 4 g/day.
Antibiotic-associated pseudomembranous colitis
PO
Adults, Elderly. 250-500 mg 3-4 times a day for 10-14 days.
Children. 30 mg/kg/day in divided doses q6h for 7-10 days.
Helicobacter pylori infections
PO
Adults, Elderly. 250-500 mg 3 times a day (in combination).
Children. 15-20 mg/kg/day in 2 divided doses.
Bacterial vaginosis
PO
Adults. 750 mg at bedtime for 7 days.
Intravaginal
Adults. One applicatorful twice a day or once a day at bedtime for 5 days.
Rosacea
Topical
Adults. Apply thin layer of lotion to affected area twice a day or cream once a day.

💲 AVAILABLE FORMS/COST
• Cap, Gel—Oral: 375 mg, 50's: **$159.58-$177.51**
• Cream—Top: 0.75%, 45 g: **$51.07-$78.63**; 1%, 30 g: **$52.49**
• Gel—Top: 0.75%, 28, 45 g: **$68.63**/45 g
• Gel—Vag: 0.75%, 70 g: **$30.42-$57.48**
• Sol, Inj—IV: 500 mg/100 ml, 100 ml: **$2.84-$30.50**
• Lotion—Top: 0.75%, 60 ml: **$78.63**
• Tab, Plain Coated—Oral: 250 mg, 100's: **$7.33-$235.09**; 500 mg, 100's: **$17.13-$428.28**
• Tab, Sus Action—Oral: 750 mg, 30's: **$232.78-$258.94**

UNLABELED USES: Treatment of bacterial vaginosis, grade III-IV decubitus ulcers with anaerobic infection, *H. pylori*–associated gastritis and duodenal ulcer, inflammatory bowel disease; topical treatment of acne rosacea

CONTRAINDICATIONS: Hypersensitivity to metronidazole or other nitroimidazole derivatives (also parabens with topical application)

PREGNANCY AND LACTATION: Pregnancy category B; use in pregnancy controversial; use in 1st trimester and single-dose therapy often avoided; use with caution during breast-feeding; if single-dose therapy is used, discontinue breast-feeding for 12-24 hr to allow excretion of the drug

SIDE EFFECTS
Frequent
Systemic: Anorexia, nausea, dry mouth, metallic taste
Vaginal: Symptomatic cervicitis and vaginitis, abdominal cramps, uterine pain
Occasional
Systemic: Diarrhea or constipation, vomiting, dizziness, erythematous rash, urticaria, reddish brown urine

Topical: Transient erythema, mild dryness, burning, irritation, stinging, tearing when applied too close to eyes
Vaginal: Vaginal, perineal, or vulvar itching; vulvar swelling
Rare
Mild, transient leukopenia; thrombophlebitis with IV therapy

SERIOUS REACTIONS
• Oral therapy may result in furry tongue, glossitis, cystitis, dysuria, pancreatitis, and flattening of T waves on EKG readings.
• Peripheral neuropathy, manifested as numbness and tingling in hands or feet, is usually reversible if treatment is stopped immediately after neurologic symptoms appear.
• Seizures occur occasionally.

INTERACTIONS
Drugs
🔢 *Carbamazepine:* Increased carbamazepine levels
🔢 *Cholestyramine, colestipol:* Reduced metronidazole absorption
🔢 *Disulfiram:* CNS toxicity
🔢 *Ethanol:* Disulfiram-like reaction
② *Fluorouracil:* Enhanced toxicity of fluorouracil
🔢 *IV phenytoin, phenobarbital, diazepam, nitroglycerine, trimethoprim-sulfamethoxazole:* Disulfiram-like reaction due to ethanol in IV preparations
② *Oral anticoagulants:* Increased hypoprothrombinemic response to warfarin
🔢 *Phenytoin:* Increased phenytoin levels
Labs
• *Interference:* Glucose
• *False decrease:* AST, zidovudine level
• *False positive increase:* Clindamycin, erythromycin, polymyxin, tetracycline, and trimethoprim assays

SPECIAL CONSIDERATIONS
• Treat sexual partner(s) for trichomoniasis
PATIENT/FAMILY EDUCATION
• Drug may cause GI upset; take with food
• Avoid alcoholic beverages during therapy and for at least 24 hr following last dose (disulfiram-like reaction possible)
• Drug may cause darkening of urine
• May cause an unpleasant metallic taste
• H_2 blocker must be prescribed with Helidac kit
MONITORING PARAMETERS
• CBC

---

metyrosine
(me-tye′roe-seen)
Rx: Demser
Chemical Class: α-methyl-L-tyrosine
Therapeutic Class: Pheochromocytoma agent

CLINICAL PHARMACOLOGY
Mechanism of Action: A tyrosine hydroxylase inhibitor that blocks conversion of tyrosine to dihydroxyphenylalanine, the rate limiting step in the biosynthetic pathway of catecholamines. *Therapeutic Effect:* Reduces levels of endogenous catecholamines.
Pharmacokinetics
Well absorbed from the gastrointestinal (GI) tract. Metabolized in the liver. Excreted primarily in the urine. **Half-life:** 7.2 hrs.
INDICATIONS AND DOSAGES
Pheochromocytoma (preoperative)
PO
Adults, Elderly. Initially, 250 mg 4 times/day. Increase by 250-500

mg/day up to 4 g/day. Maintenance: 2-4 g/day in 4 divided doses for 5-7 days.
S AVAILABLE FORMS/COST
• Cap, Gel—Oral: 250 mg, 100's: **$178.33**
UNLABELED USES: Tourette syndrome
CONTRAINDICATIONS: Hypertension of unknown etiology, hypersensitivity to metyrosine or any component of the formulation
PREGNANCY AND LACTATION: Pregnancy category C
SIDE EFFECTS
Frequent
Drowsiness, extrapyramidal symptoms, diarrhea
Occasional
Galactorrhea, edema of the breasts, nausea, vomiting, dry mouth, impotence, nasal congestion
Rare
Lower extremity edema, urinary problems, urticaria, anemia, depression, disorientation
SERIOUS REACTIONS
• Serious or life-threatening allergic reaction characterized hallucinations, hematuria, hyperstimulation after withdrawal, severe lower extremity edema, and parkinsonism.
INTERACTIONS
Drugs
3 *Phenothiazines, haloperidol:* Potentiation of EPS
Labs
• *False increase:* Urinary catecholamines (due to presence of metyrosine metabolites)
SPECIAL CONSIDERATIONS
PATIENT/FAMILY EDUCATION
• Maintain a daily liberal fluid intake
• Avoid alcohol or CNS depressants
MONITORING PARAMETERS
• Blood pressure, ECG

mexiletine

(mex-il'e-teen)

Rx: Mexitil

Chemical Class: Lidocaine derivative

Therapeutic Class: Antiarrhythmic, class IB

CLINICAL PHARMACOLOGY

Mechanism of Action: An antiarrhythmic that shortens duration of action potential and decreases effective refractory period in the His-Purkinje system of the myocardium by blocking sodium transport across myocardial cell membranes. *Therapeutic Effect:* Suppresses ventricular arrhythmias.

INDICATIONS AND DOSAGES

Arrhythmias

PO

Adults, Elderly. Initially, 200 mg q8h. Adjust dosage by 50–100 mg at 2– to 3-day intervals. Maximum: 1,200 mg/day.

$ **AVAILABLE FORMS/COST**

- Cap, Gel—Oral: 150 mg, 100's: **$42.47-$126.05**; 200 mg, 100's: **$54.44-$150.03**; 250 mg, 100's: **$123.83-$172.84**

UNLABELED USES: Treatment of diabetic neuropathy

CONTRAINDICATIONS: Cardiogenic shock, pre-existing second- or third-degree AV block, right bundle-branch block without presence of pacemaker

PREGNANCY AND LACTATION: Pregnancy category C; limited data do not suggest significant risk to the fetus; compatible with breast-feeding

SIDE EFFECTS

Frequent (greater than 10%)

GI distress, including nausea, vomiting, and heartburn; dizziness; light-headedness; tremor

Occasional (10%–1%)

Nervousness, change in sleep habits, headache, visual disturbances, paresthesia, diarrhea or constipation, palpitations, chest pain, rash, respiratory difficulty, edema

SERIOUS REACTIONS

- Mexiletine has the ability to worsen existing arrhythmias or produce new ones.
- CHF may occur and existing CHF may worsen.

INTERACTIONS

Drugs

3 *Acetazolamide, sodium bicarbonate:* Alkalinization of urine retards mexiletine elimination

3 *Phenytoin, rifampin:* Reduced mexiletine concentrations

3 *Quinidine:* Elevated mexiletine concentrations

② *Theophylline:* Elevated theophylline serum concentrations and toxicity

SPECIAL CONSIDERATIONS

- Because of proarrhythmic effects, not recommended for non-life threatening arrhythmias
- Antiarrhythmic drugs have not been shown to increase survival of patients with ventricular arrhythmias
- Initiate therapy in facilities capable of providing continuous ECG monitoring and managing life-threatening dysrhythmias

PATIENT/FAMILY EDUCATION

- Take with food or antacid

MONITORING PARAMETERS

- Therapeutic mexiletine concentrations 0.5-2 mcg/ml

miconazole

(mih-kon'-ah-zole)

Rx: *IV:* Monistat

Rx: *Top:* Micatin, Monistat-Derm, Fungoid Tincture Nail Kit

Rx: *Vag:* Monistat 3, Monistat 5, Monistat 7, Monistat Dual-Pak, Femizol-7

Chemical Class: Imidazole derivative

Therapeutic Class: Antifungal

CLINICAL PHARMACOLOGY

Mechanism of Action: An imidazole derivative that inhibits synthesis of ergosterol (vital component of fungal cell formation), damaging cell membraine. *Therapeutic Effect:* Fungistatic; may be fungicidal, depending on concentration.

Pharmacokinetics

Parenteral: Widely distributed in tissues. Metabolized in liver. Primarily excreted in urine. **Half-life:** 24 hrs. Topical: No systemic absorption following application to intact skin. Intravaginally: Small amount absorbed systemically.

INDICATIONS AND DOSAGES

Coccidioidomycosis

IV

Adults, Elderly. 1.8-3.6 g/day for 3-20 wks or longer.

Cryptococcosis

IV

Adults, Elderly. 1.2-2.4 g/day for 3-12 wks or longer.

Petriellidiosis

IV

Adults, Elderly. 0.6-3.0 g/day for 5-20 wks or longer.

Candidiasis

IV

Adults, Elderly. 0.6-1.8 g/day for 1-20 wks or longer.

Paracoccidioidomycosis

IV

Adults, Elderly. 0.2-1.2 g/day for 2-16 wks or longer.

Usual dosage for children

IV

20-40 mg/kg/day in 3 divided doses. (Do not exceed 15 mg/kg for any 1 infusion).

Vulvovaginal candidiasis

Intravaginally

Adults, Elderly. One 200 mg suppository at bedtime for 3 days; one 100 mg suppository or one applicatorful at bedtime for 7 days.

Topical fungal infections, cutaneous candidiasis

Topical

Adults, Elderly, Children 2 years and older. Apply liberally 2 times/day, morning and evening.

[$] **AVAILABLE FORMS/COST**

- Aer, Spray Powder—Top: 2%, 90, 105, 120 ml: **$4.55-$4.74**/90 ml
- Cre—Top: 2%, 15, 30, 60, 85 g: **$2.35-$20.43**/15 g
- Cre—Vag: 2%, 45 g: **$5.86-$8.73**; 4%, 15, 25 g: **$14.38**/15 g
- Sol, Inj—Intrathecal, IV: 10 mg/ml, 20 ml: **$192.35**
- Kit—Top Cre, Vag Supp: 2%-100 mg: **$16.44**; 2%-200 mg: **$10.16-$33.63**; 2%-1200 mg: **$28.74**
- Liq—Top: 2%, 30 ml: **$9.00-$18.00**
- Powder—Top: 2%, 90 g: **$3.51-$7.14**
- Supp—Vag: 100 mg, 7's: **$8.83-$22.81**; 200 mg, 3's: **$17.92-$41.95**
- Tampon—Vag: 100 mg, 5's: **$15.96**

CONTRAINDICATIONS: Children younger than 1 year old, hypersensitivity to miconazole or any component of the formulation

Topically: Children younger than 2 years old

PREGNANCY AND LACTATION:
Pregnancy category C (Top category B); unknown if excreted into breast milk

SIDE EFFECTS

Frequent

Phlebitis, fever, chills, rash, itching, nausea, vomiting

Occasional

Dizziness, drowsiness, headache, flushed face, abdominal pain, constipation, diarrhea, decreased appetite

Topical: Itching, burning, stinging, erythema, urticaria

Vaginal: Vulvovaginal burning, itching, irritation, headache, skin rash

SERIOUS REACTIONS

• Anemia, thrombocytopenia, and liver toxicity occur rarely

INTERACTIONS

Drugs

▨ *Aminoglycosides:* Decreased antibiotic peak levels

❷ *Cisapride:* Increased cisapride concentrations, toxicity and arrhythmias

▨ *Cyclosporine:* Possible increased cyclosporine levels

▨ *Felodipine:* Enhanced vasodilation, hypotension

❷ *HMG-CoA reductase inhibitors (e.g. lovastatin):* Increased toxicity, rhabdomyolysis

▨ *Loratadine:* Increased loratadine concentrations

▨ *Midazolam:* Reduced midazolam metabolism

▨ *Quinidine:* Increased quinidine concentrations

▨ *Tacrolimus:* Possible increased tacrolimus levels

▨ *Tolbutamide:* Inhibition of tolbutamide metabolism

▨ *Triazolam:* Reduced triazolam metabolism

▨ *Warfarin:* Enhanced anticoagulant effect

Labs

• The base in suppository products may interfere with latex; do not use these with contraceptive diaphragms, condoms

---

midazolam

(mid-az'zoe-lam)

Rx: Versed

Chemical Class: Benzodiazepine

Therapeutic Class: Sedative/hypnotic

DEA Class: Schedule IV

CLINICAL PHARMACOLOGY

Mechanism of Action: A benzodiazepine that enhances the action of gamma-aminobutyric acid, one of the major inhibitory neurotransmitters in the brain. *Therapeutic Effect:* Produces anxiolytic, hypnotic, anticonvulsant, muscle relaxant, and amnestic effects.

Pharmacokinetics

Route	Onset	Peak	Duration
PO	10-20 min	N/A	N/A
IV	1-5 min	5-7 min	20-30 min
IM	5-15 min	15-60 min	2-6 hr

Well absorbed after IM administration. Protein binding: 97%. Metabolized in the liver to active metabolite. Primarily excreted in urine. Not removed by hemodialysis. **Half-life:** 1-5 hr.

INDICATIONS AND DOSAGES

Preoperative sedation

PO

Children. 0.25-0.5 mg/kg. Maximum: 20 mg.

IV

Children 6-12 yr. 0.025-0.05 mg/kg.

Children 6 mo-5 yr. 0.05-0.1 mg/kg.

IM

Adults, Elderly. 0.07-0.08 mg/kg 30-60 min before surgery.

Children. 0.1-0.15 mg/kg 30-60 min before surgery. Maximum: 10 mg.

Conscious sedation for diagnostic, therapeutic, and endoscopic procedures

IV

Adults, Elderly. 1-2.5 mg over 2 min. Titrate as needed. Maximum total dose: 2.5-5 mg.

Conscious sedation during mechanical ventilation

IV

Adults, Elderly. 0.01-0.05 mg/kg; may repeat q10-15min until adequately sedated. Then continuous infusion at initial rate of 0.02-0.1 mg/kg/hr (1-7 mg/hr).

Children older than 32 wk. Initially, 1 mcg/kg/min as continuous infusion.

Children 32 wk and younger. Initially, 0.5 mcg/kg/min as continuous infusion.

Status epilepticus

IV

Children older than 2 mo. Loading dose of 0.15 mg/kg followed by continuous infusion of 1 mcg/kg/min. Titrate as needed. Range: 1-18 mcg/kg/min.

[$] **AVAILABLE FORMS/COST**

• Sol, Inj—IM, IV: 1 mg/ml, 2, 5, 10 ml: **$0.69-$5.55**/2 ml; 5 mg/ml, 1, 2, 5, 10 ml: **$3.41-$27.40**/2 ml

• Syrup—Oral: 2 mg/ml, 118 ml: **$127.15**

CONTRAINDICATIONS: Acute alcohol intoxication, acute angle-closure glaucoma, coma, shock

PREGNANCY AND LACTATION: Pregnancy category D; excreted in breast milk; use with caution in nursing mothers

SIDE EFFECTS

Frequent (10%-4%)

Decreased respiratory rate, tenderness at IM or IV injection site, pain during injection, oxygen desaturation, hiccups

Occasional (3%-2%)

Hypotension, paradoxical CNS reaction

Rare (less than 2%)

Nausea, vomiting, headache, coughing

SERIOUS REACTIONS

• Inadequate or excessive dosage or improper administration may result in cerebral hypoxia, agitation, involuntary movements, hyperactivity, and combativeness.

• A too-rapid IV rate, excessive doses, or a single large dose increases the risk of respiratory depression or arrest.

• Respiratory depression or apnea may produce hypoxia and cardiac arrest.

INTERACTIONS

Drugs

[3] *Calcium channel blockers, erythromycin, ketoconazole, itraconazole:* Increased midazolam levels; increased sedation; respiratory depression

[3] *CNS depressants:* Additive effects with other CNS depressants

midodrine

(mid'o-dreen)

Rx: ProAmatine

Chemical Class: Catecholamine, synthetic

Therapeutic Class: Vasopressor; α-adrenergic sympathomimetic amine

CLINICAL PHARMACOLOGY

Mechanism of Action: A vasopressor that forms the active metabolite desglymidodrine, an alpha$_1$-agonist, activating alpha receptors of the arteriolar and venous vasculature. *Therapeutic Effect:* Increases vascular tone and BP.

INDICATIONS AND DOSAGES
Orthostatic hypotension
PO
Adults, Elderly. 10 mg 3 times a day. Give during the day when patient is upright, such as upon arising, midday, and late afternoon. Do not give later than 6 p.m.
Dosage in renal impairment
For adults and elderly patients, give 2.5 mg 3 times a day; increase gradually, as tolerated.

AVAILABLE FORMS/COST
• Tab—Oral: 2.5 mg, 100's: **$120.10-$142.93**; 5 mg, 100's: **$241.80-$287.78**; 10 mg, 100's: **$483.60-$575.55**

CONTRAINDICATIONS: Acute renal function impairment, persistent hypertension, pheochromocytoma, severe cardiac disease, thyrotoxicosis, urine retention

PREGNANCY AND LACTATION: Pregnancy category C; unknown if excreted in breast milk

SIDE EFFECTS
Frequent (20%–7%)
Paresthesia, piloerection, pruritus, dysuria, supine hypertension
Occasional (less than 7%–1%)
Pain, rash, chills, headache, facial flushing, confusion, dry mouth, anxiety

SERIOUS REACTIONS
• None known.

INTERACTIONS
Drugs
❷ *α-adrenergic agonists:* Enhanced pressor response
❸ *α-adrenergic antagonists:* Antagonism of midodrine's effects
❸ *Cardiac glycosides, β-blockers:* Increased risk of bradycardia, AV block, arrhythmia

SPECIAL CONSIDERATIONS
• Advantages include rapid and nearly complete absorption, a long elimination t$_{1/2}$, lack of central nervous system (CNS) penetration, and minimal to no cardiac effects
• Supine hypertension has been a therapy-limiting complication

PATIENT/FAMILY EDUCATION
• To minimize supine hypertension, avoid taking drug after the evening meal

---

mifepristone
(miff-eh-pris'tone)
Rx: Mifeprex, RU-486
Chemical Class: Antiprogestational agent; progestin derivative
Therapeutic Class: Abortifacient

CLINICAL PHARMACOLOGY
Mechanism of Action: An abortifacient that has antiprogestational activity resulting from competitive interaction with progesterone. Inhibits the activity of endogenous or exogenous progesterone. Also has antiglucocorticoid and weak antiandrogenic activity. *Therapeutic Effect:* Terminates pregnancy.

INDICATIONS AND DOSAGES
Termination of pregnancy
PO
Adults. Day 1: 600 mg as single dose. Day 3: 400 mcg misoprostol. Day 14: Post-treatment examination.

AVAILABLE FORMS/COST
• Tab—Oral: 200 mg, 3's: **$250.00**

UNLABELED USES: Cushing's syndrome, endometriosis, intrauterine fetal death or nonviable early pregnancy, postcoital contraception or contragestation, unresectable meningioma

CONTRAINDICATIONS: Chronic adrenal failure, concurrent long-term steroid or anticoagulant therapy, confirmed or suspected ectopic pregnancy, intrauterine device (IUD) in place, hemorrhagic disorders, inherited porphyria

PREGNANCY AND LACTATION: Pregnancy category X; excretion in human milk unknown but likely

SIDE EFFECTS

Frequent (greater than 10%)

Headache, dizziness, abdominal pain, nausea, vomiting, diarrhea, fatigue

Occasional (10%–3%)

Uterine hemorrhage, insomnia, vaginitis, dyspepsia, back pain, fever, viral infections, rigors

Rare (2%–1%)

Anxiety, syncope, anemia, asthenia, leg pain, sinusitis, leukorrhea

SERIOUS REACTIONS

• None known.

INTERACTIONS

Drugs

▣ *Ketoconazole, itraconazole, erythromycin, grapefruit juice:* May inhibit mifepristone metabolism, raising serum levels

▣ *Rifampin, dexamethasone, St. John's Wort, phenytoin, phenobarbital, carbamazepine:* May induce mifepristone metabolism, lowering serum levels

SPECIAL CONSIDERATIONS

• Provided only to licensed physicians who sign and return a Prescriber's Agreement. Not available through pharmacies

• Patients should be given the Medication Guide and sign the Patient Agreement (Danco Laboratories, 1-877-432-7596)

• Provide medication for cramping and GI symptoms, instructions on what to do if significant bleeding or other adverse reactions occur

• Advise patient bleeding/spotting occur for average of 9-16 days; 8% have some bleeding for >30 days

• Expulsion occurs within the first 48hs in 6%, in 63-72% within 24 hr of misoprostol administration (most of these within 4 hr), surgical intervention in 4.5-8%

• Quantitative hCG levels not decisive until ≥10 days following mifepristone administration. Confirm continuing pregnancy by ultrasound scan. Uterine debris does not necessarily require surgical removal

• Report adverse events (blood transfusion, hospitalization, ongoing pregnancy) in writing to Medical Director, Danco Laboratories LLC, PO Box 4816, New York, NY 10185

• For 24 hr/day consultation contact Danco Laboratories at 1-877-432-7596

PATIENT/FAMILY EDUCATION

• Completing treatment schedule is important, including the 48 hr visit for misoprostol and the post treatment follow-up visit at 14 days

• Vaginal bleeding and uterine cramping will occur, but are not proof of complete expulsion

• There is a risk of fetal malformation if treatment fails

• Treatment failure is managed by surgical termination

• Contraception should be initiated as soon as pregnancy termination has been confirmed

milrinone

(mill're-none)

Rx: Primacor

Chemical Class: Bipyridine derivative

Therapeutic Class: Cardiac inotropic agent

CLINICAL PHARMACOLOGY

Mechanism of Action: A cardiac inotropic agent that inhibits phosphodiesterase, which increases cyclic adenosine monophosphate and potentiates the delivery of calcium to myocardial contractile systems. *Therapeutic Effect:* Relaxes vascular muscle, causing vasodilation. Increases cardiac output; decreases pulmonary capillary wedge pressure and vascular resistance.

Pharmacokinetics

Route	*Onset*	*Peak*	*Duration*
IV	5–15 min	N/A	N/A

Protein binding: 70%. Primarily excreted unchanged in urine. **Half-life:** 2.4 hr.

INDICATIONS AND DOSAGES

Short-term management of CHF

IV

Adults. Initially, 50 mcg/kg over 10 min. Continue with maintenance infusion rate of 0.375–0.75 mcg/kg/min based on hemodynamic and clinical response. Total daily dosage: 0.59–1.13 mg/kg.

Dosage in renal impairment

For patients with severe renal impairment, reduce dosage to 0.2–0.43 mcg/kg/min.

[$] AVAILABLE FORMS/COST

• Sol, Inj—IV: 1 mg/ml, 5, 10 ml: **$51.70-$52.01**/5 ml

CONTRAINDICATIONS: None known

PREGNANCY AND LACTATION: Pregnancy category C; caution with breast-feeding until more known about excretion in breast milk

SIDE EFFECTS

Occasional (3%–1%)

Headache, hypotension

Rare (less than 1%)

Angina, chest pain

SERIOUS REACTIONS

• Supraventricular and ventricular arrhythmias (12%), nonsustained ventricular tachycardia (2%), and sustained ventricular tachycardia (1%) may occur.

SPECIAL CONSIDERATIONS

MONITORING PARAMETERS

• Fluid and electrolyte changes, renal function

• Improvement in cardiac output may increase diuresis, and K^+ loss

minocycline

(mi-noe-sye'kleen)

Rx: Dynacin, Minocin

Chemical Class: Tetracycline derivative

Therapeutic Class: Antibiotic

CLINICAL PHARMACOLOGY

Mechanism of Action: A tetracycline antibiotic that inhibits bacterial protein synthesis by binding to ribosomes. *Therapeutic Effects:* Bacteriostatic.

INDICATIONS AND DOSAGES

Mild, moderate, or severe prostate, urinary tract, and CNS infections (excluding meningitis); uncomplicated gonorrhea; inflammatory acne; brucellosis; skin granulomas; cholera; trachoma; nocardiasis; yaws; and syphilis when penicillins are contraindicated

PO

Adults, Elderly. Initially, 100-200 mg, then 100 mg q12h or 50 mg q6h.

IV
Adults, Elderly. Initially, 200 mg, then 100 mg q12h up to 400 mg/day.
PO, IV
Children older than 8 yr. Initially, 4 mg/kg, then 2 mg/kg q12h.

AVAILABLE FORMS/COST
• Cap, Gel—Oral: 50 mg, 100's: **$118.40-$274.51**; 75 mg, 100's: **$197.96-$403.02**; 100 mg, 60's: **$56.30-$155.89**
• Insert—Subgingival: 1 mg, 12's: **$70.97**
• Powder, Inj—IV: 100 mg/vial: **$46.38**
• Tab—Oral: 75 mg, 100's: **$403.01**; 100 mg, 50's: **$240.58**

UNLABELED USES: Treatment of atypical mycobacterial infections, rheumatoid arthritis, scleroderma

CONTRAINDICATIONS: Children younger than 8 years, hypersensitivity to tetracyclines, last half of pregnancy

PREGNANCY AND LACTATION: Pregnancy category D; not recommended in last half of pregnancy secondary to adverse effects on fetal teeth; not recommended in breast-feeding

SIDE EFFECTS
Frequent
Dizziness, light-headedness, diarrhea, nausea, vomiting, abdominal cramps, possibly severe photosensitivity , drowsiness, vertigo
Occasional
Altered pigmentation of skin or mucous membranes, rectal or genital pruritus, stomatitis

SERIOUS REACTIONS
• Superinfection (especially fungal), anaphylaxis, and benign intracranial hypertension may occur.
• Bulging fontanelles occur rarely in infants.

INTERACTIONS
Drugs
▣ *Antacids:* Decreased effect of minocycline
▣ *Barbiturates:* Decreased effect of minocycline
❷ *Bismuth:* Inhibited antibiotic absorption
▣ *Carbamazepine:* Decreased effect of minocycline
▣ *Colestipol, cholestyramine:* Inhibited antibiotic absorption
▣ *Digoxin:* Increased digoxin levels in 10% of patients
▣ *Iron:* Decreased minocycline absorption
❷ *Methoxyflurane:* Renal toxicity
▣ *Oral contraceptives:* Decreased contraceptive efficacy
▣ *Penicillins:* Antagonizes antibacterial effect of penicillins
▣ *Warfarin:* Possible increase in hypoprothrombinemic response

SPECIAL CONSIDERATIONS
PATIENT/FAMILY EDUCATION
• May take with food
• Avoid sun exposure

---

minoxidil
(min-nox'i-dill)
Rx: *Oral:* Loniten
OTC: Rogaine
Chemical Class: Piperidinopyrimidine derivative
Therapeutic Class: Antihypertensive; direct vasodilator; hair growth stimulant (topical use)

CLINICAL PHARMACOLOGY
Mechanism of Action: An antihypertensive and hair growth stimulant that has direct action on vascular smooth muscle, producing vasodilation of arterioles. *Therapeutic Effect:* Decreases peripheral vascular resistance and BP; increases cu-

taneous blood flow; stimulates hair follicle epithelium and hair follicle growth.

Pharmacokinetics

Route	Onset	Peak	Duration
PO	0.5 hr	2–8 hr	2–5 days

Well absorbed from the GI tract; minimal absorption after topical application. Protein binding: None. Widely distributed. Metabolized in the liver to active metabolite. Primarily excreted in urine. Removed by hemodialysis. **Half-life:** 4.2 hr.

INDICATIONS AND DOSAGES

Severe symptomatic hypertension, hypertension associated with organ damage, hypertension that has failed to respond to maximal therapeutic dosages of a diuretic or two other antihypertensives

PO

Adults. Initially, 5 mg/day. Increase with at least 3-day intervals to 10 mg, then 20 mg, then up to 40 mg/day in 1–2 doses.

Elderly. Initially, 2.5 mg/day. May increase gradually. Maintenance: 10–40 mg/day. Maximum: 100 mg/day.

Children. Initially, 0.1–0.2 mg/kg (5 mg maximum) daily. Gradually increase at minimum 3-day intervals. Maintenance: 0.25–1 mg/kg/day in 1–2 doses. Maximum: 50 mg/day.

Hair regrowth

Topical

Adults. 1 ml to affected areas of scalp 2 times a day. Total daily dose not to exceed 2 ml.

$ AVAILABLE FORMS/COST

• Sol—Top: 2%, 60 ml: **$9.70-$23.50**; 5%, 60 ml: **$8.99-$25.20**

• Tab—Oral: 2.5 mg, 100's: **$22.01-$91.73**; 10 mg, 100's: **$53.50-$200.20**

CONTRAINDICATIONS: Pheochromocytoma

PREGNANCY AND LACTATION: Pregnancy category C; compatible with breast-feeding

SIDE EFFECTS

Frequent

PO: Edema with concurrent weight gain, hypertrichosis (elongation, thickening, increased pigmentation of fine body hair; develops in 80% of patients within 3–6 weeks after beginning therapy)

Occasional

PO: T-wave changes (usually revert to pretreatment state with continued therapy or drug withdrawal)

Topical: Pruritus, rash, dry or flaking skin, erythema

Rare

PO: Breast tenderness, headache, photosensitivity reaction

Topical: Allergic reaction, alopecia, burning sensation at scalp, soreness at hair root, headache, visual disturbances

SERIOUS REACTIONS

• Tachycardia and angina pectoris may occur because of increased oxygen demands associated with increased heart rate and cardiac output.

• Fluid and electrolyte imbalance and CHF may occur, especially if a diuretic is not given concurrently with minoxidil.

• Too rapid reduction in BP may result in syncope, CVA, MI, and ocular or vestibular ischemia.

• Pericardial effusion and tamponade may be seen in patients with impaired renal function who are not on dialysis.

INTERACTIONS

Drugs

❷ *Guanethidine:* Orthostatic hypotension, may be severe

Labs

• No known interactions with top sol

SPECIAL CONSIDERATIONS
• Must be used in conjunction with diuretic (except dialysis patients) and β-blocker or other sympathetic nervous system depressant (to prevent reflex tachycardia)

PATIENT/FAMILY EDUCATION
• At least 4 mo of bid application necessary before evidence of hair growth with topical solution
• Continued treatment necessary to maintain or increase hair growth with topical solution

---

mirtazapine
(mir-taz′a-peen)
Rx: Remeron
Chemical Class: Tetracyclic piperazino-azepine derivative
Therapeutic Class: Antidepressant

CLINICAL PHARMACOLOGY
Mechanism of Action: A tetracyclic compound that acts as an antagonist at presynaptic alpha$_2$-adrenergic receptors, increasing both norepinephrine and serotonin neurotransmission. Has low anticholinergic activity. *Therapeutic Effect:* Relieves depression and produces sedative effects.

Pharmacokinetics
Rapidly and completely absorbed after PO administration; absorption not affected by food. Protein binding: 85%. Metabolized in the liver. Primarily excreted in urine. Unknown if removed by hemodialysis. **Half-life:** 20-40 hr (longer in males [37 hr] than females [26 hr]).

INDICATIONS AND DOSAGES
Depression
PO
Adults. Initially, 15 mg at bedtime. May increase by 15 mg/day q1-2wk. Maximum: 45 mg/day.

Elderly. Initially, 7.5 mg at bedtime. May increase by 7.5-15 mg/day q1-2wk. Maximum: 45 mg/day.

[S] AVAILABLE FORMS/COST
• Tab—Oral: 15 mg, 30's: **$81.45-$94.59**; 30 mg, 30's: **$83.90-$97.43**; 45 mg, 30's: **$85.50-$99.30**
• Tab, Disintegrating—Oral: 15 mg, 30's: **$70.83-$78.71**; 30 mg, 30's: **$72.98-$81.10**; 45 mg, 30's: **$86.41**

CONTRAINDICATIONS: Use within 14 days of MAOIs

PREGNANCY AND LACTATION: Unknown if excreted in breast milk

SIDE EFFECTS
Frequent
Somnolence (54%), dry mouth (25%), increased appetite (17%), constipation (13%), weight gain (12%)

Occasional
Asthenia (8%), dizziness (7%), flu-like symptoms (5%), abnormal dreams (4%)

Rare
Abdominal discomfort, vasodilation, paresthesia, acne, dry skin, thirst, arthralgia

SERIOUS REACTIONS
• Mirtazapine poses a higher risk of seizures than tricyclic antidepressants, especially in those with no previous history of seizures.
• Overdose may produce cardiovascular effects, such as severe orthostatic hypotension, dizziness, tachycardia, palpitations, and arrhythmias.
• Abrupt discontinuation after prolonged therapy may produce headache, malaise, nausea, vomiting, and vivid dreams.
• Agranulocytosis occurs rarely.

INTERACTIONS
Drugs
⚠ *MAOIs:* Possible serotonin syndrome (hyperthermia, autonomic instability, seizures, death)

M

SPECIAL CONSIDERATIONS
- Chemical structure unrelated to TCAs, SSRIs, MAOIs
- Shown to be an effective antidepressant in several trials but place in therapy not yet determined
- Manufacturer recommends stopping MAOI 14 days before initiating therapy secondary to interactions between MAOIs and other antidepressants

---

misoprostol
(mis-oh-pros-toll)
Rx: Cytotec
Combinations
   Rx: with diclofenac (Arthrotec)
Chemical Class: Prostaglandin E₁ analog

Chemical Class: Prostaglandin E_1 analog
Therapeutic Class: Abortifacient; gastrointestinal protectant

CLINICAL PHARMACOLOGY
Mechanism of Action: A prostaglandin that inhibits basal, nocturnal gastric acid secretion via direct action on parietal cells. *Therapeutic Effect:* Increases production of protective gastric mucus.
Pharmacokinetics
Rapidly absorbed from gastrointestinal (GI) tract. Rapidly converted to active metabolite. Primarily excreted in urine. **Half-life:** 20-40 min.

INDICATIONS AND DOSAGES
Prevention of NSAID-induced gastric ulcer
PO
Adults. 200 mcg 4 times/day with food (last dose at bedtime). Continue for duration of NSAID therapy. May reduce dosage to 100 mcg if 200 mcg dose is not tolerable.

Elderly: 100-200 mcg 4 times/day with food.

▒ AVAILABLE FORMS/COST
- Tab—Oral: 100 mcg, 60's: **$46.80-$60.12**; 200 mcg, 60's: **$53.51-$80.46**

UNLABELED USES: Treatment of duodenal ulcer

CONTRAINDICATIONS: Pregnancy (produces uterine contractions), hypersensitivity to misoprostol or any component of the formulation

PREGNANCY AND LACTATION: Pregnancy category X; do not use in breast-feeding (possible diarrhea in infant)

SIDE EFFECTS
Frequent
Abdominal pain, diarrhea
Occasional
Nausea, flatulence, dyspepsia, headache
Rare
Vomiting, constipation

SERIOUS REACTIONS
- Overdosage may produce sedation, tremor, convulsions, dyspnea, palpitations, hypotension, and bradycardia.

INTERACTIONS
Drugs
▨ *Phenylbutazone:* Increase in adverse effects (headache, flushes, dizziness, nausea)

SPECIAL CONSIDERATIONS
- Reserve use for those patients at high risk for NSAID-induced ulcer (e.g., elderly, history of previous ulcer)
- Does not prevent NSAID-associated GI pain or discomfort

modafinil

Rx: Provigil
Chemical Class: Benzhydryl-sulfinylacetamide compound
Therapeutic Class: Central nervous system stimulant

CLINICAL PHARMACOLOGY

Mechanism of Action: An alpha$_1$-agonist that may bind to dopamine reuptake carrier sites, increasing alpha activity and decreasing delta, theta, and beta brain wave activity. *Therapeutic Effect:* Reduces the number of sleep episodes and total daytime sleep.

Pharmacokinetics

Well absorbed. Protein binding: 60%. Widely distributed. Metabolized in the liver. Excreted by the kidneys. Unknown if removed by hemodialysis. **Half-life:** 8-10 hr.

INDICATIONS AND DOSAGES

Narcolepsy, other sleep disorders
PO
Adults, Elderly. 200-400 mg/day.

S **AVAILABLE FORMS/COST**
• Tab—Oral: 100 mg, 100's: **$440.00**; 200 mg, 100's: **$609.00**

UNLABELED USES: Treatment of depression

CONTRAINDICATIONS: None known.

PREGNANCY AND LACTATION: Pregnancy category C; no mutagenic or clastogenic potential in several *in vitro* assays; *in vivo* mouse bone marrow micronucleus assays were also negative for mutagenicity; not fully evaluated; breast milk excretion unknown

SIDE EFFECTS

Frequent
Anxiety, insomnia, nausea, nervousness

Occasional
Anorexia, diarrhea, dizziness, dry mouth or skin, muscle stiffness, polydipsia, rhinitis, paraesthesia, tremor, headache, vomiting

SERIOUS REACTIONS
• Agitation, excitation, hypertension, and insomnia may occur.

SPECIAL CONSIDERATIONS

• Comparisons of modafinil with agents that have proven effective in narcolepsy, including methylphenidate, pemoline, and dextroamphetamine, are needed to clarify its relative safety and efficacy, and place in therapy

MONITORING PARAMETERS
• *Efficacy:* Daytime sleepiness, daytime sleep episodes, and overall daily performance
• *Toxicity:* Blood pressure

moexipril

(moe-ex'a-prile)
Rx: Univasc
Combinations
　Rx: with hydrochlorothiazide (Uniretic)
Chemical Class: Angiotensin-converting enzyme (ACE) inhibitor, nonsulfhydryl
Therapeutic Class: Antihypertensive

CLINICAL PHARMACOLOGY

Mechanism of Action: An ACE inhibitor that suppresses the renin-angiotensin-aldosterone system and prevents conversion of angiotensin I to angiotensin II, a potent vasoconstrictor; may also inhibit angiotensin II at local vascular and renal sites. *Therapeutic Effect:* Reduces peripheral arterial resistance and lowers BP.

Pharmacokinetics

Route	Onset	Peak	Duration
PO	1 hr	3–6 hr	24 hr

Incompletely absorbed from the GI tract. Food decreases drug absorption. Rapidly converted to active metabolite. Protein binding: 50%. Primarily recovered in feces, partially excreted in urine. Unknown if removed by dialysis. **Half-life:** 1 hr, metabolite 2–9 hr.

INDICATIONS AND DOSAGES
Hypertension
PO

Adults, Elderly. For patients not receiving diuretics, initial dose is 7.5 mg once a day 1 hr before meals. Adjust according to BP effect. Maintenance: 7.5–30 mg a day in 1–2 divided doses 1 hr before meals.

Hypertension in patients with impaired renal function
PO

Adults, Elderly. 3.75 mg once a day in patients with creatinine clearance of 40 ml/min. Maximum: May titrate up to 15 mg/day.

$ AVAILABLE FORMS/COST
• Tab—Oral: 7.5, 15 mg, 100's; all: **$87.94-$109.99**

CONTRAINDICATIONS: History of angioedema from previous treatment with ACE inhibitors

PREGNANCY AND LACTATION: Pregnancy category D; ACE inhibitors can cause fetal and neonatal morbidity and death when administered to pregnant women; when pregnancy is detected, discontinue ACE inhibitors as soon as possible

SIDE EFFECTS
Occasional

Cough, headache (6%); dizziness (4%); fatigue (3%)

Rare

Flushing, rash, myalgia, nausea, vomiting

SERIOUS REACTIONS
• Excessive hypotension (first-dose syncope) may occur in patients with CHF and in those who are severely salt or volume depleted.
• Angioedema (swelling of face and lips) and hyperkalemia occur rarely.
• Agranulocytosis and neutropenia may be noted in those with collagen vascular disease, including scleroderma and systemic lupus erythematosus, and impaired renal function.
• Nephrotic syndrome may be noted in those with history of renal disease.

INTERACTIONS
Drugs

② *Allopurinol:* Combination may predispose to hypersensitivity reactions

③ *α-adrenergic blockers:* Exaggerated first dose hypotensive reactions when added to moexipril

③ *Aspirin:* May reduce hemodynamic effects of moexipril; less likely at doses under 236 mg; less likely with nonacetylated salicylates

③ *Azathioprine:* Increased myelosuppression

③ *Cyclosporine:* Combination may cause renal insufficiency

③ *Insulin:* Moexipril may enhance insulin sensitivity

③ *Iron:* Moexipril may increase chance of systemic reaction to IV iron

③ *Lithium:* Reduced lithium clearance

③ *Loop diuretics:* Initiation of moexipril may cause hypotension and renal insufficiency in patients taking loop diuretics

③ *NSAIDs:* May reduce hemodynamic effects of moexipril

③ *Potassium-sparing diuretics:* Increased risk of hyperkalemia

[3] *Trimethoprim:* Additive risk of hyperkalemia, especially in patient predisposed to renal insufficiency

Labs

• ACE inhibition can account for approximately 0.5 mEq/L rise in serum potassium

SPECIAL CONSIDERATIONS

PATIENT/FAMILY EDUCATION

• Caution with salt substitutes containing potassium chloride
• Rise slowly to sitting/standing position to minimize orthostatic hypotension
• Dizziness, fainting, lightheadedness may occur during first few days of therapy
• May cause altered taste perception or cough; persistent dry cough usually does not subside unless medication is stopped; notify clinician if these symptoms persist

MONITORING PARAMETERS

• BUN, creatinine, potassium within 2 wk after initiation of therapy (increased levels may indicate acute renal failure)

molindone

(moe-lin-'done)

Rx: Moban

Chemical Class: Dihydroindolone derivative

Therapeutic Class: Antipsychotic

CLINICAL PHARMACOLOGY

Mechanism of Action: An indole derivative of dihydroindole compounds that reduces spontaneous locomotion and aggressiveness. *Therapeutic Effect:* Suppresses behavioral response in psychosis.

Pharmacokinetics

Rapidly absorbed from the gastrointestinal (GI) tract. Metabolized in liver. Excreted feces, and a small amount excreted via lungs as carbon dioxide. Not removed by dialysis. **Half-life:** unknown.

INDICATIONS AND DOSAGES

Schizophrenia

PO

Adults, Children 12 yrs and older. Initially, 50-75 mg/day, increased to 100 mg/day in 3-4 days. Maintenance: 5-15 mg 3-4 times/day (mild psychosis). Maintenance: 10-25 mg 3-4 times/day (moderate psychosis). Maintenance: 225 mg/day maximum in divided doses (severe psychosis).

Elderly. Start at a lower dose.

[$] **AVAILABLE FORMS/COST**

• Conc—Oral: 20 mg/ml, 120 ml: **$254.81**
• Tab—Oral: 5 mg, 100's: **$132.31**; 10 mg, 100's: **$190.19**; 25 mg, 100's: **$283.69**; 50 mg, 100's: **$378.94**; 100 mg, 100's: **$459.06**

CONTRAINDICATIONS: Severe central nervous system (CNS) depression, hypersensitivity to molindone or any component of the formulation

PREGNANCY AND LACTATION: Pregnancy category C

SIDE EFFECTS

Frequent

Blurred vision, constipation, drowsiness, headache, extrapyramidal symptoms

Occasional

Mental depression

Rare

Skin rash, hot and dry skin, inability to sweat, muscle weakness, confusion, jaundice, convulsions

SERIOUS REACTIONS

• Neuroleptic malignant syndrome or tardive dyskinesia has been reported.

INTERACTIONS

Drugs

[3] *Barbiturates:* Reduce serum levels of molindone

⬛ *Benztropine:* May inhibit therapeutic response to molindone

⬛ *Bromocriptine:* May inhibit therapeutic response to molindone; molindone may inhibit therapeutic effect of bromocriptine on hyperprolactinemia

⬛ *Carbamazepine:* Reduces serum levels of molindone

⬛ *Fluoxetine:* Increases serum levels of molindone

⬛ *Guanethidine:* Reduced antihypertensive effect of guanethidine

⬛ *Indomethacin:* May increase risk of CNS side effects of molindone

❷ *Levodopa:* Molindone reduces antiparkinsonian effects of levodopa

⬛ *Lithium:* May reduce serum levels of lithium

⬛ *Orphenadrine:* Reduces serum levels of molindone

⬛ *Paroxetine:* Increases serum levels of molindone

⬛ *Quinidine:* Increases serum levels of molindone

⬛ *Trihexyphenidyl:* May inhibit therapeutic response to molindone

SPECIAL CONSIDERATIONS

• Neuroleptic structurally different from the phenothiazines, thioxanthenes, and butyrophenones

• High potency with high incidence of EPS, but a low incidence of sedation, anticholinergic effects, and cardiovascular effects

mometasone
(mo-met'a-sone)
Rx: Elocon, Nasonex
Chemical Class: Corticosteroid, synthetic
Therapeutic Class: Corticosteroid, topical

CLINICAL PHARMACOLOGY
Mechanism of Action: An adrenocorticosteroid that inhibits the release of inlammatory cells into nasal tissue, preventing early activation of the allergic reaction. *Therapeutic Effect:* Decreases response to seasonal and perennial rhinitis.
Pharmacokinetics
Undetectable in plasma. Protein binding: 98%–99%. The swallowed portion undergoes extensive metabolism. Excreted primarily through bile and, to a lesser extent, urine.

INDICATIONS AND DOSAGES
Allergic rhinitis
Nasal spray
Adults, Elderly, Children 12 yr and older. 2 sprays in each nostril once a day.
Children 2–11 yr. 1 spray in each nostril once a day.

⬛ AVAILABLE FORMS/COST
• Cre—Top: 0.1%, 15, 45 g: **$21.95-$27.18**/15 g
• Lotion—Top: 0.1%, 30, 60 ml: **$29.45**/30 ml
• Oint—Top: 0.1%, 15, 45 g: **$24.30-$27.18**/15 g
• Spray—Nasal: 0.05 mg/inh, 17 g: **$72.16**

CONTRAINDICATIONS: Hypersensitivity to any corticosteroid, persistently positive sputum cultures for *Candida albicans*, systemic fungal infections, untreated localized infection involving nasal mucosa.

PREGNANCY AND LACTATION: Pregnancy category C; systemic corticosteroids are excreted into breast milk in quantities not likely to have deleterious effects in breast-feeding infants; no information on topical steroids

SIDE EFFECTS

Occasional

Nasal irritation, stinging

Rare

Nasal or pharyngeal candidiasis

SERIOUS REACTIONS

• An acute hypersensitivity reaction, including urticaria, angioedema, and severe bronchospasm, occurs rarely.

• Transfer from systemic to local steroid therapy may unmask previously suppressed bronchial asthma condition.

INTERACTIONS

Labs

• *Interference:* With adrenal function as assessed by corticotropin stimulation, 24-hr urine-free cortisol measurements; plasma cortisol

---

monobenzone
(mon-oh-benz-one)
Rx: Benoquin
Chemical Class: Hydroquinone derivative
Therapeutic Class: Depigmenting agent

CLINICAL PHARMACOLOGY
Mechanism of Action: The mechanism of action is not fully understood. Monobenzone may be converted to hydroquinone, which inhibits the enzymatic oxidation of tyrosine to DOPA; it may have a direct action on tyrosinase; or, it may act as an anti-oxidant to prevent SH-group oxidation so that more SH groups is available to inhibit tyrosinase. *Therapeutic Effect:* Depigmentation in extensive vitiligo.

Pharmacokinetics
Not fully understood. Initial response occurs in 1-4 months.

INDICATIONS AND DOSAGES
Vitiligo
Topical
Adults, Elderly. Apply 2-3 times/day to affected area.

$ AVAILABLE FORMS/COST
• Cre—Top: 20%, 37.5 g: **$45.21**

CONTRAINDICATIONS: History of hypersensitivity to monobenzone or any of its components.

PREGNANCY AND LACTATION: Pregnancy category C; excretion into breast milk unknown

SIDE EFFECTS
Occasional
Irritation, burning sensation, dermatitis

SERIOUS REACTIONS
• None known.

SPECIAL CONSIDERATIONS
PATIENT/FAMILY EDUCATION
• Drug is not a mild cosmetic bleach; treated areas should not be exposed to sunlight (protect with a topical sunscreen)

---

montelukast
(mon-te'loo-kast)
Rx: Singulair
Chemical Class: Cyclopropaneacetic acid derivative
Therapeutic Class: Antiasthmatic; leukotriene receptor antagonist

---

CLINICAL PHARMACOLOGY
Mechanism of Action: An antiasthmatic that binds to cysteinyl leukotriene receptors, inhibiting the effects of leukotrienes on bronchial smooth muscle. *Therapeutic Effect:* De-

M

creases bronchoconstriction, vascular permeability, mucosal edema, and mucus production.

Pharmacokinetics

Route	Onset	Peak	Duration
PO	N/A	N/A	24 hr
PO (chewable)	N/A	N/A	24 hr

Rapidly absorbed from the GI tract. Protein binding: 99%. Extensively metabolized in the liver. Excreted almost exclusively in feces. **Half-life:** 2.7–5.5 hr (slightly longer in the elderly).

INDICATIONS AND DOSAGES

Bronchial asthma

PO

Adults, Elderly, Adolescents older than 14 yr. One 10-mg tablet a day, taken in the evening.

Children 6–14 yr. One 5-mg chewable tablet a day, taken in the evening.

Children 1–5 yr. One 4-mg chewable tablet a day, taken in the evening.

Ⓢ **AVAILABLE FORMS/COST**

• Granules—Oral: 4 mg/packet, 30's: **$93.90**
• Tab, Coated—Oral: 10 mg, 90's: **$270.43**
• Tab, Chewable—Oral: 4 mg, 5 mg, 90's; all: **$270.43**

CONTRAINDICATIONS: None known.

PREGNANCY AND LACTATION: Pregnancy category B; excretion into breast milk unknown, use caution in nursing mothers

SIDE EFFECTS

Adults, Adolescents older than 14 years

Frequent (18%)

Headache

Occasional (4%)

Influenza

Rare (3%–2%)

Abdominal pain, cough, dyspepsia, dizziness, fatigue, dental pain

Children 6–14 years

Rare (less than 2%)

Diarrhea, laryngitis, pharyngitis, nausea, otitis media, sinusitis, viral infection

SERIOUS REACTIONS

• None known.

SPECIAL CONSIDERATIONS

PATIENT/FAMILY EDUCATION

• Take regularly, even during symptom-free periods

MONITORING PARAMETERS

• Pulmonary function tests

---

moricizine

(mor-iss'i-zeen)

Rx: Ethmozine

Chemical Class: Phenothiazine derivative

Therapeutic Class: Antiarrhythmic, class IA

CLINICAL PHARMACOLOGY

Mechanism of Action: An antiarrhythmic that prevents sodium current across myocardial cell membranes. Has potent local anesthetic activity and membrane stabilizing effects. Slows AV and His-Purkinje conduction and decreases action potential duration and effective refractory period. *Therapeutic Effect:* Suppresses ventricular arrhythmias.

INDICATIONS AND DOSAGES

Arrhythmias

PO

Adults, Elderly. 200–300 mg q8h. May increase by 150 mg/day at no less than 3-day intervals.

Ⓢ **AVAILABLE FORMS/COST**

• Tab, Coated—Oral: 200 mg, 100's: **$120.61**; 250 mg, 100's: **$137.14**; 300 mg, 100's: **$163.94**

UNLABELED USES: Atrial arrhythmias, complete and non-sustained ventricular arrhythmias, premature ventricular contractions (PVCs)

CONTRAINDICATIONS: Cardiogenic shock, pre-existing second- or third-degree AV block or right bundle-branch block without pacemaker

PREGNANCY AND LACTATION: Pregnancy category B; secreted into breast milk (1 patient); potential for serious adverse effects exists

SIDE EFFECTS

Frequent (15%–6%)

Dizziness, nausea, headache, fatigue, dyspnea

Occasional (5%–2%)

Nervousness, paresthesia, sleep disturbances, dyspepsia, vomiting, diarrhea

SERIOUS REACTIONS

• Moricizine may worsen existing arrhythmias or produce new ones.

• Jaundice with hepatitis occurs rarely.

• Overdosage produces vomiting, lethargy, syncope, hypotension, conduction disturbances, exacerbation of CHF, MI, and sinus arrest.

INTERACTIONS

Drugs

3 *Cimetidine:* Increases serum moricizine concentrations

3 *Theophylline:* Reduces serum theophylline levels by increasing clearance

SPECIAL CONSIDERATIONS

• Antidysrhythmic therapy has not been proven to be beneficial in terms of improving survival among patients with asymptomatic or mildly symptomatic ventricular dysrhythmias

• Studied in the CAST (Cardiac Arrhythmia Suppression Trial, I and II) with findings of excessive cardiac mortality and no benefit on long-term survival compared to placebo

• Initiate therapy in facilities capable of providing continuous ECG monitoring and managing life threatening dysrhythmias

---

morphine

(mor′feen)

Rx: Astramorph, Avinza, DepoDur, Duramorph, Infumorph, Kadian, MS Contin, MSIR, Oramorph SR, RMS, Roxanol

Chemical Class: Natural opium alkaloid; phenanthrene derivative

Therapeutic Class: Narcotic analgesic

DEA Class: Schedule II

CLINICAL PHARMACOLOGY

Mechanism of Action: An opioid agonist that binds with opioid receptors in the CNS. *Therapeutic Effect:* Alters the perception of and emotional response to pain; produces generalized CNS depression.

Pharmacokinetics

Route	Onset	Peak	Duration
Oral Solution	N/A	1 hr	3–5 hr
Tablets	N/A	1 hr	3–5 hr
Tablets (ER)	N/A	3–4 hr	8–12 hr
IV	Rapid	0.3 hr	3–5 hr
IM	5–30 min	0.5–1 hr	3–5 hr
Epidural	N/A	1 hr	12–20 hr
Subcutaneous	N/A	1.1–5 hr	3–5 hr
Rectal	N/A	0.5–1 hr	3–7 hr

Variably absorbed from the GI tract. Readily absorbed after IM or subcutaneous administration. Protein binding: 20%–35%. Widely distributed. Metabolized in the liver. Primarily excreted in urine. Removed by hemodialysis. **Half-life:** 2–3 hr. (increased in patients with hepatic disease)

INDICATIONS AND DOSAGES:
Alert Dosage should be titrated to desired effect.

Analgesia
PO (Prompt-release)
Adults, Elderly. 10–30 mg q3-4h as needed.
Children. 0.15–0.3 mg/kg q3-4h as needed.

Alert For the Kadian dosage information below, be aware that this drug is to be administered q12h or once a day only.

Alert Be aware that pediatric dosages of extended-release preparations Kadian and Avinza have not been established.

Alert For the MSContin and Oramorph SR dosage information below, be aware that the daily dosage is divided and given q8h or q12h.

PO (Extended-Release [Avinza])
Adults, Elderly. Dosage requirment should be established using prompt-release formulations and is based on total daily dose (one-half the dose is given q12h or one-third the dose is given q8h).

PO (Extended-Release [Kadian])
Adults, Elderly. Dosage requirment should be established using prompt-release formulations and is based on total daily dose. Dose is given once a day or divided and given q12h.

PO (Extended-Release [MSContin, Oramorph SR])
Adults, Elderly. Dosage requirment should be established using prompt-release formulations and is based on total daily dose. Daily dose is divided and given q8h or q12h.
Children. 0.3-0.6 mg/kg/dose q12h.
IM
Adults, Elderly. 5–10 mg q3-4h as needed.

Children. 0.1 mg/kg q3-4h as needed.
IV
Adults, Elderly. 2.5-5 mg q3-4h as needed. Note: Repeated doses (e.g. 1-2 mg) may be given more frequently (e.g. every hour) if needed.
Children. 0.05-0.1 mg/kg q3-4h as needed.
IV continuous infusion
Adults, Elderly. 0.8–10 mg/h. Range: Up to 80 mg/h.
Children. 10-30 mcg/kg/hr.
Epidural
Adults, Elderly. Initially, 1-6 mg bolus, infusion rate: 0.1-1 mg/h. Maximum: 10 mg/24 h.
Intrathecal
Adults, Elderly. One-tenth of the epidural dose: 0.2–1 mg/dose.
PCA
IV
Adults, Elderly. Loading dose: 5–10 mg. Intermittent bolus: 0.5–3 mg. Lockout interval: 5–12 min. Continuous infusion: 1–10 mg/hr. 4-hr limit: 20–30 mg.

AVAILABLE FORMS/COST
• Cap, Gel—Oral: 15 mg, 100's: **$37.19**; 30 mg, 100's: **$69.40**
• Cap, Sus Action—Oral: 20 mg, 100's: **$109.04**; 30 mg, 60's: **$135.55**; 50 mg, 100's: **$265.94**; 60 mg, 60's: **$258.18**; 100 mg, 100's: **$472.50**
• Cap, Sus Action (24 hr)—Oral: 30 mg, 100's: **$248.00**; 60 mg, 100's: **$476.00**; 90 mg, 100's: **$723.00**; 120 mg, 100's: **$845.00**
• Sol, Inj—Epidural, Intrathecal, IV: 0.5 mg/ml, 2, 10, 30 ml: **$2.53-$8.60**/10 ml; 1 mg/ml, 2, 10, 30 ml: **$7.51-$9.23**/10 ml; 10 mg/ml, 20, 30 ml: **$23.16**/30 ml; 25 mg/ml, 4, 10, 20, 30, 40, 50 ml: **$202.50**/30 ml; 50 mg/ml, 30, 50 ml: **$337.01**/30 ml
• Sol, Inj—IM; IV; SC: 0.5 mg/ml, 10 ml: **$2.41**/10 ml; 1 mg/ml, 10, 30, 60 ml: **$2.30-$7.64**/10 ml; 2 mg/ml,

1, 30 ml: **$0.72-$1.10**/1 ml; 4 mg/ml, 1 ml: **$0.70-$1.31**/1 ml; 5 mg/ml, 1, 30 ml: **$2.53-$17.00**/30 ml; 8 mg/ml, 1 ml: **$0.79-$1.24**/1 ml; 10mg/ml, 1, 3, 10, 20, 30 ml: **$0.66-$1.29**/1 ml; 15 mg/ml, 1, 10, 20 ml: **$0.90-$1.04**/1 ml

• Sol, Inj—IV: 25 mg/ml, 4, 10, 20, 40, 50 ml: **$14.13-$21.26**/10 ml; 50 mg/ml, 10, 20, 40, 50 ml: **$42.98-$286.62**/10 ml

• Sol—Oral: 10 mg/5 ml, 100, 120, 500 ml: **$8.33-$11.46**/120 ml; 20 mg/5 ml, 5, 100, 120, 500 ml: **$12.08-$15.71**/120 ml

• Conc—Oral: 20 mg/ml, 30, 120, 240 ml: **$59.50-$81.90**/120 ml

• Supp—Rect: 5 mg, 12's: **$14.35-$15.10**; 10 mg, 12's: **$14.39-$17.75**; 20 mg, 12's: **$17.02-$21.60**; 30 mg, 12's: **$21.87-$29.44**

• Tab, Coated, Sus Action—Oral: 15 mg, 100's: **$72.60-$99.63**; 30 mg, 100's: **$70.84-$189.34**; 60 mg, 100's: **$269.21-$369.44**; 100 mg, 100's: **$489.56-$546.99**; 200 mg, 100's: **$896.53-$1,001.71**

• Tab—Oral: 10 mg, 100's: **$25.79-$33.26**; 15 mg, 100's: **$12.15-$42.21**; 30mg,100's: **$31.22-$54.91**

CONTRAINDICATIONS: Acute or severe asthma, GI obstruction, severe hepatic or renal impairment, severe respiratory depressione asthma, severe liver or renal impairment

PREGNANCY AND LACTATION: Pregnancy category B; trace amounts enter breast milk; compatible with breast-feeding

SIDE EFFECTS

Frequent

Sedation, decreased BP (including orthostatic hypotension), diaphoresis, facial flushing, constipation, dizziness, somnolence, nausea, vomiting

Occasional

Allergic reaction (rash, pruritus), dyspnea, confusion, palpitations, tremors, urine retention, abdominal cramps, vision changes, dry mouth, headache, decreased appetite, pain or burning at injection site

Rare

Paralytic ileus

SERIOUS REACTIONS

• Overdose results in respiratory depression, skeletal muscle flaccidity, cold or clammy skin, cyanosis, and extreme somnolence progressing to seizures, stupor, and coma.

• The patient who uses morphine repeatedly may develop a tolerance to the drug's analgesic effect and physical dependence.

• The drug may have a prolonged duration of action and cumulative effect in those with hepatic and renal impairment.

INTERACTIONS

Drugs

③ *Amitryptylline:* Additive respiratory and CNS-depressant effects

③ *Antihistamines, chloroal hydrate, gluethimide, methocarbamol:* Enhanced depressant effects

③ *Barbiturates:* Additive respiratory and CNS-depressant effects

③ *Cimetidine:* Increased respiratory and CNS depression

③ *Cloimpramine:* Additive respiratory and CNS-depressant effects

③ *Ethanol:* Additive CNS effects

③ *MAOI's:* Markedly potentiate the actions of morphine

③ *Nortriptylline:* Additive respiratory and CNS-depressant effects

Labs

• *Increase:* Urine glucose, urine 17-ketosteroids

• False elevations of amylase and lipase

SPECIAL CONSIDERATIONS

• Treatment of overdose: Naloxone (Narcan) 0.2-0.8 mg IV

M

• Remains the strong analgesic of choice for acute, severe pain, acute MI pain, and the agent of choice for chronic cancer pain
• 200 mg Sus Action tablet for use only in opioid-tolerant patients
• Do not administer agonist/antagonist analgesics (i.e., pentazocine, nalbuphine, butorphanol, dezocine, buprenorphine) to patient who has received a prolonged course of morphine (a pure agonist). In opioid-dependent patients, mixed agonist/anagonist analgesics may precipitate withdrawal symptoms

PATIENT/FAMILY EDUCATION
• Change position slowly to avoid orthostasis
• Avoid alcohol and other CNS depressants
• Physical dependency may result
• Do not chew or crush Sus Action preparations

moxifloxacin
(moks-i-floks'a-sin)
Rx: Avelox
Chemical Class: Fluoroquinolone derivative
Therapeutic Class: Antibiotic

CLINICAL PHARMACOLOGY
Mechanism of Action: A fluoroquinolone that inhibits two enzymes, topoisomerase II and IV, in susceptible microorganisms. *Therapeutic Effect:* Interferes with bacterial DNA replication. Prevents or delays emergence of resistant organisms. Bactericidal.
Pharmacokinetics
Well absorbed from the gastrointestinal (GI) tract after PO administration. Protein binding: 50%. Widely distributed throughout body with tissue concentration often exceeding plasma concentration. Metabolized in liver. Primarily excreted in urine with a lesser amount in feces. **Half-life:** 10.7–13.3 hrs.

INDICATIONS AND DOSAGES
Acute bacterial sinusitis, community-acquired pneumonia
IV/PO
Adults, Elderly. 400 mg q24h for 10 days.
Acute bacterial exacerbation of chronic bronchitis
IV/PO
Adults, Elderly. 400 mg q24h for 5 days.
Skin and skin-structure infection
IV/PO
Adults, Elderly. 400 mg once a day for 7 days.
Topical treatment of bacterial conjunctivitis due to susceptible strains of bacteria
Ophthalmic
Adults, Elderly, Children older than 1 yr. 1 drop 3 times/day for 7 days.

[$] **AVAILABLE FORMS/COST**
• Sol—Ophth: 0.5%, 3 ml: **$48.75**
• Sol, Inj—IV (in sodium chloride): 400 mg/250 ml: **$43.75**
• Tab, Coated—Oral: 400 mg, 30's: **$294.01**

CONTRAINDICATIONS: Hypersensitivity to quinolones

PREGNANCY AND LACTATION: Pregnancy category C; excreted into breast milk, safety not established, allow 48 hr to elapse after last dose before resuming breast-feeding

SIDE EFFECTS
Frequent (8%–6%)
Nausea, diarrhea
Occasional (3%–2%)
Dizziness, headache, abdominal pain, vomiting
Ophthalmic (6%–1%): conjunctival irritation, reduced visual acuity, dry eye, keratitis, eye pain, ocular itching, swelling of tissue around cornea, eye discharge, fever, cough, pharyngitis, rash, rhinitis

Rare (1%)

Change in sense of taste, dyspepsia (heartburn, indigestion), photosensitivity

SERIOUS REACTIONS

• Pseudomembranous colitis as evidenced by fever, severe abdominal cramps or pain, and severe watery diarrhea may occur.

• Superinfection manifested as anal or genital pruritus, moderate to severe diarrhea, and stomatitis may occur.

INTERACTIONS

Drugs

◩ *Aluminum:* Reduced absorption of moxifloxacin; do not take within 4 hr of dose

◩ *Antacids:* Reduced absorption of moxifloxacin; do not take within 4 hr of dose

◩ *Antipyrine:* Inhibits metabolism of antipyrine; increased plasma antipyrine level

◩ *Calcium:* Reduced absorption of moxifloxacin; do not take within 4 hr of dose

◩ *Diazepam:* Inhibits metabolism of diazepam; increased plasma diazepam level

◩ *Didanosine:* Markedly reduced absorption of moxifloxacin; take moxifloxacin 2 hr before didanosine

◩ *Foscarnet:* Coadministration increases seizure risk

◩ *Iron:* Reduced absorption of moxifloxacin; do not take within 4 hr of dose

◩ *Magnesium:* Reduced absorption of moxifloxacin; do not take within 4 hr of dose

◩ *Metoprolol:* Inhibits metabolism of metoprolol; increased plasma metoprolol level

◩ *Morphine:* Reduced absorption of moxifloxacin; do not take within 2 hr of dose

◩ *Pentoxifylline:* Inhibits metabolism of pentoxifylline; increased plasma pentoxifylline level

◩ *Phenytoin:* Inhibits metabolism of phenytoin; increased plasma phenytoin level

◩ *Propranolol:* Inhibits metabolism of propranolol; increased plasma propranolol level

◩ *Ropinirole:* Inhibits metabolism of ropinirole; increased plasma ropinirole level

◩ *Sodium bicarbonate:* Reduced absorption of moxifloxacin; do not take within 4 hr of dose

◩ *Sucralfate:* Reduced absorption of moxifloxacin; do not take within 4 hr of dose

◩ *Warfarin:* Inhibits metabolism of warfarin; increases hypoprothrombinemic response to warfarin

◩ *Zinc:* Reduced absorption of moxifloxacin; do not take within 4 hr of dose

SPECIAL CONSIDERATIONS

PATIENT/FAMILY EDUCATION

• May be taken with or without meals

• Should be taken at least 4 hr before or 8 hr after multivitamins (containing iron or zinc), antacids (containing magnesium, calcium, or aluminum), sucralfate, or didanosine chewable/buffered tablets

• Discontinue treatment, rest and refrain from exercise, and inform prescriber if pain, inflammation, or rupture of a tendon occur

• Test reaction to this drug before operating an automobile or machinery or engaging in activities requiring mental alertness or coordination

mupirocin
(mew-peer'-oh-sin)
Rx: Bactroban
Chemical Class: Pseudomonic acid derivative
Therapeutic Class: Antibiotic, topical

CLINICAL PHARMACOLOGY
Mechanism of Action: An antibacterial agent that inhibits bacterial protein, RNA synthesis. Less effective on DNA synthesis. Nasal: Eradicates nasal colonization of MRSA. *Therapeutic Effect:* Prevents bacterial growth and replication. Bacteriostatic.
Pharmacokinetics
Metabolized in skin to inactive metabolite. Transported to skin surface; removed by normal skin desquamation.

INDICATIONS AND DOSAGES
Impetigo, infected traumatic skin lesions
Topical
Adults, Elderly, Children. Apply 3 times/day (may cover w/gauze).
Nasal colonization of resistant Staphylococcus aureus
Intranasal
Adults, Elderly, Children 12 yrs and older. Apply 2 times/day for 5 days.
[S] **AVAILABLE FORMS/COST**
• Cre—Top: 2%, 15, 30 g: **$32.74/15 g**
• Oint—Nasal: 2%, 1 g: **$5.64**
• Oint—Top: 2%, 15, 30 g: **$17.35-$32.74/15 g**
UNLABELED USES: Treatment of infected eczema, folliculitis, minor bacterial skin infections.
CONTRAINDICATIONS: Hypersensitivity to mupirocin or any component of the formulation

PREGNANCY AND LACTATION:
Pregnancy category B; excretion into breast milk unknown
SIDE EFFECTS
Frequent
Nasal: Headache, rhinitis, upper respiratory congestion, pharyngitis, altered taste
Occasional
Nasal: Burning, stinging, cough
Topical: Pain, burning, stinging, itching
Rare
Nasal: Pruritis, diarrhea, dry mouth, epistaxis, nausea, rash
Topical: Rash, nausea, dry skin, contact dermatitis
SERIOUS REACTIONS
• Superinfection may result in bacterial or fungal infections, especially with prolonged or repeated therapy.
SPECIAL CONSIDERATIONS
• Comparable efficacy to systemic semisynthetic penicillins and erythromycin in impetigo and infected wounds

mycophenolate
(my-co-fen'o-late)
Rx: CellCept, Myfortic
Chemical Class: Mycophenolic acid derivative
Therapeutic Class: Immunosuppressant

CLINICAL PHARMACOLOGY
Mechanism of Action: An immunologic agent that suppresses the immunologically mediated inflammatory response by inhibiting inosine monophosphate dehydrogenase, an enzyme that deprives lymphocytes of nucleotides necessary for DNA and RNA synthesis, thus inhibiting

the proliferation of T and B lymphocytes. *Therapeutic Effect*: Prevents transplant rejection.

Pharmacokinetics

Rapidly and extensively absorbed after PO administration (food decreases drug plasma concentration but does not affect absorption). Protein binding: 97%. Completely hydrolyzed to active metabolite mycophenolic acid. Primarily excreted in urine. Not removed by hemodialysis. **Half-life:** 17.9 hr.

INDICATIONS AND DOSAGES

Prevention of renal transplant rejection
PO, IV
Adults, Elderly. 1 g twice a day.

Prevention of heart transplant rejection
PO, IV
Adults, Elderly. 1.5 g twice a day.

Prevention of liver transplant rejection
IV
PO
Adults, Elderly. 1.5 g twice a day.
Adults, Elderly. 1 g twice a day.

Usual pediatric dosage
PO
Children. 600 mg/m^2/dose twice a day. Maximum: 2 g/dose.

AVAILABLE FORMS/COST
• Cap, Gel—Oral: 250 mg, 100's: **$308.24**
• Powder, Inj—IV: 500 mg vial, 4's: **$146.45**
• Susp—Oral: 200 mg/ml 175 ml: **$431.48**
• Tab—Oral: 500 mg, 100's: **$616.39**

UNLABELED USES: Treatment of liver transplantation rejection, mild heart transplant rejection, moderate to severe psoriasis

CONTRAINDICATIONS: Hypersensitivity to mycophenolic acid

PREGNANCY AND LACTATION: Pregnancy category C; mycophenolic acid excreted in milk; not recommended during breast-feeding

SIDE EFFECTS
Frequent (37%–20%)
UTI, hypertension, peripheral edema, diarrhea, constipation, fever, headache, nausea
Occasional (18%–10%)
Dyspepsia; dyspnea; cough; hematuria; asthenia; vomiting; edema; tremors; abdominal, chest, or back pain; oral candidiasis; acne
Rare (9%–6%)
Insomnia, respiratory tract infection, rash, dizziness

SERIOUS REACTIONS
• Significant anemia, leukopenia, thrombocytopenia, neutropenia, and leukocytosis may occur, particularly in those undergoing reanl transplant rejection.
• Sepsis and infection occur occasionally.
• GI tract hemorrhage occurs rarely.
• Patients receiving mycophenolate have an increased risk of developing neoplasms.

INTERACTIONS
Drugs
▣ *Acyclovir:* Increased serum acyclovir and mycophenolate concentrations possible
▣ *Antacids with magnesium and aluminum hydroxides:* Decreased mycophenolate bioavailability; separate administration times
▣ *Azathioprine:* Due to potential bone marrow suppression, concomitant administration not recommended
▣ *Cholestyramine:* Decreased mycophenolate bioavailability due to interruption of enterohepatic recirculation
▣ *Ganciclovir:* Increased serum ganciclovir and mycophenolate concentrations possible

M

3 *Live vaccines:* Use of live attenuated vaccines should be avoided; vaccines may be less effective

3 *Probenecid:* Increased serum mycophenolate concentrations

SPECIAL CONSIDERATIONS

• Drug can be given concurrently with cyclosporine, which may enable reduced cyclosporine doses and lower toxicity, or potential cyclosporine substitute in patients developing cyclosporine toxicity

• Drug is less likely than azathioprine to induce severe bone marrow depression, and may replace azathioprine in conventional maintenance immunosuppression regimens

• IV can be administered for up to 14 days; switch to PO as soon as possible

PATIENT/FAMILY EDUCATION

• Women of childbearing potential should use effective contraception before and during therapy and 6 weeks after therapy has stopped

MONITORING PARAMETERS

• CBC qwk × 1 mo, then q2wk × 2 mo, then monthly

---

nabumetone
(na-byu'-me-tone)
Rx: Relafen
Chemical Class: Acetic acid derivative
Therapeutic Class: NSAID; antipyretic; nonnarcotic analgesic

CLINICAL PHARMACOLOGY

Mechanism of Action: An NSAID that produces analgesic and anti-inflammatory effects by inhibiting prostaglandin synthesis. *Therapeutic Effect:* Reduces the inflammatory response and intensity of pain.

Pharmacokinetics

Readily absorbed from the GI tract. Protein binding: 99%. Widely distributed. Metabolized in the liver to active metabolite. Primarily excreted in urine. Not removed by hemodialysis. **Half-life:** 22–30 hr.

INDICATIONS AND DOSAGES

Acute or chronic rheumatoid arthritis and osteoarthritis

PO

Adults, Elderly. Initially, 1,000 mg as a single dose or in 2 divided doses. May increase up to 2,000 mg/day as a single or in 2 divided doses.

S **AVAILABLE FORMS/COST**

• Tab—Oral: 500 mg, 100's: **$129.70-$160.53**; 750 mg, 100's: **$153.17-$189.56**

CONTRAINDICATIONS: Active peptic ulcer disease, chronic inflammation of GI tract, GI bleeding or ulceration, history of hypersensitivity to aspirin or NSAIDs, history of significant renal impairment

PREGNANCY AND LACTATION: Pregnancy category C; excretion into breast milk unknown, not recommended for use in nursing mothers

SIDE EFFECTS

Frequent (14%–12%)

Diarrhea, abdominal cramps or pain, dyspepsia

Occasional (9%–4%)

Nausea, constipation, flatulence, dizziness, headache

Rare (3%–1%)

Vomiting, stomatitis, confusion

SERIOUS REACTIONS

• Overdose may result in acute hypotension and tachycardia.

• Rare reactions with long-term use include peptic ulcer disease, GI bleeding, gastritis, nephrotoxicity (dysuria, cystitis, hematuria, proteinuria, nephrotic syndrome), severe hepatic reactions (cholestasis, jaundice), and severe hypersensitivity reactions (bronchospasm, angioedema).

INTERACTIONS
Drugs
▣ *Aminoglycosides:* Reduced clearance with elevated aminoglycoside levels and potential for toxicity (especially indomethacin in premature infants; other NSAIDs probably)

▣ *Antihypertensives:* (α-blockers, angiotensin converting enzyme inhibitors, angiotensin II receptor blockers, β-blockers, diuretics) inhibition of antihypertensive and other favorable hemodynamic effects

▣ *Corticosteroids:* Increased risk of GI ulceration

▣ *Cyclosporine:* Increased nephrotoxicity risk

▣ *Lithium:* Decreased clearance of lithium (mediated via prostaglandins) resulting in elevated serum lithium levels and risk of toxicity

▣ *Methotrexate:* Decreased renal secretion of methotrexate resulting in elevated methotrexate levels and risk of toxicity

▣ *Phenylpropanolamine:* Possible acute hypertensive reaction

▣ *Potassium-Sparing Diuretics:* Additive hyperkalemia potential

▣ *Triamterene:* Acute renal failure reported with addition of indomethacin; caution with other NSAIDs

▣ *Warfarin:* Transient increase in prothrombin time due to displaced protein binding; increased risk of GI bleeding although likely less risky than other NSAIDs due to preferential action on COX-2

SPECIAL CONSIDERATIONS
• No significant advantage over other NSAIDs; cost should govern use

MONITORING PARAMETERS
• Initial hemogram and fecal occult blood test within 3 months of starting regular chronic therapy; repeat every 6-12 months (more frequently in high risk patients (>65 years, peptic ulcer disease, concurrent steroids or anticoagulants); electrolytes, creatinine, and BUN within 3 months of starting regular chronic therapy; repeat every 6-12 months

---

nadolol
(nay-doe'lole)
Rx: Corgard
Combinations
   Rx: With Bendroflumenthiazide (Corzide)
Chemical Class: β-adrenergic blocker, nonselective
Therapeutic Class: Antianginal; antiglaucoma agent; antihypertensive

N

CLINICAL PHARMACOLOGY
Mechanism of Action: A nonselective beta-blocker that blocks beta$_1$- and beta$_2$-adrenergenic receptors. Large doses increase airway resistance. *Therapeutic Effect:* Slows sinus heart rate, decreases cardiac output and BP. Decreases myocardial ischemia severity by decreasing oxygen requirements.

INDICATIONS AND DOSAGES
Mild to moderate hypertension, angina
PO
Adults. Initially, 40 mg/day. May increase by 40–80 mg at 3–7 day intervals. Maximum: 240–360 mg/day.
Elderly. Initially, 20 mg/day. May increase gradually. Range: 20–240 mg/day.

Dosage in renal impairment

Dosage is modified based on creatinine clearance.

Creatinine Clearance	% Usual Dosage
10–50 ml/min	50
less than 10 ml/min	25

§ **AVAILABLE FORMS/COST**

• Tab—Oral: 20 mg, 100's: **$73.60-$176.48**; 40 mg, 100's: **$22.34-$206.60**; 80 mg, 100's: **$118.30-$283.84**; 120 mg, 100's: **$74.93-$369.94**; 160 mg, 100's: **$78.47-$380.96**

UNLABELED USES: Treatment of arrhythmias, hypertrophic cardiomyopathy, MI, mitral valve prolapse syndrome, neuroleptic-induced akathisia, pheochromocytoma, tremors, thyrotoxicosis, vascular headaches

CONTRAINDICATIONS: Bronchial asthma, cardiogenic shock, CHF secondary to tachyarrhythmias, COPD, patients receiving MAOI therapy, second- or third-degree heart block, sinus bradycardia, uncontrolled cardiac failure

PREGNANCY AND LACTATION: Pregnancy category C; similar drug, atenolol, frequently used in the third trimester for treatment of hypertension (many studies of efficacy and safety of atenolol in pregnancy-induced hypertension); long-term use has been associated with intrauterine growth retardation; mean milk: plasma ratio, 0.80 in one study; quantity of drug ingested by breastfeeding infant unlikely to be therapeutically significant

SIDE EFFECTS

Nadolol is generally well tolerated, with transient and mild side effects.

Frequent

Diminished sexual ability, drowsiness, unusual fatigue or weakness

Occasional

Bradycardia, difficulty breathing, depression, cold hands or feet, diarrhea, constipation, anxiety, nasal congestion, nausea, vomiting

Rare

Altered taste, dry eyes, itching

SERIOUS REACTIONS

• Overdose may produce profound bradycardia and hypotension.

• Abrupt withdrawal of nadolol may result in diaphoresis, palpitations, headache, tremulousness, exacerbation of angina, MI, and ventricular arrhythmias.

• Nadolol administration may precipitate CHF and MI in patients with cardiac disease; thyroid storm in those with thyrotoxicosis; and peripheral ischemia in those with existing peripheral vascular disease.

• Hypoglycemia may occur in patients with previously controlled diabetes.

INTERACTIONS

Drugs

▣ *Adenosine:* Bradycardia aggravated

▣ *α₁-adrenergic blockers:* Potential enhanced first dose response (marked initial drop in blood pressure, particularly on standing (especially prazocin).

▣ *Amiodarone:* Symptomatic bradycardia and sinus arrest; caution in patients with bradycardia, sick sinus syndrome, or partial AV block when either amiodarone or β-blocking drug is used

▣ *Ampicillin:* Reduced nadolol bioavailability

▣ *Antacids:* Reduced nadolol absorption

▣ *Calcium channel blockers:* See dihydropyridine and verapamil

▣ *Clonidine:* Exacerbation of rebound hypertension upon discontinuation of clonidine

3 *Digoxin:* Additive prolongation of atrioventricular (AV) conduction time

3 *Dihydropyridine calcium channel blockers:* Severe hypotension or impaired cardiac performance; most prevalent with impaired left ventricular function, cardiac arrhythmias, or aortic stenosis

3 *Diltiazem:* Potentiates β-adrenergic effects; hypotension, left ventricular failure, and AV conduction disturbances problematic in elderly, patients with left ventricular dysfunction, aortic stenosis, or with large doses of either drug

3 *Dipyridamole:* Bradycardia aggravated

3 *Hypoglycemic agents:* Masked hypoglycemia, hyperglycemia

3 *Lidocaine:* Increased serum lidocaine concentrations possible

3 *Neostigmine:* Bradycardia aggravated

3 *NSAIDs:* Reduced antihypertensive effect of nadolol

3 *Physostigmine:* Bradycardia aggravated

3 *Prazosin:* First-dose response to prazosin may be enhanced by β-blockade

3 *Tacrine:* Bradycardia aggravated

2 *Theophylline:* Antagonistic pharmacodynamic effects

3 *Verapamil:* Potentiates β-adrenergic effects; hypotension, left ventricular failure, and AV conduction disturbances problematic in elderly, patients with left ventricular dysfunction, aortic stenosis, or with large doses of either drug

SPECIAL CONSIDERATIONS
• No unique advantage over less expensive β-blockers

PATIENT/FAMILY EDUCATION
• Do **not** discontinue abruptly; may require taper; rapid withdrawal may produce rebound hypertension or angina

MONITORING PARAMETERS
• Angina: reduction in nitroglycerin usage; frequency, severity, onset, and duration of angina pain; heart rate
• Arrhythmias: heart rate
• Congestive heart failure: functional status, cough, dyspnea on exertion, paroxysmal nocturnal dyspnea, exercise tolerance, and ventricular function
• Hypertension: Blood pressure
• Migraine headache: reduction in the frequency, severity, and duration of attacks
• Post myocardial infarction: left ventricular function, lower resting heart rate
• Toxicity: blood glucose, bronchospasm, hypotension, bradycardia, depression, confusion, hallucination, sexual dysfunction

N

---

nafarelin
(naf-ah-rell-in)
Rx: Synarel
Chemical Class: Gonadotropin-releasing hormone analog
Therapeutic Class: Antiendometriosis agent

CLINICAL PHARMACOLOGY
Mechanism of Action: A gonadotropin inhibitor that initially stimulates the release of the pituitary gonadotropins, luteinizing hormone and follicle-stimulating hormone, then decreases secretion of gonadal steroids. *Therapeutic Effect:* Temporarily increases ovarian steroidogenesis, abolishes the stimulatory

effect on the pituitary gland, decreases secretion of gonadal steroids.

Pharmacokinetics

Rapidly absorbed after nasal administration. Protein binding: 78%-84%, binds primarily to albumin. Metabolism: unknown. Excreted in urine. **Half-life:** 3 hrs.

INDICATIONS AND DOSAGES

Endometriosis

Intranasal

Adults. 400 mcg/day: 200 mcg (1 spray) into 1 nostril in morning, 1 spray into other nostril in evening. For patients with persistent regular menstruation after months of treatment, increase dose to 800 mcg/day (1 spray into each nostril in morning and evening).

Central precocious puberty

Intranasal

Children. 1,600 mcg/day: 400 mcg (2 sprays into each nostril in morning and evening; total 8 sprays).

S **AVAILABLE FORMS/COST**

• Sol—Nasal: 200 mcg/inh, 8 ml: **$611.26**

CONTRAINDICATIONS: Pregnancy, other agonist analogues, undiagnosed abnormal vaginal bleeding, hypersensitivity to nafarelin or any component of the formulation

PREGNANCY AND LACTATION: Pregnancy category X; not recommended in nursing mothers

SIDE EFFECTS

Frequent

Hot flashes. muscle pain, decreased breast size, myalgia

Occasional

Nasal irritation, decreased libido, vaginal dryness, headache, emotional lability, acne

Rare

Insomnia, edema, weight gain, seborrhea, depression.

SERIOUS REACTIONS

• None reported.

INTERACTIONS

Drugs

3 *Decongestants, nasal/topical:* Potential interference with absorption; allow 30 min after use of nafarelin before applying a topical decongestant

Labs

• *Interference:* Gonadal and gonadotropic function tests conducted during treatment and for 4-8 wk after treatment may be misleading

SPECIAL CONSIDERATIONS

• Alternative to danazol and oophorectomy in the treatment of endometriosis; more tolerable adverse effect profile compared to danazol for some patients

• Agent of choice in patients concerned about future fertility

• Benefits are temporary

---

nafcillin

(naph-sil′in)

Rx: Nallpen

Chemical Class: Penicillin derivative, penicillinase-resistant

Therapeutic Class: Antibiotic

CLINICAL PHARMACOLOGY

Mechanism of Action: A penicillin that acts as a bactericidal in susceptible microorganisms. *Therapeutic Effect:* Inhibits bacterial cell wall synthesis. Bactericidal.

Pharmacokinetics

Poorly absorbed from gastrointestinal (GI) tract. Protein binding: 87%-90%. Mtabolized in liver. Primarily excreted in urine. Not removed by hemodialysis. **Half-life:** 10.5-1 hr (half-life increased with imparied renal function, neonates).

INDICATIONS AND DOSAGES
Staphylococcal infections
IV

Adults, Elderly. 3-6 g/24 hrs in divided doses.

Children. 25 mg/kg 2 times/day.

Neonates 7 days and older. 75 mg/kg/day in 4 divided doses.

Neonates less than 7 days old. 50 mg/kg/day in 2-3 divided doses.

Neonates less than 7 days old. 50 mg/kg/day in 2-3 divided doses.

Adults, Elderly. 500 mg q4-6h.

Children. 25 mg/kg 2 times/day.

Neonates 7 days and older. 75 mg/kg/day in 4 divided doses.

Neonates 7 days and older. 75 mg/kg/day in 4 divided doses.

PO

Adults, Elderly. 250 mg to 1 g q4-6h.

Children. 25-50 mg/kg/day in 4 divided doses.

Ⓢ   AVAILABLE FORMS/COST
• Powder, Inj—IM, IV: 500 mg: **$0.22-$1.20**; 1 g: **$2.27-$11.50**; 2 g: **$0.67-$19.24**

UNLABELED USES: Surgical prophylaxis

CONTRAINDICATIONS: Hypersensitivity to any penicillin

PREGNANCY AND LACTATION: Pregnancy category B; excreted into breast milk

SIDE EFFECTS
Frequent
Mild hypersensitivity reaction (fever, rash, pruritus), GI effects (nausea, vomiting, diarrhea) more frequent w/oral administration

Occasional
Hypokalemia with high IV doses, phlebitis, thrombophlebitis (more common in elderly)

Rare
Extravasation with IV administration

SERIOUS REACTIONS
• Superinfections, potentially fatal antibiotic-associated colitis may result from altered bacterial balance.

• Hematologic effects (especially involving platelets, WBCs), severe hypersensitivity reactions, and anaphylaxis occur rarely.

INTERACTIONS
Drugs
▣ *Chloramphenicol:* Inhibited antibacterial activity of nafcillin; administer nafcillin 3 hr before chloramphenicol

▣ *Cyclosporine:* Reduced serum cyclosporine concentrations

▣ *Macrolide antibiotics:* Inhibited antibacterial activity of nafcillin; administer nafcillin 3 hr before macrolides

▣ *Methotrexate:* Increased serum methotrexate concentrations

▣ *Oral contraceptives:* Occasional impairment of oral contraceptive efficacy; consider use of supplemental contraception during cycles in which nafcillin is used

▣ *Tacrolimus:* Reduced serum tacrolimus concentrations

▣ *Tetracyclines:* Inhibited antibacterial activity of nafcillin; administer nafcillin 3 hr before tetracyclines

▣ *Warfarin:* May inhibit hypoprothrombinemic response to warfarin

Labs
• *Increase:* Serum protein

SPECIAL CONSIDERATIONS
MONITORING PARAMETERS
• Oral nafcillin absorption is erratic (consider alternate oral penicillinase-resistant penicillins)

• CBC, creatinine and UA for eosinophils during therapy to monitor for adverse effects

naftifine
(naf-ti-feen)
Rx: Naftin
Chemical Class: Allylamine derivative
Therapeutic Class: Antifungal

CLINICAL PHARMACOLOGY
Mechanism of Action: An antifungal that selectively inhibits the enzyme squalene epoxidase in a dose-dependent manner, which results in the primary sterol, ergosterol, within the fungal membrane not being synthesized. *Therapeutic Effect:* Results in fungal cell death. Fungistatic and fungicidal.

Pharmacokinetics
Minimal systemic absorption. Metabolized in the liver. Excreted in the urine as well as the feces and bile. **Half-life:** 48-72 hrs.

INDICATIONS AND DOSAGES
Tinea pedis, t.cruris, t.corporis
Topical
Adults, Elderly, Children 12 yrs and older. Apply cream 1 time a day for 4 weeks or until signs and symptoms significantly improve. Apply gel 2 times a day for 4 weeks or until signs and symptoms significantly improve.

$ **AVAILABLE FORMS/COST**
• Cre—Top: 1%, 15, 30, 60 g: **$42.86**/30 g
• Gel—Top: 1%, 20, 40, 60 g: **$58.82**/40 g

UNLABELED USES: Trichomycosis
CONTRAINDICATIONS: Hypersensitivity to naftifine or any of its components

PREGNANCY AND LACTATION:
Pregnancy category B; excretion into breast milk unknown

SIDE EFFECTS
Frequent
Burning, stinging

Occasional
Erythema, itching, dryness, irritation

SERIOUS REACTIONS
• Excessive irritation may indicate hypersensitivity reaction.

SPECIAL CONSIDERATIONS
• First of a new class of antifungals (allylamine derivatives) unrelated to imidazoles
• Because of fungicidal activity at low concentrations may provide quicker onset of healing, enhance patient compliance with qday therapy

nalbuphine
(nal'byoo-feen)
Rx: Nubain
Chemical Class: Opiate derivative; phenanthrene derivative
Therapeutic Class: Narcotic agonist-antagonist analgesic

CLINICAL PHARMACOLOGY
Mechanism of Action: A narcotic agonist-antagonist that binds with opioid receptors in the CNS. May displace opioid agonists and competitively inhibit their action; may precipitate withdrawal symptoms. *Therapeutic Effect:* Alters the perception of and emotional response to pain.

Pharmacokinetics

Route	Onset	Peak	Duration
IV	2- 3 min	30 min	3-6 hr
IM	less than 15 min	60 min	3-6 hr
Subcutaneous	less than 15 min	N/A	3-6 hr

Well absorbed after IM or subcutaneous administration. Protein binding: 50%. Metabolized in the liver. Primarily eliminated in feces by biliary secretion. **Half-life:** 3.5-5 hr.

INDICATIONS AND DOSAGES
Analgesia
IV, IM, Subcutaneous

Adults, Elderly. 10 mg q3-6h as needed. Do not exceed maximum single dose of 20 mg or daily dose of 160 mg. For patients receiving long-term narcotic analgesics of similar duration of action, give 25% of usual dose.

Children. 0.1-0.15 mg/kg q3–6h as needed.

Supplement to anesthesia
IV

Adults, Elderly. Induction: 0.3-3 mg/kg over 10-15 min. Maintenance: 0.25-0.5 mg/kg as needed.

$ AVAILABLE FORMS/COST
• Sol, Inj—IM, IV, SC: 10 mg/ml, 1 ml: **$2.04-$2.94**; 20 mg/ml, 1 ml: **$1.46-$2.51**

CONTRAINDICATIONS: Respiratory rate less than 12 breaths/minute

PREGNANCY AND LACTATION: Pregnancy category B

SIDE EFFECTS
Frequent (35%)

Sedation

Occasional (9%-3%)

Diaphoresis, cold and clammy skin, nausea, vomiting, dizziness, vertigo, dry mouth, headache

Rare (less than 1%)

Restlessness, emotional lability, paresthesia, flushing, paradoxical reaction

SERIOUS REACTIONS
• Abrupt withdrawal after prolonged use may produce symptoms of narcotic withdrawal, such as abdominal cramping, rhinorrhea, lacrimation, anxiety, fever, and piloerection (goose bumps).

• Overdose results in severe respiratory depression, skeletal muscle flaccidity, cyanosis, and extreme somnolence progressing to seizures, stupor, and coma.

• Repeated use may result in drug tolerance and physical dependence.

INTERACTIONS
Drugs
▣ *Barbiturates:* Additive respiratory and CNS depression

▣ *Cimetidine:* Inhibition of narcotic hepatic metabolism; additive CNS effects

▣ *Rifampin:* May reduce narcotic concentrations and precipitate withdrawal

Labs
• *Increase:* Amylase

SPECIAL CONSIDERATIONS
• Proposed, but not significant, advantages include low abuse potential, low respiratory depressant effects, low incidence of psychomimetic toxicity, and a lower incidence of hemodynamic toxicity

N

---

nalmefene
(nal'-meh-feen)

Rx: Revex

Chemical Class: Thebaine derivative

Therapeutic Class: Antidote, opiate

CLINICAL PHARMACOLOGY
Mechanism of Action: A narcotic antagonist that binds to opioid receptors. *Therapeutic Effect:* Prevents and reverses effects of opioids (respirtoary depression, sedation, hypotenstion).

Pharmacokinetics
Well absorbed. Protein binding: 45%. Metabolized primarily via glucuronidation. Excreted in urine and feces. **Half-life:** 8.5-10.8 hrs.

INDICATIONS AND DOSAGES
Solution for Injection: 100 mcg/ml ([blue label] Revex), 1000 mcg/ml ([green label] Revex)
IV/IM/Subcutaneous
Adults. Initially, 0.25 mcg/kg followed by additional 0.25 mcg doses at 2 to 5 min intervals until desired response. Cumulative doses >1 mcg/kg do not provide additional therapeutic effect.

Known or suspected opioid overdose
IV/IM/Subcutaneous
Adults. Initially, 0.5 mg/70 kg. May give 1 mg/70 kg in 2-5 min. If physical opioid dependence suspected, initial dose is 0.1 mg/70 kg.

S **AVAILABLE FORMS/COST**
• Sol—Inj: 100 mcg/ml, 1 ml: **$3.56**; 1 mg/ml, 2 ml: **$54.47**

CONTRAINDICATIONS: Hypersensitivity to nalmefene

PREGNANCY AND LACTATION: Pregnancy category B; excretion into breast milk unknown, use caution in nursing mothers

SIDE EFFECTS
Frequent
Nausea, headache, hypertension
Occasional
Postop pain, fever, dizziness, headache, chills, hypotension, vasodilation

SERIOUS REACTIONS
• Signs and symptoms of opioid withdrawal include stuffy or runny nose, tearing, yawning, sweating, tremor, vomiting, piloerection, feeling of temperature change, joint, bone or muscle pain, abdominal cramps, and feeling of skin crawling.

SPECIAL CONSIDERATIONS
• Longer duration of action than naloxone at fully reversing doses; agent of choice in instances where prolonged opioid effects are predicted, including overdose with longer-acting opioids (e.g., methadone, propoxyphene), patients given large doses of opioids, and those with liver disease or renal failure (eliminating the need for continuous infusions of naloxone and prolonged observation periods after outpatient procedures)

---

naloxone
(nal-oks´one)
Rx: Narcan
Combinations
   Rx: with pentazocine (Talwin NX); with buprenorphine (Suboxone)
Chemical Class: Thebaine derivative
Therapeutic Class: Antidote, opiate

CLINICAL PHARMACOLOGY
Mechanism of Action: A narcotic antagonist that displaces opioids at opioid-occupied receptor sites in the CNS. *Therapeutic Effect:* Reverses opioid-induced sleep or sedation, increases respiratory rate, raises BP to normal range.

Pharmacokinetics

Route	Onset	Peak	Duration
IV	1-2 min	N/A	20-60 min
IM	2-5 min	N/A	20-60 min
Subcutaneous	2-5 min	N/A	20-60 min

Well absorbed after IM or subcutaneous administration. Metabolized in the liver. Primarily excreted in urine. **Half-life:** 60-100 min.

INDICATIONS AND DOSAGES
Opioid toxicity
IV, IM, Subcutaneous
Adults, Elderly. 0.4-2 mg q2-3min as needed. May repeat q20-60min.

Children 5 yr and older and weighing 22 kg or more. 2 mg/dose; if no response, may repeat q2-3min. May need to repeat q20-60min.

Children younger than 5 yr and weighing less than 22 kg. 0.1 mg/kg; if no response, repeat q2-3min. May need to repeat q20-60min.

Postanesthesia narcotic reversal
IV

Children. 0.01 mg/kg; may repeat q2-3min.

Neonatal opioid-induced depression
IV

Neonates. may repeat q2-3min as needed. May need to repeat q1-2h.

Ⓢ **AVAILABLE FORMS/COST**
• Sol, Inj—IM, IV, SC: 0.02 mg/ml, 2 ml: **$1.14-$2.92**; 0.4 mg/ml, 1 ml: **$1.33-$3.72**; 1 mg/ml, 2 ml: **$5.24-$15.00**

UNLABELED USES: Treatment of PCP, ethanol ingestion

CONTRAINDICATIONS: Respiratory depression due to nonopioid drugs

PREGNANCY AND LACTATION: Pregnancy category B; excretion into breast milk unknown; use caution in nursing mothers

SIDE EFFECTS
None known; little or no pharmacologic effect in absence of narcotics.

SERIOUS REACTIONS
• Too-rapid reversal of narcotic-induced respiratory depression may result in nausea, vomiting, tremors, increased BP, and tachycardia.
• Excessive dosage in postoperative patients may produce significant excitement, tremors, and reversal of analgesia.
• Patients with cardiovascular disease may experience hypotension or hypertension, ventricular tachycardia and fibrillation, and pulmonary edema.

• Duration of action of some narcotics may exceed that of naloxone; repeat doses prn

MONITORING PARAMETERS
• ECG, blood pressure, respiratory rate, mental status, pupil dilation

---

naltrexone
(nal-trex'one)
Rx: ReVia
Chemical Class: Thebaine derivative
Therapeutic Class: Alcohol deterrent; antidote, opiate

CLINICAL PHARMACOLOGY
Mechanism of Action: A narcotic antagonist that displaces opioids at opioid-occupied receptor sites in the CNS. *Therapeutic Effect:* Blocks physical effects of opioid analgesics; decreases craving for alcohol and relapse rate in alcoholism.

INDICATIONS AND DOSAGES
Naloxone challenge test to determine if patient is opioid dependent
Alert

Expect to perform the naloxone challenge test if there is any question that the patient is opioid dependent. Do not administer naltrexone until the naloxone challenge test is negative.
IV

Adults, Elderly. Draw 2 ml (0.8 mg) of naloxone into syringe. Inject 0.5 ml (0.2 mg); while needle is still in vein, observe patient for 30 sec for withdrawal signs or symptoms. If no evidence of withdrawal, inject remaining 1.5 ml (0.6 mg); observe patient for additional 20 min for withdrawal signs or symptoms.

N

Subcutaneous

Adults, Elderly. Inject 2 ml (0.8 mg) of naloxone; observe patient for 45 min for withdrawal signs or symptoms.

Treatment of opioid dependence in patients who have been opioid free for at least 7-10 days

PO

Adults, Elderly. Initially, 25 mg. Observe patient for 1 hr. If no withdrawal signs or symptoms appear, give another 25 mg. May be given as 100 mg every other day or 150 mg every 3 days.

Adjunctive treatment of alcohol dependence

PO

Adults, Elderly. 50 mg once a day.

S **AVAILABLE FORMS/COST**

• Tab—Oral: 50 mg, 100's: **$427.51-$508.16**

UNLABELED USES: Treatment of eating disorders, post-concussional syndrome unresponsive to other treatments

CONTRAINDICATIONS: Acute hepatitis, acute opioid withdrawal, failed naloxone challenge test, hepatic failure, history of hypersensitivity to naltrexone, opioid dependence, positive urine screen for opioids

PREGNANCY AND LACTATION: Pregnancy category C

SIDE EFFECTS

Frequent

Alcoholism (10%-7%): Nausea, headache, depression

Narcotic addiction (10%-5%): Insomnia, anxiety, nervousness, headache, low energy, abdominal cramps, nausea, vomiting, arthralgia, myalgia

Occasional

Alcoholism (4%-2%): Dizziness, nervousness, fatigue, insomnia, vomiting, anxiety, suicidal ideation

Narcotic addiction (5%-2%): Irritability, increased energy, dizziness, anorexia, diarrhea or constipation, rash, chills, increased thirst

SERIOUS REACTIONS

• Signs and symptoms of opioid withdrawal include stuffy or runny nose, tearing, yawning, diaphoresis, tremor, vomiting, piloerection, feeling of temperature change, bone pain, arthralgia, myalgia, abdominal cramps, and feeling of skin crawling.

• Accidental naltrexone overdose produces withdrawal symptoms within 5 minutes of ingestion that may last for up to 48 hours. Symptoms include confusion, visual hallucinations, somnolence, and significant vomiting and diarrhea.

• Hepatocellular injury may occur with large doses.

SPECIAL CONSIDERATIONS

PATIENT/FAMILY EDUCATION

• Wear ID tag indicating naltrexone use

• Do not try to overcome reversal of opiate effects by self-administration of large doses of narcotic

• Do not exceed recommended dose

MONITORING PARAMETERS

• Liver function tests

nandrolone

(nan'-droe-lone)

Rx:

Decanoate:Deca-Durabolin, Hybolin Decanoate, Kabolin, Nandrolone Decanoate

Chemical Class: Anabolic steroid; testosterone derivative

Therapeutic Class: Androgen; antineoplastic

DEA Class: Schedule III

CLINICAL PHARMACOLOGY

Mechanism of Action: An anabolic steroid that promotes tissue-building processes, increases production of erythropoietin, causes protein anabolism, and increases hemoglobin and red blood cell volume. *Therapeutic Effect:* Controls metastatic breast cancer and helps manage anemia of renal insufficiency.

Pharmacokinetics

Well absorbed after IM administration (about 77%). Metabolized in liver. Primarily excreted in urine. **Half-life:** 6-8 days.

INDICATIONS AND DOSAGES

Breast cancer

IM

Adults, Elderly. 50-100 mg/week.

Anemia of renal insufficiency

IM

Adults, Elderly (male). 100-200 mg/week.

Adults, Elderly (female). 50-100 mg/week.

Children, 2-13 yrs. 25-50 mg every 3-4 weeks.

AVAILABLE FORMS/COST

• Sol, Inj (decanoate)—IM: 50 mg/ml, 2 ml: **$4.90-$14.05**; 100 mg/ml, 2 ml: **$7.50-$29.40**; 200 mg/ml, 1 ml: **$15.30-$17.00**

UNLABELED USES: Hyperlipidemia, lung cancer, male contraception, malnutrition, postmenopausal osteoporosis, rheumatoid arthritis, Sjogren's syndrome, trauma/surgery

CONTRAINDICATIONS: Nephrosis, pregnancy, carcinoma of breast or prostate, not for use in infants, hypersensitivity to nandrolone or any component of the formulation such as sesame oil

PREGNANCY AND LACTATION: Pregnancy category X, use extreme caution in nursing mothers

SIDE EFFECTS

Frequent

Male, postpubertal: Gynecomastia, acne, bladder irritability, priapism

Male, prepubertal: Acne, virilism

Females: Virilism

Occasional

Male, postpubertal/prepubertal: Insomnia, chills, decreased libido, hepatic dysfunction, nausea, diarrhea, prostatic hyperplasia (elderly), iron-deficiency anemia, suppression of clotting factors

Male, prepubertal: Chills, insomnia, hyperpigmentation, diarrhea, nausea, iron deficiency anemia, suppression of clotting factors

Female: Chills, insomnia, hypercalcemia, nausea, diarrhea, iron deficiency anemia, suppression of clotting factors, hepatic dysfunction

Rare

Hepatic necrosis, heptocellular carcinoma

SERIOUS REACTIONS

• Peliosis hepatitis of liver, spleen replaced with blood-filled cysts, hepatic neoplasms and hepatocellular carcinoma have been associated with prolonged high-dosage, anaphylactic reactions.

N

INTERACTIONS
Drugs
3 *Antidiabetic agents:* Enhanced hypoglycemic effects

2 *Cyclosporine:* Increased cyclosporine concentrations, potential for toxicity

3 *HMG-CoA reductase inhibitors (lovastatin, pravastatin):* Myositis risk increased

2 *Oral anticoagulants:* Enhanced hypoprothrombinemic response

3 *Tacrolimus:* Increased tacrolimus concentrations, potential for toxicity

SPECIAL CONSIDERATIONS
• Anabolic steroids have potential for abuse, especially in the athlete

MONITORING PARAMETERS
• Women should be observed for signs of virilization
• Liver function tests, lipids, Hct
• Growth rate in children (X-rays for bone age q6 mo)

---

naproxen
(na-prox'en)

Rx: *Sodium salt:*Anaprox, Anaprox DS, Naprelan
Rx: EC-Naprosyn
Combinations
   Rx: with lansoprazole (NapraPAC)
Chemical Class: Propionic acid derivative
Therapeutic Class: NSAID; antipyretic; nonnarcotic analgesic

CLINICAL PHARMACOLOGY
Mechanism of Action: An NSAID that produces analgesic and anti-inflammatory effects by inhibiting prostaglandin synthesis. *Therapeutic Effect:* Reduces the inflammatory response and intensity of pain.

Pharmacokinetics

Route	Onset	Peak	Duration
PO (analgesic)	less than 1 hr	N/A	7 hr or less
PO (antirheumatic)	less than 14 days	2–4 wk	N/A

Completely absorbed from the GI tract. Protein binding: 99%. Metabolized in the liver. Primarily excreted in urine. Not removed by hemodialysis. **Half-life:** 13 hr.

INDICATIONS AND DOSAGES
Rheumatoid arthritis, osteoarthritis, ankylosing spondylitis
PO

Adults, Elderly. 250–500 mg naproxen (275–550 mg naproxen sodium) twice a day or 250 mg naproxen (275 mg naproxen sodium) in morning and 500 mg naproxen (550 mg naproxen sodium) in evening. Naprelan: 750–1,000 mg once a day.

Acute gouty arthritis
PO

Adults, Elderly. Initially, 750 mg naproxen (825 mg naproxen sodium), then 250 mg naproxen (275 mg naproxen sodium) q8h until attack subsides. Naprelan: Initially, 1,000–1,500 mg, then 1,000 mg once a day until attack subsides.

Mild to moderate pain, dysmenorrhea, bursitis, tendinitis
PO

Adults, Elderly. Initially, 500 mg naproxen (550 mg naproxen sodium), then 250 mg naparoxen (275 mg naproxen sodium) q6–8h as needed. Maximum: 1.25 g/day naproxen (1.375 g/day naproxen sodium). Naprelan: 1,000 mg once a day.

Juvenile rheumatoid arthritis
PO (naproxen only)
Children. 10–15 mg/kg/day in 2 divided doses. Maximum: 1,000 mg/day.

§ AVAILABLE FORMS/COST
Naproxen
• Susp—Oral: 125 mg/5 ml, 500 ml: **$44.32**
• Tab—Oral: 250 mg, 100's: **$8.60-$110.54**; 375 mg, 100's: **$11.28-$156.61**; 500 mg, 100's: **$105.30-$173.53**
• Tab, Enteric Coated—Oral: 375 mg, 100's: **$101.21-$106.40**; 500 mg, 100's: **$124.67-$163.94**
Naproxen Sodium (Naproxen)
• Tab—Oral: 220 mg (200 mg), 100's: **$8.25-$22.00**; 275 mg (250 mg), 100's: **$11.13-$114.56**; 550 mg (500 mg), 100's: **$90.00-$178.36**
• Tab, Enteric Coated—Oral: 412.5 mg (375 mg), 100's: **$134.34**; 550 mg (500 mg), 75's: **$110.59-$122.88**

UNLABELED USES: Treatment of vascular headaches

CONTRAINDICATIONS: Hypersensitivity to aspirin, naproxen, or other NSAIDs

PREGNANCY AND LACTATION: Pregnancy category B (category D if used in 3rd trimester); could cause constriction of the ductus arteriosus *in utero,* persistent pulmonary hypertension of the newborn, or prolonged labor; passes into breast milk in small quantities; compatible with breast-feeding

SIDE EFFECTS
Frequent (9%–4%)
Nausea, constipation, abdominal cramps or pain, heartburn, dizziness, headache, somnolence
Occasional (3%–1%)
Stomatitis, diarrhea, indigestion
Rare (less than 1%)
Vomiting, confusion

SERIOUS REACTIONS
• Rare reactions with long-term use include peptic ulcer disease, GI bleeding, gastritis, severe hepatic reactions (cholestasis, jaundice), nephrotoxicity (dysuria, hematuria, proteinuria, nephrotic syndrome), and a severe hypersensitivity reaction (fever, chills, bronchospasm).

INTERACTIONS
Drugs
▣ *Aminoglycosides:* Reduced clearance with elevated aminoglycoside levels and potential for toxicity (especially indomethacin in premature infants; other NSAIDs probably)
▣ *Anticoagulants:* Excessive hypoprothrombinemia, decreased platelet aggregation with increased risk of GI bleeding
▣ *Antihypertensives (α-blockers, angiotensin-converting enzyme inhibitors, angiotensin II receptor blockers, β-blockers, diuretics):* Inhibition of antihypertensive and other favorable hemodynamic effects
▣ *Corticosteroids:* Increased risk of GI ulceration
▣ *Cyclosporine:* Increased nephrotoxicity risk
▣ *Lithium:* Decreased clearance of lithium (mediated via prostaglandins) resulting in elevated serum lithium levels and risk of toxicity
▣ *Methotrexate:* Decreased renal secretion of methotrexate resulting in elevated methotrexate levels and risk of toxicity
▣ *Phenylpropanolamine:* Possible acute hypertensive reaction
▣ *Potassium-sparing diuretics:* Additive hyperkalemia potential
▣ *Triamterene:* Acute renal failure reported with addition of indomethacin; caution with other NSAIDs

N

Labs
• *False increase:* Serum bicarbonate, urine 5-HIAA

SPECIAL CONSIDERATIONS
• No significant advantage over other NSAIDs; cost should govern use

PATIENT/FAMILY EDUCATION
• Avoid concurrent use of aspirin and alcoholic beverages
• Take with food, milk, or antacids to decrease GI upset
• Notify clinician if edema, black stools, or persistent headache occur

MONITORING PARAMETERS
• Initial hemogram and fecal occult blood test within 3 mo of starting regular chronic therapy; repeat every 6-12 mo (more frequently in high-risk patients (>65 years, peptic ulcer disease, concurrent steroids or anticoagulants); electrolytes, creatinine, and BUN within 3 mo of starting regular chronic therapy; repeat every 6-12 mo

---

naratriptan
(nare-a-trip'tan)
Rx: Amerge
Chemical Class: Serotonin derivative
Therapeutic Class: Antimigraine agent

CLINICAL PHARMACOLOGY
Mechanism of Action: A serotonin receptor agonist that binds selectively to vascular receptors producing a vasoconstrictive effect on cranial blood vessels. *Therapeutic Effect:* Relieves migraine headache.
Pharmacokinetics
Well absorbed after PO administration. Protein binding: 28%-31%. Metabolized by the liver to inactive metabolite. Eliminated primarily in urine and, to a lesser extent, in feces.

Half-life: 6 hr (increased in hepatic or renal impairment).

INDICATIONS AND DOSAGES
Acute migraine attack
PO
Adults. 1 mg or 2.5 mg. If headache improves but then returns, dose may be repeated after 4 hr. Maximum: 5 mg/24 hr.
Dosage in mild to moderate hepatic or renal impairment
A lower starting dose is recommended. Do not exceed 2.5 mg/24 hr.

Ⓢ AVAILABLE FORMS/COST
• Tab, Film Coated—Oral: 1 mg, 2.5 mg, 9's: **$187.19**

CONTRAINDICATIONS: Basilar or hemiplegic migraine, cerebrovascular or peripheral vascular disease, coronary artery disease, ischemic heart disease (including angina pectoris, history of MI, silent ischemia, and Prinzmetal's angina), severe hepatic impairment (Child-Pugh grade C), severe renal impairment (serum creatinine less than 15 ml/min), uncontrolled hypertension, use within 24 hours of ergotamine-containing preparations or another serotonin receptor agonist, use within 14 days of MAOIs

PREGNANCY AND LACTATION: Pregnancy category C; use caution in nursing mothers

SIDE EFFECTS
Occasional (5%)
Nausea
Rare (2%)
Paresthesia; dizziness; fatigue; somnolence; jaw, neck, or throat pressure

SERIOUS REACTIONS
• Corneal opacities and other ocular defects may occur.
• Cardiac reactions (including ischemia, coronary artery vasospasm, and MI) and noncardiac vasospasm-related reactions (such as hemor-

rhage and CVA), occur rarely, particularly in patients with hypertension, diabetes, or a strong family history of coronary artery disease; obese patients; smokers; males older than 40 years; and postmenopausal women.

INTERACTIONS
Drugs
⚠ *Ergotamine containing drugs:* Increased vasoconstriction

⚠ *MAO inhibitors:* Potential for decreased metabolism of naratriptan

❷ *Sibutramine:* Increased risk of serotonin syndrome

SPECIAL CONSIDERATIONS
• Longer acting than sumatriptan and zolmitriptan so recurrent headaches requiring a second dose less likely; slower onset than sumatriptan and zolmitriptan; should probably be reserved for patients who get recurrent headaches

• Safety of treating, on average, more than 4 headaches in a 30-day period has not been established

PATIENT/FAMILY EDUCATION
• Use only to treat migraine headache, not for prevention

---

natamycin
(na-ta-mye'-sin)
Rx: Natacyn
Chemical Class: Tetraene polyene derivative
Therapeutic Class: Ophthalmic antifungal

CLINICAL PHARMACOLOGY
Mechanism of Action: A polyene antifungal agent that increases cell membrane permeability in susceptible fungi. *Therapeutic Effect:* Fungicidal.

Pharmacokinetics
Minimal systemic absorption. Adheres to cornea and retained in conjunctival fornices.

INDICATIONS AND DOSAGES
Fungal keratitis, ophthalmic fungal infections
Ophthalmic
Adults, Elderly. Instill 1 drop in conjunctival sac every 1-2 hours. After 3-4 days, reduce to 1 drop 6-8 times daily. Usual course of therapy is 2-3 weeks.

Ⓢ **AVAILABLE FORMS/COST**
• Susp—Ophth: 5%, 15 ml: **$153.50**
UNLABELED USES: Oral and vaginal candidiasis, onychomycosis, pulmonary aspergillosis
CONTRAINDICATIONS: Hypersensitivity to natamycin or any component of the formulation
PREGNANCY AND LACTATION: Pregnancy category C
SIDE EFFECTS
Occasional (10%-3%)
Blurred vision, eye irritation, eye pain, photophobia
SERIOUS REACTIONS
• Vomiting and diarrhea have occurred with large doses in the treatment of systemic mycoses.
SPECIAL CONSIDERATIONS
PATIENT/FAMILY EDUCATION
• Shake well before using
MONITORING PARAMETERS
• Failure of keratitis to improve following 7-10 days of administration suggests infection not susceptible to natamycin

N

nateglinide
(na-teg'lin-ide)
Rx: Starlix
Chemical Class: Amino acid derivative; meglitinide
Therapeutic Class: Antidiabetic; hypoglycemic

CLINICAL PHARMACOLOGY
Mechanism of Action: An antihyperglycemic that stimulates release of insulin from beta cells of the pancreas by depolarizing beta cells, leading to an opening of calcium channels. Resulting calcium influx induces insulin secretion. *Therapeutic Effect:* Lowers blood glucose concentration.

INDICATIONS AND DOSAGES
Diabetes mellitus
PO
Adult, Elderly. 120 mg 3 times a day before meals. Initially, 60 mg may be given.

§ AVAILABLE FORMS/COST
• Tab—Oral: 60 mg, 100's: **$109.11**; 120 mg, 100's: **$113.36**

CONTRAINDICATIONS: Diabetic ketoacidosis, type 1 diabetes mellitus

PREGNANCY AND LACTATION: Pregnancy category C (no adequate and well-controlled studies in pregnant women); excretion into human breast milk unknown

SIDE EFFECTS
Frequent (10%)
Upper respiratory tract infection
Occasional (4%–3%)
Back pain, flu symptoms, dizziness, arthropathy, diarrhea
Rare (2%)
Bronchitis, cough

SERIOUS REACTIONS
• Hypoglycemia occurs in less than 2% of patients.

INTERACTIONS
Drugs
▣ β-blockers: Antagonistic glycemic effects, prolong hypoglycemia, mask hypoglycemia symptoms
▣ *Diazoxide:* Antagonistic effects (diazoxide causes hyperglycemia)
▣ *Epinephrine:* Antagonistic effects; combination may decrease hypoglycemic efficacy
▣ *MAOI:* MAOIs stimulate insulin secretion; additive effects; increased risk of hypoglycemia
▣ *Hypoglycemics (bioguanides, insulin):* Combination increases risk of hypoglycemia
▣ *Isoniazid:* Antagonistic effects; combination may decrease hypoglycemic efficacy
▣ *Niacin:* Antagonistic effects; combination may decrease hypoglycemic efficacy
Labs
• *Uric acid:* Increased

SPECIAL CONSIDERATIONS
• *Pharmacodynamics* (60-120 mg tid ac for 24 weeks): HbA1c change -0.5%; fasting plasma glucose change -15 mg/dL; weight change -0.3-0.9 kg

PATIENT/FAMILY EDUCATION
• Review signs and symptoms and management of hypoglycemia
• Drug administration timing (i.e., before meals)

MONITORING PARAMETERS
• Home/self blood glucose monitoring, HbA1c, signs and symptoms of hyper/hypoglycemia, complete blood count, routine blood chemistry

nedocromil

(ned-oh-crow'mil)

Rx: *Oral:*Tilade

Rx: *Ophth:*Alocril

Chemical Class: Mast cell stabilizer; pyranoquinoline dicarboxylic acid derivative

Therapeutic Class: Antiasthmatic; inhaled antiinflammatory

CLINICAL PHARMACOLOGY

Mechanism of Action: A mast cell stabilizer that prevents the activation and release of inflammatory mediators, such as histamine, leukotrienes, mast cells, eosinophils, and monocytes. *Therapeutic Effect:* Prevents both early and late asthmatic responses.

INDICATIONS AND DOSAGES

Mild to moderate asthma

Oral inhalation

Adults, Elderly, Children 6 yr and older. 2 inhalations 4 times a day. May decrease to 3 times a day then twice a day as asthma becomes controlled.

Allergic conjunctivitis

Ophthalmic

Adults, Elderly, Children 3 yr and older. 1–2 drops in each eye twice a day.

[$] **AVAILABLE FORMS/COST**

• Aer—INH: 1.75 mg/spray, 112 sprays: **$69.86**

• Sol—Ophth: 2%, 5 ml: **$64.01**

UNLABELED USES: Prevention of bronchospasm in patients with reversible obstructive airway disease

CONTRAINDICATIONS: None known.

PREGNANCY AND LACTATION: Pregnancy category B; excretion into breast milk unknown

SIDE EFFECTS

Frequent (10%–6%)

Cough, pharyngitis, bronchospasm, headache, altered taste

Occasional (5%–1%)

Rhinitis, upper respiratory tract infection, abdominal pain, fatigue

Rare (less than 1%)

Diarrhea, dizziness

SERIOUS REACTIONS

• None known.

SPECIAL CONSIDERATIONS

PATIENT/FAMILY EDUCATION

• Must be used regularly to achieve benefit, even during symptom-free periods

• Therapeutic effect may take up to 4 wk

• Not to be used to treat acute asthmatic symptoms

nefazodone

(neh-faz'oh-doan)

Rx: Serzone

Chemical Class: Phenylpiperazine derivative

Therapeutic Class: Antidepressant

CLINICAL PHARMACOLOGY

Mechanism of Action: Exact mechanism is unknown. Appears to inhibit neuronal uptake of serotonin and norepinephrine and to antagonize $alpha_1$-adrenergic receptors. *Therapeutic Effect:* Relieves depression.

Pharmacokinetics

Rapidly and completely absorbed from the GI tract; food delays absorption. Protein binding: 99%. Widely distributed in body tissues, including CNS. Extensively metabolized to active metabolites. Excreted in urine and eliminated in feces. Unknown if removed by hemodialysis. **Half-life:** 2-4 hr.

N

INDICATIONS AND DOSAGES
Depression, prevention of relapse of acute depressive episode
PO

Adults. Initially, 200 mg/day in 2 divided doses. Gradually increase by 100-200 mg/day at intervals of at least 1 wk. Range: 300-600 mg/day.
Elderly. Initially, 100 mg/day in 2 divided doses. Subsequent dosage titration based on clinical response. Range: 200-400 mg/day.
Children. 300-400 mg/day.

§ AVAILABLE FORMS/COST
• Tab—Oral: 50 mg, 60's: **$90.17-$150.28**; 100 mg, 60's: **$87.94-$102.60**; 150 mg, 60's: **$74.12-$104.53**; 200 mg, 60's: **$91.29-$106.50**; 250 mg, 60's: **$96.55-$108.48**

CONTRAINDICATIONS: Use within 14 days of MAOIs

PREGNANCY AND LACTATION: Pregnancy category C; excretion into breast milk unknown, use caution in nursing mothers

SIDE EFFECTS
Frequent

Headache (36%); dry mouth, somnolence (25%); nausea (22%); dizziness (17%); constipation (14%); insomnia, asthenia, light-headedness (10%).

Occasional

Dyspepsia, blurred vision (9%); diarrhea, infection (8%); confusion, abnormal vision (7%); pharyngitis (6%); increased appetite (5%); orthostatic hypotension, flushing, feeling of warmth (4%); peripheral edema, cough, flu-like symptoms (3%).

SERIOUS REACTIONS
• Serious reactions, such as hyperthermia, rigidity, myoclonus, extreme agitation, delirium, and coma, will occur if the patient takes an MAOI concurrently or fails to let

enough time elapse when switching from an MAOI to nefazodone or vice versa.

INTERACTIONS
Drugs
❷ *Alprazolam:* Significant increase in serum alprazolam concentrations; if coadministered reduce alprazolam dose by 50%

❸ *Atorvastatin, lovastatin, simvastatin:* Potential for development of myositis with rhabdomyolysis

❸ *Buspirone:* Significant increase in serum buspirone concentrations

❷ *Carbamazepine:* 95% decrease in serum nefazodone concentrations; concomitant use contraindicated

▲ *Cisapride, pimozide:* Theoretical potential for QT prolongation and dysrhythmia; concomitant use contraindicated

❸ *Cyclosporine, tacrolimus:* Toxic blood levels of immunosuppressives have been reported; monitor levels and adjust immunosuppressive dosage as needed

❸ *Digoxin:* Increased serum digoxin concentrations

❷ *Triazolam:* Significant increase in serum triazolam concentrations; if coadministered reduce triazolam dose by 75%

❷ *MAOIs:* Serious adverse reactions possible including hyperthermia, rigidity, myoclonus, autonomic instability, mental status changes, seizures; observe a 14-day washout period between discontinuing one drug and starting the other

SPECIAL CONSIDERATIONS
• Priapism has been reported; educate and monitor appropriately

PATIENT/FAMILY EDUCATION
• Therapeutic effect may not be apparent for several weeks
• Drug may cause drowsiness, use caution driving or performing other tasks where alertness is required

nelfinavir
(nel-fin'eh-veer)
Rx: Viracept
Chemical Class: Protease inhibitor, HIV
Therapeutic Class: Antiretroviral

CLINICAL PHARMACOLOGY
Mechanism of Action: Inhibits the activity of HIV-1 protease, the enzyme necessary for the formation of infectious HIV. *Therapeutic Effect:* Formation of immature noninfectious viral particles rather than HIV replication.

Pharmacokinetics
Well absorbed after PO administration (absorption increased with food). Protein binding: 98%. Metabolized in the liver. Highly bound to plasma proteins. Eliminated primarily in feces. Unknown if removed by hemodialysis. **Half-life:** 3.5-5 hr.

INDICATIONS AND DOSAGES
HIV infection
PO
Adults. 750 mg (three 250-mg tablets) 3 times a day or 1,250 mg twice a day in combination with nucleoside analogues (enhances antiviral activity).
Children 2-13 yr. 20-30 mg/kg/dose 3 times a day. Maximum: 750 mg q8h.

$ AVAILABLE FORMS/COST
• Powder, Reconst—Oral: 50 mg nelfinavir base per g, 144 g: **$66.48**
• Tab—Oral: 250 mg, 270's: **$692.83**

CONTRAINDICATIONS: Concurrent administration with midazolam, rifampin, or triazolam

PREGNANCY AND LACTATION: Pregnancy category B; excreted in breast milk; breast-feeding not recommended for HIV-infected women

SIDE EFFECTS
Frequent (20%)
Diarrhea
Occasional (7%-3%)
Nausea, rash
Rare (2%-1%)
Flatulence, asthenia

SERIOUS REACTIONS
• None known.

INTERACTIONS
Drugs
▣ *Barbiturates:* Increased clearance of nelfinavir; reduced clearance of barbiturates

❷ *Carbamazepine:* Increased clearance of nelfinavir; reduced clearance of carbamazepine

▲ *Cisapride:* Increased plasma levels of cisapride

▲ *Ergot alkaloids:* Increased plasma levels of ergot alkaloids

▣ *Erythromycin:* Reduced clearance of nelfinavir; nelfinavir reduces clearance of erythromycin

▲ *Lovastatin:* Nelfinavir reduces clearance of lovastatin

▲ *Midazolam:* Increased plasma levels of midazolam and prolonged effect

▣ *Nevirapine:* Reduces plasma nelfinavir levels; increase nelfinavir dose to 1000 mg tid

▣ *Oral contraceptives:* Nelfinavir may reduce efficacy

▣ *Phenytoin:* Increased clearance of nelfinavir; reduced clearance of phenytoin

❷ *Rifabutin:* Increased clearance of nelfinavir; reduced clearance of rifabutin—reduce rifabutin dose to 150 mg qday and increase nelfinavir dose to 1000 mg tid

▲ *Rifampin:* Increased clearance of nelfinavir

▣ *Ritonavir:* Decreased clearance of nelfinavir; decrease nelfinavir dose to 750 mg bid

▣ *Saquinavir:* Decreased clearance of saquinavir; reduce dose of Fortovase (saquinavir soft gel capsule) to 800 mg tid

▲ *Simvastatin:* Nelfinavir reduces clearance of simvastatin

▲ *Triazolam:* Increased plasma levels of triazolam and prolonged effect

SPECIAL CONSIDERATIONS

• Positive results of treatment are based on surrogate markers only

• Take with meal or snack

PATIENT/FAMILY EDUCATION

• Contains phenylalanine, take with food

MONITORING PARAMETERS

• CBC, electrolytes, renal function, liver enzymes, CPK

---

neomycin

(nee-oh-mye′sin)

Rx: *Oral:* Mycifradin, Neo-Fradin

OTC: *Topical:* Myciguent Combinations

   Rx: with polymyxin B (Neosporin G.U. irrigant)

   OTC: with polymyxin B, bacitracin (Neosporin, Mycitracin)

Chemical Class: Aminoglycoside

Therapeutic Class: Antibiotic

CLINICAL PHARMACOLOGY

Mechanism of Action: An aminoglycoside antibiotic that binds to bacterial microorganisms. *Therapeutic Effect:* Interferes with bacterial protein synthesis.

INDICATIONS AND DOSAGES

Preoperative bowel antisepsis

PO

Adults, Elderly. 1 g/hr for 4 doses; then 1 g q4h for 5 doses or 1 g at 1 p.m., 2 p.m., and 10 p.m. (with erythromycin) on day before surgery.

Children. 90 mg/kg/day in divided doses q4h for 2 days or 25 mg/kg at 1 p.m., 2 p.m., and 10 p.m. on day before surgery.

Hepatic encephalopathy

PO

Adults, Elderly. 4-12 g/day in divided doses q4-6h.

Children. 2.5-7 g/m²/day in divided doses q4-6h.

Diarrhea caused by Escherichia coli

PO

Adults, Elderly. 3 g/day in divided doses q6h.

Children. 50 mg/kg/day in divided doses q6h.

Minor skin infections

Topical

Adults, Elderly, Children. Usual dosage, apply to affected area 1-3 times/day.

🅢 **AVAILABLE FORMS/COST**

• Cre—Top: 0.5%, 15, 30 g: **$2.98**/15 g

• Oint—Top: 0.5%, 15, 30 g: **$2.98**/15 g

• Tab—Oral: 500 mg, 100′s: **$11.51-$124.57**

CONTRAINDICATIONS: Hypersensitivity to neomycin, other aminoglycosides (cross-sensitivity), or their components

PREGNANCY AND LACTATION: Pregnancy category D; ototoxicity has not been reported as an effect of *in utero* exposure; 8th cranial nerve toxicity in the fetus is well known following exposure to other aminoglycosides and could potentially occur with neomycin

SIDE EFFECTS
Frequent

Systemic: Nausea, vomiting, diarrhea, irritation of mouth or rectal area

Topical: Itching, redness, swelling, rash

Rare

Systemic: Malabsorption syndrome, neuromuscular blockade (difficulty breathing, drowsiness, weakness)

SERIOUS REACTIONS
• Nephrotoxicity (as evidenced by increased BUN and serum creatinine levels and decreased creatinine clearance) may be reversible if the drug is stopped at the first sign of nephrotoxic symptoms.

• Irreversible ototoxicity (manifested as tinnitus, dizziness, and impaired hearing) and neurotoxicity (as evidenced by headache, dizziness, lethargy, tremor, and visual disturbances) occur occasionally.

• Severe respiratory depression and anaphylaxis occur rarely.

• Superinfections, particularly fungal infections, may occur.

INTERACTIONS
Drugs

3 *Digitalis glycosides:* Reduced serum digoxin concentration

2 *Ethacrynic acid:* Increased risk of ototoxicity, especially in patients with renal impairment

3 *Oral anticoagulants:* Enhanced hypoprothrombinemic response; more common with large doses of neomycin, dietary vitamin K deficiency, impaired hepatic function

⚠ *Methotrexate:* Oral absorption of methotrexate reduced 30%-50%

3 *Penicillin V:* Reduced concentrations of penicillin V, possible reduced efficacy

3 *Warfarin:* Enhanced hypoprothrombinemic response

SPECIAL CONSIDERATIONS
• Inform patient and family about possible toxic effects on the 8th cranial nerve; monitor for loss of hearing, ringing or roaring in ears, or a feeling of fullness in head

PATIENT/FAMILY EDUCATION
• Drink plenty of fluids

MONITORING PARAMETERS
• Renal function, audiometric testing during extended therapy or with application to extensive burns or large surface area

---

neostigmine
Rx: Prostigmin
Chemical Class: Cholinesterase inhibitor; quaternary ammonium derivative
Therapeutic Class: Cholinergic

CLINICAL PHARMACOLOGY
Mechanism of Action: A cholinergic that prevents destruction of acetylcholine by inhibiting the enzyme acetylcholinesterase, thus enhancing impulse transmission across the myoneural junction. *Therapeutic Effect:* Improves intestinal and skeletal muscle tone; stimulates salivary and sweat gland secretions.

INDICATIONS AND DOSAGES
Myasthenia gravis
PO

Adults, Elderly. Initially, 15–30 mg 3–4 times a day. Increase as necessary. Maintenance: 150 mg/day (range of 15–375 mg).

Children. 2 mg/kg/day or 60 mg/m^2/day divided q3–4h.

IV, IM, Subcutaneous

Adults. 0.5–2.5 mg as needed.

Children. 0.01–0.04 mg/kg q2–4h.

Diagnosis of myasthenia gravis
IM
Adults, Elderly. 0.022 mg/kg. If cholinergic reaction occurs, discontinue tests and administer 0.4–0.6 mg or more atropine sulfate IV.
Children. 0.025–0.04 mg/kg preceded by atropine sulfate 0.011 mg/kg subcutaneously.

Prevention of postoperative urinary retention
IM, Subcutaneous
Adults, Elderly. 0.25 mg q4–6h for 2–3 days.

Postoperative abdominial distention and urine retention
IM, Subcutaneous
Adults, Elderly. 0.5–1 mg. Catheterize patient if voiding does not occur within 1 hr. After voiding, administer 0.5 mg q3h for 5 injections.

Reversal of neuromuscular blockade
IV
Adults, Elderly. 0.5–2.5 mg given slowly.
Children. 0.025–0.08 mg/kg/dose.
Infants. 0.025–0.1 mg/kg/dose.

$ AVAILABLE FORMS/COST
• Sol, Inj—IM, IV, SC: 1:1000 (1 mg/ml), 10 ml: **$1.13-$16.08**; 1:2000 (0.5 mg/ml), 1, 10 ml: **$1.06-$12.19**/10 ml; 1:4000 (0.25 mg/ml), 1 ml: **$1.41**
• Tab—Oral: 15 mg, 100's: **$58.19**

CONTRAINDICATIONS: GI or GU obstruction, peritonitis

PREGNANCY AND LACTATION: Pregnancy category C; transient muscle weakness occurred in 20% of infants born to mothers using neostigmine and similar drugs; ionized at physiologic pH, would not be expected to be excreted in breast milk

SIDE EFFECTS
Frequent
Muscarinic effects (diarrhea, diaphoresis, increased salivation, nausea, vomiting, abdominal cramps or pain)
Occasional
Muscarinic effects (urinary urgency or frequency, increased bronchial secretions, miosis, lacrimation)

SERIOUS REACTIONS
• Overdose produces a cholinergic crisis manifested as abdominal discomfort or cramps, nausea, vomiting, diarrhea, flushing, facial warmth, excessive salivation, diaphoresis, lacrimation, pallor, bradycardia or tachycardia, hypotension, bronchospasm, urinary urgency, blurred vision, miosis, and fasciculation (involuntary muscular contractions visible under the skin).

INTERACTIONS
Drugs
🔳 *Tacrine:* Increased cholinergic effects

SPECIAL CONSIDERATIONS
MONITORING PARAMETERS
• *Myasthenia gravis*
• Therapeutic response: Increased muscle strength, improved gait, absence of labored breathing
• Toxicity: Narrow margin between first appearance of side effects and serious toxicity

---

nesiritide
(neh-sir'i-tide)
Rx: Natrecor
Chemical Class: Recombinant human peptide
Therapeutic Class: Vasodilator

CLINICAL PHARMACOLOGY
Mechanism of Action: A brain natriuretic peptide that facilitates cardiovascular homeostasis and fluid status through counterregulation of the renin-angiotensin-aldos-

terone system, stimulating cyclic guanosine monophosphate, thereby leading to smooth-muscle cell relaxation. *Therapeutic Effect:* Promotes vasodilation, natriuresis, and diuresis, correcting CHF.

Pharmacokinetics

Route	Onset	Peak	Dura-tion
IV	15–30 min	1–2 hr	4 hr

Excreted primarily in the heart by the left ventricle. Metabolized by the natriuretic neutral endopeptidase enzymes on the vascular luminal surface. **Half-life:** 18–23 min.

INDICATIONS AND DOSAGES
Treatment of acutely decompensated CHF in patients with dyspnea at rest or with minimal activity
IV bolus

Adults, Elderly. 2 mcg/kg followed by a continuous IV infusion of 0.01 mcg/kg/min. May be incrementally increased q3h to a maximum of 0.03 mcg/kg/min.

$ AVAILABLE FORMS/COST
• Powder, Inj—IV: 1.5 mg, single use vials: **$507.60**

CONTRAINDICATIONS: Cardiogenic shock, systolic BP less than 90 mm Hg

PREGNANCY AND LACTATION: Pregnancy category C (neither animal or human studies have been done); breast milk data unavailable

SIDE EFFECTS
Frequent (11%)
Hypotension
Occasional (8%–2%)
Headache, nausea, bradycardia
Rare (1% or less)
Confusion, paresthesia, somnolence, tremor

SERIOUS REACTIONS
• Ventricular arrhythmias, including ventricular tachycardia, atrial fibrillation, AV node conduction abnormalities, and angina pectoris occur rarely.

INTERACTIONS
Drugs
3 *Angiotensin-converting enzyme inhibitors:* Added hypotensive effects
2 *Bumetanide:* Physically and/or chemically incompatible; should not be coadministered as infusions
2 *Enalaprilat:* Physically and/or chemically incompatible; should not be coadministered as infusions
2 *Ethacrynic acid:* Physically and/or chemically incompatible; should not be coadministered as infusions
2 *Furosemide:* Physically and/or chemically incompatible; should not be coadministered as infusions
2 *Heparin:* Physically and/or chemically incompatible; should not be coadministered as infusions
2 *Hydralazine:* Physically and/or chemically incompatible; should not be coadministered as infusions
2 *Insulin:* Physically and/or chemically incompatible; should not be coadministered as infusions
2 *Sodium Metabisulfite (preservative):* Incompatible; flush line between administration

SPECIAL CONSIDERATIONS
• Limited experience in administration for longer than 48 hr
• If hypotension occurs, discontinue and subsequently restart at dose reduced dose by 30% (no bolus) once patient has stabilized

MONITORING PARAMETERS
• Plasma brain natriuretic peptide concentrations, plasma aldosterone, heart failure hemodynamic mea-

N

surements, clinical symptoms of heart failure, routine blood chemistries, blood pressure

---

nevirapine
(neh-veer′a-peen)

Rx: Viramune

Chemical Class: Dipyridodiazepinone derivative; non-nucleoside reverse transcriptase inhibitor

Therapeutic Class: Antiretroviral

CLINICAL PHARMACOLOGY

Mechanism of Action: A non-nucleoside reverse transcriptase inhibitor that binds directly to HIV-1 reverse transcriptase, thus changing the shape of this enzyme and blocking RNA- and DNA-dependent polymerase activity. *Therapeutic Effect:* Interferes with HIV replication, slowing the progression of HIV infection.

Pharmacokinetics

Readily absorbed after PO administration. Protein binding: 60%. Widely distributed. Extensively metabolized in the liver. Excreted primarily in urine. **Half-life:** 45 hr (single dose), 25-30 hr (multiple doses).

INDICATIONS AND DOSAGES
HIV infection
PO

Adults. 200 mg once a day for 14 days (to reduce the risk of rash). Maintenance: 200 mg twice a day in combination with nucleoside analogues.

Children older than 8 yr. 4 mg/kg once a day for 14 days; then 4 mg/kg twice a day. Maximum: 400 mg/day.

Children 2 mos-8 yr. 4 mg/kg once a day for 14 days; then 7 mg/kg twice a day.

AVAILABLE FORMS/COST
• Cap—Oral: 200 mg, 100's: **$544.13**
• Susp—Oral: 50 mg/ml, 240 ml: **$69.05**

UNLABELED USES: To reduce the risk of transmitting HIV from infected mother to newborn

CONTRAINDICATIONS: None known.

PREGNANCY AND LACTATION: Pregnancy category C; excreted in breast milk, breast-feeding not recommended

SIDE EFFECTS
Frequent (8%-3%)
Rash, fever, headache, nausea, granulocytopenia (more common in children)
Occasional (3%-1%)
Stomatitis (burning, erythema, or ulceration of the oral mucosa; dysphagia)
Rare (less than 1%)
Paresthesia, myalgia, abdominal pain

SERIOUS REACTIONS
• Hepatitis and rash may become severe and life-threatening.

INTERACTIONS
Drugs

🔢 *Clarithromycin:* 26% increase in plasma nevirapine level by clarithromycin; 30% decrease in plasma clarithromycin level by nevirapine; dose adjustment not recommended

🔢 *Erythromycin:* Mild increase in plasma nevirapine level by erythromycin; dose adjustment not recommended

🔢 *Indinavir:* 28% decrease in indinavir AUC by nevirapine; dose adjustment not recommended

② *Ketoconazole:* 63% reduction in plasma ketoconazole level by nevirapine; 15%-30% increase in plasma nevirapine level by ketoconazole; coadministration not recommended

3 *Methadone:* Marked decrease in methadone level by nevirapine; dose adjustment recommended

3 *Nelfinavir:* 10% increase in nelfinavir AUC by nevirapine; dose adjustment not recommended

3 *Rifabutin:* 16% reduction in plasma nevirapine level by rifabutin

2 *Rifampin:* 37% reduction in plasma nevirapine level by rifampin; coadministration not recommended

3 *Ritonavir:* 11% decrease in ritonavir AUC by nevirapine; dose adjustment not recommended

3 *Saquinavir:* 25% decrease in saquinavir AUC by nevirapine; dose adjustment not recommended

3 *Troleandomycin:* Mild increase in plasma nevirapine level by troleandomycin; dose adjustment not recommended

SPECIAL CONSIDERATIONS
• 2-week lead in period with qday dosing decreases the potential for development of rash; stop therapy in any patient developing a severe rash or rash with constitutional symptoms

MONITORING PARAMETERS
• CBC, ALT, AST, renal function

---

niacin (vitamin B₃; nicotinic acid)

(nye´a-sin)

Rx: Niacor, Niaspan, Nicolor Combinations
  Rx: with lovastatin (Advicor)
Chemical Class: Vitamin B complex
Therapeutic Class: Antilipemic; vitamin

CLINICAL PHARMACOLOGY
Mechanism of Action: An antihyperlipidemic, water-soluble vitamin that is a component of two coenzymes needed for tissue respiration, lipid metabolism, and glycogenolysis. Inhibits synthesis of VLDLs. *Therapeutic Effect:* Reduces total, LDL, and VLDL cholesterol levels and triglyceride levels; increases HDL cholesterol concentration.

Pharmacokinetics
Readily absorbed from the GI tract. Widely distributed. Metabolized in the liver. Primarily excreted in urine. **Half-life:** 45 min.

INDICATIONS AND DOSAGES
Hyperlipidemia
PO (immediate-release)
Adults, Elderly. Initially, 50–100 mg twice a day for 7 days. Increase gradually by doubling dose qwk up to 1–1.5 g/day in 2–3 doses. Maximum: 3 g/day.

Children. Initially, 100–250 mg/day (maximum: 10 mg/kg/day) in 3 divided doses. May increase by 100 mg/wk or 250 mg q2–3wks. Maximum: 2,250 mg/day.

PO (timed-release)
Adults, Elderly. Initially, 500 mg/day in 2 divided doses for 1 wk; then increase to 500 mg twice a day. Maintenance: 2 g/day.

Nutritional supplement
PO
Adults, Elderly. 10–20 mg/day. Maximum: 100 mg/day.

Pellegra
PO
Adults, Elderly. 50-100 mg 3-4 times a day. Maximum: 500 mg/day.
Children. 50-100 mg 3 times a day.

$ AVAILABLE FORMS/COST
• Cap, Gel, Sus Action—Oral: 125 mg, 100's: **$4.05-$6.15**; 250 mg, 100's: **$2.70-$8.42**; 400 mg, 100's: **$6.30-$7.80**; 500 mg, 100's: **$5.09-$7.80**
• Elixir—Oral: 50 mg/5 ml, 480 ml: **$8.25**

• Tab—Oral: 50   mg,   100's: **$0.64-$4.02**; 100 mg, 100's: **$0.74-$4.21**; 250 mg, 100's: **$2.46-$3.39**; 500 mg, 100's: **$1.99-$70.66**
• Tab, Sus Action—Oral: 500 mg, 100's: **$3.52-$109.63**;   750   mg, 100's: **$7.42-$156.37**; 1000 mg, 100's: **$8.25-$195.85**

CONTRAINDICATIONS: Active peptic ulcer disease, arterial hemorrhaging, hepatic dysfunction, hypersensitivity to niacin or tartrazine (frequently seen in patients sensitive to aspirin), severe hypotension

PREGNANCY AND LACTATION: Pregnancy category A (category C if used in doses greater than recommended daily allowance); actively excreted in human breast milk; recommended daily allowance during lactation is 18-20 mg

SIDE EFFECTS
Frequent
Flushing (especially of the face and neck) occurring within 20 minutes of drug administration and lasting for 30–60 minutes, GI upset, pruritus
Occasional
Dizziness, hypotension, headache, blurred vision, burning or tingling of skin, flatulence, nausea, vomiting, diarrhea
Rare
Hyperglycemia, glycosuria, rash, hyperpigmentation, dry skin

SERIOUS REACTIONS
• Arrhythmias occur rarely.

INTERACTIONS
Drugs
3 *Lovastatin:* Isolated cases of myopathy and rhabdomyolysis have occurred, causality not established
Labs
• *Interference:* Plasma and urine catecholamines, urine glucose with Benedict's reagent

SPECIAL CONSIDERATIONS
• In 1 g doses: 10%-20% reduction of total plus LDL-cholesterol, 30%-70% reduction in triglycerides, and a 20%-35% increase in HDL-cholesterol
• Increased risk of hepatotoxicity with sustained release products

PATIENT/FAMILY EDUCATION
• Gradual dosage titration lessens flushing, adverse effects
• Avoid alcohol and hot beverages (increases flushing)
• Administer with meals and 2 glasses of water
• 125-350 mg of aspirin 20-30 min prior to dose may lessen flushing
• Do not miss any doses (flushing may return)

MONITORING PARAMETERS
• Liver function tests, blood glucose, uric acid regularly
• Fasting lipid profile q3-6 mo

---

nicardipine
(nye-card'i-peen)
Rx: Cardene, Cardene SR
Chemical Class: Dihydropyridine
Therapeutic Class: Antianginal; antihypertensive; calcium channel blocker

CLINICAL PHARMACOLOGY
Mechanism of Action: An antianginal and antihypertensive agent that inhibits calcium ion movement across cell membranes, depressing contraction of cardiac and vascular smooth muscle. *Therapeutic Effect:* Increases heart rate and cardiac output. Decreases systemic vascular resistance and BP.
Pharmacokinetics

Route	Onset	Peak	Duration
PO	N/A	1–2 hr	8 hr

Rapidly, completely absorbed from the GI tract. Protein binding: 95%. Undergoes first-pass metabolism in the liver. Primarily excreted in urine. Not removed by hemodialysis. **Half-life:** 2–4 hr.

INDICATIONS AND DOSAGES

Chronic stable (effort-associated) angina

PO

Adults, Elderly. Initially, 20 mg 3 times a day. Range: 20–40 mg 3 times a day.

Essential hypertension

PO

Adults, Elderly. Initially, 20 mg 3 times a day. Range: 20–40 mg 3 times a day.

PO (sustained-release)

Adults, Elderly. Initially, 30 mg twice a day. Range: 30–60 mg twice a day.

Short-term treatment of hypertension when oral therapy is not feasible or desirable (substitute for oral nicardipine)

IV

Adults, Elderly. 0.5 mg/hr (for patient receiving 20 mg PO q8h); 1.2 mg/hr (for patient receiving 30 mg PO q8h); 2.2 mg/hr (for patient receiving 40 mg PO q8h).

Patients not already receiving nicardipine

IV

Adults, Elderly (gradual BP decrease). Initially, 5 mg/hr. May increase by 2.5 mg/hr q15min. After BP goal is achieved, decrease rate to 3 mg/hr.

Adults, Elderly (rapid BP decrease). Initially, 5 mg/hr. May increase by 2.5 mg/hr q5min. Maximum: 15 mg/hr until desired BP attained. After BP goal achieved, decrease rate to 3 mg/hr.

Changing from IV to oral antihypertensive therapy

Adults, Elderly. Begin antihypertensives other than nicardipine when IV has been discontinued; for nicardipine, give first dose 1 hr before discontinuing IV.

Dosage in hepatic impairment

For adults and elderly pateints, initially give 20 mg twice a day; then titrate.

Dosage in renal impairment

For adults and elderly patients, initially give 20 mg q8h (30 mg twice a day [sustained-release capsules]); then titrate.

ⓢ AVAILABLE FORMS/COST

• Cap—Oral: 20 mg, 100's: **$39.25-$63.35**; 30 mg, 100's: **$62.42-$65.55**
• Cap, Gel, Sus Action—Oral: 30 mg, 60's: **$54.49**; 45 mg, 60's: **$94.30**; 60 mg, 60's: **$112.88**
• Sol, Inj—IV: 25 mg/10 ml ampul: **$81.25**

UNLABELED USES: Treatment of associated neurologic deficits, Raynaud's phenomenon, subarachnoid hemorrhage, vasospastic angina

CONTRAINDICATIONS: Atrial fibrillation or flutter associated with accessory conduction pathways, cardiogenic shock, CHF, second- or third-degree heart block, severe hypotension, sinus bradycardia, ventricular tachycardia, within several hours of IV beta-blocker therapy

PREGNANCY AND LACTATION: Pregnancy category C; significant excretion into rat maternal milk

SIDE EFFECTS

Frequent (10%–7%)

Headache, facial flushing, peripheral edema, light-headedness, dizziness

Occasional (6%–3%)

Asthenia (loss of strength, energy), palpitations, angina, tachycardia

Rare (less than 2%)
Nausea, abdominal cramps, dyspepsia, dry mouth, rash
SERIOUS REACTIONS
• Overdose produces confusion, slurred speech, somnolence, marked hypotension, and bradycardia.
INTERACTIONS
Drugs
⚂ *Cyclosporine, tacrolimus:* Increased blood concentrations of these drugs, increased risk of toxicity
⚂ *Histamine H_2-antagonists:* Increased blood levels of nicardipine with cimetidine and ranitidine
⚂ *Fentanyl:* Severe hypotension or increased fluid volume requirements
⚂ *Neuromuscular blocking agents:* Prolongation of neuromuscular blockade

---

nicotine
(nik'o-teen)
Rx: *Nasal Spray:* Nicotrol NS; *Inhaler:* Nicotrol Inhaler
Rx: *Chewing Gum:* Commit, Nicorette
Rx: *Transdermal:* Nicoderm CQ, Nicotrol, Habitrol
Chemical Class: Pyridine alkaloid
Therapeutic Class: Smoking deterrent

CLINICAL PHARMACOLOGY
Mechanism of Action: A cholinergic-receptor agonist binds to acetylcholine receptors, producing both stimulating and depressant effects on the peripheral and central nervous systems. *Therapeutic Effect:* Provides a source of nicotine during nicotine withdrawal and reduces withdrawal symptoms.

Pharmacokinetics
Absorbed slowly after transdermal administration. Protein binding: 5%. Metabolized in the liver. Excreted primarily in urine. **Half-life:** 4 hr.

INDICATIONS AND DOSAGES
Smoking cessation aid to relieve nicotine withdrawal symptoms
PO (Chewing gum)
Adults, Elderly. Usually, 10–12 pieces/day. Maximum: 30 pieces/day.
PO (Lozenge)
Alert for those who smoke the first cigarette within 30 min of waking, administer the 4 mg-lozenge; otherwise administer the 2-mg lozenge.
Adults, Elderly. One 4-mg or 2-mg lozenge q1-2h for the first 6 weeks; one lozenge q2-4h for wk 7-9; and one lozenge q4-8h for wk 10-12. Maximum: one lozenge at a time, 5 lozenges/6 hr, 20 lozenges/day.
Transdermal
Adults, Elderly who smoke 10 cigarettes or more per day. Follow the guidelines below.
Step 1: 21 mg/day for 4–6 wk.
Step 2: 14 mg/day for 2 wk.
Step 3: 7 mg/day for 2 wk.
Adults, Elderly who smoke less than 10 cigarettes per day. Follow the guidelines below.
Step 1: 14 mg/day for 6 wk.
Step 2: 7 mg/day for 2 wk.
Patients weighing less than 100 lb, patients with a history of cardiovascular disease. Initially, 14 mg/day for 4–6 wk, then 7 mg/day for 2–4wk.
Transdermal (Nicotrol)
Adults, Elderly. One patch a day for 6 wk.
Nasal
Adults, Elderly. 1–2 doses/hr (1 dose = 2 sprays [1 in each nostril] = 1 mg). Maximum: 5 doses (5 mg)/hr; 40 doses (40 mg) /day.

Inhaler (Nicotrol)

Adults, Elderly. Puff on nicotine cartridge mouthpiece for about 20 min as needed.

§ AVAILABLE FORMS/COST

• Aerosol—INH: 4 mg delivered (10 mg/cartridge), 42's: **$42.50** (Nicotrol Inhaler)

• Film, Cont Rel—Percutaneous: 7, 14, 21 mg/24 hr, 7's: all: **$24.21** (Nicoderm CQ-OTC); 7 mg/24 hr, 30's: **$109.61** (Habitrol); 14 mg/24 hr, 30's: **$139.15** (Habitrol); 15 mg/16 hr, 7's: **$22.65-$26.95** (Nicotrol-OTC); 21 mg/24 hr, 30's: **$146.42** (Habitrol)

• Sol—Nasal Spray: 0.5 mg/Inh, 10 mg/ml, 10 ml: **$42.50** (Nicotrol NS)

• Tab, Chewing Gum—Buccal: 2 mg, 48's: **$23.36-$27.36** (Nicorette-OTC); 4 mg, 48's: **$26.17-$32.07** (Nicorette-OTC)

CONTRAINDICATIONS: Immediate post MI period, life-threatening arrhythmias, severe or worsening angina

PREGNANCY AND LACTATION: Pregnancy category D; use of nicotine gum during last trimester has been associated with decreased fetal breathing movements; passes freely into breast milk; however, lower concentrations in milk can be expected with transdermal systems than cigarette smoking when used as directed

SIDE EFFECTS

Frequent

All forms: Hiccups, nausea

Gum: Mouth or throat soreness, nausea, hiccups

Transdermal: Erythema, pruritus, or burning at application site

Occasional

All forms: Eructation, GI upset, dry mouth, insomnia, diaphoresis, irritability

Gum: Hiccups, hoarseness

Inhaler: Mouth or throat irritation, cough

Rare

All forms: Dizziness, myalgia, arthralgia

SERIOUS REACTIONS

• Overdose produces palpitations, tachyarrhythmias, seizures, depression, confusion, diaphoresis, hypotension, rapid or weak pulse, and dyspnea. Lethal dose for adults is 40–60 mg. Death results from respiratory paralysis.

INTERACTIONS

Drugs

③ *Adenosine:* Increased hemodynamic and AV blocking effects of adenosine

③ *Cimetidine:* Increased blood nicotine concentration, may reduce the amount of gum or patches needed

③ *Coffee, cola:* Reduced absorption of nicotine from chewing gum

SPECIAL CONSIDERATIONS

• Drugs that may require dosage reduction with smoking cessation: acetaminophen, caffeine, imipramine, oxazepam, pentazocine, propranolol, theophylline, insulin, prazocin, labetalol

• Drugs that may require an increase in dose with smoking cessation: isoproterenol, phenylephrine

PATIENT/FAMILY EDUCATION

• Chew gum slowly until burning or tingling sensation is felt, then park gum between cheek and gum until tingling sensation goes away

• Chew <30 min/piece

• Avoid coffee and cola drinks while chewing gum or using inhaler

• **Do not smoke while utilizing nicotine replacement therapy**

• Apply new transdermal system daily

• Rotate sites; apply to non-hairy area on upper torso

N

nifedipine
(nye-fed'i-peen)
Rx: Adalat, Adalat CC, Procardia; Procardia XL
Chemical Class: Dihydropyridine
Therapeutic Class: Antianginal; antihypertensive; calcium channel blocker

CLINICAL PHARMACOLOGY
Mechanism of Action: An antianginal and antihypertensive agent that inhibits calcium ion movement across cell membranes, depressing contraction of cardiac and vascular smooth muscle. *Therapeutic Effect:* Increases heart rate and cardiac output. Decreases systemic vascular resistance and BP.

Pharmacokinetics

Route	Onset	Peak	Duration
Sublingual	1–5 min	N/A	N/A
PO	20–30 min	N/A	4–8 hr
PO (extended release)	2 hr	N/A	24 hr

Rapidly, completely absorbed from the GI tract. Protein binding: 92%–98%. Undergoes first-pass metabolism in the liver. Primarily excreted in urine. Not removed by hemodialysis. **Half-life:** 2–5 hr.

INDICATIONS AND DOSAGES
Prinzmetal's variant angina, chronic stable (effort-associated) angina
PO
Adults, Elderly. Initially, 10 mg 3 times a day. Increase at 7- to 14-day intervals. Maintenance: 10 mg 3 times a day up to 30 mg 4 times a day.
PO (extended-release)

Adults, Elderly. Initially, 30–60 mg/day. Maintenance: Up to 120 mg/day.
Essential hypertension
PO (extended-release)
Adults, Elderly. Initially, 30–60 mg/day. Maintenance: Up to 120 mg/day.

Ⓢ AVAILABLE FORMS/COST
• Cap, Gel—Oral: 10 mg, 100's: **$9.98-$79.59**; 20 mg, 100's: **$81.82-$134.20**
• Tab, Coated, Sus Action—Oral: 30 mg, 100's: **$108.14-$182.54**; 60 mg, 100's: **$216.79-$321.57**; 90 mg, 100's: **$256.15-$322.75**

UNLABELED USES: Treatment of Raynaud's phenomenon
CONTRAINDICATIONS: Advanced aortic stenosis, severe hypotension
PREGNANCY AND LACTATION: Pregnancy category C; has been used for tocolysis and as an antihypertensive agent in pregnant women; compatible with breastfeeding

SIDE EFFECTS
Frequent (30%–11%)
Peripheral edema, headache, flushed skin, dizziness
Occasional (12%–6%)
Nausea, shakiness, muscle cramps and pain, somnolence, palpitations, nasal congestion, cough, dyspnea, wheezing
Rare (5%–3%)
Hypotension, rash, pruritus, urticaria, constipation, abdominal discomfort, flatulence, sexual difficulties

SERIOUS REACTIONS
• Nifedipine may precipitate CHF and MI in patients with cardiac disease and peripheral ischemia.
• Overdose produces nausea, somnolence, confusion, and slurred speech.

INTERACTIONS
Drugs
▪ *Barbiturates, rifampin, rifabutin:* Reduced plasma concentrations of nifedipine

▪ *β-blockers:* Enhanced effects of β-blockers, hypotension; increased metoprolol and propanolol concentrations; additive negative effects on myocardial contractility

▪ *Cimetidine, ranitidine, famotidine:* Increased nifedipine concentrations possible

▪ *Digitalis glycosides:* Increased digitalis levels; increased risk of toxicity

▪ *Diltiazem:* Increased serum concentrations of nifedipine

▪ *Doxazosin:* Enhanced hypotensive effects

▪ *Fentanyl:* Severe hypotension or increased fluid volume requirements

▪ *Food:* Increased absorption of Adalat CC

▪ *Grapefruit juice:* Increased serum nifedipine concentrations

▪ *Histamine H$_2$-antagonists:* Increased blood levels of nifedipine with cimetidine

▪ *Lansoprazole:* Increased nifedipine absorption

▪ *Magnesium:* Potential for transient hypotensive effect

▪ *Phenytoin:* Increased phenytoin concentration

▪ *Quinidine:* Reduced blood concentrations of quinidine

▪ *Vincristine:* Marked increase in vincristine half-life, clinical significance unknown

SPECIAL CONSIDERATIONS
• Given the seriousness of the reported adverse events and the lack of any clinical documentation attesting to a benefit, the use of nifedipine capsules for hypertensive urgencies or emergencies should be abandoned (*JAMA* 1996; 276:1328-1331)

PATIENT/FAMILY EDUCATION
• Administer Adalat CC on an empty stomach
• Do not crush or chew sustained release dosage forms
• Empty Procardia XL tablets may appear in stool, this is no cause for concern

---

nimodipine
(nye-mode'i-peen)
Rx: Nimotop
Chemical Class: Dihydropyridine
Therapeutic Class: Calcium channel blocker; cerebral vasodilator

---

CLINICAL PHARMACOLOGY
Mechanism of Action: A cerebral vasospasm agent that inhibits movement of calcium ions across vascular smooth-muscle cell membranes. *Therapeutic Effect:* Produces favorable effect on severity of neurologic deficits due to cerebral vasospasm. Exerts greatest effect on cerebral arteries; may prevent cerebral spasm.
Pharmacokinetics
Rapidly absorbed from the GI tract. Protein binding: 95%. Metabolized in the liver. Excreted in urine; eliminated in feces. Not removed by hemodialysis. **Half-life:** terminal, 3 hr.

INDICATIONS AND DOSAGES
Improvement neurologic deficits after subarachnoid hemorrhage from ruptured congenital aneurysms
PO
Adults, Elderly. 60 mg q4h for 21 days. Begin within 96 hr of subarachnoid hemorrhage.

AVAILABLE FORMS/COST
• Cap, Elastic—Oral: 30 mg, 100's: **$799.94**

UNLABELED USES: Treatment of chronic and classic migraine, chronic cluster headaches

CONTRAINDICATIONS: Atrial fibrillation or flutter, cardiogenic shock, CHF, heart block, sinus bradycardia, ventricular tachycardia, within several hours of IV beta-blocker therapy

PREGNANCY AND LACTATION: Pregnancy category C

SIDE EFFECTS

Occasional (6% –2%)
Hypotension, peripheral edema, diarrhea, headache

Rare (less than 2%)
Allergic reaction (rash, hives), tachycardia, flushing of skin

SERIOUS REACTIONS
• Overdose produces nausea, weakness, dizziness, somnolence, confusion, and slurred speech.

INTERACTIONS

Drugs

3 *Cimetidine:* Increased serum nimodipine concentrations

3 *Omeprazole:* Increased serum nimodipine concentrations

3 *Valproic acid:* Increased oral bioavailability of nimodipine

SPECIAL CONSIDERATIONS

MONITORING PARAMETERS
• Blood pressure

---

nisoldipine
(nye-soul-dih-peen)
Rx: Sular
Chemical Class: Dihydropyridine
Therapeutic Class: Antihypertensive; calcium channel blocker

CLINICAL PHARMACOLOGY

Mechanism of Action: A calcium channel blocker that inhibits calcium ion movement across cell membrane, depressing contraction of cardiac and vascular smooth muscle. *Therapeutic Effect:* Increases heart rate and cardiac output. Decreases systemic vascular resistance and blood pressure (BP).

Pharmacokinetics

Poor absorption from the gastrointestinal (GI) tract. Food increases bioavailability. Protein binding: more than 99%. Metabolism occurs in the gut wall. Primarily excreted in urine. Not removed by hemodialysis. **Half-life:** 7-12 hrs.

INDICATIONS AND DOSAGES

Hypertension

PO

Adults. Initially, 20 mg once daily, then increase by 10 mg per week, or longer intervals until therapeutic BP response is attained.

Elderly. Initially, 10 mg once daily. Increase by 10 mg per week to therapeutic response. Maintenance: 20-40 mg once daily. Maximum: 60 mg once daily.

AVAILABLE FORMS/COST
• Tab, Coated—Oral: 10, 20 mg, 100's; all: **$132.83**; 30, 40 mg, 100's; all: **$144.11**

UNLABELED USES: Stable angina pectoris, CHF

CONTRAINDICATIONS: Sick-sinus syndrome/second- or third-degree AV block (except in presence of pacemaker), hypersensitivity to nisoldipine or any component of the formulation

PREGNANCY AND LACTATION: Pregnancy category C

SIDE EFFECTS

Frequent

Giddiness, dizziness, lightheadedness, peripheral edema, headache, flushing, weakness, nausea

Occasional

Transient hypotension, heartburn, muscle cramps, nasal congestion, cough, wheezing, sore throat, palpitations, nervousness, mood changes

Rare

Increase in frequency, intensity, duration of anginal attack during initial therapy

SERIOUS REACTIONS

• May precipitate congestive heart failure (CHF) and myocardial infarction (MI) in patients with cardiac disease and peripheral ischemia.

• Overdose produces nausea, drowsiness, confusion, and slurred speech.

INTERACTIONS

Drugs

▣ *β-adrenergic blockers:* Increased propranolol concentration

▣ *Cimetidine, famotidine, nizatidine, omeprazole, ranitidine:* Increased nisoldipine concentrations possible

▣ *Fentanyl:* Severe hypotension or increased fluid volume requirements

▣ *Food:* Increased absorption with high-fat meal or grapefruit juice

SPECIAL CONSIDERATIONS

• No significant advantages over other dihydropyridine calcium channel blockers

PATIENT/FAMILY EDUCATION

• Do not take with high-fat meal or grapefruit juice

---

nitazoxanide

(nigh-tazz-oks′ah-nide)

Rx: Alinia

Chemical Class: Benzamide derivative

Therapeutic Class: Antiprotozoal

CLINICAL PHARMACOLOGY

Mechanism of Action: An antiparasitic that interferes with the body's reaction to pyruvate ferredoxin oxidoreductase, an enzyme essential for anaerobic energy metabolism. *Therapeutic Effect:* Produces antiprotozoal activity, reducing or terminating diarrheal episodes.

Pharmacokinetics

Rapidly hydrolyzed to an active metabolite. Protein binding: 99%. Excreted in the urine, bile, and feces. **Half-life:** 2–4 hr.

INDICATIONS AND DOSAGES

Diarrhea

PO

Children 12 yr and older. 200 mg q12h.

Children 4-11 yr. 200 mg (10 ml) q12h for 3 days.

Children 12–47 mo. 100 mg (5 ml) q12h for 3 days.

Ⓢ **AVAILABLE FORMS/COST**

• Powder, Reconst—Oral: 100 mg/5 ml, 60 ml: **$60.00**

CONTRAINDICATIONS: History of sensitivity to aspirin and salicylates

PREGNANCY AND LACTATION: Pregnancy category B; excretion into breast milk unknown; use caution in nursing mothers

SIDE EFFECTS
Occasional (8%)
Abdominal pain
Rare (2%–1%)
Diarrhea, vomiting, headache
SERIOUS REACTIONS
• None known.
SPECIAL CONSIDERATIONS
• Efficacy in adults or immunocompromised patients not known
• Efficacy for *Cryptosporidium parvum* 88% (38% for placebo in controlled trial)
• Efficacy for *Giardia lamblia* 90% (equal to metronidazole)
PATIENT/FAMILY EDUCATION
• Take with food

---

nitrofurantoin
(nye-troe-fyoor′an-toyn)
Rx: Furadantin, Macrodantin
Combinations
  Rx: nitrofurantoin macrocrystals with nitrofurantoin monohydrate (Macrobid)
Chemical Class: Nitrofuran derivative
Therapeutic Class: Antibiotic

CLINICAL PHARMACOLOGY
Mechanism of Action: An antibacterial UTI agent that inhibits the synthesis of bacterial DNA, RNA, proteins, and cell walls by altering or inactivating ribosomal proteins. *Therapeutic Effect:* Bacteriostatic (bactericidal at high concentrations).
Pharmacokinetics
Microcrystalline form rapidly and completely absorbed; macrocrystalline form more slowly absorbed. Food increases absorption. Protein binding: 40%. Primarily concentrated in urine and kidneys. Metabolized in most body tissues. Primarily excreted in urine. Removed by hemodialysis. **Half-life:** 20-60 min.

INDICATIONS AND DOSAGES
Urinary tract infections (UTIs)
PO
Adults, Elderly. (Furadantin, Macrodantin): 50-100 mg q6h. (Macrobid): 100 mg 2 times/day. Maximum: 400 mg/day.
Children. (Furadantin, Macrodantin): 5-7 mg/kg/day in divided doses q6h. Maximum: 400 mg/day.
Long-term prevention of UTIs
PO
Adults, Elderly. 50-100 mg at bedtime.
Children. 1-2 mg/kg/day as a single dose. Maximum: 100 mg/day.
Ⓢ AVAILABLE FORMS/COST
• Cap—Oral: 25 mg, 100's: **$96.33**; 50 mg, 100's: **$58.20-$126.84**; 100 mg, 100's: **$98.50-$215.43**; 100 mg, 100's: **$226.48** (Macrobid)
• Susp—Oral: 25 mg/5 ml, 60, 470 ml: **$84.22-$154.87**/470 ml
UNLABELED USES: Prevention of bacterial UTIs
CONTRAINDICATIONS: Anuria, oliguria, substantial renal impairment (creatinine clearance less than 40 ml/min); infants younger than 1 mo old because of the risk of hemolytic anemia
PREGNANCY AND LACTATION: Pregnancy category B; compatible with breast-feeding in infants >1 mo
SIDE EFFECTS
Frequent
Anorexia, nausea, vomiting, dark urine
Occasional
Abdominal pain, diarrhea, rash, pruritus, urticaria, hypertension, headache, dizziness, drowsiness
Rare
Photosensitivity, transient alopecia, asthmatic exacerbation in those with history of asthma

SERIOUS REACTIONS

• Superinfection, hepatotoxicity, peripheral neuropathy (may be irreversible), Stevens-Johnson syndrome, permanent pulmonary function impairment, and anaphylaxis occur rarely.

INTERACTIONS

Labs

• *Interference:* Urine alkaline phosphatase, urine lactate dehydrogenase

• *False positive:* Urine glucose (not with glucose enzymatic tests)

• *False increase:* Serum bilirubin, serum creatinine

• *False decrease:* Serum unconjugated bilirubin

SPECIAL CONSIDERATIONS

PATIENT/FAMILY EDUCATION

• Food or milk may decrease GI upset

• May cause brown discoloration of urine

MONITORING PARAMETERS

• Periodic liver function tests during prolonged therapy

• CBC with differential and platelets during prolonged therapy

• Pulmonary review of systems

---

nitrofurazone

(nye-troe-fyoor′a-zone)

Rx: Furacin
Chemical Class: Nitrofuran derivative
Therapeutic Class: Antibiotic, topical

CLINICAL PHARMACOLOGY

Mechanism of Action: A synthetic nitrofuran that inhibits bacterial enzymes involved in carbohydrate metabolism. *Therapeutic Effect:* Inhibits a variety of enzymes. Bactericidal.

Pharmacokinetics

Not known.

INDICATIONS AND DOSAGES

Burns, catheter-related urinary tract infection, skin grafts

Topical

Adults. Apply directly on lesion with spatula or place on a piece of gauze first. Use of a bandage is optional. Preparation should remain on lesion for at least 24 hours. Dressing may be changed several times daily or left on the lesion for a longer period.

$ **AVAILABLE FORMS/COST**

• Cre—Top: 0.2%, 28 g: **$20.50**

• Oint—Top: 0.2%, 30, 454 g: **$7.80-$98.11**/454 g

• Sol—Top: 0.2%, 480 ml: **$6.48**

UNLABELED USES: Fire and ant bites, scabies, urethritis, vaginal malodor, vasectomy, wounds

CONTRAINDICATIONS: Hypersensitivity to nitrofurazone or any of its components

PREGNANCY AND LACTATION: Pregnancy category C; excretion into breast milk unknown

SIDE EFFECTS

Occasional

Itching, rash, swelling

SERIOUS REACTIONS

• Use of nitrofurazone may result in bacterial or fungal overgrowth of nonsusceptible pathogens, which may lead to secondary infection.

INTERACTIONS

Labs

• *False increase:* Urine creatinine, urine glucose via Benedict's reagent

N

nitroglycerin
(nye-troe-gli′ser-in)

Rx: *Translingual: Buccal/ Sublingual/Translingual:* Nitrolingual, Nitroquick, Nitrostat

Rx: *Oral:* Nitro-Bid, Nitrocap TD, Nitrocine, Nitrogard, Nitroglyn, Nitrong, Nitro TD, Nitro-Time

Rx: *Topical:* Nitr-Bid, Nitrol

Rx: *IV:* Nitro-Bid, Nitrostat IV, Tridil

Chemical Class: Nitrate, organic

Therapeutic Class: Antianginal; vasodilator

CLINICAL PHARMACOLOGY
Mechanism of Action: A nitrate that decreases myocardial oxygen demand. Reduces left ventricular preload and afterload. *Therapeutic Effect:* Dilates coronary arteries and improves collateral blood flow to ischemic areas within myocardium. IV form produces peripheral vasodilation.

Pharmacokinetics

Route	Onset	Peak	Duration
Sublingual	1–3 min	4–8 min	30–60 min
Translingual spray	2 min	4-10 min	30-60 min
Buccal Tablet	2–5 min	4–10 min	2 hr
PO (Extended-Release)	20–45 min	45-120 min	4–8 hr
Topical	15–60 min	30-120 min	2-12 hr
Transdermal Patch	40–60 min	60-180 min	18–24 hr
IV	1–2 min	Immediate	3–5 min

Well absorbed after PO, sublingual, and topical administration. Undergoes extensive first-pass metabolism. Metabolized in the liver and by enzymes in the bloodstream. Primarily excreted in urine. Not removed by hemodialysis. **Half-life:** 1–4 min.

INDICATIONS AND DOSAGES
Acute relief of angina pectoris, acute prophylaxis
Lingual spray
Adults, Elderly. 1 spray onto or under tongue q3–5min until relief is noted (no more than 3 sprays in 15-min period).
Sublingual
Adults, Elderly. 0.4 mg q5min until relief is noted (no more than 3 doses in 15-min period). Use prophylactically 5–10 min before activities that may cause an acute attack.
Long-term prophylaxis of angina
PO (extended-release)
Adults, Elderly. 2.5–9 mg q8–12h.
Topical
Adults, Elderly. Initially, ½ inch q8h. Increase by ½ inch with each application. Range: 1–2 inches q8h up to 4–5 inches q4h.
Transdermal patch
Adults, Elderly. Initially, 0.2–0.4 mg/hr. Maintenance: 0.4–0.8 mg/hr. Consider patch on for 12–14 hr, patch off for 10–12 hr (prevents tolerance).
CHF associated with acute MI
IV
Adults, Elderly. Initially, 5 mcg/min via infusion pump. Increase in 5-mcg/min increments at 3- to 5-min intervals until BP response is noted or until dosage reaches 20 mcg/min; then increase as needed by 10 mcg/min. Dosage may be further titrated according to clinical, therapeutic response up to 200 mcg/min.

Children. Initially, 0.25–0.5 mcg/kg/min; titrate by 0.5–1 mcg/kg/min up to 20 mcg/kg/min.

🔋 AVAILABLE FORMS/COST

• Aer Spray—SL: 0.4 mg/spray, 12 g: **$43.64**
• Cap, Gel, Sus Action—Oral: 2.5 mg, 100's: **$5.00-$17.45**; 6.5 mg, 100's: **$7.51-$24.00**; 9 mg, 100's: **$8.25-$49.80**
• Sol, Inj—IV: 5 mg/ml, 10 ml: **$1.13-$15.00**
• Oint—Percutaneous: 2%; 1, 3, 30, 60 g: **$6.48-$16.90/60 g**
• Tab, Sus Action—Buccal: 1 mg, 100's: **$37.87**; 2.6 mg, 100's: **$33.54**; 3 mg, 100's: **$43.33**; 6.5 mg, 100's: **$41.98**
• Tab—SL: 0.3 mg, 100's: **$5.68-$10.78**; 0.4 mg, 100's: **$5.68-$11.70**; 0.6 mg, 100's: **$7.36-$11.36**
• Film, Cont Rel—Transdermal: 0.1 mg/hr, 30's: **$47.40-$67.05**; 0.2 mg/hr, 30's: **$33.06-$69.51**; 0.3 mg/hr, 30's: **$67.08-$76.26**; 0.4 mg/hr, 30's: **$45.05-$76.26**; 0.6 mg/hr, 30's: **$51.30-$82.71**; 0.8 mg/hr, 30's: **$72.77-$82.71**

CONTRAINDICATIONS: Allergy to adhesives (transdermal), closed-angle glaucoma, constrictive pericarditis (IV), early MI (sublingual), GI hypermotility or malabsorption (extended-release), head trauma, hypotension (IV), inadequate cerebral circulation (IV), increased intracranial pressure, nitrates, orthostatic hypotension, pericardial tamponade (IV), severe anemia, uncorrected hypovolemia (IV)

PREGNANCY AND LACTATION: Pregnancy category C; use of SL for angina during pregnancy without fetal harm has been reported

SIDE EFFECTS

Frequent

Headache (possibly severe; occurs mostly in early therapy, diminishes rapidly in intensity, and usually disappears during continued treatment), transient flushing of face and neck, dizziness (especially if patient is standing immobile or is in a warm environment), weakness, orthostatic hypotension
Sublingual: Burning, tingling sensation at oral point of dissolution
Ointment: Erythema, pruritus
Occasional
GI upset
Transdermal: Contact dermatitis

SERIOUS REACTIONS

• Nitroglycerin should be discontinued if blurred vision or dry mouth occurs.
• Severe orthostatic hypotension may occur, manifested by fainting, pulselessness, cold or clammy skin, and diaphoresis.
• Tolerance may occur with repeated, prolonged therapy; minor tolerance may occur with intermittent use of sublingual tablets.
• High doses of nitroglycerin tend to produce severe headache.

INTERACTIONS

Drugs

❷ *Ergot alkaloids:* Opposition to coronary vasodilatory effects of nitrates
❸ *Ethanol:* Additive vasodilation could cause hypotension
❸ *Metronidazole:* Ethanol contained in IV nitroglycerine preparations could cause disulfiram-like reaction in some patients
❸ *Sildenafil:* Excessive hypotensive effects
Labs
• *False increase:* Serum triglycerides

SPECIAL CONSIDERATIONS

• 10-12 hr drug-free intervals prevent development of tolerance

PATIENT/FAMILY EDUCATION

• Avoid alcohol
• Notify clinician if persistent headache occurs

N

• Take oral nitrates on empty stomach with full glass of water
• Keep tablets and capsules in original container, keep container closed tightly
• Dissolve SL tablets under tongue, lack of burning does not indicate loss of potency, use when seated, take at 1st sign of anginal attack, activate emergency response system if no relief after 3 tablets spaced 5 min apart
• Spray translingual spray onto or under tongue, do not inhale spray
• Place buccal tablets under upper lip or between cheek and gum, permit to dissolve slowly over 3-5 min, do not chew or swallow
• Spread thin layer of ointment on skin using applicator or dose-measuring papers, do not use fingers, do not rub or massage
• Apply transdermal systems to nonhairy area on upper torso, remove for 10-12 hr/day (usually hs)

MONITORING PARAMETERS
• Blood pressure, heart rate at peak effect times

nitroprusside
(nye-troe-pruss'ide)
Rx: Nitropress
Chemical Class: Cyanonitrosylferrate derivative
Therapeutic Class: Antihypertensive

CLINICAL PHARMACOLOGY
Mechanism of Action: A potent vasodilator used to treat emergent hypertensive conditions; acts directly on arterial and venous smooth muscle. Decreases peripheral vascular resistance, preload and afterload; improves cardiac output. *Therapeutic Effect:* Dilates coronary arteries, decreases oxygen consumption, and relieves persistent chest pain.
Pharmacokinetics

Route	*Onset*	*Peak*	*Duration*
IV	1–10 min	Dependent on infusion rate	Dissipates rapidly after stopping IV

Reacts with Hgb in erythrocytes, producing cyanmethemoglobin, and cyanide ions. Primarily excreted in urine. **Half-life:** less than 10 min.

INDICATIONS AND DOSAGES
Immediate reduction of BP in hypertensive crisis; to produce controlled hypotension in surgical procedures to reduce bleeding; treatment of acute CHF
IV
Adults, Elderly, Children. Initially, 0.3 mcg/kg/min. Range: 0.5–10 mcg/kg/min. Do not exceed 10 mcg/kg/min (risk of precipitous drop in BP).

[$] **AVAILABLE FORMS/COST**
• Powder, Inj-IV: 50 mg/vial: **$1.84-$12.48**

UNLABELED USES: Control of paroxysmal hypertension before and during surgery for pheochromocytoma, peripheral vasospasm caused by ergot alkaloid overdose, treatment adjunct for MI, valvular regurgitation

CONTRAINDICATIONS: Compensatory hypertension (atrioventricular [AV] shunt or coarctation of aorta), inadequate cerebral circulation, moribund patients

PREGNANCY AND LACTATION: Pregnancy category C; excretion into breast milk is unknown, use caution in nursing mothers

SIDE EFFECTS
Occasional

Flushing of skin, increased intracranial pressure, rash, pain or redness at injection site

SERIOUS REACTIONS

• A too rapid IV infusion rate reduces BP too quickly.

• Nausea, vomiting, diaphoresis, apprehension, headache, restlessness, muscle twitching, dizziness, palpitations, retrosternal pain, and abdominal pain may occur. Symptoms disappear rapidly if rate of administration is slowed or drug is temporarily discontinued.

• Overdose produces metabolic acidosis and tolerance to therapeutic effect.

INTERACTIONS
Drugs

▣ *Clonidine:* Severe hypotensive reactions have been reported

▣ *Diltiazem:* Reduction in the dose of nitroprusside required to produce hypotension

▣ *Guanabenz, guanfacine:* Potential for severe hypotensive reactions

SPECIAL CONSIDERATIONS
MONITORING PARAMETERS

• Blood pressure, arterial blood gases, oxygen saturation, cyanide and thiocyanate concentrations, anion gap, lactate levels

---

nizatidine
(ni-za'ti-deen)
Rx: Axid
OTC: Axid AR
Chemical Class: Ethenediamine derivative
Therapeutic Class: Antiulcer agent

CLINICAL PHARMACOLOGY

Mechanism of Action: An antiulcer agent and gastric acid secretion inhibitor that inhibits histamine action at histamine 2 receptors of parietal cells. *Therapeutic Effect:* Inhibits basal and nocturnal gastric acid secretion.

Pharmacokinetics

Rapidly, well absorbed from the GI tract. Protein binding: 35%. Metabolized in the liver. Primarily excreted in urine. Not removed by hemodialysis. **Half-life:** 1–2 hr (increased with impaired renal function).

INDICATIONS AND DOSAGES
Active duodenal ulcer
PO

Adults, Elderly. 300 mg at bedtime or 150 mg twice a day.

Prevention of duodenal ulcer recurrence
PO

Adults, Elderly. 150 mg at bedtime.

Gastroesophageal reflux disease
PO

Adults, Elderly. 150 mg twice a day.

Active benign gastric ulcer
PO

Adults, Elderly. 150 mg twice a day or 300 mg at bedtime.

Dyspepsia
PO (OTC)

Adults, Elderly. 75 mg 30–60 min before meals; no more than 2 tablets a day.

Dosage in renal impairment

Dosage adjustment is based on creatinine clearance.

Creatinine Clearance	Active Ulcer	Maintenance Therapy
20–50 ml/min	150 mg at bedtime	150 mg every other day
less than 20 ml/min	150 mg every other day	150 mg q3 days

$ AVAILABLE FORMS/COST

• Cap, Gel—Oral: 75 mg, 30's (OTC): **$9.36**; 150 mg, 60's: **$120.15-$183.58**; 300 mg, 30's: **$125.37-$179.93**

UNLABELED USES: Gastric hypersecretory conditions, multiple endocrine adenoma, Zollinger-Ellison syndrome, weight gain reduction in patients taking Zyprexa

CONTRAINDICATIONS: None known

PREGNANCY AND LACTATION: Pregnancy category B; excreted in breast milk (0.1% of dose)

SIDE EFFECTS

Occasional (2%)

Somnolence, fatigue

Rare (1%)

Diaphoresis, rash

SERIOUS REACTIONS

• Asymptomatic ventricular tachycardia, hyperuricemia not associated with gout, and nephrolithiasis occur rarely.

INTERACTIONS

Drugs

▨ *Cefpodoxime, cefuroxime; enoxacin; ketoconazole:* Reduction in gastric acidity reduces absorption, decreases plasma levels, potential for therapeutic failure

▨ *Glipizide, glyburide tolbutamide:* Increased absorption of these drugs, potential for hypoglycemia

▨ *Nifedipine; Nitrendipine; nisoldipine:* Increased concentrations of these drugs

SPECIAL CONSIDERATIONS

• No advantage over other agents of this class, base selection on cost

PATIENT/FAMILY EDUCATION

• Stagger doses of nizatidine and antacids

---

norepinephrine

(nor-ep-i-nef′rin)

Rx: Levophed

Chemical Class: Catecholamine, synthetic

Therapeutic Class: Vasopressor; α- and ß-adrenergic sympathomimetic

CLINICAL PHARMACOLOGY

Mechanism of Action: A sympathomimetic that stimulates beta$_1$-adrenergic receptors and alpha-adrenergic receptors, increasing peripheral resistance. Enhances contractile myocardial force, increases cardiac output. Constricts resistance and capacitance vessels. *Therapeutic Effect:* Increases systemic BP and coronary blood flow.

Pharmacokinetics

Route	Onset	Peak	Duration
IV	Rapid	1–2 min	N/A

Localized in sympathetic tissue. Metabolized in the liver. Primarily excreted in urine.

INDICATIONS AND DOSAGES

Acute hypotension unresponsive to fluid volume replacement

IV

Adults, Elderly. Initially, administer at 0.5–1 mcg/min. Adjust rate of flow to establish and maintain desired BP (40 mm Hg below preexisting systolic pressure). Average maintenance dose: 8–12 mcg/min.

Children. Initially, 0.05–0.1 mcg/kg/min; titrate to desired effect. Maximum: 1–2 mcg/kg/min. Range: 0.5–3 mcg/min.

AVAILABLE FORMS/COST

• Sol, Inj-IV: 0.1%, 4 ml: **$10.98-$13.08**

CONTRAINDICATIONS: Hypovolemic states (unless as an emergency measure), mesenteric or peripheral vascular thrombosis, profound hypoxia

PREGNANCY AND LACTATION: Pregnancy category D

SIDE EFFECTS

Norepinephrine produces less pronounced and less frequent side effects than epinephrine.

Occasional (5%–3%)

Anxiety, bradycardia, palpitations

Rare (2%–1%)

Nausea, anginal pain, shortness of breath, fever

SERIOUS REACTIONS

• Extravasation may produce tissue necrosis and sloughing.

• Overdose is manifested as severe hypertension with violent headache (which may be the first clinical sign of overdose), arrhythmias, photophobia, retrosternal or pharyngeal pain, pallor, excessive sweating, and vomiting.

• Prolonged therapy may result in plasma volume depletion. Hypotension may recur if plasma volume is not restored.

INTERACTIONS

Drugs

❷ *Amitriptyline, desipramine, imipramine, protriptyline:* Marked enhancement of pressor response to norepinephrine

❸ *Guanadrel, guanethidine:* Exaggerated pressor response to norepinephrine

❸ *MAOIs:* Slight increase in the pressor response to norepinephrine

❸ *Methyldopa:* Prolongation in the pressor response to norepinephrine

SPECIAL CONSIDERATIONS

• Antidote for extravasation ischemia: infiltrate with 10-15 ml of saline containing 5-10 mg of phentolamine

MONITORING PARAMETERS

• Blood pressure, heart rate, ECG, urine output, peripheral perfusion

---

norethindrone

(nor-eth'-in-drone)

Rx: Micronor, Nor-Q.D.;
Acetate: Aygestin
Combinations

  Rx: with ethinyl estradiol (see oral contraceptives)

Chemical Class: 19-nortestosterone derivative; progestin derivative

Therapeutic Class: Contraceptive; progestin

CLINICAL PHARMACOLOGY

Mechanism of Action: A synthetic progestin that is used as a single agent or in combination with estrogens for the treatment of gynecological disorders. It inhibits secretion of pituitary gonadotropin (LH) which prevents follicular maturation and ovulation. *Therapeutic Effect:* Transforms endometrium from proliferative to secretory in an estrogen-primed endometrium, promotes mammary gland development, relaxes uterine smooth muscle.

Pharmacokinetics

Rapidly absorbed from the gastrointestinal (GI) tract. Widely distributed. Protein binding: 61%. Metabolized in liver. Excreted in urine and feces. **Half-life:** 4-13 hrs.

INDICATIONS AND DOSAGES
Contraception
PO
Adults. 1 tablet/day.

Amenorrhea and abnormal uterine bleeding
PO
Adults. 5-20 mg/day cyclically (21 days on; 7 days off or continuously) or for acetate salt formulation, 2.5-10 mg cyclically.

Endometriosis
PO
Adults. 10 mg/day for 2 weeks increase at increments of 5 mg/day every 2 weeks until 30 mg/day; continue for 6-9 months or until breakthrough bleeding demands temporary termination. For acetate salt formulation, 5 mg/day for 14 days increase at increments of 2.5 mg/day every 2 weeks up to 15 mg/day continue for 6-9 months or until breakthrough bleeding demands temporary termination.

🅢 AVAILABLE FORMS/COST
• Tab-Oral: 0.35 mg, 28's: **$36.53-$48.41**
• Tab (acetate)-Oral: 5 mg, 50's: **$79.64-$88.49**

UNLABELED USES: Treatment of corpus luteum dysfunction

CONTRAINDICATIONS: Acute liver disease, benign or malignant liver tumors, hypersensitivity to norethindrone and any component of the formulation, known or suspected carcinoma of the breast, known or suspected pregnancy, undiagnosed abnormal genital bleeding

PREGNANCY AND LACTATION: Pregnancy category X; compatible with breast-feeding

SIDE EFFECTS
Occasional
Breast tenderness, dizziness, headache, breakthrough bleeding, amenorrhea, menstrual irregularity, nausea, weakness
Rare
Mental depression, fever, insomnia, rash, acne, increased breast tenderness, weight gain/loss, changes in cervical erosion and secretions, cholestatic jaundice

SERIOUS REACTIONS
• Thrombophlebitis, cerebrovascular disorders, retinal thrombosis, cholestatic jaundice, and pulmonary embolism occur rarely.

SPECIAL CONSIDERATIONS
PATIENT/FAMILY EDUCATION
• Missed dose: one tablet—Take as soon as remembered, or take 2 tablets at next regular time
• Missed 2 consecutive tablets—take 2 tablets at next 2 regular times
• Three missed tablets—Discontinue, restart after menses appear or pregnancy is ruled out
NOTE: Use an additional method of contraception if 2 or more tablets are missed until menses appear or pregnancy ruled out
• Progestin only pills have slightly higher failure rate than combination oral contraceptives
• When used as contraceptive, menstrual cycle may be disrupted and irregular and unpredictable bleeding or spotting may result

norfloxacin
(nor-flox′a-sin)
Rx: Noroxin
Rx: *Ophthalmic:* Chibroxin
Chemical Class: Fluoroquinolone derivative
Therapeutic Class: Antibiotic

CLINICAL PHARMACOLOGY
Mechanism of Action: A quinolone that inhibits DNA gyrase in susceptible microorganisms, interfering with bacterial cell replication and repair. *Therapeutic Effect:* Bactericidal.

INDICATIONS AND DOSAGES
Urinary tract infections (UTIs)
PO
Adults, Elderly. 400 mg twice a day for 7-21 days.
Prostatitis
PO
Adults. 400 mg twice a day for 28 days.
Uncomplicated gonococcal infections
PO
Adults. 800 mg as a single dose.
Dosage in renal impairment
Dosage and frequency are modified based on creatinine clearance.

Creatinine Clearance	Dosage
30 ml/min or higher	400 mg twice a day
less than 30 ml/min	400 mg once a day

$ AVAILABLE FORMS/COST
• Sol-Ophth: 0.3%, 5 ml: **$22.54**
• Tab, Plain Coated-Oral: 400 mg, 100's: **$399.35**
CONTRAINDICATIONS: Children younger than 18 years because of risk arthropathy; hypersensitivity to norfloxacin, other quinolones, or their components

PREGNANCY AND LACTATION: Pregnancy category C; excretion into breast milk unknown; due to the potential for arthropathy and osteochondrosis use extreme caution in nursing mothers

SIDE EFFECTS
Frequent
Nausea, headache, dizziness
Occasional
Rare
Vomiting, diarrhea, dry mouth, bitter taste, nervousness, drowsiness, insomnia, photosensitivity, tinnitus, crystalluria, rash, fever, seizures

SERIOUS REACTIONS
• Superinfection, anaphylaxis, Stevens-Johnson syndrome, and arthropathy occur rarely.
• Hypersensitivity reactions, including photosensitivity (as evidenced by rash, pruritus, blisters, edema, and burning skin), have occurred in patients receiving fluoroquinolones.

INTERACTIONS
Drugs
🔳 *Aluminum:* Reduced absorption of norfloxacin; do not take within 4 hr of dose
🔳 *Antacids:* Reduced absorption of norfloxacin; do not take within 4 hr of dose
🔳 *Antipyrine:* Inhibits metabolism of antipyrine; increased plasma antipyrine level
🔳 *Caffeine:* Inhibits metabolism of caffeine; increased plasma caffeine level
🔳 *Calcium:* Reduced absorption of norfloxacin; do not take within 4 hr of dose
🔳 *Diazepam:* Inhibits metabolism of diazepam; increased plasma diazepam level
🔳 *Didanosine:* Markedly reduced absorption of norfloxacin; take norfloxacin 2 hr before didanosine

N

🔳 *Foscarnet:* Coadministration increase seizure risk

🔳 *Iron:* Reduced absorption of norfloxacin; do not take within 4 hr of dose

🔳 *Magnesium:* Reduced absorption of norfloxacin; do not take within 4 hr of dose

🔳 *Metoprolol:* Inhibits metabolism of metoprolol; increased plasma metoprolol level

🔳 *Pentoxifylline:* Inhibits metabolism of pentoxifylline; increased plasma pentoxifylline level

🔳 *Phenytoin:* Inhibits metabolism of phenytoin; increased plasma phenytoin level

🔳 *Propranolol:* Inhibits metabolism of propranolol; increased plasma propranolol level

🔳 *Ropinirole:* Inhibits metabolism of ropinirole; increased plasma ropinirole level

🔳 *Sodium bicarbonate:* Reduced absorption of norfloxacin; do not take within 4 hr of dose

🔳 *Sucralfate:* Reduced absorption of norfloxacin; do not take within 4 hr of dose

🔳 *Theobromine:* Inhibits metabolism of theobromine; increased plasma theobromine level

🔳 *Theophylline:* Inhibits metabolism of theophylline; cut maintenance theophylline dose in half during therapy with norfloxacin

🔳 *Warfarin:* Inhibits metabolism of warfarin; increases hypoprothrombinemic response to warfarin

🔳 *Zinc:* Reduced absorption of norfloxacin; do not take within 4 hr of dose

Labs

• *False increase:* Uroporphyrin

SPECIAL CONSIDERATIONS

PATIENT/FAMILY EDUCATION

• Administer on an empty stomach (1 hr before or 2 hr after meals)

• Drink fluids liberally

• Do not take antacids containing magnesium or aluminum or products containing iron or zinc within 4 hr before or 2 hr after dosing

• Avoid excessive exposure to sunlight

norgestrel

(nor-jes-'trel)

Rx: Ovrette
Combinations
  Rx: with ethinyl estradiol (see oral contraceptives)
Chemical Class: 19-nortestosterone derivative; progestin derivative
Therapeutic Class: Contraceptive; progestin

CLINICAL PHARMACOLOGY

Mechanism of Action: A progestin that inhibits secretion of pituitary gonadotropin (LH) which prevents follicular maturation and ovulation. *Therapeutic Effect:* Transforms endometrium from proliferative to secretory in an estrogen-primed endometrium, promotes mammary gland development, relaxes uterine smooth muscle.

Pharmacokinetics

Well absorbed from the gastrointestinal (GI) tract. Widely distributed. Protein binding: 97%. Metabolized in liver via reduction and conjugation. Primarily excreted in urine. **Half-life:** 20 hrs.

INDICATIONS AND DOSAGES

Contraception, female

PO

Adults. 0.075 mg/day.

🔳 **AVAILABLE FORMS/COST**

• Tab-Oral: 0.075 mg, 28's: **$36.81**

UNLABELED USES: Endometrial protection, endometriosis, menorrhagia

CONTRAINDICATIONS: Hypersensitivity to norgestrel or any component of the formulation, hypersensitivity to tartrazine, thromboembolic disorders, severe hepatic disease; breast cancer; undiagnosed vaginal bleeding, pregnancy

PREGNANCY AND LACTATION: Pregnancy category X; compatible with breast-feeding

SIDE EFFECTS

Frequent

Breakthrough bleeding or spotting at beginning of therapy, amenorrhea, change in menstrual flow, breast tenderness

Occasional

Edema, weight gain or loss, rash, pruritus, photosensitivity, skin pigmentation

Rare

Pain or swelling at injection site, acne, mental depression, alopecia, hirsutism

SERIOUS REACTIONS

• Thrombophlebitis, cerebrovascular disorders, retinal thrombosis, and pulmonary embolism occur rarely.

SPECIAL CONSIDERATIONS

PATIENT/FAMILY EDUCATION

• Missed dose: One tablet—Take as soon as remembered, take next tablet at regular time; Two consecutive tablets—Take 1 of the missed tablets, discard the other

• Three missed tablets—Discontinue

• Use an additional method of contraception if 2 or more tablets are missed until menses appear or pregnancy ruled out.

• Progestin only pills have slightly higher failure rate than combination oral contraceptives

• Take with food if GI upset occurs

• Menstrual cycle may be disrupted and irregular and unpredictable bleeding or spotting can result

• Based on WHO study, norgestrel (levonorgestrel) only pills preferred emergency contraception; equal efficacy and 50% less nausea, vomiting compared to combined regimen

---

nortriptyline

(nor-trip'ti-leen)

Rx: Aventyl, Pamelor

Chemical Class: Dibenzocycloheptene derivative; secondary amine

Therapeutic Class: Antidepressant, tricyclic

CLINICAL PHARMACOLOGY

Mechanism of Action: A tricyclic antidepressant that blocks reuptake of the neurotransmitters norepinephrine and serotonin at neuronal presynaptic membranes, increasing their availability at postsynaptic receptor sites. *Therapeutic Effect:* Relieves depression.

INDICATIONS AND DOSAGES

Depression

PO

Adults. 75-100 mg/day in 1-4 divided doses until therapeutic response is achieved. Reduce dosage gradually to effective maintenance level.

Elderly. Initially, 10-25 mg at bedtime. May increase by 25 mg every 3-7 days. Maximum: 150 mg/day.

Children 12 yr and older. 30-50 mg/day in 3-4 divided doses.

Children 6-11 yr. 10-20 mg/day in 3-4 divided doses.

Enuresis

PO

Children 12 yr and older. 25-35 mg/day.

Children 8-11 yr. 10-20 mg/day.

Children 6-7 yr. 10 mg/day.

N

$ AVAILABLE FORMS/COST

• Cap, Gel—Oral: 10 mg, 100's: **$5.51-$213.41**; 25 mg, 100's: **$6.95-$425.80**; 50 mg, 100's: **$13.41-$802.44**; 75 mg, 100's: **$17.59-$1,223.11**
• Sol—Oral: 10 mg/5 ml, 480 ml: **$48.50-$55.52**

UNLABELED USES: Treatment of neurogenic pain, panic disorder; prevention of migraine headache

CONTRAINDICATIONS: Acute recovery period after MI, use within 14 days of MAOIs

PREGNANCY AND LACTATION: Pregnancy category D; effect on nursing infant unknown but may be of concern, especially after prolonged exposure

SIDE EFFECTS

Frequent

Somnolence, fatigue, dry mouth, blurred vision, constipation, delayed micturition, orthostatic hypotension, diaphoresis, impaired concentration, increased appetite, urine retention

Occasional

GI disturbances (nausea, GI distress, metallic taste), photosensitivity

Rare

Paradoxical reactions (agitation, restlessness, nightmares, insomnia), extrapyramidal symptoms (particularly fine hand tremor)

SERIOUS REACTIONS

• Overdose may produce seizures; cardiovascular effects, such as severe orthostatic hypotension, dizziness, tachycardia, palpitations, and arrhythmias; andaltered temperature regulation, such as hyperpyrexia or hypothermia.

• Abrupt discontinuation after prolonged therapy may produce headache, malaise, nausea, vomiting, and vivid dreams.

INTERACTIONS
Drugs

▨ *Anticholinergics:* Excessive anticholinergic effects

▨ *Barbiturates:* Reduced serum concentrations of cyclic antidepressants

▨ *Carbamazepine, rifampin:* Reduced cyclic antidepressant serum concentrations

▨ *Chlorpropamide:* Enhanced by hypoglycemic effects of chlorpropamide

▨ *Cimetidine:* Increased serum nortriptyline concentrations

▨ *Clonidine:* Reduced antihypertensive response to clonidine; enhanced hypertensive response with abrupt clonidine withdrawal

❷ *Epinephrine:* Markedly enhanced pressor response to IV epinephrine

▨ *Ethanol:* Additive impairment of motor skills; abstinent alcoholics may eliminate cyclic antidepressants more rapidly than non-alcoholics

▨ *Fluoxetine:* Marked increases in cyclic antidepressant plasma concentrations

❷ *Guanethidine:* Inhibited antihypertensive response to guanethidine

❷ *Moclobemide:* Potential association with fatal or non-fatal serotonin syndrome

⚠ *MAOIs:* Excessive sympathetic response, mania or hyperpyrexia possible

▨ *Neuroleptics:* Increased therapeutic and toxic effects of both drugs

❷ *Norepinephrine:* Markedly enhanced pressor response to norepinephrine

▨ *Phenylephrine:* Enhanced pressor response to IV phenylephrine

▨ *Propoxyphene:* Enhanced effect of cyclic antidepressants

▨ *Quinidine:* Increased cyclic antidepressant serum concentrations

Labs
• *False increase:* Serum carbamaze-pine
SPECIAL CONSIDERATIONS
PATIENT/FAMILY EDUCATION
• Therapeutic effects may take 2-3 wk
• Avoid rising quickly from sitting to standing, especially elderly
• Avoid alcohol and other CNS depressants
• Do not discontinue abruptly after long-term use
• Wear sunscreen or large hat to prevent sunburn
MONITORING PARAMETERS
• CBC, weight, ECG, mental status (mood, sensorium, affect, suicidal tendencies)
• Determination of nortriptyline plasma concentrations is not routinely recommended but may be useful in identifying toxicity, drug interactions, or noncompliance (adjustments in dosage should be made according to clinical response not plasma concentrations), therapeutic range 50-150 ng/ml

---

nystatin
(nye-stat'in)
Rx: *Troche:* Mycostatin
Rx: *Oral:* Mycostatin, Nilstat, Nystex
Rx: *Topical:* Mycostatin, Nystex, Nystop, Pedi-Dry
Combinations
  Rx: *Topical:* with triamcino-lone (Mycolog-II, Mycomer, Mycasone, Myco Biotic II, Tri-Statin II, Mytrex, Myco-Triacet II, Mycogen II)
Chemical Class: Amphoteric polyene macrolide
Therapeutic Class: Antifungal

CLINICAL PHARMACOLOGY
Mechanism of Action: A fungistatic antifungal that binds to sterols in the fungal cell membrane. *Therapeutic Effect:* Increases fungal cell-membrane permeability, allowing loss of potassium and other cellular components.
Pharmacokinetics
PO: Poorly absorbed from the GI tract. Eliminated unchanged in feces. Topical: Not absorbed systemically from intact skin.
INDICATIONS AND DOSAGES
Intestinal infections
PO
Adults, Elderly. 500,000-1,000,000 units q8h.
Oral candidiasis
PO
Adults, Elderly, Children. 400,000-600,000 units 4 times/day.
Infants. 200,000 units 4 times/day.
Vaginal infections
Vaginal
Adults, Elderly, Adolescents. 1 tablet/day at hs for 14 days.
Cutaneous candidal infections
Topical

Adults, Elderly, Children. Apply 2-4 times/day.

S **AVAILABLE FORMS/COST**
• Cap, Gel—Oral: 500,000 U 100's: **$24.00**; 1,000,000 U 100's: **$35.00**
• Cre—Top: 100,000 U/g 15, 30 g: **$2.41-$29.71**/30 g
• Lozenge—Oral: 200,000 U, 30's: **$31.40**
• Oint—Top: 100,000 U/g, 15, 30 g: **$2.40-$3.99**/30 g
• Powder—Top: 100,000 U/g, 15, 60 g: **$26.58-$30.51**/15 g
• Susp—Oral: 100,000 U/ml, 60, 480 ml: **$5.86-$32.29**/60 ml
• Tab, Plain Coated—Oral: 500,000 U, 100's: **$21.71-$71.55**
• Tab-Vag: 100,000 U, 15's: **$5.50-$54.14**

UNLABELED USES: Prophylaxis and treatment of oropharyngeal candidiasis, tinea barbae, tinea capitis
CONTRAINDICATIONS: None known.

PREGNANCY AND LACTATION: Pregnancy category A/C; due to poor bioavailability, serum and breast milk levels do not occur

SIDE EFFECTS
Occasional
PO: None known
Topical: Skin irritation
Vaginal: Vaginal irritation

SERIOUS REACTIONS
• High dosages of oral form may produce nausea, vomiting, diarrhea, and GI distress.

SPECIAL CONSIDERATIONS
PATIENT/FAMILY EDUCATION
• Do not use troches in child <5 yr

octreotide
(ok-tree'oh-tide)
Rx: Sandostatin, Sandostatin Lar Depot
Chemical Class: Somatostatin analog
Therapeutic Class: Acromegaly agent; antidiarrheal

CLINICAL PHARMACOLOGY
Mechanism of Action: An antidiarrheal and growth hormone suppressant that suppresses the secretion of serotonin and gastroenteropancreatic peptides and enhances fluid and electrolyte absorption from the GI tract. *Therapeutic Effect:* Prolongs intestinal transit time.
Pharmacokinetics

Route	Onset	Peak	Duration
Subcutaneous	N/A	N/A	Up to 12 hr

Rapidly and completely absorbed from injection site. Excreted in urine. Removed by hemodialysis. **Half-life:** 1.5 hr.

INDICATIONS AND DOSAGES
Diarrhea
IV (Sandostatin)
Adults, Elderly. Initially, 50–100 mcg q8h. May increase by 100 mcg/dose q48h. Maximum: 500 mcg q8h.
Subcutaneous (Sandostatin)
Adults, Elderly. 50 mcg 1–2 times a day.
IV, Subcutaneous (Sandostatin)
Children. 1–10 mcg/kg q12h.
Carcinoid tumors
IV, Subcutaneous (Sandostatin)
Adults, Elderly. 100–600 mcg/day in 2–4 divided doses.
IM (Sandostatin LAR)
Adults, Elderly. 20 mg q4wk.
Vipomas
IV, Subcutaneous (Sandostatin)

Adults, Elderly. 200–300 mcg/day in 2–4 divided doses.
IM (Sandostatin LAR)
Adults, Elderly. 20 mg q4wk.
Esophageal varices
IV (Sandostatin)
Adults, Elderly. Bolus of 25–50 mcg followed by IV infusion of 25–50 mcg/hr.
Acromegaly
IV, Subcutaneous (Sandostatin)
Adults, Elderly. 50 mcg 3 times a day. Increase as needed. Maximum: 500 mcg 3 times a day.
Acromegaly
IM (Sandostatin LAR)
Adults, Elderly. 20 mg q4wk for 3 mo. Maximum: 40 mg q4wk.

S AVAILABLE FORMS/COST
• Powder, Inj (Depot)-IM: 10 mg: **$1,535.23**; 20 mg: **$1,951.23**; 30 mg: **$2,622.03**
• Sol, Inj-SC, IV: 0.05 mg/ml, 1 ml: **$10.66**; 0.1 mg/ml, 1 ml: **$19.35**; 0.2 mg/ml, 5 ml: **$213.19**; 0.5 mg/ml, 1 ml: **$99.75**; 1 mg/ml, 5 ml: **$1,049.03**

UNLABELED USES: Treatment of AIDS-associated secretory diarrhea, chemotherapy-induced diarrhea, insulinomas, small-bowel fistulas, control of bleeding esophageal varices
CONTRAINDICATIONS: None known.
PREGNANCY AND LACTATION: Pregnancy category B; breast milk excretion unknown
SIDE EFFECTS
Frequent (10%–6%, 58%–30% in acromegaly patients)
Diarrhea, nausea, abdominal discomfort, headache, injection site pain
Occasional (5%–1%)
Vomiting, flatulence, constipation, alopecia, facial flushing, pruritus, dizziness, fatigue, arrhythmias, ecchymosis, blurred vision

Rare (less than 1%)
Depression, diminished libido, vertigo, palpitations, dyspnea
SERIOUS REACTIONS
• Patients using octreotide may develop cholelithiasis or, with prolonged high dosages, hypothyroidism.
• GI bleeding, hepatitis, and seizures occur rarely.
INTERACTIONS
Drugs
❷ *Cyclosporine:* Decreased serum cyclosporine concentrations
❸ *Oral hypoglycemic agents, insulin:* Octreotide can alter glycemic control, dose adjustment of antidiabetic agents may be necessary

SPECIAL CONSIDERATIONS
• Octreotide is incompatible in TPN solutions
• Patient tolerance to ocreotide should be determined with 2 weeks SC/IV therapy before switching to depot therapy
• Only give depot intragluteally, avoid deltoid injections due to pain at injection site
• Withdraw octreotide yearly for 4 wk in acromegaly patients who have received irradiation to assess disease activity
MONITORING PARAMETERS
• Thyroid function, serum glucose (especially in drug-treated diabetics), vitamin B_{12} levels
• Heart rate (especially in persons taking β-blockers and calcium channel blockers)
• Periodic zinc levels in patients receiving TPN

ofloxacin

(o-flox'a-sin)

Rx: (Oral): Floxin;
(Ophthalmic): Ocuflox
Chemical Class: Fluoroqui-
nolone derivative
Therapeutic Class: Antibiotic

CLINICAL PHARMACOLOGY

Mechanism of Action: A fluoroquinolone antibiotic that inhibits DNA
gyrase in susceptible microorganisms, interfering with bacterial cell
replication and repair. *Therapeutic
Effect:* Bactericidal.

Pharmacokinetics

Rapidly and well absorbed from the
GI tract. Protein binding: 20%-25%.
Widely distributed (including to
CSF). Metabolized in the liver.
Primarily excreted in urine. Re-
moved by hemodialysis. **Half-life:**
4.7-7 hr (increased in impaired renal
function, cirrhosis, and the elderly).

INDICATIONS AND DOSAGES

UTIs

PO, IV

Adults. 200 mg q12h.

Pelvic inflammatory disease (PID)

PO

Adults. 400 mg q12h for 10-14 days.

*Lower respiratory tract, skin and
skin-structure infections*

PO, IV

Adults. 400 mg q12h for 10 days.

*Prostatitis, sexually transmitted
diseases (cervicitis, urethritis)*

PO

Adults. 300 mg q12h.

Prostatitis

IV

Adults. 300 mg q12h.

Sexually transmitted diseases

IV

Adults. 400 mg as a single dose.

Acute, uncomplicated gonorrhea

PO

Adults. 400 mg 1 time.

Usual elderly dosage

PO

Elderly. 200-400 mg q12-24h for 7
days up to 6 wk.

Bacterial conjunctivitis

Ophthalmic

Adults, Elderly. 1-2 drops q2-4h for
2 days, then 4 times a day for 5 days.

Corneal ulcers

Ophthalmic

Adults. 1-2 drops q30min while
awake for 2 days, then q60min while
awake for 5-7 days, then 4 times a
day.

Acute otitis media

Otic

Children 1-12 yr. 5 drops into the affected ear 2 times/day for 10 days.

Otitis externa

Otic

*Adults, Elderly, Children 12 yr and
older.* 10 drops into the affected ear
once a day for 7 days.

Children 6 mo-11 yr. 5 drops into the
affected ear once a day for 7 days.

Dosage in renal impairment

After a normal initial dose, dosage
and frequency are based on creatinine clearance.

Creatinine Clearance	Adjusted Dose	Dosage Interval
greater than 50 ml/min	None	q12h
10-50 ml/min	None	q24h
less than 10 ml/min	½	q24h

💲 AVAILABLE FORMS/COST

• Sol—Ophth: 0.3%, 5, 10 ml:
$34.55-$44.63/5 ml

• Sol-Otic: 0.3%, 5, 10 ml: **$44.37**/5
ml

• Tab, Plain Coated—Oral: 200 mg,
50's: **$239.20-$265.78**; 300 mg,
50's: **$284.66-$316.29**; 400 mg,
100's: **$600.36-$667.11**

CONTRAINDICATIONS: Children younger than 18 years, hypersensitivity to any quinolones

PREGNANCY AND LACTATION: Pregnancy category C; excreted into breast milk in quantities approximating maternal plasma concentrations; due to the potential for arthropathy and osteochondrosis, use extreme caution in nursing mothers

SIDE EFFECTS

Frequent (10%-7%)

Nausea, headache, insomnia

Occasional (5%-3%)

Abdominal pain, diarrhea, vomiting, dry mouth, flatulence, dizziness, fatigue, drowsiness, rash, pruritus, fever

Rare (less than 1%)

Constipation, paraesthesia

SERIOUS REACTIONS

• Antibiotic-associated colitis and other superinfections may occur from altered bacterial balance.

• Hypersensitivity reactions, including photosensitivity (as evidenced by rash, pruritus, blisters, edema, and burning skin), have occurred in patients receiving fluoroquinolones.

• Arthropathy (swelling, pain, and clubbing of fingers and toes, degeneration of stress-bearing portion of a joint) may occur if the drug is given to children.

INTERACTIONS

Drugs

▣ *Aluminum:* Reduced absorption of ofloxacin; do not take within 4 hr of dose

▣ *Antacids:* Reduced absorption of ofloxacin; do not take within 4 hr of dose

▣ *Calcium:* Reduced absorption of ofloxacin; do not take within 4 hr of dose

▣ *Iron:* Reduced absorption of ofloxacin; do not take within 4 hr of dose

▣ *Magnesium:* Reduced absorption of ofloxacin; do not take within 4 hr of dose

▣ *Procainamide:* Ofloxacin competitively inhibits renal tubular excretion of procainamide

▣ *Sodium bicarbonate:* Reduced absorption of ofloxacin; do not take within 4 hr of dose

▣ *Sucralfate:* Reduced absorption of ofloxacin; do not take within 4 hr of dose

▣ *Warfarin:* Inhibits metabolism of warfarin; increases hypoprothrombinemic response to warfarin

▣ *Zinc:* Reduced absorption of ofloxacin; do not take within 4 hr of dose

Labs

• *False increase:* Uroporphyrin

SPECIAL CONSIDERATIONS

PATIENT/FAMILY EDUCATION

• Administer on an empty stomach (1 hr before or 2 hr after meals)

• Drink fluids liberally

• Do not take antacids containing magnesium or aluminum or products containing iron or zinc within 4 hr before or 2 hr after dosing

• Avoid excessive exposure to sunlight

olanzapine
(oh-lan'za-peen)
Rx: Zyprexa, Zyprexa
Intramuscular
Combinations
  Rx: with fluoxetine (Symbyax)
Chemical Class: Thienbenzodiazepine derivative
Therapeutic Class: Antipsychotic

CLINICAL PHARMACOLOGY
Mechanism of Action: A dibenzepin derivative that antagonizes alpha$_1$-adrenergic, dopamine, histamine, muscarinic, and serotonin receptors. Produces anticholinergic, histaminic, and CNS depressant effects. *Therapeutic Effect:* Diminishes manifestations of psychotic symptoms.
Pharmacokinetics
Well absorbed after PO administration. Protein binding: 93%. Extensively distributed throughout the body. Undergoes extensive first-pass metabolism in the liver. Excreted primarily in urine and, to a lesser extent, in feces. Not removed by dialysis. **Half-life:** 21-54 hr
INDICATIONS AND DOSAGES
Schizophrenia
PO
Adults. Initially, 5-10 mg once daily. May increase by 10 mg/day at 5-7 day intervals. If further adjustments are indicated, may increase by 5-10 mg/day at 7 day intervals. Range: 10-30 mg/day.
Elderly. Initially, 2.5 mg/day. May increase as indicated. Range: 2.5-10 mg/day.
Children. Initially, 2.5 mg/day. Titrate as necessary up to 20 mg/day.

Bipolar mania
PO
Adults. Initially, 10-15 mg/day. May increase by 5 mg/day at intervals of at least 24 hr. Maximum: 20 mg/day.
Children. Initially, 2.5 mg/day. Titrate as necessary up to 20 mg/day.
Dosage for elderly or debilitated patients and those predisposed to hypotensive reactions
The initial dosage for these patients is 5 mg/day.
Control agitation in schizophrenic or bipolar patients
IM
Adults, Elderly. 2.5-10 mg. May repeat 2h after first dose and 4h after 2nd dose. Maximum: 30 mg/day.
$ **AVAILABLE FORMS/COST**
• Tab, Film-Coated—Oral: 2.5 mg, 60's: **$347.28**; 5 mg, 60's: **$410.16**; 7.5 mg, 60's: **$498.81**; 10 mg, 60's: **$623.46**; 15 mg, 60's: **$935.19**; 20 mg, 60's: **$1,245.10**
• Tab, Disintegrating—Oral: 5 mg, 30's: **$225.49**; 10 mg, 30's: **$324.42**; 15 mg, 100's: **$468.98**; 20 mg, 30's: **$612.72**
UNLABELED USES: Treatment of anorexia, maintenance of long-term treatment response in schizophrenic patients, nausea, vomiting
CONTRAINDICATIONS: None known.
PREGNANCY AND LACTATION: Pregnancy category C; excretion into human breast milk unknown; excreted in the milk of treated rats
SIDE EFFECTS
Frequent
Somnolence (26%), agitation (23%), insomnia (20%), headache (17%), nervousness (16%), hostility (15%), dizziness (11%), rhinitis (10%)
Occasional
Anxiety, constipation (9%); nonaggressive atypical behavior (8%); dry mouth (7%); weight gain (6%); or-

thostatic hypotension, fever, arthralgia, restlessness, cough, pharyngitis, visual changes (dim vision) (5%)
Rare
Tachycardia; back, chest, abdominal, or extremity pain; tremor
SERIOUS REACTIONS
• Rare reactions include seizures and neuroleptic malignant syndrome, a potentially fatal syndrome characterized by hyperpyrexia, muscle rigidity, irregular pulse or BP, tachycardia, diaphoresis, and cardiac arrhythmias.
• Extrapyramidal symptoms and dysphagia may also occur.
• Overdose (300 mg) produces drowsiness and slurred speech.
INTERACTIONS
Drugs
☒ *Carbamazepine:* Decreased olanzapine concentrations
☒ *Levodopa:* Antagonism of the effects of levodopa due to dopamine receptor blockade
SPECIAL CONSIDERATIONS
PATIENT/FAMILY EDUCATION
• Avoid exposure to extreme heat
MONITORING PARAMETERS
• Periodic assessment of liver transaminases in patients with significant hepatic disease

---

olsalazine
(ohl-sal'ah-zeen)
Rx: Dipentum
Chemical Class: Salicylate derivative
Therapeutic Class: Gastrointestinal antiinflammatory

CLINICAL PHARMACOLOGY
Mechanism of Action: A salicylic acid derivative that is converted to mesalamine in the colon by bacterial action. Blocks prostaglandin production in bowel mucosa. *Thera-*peutic Effect:* Reduces colonic inflammation in inflammatory bowel disease.
INDICATIONS AND DOSAGES
Maintenance of controlled ulcerative colitis
PO
Adults, Elderly. 1 g/day in 2 divided doses, preferably q12h.
AVAILABLE FORMS/COST
• Cap, Gel—Oral: 250 mg, 100's: **$156.75**
UNLABELED USES: Treatment of inflammatory bowel disease
CONTRAINDICATIONS: History of hypersensitivity to salicylates
PREGNANCY AND LACTATION: Pregnancy category C; mesalamine has produced adverse effects in a nursing infant and should be used with caution during breast-feeding, observe nursing infant closely for changes in stool consistency
SIDE EFFECTS
Frequent (10%–5%)
Headache, diarrhea, abdominal pain or cramps, nausea
Occasional (5%–1%)
Depression, fatigue, dyspepsia, upper respiratory tract infection, decreased appetite, rash, itching, arthralgia
Rare (1%)
Dizziness, vomiting, stomatitis
SERIOUS REACTIONS
• Sulfite sensitivity may occur in susceptible patients manifested by cramping, headache, diarrhea, fever, rash, hives, itching, and wheezing may occur. Discontinue drug immediately.
• Excessive diarrhea associated with extreme fatigue is noted rarely.
SPECIAL CONSIDERATIONS
PATIENT/FAMILY EDUCATION
• Take with food. Notify clinician if diarrhea occurs

MONITORING PARAMETERS
• BUN, urinalysis, serum creatinine in patients with pre-existing renal disease

---

omalizumab

Rx: Xolair
Chemical Class: Monoclonal antibody
Therapeutic Class: Antiasthmatic

CLINICAL PHARMACOLOGY
Mechanism of Action: A monoclonal antibody that selectively binds to human immunoglobulin E (IgE) preventing it from binding to the surface of mast cells and basophiles. *Therapeutic Effect:* Prevents or reduces the number of asthmatic attacks.

Pharmacokinetics
Absorbed slowly after subcutaneous administration, with peak concentration in 7–8 days. Excreted in the liver, reticuloendothelial system, and endothelial cells. **Half-life:** 26 days.

INDICATIONS AND DOSAGES
Moderate to severe persistent asthma in patients who are reactive to a perennial allergen and whose asthma symptoms have been inadequately controlled with inhaled corticosteroids
Subcutaneous
Adults, Elderly, Children 12 yr and older. 150–375 mg every 2 or 4 wk; dose and dosing frequency are individualized based on weight and pretreatment immunoglobulin E (IgE) level (as shown below).

4-week dosing table

Pre-treatment serum IgE levels (units/ml)	Weight 30–60 kg	Weight 61–70 kg	Weight 71–90 kg	Weight 91–150 kg
30 to 100	150 mg	150 mg	150 mg	300 mg
101–200	300 mg	300 mg	300 mg	See next table
201–300	300 mg	See next table	See next table	See next table

2-week dosing table

Pre-treatment serum IgE levels (units/ml)	Weight 30–60 kg	Weight 61–70 kg	Weight 71–90 kg	Weight 91–150 kg
101–200	see preceding table	see preceding table	see preceding table	225 mg
201–300	See previous table	225 mg	225 mg	300 mg
301–400	225 mg	225 mg	300 mg	Do not dose
401–500	300 mg	300 mg	375 mg	Do not dose
501–600	300 mg	375 mg	Do not dose	Do not dose
601–700	375 mg	Do not dose	Do not dose	Do not dose

AVAILABLE FORMS/COST
• Powder, Inj-SC: 150 mg/vial: **$541.25**

UNLABELED USES: Treatment of seasonal allergic rhinitis

CONTRAINDICATIONS: None known.

PREGNANCY AND LACTATION: Pregnancy category B; while omalizumab presence in human milk has not been studied, IgG is excreted in human milk and therefore it is expected that omalizumab will be present in human milk; the potential harm to the infant is unknown; caution should be exercised when administering nursing mothers

SIDE EFFECTS
Frequent (45%–11%)

Injection site ecchymosis, redness, warmth, stinging, and urticaria; viral infections; sinusitis; headache; pharyngitis

Occasional (8%–3%)

Arthralgia, leg pain, fatigue, dizziness

Rare (2%)

Arm pain, earache, dermatitis, pruritus

SERIOUS REACTIONS

• Anaphylaxis occurs within 2 hours of the first dose or subsequent doses in 0.1% of patients.

• Malignant neoplasms occur in 0.5% of patients.

INTERACTIONS
Labs

• Serum total IgE levels increase following administration due to formation of omalizumab:IgE complexes; elevated serum total IgE levels may persist for up to 1 year following discontinuation

SPECIAL CONSIDERATIONS

• In clinical studies, a reduction of asthma exacerbations was not observed in omalizumab-treated patients who had FEV1 >80% at the time of randomization; reductions in exacerbations were not seen in patients who required oral steroids as maintenance therapy

PATIENT/FAMILY EDUCATION

• Systemic or inhaled corticosteroids should not be abruptly discontinued upon initiation of omalizumab therapy

• Do not decrease the dose of, or stop taking any other asthma medications unless otherwise instructed by clinician

• Immediate improvement in asthma symptoms may not be apparent after beginning omalizumab therapy

• Because the solution is slightly viscous, the injection may take 5-10 sec to administer

• Should be stored under refrigerated conditions 2-8°C (36-46°F)

MONITORING PARAMETERS

• Patients should be observed after injection of omalizumab, and medications for the treatment of severe hypersensitivity reactions including anaphylaxis should be available

• Total IgE levels are elevated during treatment and remain elevated for up to 1 year after the discontinuation of treatment; re-testing of IgE levels during omalizumab treatment cannot be used as a guide for dose determination; dose determination after treatment interruptions lasting <1 yr should be based on serum IgE levels obtained at the initial dose determination

• Doses should be adjusted for significant changes in body weight

---

omeprazole
(om-eh-pray′zole)

Rx: Prilosec, Zegerid
OTC: Prilosec OTC
Chemical Class: Benzimidazole derivative
Therapeutic Class: Antiulcer agent; gastrointestinal antisecretory agent

CLINICAL PHARMACOLOGY

Mechanism of Action: A benzimidazole that is converted to active metabolites that irreversibly bind to and inhibit hydrogen-potassium adenosine triphosphatase, an enzyme on the surface of gastric parietal cells. Inhibits hydrogen ion transport into gastric lumen. *Therapeutic Effect:* Increases gastric pH, reduces gastric acid production.

Pharmacokinetics

Route	Onset	Peak	Dura-tion
PO	1 hr	2 hr	72 hr

Rapidly absorbed from the GI tract. Protein binding: 99%. Primarily distributed into gastric parietal cells. Metabolized extensively in the liver. Primarily excreted in urine. Unknown if removed by hemodialysis. **Half-life:** 0.5–1 hr (increased in patients with hepatic impairment).

INDICATIONS AND DOSAGES

Erosive esophagitis, poorly responsive gastroesophageal reflux disease, active duodenal ulcer, prevention and treatment of NSAID-induced ulcers

PO

Adults, Elderly. 20 mg/day.

To maintain healing of erosive esophagitis

PO

Adults, Elderly. 20 mg/day.

Pathologic hypersecretory conditions

PO

Adults, Elderly. Initially, 60 mg/day up to 120 mg 3 times a day.

Duodenal ulcer caused by Helibacter Pylori

PO

Adults, Elderly. 20 mg twice a day for 10 days.

Active benign gastric ulcer

PO

Adults, Elderly. 40 mg/day for 4–8 wk.

Usual pediatric dosage

Children older than 2 yr, weighing 20 kg and more. 20 mg/day.

Children older than 2 yr, weighing less than 20 kg. 10 mg/day.

$ **AVAILABLE FORMS/COST**

• Cap, Gel, Sus Action—Oral: 10 mg, 100's: **$369.99-$413.39**; 20 mg, 100's: **$415.27-$461.47**; 40 mg, 100's: **$594.00-$662.18**

• Tab, Sus Action-Oral: 20 mg, 14's (OTC): **$10.80**

UNLABELED USES: *H. pylori*–associated duodenal ulcer (with amoxicillin and clarithromycin), prevention and treatment of NSAID-induced ulcers, treatment of active benign gastric ulcers,

CONTRAINDICATIONS: None known

PREGNANCY AND LACTATION: Pregnancy category C; excretion into breast milk unknown, suppression of gastric acid secretion is potential effect in nursing infant, clinical significance unknown, use with caution in nursing mothers

SIDE EFFECTS

Frequent (7%)

Headache

Occasional (3%–2%)

Diarrhea, abdominal pain, nausea

Rare (2%)

Dizziness, asthenia or loss of strength, vomiting, constipation, upper respiratory tract infection, back pain, rash, cough

SERIOUS REACTIONS

• None known.

INTERACTIONS

Drugs

▧ *Benzodiazepines, carbamazepine, cyclosporine, digoxin, nifedipine, nimodipine, nisoldipine:* Increased concentrations of these drugs

▧ *Ampicillin esters, cefpodoxime, cefuroxime, cyanocobalamin, enoxacin, iron salts, itraconazole, ketoconazole:* Decreased concentrations of these drugs

▧ *Glipizide, glyburide, tolbutamide:* Increased absorption of these drugs, potential of hypoglycemia

3 *Methotrexate:* Case report of elevated methotrexate concentration
3 *Phenytoin:* Increased phenytoin concentration

SPECIAL CONSIDERATIONS

• Some patients on maintenance therapy may respond to 10 mg qday or 20 mg qod

PATIENT/FAMILY EDUCATION

• Take before eating
• Swallow capsule whole; do not open, chew, or crush

---

ondansetron

(on-dan-seh'tron)
Rx: Zofran, Zofran ODT
Chemical Class: Carbazole derivative
Therapeutic Class: Antiemetic

CLINICAL PHARMACOLOGY

Mechanism of Action: An antiemetic that blocks serotonin, both peripherally on vagal nerve terminals and centrally in the chemoreceptor trigger zone. *Therapeutic Effect:* Prevents nausea and vomiting.

Pharmacokinetics

Readily absorbed from the GI tract. Protein binding: 70%-76%. Metabolized in the liver. Primarily excreted in urine. Unknown if removed by hemodialysis. **Half-life:** 4 hr.

INDICATIONS AND DOSAGES

Prevention of chemotherapy-induced nausea and vomiting

PO

Adults, Elderly, Children older than 11 yr. 24 mg as a single dose 30 min before starting chemotherapy. Or 8 mg 30 min before chemotherapy and again 8 hr after first dose, then q12h for 1-2 days.

Children 4–11 yr. 4 mg 30 min before chemotherapy and again 4 and 8 hr after chemotherapy, then q8h for 1-2 days.

IV

Adults, Elderly, Children 4–18 yr. 32 mg as a single dose or 0.15 mg/kg/dose 30 min before chemotherapy, then 4 and 8 hr after chemotherapy.

Prevention of radiation-induced nausea and vomiting

PO

Adults, Elderly. 8 mg 3 times a day.

Prevention of postoperative nausea and vomiting

IV, IM

Adults, Elderly. 4 mg undiluted over 2-5 min.

Children weighing less than 40 kg. 0.1 mg/kg.

Children weighing 10 kg and more. 4 mg.

S AVAILABLE FORMS/COST

• Sol, Inj-IV: 2 mg/ml, 2 ml: **$26.71**; 32 mg/50 ml, 50 ml: **$1,290.06**
• Sol—Oral: 4 mg/5 ml, 50 ml: **$203.28**
• Tab, Coated—Oral: 4 mg, 30's: **$600.88**; 8 mg, 30's: **$1,000.85**; 24 mg, 1's: **$94.40**
• Tab ODT (dissolving)—Oral: 4 mg, 30's: **$566.84**; 8 mg, 30's: **$944.16**

UNLABELED USES: Treatment of postoperative nausea and vomiting

CONTRAINDICATIONS: None known.

PREGNANCY AND LACTATION: Pregnancy category B; has been used in the treatment of hyperemesis gravidarum

SIDE EFFECTS

Frequent (13%-5%)

Anxiety, dizziness, somnolence, headache, fatigue, constipation, diarrhea, hypoxia, urine retention

Occasional (4%-2%)
Abdominal pain, xerostomia, fever, feeling of cold, redness and pain at injection site, paresthesia, asthenia
Rare (1%)
Hypersensitivity reaction (including rash and pruritus), blurred vision
SERIOUS REACTIONS
• Overdose may produce a combination of CNS stimulant and depressant effects.

---

opium tincture
(oh'pee-um)

Rx: Opium Tincture
Combinations
  Rx: with belladonna alkaloids (B&O Suppositories)
Chemical Class: Natural alkaloid
Therapeutic Class: Antidiarrheal; narcotic analgesic
DEA Class: Schedule II

CLINICAL PHARMACOLOGY
Mechanism of Action: An opioid agonist that contains many narcotic alkaloids including morphine. It inhibits gastric motility due to its morphine content. *Therapeutic Effect:* Decreases digestive secretions, increases in gastrointestinal (GI) muscle tone, and reduces GI propulsion.

Pharmacokinetics
Duration of action is 4-5 hrs. Variably absorbed from the gastrointestinal (GI) tract. Protein binding: unknown. Metabolized in liver. Primarily excreted in urine. Unknown if removed by hemodialysis. **Half-life:** unknown.

INDICATIONS AND DOSAGES
Analgesia
PO
Adults, Elderly. 0.6- 1.5 ml q3-4h. Maximum: 6 ml/day.

Children. 0.01-0.02 ml/kg/dose q3-4h. Maximum: 6 doses/day.
Antidiarrheal
PO
Adults, Elderly. 0.3- 1 ml q2-6h. Maximum: 6 ml/day.
Children. 0.005-0.01 ml/kg/dose q3-4h. Maximum: 6 doses/day.

S AVAILABLE FORMS/COST
• Tincture—Oral: 10%, 118 ml: **$49.29**

UNLABELED USES: Narcotic withdrawal symptoms in neonates
CONTRAINDICATIONS: Hypersensitivity to morphine sulfate or any component of the formulation, increased intracranial pressure, severe respiratory depression, severe hepatic or renal insufficiency, pregnancy (prolonged use or high dosages near term)
PREGNANCY AND LACTATION: Pregnancy category B (category D if used for prolonged periods or in high doses at term); compatible with breast-feeding
SIDE EFFECTS
Frequent
Constipation, drowsiness, nausea, vomiting
Occasional
Paradoxical excitement, confusion, pounding heartbeat, facial flushing, decreased urination, blurred vision, dizziness, dry mouth, headache, hypotension, decreased appetite, redness, burning, pain at injection site
Rare
Hallucinations, depression, stomach pain, insomnia
SERIOUS REACTIONS
• Overdosage results in cold or clammy skin, confusion, convulsions, decreased blood pressure (BP), restlessness, pinpoint pupils, bradycardia, respiratory depression, decreased level of consciousness (LOC), and severe weakness.

• Tolerance to analgesic effect and physical dependence may occur with repeated use.

INTERACTIONS

Drugs

③ *Barbiturates:* Additive CNS depression

③ *Cimetidine:* Increased effect of narcotic analgesics

③ *Ethanol:* Additive CNS effects

③ *Neuroleptics:* Hypotension and excessive CNS depression

Labs

• *False increase:* Amylase and lipase

SPECIAL CONSIDERATIONS

• Opium has been replaced by safer, more effective analgesics and sedative/hypnotics for diagnostic or operative medication; useful as an antidiarrheal

• Do not administer agonist/antagonist analgesics (i.e., pentazocine, nalbuphine, butorphanol, dezocine, buprenorphine) to patient who has received a prolonged course of opium (a pure agonist). In opioid-dependent patients, mixed agonist/antagonist analgesics may precipitate withdrawal symptoms

PATIENT/FAMILY EDUCATION

• Drug may be addictive if used for prolonged periods

---

orlistat

(ohr′lih-stat)

Rx: Xenical

Chemical Class: Lipase inhibitor

Therapeutic Class: Weight loss

CLINICAL PHARMACOLOGY

Mechanism of Action: A gastric and pancreatic lipase inhibitor that inhibits absorption of dietary fats by inactivating gastric and pancreatic enzymes. *Therapeutic Effect:* Resulting caloric deficit may positively affect weight control.

Pharmacokinetics

Minimal absorption after administration. Protein binding: 99%. Primarily eliminated unchanged in feces. Unknown if removed by hemodialysis. **Half-life:** 1–2 hr.

INDICATIONS AND DOSAGES

Weight reduction

PO

Adults, Elderly, Children 12-16 yr. 120 mg 3 times a day.

Ⓢ **AVAILABLE FORMS/COST**

• Cap—Oral: 120 mg, 90's: **$136.13**

CONTRAINDICATIONS: Cholestasis, chronic malabsorption syndrome

PREGNANCY AND LACTATION: Pregnancy category B

SIDE EFFECTS

Frequent (30%–20%)

Headache, abdominal discomfort, flatulence, fecal urgency, fatty or oily stool

Occasional (14%–5%)

Back pain, menstrual irregularity, nausea, fatigue, diarrhea, dizziness

Rare (less than 4%)

Anxiety, rash, myalgia, dry skin, vomiting

SERIOUS REACTIONS

• None known.

INTERACTIONS

Drugs

❷ *Fat-soluble vitamins:* pharmacokinetic interaction resulting in 30-60% reduction in beta-carotene, vitamin E

❷ *Warfarin:* because fat soluble vitamins may be depleted; an exaggerated hypoprothrombinemic effect is possible

SPECIAL CONSIDERATIONS

• Standard weight loss maintained over 2 years is approximately 10% of initial weight

PATIENT/FAMILY EDUCATION
• If a meal contains no fat, the dose of orlistat can be omitted
• Supplement with fat soluble vitamin, vitamin D, and beta-carotene
• Psyllium laxative may decrease GI adverse effects

MONITORING PARAMETERS
• Lipids, weight, plasma levels of vitamins A, D, E

---

orphenadrine
(or-fen´-a-dreen)
Rx: Antiflex, Banflex, Mio-rel, Myotrol, Norflex, Orfro, Orphenate
Combinations
  Rx: with aspirin, caffeine (Norgesic, Norgesic Forte, Orphengesic, Orphengesic Forte)
Chemical Class: Tertiary amine
Therapeutic Class: Skeletal muscle relaxant

CLINICAL PHARMACOLOGY
Mechanism of Action: A skeletal muscle relaxant that is structurally related to diphenhydramine and may thought to indirectly affect skeletal muscle by central atropine-like effects. *Therapeutic Effect:* Relieves musculoskeletal pain.

Pharmacokinetics
Well absorbed after PO and IM absorption. Protein binding: low. Metabolized in liver. Primarily excreted in urine and feces. **Half-life:** 14 hrs.

INDICATIONS AND DOSAGES
Musculoskeletal pain
IM/IV
Adults, Elderly. 60 mg 2 times/day. Switch to oral form for maintenance.
PO
Adults, Elderly. 100 mg 2 times/day.

$ AVAILABLE FORMS/COST
• Sol, Inj-IM, IV: 30 mg/ml, 10 ml: **$6.25-$29.90**
• Tab, Sus Action—Oral: 100 mg, 100's: **$9.50-$257.25**

UNLABELED USES: Drug-induced extrapyramidal reactions

CONTRAINDICATIONS: Angle-closure glaucoma, myasthenia gravis, pyloric or duodenal obstruction, stenosing peptic ulcer, prostatic hypertrophy, obstruction of the bladder neck, achalasia, cardiospasm (megaesophagus), hypersensitivity to orphenadrine or any component of the formulation

PREGNANCY AND LACTATION: Pregnancy category C; excretion into breast milk unknown, use caution in nursing mothers

SIDE EFFECTS
Frequent
Drowsiness, dizziness, muscular weakness, hypotension, dry mouth, nose, throat, and lips, urinary retention, thickening of bronchial secretions
Elderly
Frequent
Sedation, dizziness, hypotension
Occasional
Flushing, visual or hearing disturbances, paresthesia, diaphoresis, chill

SERIOUS REACTIONS
• Hypersensitivity reaction, such as eczema, pruritus, rash, cardiac disturbances, and photosensitivity, may occur.
• Overdosage may vary from CNS depression, including sedation, apnea, hypotension, cardiovascular collapse, or death to severe paradoxical reaction, such as hallucinations, tremor, and seizures.

INTERACTIONS
Drugs
3 *Neuroleptics:* Lower serum neuroleptic concentrations, excessive anticholinergic effects

---

oseltamivir
(ah-suhl-tahm'ah-veer)
Rx: Tamiflu
Chemical Class: Carboxylic acid ethyl ester
Therapeutic Class: Antiviral

CLINICAL PHARMACOLOGY
Mechanism of Action: A selective inhibitor of influenza virus neuraminidase, an enzyme essential for viral replication. Acts against both influenza A and B viruses. *Therapeutic Effect:* Suppresses the spread of infection within the respiratory system and reduces the duration of clinical symptoms.
Pharmacokinetics
Readily absorbed. Protein binding: 3%. Extensively converted to active drug in the liver. Primarily excreted in urine. **Half-life:** 6-10 hr.
INDICATIONS AND DOSAGES
Influenza
PO
Adults, Elderly. 75 mg 2 times a day for 5 days.
Children weighing more than 40 kg. 75 mg twice a day.
Children weighing 24-40 kg. 60 mg twice a day.
Children weighing 15-23 kg. 45 mg twice a day.
Children weighing less than 15 kg. 30 mg twice a day.
Prevention of influenza
PO
Adults, Elderly. 75 mg once a day.
Dosage in renal impairment
PO
For adult and elderly patients, dosage is decreased to 75 mg once a day

for at least 7 days and possibly up to 6 wk.
AVAILABLE FORMS/COST
• Cap—Oral: 75 mg, 10's: **$69.70**
• Powder, Reconst—Oral: 12 mg/ml, 25, 75 ml: **$34.85**/25 ml
CONTRAINDICATIONS: None known.
PREGNANCY AND LACTATION: Pregnancy category C; excreted in breast milk of animals
SIDE EFFECTS
Frequent (5%)
Nausea, vomiting, diarrhea
Occasional (4%-1%)
Abdominal pain, bronchitis, dizziness, headache, cough, insomnia, fatigue, vertigo
SERIOUS REACTIONS
• Colitis, pneumonia, and pyrexia occur rarely.
SPECIAL CONSIDERATIONS
PATIENT/FAMILY EDUCATION
• May administer without regard for food
• When started within 40 hr of onset of symptoms, there was a 1.3 day reduction in the median time to improvement in influenza-infected subjects receiving osteltamivir compared to subjects receiving placebo

---

oxacillin
(ox-a-sill'in)
Rx: Bactrocill
Chemical Class: Penicillin derivative, penicillinase-resistant
Therapeutic Class: Antibiotic

CLINICAL PHARMACOLOGY
Mechanism of Action: A penicillin that binds to bacterial membranes. *Therapeutic Effect:* Bactericidal.

INDICATIONS AND DOSAGES
Upper respiratory tract, skin, and skin-structure infections
IV, IM

Adults, Elderly, Children weighing 40 kg or more. 250-500 mg q4-6h.
Children weighing less than 40 kg. 50 mg/kg/day in divided doses q6h. Maximum: 12 g/day.

Lower respiratory tract and other serious infections
IV, IM

Adults, Elderly, Children weighing 40 kg or more. 1 g q4-6h. Maximum: 12 g/day.
Children weighing less than 40 kg. 100 mg/kg/day in divided doses q4-6h.

S AVAILABLE FORMS/COST
• Cap, Gel—Oral: 250 mg, 100's: **$28.71-$30.50**; 500 mg, 100's: **$53.20-$56.85**

• Powder, Inj-IM, IV: 500 mg/vial: **$1.37-$3.17**; 1 g/vial: **$3.35-$11.11**; 2 g/vial: **$5.30-$25.28**; 4 g/vial: **$11.78**

• Powder, Reconst—Oral: 250 mg/5 ml, 100 ml: **$5.80-$14.58**

CONTRAINDICATIONS: Hypersensitivity to any penicillin

PREGNANCY AND LACTATION: Pregnancy category B; potential exists for modification of bowel flora in nursing infant; allergy or sensitization, and interference with interpretation of culture results if fever workup required

SIDE EFFECTS
Frequent
Mild hypersensitivity reaction (fever, rash, pruritus), GI effects (nausea, vomiting, diarrhea)
Occasional
Phlebitis, thrombophlebitis (more common in elderly), hepatotoxicity (with high IV dosage)

SERIOUS REACTIONS
• Antibiotic-associated colitis and other superinfections may result from altered bacterial balance.
• A mild to severe hypersensitivity reaction may occur in those allergic to penicillins.

INTERACTIONS
Drugs
▣ *Chloramphenicol:* Inhibited antibacterial activity of oxacillin, ensure adequate amounts of both agents are given and administer oxacillin a few hours before chloramphenicol
▣ *Methotrexate:* Increased serum methotrexate concentrations
▣ *Tetracyclines:* Inhibited antibacterial activity of oxacillin, ensure adequate amounts of both agents are given and administer oxacillin a few hours before tetracycline

SPECIAL CONSIDERATIONS
• Sodium content of 1 g = 2.8-3.1 mEq

PATIENT/FAMILY EDUCATION
• Administer on an empty stomach (1 hr before or 2 hr after meals)

MONITORING PARAMETERS
• Urinalysis, BUN, serum creatinine, CBC with differential, periodic liver function tests

---

oxaliplatin
(ahks-al-eh-plah'tin)
Rx: Eloxatin
Chemical Class: Organoplatinum complex
Therapeutic Class: Antineoplastic

CLINICAL PHARMACOLOGY
Mechanism of Action: A platinum-containing complex that cross-links with DNA strands, preventing cell

division. Cell cycle–phase nonspecific. *Therapeutic Effect:* Inhibits DNA replication.

Pharmacokinetics

Rapidly distributed. Protein binding: 90%. Undergoes rapid, extensive nonenzymatic biotransformation. Excreted in urine. **Half-life:** 70 hr.

INDICATIONS AND DOSAGES

Metastatic colon or rectal cancer in patients whose disease has recurred or progressed during or within 6 months of completing first-line therapy with bolus 5-fluorouracil (5-FU), leucovorin, and irinotecan.

IV

Adults. Day 1: Oxaliplatin 85 mg/m2 in 250-500 ml D_5W and leucovorin 200 mg/m^2, both given simultaneously over more than 2 hr in separate bags using a Y-line, followed by 5-FU 400 mg/m2 IV bolus given over 2-4 min, followed by 5-FU 600 mg/m2 in 500 ml D_5W as a 22-hr continuous IV infusion. Day 2: Leucovorin 200 mg/m2 IV infusion given over more than 2 hr, followed by 5-FU 400 mg/m^2 IV bolus given over 2-4 min, followed by 5-FU 600 mg/m^2 in 500 ml D_5W as a 22-hr continuous IV infusion.

Ovarian cancer

IV

Adults. Cisplatin 100 mg/m^2 and oxaliplatin 130 mg/m^2 every 3 wk.

S   AVAILABLE FORMS/COST

• Inj, Powder—IV: 50 mg, 1's: **$994.26**; 100 mg, 1's: **$1,988.53**
UNLABELED USES: Treatment of ovarian cancer
CONTRAINDICATIONS: History of allergy to platinum compounds
PREGNANCY AND LACTATION: Pregnancy category D; excretion into breast milk unknown; breastfeeding not recommended

SIDE EFFECTS

Frequent (76%-20%)

Peripheral or sensory neuropathy (usually occurs in hands, feet, perioral area, and throat but may present as jaw spasm, abnormal tongue sensation, eye pain, chest pressure, or difficulty walking, swallowing, or writing), nausea (occurs in 64%), fatigue, diarrhea, vomiting, constipation, abdominal pain, fever, anorexia

Occasional (14%-10%)

Stomatitis, earache, insomnia, cough, difficulty breathing, backache, edema

Rare (7%-3%)

Dyspepsia, dizziness, rhinitis, flushing, alopecia

SERIOUS REACTIONS

• Peripheral or sensory neuropathy can occur, sometimes precipitated or exacerbated by drinking or holding a glass of cold liquid during the IV infusion.

• Pulmonary fibrosis, characterized by a nonproductive cough, dyspnea, crackles, and radiologic pulmonary infiltrates, may require drug discontinuation.

• Hypersensitivity reaction (rash, urticaria, pruritus) occurs rarely.

SPECIAL CONSIDERATIONS

• Extravasation may lead to tissue necrosis

PATIENT/FAMILY EDUCATION

• Neurotoxicity may be acute and aggravated by exposure to cold

MONITORING PARAMETERS

• CBC with platelets, hepatic and renal function

oxandrolone

(ox-an'droe-lone)

Rx: Oxandrin

Chemical Class: Anabolic steroid; testosterone derivative

Therapeutic Class: Androgen

DEA Class: Schedule III

CLINICAL PHARMACOLOGY

Mechanism of Action: A synthetic testosterone derivative that promotes growth and development of male sex organs, maintains secondary sex characteristics in androgen-deficient males. *Therapeutic Effect:* Androgenic and anabolic actions.

Pharmacokinetics

Well absorbed from the gastrointestinal (GI) tract. Protein binding: 94-97%. Metabolized in liver. Primarily excreted in urine. Unknown if removed by hemodialysis. **Half-life:** 5-13 hrs.

INDICATIONS AND DOSAGES

Weight gain

Adults, Elderly. 2.5-20 mg in divided doses 2-4 times/day usually for 2-4 weeks. Course of therapy is based on individual response. Repeat intermittently as needed.

Children. Total daily dose is 0.1 mg/kg. Repeat intermittently as needed.

$ **AVAILABLE FORMS/COST**

• Tab-Oral: 2.5 mg, 100's: **$476.84**; 10 mg, 60's: **$1,048.38**

UNLABELED USES: AIDS wasting syndrome, alcoholic hepatitis, athletic performance enhancement, burns, growth hormone deficiency, hyperlipidemia, Turner syndrome

CONTRAINDICATIONS: Nephrosis, carcinoma of breast or prostate hypercalcemia, pregnancy, hypersensitivity to oxandrolone or any component of the formulation

PREGNANCY AND LACTATION: Pregnancy category X; use extreme caution in nursing mothers

SIDE EFFECTS

Frequent

Gynecomastia, acne, amenorrhea, other menstrual irregularities

Females: Hirsutism, deepening of voice, clitoral enlargement that may not be reversible when drug is discontinued

Occasional

Edema, nausea, insomnia, oligospermia, priapism, male pattern of baldness, bladder irritability, hypercalcemia in immobilized patients or those with breast cancer, hypercholesterolemia

Rare

Polycythemia with high dosage

SERIOUS REACTIONS

• Peliosis hepatitis of the liver, spleen replaced with blood-filled cysts, hepatic neoplasms and hepatocellular carcinoma have been associated with prolonged high-dosage, anaphylactic reactions.

INTERACTIONS

Drugs

[3] *Antidiabetic agents:* Enhanced hypoglycemic effects

[2] *Cyclosporine:* Increased cyclosporine concentrations, toxicity

[3] *HMG-CoA reductase inhibitors (lovastatin, pravastatin):* Myositis risk increased

[3] *Tacrolimus:* Increased tacrolimus concentrations, toxicity

[2] *Oral anticoagulants:* Enhanced hypoprothrombinemic response

SPECIAL CONSIDERATIONS

• Anabolic steroids have potential for abuse, especially in the athlete

PATIENT/FAMILY EDUCATION

• Adequate dietary intake of calories and protein essential for successful treatment

MONITORING PARAMETERS
• LFTs, lipids
• Growth rate in children (X-rays for bone age q 6 mo)
• Serum calcium in breast cancer patients

---

oxaprozin

(ox-a-pro'zin)
Rx: Daypro
Chemical Class: Propionic acid derivative
Therapeutic Class: NSAID; antipyretic; nonnarcotic analgesic

CLINICAL PHARMACOLOGY
Mechanism of Action: An NSAID that produces analgesic and anti-inflammatory effects by inhibiting prostaglandin synthesis. *Therapeutic Effect:* Reduces the inflammatory response and intensity of pain.
Pharmacokinetics
Well absorbed from the GI tract. Protein binding: 99%. Widely distributed. Metabolized in the liver. Primarily excreted in urine; partially eliminated in feces. Not removed by hemodialysis. **Half-life:** 42–50 hr.

INDICATIONS AND DOSAGES
Osteoarthritis
PO
Adults, Elderly. 1,200 mg once a day (600 mg in patients with low body weight or mild disease). Maximum: 1,800 mg/day.
Rheumatoid arthritis
PO
Adults, Elderly. 1,200 mg once a day. Range: 600–1,800 mg/day.
Juvenile rheumatoid arthritis
Children weighing more than 54 kg. 1,200 mg/day.
Children weighing 32-54 kg. 900 mg/day.

Children weighing 22-31 kg. 600 mg/day.
Dosage in renal impairment
For adults and elderly patients with renal impairment, the recommended initial dose is 600 mg/day; may be increased up to 1,200 mg/day.

S **AVAILABLE FORMS/COST**
• Tab-Oral: 600 mg, 100's: **$149.80-$263.24**
CONTRAINDICATIONS: Active peptic ulcer disease, chronic inflammation of GI tract, GI bleeding or ulceration, history of hypersensitivity to aspirin or NSAIDs
PREGNANCY AND LACTATION: Pregnancy category C (category D if used in 3rd trimester); could cause constriction of the ductus arteriosus *in utero,* persistent pulmonary hypertension of the newborn, or prolonged labor

SIDE EFFECTS
Occasional (9%–3%)
Nausea, diarrhea, constipation, dyspepsia, edema
Rare (less than 3%)
Vomiting, abdominal cramps or pain, flatulence, anorexia, confusion, tinnitus, insomnia, somnolence

SERIOUS REACTIONS
• Hypertension, acute renal failure, respiratory depression, GI bleeding, and coma occur rarely.

INTERACTIONS
Drugs
3 *Aminoglycosides:* Reduced clearance with elevated aminoglycoside levels and potential for toxicity (especially indomethacin in premature infants; other NSAIDs probably)
3 *Anticoagulants:* Excessive hypoprothrombinemia, decreased platelet aggregation with increased risk of GI bleeding

❸ *Antihypertensives (α-blockers, angiotensin-converting enzyme inhibitors, angiotensin II receptor blockers, β-blockers, diuretics):* Inhibition of antihypertensive and other favorable hemodynamic effects

❸ *Corticosteroids:* Increased risk of GI ulceration

❸ *Cyclosporine:* Increased nephrotoxicity risk

❸ *Lithium:* Decreased clearance of lithium (mediated via prostaglandins) resulting in elevated serum lithium levels and risk of toxicity

❸ *Methotrexate:* Decreased renal secretion of methotrexate resulting in elevated methotrexate levels and risk of toxicity

❸ *Phenylpropanolamine:* Possible acute hypertensive reaction

❸ *Potassium-sparing diuretics:* Additive hyperkalemia potential

❸ *Triamterene:* Acute renal failure reported with addition of indomethacin; caution with other NSAIDs

SPECIAL CONSIDERATIONS
• No significant advantage over other NSAIDs; cost should govern use

PATIENT/FAMILY EDUCATION
• Avoid aspirin and alcoholic beverages
• Take with food, milk, or antacids to decrease GI upset

MONITORING PARAMETERS
• Initial hemogram and fecal occult blood test within 3 mo of starting regular chronic therapy; repeat every 6-12 mo (more frequently in high-risk patients (>65 years, peptic ulcer disease, concurrent steroids or anticoagulants); electrolytes, creatinine, and BUN within 3 mo of starting regular chronic therapy; repeat every 6-12 mo

---

oxazepam
(ox-a′ze-pam)
Rx: Serax
Chemical Class: Benzodiazepine
Therapeutic Class: Anxiolytic
DEA Class: Schedule IV

CLINICAL PHARMACOLOGY
Mechanism of Action: A benzodiazepine that potentiates the effects of gamma-aminobutyric acid and other inhibitory neurotransmitters by binding to specific receptors in the CNS. *Therapeutic Effect:* Produces anxiolytic effect and skeletal muscle relaxation.

Pharmacokinetics
Well absorbed from the GI tract. Protein binding: 97%. Metabolized in the liver. Primarily excreted in urine. Not removed by hemodialysis. **Half-life:** 5-20 hr.

INDICATIONS AND DOSAGES
Mild to moderate anxiety
PO
Adults. 10-15 mg 3-4 times a day.
Severe anxiety
PO
Adults. 15-30 mg 3-4 times a day.
Alcohol withdrawal
PO
Adults. 15-30 mg 3-4 times a day.
Elderly. Initially, 10-20 mg 3 times a day. May gradually increase up to 30-45 mg/day.

Ⓢ **AVAILABLE FORMS/COST**
• Cap, Gel—Oral: 10 mg, 100's: **$18.40-$102.68**; 15 mg, 100's: **$23.80-$129.64**; 30 mg, 100's: **$33.80-$187.50**
• Tab—Oral: 15 mg, 100's: **$129.64**
CONTRAINDICATIONS: Angle-closure glaucoma; pre-existing CNS depression; severe, uncontrolled pain

PREGNANCY AND LACTATION:
Pregnancy category D; may cause fetal damage when administered during pregnancy; excreted into breast milk, may accumulate in breast-fed infants and is therefore not recommended

SIDE EFFECTS

Frequent

Mild, transient somnolence at beginning of therapy

Occasional

Dizziness, headache

Rare

Paradoxical CNS reactions, such as hyperactivity or nervousness in children and excitement or restlessness in the elderly or debilitated (generally noted during the first 2 weeks of therapy)

SERIOUS REACTIONS

• Abrupt or too-rapid withdrawal may result in pronounced restlessness, irritability, insomnia, hand tremor, abdominal or muscle cramps, diaphoresis, vomiting, and seizures.

• Overdose results in somnolence, confusion, diminished reflexes, and coma.

INTERACTIONS

Drugs

▣ *Ethanol:* Enhanced adverse psychomotor effects of benzodiazepines

Labs

• *False increase:* Serum glucose

SPECIAL CONSIDERATIONS

• Niche compared to other benzodiazepines: treatment of anxiety in patients with hepatic disease; consider for alcohol withdrawal

• Tablet form contains tartrazine; risk of allergic-type reactions especially in patients with aspirin hypersensitivity

PATIENT/FAMILY EDUCATION

• Avoid alcohol and other CNS depressants

• Do not discontinue abruptly after prolonged therapy

• Inform clinician if planning to become pregnant, pregnant, or become pregnant while taking this medicine

• May be habit forming

MONITORING PARAMETERS

• Periodic CBC, UA, blood chemistry analyses during prolonged therapy

---

oxcarbazepine
(oks-kar-bays'uh-peen)
Rx: Trileptal
Chemical Class: Dibenzazepine derivative
Therapeutic Class: Anticonvulsant

CLINICAL PHARMACOLOGY

Mechanism of Action: An anticonvulsant that blocks sodium channels, resulting in stabilization of hyperexcited neural membranes, inhibition of repetitive neuronal firing, and diminishing synaptic impulses. *Therapeutic Effect:* Prevents seizures.

Pharmacokinetics

Completely absorbed from GI tract and extensively metabolized in the liver to active metabolite. Protein binding: 40%. Primarily excreted in urine. **Half-life:** 2 hr; metabolite, 6-10 hr.

INDICATIONS AND DOSAGES

Adjunctive treatment of seizures

PO

Adults, Elderly. Initially, 600 mg/day in 2 divided doses. May increase by up to 600 mg/day at weekly intervals. Maximum: 2,400 mg/day.

Children 4-16 yr. 8-10 mg/kg. Maximum: 600 mg/day. Maintenance (based on weight): 1,800 mg/day for children weighing more than 39 kg;

1,200 mg/day for children weighing 29.1–39 kg; and 900 mg/day for children weighing 20-29 kg.

Conversion to monotherapy
PO

Adults, Elderly. 600 mg/day in 2 divided doses (while decreasing concomitant anticonvulsant over 3-6 wk). May increase by 600 mg/day at weekly intervals up to 2,400 mg/day.

Children. Initially, 8-10 mg/kg/day in 2 divided doses with simultaneous initial reduction of dose of concomitant antiepileptic.

Initiation of monotherapy
PO

Adults, Elderly. 600 mg/day in 2 divided doses. May increase by 300 mg/day every 3 days up to 1,200 mg/day.

Children. Initially, 8-10 mg/kg/day in 2 divided doses. Increase at 3 day intervals by 5 mg/kg/day to achieve maintenance dose by weight; (70 kg): 1500-2100 mg/day; (60-69 kg): 1200-2100 mg/day; (50-59 kg): 1200-1800 mg/day; (41-49 kg): 1200-1500 mg/day; (35-40 kg): 900-1500 mg/day; (25-34 kg): 900-1200 mg/day; (20-24 kg): 600-900 mg/day.

Dosage in renal impairment
For patients with creatinine clearance less than 30 ml/min, give 50% of normal starting dose, then titrate slowly to desired dose.

🅂 AVAILABLE FORMS/COST
• Susp—Oral: 300 mg/5 ml, 250 ml: **$100.66**
• Tab, Coated—Oral: 150 mg, 100's: **$108.69**; 300 mg, 100's: **$198.86**; 600 mg, 100's: **$365.50**
UNLABELED USES: Atypical panic disorder
CONTRAINDICATIONS: None known.

PREGNANCY AND LACTATION: Pregnancy category C, increased incidence of fetal structural abnormalities and other manifestation of developmental toxicity have been observed in the offspring of animals; no adequate and well-controlled data in humans; oxcarbazepine and MHD both excreted in human breast milk; milk:plasma ratio: 0.5 (both)

SIDE EFFECTS
Frequent (22%-13%)
Dizziness, nausea, headache
Occasional (7%-5%)
Vomiting, diarrhea, ataxia, nervousness, heartburn, indigestion, epigastric pain, constipation
Rare (4%)
Tremor, rash, back pain, epistaxis, sinusitis, diplopia

SERIOUS REACTIONS
• Clinically significant hyponatremia may occur.

INTERACTIONS
Drugs
• *Note:* Oxcarbazepine is an inhibitor of CYP2C19 and an inducer of CYP3A4 and CYP3A5
🄳 *Alcohol:* Additive CND depression and psychomotor impairment
🄳 *Barbiturates:* Decreases oxcarbazepine levels
🄳 *Benzodiazepines:* Additive CNS effects
🄳 *Calcium channel blockers (dihydropyridines):* Induction of antihypertensive metabolism; decreased antihypertensive efficacy
🄳 *Estradiol, oral contraceptives:* Induction of hepatic metabolism; decreased hormonal efficacy
🄳 *Medroxyprogesterone:* Induction of hepatic metabolism; decreased hormonal efficacy
🄳 *Lamotrigine:* Induction of hepatic metabolism; decreased lamotrigine levels by 30%

3 *Phenytoin:* Alterations in hepatic metabolism resulting in increases in phenytoin levels/risk of toxicity and decreases in oxcarbazepine

3 *Verapamil:* Decreased plasma oxcarbazepine concetrations

Labs

• *Thyroid levels:* Decreased

• *Serum sodium:* Decreased; increased risk of hyponatremia

SPECIAL CONSIDERATIONS

• Considered an alternative to carbamazepine in intolerant patients

PATIENT/FAMILY EDUCATION

• Review and reinforce prevalence of CNS adverse effects early in treatment (reason for gradual titration regimens) with tolerance developing with continued adherence

• Risk of recurrent seizures with missed doses

MONITORING PARAMETERS

• Seizure frequency and electroencephalogram changes in patients with seizure disorder; a reduction or elimination of pain in patients with trigeminal neuralgia; therapeutic serum levels not adequately established - estimates of therapeutic serum concentrations of the active metabolite (MHD) in the 50-110 μmol range; serum electrolytes (especially sodium), LFTs, blood counts, serum lipids

---

oxiconazole
(ox-i-con'a-zole)
Rx: Oxistat
Chemical Class: Imidazole derivative
Therapeutic Class: Antifungal

CLINICAL PHARMACOLOGY

Mechanism of Action: An antifungal agent that inhibits ergosterol synthesis. *Therapeutic Effect:* Destroys cytoplasmic membrane integrity of fungi. Fungicidal.

Pharmacokinetics

Low systemic absorption. Absorbed and distributed in each layer of the dermis. Excreted in the urine.

INDICATIONS AND DOSAGES

Tinea pedis

Topical

Adults, Elderly, Children 12 yrs and older. Apply 1-2 times daily for one month or until signs and symptoms significantly improve.

Tinea cruris, Tinea corporis

Topical

Adults, Elderly, Children 12 yrs and older. Apply 1-2 times daily for two weeks or until signs and symptoms significantly improve.

S AVAILABLE FORMS/COST

• Cre—Top: 1%, 15, 30, 60 g: **$38.41**/30 g

• Lotion—Top: 1% 30 ml: **$38.41**

CONTRAINDICATIONS: Not for ophthalmic use, hypersensitivity to oxiconazole or any other azole fungals

PREGNANCY AND LACTATION: Pregnancy category B; excreted in breast milk

SIDE EFFECTS

Occasional

Itching, local irritation, stinging, dryness

SERIOUS REACTIONS
• Hypersensitivity reactions characterized by rash, swelling, pruritus, maceration and a sensation of warmth may occur.

SPECIAL CONSIDERATIONS
• Niche: once daily imadazole; base choice on cost and convenience

PATIENT/FAMILY EDUCATION
• For external use only, avoid contact with eyes or vagina

---

oxtriphylline
(ox-trye′fi-lin)

Rx: Choledyl SA
Chemical Class: Xanthine derivative (64% theophylline)
Therapeutic Class: COPD agent; antiasthmatic; bronchodilator

CLINICAL PHARMACOLOGY
Mechanism of Action: A choline salt of theophylline acts as a bronchodilator by directly relaxing smooth muscle of the bronchial airway and pulmonary blood vessels. *Therapeutic Effect:* Relieves bronchospasm, increases vital capacity. Produces cardiac skeletal muscle stimulation.

Pharmacokinetics
Absorbed slowly due to extended release formulation. Protein binding: 40%. Distributed rapidly into peripheral non-adipose tissues and body water, including cerebrospinal fluid (CSF). Metabolized in liver. Eliminated in urine. **Half-life:** Adults, 6-12 hrs; Children, 1.2-7 hrs.

INDICATIONS AND DOSAGES
Asthma
PO
Adults, Elderly, Children. 400-600 mg q12h

Children (younger than 5 yrs). 24-36 mg/kg/day given in divided doses.
Children (5-9 yrs). 200-400 mg/day given in divided doses.
Children (10-14 yrs). 400-800 mg/day given in divided doses.

ⓢ AVAILABLE FORMS/COST
• Tab, Coated, Sus Action—Oral: 400 mg, 100's: **$41.15**; 600 mg, 100's: **$49.37**

CONTRAINDICATIONS: Active peptic ulcer disease, seizure disorder (unless receiving appropriate anticonvulsant medication, history of hypersensitivity to xanthines

PREGNANCY AND LACTATION: Pregnancy category C; pharmacokinetics of theophylline may be altered during pregnancy, monitor serum concentrations carefully; excreted into breast milk, may cause irritability in the nursing infant, otherwise compatible with breast-feeding

SIDE EFFECTS
Frequent
Headache, shakiness, restlessness, tachycardia, trembling
Occasional
Nausea, vomiting, epigastric pain, diarrhea, headache, mild diuresis, insomnia
Rare
Alopecia, hyperglycemia, SIADH, rash

SERIOUS REACTIONS
• Nausea, vomiting, seizures and coma can result from overdosage.

INTERACTIONS
Drugs
🔳 *Adenosine:* Inhibited hemodynamic effects of adenosine
🔳 *Allopurinol, amiodarone, cimetadine, ciprofloxacin, disulfiram, erythromycin, interferon alfa, isoniazid, methimazole, metoprolol, norfloxacin, pefloxacin, pentoxifylline, propafenone, propylthiouracil,*

radioactive iodine, tacrine, thiabendazole, ticlopidine, verapamil: Increased theophylline concentrations

3 Aminoglutethimide, barbiturates, carbamazepine, moricizine, phenytoin, rifampin, ritonavir, thyroid hormone: Reduced theophylline concentrations; decreased serum phenytoin concentrations

2 Enoxacin, fluvoxamine, mexiletine, propanolol, troleandomycin: Increased theophylline concentrations

3 Imipenem: Some patients on oxtriphylline have developed seizures following the addition of imipenem

3 Lithium: Reduced lithium concentrations

3 Smoking: Increased oxtriphylline dosing requirements

Labs
• False increase: Serum barbiturate concentrations, urinary uric acid
• False decrease: Serum bilirubin
• Interference: Plasma somatostatin

SPECIAL CONSIDERATIONS
• Touted to produce less GI side effects; if dosed equipotently based on theophylline equivalents (oxtriphylline = 64% theophylline) no difference; compare costs as well as other characteristics

PATIENT/FAMILY EDUCATION
• Avoid large amounts of caffeine-containing products (tea, coffee, chocolate, colas)

MONITORING PARAMETERS
• Serum theophylline concentrations (therapeutic level is 8-20 mcg/ml); toxicity may occur with small increase above 20 mcg/ml, especially in the elderly

oxybutynin
(ox-i-byoo'ti-nin)
Rx: Ditropan, Ditropan XL, Oxytrol
Chemical Class: Tertiary amine
Therapeutic Class: Antispasmodic; gastrointestinal; genitourinary muscle relaxant

CLINICAL PHARMACOLOGY
Mechanism of Action: An anticholinergic that exerts antispasmodic (papaverine-like) and antimuscarinic (atropine-like) action on the detrusor smooth muscle of the bladder. *Therapeutic Effect:* Increases bladder capacity and delays desire to void.

Pharmacokinetics

Route	Onset	Peak	Duration
PO	0.5–1 hr	3–6 hr	6–10 hr

Rapidly absorbed from the GI tract. Metabolized in the liver. Primarily excreted in urine. Unknown if removed by hemodialysis. **Half-life:** 1–2.3 hr.

INDICATIONS AND DOSAGES
Neurogenic bladder
PO
Adults. 5 mg 2–3 times a day up to 5 mg 4 times a day.
Elderly. 2.5–5 mg twice a day. May increase by 2.5 mg/day every 1–2 days.
Children 5 yr and older. 5 mg twice a day up to 5 mg 4 times a day.
Children 1–4 yr. 0.2 mg/kg/dose 2–4 times a day.
PO (extended release)
Adults. 5–10 mg/day up to 30 mg/day.
Transdermal
Adults. 3.9 mg applied twice a week. Apply every 3–4 days.

S AVAILABLE FORMS/COST
- Film, Cont Rel—Transdermal: 3.9 mg/24 hr: **$10.74**
- Syr—Oral: 5 mg/5 ml, 473 ml: **$33.80-$111.45**
- Tab—Oral: 5 mg, 100's: **$6.79-$144.09**
- Tab, Sus Action—Oral: 5 mg, 100's: **$311.94**; 10 mg, 100's: **$319.63**; 15 mg, 100's: **$354.00**

CONTRAINDICATIONS: GI or GU obstruction, glaucoma, myasthenia gravis, toxic megacolon, ulcerative colitis

PREGNANCY AND LACTATION: Pregnancy category B; may suppress lactation

SIDE EFFECTS
Frequent
Constipation, dry mouth, somnolence, decreased perspiration
Occasional
Decreased lacrimation or salivation, impotence, urinary hesitancy and retention, suppressed lactation, blurred vision, mydriasis, nausea or vomiting, insomnia

SERIOUS REACTIONS
- Overdose produces CNS excitation (including nervousness, restlessness, hallucinations, and irritability), hypotension or hypertension, confusion, tachycardia, facial flushing, and respiratory depression.

SPECIAL CONSIDERATIONS
- Reported anticholinergic side effects not clinically or significantly different from other agents (i.e., propantheline); compare costs

PATIENT/FAMILY EDUCATION
- Avoid prolonged exposure to hot environments, heat prostration may result
- Use caution in driving or other activities requiring alertness
- Swallow extended release tablets whole, do not chew or crush

- Extended release tablet shell not absorbable
- Apply patch to dry, intact skin on abdomen, hip, or buttock; select new side with each new patch to avoid re-application to the same site within 7 days

---

oxycodone
(ox-ee-koe′done)
Rx: Oxycontin, Oxy IR, Percolone Oxyfast, Roxicodone
Combinations
Rx: with aspirin (Percodan, Endodan, Roxiprin); with acetaminophen (Percocet, Endocet, Tylox, Roxicet, Roxilox)
Chemical Class: Opiate derivative; phenanthrene derivative
Therapeutic Class: Narcotic analgesic
DEA Class: Schedule II

CLINICAL PHARMACOLOGY
Mechanism of Action: An opioid analgesic that binds with opioid receptors in the CNS. *Therapeutic Effect:* Alters the perception of and emotional response to pain.
Pharmacokinetics

Route	Onset	Peak	Dura-tion
PO, Immediate-release	N/A	N/A	4-5 hr
PO, Controlled-release	N/A	N/A	12 hr

Moderately absorbed from the GI tract. Protein binding: 38%-45%. Widely distributed. Metabolized in the liver. Excreted in urine. Unknown if removed by hemodialysis.
Half-life: 2-3 hr (3.2 hr controlled-release).

INDICATIONS AND DOSAGES
Analgesia
PO (Controlled-Release)

Adults, Elderly. Initially, 10 mg q12h. May increase every 1-2 days by 25%-50%. Usual: 40 mg/day (100 mg/day for cancer pain).

PO (Immediate-Release)

Adults, Elderly. Initially, 5 mg q6h as needed. May increase up to 30 mg q4h. Usual: 10-30 mg q4h as needed.

Children. 0.05-0.15 mg/kg/dose q4-6h.

🆂 AVAILABLE FORMS/COST
• Cap—Oral: 5 mg, 100's: **$20.00-$39.31**
• Conc-Oral: 20 mg/ml, 30 ml: **$34.42-$46.25**
• Sol—Oral: 5 mg/5 ml, 500 ml: **$37.00-$41.65**
• Tab—Oral: 5 mg, 100's: **$31.04-$68.75**; 15 mg, 100's: **$74.94**; 30 mg, 100's: **$144.43**
• Tab, Sus Action—Oral: 10 mg, 100's: **$143.80**; 20 mg, 100's: **$275.16**; 40 mg, 100's: **$488.24**; 80 mg, 100's: **$918.14**; 160 mg, 100's: **$1,731.20**

CONTRAINDICATIONS: None known.

PREGNANCY AND LACTATION: Pregnancy category B (category D if used for prolonged periods or in high doses at term); excreted into breast milk

SIDE EFFECTS
Frequent

Somnolence, dizziness, hypotension (including orthostatic hypotension), anorexia

Occasional

Confusion, diaphoresis, facial flushing, urine retention, constipation, dry mouth, nausea, vomiting, headache

Rare

Allergic reaction, depression, paradoxical CNS hyperactivity or nervousness in children, paradoxical excitement and restlessness in elderly or debilitated patients

SERIOUS REACTIONS
• Overdose results in respiratory depression, skeletal muscle flaccidity, cold or clammy skin, cyanosis, and extreme somnolence progressing to seizures, stupor, and coma.

• Hepatotoxicity may occur with overdose of the acetaminophen component of fixed-combination products.

• The patient who uses oxycodone repeatedly may develop a tolerance to the drug's analgesic effect and physical dependence.

INTERACTIONS
Drugs

🗷 *Amitriptylline:* Additive respiratory and CNS-depressant effects

🗷 *Antihistamines, chloral hydrate, glutethimide, methocarbamol:* Enhanced depressant effects

🗷 *Barbiturates:* Additive respiratory and CNS depressant effects

🗷 *Cimetidine:* Increased respiratory and CNS depression

🗷 *Clomipramine:* Additive respiratory and CNS depressant effects

🗷 *Ethanol:* Additive CNS effects

🗷 *MAOI's:* Markedly potentiate the actions of morphine

🗷 *Nortriptylline:* Additive respiratory and CNS depressant effects

🗷 *Protease inhibitors:* Increased CNS and respiratory depression

Labs

• *False increase:* Amylase and lipase

SPECIAL CONSIDERATIONS
PATIENT/FAMILY EDUCATION
• Physical dependency may result when used for extended periods
• Change position slowly, orthostatic hypotension may occur

• Do not administer agonist/antagonist analgesics (i.e., pentazocine, nalbuphine, butorphanol, dezocine, buprenorphine) to patient who has received a prolonged course of oxycodone (a pure agonist). In opioid-dependent patients, mixed agonist/antagonist analgesics may precipitate withdrawal symptoms

oxymetazoline

(ox-ee-met-az'oh-leen)

OTC: *Nasal:* 4-way long lasting, Afrin 12-Hour, Benzedrex 12 hr, Cheracol, Dristan 12-hour, Duramist Plus, Duration, Genasal, Neo-Synephrine 12-Hour, Oxymata 12, Vicks Sinex 12-Hour Ultra Fine Mist

OTC: *Ophthalmic:* Ocu Clear, Visine L.R.

Chemical Class: Imidazoline derivative

Therapeutic Class: Decongestant

CLINICAL PHARMACOLOGY

Mechanism of Action: A direct-acting sympathomimetic amine that acts on alpha-adrenergic receptors in arterioles of the nasal mucosa to produce constriction. *Therapeutic Effect:* Causes vasoconstriction resulting in decreased blood flow and decreased nasal congestion.

Pharmacokinetics

Onset of action is about 10 min., and a duration of action is 7 hrs or more. Absorption occurs from the nasal mucosa and can produce systemic effects, primarily following overdose or excessive use. Excreted mostly in the urine as well as the feces. **Half-life:** 5-8 hrs.

INDICATIONS AND DOSAGES

Rhinitis

Intranasal

Adults, Elderly, Children older than 6 yrs. 2-3 drops/sprays (0.05% nasal solution) in each nostril q12h.

Children (2-5 yrs). 2-4 drops/sprays (0.025% nasal solution) in each nostril q12h for up to 3 days.

Conjunctivitis

Ophthalmic

Adults, Elderly, Children older than 6 yrs. 1- 2 drops (0.025% ophthalmic solution) q6h for 3- 4 days.

[$] AVAILABLE FORMS/COST

• Sol—Nasal: 0.025%, 20 ml: **$3.52-$4.82**; 0.05%, 30 ml: **$1.84**

• Spray—Nasal: 0.05%, 15, 30 ml: **$0.76-$7.60**/30 ml

• Sol—Ophth: 0.025%, 15, 30 ml: **$3.89-$5.70**/30 ml

UNLABELED USES: Otitis media surgical procedures

CONTRAINDICATIONS: Narrow-angle glaucoma or hypersensitivity to oxymetazoline or other adrenergic agents

PREGNANCY AND LACTATION: Pregnancy category C

SIDE EFFECTS

Occasional

Burning, stinging, drying nasal mucosa, sneezing, rebound congestion, insomnia, nervousness

SERIOUS REACTIONS

• Large doses may produce tachycardia, hypertension, arrhythmias, palpitations, lightheadedness, nausea, and vomiting.

SPECIAL CONSIDERATIONS

• Manage rebound congestion by stopping oxymetazoline: one nostril at a time, substitute systemic decongestant, substitute inhaled steroid

PATIENT/FAMILY EDUCATION

• Do not use for > 3-5 days or rebound congestion may occur

oxymetholone
(ox-ee-meth'oh-lone)
Rx: Anadrol-50
Chemical Class: Anabolic steroid; testosterone derivative
Therapeutic Class: Androgen; hematopoietic agent
DEA Class: Schedule III

CLINICAL PHARMACOLOGY
Mechanism of Action: An androgenic-anabolic steroid that is a synthetic derivative of testosterone synthesized to accentuate anabolic as opposed to androgenic effects. *Therapeutic Effect:* Improves nitrogen balance in conditions of unfavorable protein metabolism with adequate caloric and protein intake, stimulates erythropoiesis, suppress gonadotropic functions of pituitary and may exert a direct effect upon the testes.
Pharmacokinetics
The pharmacokinetics of oxymetholone has been studied. Metabolized in the liver via reduction and oxidation. Unchanged oxymetholone and its metabolites are excreted in urine. **Half-life:** Unknown.

INDICATIONS AND DOSAGES
Anemia, chronic renal failure, acqured aplastic anemia, chemotherapy-induced myelosuppresion, Fanconi's anemia, red cell aplasia
PO
Adults, Elderly, Children. 1 -5 mg/kg/day. Response is not immediate and a minimum of 3 – 6 months should be given.

Ⓢ   AVAILABLE FORMS/COST
• Tab—Oral: 50   mg,   100's: **$1,711.59**
UNLABELED USES: Amegakaryocytic thrombocytopenia, familial antithrombin III deficiency, heredi-tary angioedema, HIV wasting, metastatic breast cancer in women, relief of bone pain associated with osteoporosis, neutropenia, Turner's syndrome, xeroderma pigmentosum

CONTRAINDICATIONS: Cardiac impairment, hypercalcemia, pregnancy/lactation, prostatic or breast cancer in males, metastatic breast cancer in women with active hypercalcemia, nephrosis or nephritic phase nephritis, severe liver disease, hypersensitivity to oxymetholone or any of its components

PREGNANCY AND LACTATION: Pregnancy category X; use extreme caution in nursing mothers

SIDE EFFECTS
Frequent
Gynecomastia, acne, amenorrhea, menstrual irregularities
Females: Hirsutism, deepening of voice, clitoral enlargement that may not be reversible when drug is discontinued
Occasional
Edema, nausea, insomnia, oligospermia, priapism, male pattern of baldness, bladder irritability, hypercalcemia in immobilized patients or those with breast cancer, hypercholesterolemia, inflammation and pain at IM injection site
Transdermal: Itching, erythema, skin irritation
Rare
Liver damage, hypersensitivity

SERIOUS REACTIONS
• Cholestatic jaundice, hepatic necrosis and death occur rarely but have been reported in association with long-term androgenic-anabolic steroid use.

INTERACTIONS
Drugs
❸ *Antidiabetic agents:* Enhanced hypoglycemic effects

❷ *Cyclosporine:* Increased cyclosporine concentrations, toxicity

❸ *HMG-CoA reductase inhibitors (lovastatin, prevastatin):* Myositis risk increased

❸ *Tacrolimus:* Increased tacrolimus concentrations, potential for toxicity

❷ *Oral anticoagulants:* Enhanced hypoprothrombinemic response

SPECIAL CONSIDERATIONS

• Anabolic steroids have potential for abuse, especially in the athlete

• Comparative advantages include less potential for virilization in women, convenience of oral administration; disadvantage includes increased risk of hepatotoxicity

PATIENT/FAMILY EDUCATION

• Hematologic response is often not immediate, needs minimum trial of 3-6 mo

MONITORING PARAMETERS

• LFTs, lipids, Hct

• Serum calcium in breast cancer patients

• Growth rate in children (X-rays for bone age q 6 mo)

---

oxymorphone

(ox-ee-mor′fone)

Rx: Numorphan

Chemical Class: Opiate derivative; phenanthrene derivative

Therapeutic Class: Narcotic analgesic

DEA Class: Schedule II

CLINICAL PHARMACOLOGY

Mechanism of Action: An opioid agonist, similar to morphine, that binds at opiate receptor sites in the central nervous system (CNS). *Therapeutic Effect:* Reduces intensity of pain stimuli incoming from sensory nerve endings, altering pain perception and emotional response to pain; suppresses cough reflex.

Pharmacokinetics

Route	Onset	Peak	Duration
Subcutaneous	5-10min	30-90min	4-6 hrs
IM	5-10min	30-60min	3-6 hrs
IV	5-10min	15-30min	3-6 hrs
Rectal	15-30min	N/A	3-6 hrs

Well absorbed from the gastrointestinal (GI) tract, after IM administration. Widely distributed. Metabolized in liver via glucuronidation. Excreted in urine. **Half-life:** 1-2 hrs.

INDICATIONS AND DOSAGES

Analgesic, Anxiety, Preanesthesia

IV

Adults, Elderly, Children 12 yrs and older. Initially 0.5 mg.

SC/IM

Adults, Elderly, Children 12 yrs and older. 1-1.5 mg IM or SC q4-6h as needed

Rectal

Adults, Elderly, Children 12 yrs and older. 0.5-1 mg q4-6h.

Obstetrical analgesic

IM

Adults, Elderly, Children 12 yrs and older. 0.5-1 mg IM during labor.

💲 **AVAILABLE FORMS/COST**

• Sol, Inj—IM, IV, SC: 1 mg/ml, 1 ml: **$2.95**; 1.5 mg/ml, 1 ml: **$3.63**

• Supp—Rect: 5 mg, 6's: **$29.19**

UNLABELED USES: Cancer pain, intractable pain in narcotic-tolerant patients

CONTRAINDICATIONS: Paralytic ileus, acute asthma attack, pulmonary edema secondary to chemical respiratory irritant, severe respiratory depression, upper airway obstruction

PREGNANCY AND LACTATION:
Pregnancy category B (category D if used for prolonged periods or in high doses at term); use during labor produces neonatal respiratory depression

SIDE EFFECTS

Frequent

Drowsiness, dizziness, hypotension, decreased appetite, tolerance or dependence

Occasional

Confusion, diaphoresis, facial flushing, urinary retention, constipation, dry mouth, nausea, vomiting, headache, pain at injection site, abdominal cramps

Rare

Allergic reaction, depression

SERIOUS REACTIONS

• Hypotension, paralytic ileus, respiratory depression and toxic megacolon rarely occur.

• Overdosage results in respiratory depression, skeletal muscle flaccidity, cold or clammy skin, cyanosis, extreme somnolence progressing to seizures, stupor and coma.

• Tolerance to analgesic effect and physical dependence may occur with repeated use.

• Prolonged duration of action and cumulative effect may occur in patients with impaired liver or renal function.

INTERACTIONS

Drugs

❸ *Barbiturates:* Additive CNS depression

❸ *Cimetidine:* Increased effect of narcotic analgesics

❷ *Ethanol:* Additive CNS effects

❸ *Neuroleptics:* Hypotension and excessive CNS depression

Labs

• *False increase:* Amylase and lipase

SPECIAL CONSIDERATIONS

• Do not administer agonist/antagonist analgesics (i.e., pentazocine, nalbuphine, butorphanol, dezocine, buprenorphine) to patient who has received a prolonged course of oxymorphone (a pure agonist). In opioid-dependent patients, mixed agonist/antagonist analgesics may precipitate withdrawal symptoms.

PATIENT/FAMILY EDUCATION

• Physical dependency may result when used for extended periods

• Change position slowly, orthostatic hypotension may occur

---

oxytetracycline

(ox′ee-tet-tra-sye′kleen)

Rx: Terramycin

Combinations

    Rx: with polymyxin (Terek); with phenazopyridine, sulfamethizole (Urobiotic-250, Tija)

Chemical Class: Tetracycline derivative

Therapeutic Class: Antibiotic

CLINICAL PHARMACOLOGY

Mechanism of Action: A tetracycline antibiotic that inhibits bacterial protein synthesis by binding to ribosomes. Cell wall synthesis is not affected. *Therapeutic Effect:* Prevents bacterial cell growth. Bacteriostatic.

Pharmacokinetics

Poorly absorbed after IM administration. Protein binding: 27%-35%. Metabolized in liver. Excreted in urine. Eliminated in feces via biliary system. Not removed by hemodialysis. **Half-life:** 8.5-9.6 hrs (half-life is increased with impaired renal function).

INDICATIONS AND DOSAGES
Treatment of inflammatory acne, anthrax, gonorrhea, skin infections, urinary tract infection (UTI)
IM
Adults, Elderly. 250 mg/day or 300 mg/day divided q8-12h
Children 8 yrs and older. 15-25 mg/kg/day in divided doses q8-12h. Maximum: 250 mg/dose.

Dosage in renal impairment

Creatinine Clearance	Dosage Interval
less than 10 ml/min	q24h

$ **AVAILABLE FORMS/COST**
• Sol, Inj—IM: 50 mg/ml, 10 ml: **$10.34**
UNLABELED USES: Chlamydia, non-specific urethritis, peptic ulcer
CONTRAINDICATIONS: Hypersensitivity to tetracyclines or any component of the formulation, children 8 years and younger
PREGNANCY AND LACTATION: Pregnancy category D; excreted into breast milk; milk:plasma ratio: 0.6-0.8; theoretically, may cause dental staining, but usually undetectable in infant serum (<0.05 mcg/ml)

SIDE EFFECTS
Frequent
Dizziness, lightheadedness, diarrhea, nausea, vomiting, stomach cramps, increased sensitivity of skin to sunlight
Occasional
Pigmentation of skin, mucous membranes, itching in rectal or genital area, sore mouth or tongue, increased BUN, irritation at injection site

SERIOUS REACTIONS
• Superinfection (especially fungal), anaphylaxis, and increased intracranial pressure may occur.
• Bulging fontanelles occur rarely in infants.

INTERACTIONS
Drugs
❷ *Antacids:* Reduced absorption of oxytetracycline
❸ *Bismuth salts:* Reduced absorption of oxytetracycline
❸ *Calcium:* See antacids
❸ *Food:* Reduced absorption of oxytetracycline
❸ *Iron:* Reduced absorption of oxytetracycline
❸ *Magnesium:* See antacids
❷ *Methoxyflurane:* Increased risk of nephrotoxicity
❸ *Oral contraceptives:* Interruption of enterohepatic circulation of estrogens, reduced oral contraceptive effectiveness
❸ *Zinc:* Reduced absorption of oxytetracycline
Labs
• *False negative:* Urine glucose with Clinistix or TesTape
• *Interference:* Uroporphyrin
• *False increase:* Urinary and plasma catecholamines, serum bilirubin, CFS protein, urine glucose, serum uric acid, urine vanillylmandelic acid

SPECIAL CONSIDERATIONS
• Offers no significant advantage over tetracycline; shares similar spectrum of activity (may be slightly less active than tetracycline and has longer dosage interval)

PATIENT/FAMILY EDUCATION
• Avoid milk products, take with a full glass of water

oxytocin

(ox-ee-toe'sin)

Rx: Pitocin, Syntocinon
Chemical Class: Polypeptide
hormone
Therapeutic Class: Galactokinetic; oxytocic

CLINICAL PHARMACOLOGY

Mechanism of Action: An oxytocic
that affect uterine myofibril activity
and stimulates mammary smooth
muscle. *Therapeutic Effect:* Contracts uterine smooth muscle. Enhances lactation.

Pharmacokinetics

Route	Onset	Peak	Duration
IV	Immediate	N/A	1 hr
IM	3–5 min	N/A	2–3 hr

Rapidly absorbed through nasal mucous membranes. Protein binding:
30%. Distributed in extracellular
fluid. Metabolized in the liver and
kidney. Primarily excreted in urine.
Half-life: 1–6 min.

INDICATIONS AND DOSAGES
Induction or stimulation of labor
IV

Adults. 0.5-1 milliunit/min. May
gradually increase in increments of
1-2 milliunit/min. Rates of 9-10 milliunit/min are rarely required.

Abortion
IV

Adults. 10-20 milliunit/min. Maximum: 30 unit/12h dose.

Control of postpartum bleeding
IV Infusion

Adults. 10–40 units in 1 liter IV fluid
at a rate sufficient to control uterine
atony.
IM

Adults. 10 units (total dose) after delivery.

AVAILABLE FORMS/COST
• Sol, Inj—IM, IV: 10 U/ml, 1 ml:
$1.35-$3.00
CONTRAINDICATIONS: Adequate
uterine activity that fails to progress,
cephalopelvic disproportion, fetal
distress without imminent delivery,
grand multiparity, hyperactive or
hypertonic uterus, obstetric emergencies that favor surgical intervention, prematurity, unengaged fetal
head, unfavorable fetal position or
presentation, when vaginal delivery
is contraindicated, such as active
genital herpes infection, placenta
previa, or cord presentation
PREGNANCY AND LACTATION:
Nasal oxytocin contraindicated during pregnancy; only minimal
amounts pass into breast milk
SIDE EFFECTS
Occasional
Tachycardia, premature ventricular
contractions, hypotension, nausea,
vomiting
Rare
Nasal: Lacrimation or tearing, nasal
irritation, rhinorrhea, unexpected
uterine bleeding or contractions
SERIOUS REACTIONS
• Hypertonicity may occur with
tearing of the uterus, increased
bleeding, abruptio placentae, and
cervical and vaginal lacerations.
• In the fetus, bradycardia, CNS or
brain damage, trauma due to rapid
propulsion, low Apgar score at 5
minutes, and retinal hemorrhage occur rarely.
• Prolonged IV infusion of oxytocin
with excessive fluid volume has
caused severe water intoxication
with seizures, coma, and death.
SPECIAL CONSIDERATIONS
• Routinely used for the induction of
labor at term and postpartum for the
control of uterine bleeding; not the
drug of choice for induction of labor
for abortion

MONITORING PARAMETERS

• Continuous monitoring necessary for IV use (length, intensity, duration of contractions); fetal heart rate—acceleration, deceleration, fetal distress

palonosetron

Rx: Aloxi

Chemical Class: Isoquinoline derivative

Therapeutic Class: Antiemetic

CLINICAL PHARMACOLOGY

Mechanism of Action: A 5-HT_3 receptor antagonist that acts centrally in the chemoreceptor trigger zone and peripherally at the vagal nerve terminals. *Therapeutic Effect:* Prevents nausea and vomiting associated with chemotherapy.

Pharmacokinetics

Protein binding: 52%. Eliminated in urine. **Half-life:** 40 hr.

INDICATIONS AND DOSAGES

Chemotherapy-induced nausea and vomiting

IV

Adults, Elderly. 0.25 mg as a single dose 30 min before starting chemotherapy.

[$] **AVAILABLE FORMS/COST**

• Sol—IV: 0.25 mg/5 ml, 5 ml: **$324.00**

CONTRAINDICATIONS: None known.

PREGNANCY AND LACTATION: Pregnancy category B; excretion into breast milk unknown, use caution in nursing mothers

SIDE EFFECTS

Occasional (9%-5%)

Headache, constipation

Rare (less than 1%)

Diarrhea, dizziness, fatigue, abdominal pain, insomnia

SERIOUS REACTIONS

• Overdose may produce a combination of CNS stimulant and depressant effects.

INTERACTIONS

Drugs

[3] *Antiarrhythmics; diuretics; cumulative high dose anthracycline therapy; drugs that prolong QTc interval:* Increased potential for arrhythmia

SPECIAL CONSIDERATIONS

• Clinical superiority over other 5-HT_3 receptor antagonists (*e.g.,* ondansetron, dolasetron) has not been adequately demonstrated

pamidronate

(pam-id'drow-nate)

Rx: Aredia

Chemical Class: Pyrophosphate analog

Therapeutic Class: Bisphosphonate; bone resorption inhibitor

CLINICAL PHARMACOLOGY

Mechanism of Action: A bisphosphate that binds to bone and inhibits osteoclast-mediated calcium resorption. *Therapeutic Effect:* Lowers serum calcium concentrations.

Pharmacokinetics

Route	*Onset*	*Peak*	*Duration*
IV	24–48 hr	5–7 days	N/A

After IV administration, rapidly absorbed by bone. Slowly excreted unchanged in urine. Unknown if removed by hemodialysis. Half-life: bone, 300 days; unmetabolized, 2.5 hr.

INDICATIONS AND DOSAGES

Hypercalcemia

IV infusion

Adults, Elderly. Moderate hypercalcemia (corrected serum calcium level 12–13.5 mg/dl): 60–90 mg. Severe hypercalcemia (corrected serum calcium level greater than 13.5 mg/dl): 90 mg.

Paget's disease
IV infusion
Adults, Elderly. 30 mg/day for 3 days.

Osteolytic bone lesion
IV infusion
Adults, Elderly. 90 mg over 2–4 hr once a month.

AVAILABLE FORMS/COST
• Powder, Inj-IV: 30 mg, 1's: **$291.53**; 90 mg, 1's: **$839.60**
• Sol, Inj—IV: 3 mg/ml: **$290.00-$1,119.44**; 6 mg/ml: **$559.72**; 9 mg/ml: **$839.60-$872.00**

CONTRAINDICATIONS: Hypersensitivity to other bisphosphonates, such as etidronate, tiludronate, risedronate, and alendronate

PREGNANCY AND LACTATION: Pregnancy category C; caution with administration to a nursing mother

SIDE EFFECTS
Frequent (greater than 10%)
Temperature elevation (at least 1°C) 24–48 hr after administration (27%); redness, swelling, induration, pain at catheter site with in patients receiving 90 mg (18%); anorexia, nausea, fatigue
Occasional (10%–1%)
Constipation, rhinitis

SERIOUS REACTIONS
• Hypophosphatemia, hypokalemia, hypomagnesemia, and hypocalcemia occur more frequently with higher dosages.
• Anemia, hypertension, tachycardia, atrial fibrillation, and somnolence occur more frequently with 90-mg doses.
• GI hemorrhage occurs rarely.

SPECIAL CONSIDERATIONS
• "Second-generation" bisphosphonate that offers potential advantages over etidronate (as does alendronate) in that it inhibits bone resorption at doses that do not impair bone mineralization, and is less likely than etidronate to produce osteomalacia
• Allow at least 7 days between initial treatment for patients requiring retreatment for hypercalcemia

pancrelipase
(pan-kre-li'pase)
Rx: Cotazym, Cotazym-S, Creon, Ilozyme, Ku-Zyme HP, Lipram, Pancrease, Pancrease MT, Protilase, Ultrase MT, Viokase, Zymase
Chemical Class: Pancreatic enzymes
Therapeutic Class: Digestant

CLINICAL PHARMACOLOGY
Mechanism of Action: Digestive enzymes that replace endogenous pancreatic enzymes. *Therapeutic Effect:* Assist in digestion of protein, starch, and fats.

INDICATIONS AND DOSAGES
Pancreatic enzyme replacement or supplement when enzymes are absent or deficient, such as with chronic pancreatitis, cystic fibrosis, or ductal obstruction from cancer of the pancreas or common bile duct; to reduce malabsorption; treatment of steatorrhea associated with bowel resection or postgastrectomy syndrome
PO
Adults, Elderly. 1–3 capsules or tablets before or with meals or snacks. May increase to 8 tablets/dose.
Children. 1–2 tablets with meals or snacks.

AVAILABLE FORMS/COST
• Cap, Enteric Coated—Oral: 4000 U lipase/12,000 U protease/12,000

U amylase, 100's: **$27.35**; 4000/ 25,000/20,000, 100's: **$25.30-$35.73**; 5000/20,000/20,000, 100's: **$30.25**; 8000/30,000/30,000, 100's: **$22.36-$57.21**; 10,000/30,000/ 30,000, 100's: **$72.95**; 12,000/ 24,000/24,000, 100's: **$66.39**; 12,000/39,000/39,000, 100's: **$74.55-$93.19**; 16,000/48,000/ 48,000, 100's: **$93.33-$151.99**; 20,000/65,000/65,000, 100's: **$129.17-$161.45**; 20,000/75,000/ 66,400, 100's: **$146.97-$179.56**
• Powder—Oral: 16,800 U lipase/ 70,000 U protease/70,000 U amylase, 8 oz: **$118.15-$159.35**
• Tab—Oral: 8000 U lipase/30,000 U protease/30,000 U amylase, 100's: **$12.81-$38.78**; 11,000/ 30,000/30,000, 250's: **$139.23**

CONTRAINDICATIONS: Acute pancreatitis, exacerbation of chronic pancreatitis, hypersensitivity to pork protein

PREGNANCY AND LACTATION: Pregnancy category C

SIDE EFFECTS

Rare

Allergic reaction, mouth irritation, shortness of breath, wheezing

SERIOUS REACTIONS

• Excessive dosage may produce nausea, cramping, and diarrhea.
• Hyperuricosuria and hyperuricemia have occurred with extremely high dosages.

SPECIAL CONSIDERATIONS

• Substitution at dispensing should be avoided
• Enteric-coated pancreatic enzymes are more effective than regular formulations; individual variations may require trials with several enzymatic preparations
• For patients who do not respond appropriately, adding antacid or H$_2$-antagonist may provide better results
• Preparations high in lipase concentration seem to be more effective for reducing steatorrhea

PATIENT/FAMILY EDUCATION

• Advise patient to take before or with meals
• Protect enteric coating; advise patient not to crush or chew microspheres in caps or tabs

MONITORING PARAMETERS

• Growth curves in children

---

pantoprazole

(pan-toe-pra′zole)

Rx: Protonix

Chemical Class: Benzimidazole derivative

Therapeutic Class: Antiulcer agent

CLINICAL PHARMACOLOGY

Mechanism of Action: A benzimidazole that is converted to active metabolites that irreversibly bind to and inhibit hydrogen-potassium adenosine triphosphate, an enzyme on the surface of gastric parietal cells. Inhibits hydrogen ion transport into gastric lumen. *Therapeutic Effect:* Increases gastric pH and reduces gastric acid production.

Pharmacokinetics

Route	Onset	Peak	Duration
PO	N/A	N/A	24 hr

Rapidly absorbed from the GI tract. Protein binding: 98%. Primarily distributed into gastric parietal cells. Metabolized extensively in the liver. Primarily excreted in urine. Not removed by hemodialysis. **Half-life:** 1 hr.

INDICATIONS AND DOSAGES
Erosive esophagitis
PO

Adults, Elderly. 40 mg/day for up to 8 wk. If not healed after 8 wk, may continue an additional 8 wk.

IV

Adults, Elderly. 40 mg/day for 7–10 days.

Hypersecretory conditions
PO

Adults, Elderly. Initially, 40 mg twice a day. May increase to 240 mg/day.

IV

Adults, Elderly. 80 mg twice a day. May increase to 80 mg q8h.

$ AVAILABLE FORMS/COST
• Tab, Sust Action—Oral: 20 mg, 40 mg, 90's: **$344.25**
• Inj, Powder—IV: 40 mg/vial: **$27.50**

CONTRAINDICATIONS: None known

PREGNANCY AND LACTATION: Pregnancy category B; excretion into breast milk unknown, use caution in nursing mothers

SIDE EFFECTS
Rare (less than 2%)

Diarrhea, headache, dizziness, pruritus, rash

SERIOUS REACTIONS
• None known.

INTERACTIONS
Drugs

❸ *Ketoconazole:* Decreased bioavailability of ketoconazole

SPECIAL CONSIDERATIONS
PATIENT/FAMILY EDUCATION
• Caution patients not to split, crush or chew delayed-release tablets; swallow whole

MONITORING PARAMETERS
• Symptom relief, mucosal healing

---

paregoric
(par-e-gor´ik)
Rx: Paregoric
Chemical Class: Opiate (most preparations also contain camphor and ethanol)
Therapeutic Class: Antidiarrheal
DEA Class: Schedule III

CLINICAL PHARMACOLOGY
Mechanism of Action: An opioid agonist that contains many narcotic alkaloids including morphine. It inhibits gastric motility due to its morphine content. *Therapeutic Effect:* Decreases digestive secretions, increases in gastrointestinal (GI) muscle tone, and reduces GI propulsion.
Pharmacokinetics
Variably absorbed from the gastrointestinal (GI) tract. Protein binding: low. Metabolized in liver. Primarily excreted in urine primarily as morphine glucuronide conjugates and unchanged drug - morphine, codeine, papaverine, etc. Unknown if removed by hemodialysis. **Half-life:** 2-3 hrs.

INDICATIONS AND DOSAGES
Antidiarrheal
PO

Adults, Elderly. 5-10 ml 1-4 times/day.
Children. 0.25-0.5 ml/kg/dose 1- 4 times/day.

$ AVAILABLE FORMS/COST
• Liq—Oral: 2 mg/5 ml, 480 ml: **$3.12-$11.29**

UNLABELED USES: Narcotic withdrawal symptoms in neonates

CONTRAINDICATIONS: Diarrhea caused by poisoning until the toxic material is removed, hypersensitivity to morphine sulfate or any component of the formulation, pregnancy (prolonged use or high dosages near term)

P

PREGNANCY AND LACTATION:
Pregnancy category B; excreted in breast milk

SIDE EFFECTS

Frequent

Constipation, drowsiness, nausea, vomiting

Occasional

Paradoxical excitement, confusion, pounding heartbeat, facial flushing, decreased urination, blurred vision, dizziness, dry mouth, headache, hypotension, decreased appetite, redness, burning, pain at injection site

Rare

Hallucinations, depression, stomach pain, insomnia

SERIOUS REACTIONS

• Overdosage results in cold or clammy skin, confusion, convulsions, decreased blood pressure (BP), restlessness, pinpoint pupils, bradycardia, respiratory depression, decreased level of consciousness (LOC), and severe weakness.

• Tolerance to analgesic effect and physical dependence may occur with repeated use.

INTERACTIONS

Drugs

▪ *Barbiturates, rifampin:* Increased metabolism of paregoric

▪ *Cimetidine:* Decreased metabolism of paregoric

SPECIAL CONSIDERATIONS

• Contains ethanol

---

paricalcitol
(pare-i-cal′ sih-tal)
Rx: Zemplar
Chemical Class: Vitamin D analog
Therapeutic Class: Vitamin

CLINICAL PHARMACOLOGY

Mechanism of Action: A fat-soluble vitamin that is essential for absorption, utilization of calcium phosphate, and normal calcification of bone. *Therapeutic Effect:* Stimulates calcium and phosphate absorption from small intestine, promotes secretion of calcium from bone to blood, promotes renal tubule phosphate resorption, acts on bone cells to stimulate skeletal growth and on parathyroid gland to suppress hormone synthesis and secretion.

Pharmacokinetics

Protein binding: more than 99%. Metabolized in liver. Primarily eliminated in feces; minimal excretion in urine. Not removed by hemodialysis. **Half-life:** 14-15 hrs.

INDICATIONS AND DOSAGES

Hypoparathyroidism

IV

Adults, Elderly, Children. 0.04-0.1 mcg/kg (2.8-7 mcg) given as a bolus dose no more frequently than every other day at any time during dialysis; dose as high as 0.24 mcg/kg (16.8 mcg) have been administered safely. Usually start with 0.04 mcg/kg 3 times/week as a bolus, increased by 0.04 mcg/kg every 2 weeks.

Dose adjust based on serum PTH levels:

Same or increasing serum PTH level: Increase dose

Serum PTH level decreased by <30%: Increase dose

Serum PTH level decreased by >30% and <60%: Maintain dose

Serum PTH level decrease by >60%: Decrease dose

Serum PTH level 1.5-3 times upper limit of normal: Maintain dose

AVAILABLE FORMS/COST

• Inj—IV: 2 mcg/ml, 1 ml: **$11.69**; 5 mcg/ml, 1 ml: **$29.20**

CONTRAINDICATIONS: Hypercalcemia, malabsorption syndrome, vitamin D toxicity, hypersensitivity to other vitamin D products or analogs

PREGNANCY AND LACTATION: Pregnancy category C; use caution in nursing mothers

SIDE EFFECTS

Occasional

Edema, nausea, vomiting, headache, dizziness

Rare

Palpiations

SERIOUS REACTIONS

• Early signs of overdosage are manifested as weakness, headache, somnolence, nausea, vomiting, dry mouth, constipation, muscle and bone pain, and metallic taste sensation.

• Later signs of overdosage are evidenced by polyuria, polydipsia, anorexia, weight loss, nocturia, photophobia, rhinorrhea, pruritus, disorientation, hallucinations, hyperthermia, hypertension, and cardiac arrhythmias.

• Hypercalcemia occur rarely.

INTERACTIONS

Drugs

▲ *Digoxin:* Hypercalcemia produced by paricalcitol may potentiate digoxin toxicity

SPECIAL CONSIDERATIONS

• Phosphate-binding compounds may be needed to control serum phosphorus levels

PATIENT/FAMILY EDUCATION

• Adhere to a dietary regimen of calcium supplementation and phosphorus restriction; avoid excessive use of aluminum-containing compounds

MONITORING PARAMETERS

• Serum calcium and phosphorus twice weekly during initial phase of therapy, then at least monthly once dosage has been established; if an elevated calcium level or a Ca × P product > 75 is noted, immediately reduce or interrupt dosage until parameters are normalized, then reinitiate at lower dose; intact PTH assay every 3 mo (target range in CRF patients ≤ 1.5-3 × the nonuremic upper limit of normal)

---

paromomycin

(par-oh-moe-mye'sin)

Rx: Humatin

Chemical Class: Aminoglycoside

Therapeutic Class: Amebicide; antibiotic

CLINICAL PHARMACOLOGY

Mechanism of Action: An antibacterial agent that acts directly on amoebas and against normal and pathogenic organisms in the GI tract. Interferes with bacterial protein synthesis by binding to 30S ribosomal subunits. *Therapeutic Effect:* Produces amoebicidal effects.

Pharmacokinetics

Poorly absorbed from the gastrointestinal (GI) tract and most of the dose is eliminated unchanged in feces.

INDICATIONS AND DOSAGES

Intestinal amebiasis

PO

Adults, Elderly, Children. 25-35 mg/kg/day q8h for 5-10 days.

Hepatic coma
PO
Adults, Elderly. 4 g/day q6-12h for 5-6 days.

AVAILABLE FORMS/COST
• Cap, Gel—Oral: 250 mg, 100's: **$190.08-$321.78**

UNLABELED USES: Cryptosporidiosis, giardiasis, leishmaniasis, microsporidiosis, mycobacterial infections, tapeworm infestation, trichomoniasis, typhoid carriers.

CONTRAINDICATIONS: Intestinal obstruction, renal failure, hypersensitivity to paromomycin or any of its components

PREGNANCY AND LACTATION: Pregnancy category C; poor oral bioavailability and lipid solubility limit passage into breast milk

SIDE EFFECTS
Occasional
Diarrhea, abdominal cramps, nausea, vomiting, heartburn
Rare
Rash, pruritus, vertigo

SERIOUS REACTIONS
• Overdosage may result in nausea, vomiting and diarrhea.

---

paroxetine
(par-ox'e-teen)
Rx: Paxil, Paxil CR
Chemical Class: Phenylpiperidine derivative
Therapeutic Class: Antidepressant, selective serotonin reuptake inhibitor (SSRI)

CLINICAL PHARMACOLOGY
Mechanism of Action: An antidepressant, anxiolytic, and antiobsessional agent that selectively blocks uptake of the neurotransmitter serotonin at neuronal presynaptic membranes, thereby increasing its availability at postsynaptic receptor sites. *Therapeutic Effect:* Relieves depression, reduces obsessive-compulsive behavior, decreases anxiety.

Pharmacokinetics
Well absorbed from the GI tract. Protein binding: 95%. Widely distributed. Metabolized in the liver. Excreted in urine. Not removed by hemodialysis. **Half-life:** 24 hr.

INDICATIONS AND DOSAGES
Depression
PO
Adults. Initially, 20 mg/day. May increase by 10 mg/day at intervals of more than 1 wk. Maximum: 50 mg/day.
PO (Controlled-Release)
Adults. Initially, 25 mg/day. May increase by 12.5 mg/day at intervals of more than 1 wk. Maximum: 62.5 mg/day.

Generalized anxiety disorder
PO
Adults. Initially, 20 mg/day. May increase by 10 mg/day at intervals of more than 1 wk. Range: 20-50 mg/day.

Obsessive compulsive disorder
PO
Adults. Initially, 20 mg/day. May increase by 10 mg/day at intervals of more than 1 wk. Range: 20-60 mg/day.

Panic disorder
PO
Adults. Initially, 10-20 mg/day. May increase by 10 mg/day at intervals of more than 1 wk. Range: 10-60 mg/day.

Social anxiety disorder
PO
Adults. Initially 20 mg/day. Range: 20-60 mg/day.

Post traumatic stress disorder
PO
Adults. Initially, 20 mg/day. May increase by 10 mg/day at intervals of more than 1 wk. Range: 20-50 mg/day.

Premenstrual dysphoric disorder
PO
Adults. (Paxil CR) Initially, 12.5 mg/day. May increase by 12.5 mg at weekly intervals to a maximum of 25 mg/day.

Usual elderly dosage
PO: Initially, 10 mg/day. May increase by 10 mg/day at intervals of more than 1 wk. Maximum: 40 mg/day.
PO (Controlled-Release): Initially, 12.5 mg/day. May increase by 12.5 mg at intervals of more than 1 wk. Maximum: 50 mg/day.

§ AVAILABLE FORMS/COST
• Susp—Oral: 10 mg/5 ml, 250 ml: **$140.49**
• Tab, Coated—Oral: 10 mg, 100's: **$270.63**; 20 mg, 100's: **$264.35-$299.73**; 30 mg, 30's: **$81.67-$91.20**; 40 mg, 30's: **$86.28-$95.88**
• Tab, Sus Action—Oral: 12.5 mg, 30's: **$84.44**; 25 mg, 30's: **$88.10**; 37.5 mg, 30's: **$90.76**

CONTRAINDICATIONS: Use within 14 days of MAOIs
PREGNANCY AND LACTATION: Pregnancy category B; limited information; milk concentrations similar to plasma following a single oral dose; thus <1% of the daily dose would be transferred to a breast-feeding infant
SIDE EFFECTS
Frequent
Nausea (26%); somnolence (23%); headache, dry mouth (18%); asthenia (15%); constipation (15%); dizziness, insomnia (13%); diarrhea (12%); diaphoresis (11%); tremor (8%)
Occasional
Decreased appetite, respiratory disturbance (such as increased cough) (6%); anxiety, nervousness (5%); flatulence, paresthesia, yawning

(4%); decreased libido, sexual dysfunction, abdominal discomfort (3%)
Rare
Palpitations, vomiting, blurred vision, altered taste, confusion
SERIOUS REACTIONS
• None known.
INTERACTIONS
Drugs
③ β-*blockers (metroprolol, propranolol, sotalol):* Inhibition of metabolism (CYP2D6) leads to increased plasma concentrations of selective β-blockers and potential cardiac toxicity; atenolol may be safer choice
③ *Cimetidine:* Increased plasma paroxetine concentrations
③ *Cyproheptadine:* Serotonin antagonist may partially reverse antidepressant and other effects
② *Dexfenfluramine:* Duplicate effects on inhibition of serotonin reuptake; inhibition of dexfenfluramine metabolism (CYP2D6) exaggerates effect; both mechanisms increase risk of serotonin syndrome
③ *Dextromethorphan:* Inhibition of dextromethorphan's metabolism (CYP2D6) by paroxetine and additive serotonergic effects
③ *Diuretics, loop (bumetanide, furosemide, torsemide):* Possible additive hyponatremia; two fatal case reports with furosemide and paroxetine
② *Fenfluramine:* Duplicate effects on inhibition of serotonin reuptake; inhibition of dexfenfluramine metabolism (CYP2D6) exaggerates effect; both mechanisms increase risk of serotonin syndrome
⚠ *Fulazolidone:* Increased risk of serotonin syndrome
③ *Haloperidol:* Inhibition of haloperidol's metabolism (CYP2D6) may increase risks of extrapyramidal symptoms

3 *Lithium:* Neurotoxicity (tremor, confusion, ataxia, dizziness, dysarthria, and abscence seizures) reported in patients receiving this combination; mechanism unknown

A *MAOI's (isocarboxazid, phenelzine, tranylcypromine):* Increased CNS serotonergic effects have been associated with severe or fatal reactions with this combination

3 *Phenobarbital:* Decreased plasma paroxetine concentrations

3 *Phenytoin:* Decreased plasma paroxetine concentrations

A *Selegiline:* Sporadic cases of mania and hypertension

3 *Sumatriptan (and other "triptans"):* Increased incidence of adverse effects, including serotonin syndrome

3 *Theophylline:* Elevated theophylline levels have been reported

A *Thioridazine:* Increased plasma thioridazine concentrations; increased risk of ventricular arrhythmias

3 *Tramadol:* Increased risk of serotonin syndrome

3 *Tricyclic antidepressants (clomipramine, desipramine, doxepin, imipramine, nortriptyline, trazodone):* Marked increases in tricyclic antidepressant levels due to inhibition of metabolism (CYP2D6)

2 *Tryptophan:* Additive serotonergic effects

3 *Warfarin:* Increased risk of bleeding

SPECIAL CONSIDERATIONS

• Somewhat sedating compared to fluoxetine and sertraline

PATIENT/FAMILY EDUCATION

• Avoid alcohol

• May take 1-4 wk to see improvement of symptoms

pegfilgrastim
(pehg-phil-gras'tim)
Rx: Neulasta
Chemical Class: Amino acid glycoprotein
Therapeutic Class: Hematopoietic agent

CLINICAL PHARMACOLOGY
Mechanism of Action: A colony-stimulating factor that regulates production of neutrophils within bone marrow. Also a glycoprotein that primarily affects neutrophil progenitor proliferation, differentiation, and selected end-cell functional activation. *Therapeutic Effect:* Increases phagocytic ability and antibody-dependent destruction; decreases incidence of infection.

Pharmacokinetics
Readily absorbed after subcutaneous administration. **Half-life:** 15–80 hr.

INDICATIONS AND DOSAGES
Myelosuppression
Subcutaneous
Adults, Elderly. Give as a single 6-mg injection once per chemotherapy cycle.

S AVAILABLE FORMS/COST
• Inj, Sol—SC: 6 mg/0.6 ml, prefilled syringe, 1's: **$2,950.00**

CONTRAINDICATIONS: Hypersensitivity to *Escherichia coli*–derived proteins, within 14 days before and 24 hours after cytotoxic chemotherapy

PREGNANCY AND LACTATION: Pregnancy category C; breast milk excretion unknown; use caution in nursing mothers

SIDE EFFECTS
Frequent (72%–15%)
Bone pain, nausea, fatigue, alopecia, diarrhea, vomiting, constipation, anorexia, abdominal pain, ar-

thralgia, generalized weakness, peripheral edema, dizziness, stomatitis, mucositis, neutropenic fever

SERIOUS REACTIONS

• Allergic reactions, such as anaphylaxis, rash, and urticaria, occur rarely.

• Cytopenia resulting from an antibody response to growth factors occurs rarely.

• Splenomegaly occurs rarely; assess for left upper abdominal or shoulder pain.

• Adult respiratory distress syndrome (ARDS) may occur in patients with sepsis.

INTERACTIONS

Drugs

[3] *Lithium:* Enhanced leukocytosis

SPECIAL CONSIDERATIONS

• Do not administer in the period between 14 days before and 24 hr after administration of cytotoxic chemotherapy

• Reduces duration of severe neutropenia from 6 days to 2 days, and incidence of febrile neutropenia from 30-40% to 10-20%

MONITORING PARAMETERS

• CBC with platelets

peginterferon alfa-2a

Rx: Pegasys

Chemical Class: Recombinant interferon

Therapeutic Class: Antiviral

CLINICAL PHARMACOLOGY

Mechanism of Action: An immunomodulator that binds to specific membrane receptors on the cell surface, inhibiting viral replication in virus-infected cells, suppressing cell proliferation, and producing reversible decreases in leukocyte and platelet counts. *Therapeutic Effect:* Inhibits hepatitis C virus.

Pharmacokinetics

Readily absorbed after subcutaneous administration. Excreted by the kidneys. **Half-life:** 80 hr.

INDICATIONS AND DOSAGES

Hepatitis C

Subcutaneous

Adults 18 yr and older, Elderly. 180 mcg (1 ml) injected in abdomen or thigh once weekly for 48 wk.

Dosage in renal impairment

For patients who require hemodialysis, dosage is 135 mg injected in abdomen or thigh once weekly for 48 wk.

Dosage in hepatic impairment

For patients with progressive ALT(SGPT) increases above baseline values, dosage is 90 mcg injected in abdomen or thigh once weekly for 48 wk.

[$] AVAILABLE FORMS/COST

• Sol, Inj—SC: 180 mcg/ml: **$381.94**

CONTRAINDICATIONS: Autoimmune hepatitis, decompensated hepatic disease, infants, neonates

PREGNANCY AND LACTATION: Pregnancy category C (category X when used with ribavirin); breast milk excretion unknown

SIDE EFFECTS

Frequent (54%)

Headache

Occasional (23%–13%)

Alopecia, nausea, insomnia, anorexia, dizziness, diarrhea, abdominal pain, flu-like symptoms, psychiatric reactions (depression, irritability, anxiety), injection site reaction

Rare (8%–5%)

Impaired concentration, diaphoresis, dry mouth, nausea, vomiting

SERIOUS REACTIONS

• Serious, acute hypersensitivity reactions, such as urticaria, angioedema, bronchoconstriction, and anaphylaxis, may occur. Other rare reactions include pancreatitis, colitis, hyperthyroidism or hypothyroidism, ophthalmologic disorders, and pulmonary disorders.

INTERACTIONS

Drugs

• *(note additional interactions occur when peginterferon combined with ribavirin; see ribavirin monograph)*

3 *Theophylline:* Peginterferon increases plasma theophylline level by up to 25%

SPECIAL CONSIDERATIONS

• Weekly administration of peginterferon alfa-2a equivalent to 3 times weekly administration of interferon alfa-2a for hepatitis C

• Sustained viral response rates substantially better when combined with ribavirin (genotype 1: 40-50%; genotype 2 or 3: 70-80% for combination therapy; overall response rate 40% for monotherapy)

PATIENT/FAMILY EDUCATION

• Effective contraception required; when used with ribavirin, effective contraception also required in female partners of male patients undergoing treatment

MONITORING PARAMETERS

• Availability of expert consultation for management of toxicity is essential

• *Baseline tests:* CBC, hepatic function, pregnancy test, TSH, renal function, uric acid, HCV RNA level. Exclusions to treatment: platelet count <90,000 cells/mm^3 (as low as 75,000 cells/mm^3 in patients with cirrhosis); absolute neutrophil count <1500 cells/mm^3; serum creatinine concentration >1.5 × upper limit of normal; abnormal thyroid function

• CBC q2weeks

• ALT, bilirubin q4weeks; if ALT rises persistently above baseline values, reduce dose to 135 mcg per week, if ALT increases are progressive despite dose reduction or accompanied by increased bilirubin or evidence of hepatic decompensation, therapy should be immediately discontinued

• TSH q12weeks

• Depression, evaluated q2weeks for weeks 1-8 of treatment; may require dose reduction

• All patients should receive an eye examination at baseline; patients with preexisting ophthalmologic disorders (*e.g.,* diabetic or hypertensive retinopathy) should receive periodic ophthalmologic exams during interferon alpha treatment

• HCV RNA (early virologic response defined as HCV RNA undetectable or >2 $\log_{10}$ lower than baseline at 12 weeks and 24 weeks); for patients who lack an early viral response at 12 weeks, chance of sustained viral response is 13%; for patients who lack an early viral response at 24 weeks, chance of sustained viral response is near zero; in consultation with experts, consider stopping peginterferon therapy if virologic response absent at 12-24 weeks

---

pemoline
(pem'oh-leen)

Rx: Cylert

Chemical Class: Oxazolidinone derivative

Therapeutic Class: Anorexiant; central nervous system stimulant

DEA Class: Schedule IV

CLINICAL PHARMACOLOGY

Mechanism of Action: A CNS stimulant that blocks the reuptake mechanism present in dopaminergic neurons in the cerebral cortex and subcortical structures. *Therapeutic Effect:* Reduces motor restlessness and fatigue, increases alertness, elevates mood.

INDICATIONS AND DOSAGES
ADHD
PO

Children 6 yr and older. Initially, 37.5 mg/day as a single dose in morning. May increase by 18.75 mg at weekly intervals until therapeutic response is achieved. Range: 56.25-75 mg/day. Maximum: 112.5 mg/day.

$ AVAILABLE FORMS/COST
• Tab, Chewable—Oral: 37.5 mg, 100's: **$136.81-$201.84**
• Tab—Oral: 18.75 mg, 100's: **$87.07-$117.80**; 37.5 mg, 100's: **$136.88-$185.15**; 75 mg, 100's: **$236.28-$319.73**

CONTRAINDICATIONS: Family history of Tourette syndrome, hepatic impairment, motor tics
PREGNANCY AND LACTATION: Pregnancy category B
SIDE EFFECTS
Frequent
Anorexia, insomnia
Occasional
Nausea, abdominal discomfort, diarrhea, headache, dizziness, somnolence
SERIOUS REACTIONS
• Visual disturbances, rash, and dyskinetic movements of the tongue, lips, face, and extremities have occurred.
• Large doses of pemoline may produce extreme nervousness and tachycardia.
• Hepatic effects, such as hepatitis and jaundice, appear to be reversible when the drug is discontinued.
• Prolonged administration to children with ADHD may temporarily delay growth.

SPECIAL CONSIDERATIONS
MONITORING PARAMETERS
• LFTs periodically

---

penbutolol
(pen-beaut-oh-lol)
Rx: Levatol
Chemical Class: β-adrenergic blocker, nonselective
Therapeutic Class: Antianginal; antihypertensive

CLINICAL PHARMACOLOGY
Mechanism of Action: An antihypertensive that possesses nonselective beta-blocking. Has moderate intrinsic sympathomimetic activity. *Therapeutic Effect:* Reduces cardiac output, decreases blood pressure (BP), increases airway resistance, and decreases myocardial ischemia severity.
Pharmacokinetics
Rapidly and extensively absorbed from the gastrointestinal (GI) tract. Protein binding: 80%-90%. Metabolized in liver. Excreted primarily via urine. **Half-life:** 17-26 hrs.

INDICATIONS AND DOSAGES
Hypertension
PO

Adults. Initially, 20 mg/day as a single dose. May increase to 40-80 mg/day.
Elderly. Initially, 10 mg/day.
$ AVAILABLE FORMS/COST
• Tab—Oral: 20 mg, 100's: **$173.06**

CONTRAINDICATIONS: Bronchial asthma or related bronchospastic conditions, cardiogenic shock, pulmonary edema, second- or third-degree atrioventricular (AV) block, severe bradycardia, overt cardiac failure, hypersensitivity to penbutolol or any component of the formulation
PREGNANCY AND LACTATION: Pregnancy category C

P

SIDE EFFECTS

Frequent

Decreased sexual ability, drowsiness, trouble sleeping, unusual tiredness/weakness

Occasional

Diarrhea, bradycardia, depression, cold hands/feet, constipation, anxiety, nasal congestion, nausea, vomiting

Rare

Altered taste, dry eyes, itching, numbness of fingers, toes, scalp

SERIOUS REACTIONS

• Abrupt withdrawal may result in sweating, palpitations, headache, and tremulousness.

• Hypoglycemia may occur in patients with previously controlled diabetes.

INTERACTIONS

Drugs

▣ *Adenosine:* Bradycardia aggravated

▣ *Amiodarone:* Bradycardia, cardiac arrest, ventricular arrhythmia risk after initiation of penbutolol

▣ *Antacids:* Reduced penbutolol absorption

▣ *Calcium channel blockers:* See dihydropyridine calcium channel blockers and verapamil

▣ *Clonidine, guanabenz, guanfacine:* Exacerbation of rebound hypertension upon discontinuation of clonidine

▣ *Cocaine:* Cocaine-induced vasoconstriction potentiated; reduced coronary blood flow

▣ *Contrast media:* Increased risk of anaphylaxis

▣ *Digitalis:* Enhances bradycardia

▣ *Dihydropyridine, calcium channel blockers:* Additive pharmacodynamic effects

▣ *Dipyridamole:* Bradycardia aggravated

❷ *Epinephrine, isoproterenol, phenylephrine:* Potentiates pressor response; resultant hypertension and bradycardia

▣ *Flecainide:* Additive negative inotropic effects

▣ *Fluoxetine:* Increased β-blockade activity

▣ *Fluoroquinolones:* Reduced clearance of penbutolol

❷ *Glimepiride, glipizide, gutbruide:* Prolong gypoglycemia reactions

❷ *Insulin:* Altered response to hypoglycemia; increased blood glucose concentrations; impaired peripheral circulation

▣ *Lidocaine:* Increased serum lidocaine concentrations possible

▣ *Neostigmine:* Bradycardia aggravated

▣ *Neuroleptics:* Both drugs inhibit each other's metabolism; additive hypotension

▣ *NSAIDs:* Reduced antihypertensive effect of penbutolol

▣ *Physostigmine:* Bradycardia aggravated

▣ *Prazosin:* First-dose response to prazosin may be enhanced by β-blockade

▣ *Tacrine:* Bradycardia aggravated

❷ *Terbutaline:* Antagonized bronchodilating effects of terbutaline

❷ *Theophylline:* Antagonistic pharmacodynamic effects

▣ *Verapamil:* Enhanced effects of both drugs; particularly AV nodal conduction slowing; reduced penbutolol clearance

SPECIAL CONSIDERATIONS

• Exacerbation of ischemic heart disease following abrupt withdrawal due to rebound sensitivity to catecholamines possible

• Comparative trials indicate that penbutolol is as effective as propranolol and atenolol in the treatment of hypertension; may have fewer adverse CNS effects than propranolol

---

penciclovir
(pen-sye′-kloe-veer)
Rx: Denavir
Chemical Class: Acyclic purine nucleoside analog
Therapeutic Class: Antiviral

CLINICAL PHARMACOLOGY
Mechanism of Action: Penciclovir triphosphate inhibits HSV polymerase competitively with deoxyguanosine triphosphate. Consequently, herpes viral DNA synthesis and, therefore, replication are selectively inhibited. *Therapeutic Effect:* An antiviral compound that has inhibitory activity against herpes simplex virus types 1 (HSV-1) and 2 (HSV-2).
Pharmacokinetics
Measurable penciclovir concentrations were not detected in plasma or urine. The systemic absorption of penciclovir following topical administration has not been evaluated.
INDICATIONS AND DOSAGES
Herpes labialis (cold sores)
Topical
Adolescents, Adults. Penciclovir should be applied every 2 hours during waking hours for a period of 4 days. Treatment should be started as early as possible (i.e., during the prodrome or when lesions appear).
$ **AVAILABLE FORMS/COST**
• Cre—Top: 10 mg/g (1%), 1.5 g: **$26.45**
UNLABELED USES: Varicellazoster virus

CONTRAINDICATIONS: Hypersensitivity to penciclovir or any of its components.
PREGNANCY AND LACTATION: Pregnancy category B; no data in nursing mothers, but milk concentrations should be low due to apparent lack of systemic absorption
SIDE EFFECTS
Frequent
Headache
Occasional
Change in sense of taste; decreased sensitivity of skin, particularly to touch; redness of the skin; skin rash (maculopapular, erythematous) local edema, skin discoloration; pruritis; hypoesthesia; parathesias; parosmia; urticaria; oral/pharyngeal edema
Rare
Mild pain, burning, or stinging
SPECIAL CONSIDERATIONS
• In clinical trials, shortened the duration of lesions by approximately ½ day compared to placebo (4½ vs. 5 days); duration of pain was also shortened by approximately ½ day

---

P

penicillamine
(pen-i-sil-a-meen)
Rx: Cuprimine, Depen
Chemical Class: Thiol derivative
Therapeutic Class: Antidote, heavy metal; disease-modifying antirheumatic drug (DMARD)

CLINICAL PHARMACOLOGY
Mechanism of Action: A heavy metal antagonist that chelates copper, iron, mercury, lead to form complexes, promoting excretion of copper. Combines with cystine-forming complex, thus reducing concentration of cystine to below levels for formation of cystine stones. Exact

mechanism for rheumatoid arthritis is unknown. May decrease cell-mediated immune response. May inhibit collagen formation. *Therapeutic Effect:* Promotes excretion of copper, prevents renal calculi, dissolves existing stones, acts as anti-inflammatory drug

Pharmacokinetics

Moderately absorbed from the gastrointestinal (GI) tract. Protein binding: 80% to albumin. Metabolized in small amounts in liver. Excreted unchanged in urine. **Half-life:** 1.7-3.2 hrs.

INDICATIONS AND DOSAGES

Wilson's disease

PO

Adults, Elderly, Children. Initially, 250 mg 4 times/day (some pts may begin at 250 mg/day; gradually increase). Dosages of 750-1,500 mg/day that produce initial 24 hr cupruresis >2 mg should be continued for 3 mos. Maintenance: Based on serum-free copper concentration (<10 mcg/dl indicative of adequate maintenance). Maximum: 2 g/day.

Cystinuria

PO

Adults, Elderly. Initially, 250 mg/day. Gradually increase dose. Maintenance: 2 g/day. Range: 1-4 g/day.

Children. 30 mg/kg/day.

Rheumatoid arthritis

PO

Adults, Elderly. Initially, 125-250 mg/day. May increase by 125-250 mg/day at 1-3 mo intervals. Maintenance: 500-750 mg/day. After 2-3 mos with no improvement or toxicity, may increase by 250 mg/day at 2-3 mo intervals until remission or toxicity. Maximum: 1 g up to 1.5 g/day.

$ AVAILABLE FORMS/COST

• Cap, Gel—Oral: 125 mg, 100's: **$81.19**; 250 mg, 100's: **$115.93**

• Tab, Coated—Oral: 250 mg, 100's: **$315.47**

UNLABELED USES: Treatment of rheumatoid vasculitis, heavy metal toxicity.

CONTRAINDICATIONS: History of penicillamine-related aplastic anemia or agranulocytosis, rheumatoid arthritis patients with history or evidence of renal insufficiency, pregnancy, breast-feeding

PREGNANCY AND LACTATION: Pregnancy category D (continued therapy in Wilson's disease and cystinuria probably OK, not rheumatoid arthritis)

SIDE EFFECTS

Frequent

Rash (pruritic, erythematous, maculopapular, morbilliform), reduced/altered sense of taste (hypogeusia), GI disturbances (anorexia, epigastric pain, nausea, vomiting, diarrhea), oral ulcers, glossitis

Occasional

Proteinuria, hematuria, hot flashes, drug fever

Rare

Alopecia, tinnitus, pemphigoid rash (water blisters)

SERIOUS REACTIONS

• Aplastic anemia, agranulocytosis, thrombocytopenia, leukopenia, myasthenia gravis, bronchiolitis, erythematouslike syndrome, evening hypoglycemia, skin friability at sites of pressure/trauma producing extravasation or white papules at venipuncture, surgical sites reported.

• Iron deficiency (particularly children, menstruating women) may develop.

INTERACTIONS

Drugs

3 *Antacids:* Magnesium-aluminum hydroxides reduce bioavailability

[3] *Digoxin:* Reduced digoxin concentrations

[3] *Iron:* Oral iron substantially reduces plasma penicillamine concentration, with reduced therapeutic response

Labs

• *Cholesterol:* Decreased serum levels

• *Fructoseamine:* Decreased serum levels

• *Iron:* Decreased serum levels

• *Ketones:* Increased false-positive reactions with legal reaction

SPECIAL CONSIDERATIONS

• Because penicillamine can cause severe adverse reactions, restrict its use in rheumatoid arthritis to patients who have severe, active disease and who have failed to respond to an adequate trial of conventional therapy

PATIENT/FAMILY EDUCATION

• Should be administered on empty stomach, ½-1 hr before meals or at least 2 hr after meals

• Urine may become discolored (red)

• Patients with cystinuria should drink large amounts of water

• Therapeutic effect may take 1-3 mo

MONITORING PARAMETERS

• Hepatic, renal studies: CBC, urinalysis, skin for rash

• Urinary copper excretion

penicillin
(pen-i-sil'-in)

Rx: *Penicillin G (Aqueous Pen G:)* Pfizerpen

Rx: *Penicillin G:* Pentids

Rx: *Penicillin V:* (Phenoxy-methyl Penicillin), Beepen VK, Pen-V, Pen-Vee K, Truxcillin VK, Veetids

Rx: *Penicillin G Benzathine:* Bicillin L-A, Permapen

Rx: *Penicillin G Procaine:* Crysticillin, Wycillin

Rx: *Penicillin G Benzathine and Procaine combined:* Bicillin C-R

Chemical Class: Penicillin, natural

Therapeutic Class: Antibiotic

CLINICAL PHARMACOLOGY

Mechanism of Action: Penicillins bind to bacterial cell wall, inhibiting bacterial cell wall synthesis. *Therapeutic Effect:* Inhibits bacterial cell wall synthesis.

Beta-lactamase inhibitors: inhibit the action of bacterial beta-lactamase. *Therapeutic Effect:* Protects the penicillin from enzymatic degradation.

Pharmacokinetics

Penicillins are generally well absorbed from the gastrointestinal (GI) tract after oral administration. Widely distributed to most tissues and body fluids. Protein binding: 20%. Partially metabolized in liver. Primarily excreted in urine. **Half-life:** varies (half-life increased in reduced renal function). AVAILABILITY

INDICATIONS AND DOSAGES: Penicillins may be used to treat a large number of infections, including pneumonia and other respiratory diseases, urinary tract infections, septicemia, meningitis, intraabdominal infections, gonorrhea, syphilis, and bone and joint infections.

Doses vary depending on the drug used. In general, penicillins should be taken on an empty stomach. Patients with impaired renal function may required dose adjustment.

§ AVAILABLE FORMS/COST

Penicillin G Potassium
• Powder, Inj—IV: 1,000,000 U/vial: **$0.93**; 5,000,000 U/vial: **$3.14-$34.44**; 20,000,000 U/vial: **$10.09**
• Sol, Inj-IV: 2,000,000 U, 50 ml: **$13.74**; 3,000,000 U, 50 ml: **$14.26**
Penicillin G Sodium
• Powder, Inj-IM, IV: 5,000,000 U/vial: **$42.18**
Penicillin V
• Powder, Reconst—Oral: 125 mg/5 ml, 100, 200 ml: **$2.16-$6.25**/100 ml; 250 mg/5 ml, 100, 150, 200 ml: **$2.60-$6.57**/100 ml
• Tab—Oral: 250 mg, 100's: **$5.50-$23.48**; 500 mg, 100's: **$9.90-$39.90**
Penicillin G Benzathine
• Susp, Inj—IM: 300,000 U/ml, 1 ml: **$3.80**; 600,000 U/ml, 1 ml: **$20.80**
Penicillin G Procaine
• Sol, Inj—IM: 600,000 U/ml, 1 ml: **$9.53-$10.90**
Penicillin G Benzathine and Procaine Combined
• Susp, Inj—IM: 150,000 U-150,000 U/ml, 1 ml: **$2.62**; 300,000 U-300,000 U/ml, 2 ml: **$28.73**; 900,000 U-300,000 U/2 ml, 2 ml: **$25.64**

UNLABELED USES: Some penicillins, such as amoxicillin, have been use in the treatment of Lyme disease and typhoid fever.

CONTRAINDICATIONS: Hypersensitivity to any penicillin, infectious mononucleosis

PREGNANCY AND LACTATION: Pregnancy category B; may cause diarrhea, candidiasis, or allergic response in nursing infant

SIDE EFFECTS

Frequent

Gastrointestinal (GI) disturbances (mild diarrhea, nausea, or vomiting), headache, oral or vaginal candidiasis

Occasional

Generalized rash, urticaria

SERIOUS REACTIONS

• Altered bacterial balance may result in potentially fatal superinfections and antibiotic-associated colitis as evidenced by abdominal cramps, watery or severe diarrhea, and fever.

• Severe hypersensitivity reactions, including anaphylaxis and acute interstitial nephritis occur rarely.

INTERACTIONS

Drugs

3 *Chloramphenicol:* Inhibited antibacterial activity of penicillin; administer penicillin 3 hr before chloramphenicol

3 *Macrolide antibiotics:* Inhibited antibacterial activity of penicillin; administer penicillin 3 hr before macrolides

3 *Methotrexate:* Penicillin in large doses may increase serum methotrexate concentrations

3 *Oral contraceptives:* Occasional impairment of oral contraceptive efficacy; consider use of supplemental contraception during cycles in which penicillin is used

3 *Tetracyclines:* Inhibited antibacterial activity of penicillin; administer penicillin 3 hr before tetracyclines

Labs

• *Albumin:* Decreased serum levels at very high penicillin levels

- *Aminoglycosides:* Decreased serum levels if specimen stored for a prolonged period of time
- *Folate:* Decreased serum levels
- *17-ketogenic steroids:* Increased urine concentrations
- *17-ketosteroids:* Increased urine concentrations
- *Protein:* Increased CSF concentrations
- *Protein electrophoresis:* False positives; causes bisalbuminemia
- *Sugar:* False positive with copper reduction procedures
- *Piperacillin:* False positive in the presence of penicillin V
- *Amdinocillin:* False positive in the presence of penicillin G
- *Methicillin:* False positive in the presence of penicillin G

SPECIAL CONSIDERATIONS

- Cross reactivity with cephalosporins is approx 10%

---

pentamidine
(pen-tam'i-deen)
Rx: NebuPent, Pentam
Chemical Class: Aromatic diamidine derivative
Therapeutic Class: Antiprotozoal

CLINICAL PHARMACOLOGY
Mechanism of Action: An anti-infective, that interferes with nuclear metabolism and incorporation of nucleotides, inhibiting DNA, RNA, phospholipid, and protein synthesis. *Therapeutic Effect:* Produces antibacterial and antiprotozoal effects.
Pharmacokinetics
Well absorbed after IM administration; minimally absorbed after inhalation. Widely distributed. Primarily excreted in urine. Minimally re-

moved by hemodialysis. **Half-life:** 6.5 hr (increased in impaired renal function).

INDICATIONS AND DOSAGES
Pneumocystis carinii pneumonia (PCP)
IV, IM
Adults, Elderly. 4 mg/kg/day once a day for 14-21 days.
Children. 4 mg/kg/day once a day for 10-14 days.
Prevention of PCP
Inhalation
Adults, Elderly. 300 mg once q4wk.
Children 5 yr and older. 300 mg q3-4wks.
Children younger than 5 yr. 8 mg/kg/dose once q3-4wk.

AVAILABLE FORMS/COST
- Powder, Reconst—INH: 300 mg, 1's: **$98.75**
- Powder, Inj—IV: 300 mg, 1's: **$47.20-$98.75**

UNLABELED USES: Treatment of African trypanosomiasis, cutaneous or visceral leishmaniasis

CONTRAINDICATIONS: Concurrent use with didanosine

PREGNANCY AND LACTATION: Pregnancy category C; since aerosolized pentamidine results in very low systemic concentrations, fetal exposure to the drug is probably negligible; breast milk levels following aerosolized administration are likely nil

SIDE EFFECTS
Frequent
Injection (greater than 10%): Abscess, pain at injection site
Inhalation (greater than 5%): Fatigue, metallic taste, shortness of breath, decreased appetite, dizziness, rash, cough, nausea, vomiting, chills
Occasional
Injection (10%-1%): Nausea, decreased appetite, hypotension, fever, rash, altered taste, confusion

Inhalation (5%-1%): Diarrhea, headache, anemia, muscle pain

Rare

Injection (less than 1%): Neuralgia, thrombocytopenia, phlebitis, dizziness

SERIOUS REACTIONS

• Rare reactions include life-threatening or fatal hypotension, arrhythmias, hypoglycemia, leukopenia, nephrotoxicity or renal failure, anaphylactic shock, Stevens-Johnson syndrome, and toxic epidural necrolysis.

• Hyperglycemia and insulin-dependent diabetes mellitus (often permanent) may occur even months after therapy has stopped.

SPECIAL CONSIDERATIONS

• Considered 2nd line for *P. carinii* pneumonia, following cotrimoxazole (unresponsive to or intolerant of cotrimoxazole)

MONITORING PARAMETERS

• BUN, serum creatinine, blood glucose daily

• CBC and platelets; liver function tests, including bilirubin, alkaline phosphatase, AST, and ALT; and serum calcium before, during, and after therapy

• ECG at regular intervals

pentazocine

(pen-tah-zoe-seen)

Rx: Talwin, Talwin NX (with Naloxone)

Combinations

Rx: with ASA (Talwin Compound) with APAP (Talacen)

Chemical Class: Benzomorphan; opiate derivative

Therapeutic Class: Narcotic agonist-antagonist analgesic

DEA Class: Schedule IV

CLINICAL PHARMACOLOGY

Mechanism of Action: An opioid antagonist that binds with opioid receptors within CNS. *Therapeutic Effect:* Alters processes affecting pain perception, emotional response to pain.

Pharmacokinetics

Well absorbed after administration. Widely distributed including CSF. Metabolized in liver via oxidative and glucuronide conjugation pathways, extensive first-pass effect. Excreted in small amounts as unchanged drug. **Half-life:** 2-3 hrs, prolonged with hepatic impairment.

INDICATIONS AND DOSAGES

Analgesia

PO

Adults. 50 mg q3-4h. May increase to 100 mg q3-4h, if needed. Maximum: 600 mg/day.

Elderly. 50 mg q4h.

Subcutaneous/IM/IV

Adults. 30 mg q3-4h. Do not exceed 30 mg IV or 60 mg subcutaneous/IM per dose. Maximum: 360 mg/day.

IM

Elderly. 25 mg q4h.

Obstetric labor

IM

Adults. 30 mg as a single dose.

IV
Adults. 20 mg when contractions are regular. May repeat 2-3 times q2-3h.

§ **AVAILABLE FORMS/COST**
• Sol, Inj—IV, IM, SC: 30 mg/ml, 10 ml: **$43.79-$46.21**
• Tab—Oral: 50 mg pentazocine-0.5 mg naloxone, 100's: **$93.99-$145.33**

CONTRAINDICATIONS: Hypersensitivity to pentazocine or any component of the formulation

PREGNANCY AND LACTATION: Pregnancy category B (category D if used for prolonged periods or in high doses at term); use during labor may produce neonatal respiratory depression

SIDE EFFECTS
Frequent
Drowsiness, euphoria, nausea, vomiting
Occasional
Allergic reaction, histamine reaction (decreased BP, increased sweating, flushing, wheezing), decreased urination, altered vision, constipation, dizziness, dry mouth, headache, hypotension, pain/burning at injection site

SERIOUS REACTIONS
• Overdosage results in severe respiratory depression, skeletal muscle flaccidity, cyanosis, extreme somnolence progressing to convulsions, stupor, and coma.
• Abrupt withdrawal after prolonged use may produce symptoms of narcotic withdrawal (abdominal cramps, rhinorrhea, lacrimation, nausea, vomiting, restlessness, anxiety, increased temperature, piloerection).

INTERACTIONS
Drugs
⊠ *Aspirin:* Increased risk of papillary necrosis
⊠ *Barbiturates:* Additive CNS depression
⊠ *Phenothiazines:* Additive CNS depression
Labs
• *Increase:* Amylase

SPECIAL CONSIDERATIONS
• Naloxone 0.5 mg added to oral tablets to discourage misuse via parenteral inj
• Less effective compared to morphine, but less respiratory depression and opposite cardiovascular pharmacodynamics; increases pulmonary, arterial, and central venous pressure

PATIENT/FAMILY EDUCATION
• Report any symptoms of CNS changes, allergic reactions
• Physical dependency may result when used for extended periods
• Change position slowly, orthostatic hypotension may occur
• Avoid hazardous activities if drowsiness or dizziness occurs
• Avoid alcohol, other CNS depressants unless directed by clinician

---

pentobarbital
(pen-toe-bar'bi-tal)
Rx: Nembutal
Chemical Class: Barbituric acid derivative
Therapeutic Class: Anticonvulsant; sedative/hypnotic
DEA Class: Schedule II; Schedule III

P

CLINICAL PHARMACOLOGY
Mechanism of Action: A barbiturate that binds at the GABA receptor complex, enhancing GABA activity. *Therapeutic Effect:* Depresses central nervous system (CNS) activity and reticular activating system.
Pharmacokinetics
Well absorbed after PO, parenteral administration. Protein binding: 35%-55%. Rapidly, widely distrib-

uted. Metabolized in liver. Primarily excreted in urine. Removed by hemodialysis. **Half-life:** 15-48 hrs.

INDICATIONS AND DOSAGES
Preanesthetic
PO
Adults, Elderly. 100 mg.
Children. 2-6 mg/kg. Maximum: 100 mg/dose.
IM
Adults, Elderly. 150-200 mg.
Children. 2-6 mg/kg. Maximum: 100 mg/dose.
Rectal
Children 12-14 yrs. 60 or 120 mg.
Children 5-12 yrs. 60 mg.
Children 1-4 yrs. 30-60 mg.
Children 1 yr-2 mos. 30 mg.

Hypnotic
PO
Adults, Elderly. 100 mg at bedtime.
IM
Adults, Elderly. 150-200 mg at bedtime.
Children. 2-6 mg/kg. Maximum: 100 mg/dose at bedtime.
IV
Adults, Elderly. 100 mg initially then, after 1 minute, may give additional small doses at 1 minute intervals, up to 500 mg total.
Children. 50 mg initially then, after 1 minute, may give additional small doses at 1 minute intervals, up to desired effect.
Rectal
Adults, Elderly. 120-200 mg at bedtime.
Children 12-14 yrs. 60 or 120 mg at bedtime.
Children 5-12 yrs. 60 mg at bedtime.
Children 1-4 yrs. 30-60 mg at bedtime.
Children 2 mos-1 yr. 30 mg at bedtime.

Anticonvulsant
IV
Adults, Elderly. 2-15 mg/kg loading dose given slowly over 1-2 hours.

Maintenance infusion: 0.5-5 mg/kg/hr.
Children. 5-15 mg/kg loading dose given slowly over 1-2 hours. Maintenance infusion: 0.5-3 mg/kg/hr.

AVAILABLE FORMS/COST
• Cap, Gel—Oral: 100 mg, 100's: **$272.05**
• Sol, Inj—IM, IV: 50 mg/ml, 2 ml: **$2.65**
• Supp—Rect: 30 mg, 12's: **$44.58**; 60 mg, 12's: **$62.53**; 120 mg, 12's: **$58.33**; 200 mg, 12's: **$85.75**

UNLABELED USES: Intracranial hypertension, psychiatric interviews, sedative withdrawal, drug abuse withdrawal

CONTRAINDICATIONS: Porphyria, hypersensitivity to barbiturates

PREGNANCY AND LACTATION: Pregnancy category D; excreted in breast milk; effect on nursing infant unknown

SIDE EFFECTS
Occasional
Agitation, confusion, dizziness, somnolence
Rare
Confusion, paradoxical CNS hyperactivity or nervousness in children, excitement or restlessness in elderly

SERIOUS REACTIONS
• Agranulocytosis, megaloblastic anemia, apnea, hypoventilation, bradycardia, hypotension, syncope, hepatic damage and Stevens-Johnson syndrome occur rarely.
• Abrupt withdrawal after prolonged therapy may produce effects ranging from markedly increased dreaming, nightmares or insomnia, tremor, sweating and vomiting, to hallucinations, delirium, seizures and status epilepticus.
• Skin eruptions appear as hypersensitivity reactions.

• Overdosage produces cold or clammy skin, hypothermia, severe CNS depression, cyanosis and rapid pulse.

INTERACTIONS

Drugs

▣ *Acetaminophen:* Enhanced hepatotoxic potential of acetaminophen overdoses

▣ *Antidepressants, cyclic:* Reduced serum concentrations of cyclic antidepressants

▣ *β-adrenergic blockers:* Reduced serum concentrations of β-blockers which are extensively metabolized

▣ *Calcium channel blockers:* Reduced serum concentrations of verapamil and dihydropyridines

▣ *Chloramphenicol:* Increased barbiturate concentrations; reduced serum chloramphenicol concentrations

▣ *Corticosteroids:* Reduced serum concentrations of corticosteroids; may impair therapeutic effect

▣ *Cyclosporine:* Reduced serum concentration of cyclosporine

▣ *Digitoxin:* Reduced serum concentration of digitoxin

▣ *Disopyramide:* Reduced serum concentration of disopyramide

▣ *Doxycycline:* Reduced serum doxycycline concentrations

▣ *Estrogen:* Reduced serum concentration of estrogen

▣ *Ethanol:* Excessive CNS depression

▣ *Griseofulvin:* Reduced griseofulvin absorption

▣ *Methoxyflurane:* Enhanced nephrotoxic effect

▣ *MAOIs:* Prolonged effect of barbiturates

▣ *Narcotic analgesics:* Increased toxicity of meperidine; reduced effect of methadone; additive CNS depression

▣ *Neuroleptics:* Reduced effect of either drug

❷ *Oral anticoagulants:* Decreased hypoprothrombinemic response to oral anticoagulants

▣ *Oral contraceptives:* Reduced efficacy of oral contraceptives

▣ *Phenytoin:* Unpredictable effect on serum phenytoin levels

▣ *Propafenone:* Reduced serum concentration of propafenone

▣ *Quinidine:* Reduced quinidine plasma concentration

▣ *Tacrolimus:* Reduced serum concentration of tacrolimus

▣ *Theophylline:* Reduced serum theophylline concentrations

▣ *Valproic acid:* Increased serum concentrations of amobarbital

▣ *Warfarin:* See oral anticoagulants

SPECIAL CONSIDERATIONS

PATIENT/FAMILY EDUCATION

• Avoid driving or other activities requiring alertness

• Avoid alcohol ingestion or CNS depressants

• Do not discontinue medication abruptly after long-term use

MONITORING PARAMETERS

• Excessive usage; hypnotic hangover

---

pentosan polysulfate
(pen-toe-san)

Rx: Elmiron

Chemical Class: Glycosaminoglycan, sulfated; heparin derivative

Therapeutic Class: Anticoagulant; fibrinolytic

CLINICAL PHARMACOLOGY

Mechanism of Action: A negatively-charged synthetic sulfated polysaccharide with heparin-like properties that appears to adhere to bladder wall mucosal membrane, may act as a buffering agent to control cell permeability preventing irritating solutes in the urine. Has anticoagulant/fibrinolytic effects. *Therapeutic Effect:* Relieves bladder pain.

Pharmacokinetics

Poorly and erratically absorbed from the gastrointestinal tract. Distributed in uroepithelium of GU tract with lesser amount found in the liver, spleen, lung, skin, periosteum and bone marrow. Metabolized in liver and kidney (secondary). Eliminated in the urine. **Half-life:** 4.8 hrs.

INDICATIONS AND DOSAGES

Interstitial cystitis

PO

Adults, Elderly. 100 mg 3 times/day.

$ AVAILABLE FORMS/COST

• Cap—Oral: 100 mg, 100's: **$240.68**

UNLABELED USES: Urolithiasis

CONTRAINDICATIONS: Hypersensitivity to pentosan polysulfate sodium or structurally related compounds

PREGNANCY AND LACTATION: Pregnancy category B; no data in nursing mothers

SIDE EFFECTS

Frequent

Alopecia areata (a single area on the scalp), diarrhea, nausea, headache, rash, abdominal pain, dyspepsia.

Occasional

Dizziness, depression, increased liver function tests.

SERIOUS REACTIONS

• Ecchymosis, epistaxis, gum hemorrhage have been reported (drug produces weak anticoagulant effect).

• Overdose may produce liver function abnormalities.

---

pentoxifylline
(pen-tox-if'ih-lin)

Rx: Pentopak, Pentoxil, Pentoxyphylline, Trental
Chemical Class: Dimethylxanthine derivative
Therapeutic Class: Hemorrheologic agent

CLINICAL PHARMACOLOGY

Mechanism of Action: A blood viscosity-reducing agent that alters the flexibility of RBCs; inhibits production of tumor necrosis factor, neutrophil activation, and platelet aggregation. *Therapeutic Effect:* Reduces blood viscosity and improves blood flow.

Pharmacokinetics

Well absorbed after oral administration. Undergoes first-pass metabolism in the liver. Primarily excreted in urine. Unknown if removed by hemodialysis. **Half-life:** 24–48 min; metabolite, 60–90 min.

INDICATIONS AND DOSAGES

Intermittent claudication

PO

Adults, Elderly. 400 mg 3 times a day. Decrease to 400 mg twice a day if GI or CNS adverse effects occur. Continue for at least 8 wk.

$ AVAILABLE FORMS/COST

• Tab, Coated, Sus Action—Oral: 400 mg, 100's: **$12.77-$91.78**

CONTRAINDICATIONS: History of intolerance to xanthine derivatives, such as caffeine, theophylline, or theobromine; recent cerebral or retinal hemorrhage

PREGNANCY AND LACTATION: Pregnancy category C; excreted in breast milk

SIDE EFFECTS

Occasional (5%–2%)

Dizziness, nausea, altered taste, dyspepsia, marked by heartburn, epigastric pain, and indigestion

Rare (less than 2%)

Rash, pruritus, anorexia, constipation, dry mouth, blurred vision, edema, nasal congestion, anxiety

SERIOUS REACTIONS

• Angina and chest pain occur rarely and may be accompanied by palpitations, tachycardia, and arrhythmias.

• Signs and symptoms of overdose, such as flushing, hypotension, nervousness, agitation, hand tremor, fever, and somnolence, appear 4–5 hours after ingestion and last for 12 hours.

INTERACTIONS

Drugs

◼ *Fluoroquinolones (ciprofloxin, enoxacin, norfloxacin, pefloxacin, pipemidic acid):* Increased pentoxyphylline concentrations with subsequent side effects

◼ *Theophylline:* Increased plasma theophylline concentrations

SPECIAL CONSIDERATIONS

• Statistically, but not always, clinically significant effects in intermittent claudication, however, other drugs less impressive; will not replace surgical options

PATIENT/FAMILY EDUCATION

• Therapeutic effect may require 2-4 wk

• Stop smoking

---

pergolide

(per´go-lide)

Rx: Permax

Chemical Class: Ergoline derivative

Therapeutic Class: Anti-Parkinson's agent; dopaminergic

CLINICAL PHARMACOLOGY

Mechanism of Action: A centrally active dopamine agonist that directly stimulates dopamine receptors. *Therapeutic Effect:* Decreases signs and symptoms of Parkinson's disease.

Pharmacokinetics

Well absorbed from the GI tract. Protein binding: 90%. Undergoes extensive first-pass metabolism in the liver. Primarily excreted in urine. Unknown if removed by hemodialysis.

INDICATIONS AND DOSAGES

Parkinsonism

PO

Adults, Elderly. Initially, 0.05 mg/day for 2 days. May increase by 0.1-0.15 mg/day every 3 days over the next 12 days; afterward may increase by 0.25 mg/day every 3 days. Range: 2-3 mg/day in 3 divided doses. Maximum: 5 mg/day.

◼ **AVAILABLE FORMS/COST**

• Tab—Oral: 0.05 mg, 30's: **$37.38-$112.32**; 0.25 mg, 100's: **$186.25-$207.00**; 1 mg, 100's: **$381.34-$446.29**

CONTRAINDICATIONS: Hypersensitivity to pergolide or other ergot derivatives

PREGNANCY AND LACTATION: Pregnancy category B; may interfere with lactation

SIDE EFFECTS

Frequent (24%-10%)

Nausea, dizziness, hallucinations, constipation, rhinitis, dystonia, confusion, somnolence

Occasional (9%-3%)

Orthostatic hypotension, insomnia, dry mouth, peripheral edema, anxiety, diarrhea, dyspepsia, abdominal pain, headache, abnormal vision, anorexia, tremor, depression, rash

Rare (less than 2%)

Urinary frequency, vivid dreams, neck pain, hypotension, vomiting

SERIOUS REACTIONS

• Symptoms of overdose may vary from CNS depression, characterized by sedation, apnea, cardiovascular collapse, and death, to severe paradoxical reactions, such as hallucinations, tremor, and seizures.

INTERACTIONS

Drugs

③ *Lisinopril:* Additive hypotension

③ *Neuroleptics:* Potentially antagonistic pharmacodynamic effects

SPECIAL CONSIDERATIONS

• Adjunct to levodopa/carbidopa in Parkinson's disease; longer acting than bromocriptine

PATIENT/FAMILY EDUCATION

• Hypotensive cautions

---

perindopril
(per-in'doh-pril)
Rx: Aceon
Chemical Class: Angiotensin-converting enzyme (ACE) inhibitor, nonsulfhydryl
Therapeutic Class: Antihypertensive

CLINICAL PHARMACOLOGY

Mechanism of Action: An ACE inhibitor that suppresses the renin-angiotensin-aldosterone system and prevents conversion of angiotensin I to angiotensin II, a potent vasoconstrictor; may also inhibit angiotensin II at local vascular and renal sites. *Therapeutic Effect:* Reduces peripheral arterial resistance and BP.

INDICATIONS AND DOSAGES

Hypertension

PO

Adults, Elderly. 2-8 mg/day as single dose or in 2 divided doses. Maximum: 16 mg/day.

Ⓢ AVAILABLE FORMS/COST

• Tab, Scored—Oral: 2 mg, 100's: **$132.49**; 4 mg, 100's: **$145.73**; 8 mg, 30's: **$185.55**

UNLABELED USES: Management of heart failure

CONTRAINDICATIONS: History of angioedema from previous treatment with ACE inhibitors

PREGNANCY AND LACTATION: Pregnancy category C (1st trimester); category D (2nd and 3rd trimesters); associated with fetal and neonatal injury including hypotension, neonatal skull hypoplasia, anuria, reversible or irreversible renal effects and death; oligohydramnios; possibly hypoplastic lung development, IUGR, PDA

SIDE EFFECTS

Occasional (5%-1%)

Cough, back pain, sinusitis, upper extremity pain, dyspepsia, fever, palpitations, hypotension, dizziness, fatigue, syncope

SERIOUS REACTIONS

• Excessive hypotension (first-dose syncope) may occur in patients with CHF and in those who are severely salt or volume depleted.

• Angioedema (swelling of face and lips) and hyperkalemia occur rarely.

• Agranulocytosis and neutropenia may be noted in those with collagen vascular disease, including scleroderma and systemic lupus erythematosus, and impaired renal function.

• Nephrotic syndrome may be noted in those with history of renal disease.

INTERACTIONS
Drugs

▣ *Azathioprine:* Increased myelosuppression

▣ *Cyclosporine, tacrolimus:* Additive effects; increased risk of hyperkalemia, nephrotoxicity

▣ *Diuretics:* Excessive hypotension, hypoperfusion

▣ *Heparin:* Hyperkalemia

▣ *Insulin, sulfonylureas:* Additive hypoglycemia

▣ *Lithium:* Increase lithium levels

▣ *Nonsteroidal antiinflammatory drugs:* Decreased antihypertensive efficacy, increased risk of nephrotoxicity

❷ *Potassium supplements, potassium sparing diuretics, potassium salt substitutes:* Hyperkalemia

▣ *Trimethoprim:* Additive risk of hyperkalemia, especially in patient predisposed to renal insufficiency

▣ *Interferon alfa 2a:* Increased myelosupression

Labs

• ACE inhibition can account for an approximately 0.5 mEq/L rise in serum potassium

SPECIAL CONSIDERATIONS
PATIENT/FAMILY EDUCATION

• Caution with salt substitutes containing potassium chloride

• Rise slowly to sitting/standing position to minimize orthostatic hypotension

• Dizziness, fainting, lightheadedness may occur during 1st few days of therapy

• May cause altered taste perception or cough; persistent dry cough usually does not subside unless medication is stopped; notify clinician if these symptoms persist

• Warnings regarding angioedema (swelling of face, extremities, eyes, lips, tongue, hoarseness, or difficulty swallowing or breathing) especially following first dose

MONITORING PARAMETERS

• Baseline electrolytes, renal function tests, and urinalysis baseline and at least BUN, creatinine, potassium within 2 weeks after initiation of therapy (increased levels may indicate acute renal failure)

• Serial orthostatic blood pressures and pulse rates

---

permethrin
(per-meth'ren)
Rx: Acticin, Elimite
OTC: Nix
Chemical Class: Pyrethroid derivative
Therapeutic Class: Pediculicide; scabicide

CLINICAL PHARMACOLOGY
Mechanism of Action: An antiparasitic agent that inhibits sodium influx through nerve cell membrane channels. *Therapeutic Effect:* Results in delayed repolarization, paralysis and death of parasites.

Pharmacokinetics

Less than 2% absorption after topical application. Detected in residual amounts on hair for at least 10 days following treatment. Metabolized by liver to inactive metabolites. Excreted in urine.

INDICATIONS AND DOSAGES
Head lice
Shampoo
Adults, Elderly, Children 2 mos and older. Shampoo hair, towel dry, apply to scalp, leave on for 10 minutes and rinse. Remove nits with nit comb. Repeat application if live lice present 7 days after initial treatment.

P

Scabies
Topical
Adults, Elderly, Children 2 mos and older. Apply from head to feet, leave on for 8-14 hrs. Wash with soap and water. Repeat application if living mites present 14 days after initial treatment.

S AVAILABLE FORMS/COST
• Cre—Top: 5%, 60 g: **$29.15-$32.75**
• Liq—Top: 1%, 60 ml: **$8.19**

UNLABELED USES: Demodicidosis, insect bite prophylaxis, leishmaniasis prophylaxis, malaria prophylaxis

CONTRAINDICATIONS: Infants less than 2 months of age, hypersensitivity to pyrethyroid, pyrethrin, chrysanthemums or any component of the formulation

PREGNANCY AND LACTATION: Pregnancy category B; excretion into breast milk unknown

SIDE EFFECTS
Occasional
Burning, pruritus, stinging, erythema, rash, swelling

SERIOUS REACTIONS
• Shortness of breath and difficulty breathing have been reported.

SPECIAL CONSIDERATIONS
PATIENT/FAMILY EDUCATION
• For external use only; shake well
• Avoid contact with eyes, mucous membranes
• Itching may be temporarily aggravated following application
• Do not repeat administration sooner than 1 wk
• Itching from allergic reaction caused by mite may persist for several weeks even though infestation is cured

perphenazine
(per-fen-ah-zeen)
Rx: Trilafon
Chemical Class: Piperidine phenothiazine derivative
Therapeutic Class: Antiemetic; antipsychotic

CLINICAL PHARMACOLOGY
Mechanism of Action: An antipsychotic agent and antiemetic that blocks postsynaptic dopamine receptor sites in the brain. *Therapeutic Effect:* Suppresses behavioral response in psychosis, and relieves nausea and vomiting.

INDICATIONS AND DOSAGES
Severe schizophrenia
PO
Adults. 4-16 mg 2-4 times/day. Maximum: 64 mg/day.
Elderly. Initially, 2-4 mg/day. May increase at 4-7 day intervals by 2-4 mg/day up to 32 mg/day.
Severe nausea and vomiting
PO
Adults. 8-16 mg/day in divided doses up to 24 mg/day.

S AVAILABLE FORMS/COST
• Sol, Inj—IM, IV: 5 mg/ml, 1 ml: **$7.83**
• Conc—Oral: 16 mg/5 ml, 120 ml: **$39.73-$44.64**
• Tab, Coated—Oral: 2 mg, 100's: **$10.03-$86.03**; 4 mg, 100's: **$13.74-$117.71**; 8 mg, 100's: **$12.23-$142.81**; 16 mg, 100's: **$27.71-$192.13**

CONTRAINDICATIONS: Coma, myelosuppression, severe cardiovascular disease, severe CNS depression, subcortical brain damage

PREGNANCY AND LACTATION: Pregnancy category C; has been used as an antiemetic during normal labor without producing any observable effect on newborn; excreted into human breast milk; effects on nursing infant unknown, but may be of concern

SIDE EFFECTS

Occasional

Marked photosensitivity, somnolence, dry mouth, blurred vision, lethargy, constipation or diarrhea, nasal congestion, peripheral edema, urine retention

Rare

Ocular changes, altered skin pigmentation, hypotension, dizziness, syncope

SERIOUS REACTIONS

• Extrapyramidal symptoms appear to be dose-related and are divided into 3 categories: akathisia (characterized by inability to sit still, tapping of feet), parkinsonian symptoms (including masklike face, tremors, shuffling gait, hypersalivation), and acute dystonias (such as torticollis, opisthotonos, and oculogyric crisis).

• Tardive dyskinesia occurs rarely.

• Abrupt withdrawal after longterm therapy may precipitate nausea, vomiting, gastritis, dizziness, and tremors.

INTERACTIONS

Drugs

3 *Amodiaquine, chloroquine, sulfadoxine-pyrimethamine:* Increased neuroleptic concentrations

3 *Anticholinergics:* May inhibit neuroleptic response; excess anticholinergic effects

3 *Antidepressants:* Potential for increased therapeutic and toxic effects from increased levels of both drugs

3 *Barbiturates:* Decreased neuroleptic levels

3 *Clonidine, guanadrel, granethidine:* Severe hypotensive episodes possible

3 *Epinephrine:* Blunted pressor response to epinephrine

3 *Ethanol:* Additive CNS depression

2 *Levodopa:* Inhibited antiparkinsonian effect of levodopa

3 *Lithium:* Lowered levels of both drugs, rarely neurotoxicity in acute mania

3 *Narcotic analgesics:* Hypotension and increased CNS depression

3 *Orphenadrine:* Lowered neuroleptic concentrations, excessive anticholinergic effects

3 *Propranolol:* Increased plasma

Labs

• *Creatinine:* Decreased serum levels

SPECIAL CONSIDERATIONS

PATIENT/FAMILY EDUCATION

• Arise slowly from reclining position

• Do not discontinue abruptly

• Use a sunscreen during sun exposure to prevent burns, take special precautions to stay cool in hot weather

• Concentrate may be diluted just prior to administration with distilled water, acidified tap water, orange or grape juice

MONITORING PARAMETERS

• Observe closely for signs of tardive dyskinesia (abnormal involuntary movement scale)

• Periodic CBC with platelets, hepatic and renal function during prolonged therapy

P

phenazopyridine

(fen-az'o-peer'i-deen)

Rx: Azo-Standard, Baridium, Eridium, Geridium, Phenazodine, Pyridiate, Pyridium, Urodine, Urogesic

Combinations

Rx: with sulfamethoxazole (Azo-Gantanol); with sulfisoxazole (Azo-Gantrisin)

Chemical Class: Azo dye
Therapeutic Class: Urinary tract analgesic

CLINICAL PHARMACOLOGY

Mechanism of Action: An interstitial cystitis agent that exerts topical analgesic effect on urinary tract mucosa. *Therapeutic Effect:* Relieves urinary pain, burning, urgency, and frequency.

Pharmacokinetics

Well absorbed from the GI tract. Partially metabolized in the liver. Primarily excreted in urine.

INDICATIONS AND DOSAGES

Urinary analgesic

PO

Adults. 100–200 mg 3–4 times a day. *Children 6 yr and older.* 12 mg/kg/day in 3 divided doses for 2 days.

Dosage in renal impairment

Dosage interval is modified based on creatinine clearance.

Creatinine Clearance	Interval
50–80 ml/min	Usual dose q8–16h
less than 50 ml/min	Avoid use.

$ AVAILABLE FORMS/COST

• Tab, Coated—Oral: 100 mg, 100's: **$1.49-$69.48**; 200 mg, 100's: **$2.09-$140.60**

CONTRAINDICATIONS: Hepatic or renal insufficiency

PREGNANCY AND LACTATION: Pregnancy category B

SIDE EFFECTS

Occasional

Headache, GI disturbance, rash, pruritus

SERIOUS REACTIONS

• Overdose may lead to hemolytic anemia, nephrotoxicity, or hepatotoxicity. Patients with renal impairment or severe hypersensitivity to the drug may also develop these reactions.

• A massive and acute overdose may result in methemoglobinemia.

INTERACTIONS

Labs

• *Albumin:* Increased serum concentrations

• *Bacteria:* False negatives on Microstix

• *Bile:* False positive with Ictotest, BiliLabstix

• *Bilirubin, conjugated:* False elevations in serum

• *Bilirubin, unconjugated:* False serum concentration elevations

• *BSP Retention:* False negatives

• *Cholinesterase:* Adds 34% negative bias to Ectachem method

• *Urine:* Yellow-orange color

• *Feces:* Orange-red color

• *Glucose:* Decreased serum levels

• *17-ketogenic steroids:* False positives in urine

• *Ketones:* Nitroprusside reactions masked by color; false negatives

• *17-ketosteroids:* Increase in urine

• *Porphyrins:* False positive

• *Pregnanediol:* Increased urine levels

• *Protein:* Increased serum levels

• *PSP excretion:* False positive in alkaline pH

• *Urobilinogen:* False positive urine test

• *Vanillylmandelic acid:* Increased urine concentrations

• *Xylose excretion:* Increased urine concentrations

SPECIAL CONSIDERATIONS
PATIENT/FAMILY EDUCATION
• May cause GI upset
• Take after meals
• May cause reddish-orange discoloration of urine; may stain fabric; may also stain contact lenses

---

phendimetrazine
(fen-dye-me'tra-zeen)
Rx: Bontril, Melfiat, Prelu-2
Chemical Class: Morpholine
Therapeutic Class: Anorexiant
DEA Class: Schedule III;
Schedule IV

CLINICAL PHARMACOLOGY
Mechanism of Action: A phenylalkylamine sympathomimetic with activity similar to amphetamines that stimulates the central nervous system (CNS) and elevates blood pressure (BP) most likely mediated via norepinephrine and dopamine metabolism. Causes stimulation of the hypothalamus. *Therapeutic Effect:* Decreases appetite.
Pharmacokinetics
The pharmacokinetics of phendimetrazine tartrate has not been well established. Metabolized to active metabolite, phendimetrazine. Excreted in urine. **Half-life:** 2-4 hrs.

INDICATIONS AND DOSAGES
Obesity
PO
Adults, Elderly. 105 mg/day in the morning or before the morning meal (sustained-release); 35 mg 2-3 times/day (immediate-release). Maximum: 70 mg 3 times/day.

$ AVAILABLE FORMS/COST
• Cap, Gel, Sus Action—Oral: 105 mg, 100's: **$98.54-$135.76**

• Tab—Oral: 35 mg, 100's: **$5.90-$40.00**

CONTRAINDICATIONS: Advanced arteriosclerosis, agitated states, glaucoma, history of drug abuse, history of hypersensitivity to sympathomimetic amines, hyperthyroidism, moderate to severe hypertension, symptomatic cardiovascular disease, use within 14 days of discontinuation MAOI, hypersensitivity to phendimetrazine or sympathomimetics

PREGNANCY AND LACTATION: Pregnancy category C

SIDE EFFECTS
Occasional
Constipation, nausea, diarrhea, dry mouth, dysuria, libido changes, flushing, hypertension, insomnia, nervousness, headache, dizziness, irritability, agitation, restlessness, palpitations, increased heart rate, sweating, tremor, urticaria

SERIOUS REACTIONS
• Multivalvular heart disease, primary pulmonary hypertension and arrhythmias occur rarely.
• Overdose may produce flushing, arrhythmias, and psychosis.
• Abrupt withdrawal following prolonged administration of high doses may produce extreme fatigue and depression.

SPECIAL CONSIDERATIONS
PATIENT/FAMILY EDUCATION
• May cause insomnia; avoid taking late in the day
• Weight reduction requires strict adherence to caloric restriction
• Do not discontinue abruptly

P

phenelzine
(fen'el-zeen)
Rx: Nardil
Chemical Class: Hydrazine derivative
Therapeutic Class: Antidepressant, monoamine oxidase inhibitor (MAOI)

CLINICAL PHARMACOLOGY
Mechanism of Action: An MAOI that inhibits the activity of the enzyme monoamine oxidase at CNS storage sites, leading to increased levels of the neurotransmitters epinephrine, norepinephrine, serotonin, and dopamine at neuronal receptor sites. *Therapeutic Effect:* Relieves depression.

INDICATIONS AND DOSAGES
Depression refractory to other antidepressants or electroconvulsive therapy
PO
Adults. 15 mg 3 times a day. May increase to 60-90 mg/day.
Elderly. Initially, 7.5 mg/day. May increase by 7.5-15 mg/day q3-4wk up to 60 mg/day in divided doses.

§ AVAILABLE FORMS/COST
• Tab, Sugar Coated—Oral: 15 mg, 100's: **$54.15**

UNLABELED USES: Treatment of panic disorder, vascular or tension headaches

CONTRAINDICATIONS: Cardiovascular or cerebrovascular disease, hepatic or renal impairment, pheochromocytoma

PREGNANCY AND LACTATION: Pregnancy category C

SIDE EFFECTS
Frequent
Orthostatic hypotension, restlessness, GI upset, insomnia, dizziness, headache, lethargy, asthenia, dry mouth, peripheral edema

Occasional
Flushing, diaphoresis, rash, urinary frequency, increased appetite, transient impotence
Rare
Visual disturbances

SERIOUS REACTIONS
• Hypertensive crisis occurs rarely and is marked by severe hypertension, occipital headache radiating frontally, neck stiffness or soreness, nausea, vomiting, diaphoresis, fever or chilliness, clammy skin, dilated pupils, palpitations, tachycardia or bradycardia, and constricting chest pain.

INTERACTIONS
Drugs
⚠ *Amphetamines, alcoholic beverages containing tyramine, metaraminol, phenylephrine, phenylpropanolamine, pseudoephedrine, tyramine:* Severe hypertensive reaction
❷ *Antidepressants, cyclic:* Excessive sympathetic response, mania, hyperpyrexia
❸ *Barbiturates:* Prolonged effect of some barbiturates
⚠ *Clomipramine:* Death
⚠ *Dexfenfluramine, dextromethorphan, fenfluramine, meperidine:* Agitation, blood pressure changes, hyperpyrexia, convulsions
⚠ *Fluoxetine, Sertraline:* Hypomania, confusion, hypertension, tremor
⚠ *Food:* Foods containing large amounts of tyramine can result in hypertensive reactions
❸ *Guanadrel, guanethidine:* May inhibit antihypertensive effects
❸ *Levodopa:* Severe hypertensive reaction
❷ *Lithium:* Malignant hyperpyrexia
❸ *Neuromuscular blocking agents:* Prolonged muscle relaxation caused by succinylcholine

3 *Reserpine:* Hypertensive reaction

3 *Sumatriptan:* Increased sumatriptan plasma concentrations

Labs

• *Aspartate aminotransferase:* Increased serum levels

• *Bilirubin:* False-positive increases in serum

• *Uric acid:* False-positive increases in serum

SPECIAL CONSIDERATIONS
PATIENT/FAMILY EDUCATION

• Avoid tyramine-containing foods, beverages, and OTC products containing decongestants or dextromethorphan and products such as diet aids

• May cause drowsiness, dizziness, blurred vision

• Use caution driving or performing other tasks requiring alertness

• Arise slowly from reclining position

• Therapeutic effect may require 4-8 wk

---

phenobarbital
(fee-noe-bar′bi-tal)

Rx: Luminal, Solfoton

Combinations

Rx: with atropine, hyoscyamine, scopolamine (Donnatal); with belladonna, ergotamine (Bellergal Spacetabs)

Chemical Class: Barbituric acid derivative

Therapeutic Class: Anticonvulsant; sedative/hypnotic

DEA Class: Schedule IV

CLINICAL PHARMACOLOGY
Mechanism of Action: A barbiturate that enhances the activity of gamma-aminobutyric acid (GABA) by binding to the GABA receptor complex. *Therapeutic Effect:* Depresses CNS activity.

Pharmacokinetics

Route	Onset	Peak	Duration
PO	20-60 min	N/A	6-10 hr
IV	5 min	30 min	4-10 hr

Well absorbed after PO or parenteral administration. Protein binding: 35%-50%. Rapidly and widely distributed. Metabolized in the liver. Primarily excreted in urine. Removed by hemodialysis. **Half-life:** 53-118 hr.

INDICATIONS AND DOSAGES
Status epilepticus

IV

Adults, Elderly, Children, Neonates. Loading dose of 15-20 mg/kg as a single dose or in divided doses.

Seizure control

PO, IV

Adults, Elderly, Children 12 yr and older. 1-3 mg/kg/day.

Children 6-12 yr. 4-6 mg/kg/day.

Children 1-5 yr. 6-8 mg/kg/day.

Children younger than 1 yr. 5-6 mg/kg/day.

Neonates. 3-4 mg/kg/day.

Sedation

PO, IM

Adults, Elderly. 30-120 mg/day in 2-3 divided doses.

Children. 2 mg/kg 3 times a day.

Hypnotic

PO, IV, IM, Subcutaneous

Adults, Elderly. 100-320 mg at bedtime.

Children. 3-5 mg/kg at bedtime.

$ **AVAILABLE FORMS/COST**

• Elixir—Oral: 20 mg/5 ml, 480 ml: **$3.65-$8.18**

• Sol, Inj—IM, IV: 30 mg/ml, 1 ml: **$2.24**; 60 mg/ml, 1 ml: **$4.95**; 65 mg/ml, 1 ml: **$1.70**; 130 mg/ml, 1 ml: **$3.67-$4.31**

P

• Tab—Oral: 15 mg, 100's: **$0.54-$4.41**; 30 mg, 100's: **$0.64-$4.49**; 60 mg, 100's: **$2.24-$6.66**; 100 mg, 100's: **$3.31-$8.44**; 16.2 mg, 90's: **$3.15**; 32.4 mg, 90's: **$3.15**; 64.8 mg, 60's: **$4.60**; 97.2 mg, 1000's: **$62.55**

UNLABELED USES: Prevention and treatment of hyperbilirubinemia

CONTRAINDICATIONS: Porphyria, pre-existing CNS depression, severe pain, severe respiratory disease

PREGNANCY AND LACTATION: Pregnancy category D; risks to fetus include minor congenital defects, hemorrhage at birth, addiction; risk to mother may be greater if seizure control is lost due to stopping drug; use at lowest possible level to control seizures; excreted into breast milk, has caused major adverse effects in some nursing infants, use caution in nursing women

SIDE EFFECTS

Occasional (3%-1%)

Somnolence

Rare (less than 1%)

Confusion; paradoxical CNS reactions, such as hyperactivity or nervousness in children and excitement or restlessness in the elderly (generally noted during first 2 weeks of therapy, particularly in presence of uncontrolled pain)

SERIOUS REACTIONS

• Abrupt withdrawal after prolonged therapy may produce increased dreaming, nightmares, insomnia, tremor, diaphoresis, and vomiting, hallucinations, delirium, seizures, and status epilepticus.

• Skin eruptions may be a sign of a hypersensitivity reaction.

• Blood dyscrasias, hepatic disease, and hypocalcemia occur rarely.

• Overdose produces cold or clammy skin, hypothermia, severe CNS depression, cyanosis, tachycardia, and Cheyne-Stokes respirations.

• Toxicity may result in severe renal impairment.

INTERACTIONS

Drugs

▪ *Acetaminophen:* Enhanced hepatotoxic potential of acetaminophen overdoses

▪ *Antidepressants:* Reduced serum concentrations of cyclic antidepressants

▪ *β-blockers:* Reduced serum concentrations of β-blockers, which are extensively metabolized (metoprolol, propranolol, sotalol)

▪ *Calcium channel blockers:* Reduced concentrations of verapamil and nifedipine

▪ *Chloramphenicol:* Increased barbiturate concentrations; reduced serum chloramphenicol concentrations

▪ *Corticosteroids:* Reduced serum concentrations of corticosteroids, may impair therapeutic effect

▪ *Cyclosporine:* Reduced serum concentration of cyclosporine

▪ *Digitoxin:* Reduced serum concentration of digitoxin

▪ *Disopyramide:* Reduced serum concentration of disopyramide

▪ *Doxycycline:* Reduced serum doxycycline concentrations

▪ *Estrogen:* Reduced serum concentration of estrogen

▪ *Ethanol:* Excessive CNS depression

▪ *Felbamate:* Increased phenobarbital concentrations; increased risk of toxicity

▪ *Furosemide:* Decreased diuretic effect

▪ *Griseofulvin:* Reduced griseofulvin absorption

3 *Lamotrigine:* Lower lamotrigine plasma levels and decreased elimination t½
3 *Methoxyflurane:* Enhanced nephrotoxic effect
3 *Narcotic analgesics:* Increased toxicity of meperidine; reduced effect of methadone; additive CNS depression
3 *Neuroleptics:* Reduced effect of either drug
2 *Oral anticoagulants:* Decreased hypoprothrombinemic response to oral anticoagulants
3 *Oral contraceptives:* Reduced efficacy of oral contraceptives
3 *Phenytoin:* Unpredictable effect on serum phenytoin levels
3 *Primidone:* Excessive phenobarbital concentrations
3 *Propafenone:* Reduced serum concentration of propafenone
3 *Quinidine:* Reduced quinidine plasma concentration
3 *Tacrolimus:* Reduced serum concentration of tacrolimus
3 *Theophylline:* Reduced serum theophylline concentrations
3 *Valproic acid:* Increased serum phenobarbital concentrations
Labs
• *Amino acids:* Increase in urine collection measurements
• *Calcium:* False increases with Technicon SRA-2000
• *Glucose:* False negatives with Clinistix, Diastix
• *5-Hydroxyindoleacetic acid:* False high colorimetric values
• *Lactate dehydrogenase:* Increased serum levels
• *Protein:* False elevations at high concentrations

SPECIAL CONSIDERATIONS
PATIENT/FAMILY EDUCATION
• Avoid driving or other activities requiring alertness
• Avoid alcohol ingestion or CNS depressants
• Do not discontinue medication abruptly after long-term use

MONITORING PARAMETERS
• Periodic CBC, liver and renal function tests, serum folate, vitamin D during prolonged therapy
• Serum phenobarbital concentration (therapeutic range for seizure disorders 20-40 mcg/ml)

---

phenoxybenzamine
(fen-ox-ee-ben′za-meen)
Rx: Dibenzyline
Chemical Class: Haloalkylamine derivative
Therapeutic Class: Pheochromocytoma agent; sympatholytic

CLINICAL PHARMACOLOGY
Mechanism of Action: An antihypertensive that produces long-lasting noncompetitive alpha-adrenergic blockade of postganglionic synapses in exocrine glands and smooth muscles. Relaxes urethra and increases opening of the bladder.
Therapeutic Effect: Controls hypertension.

Pharmacokinetics
Well absorbed from the gastrointestinal (GI) tract. Distributed into fatty tissue. Metabolized in liver. Eliminated in urine and feces. Not removed by hemodialysis. **Half-life:** 24 hours.

INDICATIONS AND DOSAGES
Pheochromocytoma
PO
Adults. Initially, 10 mg twice daily. May increase dose every other day to 20-40 mg 2-3 times/day
Children. 1-2 mg/kg/day in divided doses.

💲 AVAILABLE FORMS/COST
• Cap, Gel—Oral: 10 mg, 100's: **$662.59**

UNLABELED USES: Bladder instability, complex regional pain syndrome (CRPS), contraception, prostatic obstruction, Raynaud's disease

CONTRAINDICATIONS: Any condition compromised by hypotension, hypersensitivity to phenoxybenzamine or any component of the formulation

PREGNANCY AND LACTATION: Pregnancy category C; indicated in hypertension secondary to pheochromocytoma during pregnancy, especially after 24 wk gestation when surgical intervention is associated with high rates of maternal and fetal mortality; no adverse fetal effects due to this treatment have been observed

SIDE EFFECTS

Frequent

Headache, lethargy, confusion, fatigue

Occasional

Nausea, postural hypotension, syncope, dry mouth

Rare

Palpitations, diarrhea, constipation, inhibition of ejaculation, weakness, altered vision, dizziness

SERIOUS REACTIONS

• Overdosage produces severe hypotension, irritability, lethargy, tachycardia, dizziness and shock.

SPECIAL CONSIDERATIONS

PATIENT/FAMILY EDUCATION

• Avoid alcohol; avoid sudden changes in posture, dizziness may result

• Avoid cough, cold, or allergy medications containing sympathomimetics

phentermine

Rx: Adipex-P, Ionamin, Pro-Fast SA

Chemical Class: Phenethylamine analog (amphetamine-like)

Therapeutic Class: Anorexiant

DEA Class: Schedule IV

CLINICAL PHARMACOLOGY

Mechanism of Action: A sympathomimetic amine structurally similar to dextroamphetamine and is most likely mediated via norephinephrine and dopamine metabolism. Causes stimulation of the hypothalamus. *Therapeutic Effect:* Decreased appetite.

Pharmacokinetics

Well absorbed from the gastrointestinal (GI) tract; resin absorbed slower. Excreted unchanged in urine. **Half-life:** 20 hrs.

INDICATIONS AND DOSAGES

Obesity

PO

Adults, Children older than 16 yrs.

Adipex-P: 37.5 mg as a single daily dose or in divided doses.

Ionamin: 15-37.5 mg/day before breakfast or 1-2 hrs. after breakfast.

Fastin: 30mg/day taken in the morning

§ **AVAILABLE FORMS/COST**

• Cap—Oral: 15 mg, 100's: **$68.48-$112.58**; 18.75 mg, 100's: **$30.95-$66.84**; 30 mg, 100's: **$11.96-$130.65**; 37.5 mg, 100's: **$38.95-$181.75**

• Cap, Sus Action—Oral: 15 mg, 100's: **$106.25**; 30 mg, 100's: **$242.44**

• Tab—Oral: 8 mg, 100's: **$15.65-$54.07**; 37.5 mg, 100's: **$23.00-$178.55**

CONTRAINDICATIONS: Advanced arteriosclerosis, agitated states, cardiovascular disease, concurrent use or within 14 days of discontinuation of MAOI therapy, glaucoma, history of drug abuse, hypertension (moderate-to-severe), hyperthyroidism, hypersensitivity to phentermine or sympathomimetic amines

PREGNANCY AND LACTATION: Pregnancy category C

SIDE EFFECTS
Occasional
Restlessness, insomnia, tremor, palpitations, tachycardia, elevation in blood pressure, headache, dizziness, dry mouth, unpleasant taste, diarrhea or constipation, changes in libido

SERIOUS REACTIONS
• Primary pulmonary hypertension (PPH), psychotic episodes, and valvular heart disease rarely occur.
• Anorectic agents have been associated with regurgitant multivalvular heart disease involving mitral, aortic, and/or tricuspid valves.
• Prolonged use may cause physical or psychological dependence.

INTERACTIONS
Drugs
3 *Furazolidone:* Increased pressor response
3 *Guanethidine:* Decreased hypotensive effect
⚠ *MAO Inhibitors:* Increased pressor response
3 *Tricyclic antidepressants:* Decreased anorexiant effect
Labs
• *Drugs of abuse:* Urine screen; false positive for amphetamines
• *Phenmetrazine:* False positive urine
• *Quinine:* False positive urine

phentolamine
(fen-tole'a-meen)
Rx: Regitine
Chemical Class: Imidazoline derivative
Therapeutic Class: Pheochromocytoma agent; sympatholytic

CLINICAL PHARMACOLOGY
Mechanism of Action: An alpha-adrenergic blocking agent which produces peripheral vasodilation and cardiac stimulation. *Therapeutic Effect:* Decreases blood pressure (BP).
Pharmacokinetics
Poorly absorbed from the gastrointestinal (GI) tract. Protein binding: 72%. Metabolized in liver. Eliminated in urine and feces. Not removed by hemodialysis. **Half-life:** 19 min.

INDICATIONS AND DOSAGES
Extravasation - norepinephrine
SC
Adults, Elderly. Infiltrate area with a small amount (1 ml) of solution (made by diluting 5-10 mg in 10 ml of NS) within 12 hours of extravasation. Do not exceed 0.1-0.2 mg/kg or 5 mg total. If dose is effective, normal skin color should return to the blanched area within 1 hour.
Children. Infiltrate area with a small amount (1 ml) of solution (made by diluting 5-10 mg in 10 ml of NS)

P

within 12 hours of extravasation. Do not exceed 0.1-0.2 mg/kg or 5 mg total.

Diagnosis of pheochromocytoma
IM/IV

Adults, Elderly. 5 mg as a single dose.

Children. 0.05-0.1 mg/kg/dose. Maximum single dose: 5 mg.

Surgery for pheochromocytoma: Hypertension
IM/IV

Adults, Elderly. 5 mg given 1-2 hours before procedure and repeated as needed every 2-4 hours.

Children. 0.05-0.1 mg/kg/dose given 1-2 hours before procedure. Repeat as needed every 2-4 hours until hypertension is controlled. Maximum single dose: 5 mg.

Hypertensive crisis
IV

Adults, Elderly. 5-20 mg as a single dose.

$ AVAILABLE FORMS/COST
• Powder, Inj—IM, IV: 5 mg/vial: **$35.00**

UNLABELED USES: Treatment of pralidoxime-induced hypertension, arrhythmias, asthma, bladder instability, cardiac diseases, diabetes mellitus, erectile dysfunction, extravasation (of dopamine and epinephrine), hyperhidrosis, myocardial infarction, Raynaud's phenomenon, surgery, sympathetic pain

CONTRAINDICATIONS: Renal impairment, coronary or cerebral arteriosclerosis, concurrent use with phosphodiesterase-5 (PDE-5) inhibitors including sildenafil (>25 mg), tadalafil, or vardenafil, hypersensitivity to phentolamine or related compounds.

PREGNANCY AND LACTATION: Pregnancy category C; unknown if excreted in breast milk

SIDE EFFECTS
Occasional

Hypotension, tachycardia, arrhythmia, flushing, orthostatic hypotension, weakness, dizziness, nausea, vomiting, diarrhea, nasal congestion, pulmonary hypertension

SERIOUS REACTIONS
• Symptoms of overdosage include tachycardia, shock, vomiting, and dizziness.

• Mixed agents, such as epinephrine, may cause more hypotension.

INTERACTIONS
Drugs

▣ *Epinepherine, ephedrine:* Vasoconstricting and hypertensive effects of these drugs are antagonized

Labs

• *5-hydroxyindoleacetic acid:* Urine, falsely high colorimetric values

SPECIAL CONSIDERATIONS
• Urinary catecholamines preferred over phentolamine for screening for pheochromocytoma

phenylephrine (systemic)

Rx: Neo-Synephrine, AH-Chew D

Combinations

Rx: with chlorpheniramine (Ed A-Hist, Prehist, Histatab); with brompheniramine (Dimetane); with chlorpheniramine, phenylpropanolamine (Hista-Vadrin); with chlorpheniramine, phenyltoloxamine (Comhist); with brompheniramine, phenylpropanolamine (Bromophen T.D., Tamine S.R.); with chlorpheniramine, phenyltoloxamine, phenylpropanolamine (Decongestabs, Naldecon, Nalgest, Tri-phen, Uni-decon); with chlorpheniramine, pyrilamine, phenylpropanolamine (Vanex, Histalet); with chlorpheniramine, pyrilamine (R-tannate, Rhinatate, R-tannamine, Rynatan, Tanoral, Triotann, Tritan, Tri-tannate)

Chemical Class: Substituted phenylethylamine
Therapeutic Class: Vasopressor

CLINICAL PHARMACOLOGY
Mechanism of Action: Phenylephrine is a powerful postsynaptic alpha-receptor stimulant with little effect on the beta receptors of the heart, lacking chronotropic and inotropic actions on the heart. *Therapeutic effect:* Vasoconstriction, decreases heart rate, increases stroke output, increases blood pressure

Pharmacokinetics
Phenylephrine is irregularly absorbed from and readily metabolized in the GI tract. After IV administration, a pressor effect occurs almost immediately and persists for 15-20 minutes. After IM administration, a pressor effect occurs within 10-15 minutes and persists for 50 minutes to 1 hour. After oral inhalation of phenylephrine in combination with isoproterenol, pulmonary effects occur within a few minutes and persist for about 3 hours. The pharmacologic effects of phenylephrine are terminated at least partially by the uptake of the drug into the tissues. Phenylephrine is metabolized in the liver and intestine by the enzyme monoamine oxidase (MAO). The metabolites and their route and rate of excretion have not been identified.

INDICATIONS AND DOSAGES
Paroxysmal supraventricular tachycardia (PSVT)
Adults. The initial dose, given by rapid IV injection, should not exceed 0.5 mg. Subsequent doses may be increased in increments of 0.1 to 0.2 mg. Maximum single dose is 1 mg IV.

Children. 5 to 10 mcg/kg IV over 20-30 seconds.

Mild to Moderate Hypotension
SC/IM

Adults. 2-5 mg IM or SC (range 1-10 mg), repeated no more than every 10-15 minutes. Maximum initial IM or SC dose is 5 mg.

Children. 0.1 mg/kg IM or SC every 1-2 hours as needed. Maximum dose is 5 mg.

IV

Adults. 0.2 mg IV (range 0.1 to 0.5 mg), given no more frequently than every 10-15 minutes. Maximum initial IV dose is 0.5 mg.

P

Severe Hypotension or Shock
IV

Adults. Initially, 100-180 mcg/min IV infusion, with dose titration to the desired MAP and SVR. A maintenance infusion rate of 40-60 mcg/min IV is usually adequate after blood pressure stabilizes. If necessary to produce the desired pressor response, additional phenylephrine in increments of 10 mg or more may be added to the infusion solution and the rate of flow adjusted according to the response of the patient.

Children. 5-20 mcg/kg IV bolus, followed by an initial IV infusion of 0.1 to 0.5 mcg/kg/min, titrated to desired effect. Doses up to 3-5 mcg/kg/min IV may be required.

Hypotensive emergencies during spinal anesthesia
IV

Adults. Initially, 0.2 mg IV. Subsequent doses should not exceed the previous dose by more than 0.1 to 0.2 mg. Maximum of 0.5 mg per dose.

Hypotension during spinal anesthesia in children
IM/SC

Children. A dose of 0.044 to 0.088 mg/kg IM or SC is recommended by the manufacturer.

Hypotension prophylaxis during spinal anesthesia
IM/SC

Adults. 2 to 3 mg SC or IM, 3 or 4 minutes before anesthesia. A dose of 2 mg SC or IM is usually adequate with low spinal anesthesia, 3 mg IM or SC may be necessary with high spinal anesthesia.

Vasoconstriction in regional anesthesia
IV

Adults. The manufacturer states that the optimum concentration of phenylephrine HCl is 0.05 mg/ml (1:20,000). Solutions may be prepared for regional anesthesia by adding 1 mg of phenylephrine HCl to each 20 ml of local anesthesia solution. Some pressor response can be expected when at least 2 mg is injected.

Prolongation of spinal anesthesia.
IV

Adults. The addition of 2-5 mg added to the anesthetic solution increases the duration of motor block by as much as 50% without an increase in the incidence of complications such as nausea, vomiting, or blood pressure disturbances.

Hypotension during special anesthesia in children.
IM/SC

Children. A dose of 0.5 mg to 1 mg per 25 pounds body weight, administered subcutaneously or IM, is recommended.

AVAILABLE FORMS/COST
• Sol, Inj—IM, IV, SC: 10 mg/ml, 1 ml: **$0.75-$4.39**
• Liq—Oral: 5 mg/5 ml, 120 ml: **$10.98**
• Supp—Rect: 0.25% 12's: **$5.50**
• Tab, chewable—Oral: 10 mg, 100's: **$76.80**

CONTRAINDICATIONS: Phenylephrine HCl injection should not be used with patients with severe hypertension, ventricular tachycardia or fibrillation, acute myocardial infarction (MI), atrial flutter or fibrillation, cardiac arrhythmias, cardiac disease, cardiomyopathy, closed-angle glaucoma, coronary artery disease, women who are in labor, during obstetric delivery, or in patients who have a known hypersensitivity to phenylephrine, sulfitres, or to any one of its components.

PREGNANCY AND LACTATION: Pregnancy category C; unknown if excreted in breast milk

SIDE EFFECTS
Occasional

Headache, reflex bradycardia, excitability, restlessness, and rarely arrhythmias.

SERIOUS REACTIONS

• Overdose may induce ventricular extrasystoles and short paroxysms of ventricular tachycardia, a sensation of fullness in the head and tingling of the extremities. Should an excessive elevation of blood pressure occur, it may be immediately relieved by an α-adrenergic blocking agent, e.g., phentolamine. The oral LD_{50} in the rat is 350 mg/kg, in the mouse 120 mg/kg.

INTERACTIONS
Drugs

▣ *β-Blockers (non-selective):* Predisposed to hypertensive episodes

▣ *Guanethidine:* Enhanced pupillary response to phenylephrine

▣ *Imipramine:* Enhanced pressor response

⚠ *MAOIs:* Hypertensive episodes

Labs

• *Amino acids:* Increased in urine
• *Metanephrines, total:* Increased in urine

SPECIAL CONSIDERATIONS

• Antidote to extravasation: 5-10 ml phentolamine in 10-15 ml saline infiltrated throughout ischemic area
• Not indicated for hypotension secondary to hypovolemia
• As not bioavailable orally (see pharmacokinetics), combination products essentially lack decongestant. Only available by prescription, as lack effectiveness data required by FDA OTC panels

phenylephrine (topical)

Rx: *Ophthalmic:* Ak-Dilate, Ak-Nefrin, Mydfrin, Neo-Synephrine, Prefrin Liquifilm, Relief
OTC: *Nasal:* Afrin Children's Pump Mist, 4-way Fast Acting Vicks Sinex, Little Noses Gentle formula, Neo-Synephrine, Rhinall
OTC: *Anorectal:* Medicone, Hem-Prep
Combinations
  Rx: (Nasal): with zinc (Zincfrin); with pheniramine (Dristan Nasal);
  Rx: (Ophthalmic); with tropicamide (Diophenyl-t); with pyrilamine (Prefrin-A)
Chemical Class: Substituted phenylethylamine
Therapeutic Class: Decongestant; mydriatic

CLINICAL PHARMACOLOGY

Mechanism of Action: Phenylephrine HCl is an alpha receptor sympathetic agonist used in local ocular disorders because of its vasoconstrictor and mydriatic action. It exhibits rapid and moderately prolonged action, and it produces little rebound vasodilatation. Systemic side effects are uncommon. *Therapeutic effect:* Vasoconstriction and pupil dilation.

Pharmacokinetics

Some absorption systemically. The duration of action of intranasal administration ranges from 30 minutes to 4 hours. The duration of the mydriatic effect is roughly 3 hours after administration of the 2.5% solution but may be as long as 7 hours after the 10% solution.

INDICATIONS AND DOSAGES
Mydriasis induction (ophthalmic)
Topical

Adults, Adolescents, Elderly. Instill 1 or 2 drops of a 2.5% or 10% solution in eye before procedure. May be repeated in 10-60 minutes if needed. In general, the 2.5% solution is preferred in the elderly to avoid cardiac reactions.

Children. Instill 1 or 2 drops of a 2.5% solution in the eye before procedure. May be repeated in 10-60 minutes if needed.

Infants < 1 year. 1 drop of 2.5% solution 15-30 minutes before procedure.

Uveitis (Posterior Synechia)
Topical

Adults, Elderly. Instill 1 drop of 10% solution in eye 3 or more times daily with atropine sulfate. In general, the 2.5% solution is preferred in elderly to avoid adverse cardiac reactions.

Adults and children over age 12 (intranasal): Apply 2-3 drops or 1-2 sprays of a 0.25% to 0.5% solution instilled in each nostril or a small quantity of 0.5% nasal jelly applied into each nostril. Apply every 4 hours as needed. The 1% solution may be used in adults with severe congestion.

Children 6-12 years (intranasal): 2-3 drops of the 0.25% solution in each nostril every 4 hours as needed.

Children < 6 years (intranasal): Apply 2-3 drops or sprays of a 0.125% or 0.16% solution in each nostril every 4 hours as needed.

Infants > 6 months (intranasal): 1 to 2 drops of the 0.16% solution in each nostril every 3 hours.

Conjunctival Congestion
Topical

Adults, Elderly.: 1 to 2 drops of a 0.12% to 0.25% solution applied to the conjunctiva every 3 to 4 hours as needed. In general, the 2.5% solution is preferred in elderly to avoid cardiac reactions.

Postoperative Malignant Glaucoma
Topical

Adults, Elderly. Instill 1 drop of a 10% solution with 1 drop of a 1% to 4% solution 3 or more times per day. In general, the 2.5% solution is preferred in elderly to avoid cardiac reactions.

Vasoconstriction and Pupil Dilatation
Topical

Adults. A drop of a suitable topical anesthetic may be applied, followed in a few minutes by 1 drop of the on the upper limbus.

Surgery
Topical

Adults. When a short-acting mydriatic is needed for wide dilatation of the pupil before intraocular surgery, phenylephrine HCl 2.5% (or the 10%) may be applied topically from 30 to 60 minutes before the operation.

Cycloplegia
Topical

Adults. One drop of the preferred cycloplegic is placed in each eye, followed in 5 minutes by one drop of phenylephrine HCl 2.5%.

Children. For a "one application method," phenylephrine HCl 2.5% may be combined with one of the preferred rapid acting cycloplegics to produce adequate cycloplegia.

Ophthalmoscopic Examination
Topical

Adults. One drop of phenylephrine HCl 2.5% is placed in each eye.

Blanching Test
Topical

Adults. One or two drops of phenylephrine HCl 2.5% should be applied to the injected eye.

Glaucoma
Topical

Adults. In certain patients with glaucoma, temporary reduction of intraocular tension may be attained by producing vasoconstriction of the intraocular vessels; this may be accompanied by placing 1 drop of the 10 % solution on the upper surface of the cornea. This treatment may be repeated as often as necessary.

Nasal Congestion
Intranasal

Adults, Children 12 and older. Use 2 or 3 drops or sprays of a 0.25 to 0.5% solution in the nose every 4 hours as needed

Children 6 to 12 years. Use 2 or 3 drops or sprays of a 0.25% solution in the nose every 4 hours as needed.

Children 2 to 6 years. Use 2 or 3 drops of a 0.125 to 0.16% solution in the nose every 4 hours as needed.

Ⓢ AVAILABLE FORMS/COST

• Sol—Nasal: 0.125% drops, 15 ml: **$3.38**; 0.25% drops, 15 ml: **$3.49-$5.36**; 0.5% drops, 15 ml: **$3.49**; 0.5% spray, 15 ml: **$3.49-$5.58**; 1% drops, 15 ml: **$3.95**
• Sol—Ophth: 0.125%, 15 ml: **$3.56-$10.00**; 2.5%, 5 ml: **$2.63-$18.00**; 10%, 5 ml: **$3.00-$29.15**

CONTRAINDICATIONS: Ophthalmic solutions, (both strengths), of phenylephrine HCl are contraindicated in patients with anatomically narrow angles or narrow angle glaucoma, some low birth weight infants and some elderly adults with severe arteriosclerotic cardiovascular or cerebrovascular disease, use during intraocular operative procedures when the corneal epithelial barrier has been disturbed, and in persons with a known sensitivity to phenylephrine, sulfites, or any of its components including preservatives. The 10% solution is contraindicated in infants and in patients with aneurysms.

PREGNANCY AND LACTATION: Pregnancy category C; no breastfeeding data, use caution

SIDE EFFECTS
Frequent

Burning or stinging or eyes, headache or browache, sensitivity to light, watering of the eyes, increase in runny or stuffy nose, burning, stinging, dryness of inside the nose

Occasional

Rare

Irritation, dizziness, fast and/or irregular and/or pounding heartbeat, increased sweating, increase in blood pressure, paleness, trembling, headache, nervousness, trouble sleeping

SERIOUS REACTIONS

• There have been reports associating the use of phenylephrine HCl 10% ophthalmic solutions with the development of serious cardiovascular reactions, including ventricular arrhythmias and myocardial infarctions. These episodes, some ending fatally, have usually occurred in elderly patients with preexisting cardiovascular diseases.

INTERACTIONS

• See interactions under systemic phenylephrine; interactions less likely than with systemic administration if given in proper dosage

SPECIAL CONSIDERATIONS

• Do not administer for more than 3-5 days (nasal product) or 2-3 days (ocular product used as decongestant) due to rebound congestion

P

phenytoin/ fosphenytoin

(fen'-i-toy-in / fos-fen'-i-toy-in)

Rx: Dilantin (phenytoin)
Rx: Cerebyx (fosphenytoin)
Chemical Class: Hydantoin derivative
Therapeutic Class: Anticonvulsant

CLINICAL PHARMACOLOGY

Mechanism of Action: An anticonvulsant and antiarrhythmic agent that stabilizes neuronal membranes in motor cortex, and decreases abnormal ventricular automaticity. *Therapeutic Effect:* Limits spread of seizure activity. Stabilizes threshold against hyperexcitability. Decreases posttetanic potentiation and repetitive discharge. Shortens refractory period, QT interval, and action potential duration.

Pharmacokinetics

Phenytoin

Slowly, variably absorbed after PO administration; slow but completely absorbed after IM administration. Protein binding: 90%-95%. Widely distributed. Metabolized in liver. Primarily excreted in urine. Not removed by hemodialysis. **Half-life:** 22 hrs.

Fosphenytoin

Completely absorbed after IM administration. Protein binding: 95%-99%. After IM or IV administration, rapidly and completely hydrolyzed to phenytoin. Time of complete conversion to phenytoin: IM: 4 hrs after injection; IV: 2 hrs after the end of infusion. **Half-life** for conversion to phenytoin: 8-15 min.

INDICATIONS AND DOSAGES

Phenytoin

Status epilepticus. IV: *Adults, Elderly, Children.* Loading dose: 15-18 mg/kg. Maintenance dose: 300 mg/day in 2-3 divided doses. *Children 10-16 yrs.* Loading dose: 15-18 mg/kg. Maintenance dose: 6-7 mg/kg/day. *Children 7-9 yrs.* Loading dose: 15-18 mg/kg. Maintenance dose 7-8 mg/kg/day. *Children 4-6 yrs.* Loading dose: 15-18 mg/kg. Maintenance dose: 7.5-9 mg/kg/day. *Children 6 mos-3 yrs.* Loading dose 15-18 mg/kg. Maintenance dose: 8-10 mg/kg/day. Neonates. Loading dose: 15-20 mg/kg. Maintenance dose: 5-8 mg/kg/day.

Fosphenytoin

IV

Adults. Loading dose: 15-20 mg PE/kg infused at rate of 100-150 mg PE/min.

Nonemergent seizures: IV: *Adults.* Loading dose: 10-20 mg PE/kg. Maintenance: 4-6 mg PE/kg/day.

Anticonvulsant: PO: *Adults, Elderly, Children.* Loading dose: 15-20 mg/kg in 3 divided doses 2-4 hrs apart. Maintenance dose: Same as above.

Arrhythmias: IV: *Adults, Elderly, Children.* Loading dose: 1.25 mg/kg q5min. May repeat to total dose of 15 mg/kg. PO: *Adults, Elderly.* Maintenance Dose: 250 mg 4 times/day for 1 day, then 250 mg 2 times/day for 2 days, then 300-400 mg/day in divided doses 1-4 times/day. PO/IV: *Children.* Maintenance dose: 5-10 mg/kg/day in 2-3 divided doses.

$ AVAILABLE FORMS/COST

Phenytoin

• Cap, Gel—Oral: 100 mg, 100's: **$19.80-$21.72**

• Cap, Sus Action: 30 mg, 100's: **$27.46**; 100 mg, 100's: **$29.88-$44.90**; 200 mg, 100's: **$56.75**; 300 mg, 100's: **$85.12**

• Sol, Inj—IM, IV: 50 mg/ml, 2 ml: **$1.51-$2.38**

• Susp—Oral: 125 mg/5 ml, 240 ml: **$33.30-$34.10**

• Tab, Chewable—Oral: 50 mg, 100's: **$28.48**

Fosphenytoin

• Sol, Inj—IV, IM: 150 mg (100 mg phenytoin sodium)/2 ml: **$21.98**

UNLABELED USES: Phenytoin Adjunct in treatment of tricyclic antidepressant toxicity, muscle relaxant in treatment of muscle hyperirritability, treatment of digoxin-induced arrhythmias and trigeminal neuralgia

CONTRAINDICATIONS: Hydantoin hypersensitivity, seizures due to hypoglycemia, Adam-Stokes syndrome, second- and third-degree heart block, sinoatrial block, sinus bradycardia

PREGNANCY AND LACTATION: Pregnancy category D (risk of congenital defects increased 2-3 times; fetal hydantoin syndrome includes craniofacial abnormalities, hypoplasia, ossification of distal phalanges; may also be transplacental carcinogen); compatible with breastfeeding

SIDE EFFECTS

Frequent

Drowsiness, lethargy, confusion, slurred speech, irritability, gingival hyperplasia, hypersensitivity reaction, including fever, rash, and lymphadenopathy, constipation, dizziness, nausea

Occasional

Headache, hair growth, insomnia, muscle twitching

SERIOUS REACTIONS

• Abrupt withdrawal may precipitate status epilepticus.

• Blood dyscrasias, lymphadenopathy, and osteomalacia, caused by interference of vitamin D metabolism, may occur.

• Toxic phenytoin blood concentration of 25 mcg/ml may produce ataxia, characterized by muscular incoordination, nystagmus or rhythmic oscillation of eyes, and double vision. As level increases, extreme lethargy to comatose states occur.

INTERACTIONS

Drugs

③ *Acetaminophen:* Enhances the hepatotoxic potential of acetaminophen overdoses; may reduce the therapeutic response to acetaminophen

③ *Acetazolamide:* Osteomalacia

③ *Amiodarone:* Increased phenytoin levels; decreased amiodarone levels

③ *Azole-antifungals (fluconazole):* Phenytoin induces metabolism (CYP3A4) reducing antifungal effects

③ *Benzodiazepines (alprazolam, diazepam, midazolam, triazolam):* Enhanced metabolism (CYP3A4) phenytoin reduces benzodiazepine effects

③ *Carbamazepine:* Combined use usually decreases levels of both drugs

③ *Chloramphenicol, disulfiram, fluoxetine, isoniazid, omeprazole, sulfonamides:* Increased phenytoin levels

③ *Cimetidine, cisplatin, diazoxide, folate, rifampin:* Decreased phenytoin levels

③ *Clozapine:* Reduced levels via phenytoin induced enhanced metabolism

③ *Corticosteroids:* Decreased therapeutic effect of steroids

③ *Cyclic antidepressants:* Increased antidepressant levels

P

③ *Cyclosporine:* Reduced cyclosporine levels

③ *Dicumarol:* Increased anticoagulant effect, increased phenytoin levels

③ *Digitalis glycosides:* Lower digitalis levels

③ *Disopyramide:* Reduced efficacy, increased toxicity of disopyramide

③ *Dopamine:* More susceptible to hypotension after IV phenytoin

③ *Doxycycline:* Reduced doxycycline concentrations

③ *Felbamate:* Felbamate consistently increases phenytoin levels

③ *Furosemide:* Decreased diuretic effect

② *Itraconazole:* Phenytoin induces metabolism (CYP3A4) reducing antifungal effects

③ *Lamotrigine:* Phenytoin stimulates metabolism-lower plasma levels; decreased $t_{1/2}$

③ *Levodopa:* Decreased antiparkinsonian effect

③ *Lithium:* Increased risk of lithium intoxication; causal explanation not known

② *Mebendazole in high doses:* Decreased mebendazole levels

② *Methadone:* Withdrawal

③ *Metyrapone:* Invalidates test

③ *Mexiletine:* Decreased mexiletine levels

③ *Oral contraceptives:* Decreased contraceptive effect

③ *Primidone:* Enhanced conversion to phenobarbital

③ *Pyridoxine:* Large doses may decrease phenytoin levels

③ *Quinidine:* Decreased quinidine levels

③ *Quinolone antibiotics (ciprofloxacin, enoxacin, norfloxacin):* Elevates phenytoin concentrations

③ *Sucralfate:* Phenytoin reduces GI absorption

③ *Tacrolimus:* Reduced tacrolimus levels

③ *Theophylline:* Reduced theophylline levels

③ *Thyroid hormone:* Increased thyroid replacement dose requirements

③ *Tolbutamide:* Phenytoin inhibits insulin release, may result in hyperglycemia; tolbutamide displaces phenytoin from protein-binding sites; monitor for alterations in glucose control

③ *Trimethoprim:* Increased phenytoin concentrations

③ *Valproic acid:* Variable effects on phenytoin levels; decreased valproic acid levels

③ *Warfarin:* Transient increased hypoprothrombinemic response followed by inhibition of hypoprothrombinemic response

Labs

• *False positive:* Barbiturates, urine
• *Increased:* Cholesterol, serum; thyroxine, serum

SPECIAL CONSIDERATIONS

• Pro-drug, fosphenytoin rapidly converted to phenytoin *in vivo:* minimal activity before conversion; water soluble, thus more suitable for parenteral applications: does not require cardiac monitoring; can be administered at faster rate; no IV filter required; compatible with both saline and dextrose mixtures; requires refrigeration

MONITORING PARAMETERS

• Therapeutic range 10-20 mcg/ml; nystagmus appears at 20 mcg/ml, ataxia at 30 mcg/ml, dysarthria and lethargy at levels above 40 mcg/ml; lethal dose 2-5 g

phosphorated carbohydrate solution

OTC: Emetrol, Formula EM, Nausea Relief, Nausetrol
Chemical Class: Hyperosmolar carbohydrate with phosphoric acid
Therapeutic Class: Antiemetic

CLINICAL PHARMACOLOGY
Mechanism of Action: An antiemetic whose mechanism of action has not been determined. Phosphorated carbohydrate solution consists of fructose, dextrose, and phosphoric acid, and may directly act on the wall of the gastrointestinal (GI) tract and reduce smooth muscle contraction and delays gastric emptying time through high osmotic pressure exerted by the solution of simple sugars. *Therapeutic Effect:* Relieves nausea and vomiting.
Pharmacokinetics
Fructose
Fructose is slowly absorbed from the gastrointestinal (GI) tract. Metabolized in liver by phosphorylation and partly converted to liver glycogen and glucose. Excreted in urine.
Dextrose
Dextrose is rapidly absorbed from GI tract. Distributed and stored throughout tissues. Metabolized in liver to carbon dioxide and water.

INDICATIONS AND DOSAGES
Antiemetic
PO
Adults, Elderly. 15-30 ml initially. May repeat dose every 15 minutes until distress subsides. Maximum: 5 doses in a 1 hr period

Children 3 yrs and older. 5-15 ml initially. May repeat dose every 15 minutes until distress subsides. Maximum: 5 doses in a 1 hr period

§ **AVAILABLE FORMS/COST**
• Sol—Oral: 1.87 g dextrose/1.87 g fructose/21.5 mg phosphoric acid; 120, 236, 473 ml: **$2.06-$50.50**/120 ml

CONTRAINDICATIONS: Symptoms of appendicitis or inflamed bowel, hereditary fructose intolerance, hypersensitivity to any component of the formulation
PREGNANCY AND LACTATION: Pregnancy category B; used to treat morning sickness
SIDE EFFECTS
Frequent
Diarrhea, abdominal pain
SERIOUS REACTIONS
• Fructose intolerance includes symptoms of fainting, swelling of face, arms and legs, unusual bleeding, vomiting, weight loss, and yellow eyes and skin.
SPECIAL CONSIDERATIONS
PATIENT/FAMILY EDUCATION
• Seek medical attention if symptoms are not relieved or recur frequently

physostigmine
(fi-zoe-stig'meen)
Rx: Antilirium
Chemical Class: Alkaloid; cholinesterase inhibitor; tertiary ammonium compound
Therapeutic Class: Antiglaucoma agent; cholinergic; miotic; ophthalmic cholinergic

CLINICAL PHARMACOLOGY
Mechanism of Action: A cholinergic that inhibits destruction of acetylcholine by enzyme acetylcho-

linesterase, thus enhancing impulse transmission across the myoneural junction. *Therapeutic Effect:* Improves skeletal muscle tone, stimulates salivary and sweat gland secretions.

INDICATIONS AND DOSAGES

To reverse CNS effects of anticholinergic drugs and tricyclic antidepressants

IV, IM

Adults, Elderly. Initially, 0.5–2 mg. If no response, repeat q20min until response or adverse cholinergic effects occur. If initial response occurs, may give additional doses of 1–4 mg q30-60min as life-threatening signs, such as arrhythmias, seizures, and deep coma, recur.

Children. 0.01–0.03 mg/kg. May give additional doses q5-10min until response or adverse cholinergic effects occur or total dose of 2 mg given.

Ⓢ **AVAILABLE FORMS/COST**

• Sol, Inj—IM, IV: 1 mg/ml, 2 ml: **$4.86**

UNLABELED USES: Treatment of hereditary ataxia

CONTRAINDICATIONS: Active uveal inflammation, angle-closure glaucoma before iridectomy, asthma, cardiovascular disease, concurrent use of ganglionic-blocking agents, diabetes, gangrene, glaucoma associated with iridocyclitis, hypersensitivity to cholinesterase inhibitors or their components, mechanical obstruction of intestinal or urogenital tract, vagotonic state

PREGNANCY AND LACTATION: Pregnancy category C; no data on breast-feeding available

SIDE EFFECTS

Expected

Miosis, increased GI and skeletal muscle tone, bradycardia

Occasional

Marked drop in BP (hypertensive patients)

Rare

Allergic reaction

SERIOUS REACTIONS

• Parenteral overdose produces a cholinergic crisis manifested as abdominal discomfort or cramps, nausea, vomiting, diarrhea, flushing, facial warmth, excessive salivation, diaphoresis, urinary urgency, and blurred vision. If overdose occurs, stop all anticholinergic drugs and immediately and administer 0.6–1.2 mg atropine sulfate IM or IV for adults, or 0.01 mg/kg for infants and children younger than 12 years.

INTERACTIONS

Drugs

③ *β-blockers:* Additive bradycardia

SPECIAL CONSIDERATIONS

• Atropine is antidote

---

phytonadione; vitamin K$_1$

(fye-toe-na-dye′one)

Rx: AquaMEPHYTON, Mephyton

Chemical Class: Naphthoquinone derivative

Therapeutic Class: Antihemorrhagic; vitamin

CLINICAL PHARMACOLOGY

Mechanism of Action: A fat-soluble vitamin that promotes hepatic formation of coagulation factors II, VII, IX, and X. *Therapeutic Effect:* Essential for normal clotting of blood.

Pharmacokinetics

Readily absorbed from the GI tract (duodenum) after IM or subcutaneous administration. Metabolized in the liver. Excreted in urine; eliminated by biliary system. Onset of action: with PO form, 6-10 hr; with parenteral form, hemorrhage controlled in 3–6 hr and PT returns to normal in 12–14 hr.

INDICATIONS AND DOSAGES
Oral anticoagulant overdose
PO, IV, Subcutaneous

Adults, Elderly. 2.5–10 mg/dose. May repeat in 12–48 hr if given orally and in 6–8 hr if given by IV or subcutaneous route.

Children. 0.5–5 mg depending on need for further anticoagulation and severity of bleeding.

Vitamin K deficiency
PO

Adults, Elderly. 2.5–25 mg/24 hr.
Children. 2.5–5 mg/24 hr.

IV, IM, Subcutaneous
Adults, Elderly. 10 mg/dose.
Children. 1–2 mg/dose.

Hemorrhagic disease of newborn
IM, Subcutaneous

Neonate. Treatment: 1–2 mg/dose/day. Prophylaxis: 0.5–1 mg within 1 hr of birth; may repeat in 6–8 hr if necessary.

$ AVAILABLE FORMS/COST
• Emulsion, Inj—IM, IV, SC: 1 mg/0.5 ml: **$2.58-$2.71**; 10 mg/ml, 1 ml: **$5.02-$5.18**
• Tab—Oral: 5 mg, 100's: **$65.33**

CONTRAINDICATIONS: None known.

PREGNANCY AND LACTATION: Pregnancy category C; oral supplementation of women on anticonvulsants during last 2 weeks of pregnancy has been done to prevent HDN, but effectiveness unproven; compatible with breast-feeding

SIDE EFFECTS
Occasional

Pain, soreness, and swelling at IM injection site; pruritic erythema (with repeated injections); facial flushing; unusual taste

SERIOUS REACTIONS
• Newborns (especially premature infants) may develop hyperbilirubinemia.
• A severe reaction (cramplike pain, chest pain, dyspnea, facial flushing, dizziness, rapid or weak pulse, rash, diaphoresis, hypotension progressing to shock, cardiac arrest) occurs rarely just after IV administration.

INTERACTIONS
Drugs
③ *Oral anticoagulants:* Decreased anticoagulant effect

SPECIAL CONSIDERATIONS
• IV doses should be diluted and infused slowly over 20-30 min

---

pilocarpine hydrochloride
(pye-loe-kar'peen)

Rx: *Ophthalmic:* Akarpine, Isopto Carpine, Ocusert Piol-20Pilocar, Pilopine-HS

Rx: *Oral:* Salagen
Combinations
  Rx: with epinephrine (E-Pilo-6)

Chemical Class: Choline ester
Therapeutic Class: Antiglaucoma agent; miotic; ophthalmic cholinergic; salivation stimulant

---

CLINICAL PHARMACOLOGY
Mechanism of Action: A cholinergic that increases exocrine gland secretions by stimulating cholinergic receptors. *Therapeutic Effect:* Improves symptoms of dry mouth in patients with salivary gland hypofunction.

Pharmacokinetics

Route	Onset	Peak	Duration
PO	20 min	1 hr	3–5 hrs

P

Absorption decreased if taken with a high-fat meal. Inactivation of pilocarpine thought to occur at neuronal synapses and probably in plasma. Excreted in urine. **Half-life:** 4-12 hr.

INDICATIONS AND DOSAGES
Dry mouth associated with radiation treatment for head and neck cancer
PO
Adults, Elderly. 5 mg three times a day. Range: 15-30 mg/day. Maximum: 2 tablets/dose.

Dry mouth associated with Sjögren's syndrome
PO
Adults, Elderly. 5 mg four times a day. Range: 20–40 mg/day.

Dosage in hepatic impairment
Dosage decreased to 5 mg twice a day for adults and elderly with hepatic impairment.

$ AVAILABLE FORMS/COST
• Gel—Ophth: 4%, 3.5 g: **$41.00**
• Insert—Ophth: 20 mcg/hr, 8's: **$51.55**; 40 mcg/hr, 8's: **$45.13**
• Sol, Ophth: 0.25%, 15 ml: **$17.25**; 0.5%, 15 ml: **$1.68-$11.62**; 1%, 15 ml: **$1.95-$23.81**; 2%, 15 ml: **$2.02-$24.31**; 3%, 15 ml: **$2.17-$12.75**; 4%, 15 ml: **$2.35-$25.63**; 5%, 15 ml: **$2.60-$10.00**; 6%, 15 ml: **$2.95-$21.35**; 8%, 15 ml: **$28.92**
• Tab, Coated—Oral: 5 mg, 100's: **$162.00**

CONTRAINDICATIONS: Conditions in which miosis is undesirable, such as acute iritis and angle-closure glaucoma; uncontrolled asthma

PREGNANCY AND LACTATION: Pregnancy category C

SIDE EFFECTS
Frequent (29%)
Diaphoresis
Occasional (11%–05%)
Headache, dizziness, urinary frequency, flushing, dyspepsia, nausea, asthenia, lacrimation, visual disturbances

Rare (less than 4%)
Diarrhea, abdominal pain, peripheral edema, chills

SERIOUS REACTIONS
• Patients with diaphoresis who do not drink enough fluids may develop dehydration.

SPECIAL CONSIDERATIONS
• Antidote is atropine

PATIENT/FAMILY EDUCATION
• Miotics cause poor dark adaptation; use caution with night driving

---

pimecrolimus
(pim-eh-crow-leh-mus)
Rx: Elidel
Chemical Class: Ascomycin derivative
Therapeutic Class: Immunosuppressant

CLINICAL PHARMACOLOGY
Mechanism of Action: An immunomodulator that inhibits release of cytokine, an enzyme that produces an inflammatory reaction. *Therapeutic Effect:* Produces anti-inflammatory activity.

Pharmacokinetics
Minimal systemic absorption with topical application. Metabolized in liver. Excreted in feces.

INDICATIONS AND DOSAGES
Atopic dermatitis (eczema)
Topical
Adults, Elderly, Children 2-17 yrs. Apply to affected area twice daily for up to 3 weeks (up to 6 weeks in adolescents, children 2-17 yrs). Rub in gently and completely.

$ AVAILABLE FORMS/COST
• Cre—Top: 1%, 15, 30, 60, 100 g: **$53.95**/30 g

UNLABELED USES: Allergic contact dermatitis, irritant contact dermatitis, psoriasis

CONTRAINDICATIONS: Hypersensitivity to pimecrolimus or any component of the formulation, Netherton's Syndrome (potential for increased systemic absorption), application to active cutaneous viral infections.

PREGNANCY AND LACTATION: Pregnancy category C; excretion into breast milk unknown, use caution in nursing mothers

SIDE EFFECTS

Rare

Transient application-site sensation of burning or feeling of heat

SERIOUS REACTIONS

• Lymphadenopathy and phototoxicity occur rarely.

INTERACTIONS

Drugs

③ Erythromycin, itraconazole, ketoconazole, fluconazole, calcium channel blockers, cimetidine: Theoretical increase in pimecrolimus concentrations

SPECIAL CONSIDERATIONS

• May be associated with increased risk of varicella zoster virus infection, herpes simplex virus infection or eczema herpeticum

PATIENT/FAMILY EDUCATION

• Do not use with occlusive dressings

---

pimozide
(pi'moe-zide)
Rx: Orap
Chemical Class: Diphenylbutylpiperidine derivative
Therapeutic Class: Antipsychotic

CLINICAL PHARMACOLOGY

Mechanism of Action: A diphenylbutylpiperidine that blocks dopamine at postsynaptic receptor sites in the brain. *Therapeutic Effect:* Suppresses behavioral response in psychosis.

INDICATIONS AND DOSAGES

Tourette's disorder

PO

Adults, Elderly. 1-2 mg/day in divided doses 3 times/day. Maximum: 10 mg/day.

Children older than 12 yrs. Initially, 0.5 mg/kg/day. Maximum: 10 mg/day.

Ⓢ **AVAILABLE FORMS/COST**

• Tab—Oral: 1 mg, 100's: **$89.23**; 2 mg, 100's: **$118.96**

CONTRAINDICATIONS: Aggressive schizophrenics when sedation is required, concurrent administration of pemoline, methylphenidate or amphetamines, concurrent administration with dofetilide, sotalol, quinidine, other Class IA and III anti-arrhythmics, mesoridazine, thioridazine, chlorpromazine, droperidol, sparfloxacin, gatifloxacin, moxifloxacin, halofantrine, mefloquine, pentamidine, arsenic trioxide, levomethadyl acetate, dolasetron mesylate, probucol, tacrolimus, ziprasidone, sertraline, macrolide antibiotics, drugs that cause QT prolongation, and less potent inhibitors of CYP3A, congenital or drug-induced long QT syndrome, doses greater than 10 mg daily day, history of cardiac arrhythmias, Parkinson's disease, patients with known hypokalemia or hypomagnesemia, severe central nervous system depression, simple tics or tics not associated with Tourette's syndrome, hypersensitivity to pimozide or any of its components

PREGNANCY AND LACTATION: Pregnancy category C

SIDE EFFECTS

Occasional

Akathisia, dystonic extrapyramidal effects, parkinsonian extrapyramidal effects, tardive dyskinesia, blurred vision, ocular changes, constipation, decreased sweating, dry mouth, nasal congestion, dizziness, drowsiness, orthostatic hypotension, urinary retention, somnolence

Rare

Rash, cholestatic jaundice, priapism

SERIOUS REACTIONS

• Serious reactions such as blood dyscrasias, agranulocytosis, leukocytopenia, thrombocytopenia, cholestatic jaundice, neuroleptic malignant syndrome (NMS), constipation or paralytic ileus, priapism, QT prolongation and torsades de pointes, seizure, systemic lupus erythematosus-like syndrome, and temperature regulation dysfunction (heatstroke or hypothermia) occur rarely.

• Abrupt withdrawal following long-term therapy may precipitate nausea, vomiting, gastritis, dizziness, and tremors.

INTERACTIONS

Drugs

▣ *Anticholinergics (benztropine, trihexyphenidyl):* Antagonistic pharmacodynamic effects; excessive anticholinergic effects

❷ *Azole antifungals (itraconazole, ketoconazole):* QT prolongation

▣ *Bromocriptine:* Antagonistic pharmacodynamic effects

▣ *Carbamazepine:* Decreased antipsychotic drug concentrations; decreased therapeutic response

▣ *Clonidine:* Exaggerated hypotension

▣ *Fluoxetine:* Increased risk of extrapyramidal symptoms

▣ *Indomethacin:* Exaggerated side effects: drowsiness, tiredness, confusion

❷ *Levodopa:* Antagonistic effects on the antiparkinsonian effects

▣ *Lithium:* Reduced serum concentrations of both drugs; neurotoxic reactions reported in manic patients (delirium, seizures, encephalopathy, extrapyramidal symptoms)

▣ *Macrolide antibiotics (clarithromycin, erythrmycin, azithromycin, dirithromycin):* QT prolongation

▣ *Meperidine:* Excessive hypotension and CNS depression

▣ *Paroxetine:* Increased risk of extrapyramidal symptoms

▣ *Phenobarbital:* Reduced pimozide concentrations; increased risk of hyperthermia associated with phenobarbital withdrawal

▣ *Protease inhibitors (ritonavir, saquinavir, indinivir, nelfinavir):* QT prolongation

▣ *Quinidine:* Increased pimozide concentrations and risk or subsequent toxicity

▣ *Trazodone:* Additive hypotension

---

pindolol
(pin′doe-loll)
Rx: Visken
Chemical Class: β-adrenergic blocker, nonselective
Therapeutic Class: Antianginal; antihypertensive

CLINICAL PHARMACOLOGY

Mechanism of Action: A nonselective beta blocker that blocks beta$_1$- and beta$_2$-adrenergic receptors. *Therapeutic Effect:* Slows heart rate, decreases cardiac output, decreases blood pressure (BP), and exhibits antiarrhythmic activity. Decreases myocardial ischemia severity by decreasing oxygen requirements.

Pharmacokinetics
Completely absorbed from GI tract. Metabolized in liver. Primarily excreted in urine. **Half-life:** 3-4 hrs (half-life increased with imparied renal function, elderly).

INDICATIONS AND DOSAGES
Mild to moderate hypertension
PO
Adults. Initially, 5 mg 2 times/day. Gradually increase dose by 10 mg/day at 2-4 week intervals. Maintenance: 10-30 mg/day in 2-3 divided doses. Maximum: 60 mg/day.
Usual elderly dosage:
PO
Initially, 5 mg/day. May increase by 5 mg q3-4 wks.

[$] **AVAILABLE FORMS/COST**
• Tab—Oral: 5 mg, 100's: **$58.00-$72.80**; 10 mg, 100's: **$17.46-$99.20**

UNLABELED USES: Treatment of chronic angina pectoris, hypertrophic cardiomyopathy, tremors, and mitral valve prolapse syndrome. Increases antidepressant effect with fluoxetine and other SSRIs.

CONTRAINDICATIONS: Bronchial asthma, COPD, uncontrolled cardiac failure, sinus bradycardia, heart block greater than first degree, cardiogenic shock, CHF, unless secondary to tachyarrhythmias

PREGNANCY AND LACTATION: Pregnancy category B; similar drug, atenolol, frequently used in the third trimester for treatment of hypertension (many studies of efficacy and safety of atenolol in pregnancy-induced hypertension); long-term use has been associated with intrauterine growth retardation; enters breast milk in measurable amounts; observe for signs of β-blockade

SIDE EFFECTS
Frequent
Decreased sexual ability, drowsiness, trouble sleeping, unusual tiredness/weakness
Occasional
Bradycardia, depression, cold hands/feet, diarrhea, constipation, anxiety, nasal congestion, nausea, vomiting
Rare
Altered taste, dry eyes, itching, numbness of fingers, toes and scalp

SERIOUS REACTIONS
• Overdosage may produce profound bradycardia and hypotension.
• Abrupt withdrawal may result in sweating, palpitations, headache, and tremulousness.
• May precipitate congestive heart failure (CHF) or myocardial infarction (MI) in patients with heart disease; thyroid storm in those with thyrotoxicosis; or peripheral ischemia in those with existing peripheral vascular disease.
• Hypoglycemia may occur in previously controlled diabetics.
• Signs of thrombocytopenia, such as unusual bleeding or bruising, occur rarely.

INTERACTIONS
Drugs
[3] *Adenosine:* Bradycardia aggravated
[3] *Amiodarone:* Additive prolongation of atrioventricular (AV) conduction time; symptomatic bradycardia and sinus arrest
[3] *Antacids:* Reduced pindolol absorption
[3] *Calcium channel blockers:* See dihydropyridine calcium channel blockers and verapamil
[3] *Cimetidine:* Renal clearance reduced; AUC increased with cimetidine coadministration

P

◪ *Clonidine, guanabenz, guanfacine:* Exacerbation of rebound hypertension upon discontinuation of clonidine

◪ *Cocaine:* Cocaine-induced vasoconstriction potentiated; reduced coronary blood flow

◪ *Contrast media:* Increased risk of anaphylaxis

◪ *Digitalis:* Enhances bradycardia:

◪ *Digoxin:* Additive prolongation of atrioventricular (AV) conduction time

◪ *Dihydropyridine calcium channel blockers:* Additive pharmacodynamic effects:

◪ *Disopyramide:* Additive decreases in cardiac output

◪ *Dipyridamole:* Bradycardia aggravated

◪ *Diltiazem:* Potentiates pharmacologic effects of β-adrenergic blocker, hypotension, left ventricular failure, and AV conduction disturbances reported; more likely in the elderly and in patients with left ventricular dysfunction, aortic stenosis, or large doses

◪ *Epinephrine, isoproterenol, phenylephrine:* Potentiates pressor response; resultant hypertension and bradycardia

◪ *Flecainide:* Additive negative inotropic effects

◪ *Fluoxetine:* Increased β-blockade activity

◪ *Fluoroquinolones:* Reduced clearance of pindolol

◪ *Insulin:* Altered response to hypoglycemia; increased blood glucose concentrations; impair peripheral circulation

◪ *Lidocaine:* Increased serum lidocaine concentrations possible

◪ *Neostigmine:* Bradycardia aggravated

◪ *Neuroleptics:* Both drugs inhibit each other's metabolism; additive hypotension

◪ *NSAIDs:* Reduced antihypertensive effect of pindolol

◪ *Physostigmine:* Bradycardia aggravated

◪ *Prazosin:* First-dose response to prazosin may be enhanced by β-blockade

◪ *Prazosin, terazosin, doxazosin:* Potential enhanced first dose response (marked initial drop in blood pressure) particularly on standing (especially prazosin)

◪ *Tacrine:* Bradycardia aggravated

❷ *Terbutaline:* Antagonized bronchodilating effects of terbutaline

❷ *Theophylline:* Antagonistic pharmacodynamic effects

◪ *Verapamil:* Enhanced effects of both drugs; particularly AV nodal conduction slowing; reduced pindolol clearance

Labs

• *Alkaline phosphatase:* Increased serum levels

• *Aspartate aminotransferase:* Decreased serum levels

• *Bilirubin:* Decreased serum level

• *Creatine kinase:* Decreased serum level

SPECIAL CONSIDERATIONS

• Abrupt discontinuation may precipitate angina; taper over 1-2 wk

• Effective antihypertensive and probably antianginal agent (though not approved for this indication), especially for patients who develop symptomatic bradycardia with β-blockade

MONITORING PARAMETERS

• Angina: Reduction in nitroglycerin usage; frequency, severity, onset, and duration of angina pain; heart rate

• Hypertension: Blood pressure

• Toxicity: Blood glucose, broncho-spasm, hypotension, bradycardia, depression, confusion, hallucination, sexual dysfunction

---

pioglitazone
(pye-oh-gli′ta-zone)
Rx: Actos
Chemical Class: Thiazo-lidinedione
Therapeutic Class: Antidia-betic; hypoglycemic; insulin resistance reducer

---

CLINICAL PHARMACOLOGY
Mechanism of Action: An antidia-betic that improves target-cell re-sponse to insulin without increasing pancreatic insulin secretion. De-creases hepatic glucose output and increases insulin-dependent glu-cose utilization in skeletal muscle. *Therapeutic Effect:* Lowers blood glucose concentration.
Pharmacokinetics
Rapidly absorbed. Highly protein bound (99%), primarily to albumin. Metabolized in the liver. Excreted in urine. Unknown if removed by he-modialysis. **Half-life:** 16–24 hr.
INDICATIONS AND DOSAGES
Diabetes mellitus, combination therapy
PO
Adult, Elderly. With insulin: Ini-tially, 15–30 mg once a day. Initially continue current insulin dosage; then decrease insulin dosage by 10% to 25% if hypoglycemia occurs or plasma glucose level decreases to less than 100 mg/dl. Maximum: 45 mg/day. With sulfonylureas: Ini-tially, 15–30 mg/day. Decrease sul-fonylurea dosage if hypoglycemia occurs. Wtih metformin: Initially, 15–30 mg/day. As monotherapy: Monotherapy is not to be used if pa-tient is well controlled with diet and exercise alone. Initially, 15–30 mg/day. May increase dosage in in-crements until 45 mg/day is reached.
§ AVAILABLE FORMS/COST
• Tab, Coated—Oral: 15 mg, 90's: **$311.36**; 30 mg, 90's: **$498.55**; 45 mg, 90's: **$540.80**
CONTRAINDICATIONS: Active hepatic disease; diabetic ketoacido-sis; increased serum transaminase levels, including ALT(SGPT) greater than 2.5 times normal serum level; type 1 diabetes mellitus
PREGNANCY AND LACTATION: Pregnancy category C; abnormally high glucose levels during preg-nancy associated with higher inci-dence of congenital anomalies, mor-bidity, and mortality; insulin mono-therapy or sulfonylurea preferred agents; breast milk excretion un-known
SIDE EFFECTS
Frequent (13%–9%)
Headache, upper respiratory tract infection
Occasional (6%–5%)
Sinusitis, myalgia, pharyngitis, ag-gravated diabetes mellitus
SERIOUS REACTIONS
• None known.
INTERACTIONS
Drugs
▣ *Combination oral contracep-tives:* May reduce estrogen and progestin levels (another thiazo-lidinedione reduced both hormones 30%)
▣ *Fenugreek, ginseng, glucoman-nan, guar gum:* Pharmacodynamic interaction as both pioglitazone and listed natural products both possess hypoglycemic effects
Labs
• Possible elevations of AST, ALT, bilirubin, LDH; increases in LDL-cholesterol (15%) and HDL-choles-

P

terol (15%); decreased in hematocrit, hemoglobin; decreased alkaline phosphatase

SPECIAL CONSIDERATIONS

• Expected hypoglycemic effects: Decreases in serum glucose: 50-75 mg/dL; decreases in hemoglobin A1c: 1.2-1.5%

PATIENT/FAMILY EDUCATION

• Caloric restriction, weight loss, and exercise are essential adjuvant therapy

• Blood draws for LFT monitoring along with routine diabetes mellitus labs. Review symptoms of hepatitis (unexplained nausea, vomiting, abdominal pain, fatigue, anorexia or dark urine)

• Notify clinician for rapid increases in weight or edema or symptoms of heart failure (shortness of breath, nocturia)

• Review hypoglycemia risks and symptoms when added to other hypoglycemic agents

MONITORING PARAMETERS

• Diabetes mellitus symptoms, periodic serum glucose and HbA1c measurements; LFT (AST, ALT) prior to initiation of therapy and periodically thereafter; hemoglobin/hematocrit, signs and symptoms of heart failure

piperacillin; piperacillin/ tazobactam

Rx: Pipracil (piperacillin); Zosyn, (piperacillin/tazobactam)
Chemical Class: Penicillin derivative, extended-spectrum; β-lactamase inhibitor (tazobactam)
Therapeutic Class: Antibiotic

CLINICAL PHARMACOLOGY

Mechanism of Action: Piperacillin inhibits cell wall synthesis by binding to bacterial cell membranes. Tazobactam inactivates bacterial beta-lactamase. *Therapeutic Effect:* Piperacillin is bactericidal in susceptible organisms. Tazobactam protects piperacillin from enzymatic degradation, extends its spectrum of activity, and prevents bacterial overgrowth.

Pharmacokinetics

Protein binding: 16%-30%. Widely distributed. Primarily excreted unchanged in urine. Removed by hemodialysis. **Half-life:** 0.7-1.2 hr (increased in hepatic cirrhosis and impaired renal function).

INDICATIONS AND DOSAGES

Severe infections

IV

Adults, Elderly, Children 12 yr and older. 4 g/0.5 g q8h or 3 g/0.375 g q6h. Maximum: 18 g/2.25 gdaily.

Moderate infections

IV

Adults, Elderly, Children 12 yr and older. 2 g/0.225g q6–8h.

Dosage in renal impairment

Dosage and frequency are modified based on creatinine clearance.

Creatinine Clearance	Dosage
20-40 ml/min	8 g/1 g/day (2.25 g q6h)
less than 20 ml/min	6 g/0.75 g/day (2.25 g q8h)

Dosage in hemodialysis patients
IV

Adults, Elderly. 2.25 g q8h with additional dose of 0.75 g after each dialysis session.

$\boxed{S}$ AVAILABLE FORMS/COST
Piperacillin
• Powder, Inj—IM, IV: 2 g/vial: **$8.35**; 3 g/vial: **$12.53**; 4 g/vial: **$16.70**

Piperacillin/Tazobactam
• Powder, Inj—IV: 2 g-0.25 mg: **$11.32**; 3 g-0.375 mg: **$16.98**; 4 g-0.5 mg: **$21.52**

CONTRAINDICATIONS: Hypersensitivity to any penicillin

PREGNANCY AND LACTATION: Pregnancy category B; excreted in breast milk in small concentrations

SIDE EFFECTS
Frequent

Diarrhea, headache, constipation, nausea, insomnia, rash

Occasional

Vomiting, dyspepsia, pruritus, fever, agitation, candidiasis, dizziness, abdominal pain, edema, anxiety, dyspnea, rhinitis

SERIOUS REACTIONS
• Antibiotic-associated colitis and other superinfections may result from altered bacterial balance.

• Seizures and other neurologic reactions are more likely to occur in patients with renal impairment and those who have received an overdose.

• Severe hypersensitivity reactions, including anaphylaxis, occur rarely.

INTERACTIONS
Drugs

$\boxed{3}$ *Aminoglycosides:* Carbenicillin and other piperacillins can inactivate aminoglycosides in vitro and in certain patients with renal dysfunction

$\boxed{3}$ *Chloramphenicol:* Inhibited antibacterial activity of piperacillin; administer piperacillin 3 hr before chloramphenicol

$\boxed{3}$ *Macrolide antibiotics:* Inhibited antibacterial activity of piperacillin; administer piperacillin 3 hr before macrolides

$\boxed{3}$ *Methotrexate:* Piperacillin in large doses may increase serum methotrexate concentrations

$\boxed{3}$ *Oral contraceptives:* Occasional impairment of oral contraceptive efficacy; consider use of supplemental contraception during cycles in which piperacillin is used

$\boxed{3}$ *Tetracyclines:* Inhibited antibacterial activity of piperacillin; administer piperacillin 3 hr before tetracyclines

Labs

• *Cephalothin:* False positive serum
• *Penicillin G:* False positive serum
• *Protein:* False positive urine

SPECIAL CONSIDERATIONS
• Preferred over mezlocillin, more effective against *Pseudomonas,* reserve for carbenicillin- or ticarcillin-resistant *P. aeruginosa* infections in combination with an aminoglycoside

P

pirbuterol
(peer-beut-er-all)
Rx: Maxair
Chemical Class: Sympathomimetic amine; β_2-adrenergic agonist
Therapeutic Class: Antiasthmatic; bronchodilator

CLINICAL PHARMACOLOGY
Mechanism of Action: A sympathomimetic, adrenergic agonist, that stimulates beta2-adrenergic receptors in the lungs, resulting in relaxation of bronchial smooth muscle. *Therapeutic Effect:* Relieves bronchospasm, reduces airway resistance.
Pharmacokinetics
Absorbed from bronchi following inhalation. Metabolized in liver. Primarily excreted in urine. Unknown if removed by hemodialysis. **Half-life:** 2-3 hrs.

INDICATIONS AND DOSAGES
Prevention of bronchospasm
Inhalation
Adults, Elderly, Children 12 yrs and older. 2 inhalations q4-6h. Maximum: 12 inhalations daily.
Treatment of bronchospasm
Inhalation
Adults, Elderly, Children 12 yrs and older. 2 inhalations separated by at least 1-3 minutes, followed by a third inhalation. Maximum: 12 inhalations daily.

$ AVAILABLE FORMS/COST
• MDI—INH: 0.2 mg/puff, 14 g: **$79.69**; 0.2 mg/puff, 25.6 g: **$50.52**
CONTRAINDICATIONS: History of hypersensitivity to pirbuterol, albuterol or any of its components
PREGNANCY AND LACTATION: Pregnancy category C

SIDE EFFECTS
Occasional (7%-1%)
Nervousness, tremor, headache, palpitations, nausea, dizziness, tachycardia, cough
SERIOUS REACTIONS
• Excessive sympathomimetic stimulation may produce palpitations, extrasystoles, tachycardia, chest pain, slight increases in BP followed by a substantial decrease, chills, sweating and blanching of skin.
• Too frequent or excessive use may lead to loss of bronchodilating effectiveness and severe, paradoxical bronchoconstriction.
INTERACTIONS
Drugs
❷ β-*blockers:* Decreased action of pirbuterol, cardioselective agents preferable if concurrent use necessary
❸ *Furosemide:* Potential for additive hypokalemia
SPECIAL CONSIDERATIONS
• No significant advantage over other selective β_2-agonists
PATIENT/FAMILY EDUCATION
• Initial and periodic reviews of metered dose inhaler technique

piroxicam
(peer-ox′i-kam)
Rx: Feldene
Chemical Class: Oxicam derivative
Therapeutic Class: NSAID; antipyretic; nonnarcotic analgesic

CLINICAL PHARMACOLOGY
Mechanism of Action: An NSAID that produces analgesic and anti-inflammatory effects by inhibiting prostaglandin synthesis. *Therapeu-

tic Effect: Reduces inflammatory response and intensity of pain.

INDICATIONS AND DOSAGES

Acute or chronic rheumatoid arthritis and osteoarthritis

PO

Adults, Elderly. Initially, 10–20 mg/day as a single dose or in divided doses. Some patients may require up to 30–40 mg/day.

Children. 0.2–0.3 mg/kg/day. Maximum: 15 mg/day.

[$] **AVAILABLE FORMS/COST**

• Cap, Gel—Oral: 10 mg, 100's: **$86.39-$179.66**; 20 mg, 100's: **$140.43-$337.93**

UNLABELED USES: Treatment of acute gouty arthritis, ankylosing spondylitis, dysmenorrhea

CONTRAINDICATIONS: Active peptic ulcer disease, chronic inflammation of the GI tract, GI bleeding or ulceration, history of hypersensitivity to aspirin or NSAIDs

PREGNANCY AND LACTATION: Pregnancy category B (avoid administration near term); excreted into breast milk; approximately 1% of mother's serum levels; should not present a risk to nursing infant

SIDE EFFECTS

Frequent (9%–4%)

Dyspepsia, nausea, dizziness

Occasional (3%–1%)

Diarrhea, constipation, abdominal cramps or pain, flatulence, stomatitis

Rare (less than 1%)

Hypertension, urticaria, dysuria, ecchymosis, blurred vision, insomnia, phototoxicity

SERIOUS REACTIONS

• Rare reactions with long-term use include peptic ulcer disease, GI bleeding, gastritis,severe hepatic reaction (cholestasis, jaundice), nephrotoxicity (dysuria, hematuria, proteinuria, nephrotic syndrome), hematologic sensitivity (anemia, leukopenia, eosinophilia, thrombocytopenia), and a severe hypersensitivity reaction (fever, chills, bronchospasm).

INTERACTIONS

Drugs

[3] *Aminoglycosides:* Reduced clearance with elevated aminoglycoside levels and potential for toxicity (especially indomethacin in premature infants; other NSAIDs probably)

[3] *Anticoagulants:* Excessive hypoprothrombinemia, decreased platelet aggregation with increased risk of GI bleeding

[3] *Antihypertensives (α-blockers, angiotensin-converting enzyme inhibitors, angiotensin II receptor blockers, β-blockers, diuretics):* Inhibition of antihypertensive and other favorable hemodynamic effects

[3] *Corticosteroids:* Increased risk of GI ulceration

[3] *Cyclosporine:* Increased nephrotoxicity risk

[3] *Lithium:* Decreased clearance of lithium (mediated via prostaglandins) resulting in elevated serum lithium levels and risk of toxicity

[3] *Methotrexate:* Decreased renal secretion of methotrexate resulting in elevated methotrexate levels and risk of toxicity

[3] *Phenylpropanolamine:* Possible acute hypertensive reaction

[3] *Potassium-sparing diuretics:* Additive hyperkalemia potential

[3] *Triamterene:* Acute renal failure reported with addition of indomethacin; caution with other NSAIDs

SPECIAL CONSIDERATIONS

• Similar in efficacy to the other NSAIDs but has the advantage and disadvantage of an extended $t_{1/2}$; high GI toxicity potential

MONITORING PARAMETERS

• Initial hemogram and fecal occult blood test within 3 mo of starting regular chronic therapy; repeat every 6-12 mo (more frequently in high-risk patients (>65 years, peptic ulcer disease, concurrent steroids or anticoagulants); electrolytes, creatinine, and BUN within 3 mo of starting regular chronic therapy; repeat every 6-12 mo

---

plicamycin
(plik-a-mi'sin)
Rx: Mithracin
Chemical Class: Crystalline aglycone
Therapeutic Class: Antihypercalcemic; antineoplastic

CLINICAL PHARMACOLOGY

Mechanism of Action: An antibiotic that forms complexes with DNA, inhibiting DNA-directed RNA synthesis. May inhibit parathyroid hormone effect on osteoclasts and inhibit bone resorption. *Therapeutic Effect:* Lowers serum calcium and phosphate levels. Blocks hypercalcemic action of vitamin D and action of parathyroid hormone. Decreases serum calcium.

Pharmacokinetics

Route	Onset	Peak	Duration
IV	1-2 days	2-3 days	3-15 days

Protein binding: None. Greatest concentrations in liver, kidney, and formed bone surfaces. Crosses the blood-brain barrier and enters CSF. Primarily excreted in urine.

INDICATIONS AND DOSAGES
Testicular tumors
IV
Adults, Elderly. 25-30 mcg/kg/day for 8-10 days. Repeat at monthly intervals.

Hypercalcemia, hyperuricemia
IV
Adults, Elderly. 25 mcg/kg as a single dose; may repeat in 48 hr if no response occurs. Or give 25 mcg/kg/day for 3-4 days or 25-50 mcg/kg/dose every other day for 3-8 doses.

Paget's disease
IV
Adults, Elderly. 15 mcg/kg/day for 10 days.

AVAILABLE FORMS/COST
• Powder, Inj—IV: 2.5 mg/vial: **$98.74**

UNLABELED USES: Treatment of Paget's disease refractory to other therapy

CONTRAINDICATIONS: Pre-existing coagulation disorders, thrombocytopathy, thrombocytopenia, impaired bone marrow function, or tendency to hemorrhage

PREGNANCY AND LACTATION: Pregnancy category X

SIDE EFFECTS
Frequent
Nausea, vomiting, anorexia, diarrhea, stomatitis
Occasional
Fever, drowsiness, weakness, lethargy, malaise, headache, depression, nervousness, dizziness, rash, acne

SERIOUS REACTIONS
• The risk of hematologic toxicity (characterized by marked facial flushing, persistent nosebleeds, hemoptysis, purpura, ecchymosis, leukopenia, and thrombocytopenia) increases with administration of high dosages or more than 10 doses.
• Electrolyte imbalances may occur.

INTERACTIONS
Drugs
⬛ *Bisphosphonates, calcitonin, foscarnet, glucagon:* Additive hypocalcemic effect

SPECIAL CONSIDERATIONS

• Effective but also toxic; use is therefore limited; additive with other calcium lowering therapies

MONITORING PARAMETERS

• CBC, differential, platelet count q wk; withhold drug if WBC is <4000/mm^3 or platelet count is <50,000/mm^3

• Renal function studies: BUN, serum uric acid, urine CrCl, electrolytes, input and output ratio

• Liver function tests: bilirubin, AST, ALT, alk phosphatase before and during therapy

---

podofilox
(po-doe-fil′ox)

Rx: Condylox
Chemical Class: Podophyllum derivative
Therapeutic Class: Keratolytic

CLINICAL PHARMACOLOGY

Mechanism of Action: An active component of podophyllin resin that binds to tubulin to prevent formation of microtubules resulting in mitotic arrest. Exercises many biological effects such as damages endothelium of small blood vessels, attenuates nucleoside transport, suppresses immune responses, inhibits macrophage metabolism, induces interleukin-1 and interleukin-2, decreases lymphocytes response to mitogens and enhances macrophage growth. *Therapeutic Effect:* Removes genital warts.

Pharmacokinetics
Time to peak occurs in 1 to 2 hours. Some degree of absorption. **Half-life:** 1-4.5 hrs.

INDICATIONS AND DOSAGES
Anogenital warts
Topical
Adults. Apply 0.5% gel for 3 days, then withhold for 4 days. Repeat cycle up to 4 times.
Genital warts (condylomata acuminate)
Topical
Adults. Apply 0.5% solution or gel q12h in the morning and evening for 3 days, then withhold for 4 days. Repeat cycle up to 4 times.

S AVAILABLE FORMS/COST
• Gel—Top: 0.5%, 3.5 g: **$169.93**
• Sol—Top: 0.5%, 3.5 ml: **$99.48-$121.58**

UNLABELED USES: Systemic: Treatment of fungal pneumonia, prostate cancer, septicemia

CONTRAINDICATIONS: Bleeding warts, moles, birthmarks or unusual warts with hair, diabetes, poor blood circulation, pregnancy, steroid use, hypersensitivity to podofilox or any component of its formulation

PREGNANCY AND LACTATION: Pregnancy category C

SIDE EFFECTS
Occasional
Erosion, inflammation, itching, pain, burning
Rare
Nausea, vomiting

SERIOUS REACTIONS
• Nausea and vomiting occur rarely and usually after cumulative doses.

SPECIAL CONSIDERATIONS
• Safety preferred over podophyllum resin

podophyllum
(po-dof-fil-um rez-in)
Rx: Podocon-25 (75%
benzoin), Podofin
Chemical Class: Podophyllum
derivative
Therapeutic Class: Keratolytic

CLINICAL PHARMACOLOGY
Mechanism of Action: A cytotoxic
agent that directly affects epithelial
cell metabolism by arresting mitosis
through binding to a protein subunit
of spindle microtubules. *Therapeutic Effect:* Removes soft genital
warts.
Pharmacokinetics
Topical podophyllum is systemically absorbed. Absorption may be
increased if applied to bleeding, fri-
able, or recently biopsied warts.

INDICATIONS AND DOSAGES
*Genital   warts   (condylomata
acuminate)*
Topical
Adults, Elderly, Children. Apply
10%-25% solution in compound
benzoin tincture to dry surface. Use
1 drop at a time allowing drying between drops until area is covered.
Total volume should be limited to
less than 0.5 ml per treatment session.

$ AVAILABLE FORMS/COST
• Liq—Top: 25%, 5, 15 ml: **$42.34-
$55.60**/15 ml

UNLABELED USES: Epithelioma-
tosis, laryngeal papilloma

CONTRAINDICATIONS: Diabetes
mellitus, concomitant steroids therapy, circulation disorders, bleeding
warts, moles, birthmarks or unusual
warts with hair growing from them,
pregnancy,   hypersensitivity   to
podophyllum resin preparations

PREGNANCY AND LACTATION:
Pregnancy category X; excretion
into breast milk unknown, use caution in nursing mothers

SIDE EFFECTS
Occasional (10%-1%)
Pruritus, nausea, vomiting, abdomi-
nal pain, diarrhea

SERIOUS REACTIONS
• Paresthesia, polyneuritis, paralytic ileus, pyrexia, leukopenia,
thrombocytopenia, coma and death
have been reported with podophyllum resin use.

SPECIAL CONSIDERATIONS
• Not to be dispensed to the patient,
professional application only
• Because of the potential for toxicity, cryotherapy should be attempted
1st or podofilox substituted

polymyxin B

(polly-mix-in)

Rx: Aerosporin

Combinations

Rx: *Ophth:* with bacitracin (Polysporin); with dexamethasone, neomycin (Dexacidin, Maxitrol); with hydrocortisone, neomycin (Cortisporin); with neomycin, bacitracin (Neosporin, Ocutricin); with neomycin, gramicidin (Neosporin); with oxytetracycline (Terak); with prednisolone, neomycin (Poly-Pred); with trimethoprim (Polytrim); *Topical:* with bacitracin, hydrocortisone, neomycin (Cortisporin); with dexamethasone, neomycin (Dioptrol, Maxitrol); with hydrocortisone, neomycin (Cortisporin)

OTC: *Topical:* with bacitracin (Bacimyxin, Polysporin); with bacitracin, neomycin (Neosporin, Triple Antibiotic); with bacitracin, neomycin, lidocaine (Lanabiotic, Spectrocin); with gramicidin (Polysporin); with gramicidin, lidocaine (Lidosporin, Polysporin Burn Formula); with gramicidin, neomycin (Neosporin)

Chemical Class: Polymyxin derivative

Therapeutic Class: Antibiotic; ophthalmic antibiotic

CLINICAL PHARMACOLOGY

Mechanism of Action: An antibiotic that alters cell membrane permeability in susceptible microorganisms. *Therapeutic Effect:* Bactericidal activity.

Pharmacokinetics

Negligible absorption. Protein binding: low. Excreted in urine. Poor removal in hemodialysis. **Half-life:** 6 hrs.

INDICATIONS AND DOSAGES

Mild to moderate infections

IV

Adults, Elderly, Children 2 yrs and older. 15,000-25,000 units/kg/day in divided doses q12h.

Infants. Up to 40,000 units/kg/day.

IM

Adults, Elderly, Children 2 yrs and older. 25,000-30,000 units/kg/day in divided doses q4-6h.

Infants. Up to 40,000 units/kg/day.

Usual irrigation dosage

Continuous Bladder Irrigation

Adults, Elderly. 1 ml urogenital concentrate (contains 200,000 units polymyxin B, 57 mg neomycin) added to 1,000 ml 0.9% NaCl. Give each 1,000 ml >24 hrs for up to 10 days (may increase to 2,000 ml/day when urine output >2 L/day).

Usual ophthalmic dosage

Ophthalmic

Adults, Elderly, Children. 1 drop q3-4h.

[$] **AVAILABLE FORMS/COST**

• Powder, Inj—IM, IV, IT: 500,000 U/vial: **$5.25-$13.13**

CONTRAINDICATIONS: Hypersensitivity to polymyxin B or any component of the formulation

PREGNANCY AND LACTATION: Pregnancy category B

SIDE EFFECTS

Frequent

Severe pain, irritation at IM injection sites, phlebitis, thrombophlebitis with IV administration

Occasional

Fever, urticaria

P

SERIOUS REACTIONS

• Nephrotoxicity, especially with concurrent/sequential use of other nephrotoxic drugs, renal impairment, concurrent/sequential use of muscle relaxants.

• Superinfection, especially with fungi, may occur.

INTERACTIONS

Drugs

❷ Anesthetics, neuromuscular blockers (e.g., gallamine, pancuronium, succinylcholine, tubocurarine): Increased skeletal muscle relaxation

SPECIAL CONSIDERATIONS

• Generally replaced by the aminoglycosides or extended-spectrum penicillins for serious infections; still used for bladder irrigation and gut decontamination; used in combination with other antibiotics and/or corticosteroids topically to treat infections of the eye and skin

MONITORING PARAMETERS

• Intake and output, BUN, creatinine, urinalysis

---

polythiazide
(poly-thi′a-zide)
Rx: Renese
Combinations
 Rx: with prazosin (Minizide); with reserpine (Renese-R)
Chemical Class: Sulfonamide derivative
Therapeutic Class: Antihypertensive; diuretic, thiazide

CLINICAL PHARMACOLOGY

Mechanism of Action: A sulfonamide derivative that acts as a thiazide diuretic and antihypertensive. As a diuretic blocks reabsorption of water, sodium and potassium at cortical diluting segment of distal tubule. As an antihypertensive it reduces plasma and extracellular fluid volume and decreases peripheral vascular resistance (PVR) by direct effect on blood vessels. *Therapeutic Effect:* Promotes diuresis, reduces blood pressure (BP).

Pharmacokinetics

Rapidly absorbed from the gastrointestinal (GI) tract. Primarily excreted unchanged in urine. Not removed by hemodialysis. **Half-life:** 25.7 hrs.

INDICATIONS AND DOSAGES

Edema

PO

Adults. 1- 4 mg/day.

Hypertension

PO

Adults. 2- 4 mg/day.

S **AVAILABLE FORMS/COST**

• Tab—Oral: 2 mg, 100's: **$64.50**

UNLABELED USES: Prevention of calcium-containing renal stones

CONTRAINDICATIONS: Anuria, history of hypersensitivity to sulfonamides or thiazide diuretics, renal decompensation

PREGNANCY AND LACTATION: Pregnancy category D; therapy for preexisting hypertension can be continued throughout pregnancy with minimal risk; initiating for simple edema not recommended; few unequivocal indications for diuretic therapy in pregnancy except for pulmonary edema or congestive heart failure; excreted in breast milk in low concentrations; compatible with breast-feeding

SIDE EFFECTS

Expected

Increase in urine frequency and volume

Frequent

Potassium depletion

Occasional

Postural hypotension, headache, gastrointestinal (GI) disturbances, photosensitivity reaction

SERIOUS REACTIONS

• Vigorous diuresis may lead to profound water loss and electrolyte depletion, resulting in hypokalemia, hyponatremia, and dehydration.
• Acute hypotensive episodes may occur.
• Hyperglycemia may be noted during prolonged therapy.
• GI upset, pancreatitis, dizziness, paresthesias, headache, blood dyscrasias, pulmonary edema, allergic pneumonitis, and dermatologic reactions occur rarely.
• Overdosage can lead to lethargy and coma without changes in electrolytes or hydration.

INTERACTIONS

Drugs

❷ *Angiotensin-converting enzyme inhibitors:* Risk of postural hypotension when added to ongoing diuretic therapy; more common with loop diuretics; first dose hypotension possible in patients with sodium depletion or hypovolemia due to diuretics or sodium restriction; hypotensive response is usually transient; hold diuretic day of first dose

❸ *Calcium:* With large doses can result in milk-alkali syndrome

❸ *Carbenoxolone:* Additive potassium wasting; severe hypokalemia

❸ *Cholestyramine, colestipol:* Reduced absorption

❸ *Corticosteroids:* Concomitant therapy may result in excessive potassium loss

❸ *Diazoxide:* Hyperglycemia

❸ *Digitalis glycosides:* Diuretic-induced hypokalemia increases risk of digitalis toxicity

❸ *Hypoglycemic agents:* Increased dosage requirements due to increased glucose levels

❸ *Lithium:* Increased lithium levels, potential toxicity

❸ *Methotrexate:* Additive bone marrow suppression

❸ *Nonsteroidal antiinflammatory drugs:* Concurrent use may reduce diuretic and antihypertensive effects

Labs

• *False decrease:* Urine estriol

SPECIAL CONSIDERATIONS

• Doses above 1 mg provide no further blood pressure reduction, but are more likely to induce metabolic disturbance (i.e., hypokalemia, hyperuricemia, etc.)
• May protect against osteoporotic hip fractures
• Loop diuretics or metolazone more effective if CrCl <40-50 ml/min

PATIENT/FAMILY EDUCATION

• Will increase urination temporarily (approx. 3 wk); take early in the day to prevent sleep disturbance
• May cause sensitivity to sunlight; avoid prolonged exposure to the sun and other ultraviolet light
• May cause gout attacks; notify clinician if sudden joint pain occurs

MONITORING PARAMETERS

• Weight, urine output, serum electrolytes, BUN, creatinine, CBC, uric acid, glucose, lipids

P

---

poractant alfa
(poor-ak'tant)
Rx: Curosurf
Chemical Class: Phospholipid
Therapeutic Class: Lung surfactant, porcine

CLINICAL PHARMACOLOGY
Mechanism of Action: A pulmonary surfactant that reduces alveolar surface tension during ventilation and stabilizes the alveoli against collapse that may occur at resting transpulmonary pressures. *Thera-*

peutic Effect: Improves lung compliance and respiratory gas exchange.

INDICATIONS AND DOSAGES
Respiratory distress syndrome (RDS)
Intratracheal

Infants. Initially, 2.5 ml/kg of birth weight. May give up to 2 subsequent doses of 1.25 ml/kg of birth weight at 12-hr intervals. Maximum: 5 ml/kg (total dose).

Ⓢ AVAILABLE FORMS/COST
• Susp—Intratracheal: 80 mg/ml 1.5, 3 ml vial: **$312.00**/1.5 ml

UNLABELED USES: Adult RDS due to viral pneumonia or near-drowning, *Pneumocystis carinii* pneumonia in HIV-infected patients, prevention of RDS

CONTRAINDICATIONS: None known.

SIDE EFFECTS
Frequent
Transient bradycardia, oxygen (O_2) desaturation, increased carbon dioxide (CO_2) retention
Occasional
Endotracheal tube reflux
Rare
Apnea, endotracheal tube blockage, hypotension or hypertension, pallor, vasoconstriction

SERIOUS REACTIONS
• None known.

SPECIAL CONSIDERATIONS
MONITORING PARAMETERS
• Continuous ECG and transcutaneous O_2 saturation; pCO_2; lung compliance; respiratory rate

---

potassium iodide
Rx: Pima, SSKI, Strong Iodine Solution (Lugol's Solution)
Chemical Class: Iodine product
Therapeutic Class: Antithyroid agent; expectorant

CLINICAL PHARMACOLOGY
Mechanism of Action: An agent that reduces viscosity of mucus by increasing respiratory tract secretions. Inhibits secretion of thyroid hormone, fosters colloid accumulation in thyroid follicles. *Therapeutic Effect:* Blocks thyroid radioiodine uptake.
Pharmacokinetics
Oral onset 24- 48 hrs, peak 10- 15 days, duration 6 weeks. Primarily excreted in the urine.

INDICATIONS AND DOSAGES
Expectorant
PO

Adults, Elderly, Children 3 yrs and older. 325-650 mg q8h (Pima); 300-600 mg 3-4 times/day (SSKI).
Children less than 3 yrs. 162 mg q8h.

Preoperative thyroidectomy
PO

Adults, Elderly, Children. 0.1-0.3 ml (3-5 drops of Lugol's solution) q8h or 50-250 mg (1-5 drops of SSKI) q8h. Administer 10 days before surgery.

Radiation protectant to radioactive isotopes of iodine
PO

Adults, Elderly. 195 mg/day (Pima) for 10 days. Start 24 hours prior to exposure.
Children more than 1 yr. 130 mg/day for 10 days. Start 24 hours prior to exposure.
Children less than 1 yr. 65 mg/day for 10 days. Start 24 hours prior to exposure.

Reduce risk of thyroid cancer following nuclear accident
PO

Adults, Elderly, Children more than 68 kg. 130 mg/day

Children 3-18 yrs. 65 mg/day.

Children 1 mos. - 3 yrs. 32 mg/day.

Children 1 mo. and younger. 16 mg/day.

Sporotrichosis
PO

Adults, Elderly. Initally, 5 drops (SSKI) q8h and increase to 40-50 drops q8h as tolerated for 3-6 months.

Thyrotoxic crisis
PO

Adults, Elderly. 300-500 mg (6-19 drops SSKI) q8h or 1 ml (Lugol's solution) q8h.

S AVAILABLE FORMS/COST
• Sol—Oral: 1 g/ml, 30, 240 ml: **$5.35-$12.10**/30 ml

• Syr—Oral: 325 mg/5 ml, 480 ml: **$22.90**

CONTRAINDICATIONS: Hypersensitivity to potassium, iodine compounds, or any of its component, pulmonary edema, hyperkalemia, impaired renal function, hyperthyroidism, iodine-induced goiter, pregnancy

PREGNANCY AND LACTATION: Pregnancy category D; use of iodides as expectorants during pregnancy is contraindicated; concentrated in breast milk, may affect infant's thyroid activity but considered compatible with breast-feeding

SIDE EFFECTS

Occasional

Irregular heart beat, confusion, drowsiness, fever, rash, diarrhea, GI bleeding, metallic taste, nausea, stomach pain, vomiting, numbness, tingling, weakness

Rare

Goiter, salivary gland swelling and tenderness, thyroid adenoma, swelling of the throat and neck, myxedema, lymph node swelling,

SERIOUS REACTIONS

• Hypersensitivity symptoms include angioedema, muscle weakness, parlysis, peaked T-waves, flattened P-waves, prolongation of QRS complex, ventricular arrhythmias.

INTERACTIONS

Drugs

3 *Lithium:* Increased likelihood of hypothyroidism

SPECIAL CONSIDERATIONS

PATIENT/FAMILY EDUCATION

• Dilute sol with water or fruit juice to improve taste, drink sol through straw

• Administer with food or milk

MONITORING PARAMETERS

• Thyroid function tests if used for thyroid-related conditions

P

potassium salts

Rx: *Potassium chloride:* Cena-K, Gen K, K+ Care, K+10, Kaochlor, Kaon-Cl, Kato, Kay Ciel, K-Dur, K-Lease, K-lor, Klor-Con, Klorvess, Klotrix, K·Lyte/Cl, K-Norm, K-tab, Micro-K, Potasalan, Rum-K, Slow-K, Ten-K

Rx: *Potassium gluconate:* Kaon, Kaylixir, K-G Elixer

Rx: *Combinations of potassium salts:* Effer-K, K·Lyte, Klor-Con EF (as bicarbonate, citrate), K+ Care ET (as bicarbonate), Klorvess Effervescent Granules (as bicarbonate, chloride, citrate); K-Lyte/Cl (as bicarbonate, chloride), Kolyum (as chloride, gluconate); Tri-K, (as acetate, bicarbonate, citrate); Twin-K (as gluconate, citrate)

Chemical Class: Monovalent cation

Therapeutic Class: Electrolyte supplement

CLINICAL PHARMACOLOGY

Mechanism of Action: An electrolyte that is necessary for multiple cellular metabolic processes. Primary action is intracellular. *Therapeutic Effect:* Is necessary for nerve impulse conduction and contraction of cardiac, skeletal, and smooth muscle; maintains normal renal function and acid-base balance.

Pharmacokinetics

Well absorbed from the GI tract. Enters cells by active transport from extracellular fluid. Primarily excreted in urine.

INDICATIONS AND DOSAGES

Prevention of hypokalemia (in patients on diuretic therapy)

PO

Adults, Elderly. 20–40 mEq/day in 1–2 divided doses.

Children. 1–2 mEq/kg/day in 1–2 divided doses.

Treatment of hypokalemia

PO

Adults, Elderly. 40–80 mEq/day; further doses based on laboratory values.

Children. 2-5 mEq/day; further doses based on laboratory values.

IV

Adults, Elderly. 5–10 mEq/hr. Maximum: 400 mEq/day.

Children. 1 mEq/kg over 1–2 hr.

$ AVAILABLE FORMS/COST

Potassium Acetate

• Sol, Inj—IV: 2 mEq/ml, 20 ml: **$1.60-$2.39**; 4 mEq/ml, 50 ml: **$6.25-$6.46**

Potassium Bicarbonate

• Tab, Effervescent—Oral: 25 mEq, 30's: **$7.98-$21.78**

Potassium Chloride

• Cap, Gel, Sus Action—Oral: 8 mEq, 100's: **$32.49**; 10 mEq, 100's: **$14.20-$35.96**

• Inj, Conc—Sol: 2 mEq/ml, 10 ml: **$0.54-$1.40**

• Liq—Oral: 20 mEq/15 ml, 480 ml: **$1.49-$48.00**; 30 mEq/15 ml, 480 ml: **$23.60**; 40 mEq/15 ml, 480 ml: **$3.02-$26.94**

• Powder, Reconst—Oral: 20 mEq/pkg, 30's: **$4.92-$53.26**; 25 mEq/pkg, 30's: **$7.41**

• Tab, Coated, Sus Action—Oral: 8 mEq, 100's: **$7.00-$46.12**; 10 mEq, 100's: **$10.50-$52.45**; 15 mEq, 100's: **$45.94**; 20 mEq, 100's: **$41.12-$63.95**

• Tab, Effervescent—Oral: 25 mEq, 100's: **$127.47**; 50 mEq, 30's: **$77.51**

Potassium Gluconate
• Elixir—Oral: 20 mEq/15 ml, 480 ml: **$5.49-$29.90**

CONTRAINDICATIONS: Concurrent use of potassium-sparing diuretics, digitalis toxicity, heat cramps, hyperkalemia, postoperative oliguria, severe burns, severe renal impairment, shock with dehydration or hemolytic reaction, untreated Addison's disease

SIDE EFFECTS
Occasional
Nausea, vomiting, diarrhea, flatulence, abdominal discomfort with distention, phlebitis with IV administration (particularly when potassium concentration of greater than 40 mEq/L is infused)
Rare
Rash

SERIOUS REACTIONS
• Hyperkalemia (more common in elderly patients and those with impaired renal function) may be manifested as paresthesia, feeling of heaviness in the lower extremities, cold skin, grayish pallor, hypotension, confusion, irritability, flaccid paralysis, and cardiac arrhythmias.

INTERACTIONS
Drugs
3 *ACE inhibitors:* Hyperkalemia
3 *Disopyramide:* Increased potassium concentrations can enhance disopyramide effects
3 *Hypoglycemics:* Correction of hypokalemia may result in hypoglycemia
2 *Potassium-sparing diuretics:* Hyperkalemia

SPECIAL CONSIDERATIONS
• Avoid use of compressed tablets or enteric-coated tablets (i.e., non-sustained release or effervescent tablets for sol) due to significant ulcerogenic tendency and propensity to cause significant local tissue destruction

• Sol, powder, and oral susp: dilute or dissove in 120 ml cold water or juice
• Extended release caps and tabs: do not crush; take with food; swallow with full glass of liquid
• Injectable potassium products must be diluted prior to administration; direct inj of potassium concentrate may be fatal
• Central line preferable for IV infusions concentrated >40 mEq/L

MONITORING PARAMETERS
• ECG monitoring advisable for IV infusion rate >10 mEq/hr
• Normal serum potassium level 3.5-5.0 mEq/L (higher, to 7.7 mEq/L in neonates)

---

pralidoxime
(pra-li-doks-eem)
Rx: Protopam
Chemical Class: Quaternary ammonium derivative
Therapeutic Class: Antidote, anticholinesterase

CLINICAL PHARMACOLOGY
Mechanism of Action: Reactivates cholinesterase activity by 2-formyl-1-methylpyridinium ion. *Therapeutic Effect:* Restores cholinesterase activity following organophosphate anticholinesterase poisoning.

Pharmacokinetics
Onset of activity is 1 hour and duration of action is short, which may require readministration. Not protein bound. Excreted in urine. **Half-life:** 1.2-2.6 hrs.

INDICATIONS AND DOSAGES
Anticholinesterase overdosage
IV

Adults, Elderly. 1-2 g initially, followed by increments of 250 mg q5min until response is observed.

Organophosphate poisoning
IV

Adults, Elderly. 1-2 g initially in 100 ml 0.9 NaCl infused over 15-30 minutes or 5% solution in sterile water for injection over not less than 5 minutes. Repeat 1-2 g in 1 hour if muscle weakness persists.

Children. 25-50 mg/kg/dose. Repeat in 1-2 hours if muscle weakness has not been relieved, then at 8-12 hour intervals if cholinergic signs recur.

§ **AVAILABLE FORMS/COST**
• Powder, Inj—IM, IV, SC: 1 g/vial: **$108.37**

CONTRAINDICATIONS: Use of aminophylline, morphine, therophylline and succinylcholine, hypersensitivity to pralidoxime or any of its components

PREGNANCY AND LACTATION: Pregnancy category C

SIDE EFFECTS

Occasional
Blurred vision, dizziness, headache, laryngospasm, hyperventilation, nausea, tachycardia, hypertension, pain at injection site

Rare
Rash, muscle rigidity, decreased renal function

SERIOUS REACTIONS
• Excessive doses may cause blurred vision, nausea, tachycardia and dizziness.

SPECIAL CONSIDERATIONS

MONITORING PARAMETERS
• CBC; plasma cholinesterase activity may help confirm diagnosis and follow course of illness

pramipexole
(pram-eh-pex'ol)
Rx: Mirapex
Chemical Class: Benzothiazolamine derivative
Therapeutic Class: Anti-Parkinson's agent; dopaminergic

CLINICAL PHARMACOLOGY
Mechanism of Action: An antiparkinson agent that stimulates dopamine receptors in the striatum. *Therapeutic Effect:* Relieves signs and symptoms of Parkinson's disease.

Pharmacokinetics
Rapidly and extensively absorbed after PO administration. Protein binding: 15%. Widely distributed. Steady-state concentrations achieved within 2 days. Primarily eliminated in urine. Not removed by hemodialysis. **Half-life:** 8 hr (12 hr in patients older than 65 yr).

INDICATIONS AND DOSAGES
Parkinson's disease
PO

Adults, Elderly. Initially, 0.375 mg/day in 3 divided doses. Don't increase dosage more frequently than every 5-7 days. Maintenance: 1.5-4.5 mg/day in 3 equally divided doses.

Dosage in renal impairment
Dosage and frequency are modified based on creatinine clearance.

Creatinine Clearance	Initial Dose	Maximum Dose
Greater than 60 ml/min	0.125 mg 3 times a day	1.5 mg 3 times a day
35-59 ml/min	0.125 mg twice a day	1.5 mg twice a day
15-34 ml/min	0.125 mg once a day	1.5 mg once a day

§ **AVAILABLE FORMS/COST**
• Tab—Oral: 0.125 mg, 63's: **$64.98**; 0.25 mg, 90's: **$118.23**; 0.5 mg, 1 mg, 1.5 mg, 90's: **$208.64**

CONTRAINDICATIONS: History of hypersensitivity to pramipexole
PREGNANCY AND LACTATION: Pregnancy category C; inhibits prolactin secretion; excretion into breast milk unknown
SIDE EFFECTS
Frequent
Early Parkinson's disease (28%-10%): Nausea, asthenia, dizziness, somnolence, insomnia, constipation
Advanced Parkinson's disease (53%-17%): Orthostatic hypotension, extrapyramidal reactions, insomnia, dizziness, hallucinations
Occasional
Early Parkinson's disease (5%-2%): Edema, malaise, confusion, amnesia, akathisia, anorexia, dysphagia, peripheral edema, vision changes, impotence
Advanced Parkinson's disease (10%-7%): Asthenia, somnolence, confusion, constipation, abnormal gait, dry mouth
Rare
Advanced Parkinson's disease (6%-2%): General edema, malaise, chest pain, amnesia, tremor, urinary frequency or incontinence, dyspnea, rhinitis, vision changes
SERIOUS REACTIONS
• None known.
INTERACTIONS
Drugs
◼ *Cimetidine:* 50% increase in pramipexole AUC and 40% increase in $t_{1/2}$
◼ *Dopamine antagonists (phenothiazines, butyrophenones, thioxanthenes, metoclopramide):* May diminish effectiveness of pramipexole
◼ *Levodopa:* 40% increase in levodopa concentrations

SPECIAL CONSIDERATIONS
• At least as effective as bromocriptine in the treatment of advanced parkinsonian patients with levodopa-related motor fluctuations; adverse effects similar in incidence and severity; appears to lack some of the toxicity seen with bromocriptine, pergolide, and cabergoline (e.g., pleuropulmonary disease); may be a useful alternative in patients with intolerable adverse effects due to ergot derivatives
MONITORING PARAMETERS
• United Parkinson's Disease Rating Scale (UPDRS) useful for monitoring efficacy endpoints

pramoxine
(pra-mox'-een)
OTC: Itch-X, PrameGel, Prax, ProctoFoam-NS, Tronolane, Tronothane
Chemical Class: Morpholine derivative
Therapeutic Class: Anesthetic, topical

P

CLINICAL PHARMACOLOGY
Mechanism of Action: A surface or local anesthetic which is not chemically related to the "caine" types of local anesthetics. Decreases the neuronal membranes permeability to sodium ions, blocking both initiation and conduction of nerve impulses, therefore inhibiting depolarization of the neuron. *Therapeutic effect:* Temporarily relieves pain and itching associated with anogenital pruritus or irritation.
Pharmacokinetics
Onset of action occurs within a few minutes of application. Peak effect is reached in 3-5 minutes. Duration is several days.

INDICATIONS AND DOSAGES
Anogenital pruritus or irritation, dermatosis, minor burns, hemorrhoids
Topical
Adults, Elderly: Apply of affected area 3 or 4 times daily.
S **AVAILABLE FORMS/COST**
• Foam—Rect: 1%, 15 g: **$29.66**
• Cre—Rect, Top: 1%, 15, 30, 60 g: **$1.62-$10.00**/30 g
• Cre—Top: 1%, 30 g: **$10.58**
• Gel—Top: 1%, 35.4, 120 g: **$8.11**/120 g
• Lotion—Top: 1%, 15, 120, 240 ml: **$3.66**/15 ml
• Spray—Top: 1%, 59 ml: **$4.32**
CONTRAINDICATIONS: Hypersensitivity to any component of the product.
PREGNANCY AND LACTATION: Pregnancy category C; excretion into breast milk unknown
SIDE EFFECTS
Occassional
Angioedema, contact dermatitis, burning, itching, irritation, stinging
Rare
Dryness, folliculitis, hypopigmentation, perioral dermatitis, maceration of the skin, secondary infection, skin atrophy, striae, miliaria.
SERIOUS REACTIONS
• None known.
SPECIAL CONSIDERATIONS
• Cross-sensitization with other local anesthetics unlikely
PATIENT/FAMILY EDUCATION
• Do not use near eyes or nose
• Contact clinician if condition fails to improve after 3-4 days or worsens
• Do not apply to large areas
• Do not apply to unaffected areas

---

pravastatin
(prav-i-sta'tin)
Rx: Pravachol
Chemical Class: Substituted hexahydronaphthalene
Therapeutic Class: HMG-CoA reductase inhibitor; antilipemic

CLINICAL PHARMACOLOGY
Mechanism of Action: An HMG-CoA reductase inhibitor that interferes with cholesterol biosynthesis by preventing the conversion of HMG-CoA reductase to mevalonate, a precursor to cholesterol. *Therapeutic Effect:* Lowers serum LDL and VLDL cholesterol and plasma triglyceride levels; increases serum HDL concentration.
Pharmacokinetics
Poorly absorbed from the GI tract. Protein binding: 50%. Metabolized in the liver (minimal active metabolites). Primarily excreted in feces via the biliary system. Not removed by hemodialysis. **Half-life:** 2.7 hr.
INDICATIONS AND DOSAGES
Hyperlipidemia, primary and secondary prevention of cardiovascular events in patient with elevated cholesterol levels
PO
Adults, Elderly. Initially, 40 mg/day. Titrate to desired response. Range: 10–80 mg/day.
Children 14–18 yr. 40 mg/day.
Children 8–13 yr. 20 mg/day.
Dosage in hepatic and renal impairment
For adults, give 10 mg/day initially. Titrate to desired response.
S **AVAILABLE FORMS/COST**
• Tab—Oral: 10 mg, 100's: **$168.79**; 20 mg, 100's: **$249.83**; 40 mg, 80 mg, 90's: **$406.84**

CONTRAINDICATIONS: Active hepatic disease or unexplained, persistent elevations of liver function test results

PREGNANCY AND LACTATION: Pregnancy category X; small amounts excreted in breast milk; should probably not be used by women who are nursing

SIDE EFFECTS

Pravastatin is generally well tolerated. Side effects are usually mild and transient.

Occasional (7%–4%)

Nausea, vomiting, diarrhea, constipation, abdominal pain, headache, rhinitis, rash, pruritus

Rare (3%–2%)

Heartburn, myalgia, dizziness, cough, fatigue, flu-like symptoms

SERIOUS REACTIONS

• Malignancy and cataracts may occur.

• Hypersensitivity occurs rarely.

INTERACTIONS

Drugs

❷ *Azole antifungals (fluconazole, itraconazole, ketoconazole, miconazole):* Increased plasma pravastatin levels via inhibition of metabolism with increased risk of rhabdomyolysis

❸ *Cholestyramine, colestipol:* Reduced bioavailability of pravastatin; give pravastatin 1 hr before or 4 hr following a bile acid sequestrant

❸ *Clarithromycin:* Increased plasma pravastatin levels via inhibition of metabolism with increased risk of rhabdomyolysis

❷ *Clofibrate:* Small increased risk of myopathy with combination

❸ *Cyclosporine:* Concomitant administration increases risk of severe myopathy or rhabdomyolysis; if used together, initiate pravastatin at 10 mg qhs and titrate cautiously, usual max is 20 mg/day

❸ *Danazol:* Increased plasma pravastatin levels via inhibition of metabolism with increased risk of rhabdomyolysis

❸ *Erythromycin:* Increased pravastatin levels via inhibition of metabolism with increased risk of rhabdomyolysis

❸ *Fluoxetine:* Increased pravastatin levels via inhibition of metabolism with increased risk of rhabdomyolysis

❷ *Gemfibrozil:* Small increased risk of myopathy with combination, especially at high doses of statin

❸ *Isradipine:* May decrease pravastatin plasma concentrations

❸ *Niacin:* Concomitant administration increases risk of severe myopathy or rhabdomyolysis

❸ *Nefazodone:* May inhibit hepatic metabolism of pravastatin with risk of rhabdomyolysis

❸ *Troleandomycin:* Increased pravastatin levels via inhibition of metabolism with increased risk of rhabdomyolysis

SPECIAL CONSIDERATIONS

• Statin selection based on lipid-lowering prowess, cost, and availability

PATIENT/FAMILY EDUCATION

• Avoid prolonged exposure to sunlight and other UV light

• Promptly report any unexplained muscle pain, tenderness, or weakness, especially if accompanied by fever or malaise

• Strictly adhere to low cholesterol diet

• Take daily doses in the evening for increased effect

MONITORING PARAMETERS

• ALT and AST at baseline, and at 12 weeks of therapy. If no change at 12 weeks, no further monitoring necessary (discontinue if elevations persist at >3 times upper limit of normal)

P

• CPK in any patient complaining of diffuse myalgia, muscle tenderness, or weakness
• Fasting lipid profile

---

praziquantel
(pray-zih-kwon-tel)
Rx: Biltricide
Chemical Class: Pyrazinoisoquinoline derivative
Therapeutic Class: Antihelmintic

CLINICAL PHARMACOLOGY
Mechanism of Action: An antihelmintic that increases cell permeability in susceptible helminths resulting in loss of intracellular calcium, massive contractions and paralysis of their musculature, followed by attachment of phagocytes to the parasites. *Therapeutic Effect:* Vermicidal. Dislodges the dead and dying worms.

Pharmacokinetics
Well absorbed from gastrointestinal (GI) tract. Protein binding: 80%. Widely distributed including CSF. Metabolized in liver. Primarily excreted in urine. Not removed by hemodialysis. **Half-life:** 4-5 hrs.

INDICATIONS AND DOSAGES
Schistosomiasis
PO
Adults, Elderly. 3 doses of 20 mg/kg as 1 day treatment. Do not give doses less than 4 hours or more than 6 hours apart.

Clonorchiasis/opisthorchiasis
PO
Adults, Elderly. 3 doses of 25 mg/kg as 1 day treatment.

Ⓢ AVAILABLE FORMS/COST
• Tab, Plain Coated—Oral: 600 mg, 6's: **$71.41**

CONTRAINDICATIONS: Ocular cysticercosis, hypersensitivity to praziquantel or any component of the formulation

PREGNANCY AND LACTATION: Pregnancy category B; do not nurse on day of treatment and during the subsequent 72 hr

SIDE EFFECTS
Frequent
Headache, dizziness, malaise, abdominal pain
Occasional
Anorexia, vomiting, diarrhea, severe cramping abdominal pain may occur within 1 hour of administration w/fever, sweating, bloody stools
Rare
Giddiness, urticaria

SERIOUS REACTIONS
• Overdose should be treated with fast-acting laxative.

INTERACTIONS
Drugs
🔳 *Chloroquine and hydroxychloroquine:* Reduces plasma level of praziquantel
🔳 *Cimetidine:* Increases plasma level of praziquantel

SPECIAL CONSIDERATIONS
PATIENT/FAMILY EDUCATION
• Swallow tablets unchewed with some liquid during meals
• May cause drowsiness
• Use caution driving or performing other tasks requiring alertness

prazosin
(pra'zoe-sin)
Rx: Minipress
Combinations
  Rx: with polythiazide (Minizide)
Chemical Class: Quinazoline derivative
Therapeutic Class: Antihypertensive; α_1-adrenergic blocker

CLINICAL PHARMACOLOGY
Mechanism of Action: An antidote, antihypertensive, and vasodilator that selectively blocks alpha$_1$-adrenergic receptors, decreasing peripheral vascular resistance. *Therapeutic Effect:* Produces vasodilation of veins and arterioles, decreases total peripheral resistance, and relaxes smooth muscle in bladder neck and prostate.

INDICATIONS AND DOSAGES
Mild to moderate hypertension
PO
Adults, Elderly. Initially, 1 mg 2–3 times a day. Maintenance: 3–15 mg/day in divided doses. Maximum: 20 mg/day.
Children. 5 mcg/kg/dose q6h. Gradually increase up to 25 mcg/kg/dose.

AVAILABLE FORMS/COST
• Cap, Gel—Oral: 1 mg, 100's: **$8.84-$48.04**; 2 mg, 100's: **$10.74-$72.41**; 5 mg, 100's: **$19.72-$93.98**
UNLABELED USES: Treatment of benign prostate hyperplasia, CHF, ergot alkaloid toxicity, pheochromocytoma, Raynaud's phenomenon

CONTRAINDICATIONS: None known
PREGNANCY AND LACTATION: Pregnancy category C

SIDE EFFECTS
Frequent (10%–7%)
Dizziness, somnolence, headache, asthenia (loss of strength, energy)
Occasional (5%–4%)
Palpitations, nausea, dry mouth, nervousness
Rare (less than 1%)
Angina, urinary urgency

SERIOUS REACTIONS
• First-dose syncope (hypotension with sudden loss of consciousness) may occur 30 to 90 minutes following initial dose of more than 2 mg, a too rapid increase in dosage, or addition of another antihypertensive agent to therapy. First-dose syncope may be preceded by tachycardia (pulse rate of 120–160 beats/minute).

INTERACTIONS
Drugs
▨ *ACE inhibitors:* Exaggerated first-dose response to prazosin
▨ *β-adrenergic blockers:* Exaggerated first-dose response to prazosin
▨ *NSAIDs:* Inhibits antihypertensive response to prazosin
▨ *Verapamil:* Reduces first pass metabolism of prazosin
Labs
• False positive urinary metabolites of norepinephrine and VMA
• No effect on prostate specific antigen (PSA)

SPECIAL CONSIDERATIONS
• The doxazosin arm of the ALLHAT study was stopped early; the doxazosin group had a 25% greater risk of combined cardiovascular disease events which was primarily accounted for by a doubled risk of CHF vs the chlorthalidone group; doxazosin was also found to be less effective at controlling systolic BP an average of 3 mm Hg; may want to

consider primary antihypertensives in addition to α-blockers for BPH symptoms

• Use as single antihypertensive agent limited by tendency to cause sodium and water retention and increased plasma volume

PATIENT/FAMILY EDUCATION

• Alert patients to the possibility of syncopal and orthostatic symptoms, especially with the 1st dose ("1st-dose syncope")

• Initial dose should be administered at bedtime in the smallest possible dose

---

prednisolone
(pred-niss'oh-lone)
Rx: Prelone; (acetate) Key-Pred, Predacort, Key-Pred-SP (sodium phosphate), Pediapred; Ophthalmic: (acetate) Econopred, Econopred Plus, Pred Mild, Pred Forte; (sodium phosphate) AK-Pred, Inflamase Mild, Inflamase Forte, Prednisol
Chemical Class: Glucocorticoid, synthetic
Therapeutic Class: Corticosteroid, ophthalmic; corticosteroid, systemic

---

CLINICAL PHARMACOLOGY
Mechanism of Action: An adrenocortical steroid that inhibits accumulation of inflammatory cells at inflammation sites, phagocytosis, lysosomal enzyme release and synthesis, and release of mediators of inflammation. *Therapeutic Effect:* Prevents or suppresses cell-mediated immune reactions. Decreases or prevents tissue response to inflammatory process.

INDICATIONS AND DOSAGES
Substitution therapy for deficiency states: acute or chronic adrenal insufficiency, congenital adrenal hyperplasia, and adrenal insufficiency secondary to pituitary insufficiency; nonendocrine disorders: arthritis; rheumatic carditis; allergic, collagen, intestinal tract, liver, ocular, renal, skin diseases; bronchial asthma; cerebral edema; malignancies
PO
Adults, Elderly. 5–60 mg/day in divided doses.
Children. 0.1–2 mg/kg/day in 1-4 divided doses.
Treatment of conjuctivitis and corneal injury
Ophthalmic
Adults, Elderly. 1-2 drops every hr during day and q2h during night. After response, decrease dosage to 1 drop q4h, then 1 drop 3-4 times a day.

§ **AVAILABLE FORMS/COST**

• Susp, Inj—IM (acetate): 25 mg/ml, 10, 30 ml: **$6.50-$7.75**/30 ml; 50 mg/ml, 10, 30 ml: **$6.98-$18.55**/30 ml

• Susp, Depot—Inj (acetate): 40 mg/ml, 10 ml: **$14.95**; 80 mg/ml, 5 ml: **$14.95**

• Sol—Ophth (sodium phosphate): 0.125%, 5, 10 ml: **$1.73-$18.56**/5 ml; 1%, 5, 10, 15 ml: **$1.72-$18.69**/5 ml; 0.25%, 5, 10 ml: **$16.06-$23.23**/5 ml

• Susp—Ophth (acetate): 0.12%, 5, 10 ml: **$24.78**/5 ml; 0.125%, 5 ml: **$4.75**/5 ml; 1%, 5, 10, 15 ml: **$1.80-$31.00**/5 ml

• Liq-Oral (acetate): 5 mg/5 ml, 120 ml: **$17.35-$21.74**

• Liq-Oral (sodium phosphate): 5 mg/5 ml, 120 ml: **$15.49-$35.70**

• Syr—Oral (acetate): 15 mg/5 ml, 60, 120, 240, 480 ml: **$11.81-$74.50**/60 ml

• Tab—Oral (acetate): 5 mg, 100's: **$2.66-$13.75**

CONTRAINDICATIONS: Acute superficial herpes simplex keratitis, systemic fungal infections, varicella

PREGNANCY AND LACTATION: Pregnancy category B; compatible with breast-feeding

SIDE EFFECTS

Frequent

Insomnia, heartburn, nervousness, abdominal distention, increased sweating, acne, mood swings, increased appetite, facial flushing, delayed wound healing, increased susceptibility to infection, diarrhea or constipation

Occasional

Headache, edema, change in skin color, frequent urination

Rare

Tachycardia, allergic reaction (such as rash and hives), psychological changes, hallucinations, depression Ophthalmic: stinging or burning, posterior subcapsular cataracts

SERIOUS REACTIONS

• Long-term therapy may cause hypocalcemia, hypokalemia, muscle wasting (especially in the arms and legs), osteoporosis, spontaneous fractures, amenorrhea, cataracts, glaucoma, peptic ulcer disease, and CHF.

• Abruptly withdrawing the drug after long-term therapy may cause anorexia, nausea, fever, headache, severe or sudden joint pain, rebound inflammation, fatigue, weakness, lethargy, dizziness, and orthostatic hypotension.

• Suddenly discontinuing prednisolone may be fatal.

INTERACTIONS

Drugs

3 *Aminoglutethamide:* Increased clearance of prednisolone; doubling of dose may be required

3 *Antidiabetics:* Increased blood glucose

3 *Barbiturates:* Increased clearance of prednisolone

3 *Cholestyramine, colestipol:* Reduced absorption of prednisolone

3 *Clarithromycin, erythromycin, troleandomycin, ketoconazole:* Possible enhanced steroid effect

3 *Estrogens, oral contraceptives:* Enhanced effects of corticosteroids

3 *Intrauterine devices:* Decreased contraceptive effect (possibly secondary inhibition of inflammatory reaction)

3 *Isoniazid:* Reduced plasma concentrations of isoniazid; (rapid isoniazid acetylators at increased risk)

3 *NSAIDs:* Increased risk GI ulceration

3 *Rifampin:* May reduce hepatic clearance of prednisolone

3 *Salicylates:* Increased salicylate clearance

Labs

• *False increase:* Cortisol, digoxin, theophylline

• *False decrease:* Urine glucose (Clinistix, Diastix only, Testape no effect)

• *False negative:* Skin allergy tests

SPECIAL CONSIDERATIONS

PATIENT/FAMILY EDUCATION

• May cause GI upset

• Take single daily doses in am

• Increased dose of rapidly acting corticosteroids may be necessary in patients subjected to unusual stress

• Signs of adrenal insufficiency include fatigue, anorexia, nausea, vomiting, diarrhea, weight loss, weakness, dizziness, and low blood sugar

• Avoid abrupt withdrawal of therapy following high-dose or long-term therapy. Relative insufficiency may exist for up to 1 yr after discontinuation

• Patients on chronic steroid therapy should wear medical alert bracelet
• Do not give live virus vaccines to patients on prolonged therapy

MONITORING PARAMETERS

• Potassium and blood sugar during long-term therapy
• Edema, blood pressure, cardiac symptoms, mental status, weight
• Observe growth and development of infants and children on prolonged therapy
• Check intraocular pressure and lens frequently during prolonged use of ophthalmic preparations

prednisone

(pred'ni-sone)

Rx: Deltasone, Liquid Pred, Meticorten, Pred-Pak 45, Pred-Pak 79, Prednisone Intensol Concentrate, Sterapred, Sterapred DS

Chemical Class: Glucocorticoid, synthetic

Therapeutic Class: Corticosteroid, systemic

CLINICAL PHARMACOLOGY

Mechanism of Action: An adrenocortic al steroid that inhibits accumulation of inflammatory cells at inflammation sites, phagocytosis, lysosomal enzyme release and synthesis, and release of mediators of inflammation. *Therapeutic Effect:* Prevents or suppresses cell-mediated immune reactions. Decreases or prevents tissue response to inflammatory process.

Pharmacokinetics

Well absorbed from the GI tract. Protein binding: 70%–90%. Widely distributed. Metabolized in the liver and converted to prednisolone. Primarily excreted in urine. Not removed by hemodialysis. **Half-life:** 3.4–3.8 hr.

INDICATIONS AND DOSAGES

Substitution therapy in deficiency states: acute or chronic adrenal insufficiency, congenital adrenal hyperplasia, and adrenal insufficiency secondary to pituitary insufficiency; nonendocrine disorders: arthritis; rheumatic carditis; allergic, collagen, intestinal tract, liver, ocular, renal, skin diseases; bronchial asthma; cerebral edema; malignancies

PO

Adults, Elderly. 5–60 mg/day in divided doses.

Children. 0.05–2 mg/kg/day in 1-4 divided doses.

[$] **AVAILABLE FORMS/COST**

• Sol—Oral: 5 mg/5 ml, 60, 120, 500 ml: **$7.02**/60 ml
• Tab—Oral: 1 mg, 100's: **$3.16-$29.37**; 2.5 mg, 100's: **$6.53**; 5 mg, 100's: **$1.09-$15.52**; 10 mg, 100's: **$4.95-$21.00**; 20 mg, 100's: **$6.69-$21.84**; 50 mg, 100's: **$17.63-$30.76**

CONTRAINDICATIONS: Acute superficial herpes simplex keratitis, systemic fungal infections, varicella

PREGNANCY AND LACTATION: Pregnancy category B; compatible with breast-feeding

SIDE EFFECTS

Frequent

Insomnia, heartburn, nervousness, abdominal distention, increased sweating, acne, mood swings, increased appetite, facial flushing, delayed wound healing, increased susceptibility to infection, diarrhea or constipation

Occasional

Headache, edema, change in skin color, frequent urination

Rare

Tachycardia, allergic reaction (including rash and hives), psychological changes, hallucinations, depression

SERIOUS REACTIONS

• Long-term therapy may cause muscle wasting in the arms and legs, osteoporosis, spontaneous fractures, amenorrhea, cataracts, glaucoma, peptic ulcer disease, and CHF.

• Abruptly withdrawing the drug following long-term therapy may cause anorexia, nausea, fever, headache, sudden or severe joint pain, rebound inflammation, fatigue, weakness, lethargy, dizziness, and orthostatic hypotension.

• Suddenly discontinuing prednisone may be fatal.

INTERACTIONS

Drugs

▪ *Aminoglutethamide:* Increased clearance of prednisone; doubling of dose may be necessary

▪ *Antidiabetics:* Increased blood glucose

▪ *Barbiturates, carbamazepine:* Increased clearance of prednisone

▪ *Cholestyramine, colestipol:* Possible reduced absorption of corticosteroids

▪ *Cyclosporine:* Possible increased concentration of both drugs, seizures

▪ *Erythromycin, troleandomycin, clarithromycin, ketoconazole:* Possible enhanced steroid effect

▪ *Estrogens, oral contraceptives:* Enhanced effects of corticosteroids

▪ *IUD's:* Inhibition of inflammation may decrease contraceptive effect

▪ *Isoniazid:* Reduced plasma concentrations of isoniazid

▪ *NSAIDs:* Increased risk GI ulceration

▪ *Rifampin:* May reduce hepatic clearance of prednisone

▪ *Salicylates:* Increased salicylate clearance

Labs

• *False increase:* Cortisol, digoxin, theophylline

• *False decrease:* Urine glucose (Clinistix, Diastix only, Testape no effect)

• *False negative:* Skin allergy tests

SPECIAL CONSIDERATIONS

PATIENT/FAMILY EDUCATION

• May cause GI upset, teach patient to take with meals or snacks

• May mask infections

• Take single daily doses in am

• Increased dose of rapidly acting corticosteroids may be necessary in patients subjected to unusual stress

• Signs of adrenal insufficiency include fatigue, anorexia, nausea, vomiting, diarrhea, weight loss, weakness, dizziness, and low blood sugar

• Avoid abrupt withdrawal of therapy following high-dose or long-term therapy; relative insufficiency may exist for up to 1 yr after discontinuation

• Patients on chronic steroid therapy should wear medical alert bracelet

• Do not give live virus vaccines to patients on prolonged therapy

MONITORING PARAMETERS

• Serum K and glucose

• Edema, blood pressure, CHF symptoms, mental status, weight

• Growth in children on prolonged therapy

P

primaquine
(prim-a-kween)
Rx: Primaquine
Chemical Class: 8-amino-quinoline derivative
Therapeutic Class: Antimalarial

CLINICAL PHARMACOLOGY
Mechanism of Action: An antimalarial and antirheumatic that eliminates tissue exoerythrocytic forms of Plasmodium falciparum. Disrupts mitochondria and binds to DNA. *Therapeutic Effect:* Inhibits parasite growth.
Pharmacokinetics
Well absorbed. Metabolized in the liver to the active metabolite, carboxyprimaquine. Excreted in the urine in small amounts as unchanged drug. **Half-life:** 4-6 hrs

INDICATIONS AND DOSAGES
Treatment of malaria
PO
Adults, Elderly. 15 mg base daily for 14 days.
Children. 0.3 mg base/kg/wk once daily for 14 days.
Malaria prophylaxis
Adults, Elderly. 30 mg base daily. Begin 1 day before departure and continue for 7 days after leaving malarious area.

$ AVAILABLE FORMS/COST
• Tab—Oral: 26.3 mg, 100's: **$103.79**

CONTRAINDICATIONS: Concomitant medications which cause bone marrow suppression, rheumatoid arthritis, lupus erythematosus, glucose-6-phosphate dehydrogenase (G-6-PD) deficiency, pregnancy, hypersensitivity to primaquine or any of its components

PREGNANCY AND LACTATION: Pregnancy category C; if possible, withhold until after delivery; however, if prophylaxis or treatment is required, primaquine should not be withheld

SIDE EFFECTS
Frequent
Abdominal pain, nausea, vomiting
Rare
Leukopenia, hemolytic anemia, methemoglobinemia

SERIOUS REACTIONS
• Leukopenia, hemolytic anemia, methemoglobinemia occur rarely.
• Overdosage include symptoms of abdominal cramps, vomiting, burning epigastric distress, central nervous system and cardiovascular disturbances, cyanosis, methemoglobinemia, moderate leukocytosis or leukopenia, and anemia.
• Acute hemolysis occurs, but patients recover completely if the dosage is discontinued.

SPECIAL CONSIDERATIONS
PATIENT/FAMILY EDUCATION
• Take with food if GI upset occurs, notify clinician if GI distress continues
• Urine may turn brown

MONITORING PARAMETERS
• CBC periodically during therapy, discontinue if marked darkening of urine or sudden decrease in hemoglobin concentrations or leukocyte count occurs

primidone
(pri'mi-done)
Rx: Mysoline
Chemical Class: Pyrimidinedione
Therapeutic Class: Anticonvulsant
DEA Class: Schedule IV

CLINICAL PHARMACOLOGY
Mechanism of Action: A barbiturate that decreases motor activity from electrical and chemical stimulation and stabilizes the seizure threshold against hyperexcitability.
Therapeutic Effect: Reduces seizure activity.

INDICATIONS AND DOSAGES
Seizure control
PO
Adults, Elderly, Children 8 yr and older. 125-150 mg/day at bedtime. May increase by 125-250 mg/day every 3-7 days. Maximum: 2 g/day.
Children younger than 8 yr. Initially, 50-125 mg/day at bedtime. May increase by 50-125 mg/day every 3-7 days. Usual dose: 10-25 mg/kg/day in divided doses.
Neonates. 12-20 mg/kg/day in divided doses.

$ AVAILABLE FORMS/COST
• Tab—Oral: 50 mg, 100's: **$36.84-$51.71**; 250 mg, 100's: **$7.95-$186.65**

UNLABELED USES: Treatment of essential tremor

CONTRAINDICATIONS: History of bronchopneumonia, porphyria

PREGNANCY AND LACTATION: Pregnancy category D; reported association between use of other anticonvulsants (phenobarbital and phenytoin) and increased incidence of birth defects; should not be discontinued abruptly in patients who become pregnant when the drug is being used to prevent major seizures because of possibility of precipitating status epilepticus with attendant hypoxia and threat to life; the majority of mothers on anticonvulsant medication deliver normal infants; neonatal hemorrhage, with a coagulation defect resembling vitamin K deficiency, has been described in newborns whose mothers were taking primidone; pregnant women on primidone should receive prophylactic vitamin K_1 therapy for 1 month before, and during, delivery; excreted in breast milk in percentages of maternal serum concentration as high as 106.9% for primidone and 56.9% for phenobarbital

SIDE EFFECTS
Frequent
Ataxia, dizziness
Occasional
Anorexia, drowsiness, mental changes, nausea, vomiting, paradoxical excitement
Rare
Rash

SERIOUS REACTIONS
• Abrupt withdrawal after prolonged therapy may produce effects ranging from increased dreaming, nightmares, insomnia, tremor, diaphoresis, and vomiting to hallucinations, delirium, seizures, and status epilepticus.
• Skin eruptions may may be a sign of a hypersensitivity reaction.
• Blood dyscrasias, hepatic disease, and hypocalcemia occur rarely.
• Overdose produces cold or clammy skin, hypothermia, and severe CNS depression, followed by high fever and coma.

INTERACTIONS
Drugs
▣ *Acetazolamide:* Decreased absorption, hence decreased anticonvulsant efficacy

P

② *Anticoagulants (anisindione, dicumarol, warfarin):* Decreased anticoagulant effectiveness

② *Barbiturates:* Additive CNS and respiratory depressant effects

② *Benzodiazepines:* Additive CNS and respiratory depressant effects

③ *Betamethasone:* Decreased betamethasone effectiveness

③ *Cannabis:* Increased CNS depression

③ *Carbamazepine:* Decreased carbamazepine effectiveness with loss of seizure control

③ *Centrally acting muscle relaxants:* Additive respiratory depression

② *Chloral hydrate:* Additive respiratory depression

③ *Cortisone:* Decreased cortisone effectiveness

③ *Dexamethasone:* Decreased dexamethasone effectiveness

② *Dexmethylphenidate:* Inhibits metabolism; increased primidone plasma concentrations

③ *Estradiol:* Estrogen effects decreased; increased doses of estrogen may be needed

③ *Ethanol:* Excessive CNS depression

③ *Ethchlorvynol:* Additive CNS and respiratory effects

② *Ethinyl estradiol:* Decreased contraceptive effectiveness

③ *Fosphenytoin:* Increased phenobarbital levels

③ *Ginkgo:* Decreased effectiveness of primidone due to presence of seizure-provoking contaminant in some ginkgo preparations

③ *Hydrocortisone:* Decreased hydrocortisone effectiveness

③ *Isoniazid:* Isoniazid inhibits primidone metabolism with elevations of primidone plasma concentrations as well as prolonging $t_{1/2}$

③ *Lamotrigine:* Decreased lamotrigine efficacy (40% decreases in lamotrigine concentrations)

③ *Leucovorin:* Antiepileptic effect counteracted; decreased primidone efficacy

② *Levonorgestrel:* Decreased contraceptive effectiveness

③ *Mesoridazine:* Decreased levels of antipsychotic via induced metabolism (25-40%)

② *Mestranol:* Decreased contraceptive effectiveness

③ *Methylprednisolone:* Decreased methylprednisolone effectiveness

③ *Methsuximide:* Competitive inhibition of hydroxylation; increased phenobarbital and primidone plasma concentrations

③ *Norethindrone:* Decreased contraceptive effectiveness

③ *Norgestrel:* Decreased contraceptive effectiveness

③ *Opioid analgesics:* Additive CNS and respiratory effects

③ *Phenytoin:* Increased phenobarbital levels

③ *Prednisolone, prednisone:* Decreased corticosteroid effectiveness

③ *Rifabutin:* Reduced primidone effectiveness

③ *Sodium oxybate:* Additive CNS and respiratory depression

② *Theophylline:* Decreased serum levels and concentration of theophylline via hepatic microsomal enzyme induction

③ *Triamcinolone:* Decreased triamcinolone effectiveness

③ *Tricyclic antidepressants:* Decreased tricyclic antidepressant serum concentrations

② *Valproic acid:* Additive respiratory and CNS depression

② *Warfarin:* Decreased anticoagulant effectiveness

SPECIAL CONSIDERATIONS
• Second-line anticonvulsant for treatment of generalized tonic-clonic seizures (or alternative to phenobarbital, which probably accounts for most of the anticonvulsant activity)
• Most effective anti-essential tremor medication, but sedative side effects troublesome; usually used second line to β-adrenergic blocking agents (non-selective)

PATIENT/FAMILY EDUCATION
• Importance of effective contraception, and considerations surrounding pregnancy
• Importance of adherence to regimen and risk associated with abrupt discontinuance of anticonvulsant
• Sedative liabilities regarding driving and operating heavy machinery

MONITORING PARAMETERS
• Therapeutic drug concentration for seizure control: 5-12 mcg/ml; serum concentrations should also include phenobarbital determinations (therapeutic: 20-40 mcg/ml)
• Periodic CBC, liver and renal function tests, serum folate, vitamin D during prolonged therapy

probenecid
(proe-ben'e-sid)
Rx: Benemid, Probalan
Combinations
  Rx: with colchicine (Colbenemid Proben-C); with ampicillin (Polycillin-PRB, Probampacin)
Chemical Class: Sulfonamide derivative
Therapeutic Class: Antigout agent; uricosuric

CLINICAL PHARMACOLOGY
Mechanism of Action: An uricosuric that competitively inhibits reabsorption of uric acid at the proximal convoluted tubule. Also, inhibits renal tubular secretion of weak organic acids, such as penicillins. *Therapeutic Effect:* Promotes uric acid excretion, reduces serum uric acid level, and increases plasma levels of penicillins and cephalosporins.

INDICATIONS AND DOSAGES
Gout
PO
Adults, Elderly. Initially, 250 mg twice a day for 1 wk; then 500 mg twice a day. May increase by 500 mg q4wk. Maximum: 2–3 g/day. Maintenance: Dosage that maintains normal uric acid level.
As adjunct to penicillin or cephalosporin therapy to prolong antibiotic plasma levels
PO
Adults, Elderly. 2 g/day in divided doses.
Children weighing more than 50 kg. Receive adult dosage.
Children 2–14 yr. Initially, 25 mg/kg. Maintenance: 40 mg/kg/day in 4 divided doses.

Gonorrhea

PO

Adults, Elderly. 1 g 30 min before penicillin, ampicillin, or amoxicillin.

$ AVAILABLE FORMS/COST

• Tab, Plain Coated—Oral: 500 mg, 100's: **$9.00-$98.33**

• Tab—Oral: 0.5 mg colchicine-500 mg probenecid 100's: **$18.50-$84.34**

CONTRAINDICATIONS: Blood dyscrasias, children younger than 2 years, concurrent high-dose aspirin therapy, severe renal impairment, uric acid calculi

PREGNANCY AND LACTATION: Pregnancy category B; has been used during pregnancy without causing adverse effects in fetus or infant

SIDE EFFECTS

Frequent (10%–6%)

Headache, anorexia, nausea, vomiting

Occasional (5%–1%)

Lower back or side pain, rash, hives, itching, dizziness, flushed face, frequent urge to urinate, gingivitis

SERIOUS REACTIONS

• Severe hypersensitivity reactions, including anaphylaxis, occur rarely and usually within a few hours after administration following previous use. If severe hypersensitivity reactions develop, discontinue the drug immediately and contact the physician.

• Pruritic maculopapular rash, possibly accompanied by malaise, fever, chills, arthralgia, nausea, vomiting, leukopenia, and aplastic anemias hould be considered a toxic reaction.

INTERACTIONS

Drugs

3 *Dapsone:* Increased serum dapsone concentrations

3 *Dyphylline:* Increased serum dyphylline concentrations

2 *Methotrexate:* Marked increases in serum methotrexate concentrations

3 *Salicylates:* Inhibition of uricosuric effect if used regularly

3 *Thiopental:* Prolonged anesthesia

3 *Zidovudine:* Increased plasma zidovudine concentrations

Labs

• *False positive:* Urine glucose (Ames Clinitest tablet, no effect on Ames Keto-Diastix, Diastix, Multistix, Clinistix)

• *False increase:* Free T_4 (Boehringer-Mannheim Enzymum procedure)

SPECIAL CONSIDERATIONS

PATIENT/FAMILY EDUCATION

• Avoid aspirin or other salicylates

• Take with food or antacids

• Drink 48-64 oz water daily to prevent development of kidney stones

MONITORING PARAMETERS

• Serum uric acid concentrations: continue the probenecid dose that maintains normal concentrations

• Renal function tests

---

procainamide

(proe-kane'a-mide)

Rx: Procan SR, Pronestyl, Pronestyl-SR

Chemical Class: Para-aminobenzoic acid derivative

Therapeutic Class: Antiarrhythmic, class IA

CLINICAL PHARMACOLOGY

Mechanism of Action: An antiarrhythmic that increases the electrical stimulation threshold of the ventricles and His-Purkinje system. Decreases myocardial excitability and conduction velocity and depresses myocardial contractility. Exerts direct cardiac effects. *Therapeutic Effect:* Suppresses arrhythmias.

Pharmacokinetics

Rapidly, completely absorbed from the GI tract. Protein binding: 15%–20%. Widely distributed. Metabolized in the liver to active metabolite. Primarily excreted in urine. Removed by hemodialysis. **Half-life:** 2.5–4.5 hr; metabolite, 6 hr.

INDICATIONS AND DOSAGES

Maintenance of normal sinus rhythm after conversion of atrial fibrillation or flutter; treatment of premature ventricular contractions, paroxysmal atrial tachycardia, atrial fibrillation, and ventricular tachycardia

PO

Adults, Elderly. 250–500 mg of immediate-release tablets q3–6h. 0.5–1 g of sustained-release tablets q6h. 1–2 g of Procanbid q12h.

Children. 15–50 mg/kg/day of immediate-release tablets in divided doses q3–6h. Maximum: 4 g/day.

IV

Adults, Elderly. Loading dose: 50–100 mg. May repeat q5–10min or 15–18 mg/kg (maximum: 1–1.5 g). Then maintenance infusion of 3–4 mg/min. Range: 1–6 mg/min.

Children. Loading dose: 3–6 mg/kg over 5 min (maximum: 100 mg). May repeat q5–10min to maximum total dose of 15 mg/kg. Then maintenance dose of 20–80 mcg/kg/min. Maximum: 2 g/day.

Dosage in renal impairment

Dosag interval is modified based on creatinine clearance.

Creatinine Clearance	Dosage Interval
10–50 ml/min	q6–12h
less than 10 ml/min	q8–24h

AVAILABLE FORMS/COST

• Cap, Gel—Oral: 250 mg, 100's: **$7.20-$88.21**; 375 mg, 30's: **$9.30-$88.00**; 500 mg, 100's: **$9.20-$95.10**

• Sol, Inj—IM, IV: 100 mg/ml, 10 ml: **$4.00**; 500 mg/ml, 2 ml: **$1.81-$5.63**

• Tab, Sugar Coated—Oral: 250 mg, 100's: **$74.48**; 375 mg, 100's: **$103.28**; 500 mg, 100's: **$143.34**

• Tab, Coated, Sus Action—Oral: 250 mg, 100's: **$17.50**; 500 mg, 100's: **$27.50-$86.78**; 750 mg, 100's: **$45.00-$54.69**; 1000 mg, 100's: **$47.50-$100.00**

UNLABELED USES: Conversion and management of atrial fibrillation

CONTRAINDICATIONS: Complete heart block, myasthenia gravis, pre-existing QT prolongation, second-degree heart block, systemic lupus erythematosus, torsades de pointes

PREGNANCY AND LACTATION: Pregnancy category C; compatible with breast-feeding, however long-term effects in nursing infant unknown

SIDE EFFECTS

Frequent

PO: Abdominal pain or cramping, nausea, diarrhea, vomiting

Occasional

Dizziness, giddiness, weakness, hypersensitivity reaction (rash, urticaria, pruritus, flushing)

IV: Transient, but at times, marked hypotension

Rare

Confusion, mental depression, psychosis

SERIOUS REACTIONS

• Paradoxical, extremely rapid ventricular rate may occur during treatment of atrial fibrillation or flutter.

• Systemic lupus erythematosus-–like syndrome (fever, myalgia, pleuritic chest pain) may occur with prolonged therapy.

• Cardiotoxic effects occur most commonly with IV administration and appear as conduction changes (50% widening of QRS complex, frequent ventricular premature contractions, ventricular tachycardia, and complete AV block).

• Prolonged PR and QT intervals and flattened T waves occur less frequently.

INTERACTIONS

Drugs

▣ *Amiodarone, cimetidine, trimethoprim:* Increased procainamide concentrations

▣ *Cholinergic drugs:* Antagonism of cholinergic actions on skeletal muscle

▣ *Procaine:* Interferes with procainamide concentration assay

Labs

• *False decrease:* Cholinesterase
• *False increase:* Potassium

SPECIAL CONSIDERATIONS

PATIENT/FAMILY EDUCATION

• Strict compliance to dosage schedule imperative

• Empty wax core from sustained release tablets may appear in stool; this is harmless

• Initiate therapy in facilities capable of providing continuous ECG monitoring and managing life-threatening dysrhythmias

MONITORING PARAMETERS

• CBC with differential and platelets qwk for first 3 mo, periodically thereafter

• ECG: R/O overdosage if QRS widens >25% or QT prolongation occurs; reduce dosage if QRS widens >50%

• ANA titer increases may precede clinical symptoms of lupoid syndrome

• Serum creatinine, urea nitrogen

• Plasma procainamide concentration (therapeutic range 3-10 mcg/ml; 10-30 mcg/ml NAPA)

---

procaine

(proe'-kane)

Rx: Novocain, Mericaine
Chemical Class: Benzoic acid derivative
Therapeutic Class: Anesthetic, local

CLINICAL PHARMACOLOGY

Mechanism of Action: Procaine causes a reversible blockade of nerve conduction by decreasing nerve membrane permeability to sodium. *Therapeutic effect:* Local anesthesia.

Pharmacokinetics

Highly plasma protein-bound and distributed to all body tissues. Excreted in the urine (80%). **Half-life:** 40 ± 9 seconds in adults, 84 ± 30 seconds in neonates.

INDICATIONS AND DOSAGES

Spinal anesthesia

Intrathecal

Adults. 0.5-1 ml of a 10% solution (50-100 mg) mixed with an equal volume of diluent injected into the third or fourth lumber interspace (perineum and lower extremities). 2 ml of a 10% solution (200 mg) mixed with 1 ml of diluent injected into the second, third or fourth interspace.

Infiltration anesthesia, dental anesthesia, control of severe pain (post-herpetic neuralgia, cancer pain, or burns)

Topical

Adults. A single dose of 350-600 mg using a 0.25 or 0.5% solution. Use 0.9% sodium chloride for dilution.

Children. 15 mg/kg of a 0.5% solution is the maximum recommended dose.

Peripheral or sympathetic nerve block (regional anesthesia)
Topical

Adults. Up to 200 ml of a 0.5% solution (1 g), 100 ml of a 1% solution (1 g), or 50 ml of a 2% solution (1 g). The 2% solution should only be used when a small volume of anesthetic is required.

S AVAILABLE FORMS/COST
• Sol, Inj—Infiltration: 1%, 30 ml: **$3.50**; 2%, 30 ml: **$2.50-$4.80**

UNLABELED USES: Severe pain

CONTRAINDICATIONS: Hypersensitivity to ester local anesthetics, sulfites, PABA, patients on anticoagulant therapy, and in patients with coagulopathy, infection, thrombocytopenia. Should not be given intraarterial, intrathecal, or intravenous.

PREGNANCY AND LACTATION: Pregnancy category C; use caution in nursing mothers

SIDE EFFECTS
Frequent
Numbness or tingling of the face or mouth, pain at the injection site, dizziness, drowsiness, lightheadedness, nausea, vomiting, back pain, headache

Rare
Anxiety, restlessness, difficulty breathing, shortness of breath, seizures (convulsions), skin rash, itching (hives), slow irregular heartbeat (palpitations), swelling of the face or mouth, tremors, QT prolongation, PR prolongation, atrial fibrillation, sinus bradycardia, hypotension, angina, cardiovascular collapse, fecal or urinary incontinence, loss of perineal sensation and sexual function, persistent motor, sensory, and/or autonomic (sphincter control) deficit

SERIOUS REACTIONS
• Procaine-induced CNS toxicity usually presents with symptoms of stimulation such as anxiety, apprehension, restlessness, nervousness, disorientation, confusion, dizziness, blurred vision, tremor, nausea/vomiting, shivering, or seizures. Subsequently, depressive symptoms can occur including drowsiness, unconsciousness, and respiratory arrest.
• If higher concentrations are introduced into the blood stream, depression of cardiac excitability and contractility may cause AV block, ventricular arrhythmias, or cardiac arrest. CNS toxicity including dizziness, tongue numbness, visual impairment and disturbances, and muscular twitching appear to occur before cardiotoxic effects.

Alert
• Procaine should be used with caution in patients that have asthma since there is the increased risk of anaphylactoid reactions including bronchospasm and status asthmaticus.

Alert
• Local anesthetics cab cause varying degrees of maternal, fetal, and neonatal toxicities during labor and obstetric delivery. Fetal heart rate should be monitored as well as the presence of symptoms indicating fetal bradycardia, fetal acidosis, and maternal hypotension. Epidural procaine may cause decreased uterine contractility or maternal expulsion efforts and alter the forces of parturition.

Alert
• Unintentional fetal intracranial injection of procaine occurring during pudendal or paracervical block has been shown to lead to neonatal depression at birth and can lead to seizures within 6 hours as a result of high serum concentrations.

P

INTERACTIONS
Drugs
3 β-blockers: Acute discontinuation of β-blockers before local anesthesia increases the risk of hypertensive reactions
Labs
• False increase: CSF protein, urine porphobilinogen, urobilinogen
SPECIAL CONSIDERATIONS
• Esther-type local anesthetic
MONITORING PARAMETERS
• Blood pressure, pulse, respiration during treatment, ECG
• Fetal heart tones if used during labor

---

prochlorperazine
(proe-klor-per′a-zeen)
Rx: Compazine
Chemical Class: Piperazine phenothiazine derivative
Therapeutic Class: Antiemetic; antipsychotic

CLINICAL PHARMACOLOGY
Mechanism of Action: A phenothiazine that acts centrally to inhibit or block dopamine receptors in the chemoreceptor trigger zone and peripherally to block the vagus nerve in the GI tract. *Therapeutic Effect:* Relieves nausea and vomiting and improves psychotic conditions.

Pharmacokinetics

Route	Onset*	Peak	Duration
Tablets, oral solution	30-40 min	N/A	3-4 hr
Capsules (Extended-Release)	30-40 min	N/A	10-12 hr
Rectal	60 min	N/A	3-4 hr

* As an antiemetic

Variably absorbed after PO administration. Widely distributed. Metabolized in the liver and GI mucosa. Primarily excreted in urine. Unknown if removed by hemodialysis. **Half-life:** 23 hr.

INDICATIONS AND DOSAGES
Nausea and vomiting
PO
Adults, Elderly. 5-10 mg 3-4 times a day.
Children. 0.4 mg/kg/day in 3-4 divided doses.
PO (Extended-Release)
Adults, Elderly. 10 mg twice a day or 15 mg once a day.
IV
Adults, Elderly. 2.5-10 mg. May repeat q3-4h.
Children. 0.1-0.15 mg/kg/dose q8-12h. Maximum: 40 mg/day.
IM
Adults, Elderly. 5-10 mg q3-4h.
Children. 0.1-0.15 mg/kg/dose q8-12h. Maximum: 40 mg/day.
Rectal
Adults, Elderly. 25 mg twice a day.
Children. 0.4 mg/kg/day in 3-4 divided doses.

Psychosis
PO
Adults, Elderly. 5-10 mg 3-4 times a day. Maximum: 150 mg/day.
Children. 2.5 mg 2-3 times a day. Maximum: 25 mg for children 6-12 yr; 20 mg for children 2-5 yr.
IM
Adults, Elderly. 10-20 mg q4h.
Children. 0.13 mg/kg/dose.

§ AVAILABLE FORMS/COST
• Cap, Gel, Sus Action—Oral: 10 mg, 20's: **$31.94**
• Sol, Inj—IM, IV: 5 mg/ml, 2 ml: **$2.39-$3.75**
• Supp—Rect: 2.5 mg, 12's: **$28.30-$38.14**; 5 mg, 12's: **$31.40**; 25 mg, 12's: **$24.55-$60.25**
• Syr—Oral: 5 mg/5 ml, 120 ml: **$24.29**

• Tab, Plain Coated—Oral: 5 mg, 100's: **$12.50-$95.00**; 10 mg, 100's: **$17.50-$102.24**; 25 mg, 100's: **$19.50**

CONTRAINDICATIONS: Angle-closure glaucoma, CNS depression, coma, myelosuppression, severe cardiac or hepatic impairment, severe hypotension or hypertension

PREGNANCY AND LACTATION: Pregnancy category C; majority of evidence indicates safety for both mother and fetus if used occasionally in low doses; excretion into breast milk should be expected; sedation is a possible effect in nursing infant

SIDE EFFECTS

Frequent

Somnolence, hypotension, dizziness, fainting (commonly occurring after first dose, occasionally after subsequent doses, and rarely with oral form)

Occasional

Dry mouth, blurred vision, lethargy, constipation, diarrhea, myalgia, nasal congestion, peripheral edema, urine retention

SERIOUS REACTIONS

• Extrapyramidal symptoms appear to be dose relatedand are divided into three categories: akathisia (marked by inability to sit still, tapping of feet), parkinsonian symptoms (including masklike face, tremors, shuffling gait, hypersalivation), and acute dystonias (such as torticollis, opisthotonos, and oculogyric crisis. A dystonic reaction may also produce diaphoresis or pallor.

• Tardive dyskinesia, manifested as tongue protrusion, puffing of the cheeks, and puckering of the mouth, is a rare reaction that may be irreversible.

• Abrupt withdrawal after long-term therapy may precipitate nausea, vomiting, gastritis, dizziness, and tremors.

• Blood dyscrasias, particularly agranulocytosis and mild leukopenia, may occur.

• Prochlorperazine use may lower the seizure threshold.

INTERACTIONS

Drugs

③ *Anticholinergics:* Inhibited therapeutic response to antipsychotic; enhanced anticholinergic side effects

③ *Antidepressants:* Increased serum concentrations of some cyclic antidepressants

③ *Attapulgite:* Inhibition of phenothiazine absorption

③ *Barbiturates:* Reduced effect of antipsychotic

③ *Bromocriptine, lithium:* Reduced effects of both drugs

③ *β-blockers:* Enhanced effects of both drugs (interaction less likely with atenolol, nadolol)

③ *Chloroquine, amodiaquine, pyrimethamine:* Possible increased phenothiazine concentrations

③ *Cigarettes:* Possible enhanced metabolism of neuroleptic

③ *Clonidine:* Possible enhanced hypotensive effect

③ *Epinephrine:* Reversed pressor response to epinephrine

③ *Ethanol:* Enhanced ethanol effects

③ *Guanethidine:* Inhibited antihypertensive response to guanethidine

③ *Indomethacin:* Possible increased CNS effects, other NSAIDs less likely to have effect

③ *Narcotic analgesics:* Excessive CNS depression, hypotension, respiratory depression

② *Levodopa:* Inhibited effect of levodopa on Parkinson's disease

P

§ *Orphenadrine:* Reduced serum neuroleptic concentrations, excessive anticholinergic effects

§ *Procarbazine:* Increased sedation, EPS effects

§ *SSRIs:* Increased risk EPS effects

§ *Trazadone:* Possible increased risk hypotension

Labs

• *False positive:* Phenylketones

SPECIAL CONSIDERATIONS

PATIENT/FAMILY EDUCATION

• Arise slowly from reclining position

• Do not discontinue abruptly

• Use a sunscreen during sun exposure to prevent burns; take special precautions to stay cool in hot weather

• May cause drowsiness

MONITORING PARAMETERS

• Observe closely for signs of tardive dyskinesia

• Treat acute dystonic reactions with parenteral diphenhydramine (2 mg/kg to max 50 mg) or benztropine (2 mg)

• Periodic CBC with platelets during prolonged therapy

---

procyclidine
(proe-sye-kli-deen)

Rx: Kemadrin
Chemical Class: Tertiary amine
Therapeutic Class: Anti-Parkinson's agent; anticholinergic

CLINICAL PHARMACOLOGY

Mechanism of Action: An anticholinergic agent that exerts an atropine-like action and produces an antispasmodic effect on smooth muscle, is a potent mydriatic, and inhibits salivation. *Therapeutic Effect:* Relieves symptoms of Parkinson's disease and drug-induced extrapyramidal symptoms.

Pharmacokinetics

Well absorbed from the gastrointestinal (GI) tract. Protein binding: extensive. Metabolized in liver—undergoes extensive first-pass effect. Primarily excreted in urine. Unknown if removed by hemodialysis. **Half-life:** 7.7-16.1 hrs.

INDICATIONS AND DOSAGES

Drug-induced extrapyramidal reactions

PO

Adults, Elderly. Initially, 2.5 mg 3 times/day. May increase by 2.5 mg daily as needed. Maintenance: 10-20 mg/day in divided doses 3 times/day.

Parkinson's disease

PO

Adults, Elderly. Initially, 2.5 mg 3 times/day after meals. Maintenance: 2.5-5 mg mg/day in divided doses 3 times/day after meals.

Hepatic function impairment

PO

Adults, Elderly. 2.5-5 mg mg/day in divided doses twice a day after meals

§ **AVAILABLE FORMS/COST**

• Tab—Oral: 5 mg, 100's: **$75.43**

CONTRAINDICATIONS: Angle-closure glaucoma

PREGNANCY AND LACTATION: Pregnancy category C; nursing infants may be particularly sensitive to anticholinergic effects

SIDE EFFECTS

Frequent

Blurred vision, mydriasis, disorientation, lightheadedness, nausea, vomiting dry mouth, nose, throat, and lips

SERIOUS REACTIONS

• Overdosage may vary from severe anticholinergic effects, such as unsteadiness, severe drowsiness, severe dryness of mouth, nose, or throat, tachycardia, shortness of breath, and skin flushing.

• Also produces severe paradoxical reaction, marked by hallucinations, tremor, seizures, and toxic psychosis.

INTERACTIONS
Drugs
▣ *Amantadine:* Potentiates CNS side effects of amantadine

▣ *Anticholinergic:* Increased anticholinergic side effects

▣ *Antipsychotic agents:* Possible worsening of psychosis, increased anticholinergic side effects

▣ *Digoxin (slow dissolution tab):* Increased digoxin concentration

▣ *Tacrine:* Reduced therapeutic effects of both drugs

SPECIAL CONSIDERATIONS
PATIENT/FAMILY EDUCATION
• Do not discontinue this drug abruptly

• Hard candy, frequent drinks, sugarless gum to relieve dry mouth

• Take with or after meals to prevent GI upset

• Use caution in hot weather, may increase susceptibility to heat stroke

---

progesterone
(proe-jess'ter-one)
Rx: Crinone (gel),
Prometrium Progestasert
(IUD)
Chemical Class: Progestin,
natural
Therapeutic Class: Contraceptive; progestin

CLINICAL PHARMACOLOGY
Mechanism of Action: A natural steroid hormone that promotes mammary gland development and relaxes uterine smooth muscle.
Therapeutic Effect: Decreases abs-normal uterine bleeding; transforms endometrium from proliferative to secretory in an estrogen-primed endometrium.

INDICATIONS AND DOSAGES
Amenorrhea
PO

Adults. 400 mg daily in evening for 10 days.
IM

Adults. 5–10 mg for 6–8 days. Withdrawal bleeding expected in 48–72 hr if ovarian activity produced proliferative endometrium.
Vaginal

Adults. Apply 45 mg (4% gel) every other day for 6 or fewer doses.
Abnormal uterine bleeding
IM

Adults. 5–10 mg for 6 days. When estrogen given concomitantly, begin progesterone after 2 wk of estrogen therapy; discontinue when menstrual flow begins.
Prevention of endometrial hyperplasia
PO

Adults. 200 mg in evening for 12 days per 28-day cycle in combination with daily conjugated estrogen.
Infertility
Vaginal

Adults. 90 mg (8% gel) once a day (2 twice a day in women with partial or complete ovarian failure).

Ⓢ **AVAILABLE FORMS/COST**
• Sol, Inj—IM: 50 mg/ml, 10 ml: **$10.20-$38.75**

• Gel—Vag: 4% 6 applicators: **$30.00-$39.96**; 8% 6 applicators: **$60.00**

• Cap—Oral: 100 mg, 100's: **$103.30**; 200 mg 100's: **$196.29**
UNLABELED USES: Treatment of corpus luteum dysfunction
CONTRAINDICATIONS: Breast cancer; history of active cerebral

apoplexy; thromboembolic disorders or thrombophlebitis; missed abortion; severe hepatic dysfunction; undiagnosed vaginal bleeding; use as a pregnancy test

PREGNANCY AND LACTATION: Pregnancy category D; possible increase in limb reduction defects, hypospadias in male fetuses and mild virilization of female fetuses

SIDE EFFECTS

Frequent

Breakthrough bleeding or spotting at beginning of therapy, amenorrhea, change in menstrual flow, breast tenderness

Gel: drowsiness

Occasional

Edema, weight gain or loss, rash, pruritus, photosensitivity, skin pigmentation

Rare

Pain or swelling at injection site, acne, depression, alopecia, hirsutism

SERIOUS REACTIONS

• Thrombophlebitis, cerebrovascular disorders, retinal thrombosis, and pulmonary embolism occur rarely.

INTERACTIONS

Drugs

3 *Aminoglutethimide:* Possible decreased progestin effect

Labs

• *Increase:* Alk phosphatase, pregnanediol, liver function tests

• *Decrease:* Glucose tolerance test, HDL

SPECIAL CONSIDERATIONS

• Gel provides enhanced uterine delivery compared with IM administration

PATIENT/FAMILY EDUCATION

• Diabetic patients may note decreased glucose tolerance

• No evidence that use for habitual or threatened abortion is effective

• Notify clinician of abnormal or excessive bleeding, severe cramping, abnormal or odorous vaginal discharge, missed period (IUD)

• Cost and risk of infection (greatest in first months after insertion) less for non hormonal IUDs (e.g. ParaGard)

---

promethazine

(proe-meth'a-zeen)

Rx: Phenergan

Combinations

Rx: with codeine (Phenergan with Codeine Syrup); with dextromethorphan (Phenergan with Dextromethorphan Syrup)

Chemical Class: Ethylamine phenothiazine derivative

Therapeutic Class: Antiemetic; antihistamine; antitussive; antivertigo agent; sedative

DEA Class: Schedule V

CLINICAL PHARMACOLOGY

Mechanism of Action: A phenothiazine that acts as an antihistamine, antiemetic, and sedative-hypnotic. As an antihistamine, inhibits histamine at histamine receptor sites. As an antiemetic, diminishes vestibular stimulation, depresses labyrinthine function, and act on the chemoreceptor trigger zone. As a sedative-hypnotic, produces CNS depression by decreasing stimulation to the brain stem reticular formation. *Therapeutic Effect:* Prevents allergic responses mediated by histamine, such as rhinitis, urticaria, and pruritus. Prevents and relieves nausea and vomiting.

Pharmacokinetics

Route	Onset	Peak	Dura-tion
PO	20 min	N/A	2–8 hr
IV	3–5 min	N/A	2–8 hr
IM	20 min	N/A	2–8 hr
Rectal	20 min	N/A	2–8 hr

Well absorbed from the GI tract after IM administration. Widely distributed. Metabolized in the liver. Primarily excreted in urine. Not removed by hemodialysis. **Half-life:** 16–19 hr.

INDICATIONS AND DOSAGES
Allergic symptoms
PO

Adults, Elderly. 6.25–12.5 mg 3 times a day plus 25 mg at bedtime.
Children. 0.1 mg/kg/dose (maximum: 12.5 mg) 3 times a day plus 0.5 mg/kg/dose (maximum: 25 mg) at bedtime.
IV, IM

Adults, Elderly. 25 mg. May repeat in 2 hr.

Motion sickness
PO

Adults, Elderly. 25 mg 30–60 min before departure; may repeat in 8–12 hr, then every morning on rising and before evening meal.
Children. 0.5 mg/kg 30–60 min before departure; may repeat in 8–12 hr, then every morning on rising and before evening meal.

Prevention of nausea, and vomiting
PO, IV, IM, Rectal

Adults, Elderly. 12.5–25 mg q4–6h as needed.
Children. 0.25–1 mg/kg q4–6h as needed.

Preoperative and postoperative sedation; adjunct to analgesics
IV, IM

Adults, Elderly. 25–50 mg.
Children. 12.5–25 mg.

Sedative
PO, IV, IM, Rectal

Adults, Elderly. 25-50 mg/dose. May repeat q4-6h as needed.
Children. 0.5-1 mg/kg/dose q6h as needed. Maximum: 50 mg/dose.

AVAILABLE FORMS/COST
• Sol, Inj—IM, IV: 25 mg/ml, 1, 10 ml: **$0.80-$3.67**/ml; 50 mg/ml, 1, 10 ml: **$1.00-$3.83**/ml
• Supp—Rect: 12.5 mg, 12's: **$30.50-$53.71**; 25 mg, 12's: **$33.25-$60.93**; 50 mg, 12's: **$44.81-$77.08**
• Syr—Oral: 6.25 mg/5 ml, 120, 240, 480 ml: **$1.80-$22.04**/480 ml; 25 mg/5 ml, 480 ml: **$10.99**
• Tab—Oral: 12.5 mg, 100's: **$33.44**; 25 mg, 100's: **$3.15-$67.91**; 50 mg, 100's: **$4.65-$90.54**

CONTRAINDICATIONS: Angle-closure glaucoma, GI or GU obstruction, severe CNS depression or coma

PREGNANCY AND LACTATION: Pregnancy category C; passage of drug into breast milk should be expected

SIDE EFFECTS
Expected
Somnolence, disorientation; in elderly, hypotension, confusion, syncope
Frequent
Dry mouth, nose, or throat; urine retention; thickening of bronchial secretions
Occasional
Epigastric distress, flushing, visual disturbances, hearing disturbances, wheezing, paraesthesia, diaphoresis, chills
Rare
Dizziness, urticaria, photosensitivity, nightmares

SERIOUS REACTIONS

- Children may experience paradoxical reactions, such as excitation, nervousness, tremor, hyperactive reflexes, and seizures.
- Infants and young children have experienced CNS depression manifested as respiratory depression, sleep apnea, and sudden infant death syndrome.
- Long-term therapy may produce extrapyramidal symptoms, such as dystonia (abnormal movements), pronounced motor restlessness (most frequently in children), and parkinsonian (most frequently in elderly patients).
- Blood dyscrasias, particularly agranulocytosis, occur rarely.

INTERACTIONS

Drugs

[3] *CNS depressants:* Additive sedative action

Labs

- *False increase:* Tricyclic antidepressant

SPECIAL CONSIDERATIONS

PATIENT/FAMILY EDUCATION

- Avoid prolonged exposure to sunlight

propafenone

(proe-pa-fen'one)

Rx: Rythmol

Chemical Class: 3-phenylpropiophenone derivative

Therapeutic Class: Antiarrhythmic, class IC

CLINICAL PHARMACOLOGY

Mechanism of Action: An antiarrhythmic that decreases the fast sodium current in Purkinje or myocardial cells. Decreases excitability and automaticity; prolongs conduction velocity and the refractory period. *Therapeutic Effect:* Suppresses arrhythmias.

INDICATIONS AND DOSAGES

Documented, life-threatening ventricular arrhythmias, such as sustained ventricular tachycardia

PO, prompt-release

Adults, Elderly. Initially, 150 mg q8h; may increase at 3-to 4-day intervals to 225 mg q8h, then to 300 mg q8h. Maximum: 900 mg/day.

PO, extended-release

Adults, Elderly. Initially, 225 mg q12h. May increase at 5 day intervals. Maximum: 425 mg q12h.

[$] **AVAILABLE FORMS/COST**

- Tab, Coated—Oral: 150 mg, 100's: **$163.58-$293.75**; 225 mg, 100's: **$232.93-$386.25**; 300 mg, 100's: **$296.99-$386.25**

UNLABELED USES: Treatment of supraventricular arrhythmias

CONTRAINDICATIONS: Bradycardia; bronchospastic disorders; cardiogenic shock; electrolyte imbalance; sinoatrial, AV, and intraventricular impulse generation or conduction disorders, such as sick sinus syndrome or AV block, without the presence of a pacemaker; uncontrolled CHF

PREGNANCY AND LACTATION: Pregnancy category C

SIDE EFFECTS

Frequent (13%–7%)

Dizziness, nausea, vomiting, altered taste, constipation

Occasional (6%–3%)

Headache, dyspnea, blurred vision, dyspepsia (heartburn, indigestion, epigastric pain)

Rare (less than 2%)

Rash, weakness, dry mouth, diarrhea, edema, hot flashes

SERIOUS REACTIONS

- Propafenone may produce or worsen existing arrhythmias.

• Overdose may produce hypotension, somnolence, bradycardia, and atrioventricular conduction disturbances.

INTERACTIONS

Drugs

[3] *β-blockers:* Increased metoprolol or propranolol concentrations

[3] *Cimetidine:* Increased propafenone concentrations

[3] *Digitalis glycosides:* Increased serum digoxin concentrations

[3] *Food:* Increased peak serum propafenone concentrations

[3] *Oral anticoagulants:* Increased serum warfarin concentrations, prolonged protime

[3] *Quinidine:* Increased propafenone concentrations but reduced concentrations of its active metabolite; net effect uncertain (toxicity vs reduced efficacy)

[3] *Rifampin, phenobarbital, rifabutin:* Reduced serum propafenone concentrations

[3] *Theophylline:* Increased plasma theophylline concentrations

SPECIAL CONSIDERATIONS

PATIENT/FAMILY EDUCATION

• Signs of overdosage include hypotension, excessive drowsiness, decreased heart rate, or abnormal heartbeat

MONITORING PARAMETERS

• ECG, consider dose reduction in patients with significant widening of the QRS complex or 2nd- or 3rd-degree AV block

• ANA, carefully evaluate abnormal ANA test, consider discontinuation if persistent or worsening ANA titers are detected

propantheline

(proe-pan-the-leen)

Rx: Propantheline

Chemical Class: Quaternary ammonium derivative

Therapeutic Class: Antispasmodic; antiulcer agent (adjunct); gastrointestinal

CLINICAL PHARMACOLOGY

Mechanism of Action: A quaternary ammonium compound which has anticholinergic properties and that inhibits action of acetylcholine at postganglionic parasympathetic sites. *Therapeutic Effect:* Reduces gastric secretions and urinary frequency, urgency and urge incontinence.

Pharmacokinetics

Onset occurs within 90 min but less than 50% is absorbed from gastrointestinal (GI) tract. Extensive hepatic metabolism. Excreted in the urine and feces. **Half-life:** 2.9 hrs.

INDICATIONS AND DOSAGES

Peptic ulcer

PO

Adults, Elderly. 15 mg 3 times/day 30 min. before meals and 30 mg at bedtime.

Children. 1-2 mg/kg/day, divided q4-6h and at bedtime.

[$] **AVAILABLE FORMS/COST**

• Tab, Sugar Coated—Oral: 7.5 mg, 100's: **$42.66**; 15 mg, 100's: **$3.67-$83.58**

CONTRAINDICATIONS: GI or genitourinary (GU) obstruction, myasthenia gravis, narrow-angle glaucoma, toxic megacolon, severe ulcerative colitis, unstable cardiovascular adjustment in acute hemorrhage, hypersensitivity to propantheline or other anticholinergics

P

PREGNANCY AND LACTATION:
Pregnancy category C; excretion into breast milk unknown, although would be expected to be minimal due to quaternary structure

SIDE EFFECTS

Frequent

Dry mouth, decreased sweating, constipation

Occasional

Blurred vision, intolerance to light, urinary hesitancy, drowsiness, agitation, excitement

Rare

Confusion, increased intraocular pressure, orthostatic hypotension, tachycardia

SERIOUS REACTIONS

• Overdosage may produce temporary paralysis of ciliary muscle, pupillary dilation, tachycardia, palpitations, hot, dry, or flushed skin, absence of bowel sounds, hyperthermia, increased respiratory rate, EKG abnormalities, nausea, vomiting, rash over face or upper trunk, CNS stimulation, and psychosis, marked by agitation, restlessness, rambling speech, visual hallucinations, paranoid behavior, and delusions, followed by depression.

INTERACTIONS

Drugs

3 *Tricyclic antidepressants:* Additive anticholinergic effects

Labs

• *False increase:* Bicarbonate, chloride

SPECIAL CONSIDERATIONS

PATIENT/FAMILY EDUCATION

• Avoid driving or other hazardous activities until stabilized on medication

• Avoid alcohol or other CNS depressants

• Avoid hot environments, heat stroke may occur

• Use sunglasses when outside to prevent photophobia, may cause blurred vision

---

propoxyphene

Rx: Darvon, Dolene; Darvon-N

Combinations

  Rx: with acetaminophen (Darvocet, Propacet, Wygesic)

Chemical Class: Diphenylheptane derivative; opiate derivative

Therapeutic Class: Narcotic analgesic

DEA Class: Schedule IV

CLINICAL PHARMACOLOGY

Mechanism of Action: An opioid agonist that binds with opioid receptors in the CNS. *Therapeutic Effect:* Alters the perception of and emotional response to pain.

Pharmacokinetics

Route	Onset	Peak	Duration
PO	15–60 min	N/A	4-6 hr

Well absorbed from the GI tract. Protein binding: High. Widely distributed. Metabolized in the liver. Primarily excreted in urine. Not removed by hemodialysis. **Half-life:** 6-12 hr; metabolite: 30-36 hr.

INDICATIONS AND DOSAGES

Mild to moderate pain

PO (propoxyphene hydrochloride)

Adults, Elderly. 65 mg q4h as needed. Maximum: 390 mg/day.

PO (propoxyphene napsylate)

Adults, Elderly. 100 mg q4h as needed. Maximum: 600 mg/day.

§ AVAILABLE FORMS/COST

• Cap, Gel—Oral (hydrochloride): 65 mg, 100's: **$7.35-$68.96**

• Tab—Oral (napsylate): 100 mg, 100's: **$100.30**

CONTRAINDICATIONS: None known.

PREGNANCY AND LACTATION: Pregnancy category C (category D if used for prolonged periods or in high doses at term); withdrawal could theoretically occur in infants exposed *in utero* to prolonged maternal ingestion; compatible with breast-feeding

SIDE EFFECTS
Frequent

Dizziness, somnolence, dry mouth, euphoria, hypotension (including orthostatic hypotension), nausea, vomiting, fatigue

Occasional

Allergic reaction (including decreased BP), diaphoresis, flushing, and wheezing), trembling, urine retention, vision changes, constipation, headache

Rare

Confusion, increased BP, depression, abdominal cramps, anorexia

SERIOUS REACTIONS

• Overdose results in respiratory depression, skeletal muscle flaccidity, cold or clammy skin, cyanosis, and extreme somnolence progressing to seizures, stupor, and coma.

• Hepatotoxicity may occur with overdose of the acetaminophen component of fixed-combination products.

• The patient who uses propoxyphene repeatedly may develop a tolerance to the drug's analgesic effect and physical dependence.

INTERACTIONS
Drugs

3 *Anticoagulants:* Potentiation of warfarin's anticoagulant effect

3 *Antidepressants:* Increased cyclic antidepressant serum concentrations

3 *Antihistamines, chloral hydrate, glutethimide, methocarbamol:* Enhanced depressant effects

3 *Barbiturates:* Additive respiratory and CNS depressant effects

3 *β-blockers:* Increased concentrations of highly metabolized β-blockers (metoprolol, propranolol)

2 *Carbamazepine:* Marked increases in plasma carbamazepine concentrations

3 *Ethanol:* Additive CNS effects

3 *Protease inhibitors:* Increased respiratory and CNS depression

Labs

• *False increase:* Amylase and lipase

SPECIAL CONSIDERATIONS
PATIENT/FAMILY EDUCATION

• May cause drowsiness, dizziness or blurred vision

• Use caution driving or engaging in other activities requiring alertness

• Avoid alcohol

P

propranolol
(proe-pran'oh-lole)

Rx: Inderal, Inderal LA
Combinations
  Rx: with HCTZ (Inderide)
Chemical Class: β-adrenergic blocker, nonselective
Therapeutic Class: Antianginal; antiarrhythmic, class II; antiglaucoma agent; antihypertensive; antimigraine agent

CLINICAL PHARMACOLOGY

Mechanism of Action: An antihypertensive, antianginal, antiarrhythmic, and antimigraine agent that blocks beta$_1$- and beta$_2$-adrenergic receptors. Decreases oxygen requirements. Slows AV conduction and increases refractory period in AV node. Large doses increase airway resistance. *Therapeutic Effect:* Slows sinus heart rate; decreases cardiac output, BP, and myocardial ischemia severity. Exhibits antiarrhythmic activity.

Pharmacokinetics

Route	Onset	Peak	Duration
PO	1–2 hr	N/A	6 hr

Well absorbed from the GI tract. Protein binding: 93%. Widely distributed. Metabolized in the liver. Primarily excreted in urine. Not removed by hemodialysis. **Half-life:** 3–5 hr.

INDICATIONS AND DOSAGES

Hypertension

PO

Adults, Elderly. Initially, 40 mg twice a day. May increase dose q3-7 days. Range: Up to 320 mg/day in divided doses. Maximum: 640 mg/day.

Children. Initially, 0.5–1 mg/kg/day in divided doses q6-12h. May increase at 3- to 5-day intervals. Usual dose: 1–5 mg/kg/day. Maximum: 16 mg/kg/day.

Angina

PO

Adults, Elderly. 80–320 mg/day in divided doses. (long acting): Initially, 80 mg/day. Maximum: 320 mg/day.

Arrhythmias

IV

Adults, Elderly. 1 mg/dose. May repeat q5min. Maximum: 5 mg total dose.

Children. 0.01–0.1 mg/kg. Maximum: infants, 1 mg; children, 3 mg.

PO

Adults, Elderly. Initially, 10–20 mg q6-8h. May gradually increase dose. Range: 40–320 mg/day.

Children. Initially, 0.5–1 mg/kg/day in divided doses q6-8h. May increase q3-5 days. Usual dosage: 2–4 mg/kg/day. Maximum: 16 mg/kg/day or 60 mg/day.

Life-threatening arrhythmias

IV

Adults, Elderly. 0.5–3 mg. Repeat once in 2 min. Give additional doses at intervals of at least 4 hr.

Children. 0.01–0.1 mg/kg.

Hypertrophic subaortic stenosis

PO

Adults, Elderly. 20–40 mg in 3–4 divided doses. Or 80–160 mg/day as extended-release capsule.

Adjunct to alpha-blocking agents to treat pheochromocytoma

PO

Adults, Elderly. 60 mg/day in divided doses with alpha-blocker for 3 days before surgery. Maintenance (inoperable tumor): 30 mg/day with alpha-blocker.

Migraine headache

PO

Adults, Elderly. 80 mg/day in divided doses. Or 80 mg once daily as extended-release capsule. Increase up to 160–240 mg/day in divided doses.

Children. 0.6–1.5 mg/kg/day in divided doses q8h. Maximum: 4 mg/kg/day.

Reduction of cardiovascular mortality and reinfarction in patients with previous MI

PO

Adults, Elderly. 180–240 mg/day in divided doses.

Essential tremor

PO

Adults, Elderly. Initially, 40 mg twice a day increased up to 120–320 mg/day in 3 divided doses.

$ AVAILABLE FORMS/COST

• Cap, Gel, Sus Action—Oral: 60 mg, 100's: **$62.55-$164.74**; 80 mg, 100's: **$73.55-$181.48**; 120 mg, 100's: **$90.90-$239.27**; 160 mg, 100's: **$118.90-$241.25**

• Sol, Inj—IV: 1 mg/ml, 1 ml: **$7.00-$18.56**

- Sol—Oral: 20 mg/5 ml, 500 ml: **$40.17**; 40 mg/5 ml, 500 ml: **$49.51**
- Conc—Oral: 80 mg/ml, 30 ml: **$33.53**
- Tab—Oral: 10 mg, 100's: **$2.25-$46.31**; 20 mg, 100's: **$2.50-$65.00**; 40 mg, 100's: **$3.00-$84.38**; 60 mg, 100's: **$4.25-$116.69**; 80 mg, 100's: **$3.75-$129.50**

UNLABELED USES: Treatment adjunct for anxiety, mitral valve prolapse syndrome, thyrotoxicosis

CONTRAINDICATIONS: Asthma, bradycardia, cardiogenic shock, COPD, heart block, Raynaud's syndrome, uncompensated CHF

PREGNANCY AND LACTATION: Pregnancy category C; similar drug, atenolol, frequently used in the third trimester for treatment of hypertension (many studies of efficacy and safety of atenolol in pregnancy-induced hypertension); long-term use has been associated with intrauterine growth retardation; milk levels approximately half of peak plasma levels; considered insignificant; compatible with breast-feeding

SIDE EFFECTS

Frequent

Diminished sexual ability, drowsiness, difficulty sleeping, unusual fatigue or weakness

Occasional

Bradycardia, depression, sensation of coldness in extremities, diarrhea, constipation, anxiety, nasal congestion, nausea, vomiting

Rare

Altered taste, dry eyes, pruritus, paraesthesia

SERIOUS REACTIONS

- Overdose may produce profound bradycardia and hypotension.
- Abrupt withdrawal may result in sweating, palpitations, headache, and tremulousness.

- Propranolol administration may precipitate CHF and MI in patients with cardiac disease; thyroid storm in those with thyrotoxicosis; and peripheral ischemia in those with existing peripheral vascular disease.
- Hypoglycemia may occur in patients with previously controlled diabetes.

INTERACTIONS

Drugs

▣ α_1-*adrenergic blockers:* Potential enhanced first dose response (marked initial drop in blood pressure), particularly on standing (especially prazosin)

▣ *Amiodarone:* Bradycardia, cardiac arrest, ventricular dysrhythmia shortly after initiation of β-blocker

▣ *Antidiabetics:* Masked symptoms of hypoglycemia, prolonged recovery of normoglycemia

▣ *Barbiturates, rifampin:* Reduced concentrations of propranolol

▣ *Antipyrine:* Increased antipyrine concentrations

▣ β-*agonists:* Antagonistic effects

▣ *Calcium channel blockers:* Increased concentrations of propranolol; increased bioavailability of nifedipine

▣ *Chlorpromazine:* Additive hypotensive effects and grand mal seizures; chlorpromazine decreases the clearance of oral propranolol by 25% to 32%, resulting in increased propranolol bioavailability

▣ *Cimetidine, etintidine, fluoxetine, propoxyphene, propafenone, quinidine, quinolones:* Increased propranolol concentrations

▣ *Clonidine, guanabenz, guanfacine:* Exacerbation of hypertension upon withdrawal of clonidine

▣ *Cocaine:* Potentiation of cocaine-induced coronary vasospasm

▣ *Contrast media:* Increased risk anaphylaxis

P

🔢 *Digitalis glycosides:* Increased digoxin concentrations

🔢 *Dihydroergotamine, ergotamine:* May result in excessive vasoconstriction

🔢 *Epinephrine:* Enhanced pressor response to epinephrine

🔢 *Fluvoxamine:* Increased propranolol serum concentrations; increased risk of bradycardia and hypotension

🔢 *Flecainide:* Increased propranolol and flecainide concentrations; additive negative inotropic effects

🔢 *Hydralazine:* Increases oral bioavailability of propranolol (high clearance and lipophilic β-blockers) increasing risk of adverse effects

🔢 *Hydrochlorothiazide:* Exaggerated hyperglycemic response

🔢 *Lidocaine:* Increased lidocaine concentrations

🔢 *Local anesthetics:* Enhanced sympathomimetic side effects of epinephrine-containing local anesthetics

🔢 *Neostigmine, physostigmine, tacrine:* Additive bradycardia

🔢 *Neuroleptics:* Increased plasma concentrations of both drugs

🔢 *NSAIDs:* Reduced hypotensive effect of propranolol

🔢 *Phenylephrine:* Predisposition to acute hypertensive episodes

➋ *Theophylline:* Increased theophylline concentrations; antagonistic pharmacodynamic effects

Labs
• *False increase:* Bilirubin

SPECIAL CONSIDERATIONS
PATIENT/FAMILY EDUCATION
• Do not discontinue abruptly, may require taper; rapid withdrawal may produce rebound hypertension or angina

MONITORING PARAMETERS
• Angina: Reduction in nitroglycerin usage; frequency, severity, onset, and duration of angina pain; heart rate
• Arrhythmias: Heart rate
• Congestive heart failure: Functional status, cough, dyspnea on exertion, paroxysmal nocturnal dyspnea, exercise tolerance, and ventricular function
• Hypertension: Blood pressure
• Migraine headache: Reduction in the frequency, severity, and duration of attacks
• Postmyocardial infarction: Left ventricular function, lower resting heart rate
• Toxicity: Blood glucose, bronchospasm, hypotension, bradycardia, depression, confusion, hallucination, sexual dysfunction

---

propylthiouracil
(proe-pill-thye-oh-yoor′a-sill)
Chemical Class: Thioamide derivative
Therapeutic Class: Antithyroid agent

CLINICAL PHARMACOLOGY
Mechanism of Action: A thiourea derivative that blocks oxidation of iodine in the thyroid gland and blocks synthesis of thyroxine and triiodothyronine. *Therapeutic Effect:* Inhibits synthesis of thyroid hormone.
INDICATIONS AND DOSAGES
Hyperthyroidism
PO
Adults, Elderly. Initially: 300–450 mg/day in divided doses q8h. Maintenance: 100–150 mg/day in divided doses q8–12h.

Children. Initially: 5–7 mg/kg/day in divided doses q8h. Maintenance: 33%-66% of initial dose in divided doses q8-12h.

Neonates. 5–10 mg/kg/day in divided doses q8h.

§ **AVAILABLE FORMS/COST**
• Tab—Oral: 50 mg, 100's: **$2.25-$15.75**

CONTRAINDICATIONS: None known

PREGNANCY AND LACTATION: Pregnancy category D; considered drug of choice for medical treatment of hyperthyroidism during pregnancy; excreted into breast milk in low amounts; compatible with breast-feeding

SIDE EFFECTS

Frequent

Urticaria, rash, pruritus, nausea, skin pigmentation, hair loss, headache, paraesthesia

Occasional

Somnolence, lymphadenopathy, vertigo

Rare

Drug fever, lupus-like syndrome

SERIOUS REACTIONS
• Agranulocytosis as long as 4 months after therapy, pancytopenia, and fatal hepatitis have occurred.

INTERACTIONS

Drugs

3 *Oral anticoagulants:* Reduced hypoprothrombinemic response to oral anticoagulants

3 *Theophylline:* Physiologic response to antithyroid drug will increase theophylline concentrations via decreased clearance

Labs
• *False increase:* Glucose

SPECIAL CONSIDERATIONS

PATIENT/FAMILY EDUCATION
• Notify clinician of fever, sore throat, unusual bleeding or bruising, rash, yellowing of skin, vomiting

MONITORING PARAMETERS
• CBC periodically during therapy (especially during initial 3 mo), TSH

---

protamine
(proe'ta-meen)
Rx: Protamine
Chemical Class: Basic protein
Therapeutic Class: Antidote, heparin

CLINICAL PHARMACOLOGY

Mechanism of Action: A protein that complexes with heparin to form a stable salt. *Therapeutic Effect:* Reduces anticoagulant activity of heparin.

INDICATIONS AND DOSAGES

Heparin oversode (antidote and treatment)

IV

Adults, Elderly. 1 mg protamine sulfate neutralizes 90–115 units of heparin. Heparin disappears rapidly from circulation, reducing the dosage demand for protamine as time elapses.

§ **AVAILABLE FORMS/COST**
• Sol, Inj—IV: 10 mg/ml, 25 ml: **$20.00**

UNLABELED USES: Treatment of enoxaparin toxicity

CONTRAINDICATIONS: None known.

PREGNANCY AND LACTATION: Pregnancy category C

SIDE EFFECTS

Frequent

Decreased BP, dyspnea

Occasional

Hypersensitivity reaction (urticaria, angioedema); nausea and vomiting, which generally occur in those sensitive to fish and seafood, vasecto-

P

mized men, infertile men, those on isophane (NPH) insulin, or those previously on protamine therapy

Rare

Back pain

SERIOUS REACTIONS

• Too rapid IV administration may produce acute hypotension, bradycardia, pulmonary hypertension, dyspnea, transient flushing, and feeling of warmth.

• Heparin rebound may occur several hours after heparin has been neutralized (usually 8–9 hours after protamine administration). Heparin rebound occurs most often after arterial or cardiac surgery.

SPECIAL CONSIDERATIONS

• Will not reliably inactivate low-molecular-weight heparin

MONITORING PARAMETERS

• Activated partial thromboplastin time (aPTT) or protamine activated clotting time (ACT) 15 min after dose, then in several hr

---

protriptyline

(proe-trip′-ti-leen)

Rx: Vivactil

Chemical Class: Dibenzocycloheptene derivative; secondary amine

Therapeutic Class: Antidepressant, tricyclic

CLINICAL PHARMACOLOGY

Mechanism of Action: A tricyclic antidepressant that increases synaptic concentration of norepinephrine and/or serotonin by inhibiting their reuptake by presynaptic membranes. *Therapeutic Effect:* Produces antidepressant effect.

Pharmacokinetics

Well absorbed from the gastrointestinal (GI) tract. Protein binding: 92%. Widely distributed. Exten-

sively metabolized in liver. Excreted in urine. Not removed by hemodialysis. **Half-life:** 54-92 hrs.

INDICATIONS AND DOSAGES

Depression

PO

Adults. 15-40 mg/day divided into 3-4 doses/day. Maximum: 600 mg/day.

Elderly. 5 mg 3 times/day. May increase gradually.

Ⓢ AVAILABLE FORMS/COST

• Tab, Plain Coated—Oral: 5 mg, 100's: **$42.89-$94.51**; 10 mg, 100's: **$62.17-$136.98**

UNLABELED USES: Narcolepsy, sleep apnea, sleep hypoxemia

CONTRAINDICATIONS: Acute recovery period after myocardial infarction, coadministration with cisapride, use of MAOIs within 14 days, hypersensitivity to protriptyline or any component of the formulation

PREGNANCY AND LACTATION: Pregnancy category C

SIDE EFFECTS

Frequent

Drowsiness, weight gain, fatigue, dry mouth, blurred vision, constipation, delayed micturition, postural hypotension, diaphoresis, disturbed concentration, increased appetite, urinary retention

Occasional

Gastrointestinal (GI) disturbances, such as nausea, diarrhea, GI distress, metallic taste sensation

Rare

Paradoxical reaction, marked by agitation, restlessness, nightmares, insomnia, extrapyramidal symptoms, particularly fine hand tremor

SERIOUS REACTIONS

• High dosage may produce confusion, seizures, severe drowsiness, arrhythmias, fever, hallucinations, agitation, shortness of breath, vomiting, and unusual tiredness or weakness.

• Abrupt withdrawal from prolonged therapy may produce severe headache, malaise, nausea, vomiting, and vivid dreams.

INTERACTIONS
Drugs
§ *Altretamine:* Orthostatic hypotension

§ *Amphetamines:* Theoretical increase in effect of amphetamines, clinical evidence lacking

§ *Antidiabetics:* Monitor for enhanced hypoglycemia

§ *Barbiturates, rifampin, carbamazepine:* Reduced cyclic antidepressant concentrations

§ *β-agonists (especially isoproterenol):* Cardiac arrhythmia risk increased

② *Bethanidine, clonidine, guanethidine, guanabenz, guanfacine, guanadrel, debrisoquen:* Reduced antihypertensive effect

② *Epinephrine, norepinephrine:* Markedly enhanced pressor response to IV administration

§ *Ethanol:* Additive impairment of motor skills; abstinent alcoholics may eliminate cyclic antidepressants more rapidly than non-alcoholics

§ *Fluoxetine, paroxetine:* Marked increases in cyclic antidepressant plasma concentrations

§ H_2 *blockers (especially cimetidine), calcium channel blockers:* Increased cyclic concentrations

§ *Lithium:* Increased risk neurotoxicity (especially in elderly)

§ *MAOIs:* Excessive sympathetic response, mania, or hyperpyrexia possible

§ *Neuroleptics:* Increased therapeutic and toxic effects of both drugs

§ *Phenylephrine:* Enhanced pressor response

§ *Propantheline:* Enhanced anticholinergic effects

§ *Propoxyphene:* Enhanced effect of cyclic antidepressants

§ *Quinidine:* Increased cyclic antidepressant serum concentrations

§ *Ritonavir, indinavir:* Possible increased cyclic concentrations, toxicity

Labs
• *Increase:* Serum bilirubin, blood glucose, alk phosphatase
• *Decrease:* VMA, 5-HIAA
• *False increase:* Urinary catecholamines

SPECIAL CONSIDERATIONS
PATIENT/FAMILY EDUCATION
• Therapeutic effects may take 2-3 wk
• Use caution in driving or other activities requiring alertness
• Avoid rising quickly from sitting to standing, especially elderly
• Avoid alcohol and other CNS depressants
• Do not discontinue abruptly after long-term use
• Wear sunscreen or large hat to prevent photosensitivity

MONITORING PARAMETERS
• CBC, weight, ECG, mental status (mood, sensorium, affect, suicidal tendencies)

pseudoephedrine

(soo-doe-e-fed'rin)

OTC: Cenafed, Decofed, Efidac Genaphed, PediaCare Infants' Decongestant, Seudotabs, Sudafed, Sudafed 12 Hour Caplets (Pseudoephedrine is available in many prescription and over-the-counter combinations; the following list is not all-inclusive)

Combinations

Rx: with azatadine (Trinalin Repetabs); brompheniramine (Bromfed); carbinoxamine (Rondec); chlorpheniramine (Deconamine SR, Novafed A); codeine (Nucofed); guaifenesin and codeine (Novagest Expectorant); loratadine (Claritin-D)

OTC: with acetaminophen (Dristan Cold); chlorpheniramine (Chlor-Trimeton 12 Hour Relief); dexbrompheniramine (Drixoral Cold and Allergy); dextromethorphan (Thera-Flu Non-Drowsy Formula); diphenhydramine (Actifed Allergy); ibuprofen (Advil Cold & Sinus, Dristan Sinus); triprolidine (Actifed)

Chemical Class: Sympathomimetic amine

Therapeutic Class: Decongestant

CLINICAL PHARMACOLOGY

Mechanism of Action: A sympathomimetic that directly stimulates alpha-adrenergic and beta-adrenergic receptors. *Therapeutic Effect:* Produces vasoconstriction of respiratory tract mucosa; shrinks nasal mucous membranes; reduces edema, and nasal congestion.

Pharmacokinetics

Route	Onset	Peak	Duration
PO (tablets, syrup)	15–30 min	N/A	4–6 hr
PO (extended-release)	N/A	N/A	8–12 hr

Well absorbed from the GI tract. Partially metabolized in the liver. Primarily excreted in urine. Not removed by hemodialysis. **Half-life:** 9–16 hr (children, 3.1 hr).

INDICATIONS AND DOSAGES

Decongestant

PO

Adults, Children 12 yr and older. 60 mg q4–6h. Maximum: 240 mg/day.

Children 6–11 yr. 30 mg q6h. Maximum: 120 mg/day.

Children 2–5 yr. 15 mg q6h. Maximum: 60 mg/day.

Children younger than 2 yr. 4 mg/kg/day in divided doses q6h.

Elderly. 30–60 mg q6h as needed.

PO (Extended-Release)

Adults, Children 12 yr and older. 120 mg q12h.

$ AVAILABLE FORMS/COST

• Drops—Oral: 7.5 mg/0.8 ml, 15 ml: **$3.47-$5.18**

• Syr—Oral: 15 mg/5 ml, 120 ml: **$2.50-$5.69**; 30 mg/5 ml, 480 ml: **$2.25-$7.42**/480 ml

• Tab, Chewable—Oral: 15 mg, 18's: **$4.71**

• Tab—Oral: 30 mg, 100's: **$1.35-$21.95**; 60 mg, 100's: **$1.24-$20.38**

• Tab, Sus Action—Oral: 120 mg, 20's: **$7.99**; 240 mg, 12's: **$6.77**

CONTRAINDICATIONS: Breastfeeding women, coronary artery disease, severe hypertension, use within 14 days of MAOIs

PREGNANCY AND LACTATION:
Pregnancy category C; not compatible with breast-feeding

SIDE EFFECTS
Occasional (10%–5%)
Nervousness, restlessness, insomnia, tremor, headache
Rare (4%–1%)
Diaphoresis, weakness

SERIOUS REACTIONS
• Large doses may produce tachycardia, palpitations (particularly in patients with cardiac disease), light-headedness, nausea, and vomiting.
• Overdose in patients older than 60 years may result in hallucinations, CNS depression, and seizures.

INTERACTIONS
Drugs
■ *Antacids:* Sodium bicarbonate doses sufficient to alkalinize urine can inhibit elimination of pseudoephedrine
▲ *MAOIs:* Hypertensive crisis
Labs
• *False increase:* Theophylline

SPECIAL CONSIDERATIONS
PATIENT/FAMILY EDUCATION
• May cause wakefulness or nervousness
• Take last dose 4-6 hr prior to hs, notify clinician of insomnia, dizziness, weakness, tremor, or irregular heart beat

psyllium
(sill'ee-yum)
OTC: Fiberall, Hydrocil, Konsyl, Metamucil, Modane Bulk, Perdiem Fiber, Reguloid, Serutan, Syllact, V-Lax
Combinations
  OTC: with senna (Perdiem)
Chemical Class: Psyllium colloid
Therapeutic Class: Laxative

CLINICAL PHARMACOLOGY
Mechanism of Action: A bulk-forming laxative that dissolves and swells in water providing increased bulk and moisture content in stool.
Therapeutic Effect: Promotes peristalsis and bowel motility.

Pharmacokinetics

Route	Onset	Peak	Duration
PO	12–24 hr	2–3 days	N/A

Acts in small and large intestines.

INDICATIONS AND DOSAGES
Constipation, irritable bowel syndrome
PO
Alert: 3.4 g powder equals 1 rounded tsp, 1 packet, or 1 wafer.
Adults, Elderly. 2-5 capsules/dose 1-3 times a day. 1-2 tsp granules 1-2 times a day. 1 rounded tsp or 1 tbsp of powder 1-3 times a day. 2 wafers 1-3 times a day.
Children 6–11 yr. One half–1 tsp powder in water 1–3 times a day.

$ AVAILABLE FORMS/COST
• Cap—Oral: 500 mg, 100's: **$9.46**
• Granules—Oral: 2.5-4.03 g/rounded teaspoon, 100, 180, 250, 480, 540 g: **$12.63/250 g**
• Powder, Effervescent—Oral: 3.4 g/dose, 30's (packets) and 300 g (bulk): **$5.16-$7.71**

P

• Powder, Hydrophilic—Oral: 3.5 g/rounded teaspoon, 300, 500 g: **$11.84**/300 g
• Powder—Oral: 50% psyllium and 50% dextrose/dose, 120, 396, 420, 480, 630 g: **$3.50-$8.86**
• Tab—Oral: 500 mg, 200's: **$5.99**
• Wafer, Chewable—Oral: 1.7 g, 24's: **$3.92-$4.17**

CONTRAINDICATIONS: Fecal impaction, GI obstruction

PREGNANCY AND LACTATION: Pregnancy category C; not systemically absorbed; exposure of fetus or nursing infant unlikely

SIDE EFFECTS

Rare

Some degree of abdominal discomfort, nausea, mild abdominal cramps, griping, faintness

SERIOUS REACTIONS

• Esophageal or bowel obstruction may occur if administered less than 250 ml of liquid.

SPECIAL CONSIDERATIONS

PATIENT/FAMILY EDUCATION

• Maintain adequate fluid consumption
• Do not use in presence of abdominal pain, nausea, or vomiting
• Avoid inhaling dust from powder preparations; can cause runny nose, watery eyes, wheezing

pyrantel

(pi-ran'tel)

OTC: Antiminth, Pin-Rid, Pin-X, Reese's Pinworm

Chemical Class: Pyrimidine derivative

Therapeutic Class: Antihelmintic

CLINICAL PHARMACOLOGY

Mechanism of Action: A depolarizing neuromuscular blocking agent that causes the release of acetylcholine and inhibits cholinesterase. *Therapeutic Effect:* Results in a spastic paralysis of the worm and consequent expulsion from the host's intestinal tract.

Pharmacokinetics

Poorly absorbed through gastrointestinal (GI) tract. Time to peak occurs in 1-3 hrs. Partially metabolized in liver. Primarily excreted in feces; minimal elimination in urine.

INDICATIONS AND DOSAGES

Enterobiasis vermicularis (pinworm)

PO

Adults, Elderly, Children older than 2 yrs. 11 mg base/kg once. Repeat in 2 wks. Maximum: 1 g/day.

[$] **AVAILABLE FORMS/COST**

• Susp—Oral: 50 mg/ml, 30, 60 ml: **$7.70**/30 ml; 144 mg/ml, 30, 60 ml: **$5.28-$9.49**/30 ml
• Tab—Oral: 180 mg, 24's: **$5.65**

CONTRAINDICATIONS: Hypersensitivity to pyrantel or any of its components

PREGNANCY AND LACTATION: Pregnancy category C

SIDE EFFECTS

Occasional

Nausea, vomiting, headache, dizziness, drowsiness, GI distress, weakness

SERIOUS REACTIONS

• Overdosage includes symptoms of anorexia, nausea, abdominal cramps, vomiting, diarrhea, and ataxia.

INTERACTIONS

Drugs

[2] *Piperazine:* Mutual antagonism

SPECIAL CONSIDERATIONS

PATIENT/FAMILY EDUCATION

• Take with food or milk
• Using a laxative to facilitate expulsion of worms is not necessary
• All family members in close contact with patient should be treated

- Strict hygiene is essential to prevent reinfection
- Shake suspension well before pouring

---

pyrazinamide

(pye-ra-zin′a-mide)
Rx: Pyrazinamide
Chemical Class: Niacinamide derivative
Therapeutic Class: Antituberculosis agent

CLINICAL PHARMACOLOGY
Mechanism of Action: An antitubercular whose exact mechanism of action is unknown. *Therapeutic Effect:* Either bacteriostatic or bactericidal, depending on the drug's concentration at the infection site and the susceptibility of infecting bacteria.

INDICATIONS AND DOSAGES
Tuberculosis (in combination with other antituberculars)
PO
Adults. 15-30 mg/kg/day in 1-4 doses. Maximum: 3 g/day.
Children. 20-40 mg/kg/day in 1 or 2 doses. Maximum: 2 g/day.

AVAILABLE FORMS/COST
- Tab—Oral: 500 mg, 100's: **$109.97-$120.55**

CONTRAINDICATIONS: Severe hepatic dysfunction

PREGNANCY AND LACTATION: Pregnancy category C; excreted into human milk

SIDE EFFECTS
Frequent
Arthralgia, myalgia (usually mild and self-limiting)
Rare
Hypersensitivity reaction (rash, pruritus, urticaria), photosensitivity, gouty arthritis

SERIOUS REACTIONS
- Hepatotoxicity, gouty arthritis, thrombocytopenia, and anemia occur rarely.

INTERACTIONS
Drugs
③ *Cyclosporine:* Decreased concentrations cyclosporine
③ *Tacrolimus:* Decreased concentrations of tacrolimus
Labs
- *False positive:* Urine ketone tests

SPECIAL CONSIDERATIONS
PATIENT/FAMILY EDUCATION
- Compliance with full course is essential
- Notify clinician of fever, loss of appetite, malaise, nausea and vomiting, darkened urine, yellowish discoloration of skin and eyes, pain or swelling of joints

MONITORING PARAMETERS
- Liver function tests, serum uric acid at baseline and periodically throughout therapy

---

pyridostigmine

(peer-id-oh-stig′meen)
Rx: Mestinon, Mestinon Timespan, Regonol
Chemical Class: Cholinesterase inhibitor; quaternary ammonium derivative
Therapeutic Class: Cholinergic

CLINICAL PHARMACOLOGY
Mechanism of Action: A cholinergic that prevents destruction of acetylcholine by inhibiting the enzyme acetylcholinesterase, thus enhancing impulse transmission across the myoneural junction. *Therapeutic Effect:* Produces miosis; increases tone of intestinal, skeletal muscle tone; stimulates salivary and sweat gland secretions.

INDICATIONS AND DOSAGES
Myasthenia gravis
PO
Adults, Elderly. Initially, 60 mg 3 times a day. Dosage increased at 48 hr intervals. Maintenance: 60 mg –1.5 g a day.
PO (Extended-Release)
Adults, Elderly. 180-540 mg once or twice a day with at least a 6 hr interval between doses.
IV, IM
Adults, Elderly. 2 mg q2–3h.
Children, Neonates. 0.05–0.15 mg/kg/dose. Maximum single dose: 10 mg.
Reversal of nondepolarizing neuromuscular blockade
IV
Adults, Elderly. 10–20 mg with, or shortly after, 0.6–1.2 mg atropine sulfate or 0.3–0.6 mg glycopyrrolate.
Children. 0.1–0.25 mg/kg/dose preceded by atropine or glycopyrrolate.

AVAILABLE FORMS/COST
• Sol, Inj—IM; IV: 5 mg/ml, 2 ml: **$5.78-$6.87**
• Syr—Oral: 60 mg/5 ml, 480 ml: **$58.10**
• Tab—Oral: 60 mg, 100's: **$54.80-$69.99**
• Tab, Coated, Sus Action—Oral: 180 mg, 100's: **$95.50**
CONTRAINDICATIONS: Mechanical GI or urinary tract obstruction
PREGNANCY AND LACTATION: Pregnancy category C; would not be expected to cross the placenta because it is ionized at physiologic pH; although apparently safe for the fetus, may cause transient muscle weakness in the newborn; compatible with breast-feeding
SIDE EFFECTS
Frequent
Miosis, increased GI and skeletal muscle tone, bradycardia, constriction of bronchi and ureters, diaphoresis, increased salivation
Occasional
Headache, rash, temporary decrease in diastolic BP with mild reflex tachycardia, short periods of atrial fibrillation (in hyperthyroid patients), marked drop in BP (in hypertensive patients)

SERIOUS REACTIONS
• Overdose may produce a cholinergic crisis, manifested as increasingly severe muscle weakness that appears first in muscles involving chewing and swallowing and is followed by muscle weakness of the shoulder girdle and upper extremities, respiratory muscle paralysis, and pelvis girdle and leg muscle paralysis. If overdose occurs, stop all cholinergic drugs and immediately administer 1–4 mg atropine sulfate IV for adults or 0.01 mg/kg for infants and children younger than 12 years.

INTERACTIONS
Drugs
▣ *β-blockers:* Additive bradycardia
▣ *Tacrine:* Increased anticholinergic effects
Labs
• *False increase:* Serum bicarbonate, chloride

SPECIAL CONSIDERATIONS
PATIENT/FAMILY EDUCATION
• Do not crush or chew sustained release preparations
MONITORING PARAMETERS
• Therapeutic response: increased muscle strength, improved gait, absence of labored breathing (if severe)
• Appearance of side effects (narrow margin between 1st appearance of side effects and serious toxicity)

• Symptoms of increasing muscle weakness may be due to cholinergic crisis (overdosage) or myasthenic crisis (increased disease severity). If crisis is myasthenia, patient will improve after 1-2 mg edrophonium; if cholinergic withdraw pyridostigmine and administer atropine

---

pyridoxine (vitamin B₆)

(peer-i-dox'een)
Rx: Doxine, Rodex, Vitabee 6 (Injection)
OTC: Nestrex
Chemical Class: Vitamin B complex
Therapeutic Class: Antidote, hydralazine/isoniazid; vitamin

CLINICAL PHARMACOLOGY
Mechanism of Action: Acts as a coenzyme for various metabolic functions, including metabolism of proteins, carbohydrates, and fats. Aids in the breakdown of glycogen and in the synthesis of gamma-aminobutyric acid in the CNS. *Therapeutic Effect:* Prevents pyridoxine deficiency. Increases the excretion of certain drugs, such as isoniazid, that are pyridoxine antagonists.

Pharmacokinetics
Readily absorbed primarily in jejunum. Stored in the liver, muscle, and brain. Metabolized in the liver. Primarily excreted in urine. Removed by hemodialysis. **Half-life:** 15–20 days.

INDICATIONS AND DOSAGES
Pyridoxine deficiency
PO
Adults, Elderly. Initially, 2.5–10 mg/day; then 2.5 mg/day when clinical signs are corrected.

Children. Initially, 5–25 mg/day for 3 wk, then 1.5–2.5 mg/day.
Pyridoxine dependent seizures
PO, IV, IM
Infants. Initially, 10–100 mg/day. Maintenance: PO: 50–100 mg/day.
Drug-induced neuritis
PO (treatment)
Adults, Elderly. 100–300 mg/day in divided doses
Children. 10-50 mg/day.
PO (prophylaxis)
Adults, Elderly. 25–100 mg/day.
Children. 1-2 mg/kg/day.

🛇 **AVAILABLE FORMS/COST**
• Sol, Inj—IM, IV: 100 mg/ml, 10, 30 ml: **$3.40-$6.45/10 ml**
• Tab—Oral: 25, 50, 100 mg, 100's; all: **$1.58-$11.07**

CONTRAINDICATIONS: None known.

PREGNANCY AND LACTATION: Pregnancy category A (category C if used in doses above RDA); deficiency during pregnancy is common in unsupplemented women; excreted in human breast milk; RDA for lactating women is 2.3-2.5 mg

SIDE EFFECTS
Occasional
Stinging at IM injection site
Rare
Headache, nausea, somnolence; sensory neuropathy (paraesthesia, unstable gait, clumsiness of hands) with high doses

SERIOUS REACTIONS
• Long-term megadoses (2-6 g over more than 2 mo) may produce sensory neuropathy (reduced deep tendon reflexex, profound impairment of sense of position in distal limbs, gradual sensory ataxia). Toxic symptoms subside when drug is discontinued.

P

• Seizures have occurred after IV megadoses.

INTERACTIONS
Drugs
■ *Levodopa:* Inhibited antiparkinsonian effect of levodopa; concurrent use of carbidopa negates the interaction

■ *Phenytoin:* Reduced phenytoin concentrations

SPECIAL CONSIDERATIONS
PATIENT/FAMILY EDUCATION
• Avoid doses exceeding RDA unless directed by clinician
MONITORING PARAMETERS
• Respiratory rate, heart rate, blood pressure during large IV doses

---

pyrimethamine
(pye-ri-meth´-a-meen)

Rx: Daraprim
Combinations
  Rx: with sulfadoxine (Fansidar)
Chemical Class: Aminopyrimidine derivative
Therapeutic Class: Antimalarial

CLINICAL PHARMACOLOGY
Mechanism of Action: An antiprotozoal with blood and some tissue schizonticidal activity against malaria parasites of humans. Highly selective activity against plasmodia and *Toxoplasma gondii*. *Therapeutic Effect:* Inhibition of tetrahydrofolic acid synthesis.

Pharmacokinetics
Well absorbed, peak levels occurring between 2-6 hours following administration. Protein binding: 87%. Eliminated slowly. **Half-life:** approximately 96 hours.

INDICATIONS AND DOSAGES
Toxoplasmosis
PO
Adults. Initially, 50-75 mg daily, with 1-4 g daily of a sulfonamide of the sulfapyrimidine type (e.g., sulfadoxine). Continue for 1-3 weeks, depending on response of patient and tolerance to therapy then reduce dose to one-half that previously given for each drug and continue for additional 4-5 weeks.
Children. 1 mg/kg/day divided into 2 equal daily doses; after 2-4 days reduce to one-half and continue for approximately 1 month. The usual pediatric sulfonamide dosage is used in conjunction with pyrimethamine.

Acute malaria
PO
Adults (in combination with sulfonamide). 25 mg daily for 2 days with a sulfonamide
Adults (without concomitant sulfonamide). 50 mg for 2 days
Children 4-10 yrs. 25 mg daily for 2 days.

Chemoprophylaxis of malaria
PO
Adults and pediatric patients over 10 years: 25 mg once weekly.
Children 4-10 years: 12.5 mg once weekly.
Infants and children under 4 years: 6.25 mg once weekly.

☒ AVAILABLE FORMS/COST
• Tab—Oral: 25 mg, 100's: **$57.71**
• Tab—Oral: 25 mg-500 mg sulfadoxine, 25's: **$98.08**

UNLABELED USES: Prophylaxis for first episode and recurrence of *Pneumocystis carinii* pneumonia and *Toxoplasma gondii* in HIV-infected patients.

CONTRAINDICATIONS: Hypersensitivity to pyrimethamine, megaloblastic anemia due to folate deficiency, monotherapy for treatment of acute malaria.

PREGNANCY AND LACTATION: Pregnancy category C; most studies have found pyrimethamine to be safe in pregnancy; folic acid supplementation should be given to prevent folate deficiency; compatible with breast-feeding

SIDE EFFECTS

Frequent

Anorexia, vomiting

Occasional

Hypersensitivity reactions, Stevens-Johnson syndrome, toxic epidermal necrolysis, erythema multiforme, anaphylaxis, hyperphenylalaninemia, megaloblastic anemia, leukopenia, thrombocytopenia, pancytopenia, atrophic glossitis, hematuria, and disorders of cardiac rhythm

Rare

Pulmonary eosinophilia

SERIOUS REACTIONS

• None known.

INTERACTIONS

Drugs

❷ *Folic acid:* Decreased efficacy of pyrimethamine

SPECIAL CONSIDERATIONS

• Discontinue if folate deficiency develops; administer leucovorin 5-15 mg IM qd for ≥3 days when recovery slow

PATIENT/FAMILY EDUCATION

• Take with food

• Discontinue at 1st sign of rash

MONITORING PARAMETERS

• CBC with platelets semi-weekly during therapy for toxoplasmosis, less frequently for malaria-related indications

quazepam
(kwaz-'ze-pam)
Rx: Doral
Chemical Class: Benzodiazepine
Therapeutic Class: Hypnotic
DEA Class: Schedule IV

CLINICAL PHARMACOLOGY

Mechanism of Action: A BZ-1 receptor selective benzodiazepine with sedative properties. *Therapeutic Effect:* Produces sedative effect from its central nervous system (CNS) depressant action.

Pharmacokinetics

Rapidly absorbed from gastrointestinal (GI) tract. Food increases absorption. Protein binding: 95%. Extensively metabolized in liver. Excreted in urine and feces. Unknown if removed by hemodialysis. **Half-life:** 25-41 hrs.

INDICATIONS AND DOSAGES

Insomnia

PO

Adults (older than 18 yrs). Initially, 15 mg at bedtime. Adjust dose up or down from 7.5 mg to 30 mg at bedtime depending on initial response.

Elderly, debilitated, liver disease. Initially, 7.5-15 mg at bedtime. Adjust dose depending on initial response.

S **AVAILABLE FORMS/COST**

• Tab, Coated—Oral: 7.5 mg, 100's: **$314.39**; 15 mg, 100's: **$367.63**

CONTRAINDICATIONS: Pregnancy, sleep apnea, hypersensitivity to quazepam or any component of the formulation

PREGNANCY AND LACTATION: Pregnancy category X; may cause fetal damage when administered during pregnancy; excreted into breast milk; may accumulate in breast-fed infants and is therefore not recommended

SIDE EFFECTS

Frequent

Muscular incoordination (ataxia), lightheadedness, transient mild drowsiness, slurred speech (particularly in elderly or debilitated patients)

Occasional

Confusion, depression, blurred vision, constipation, diarrhea, dry mouth, headache, nausea

Rare

Behavioral problems such as anger, impaired memory, paradoxical reactions such as insomnia, nervousness, or irritability

SERIOUS REACTIONS

• Abrupt or too rapid withdrawal may result in pronounced restlessness, irritability, insomnia, hand tremors, abdominal and muscle cramps, sweating, vomiting, and seizures.

• Overdosage results in somnolence, confusion, diminished reflexes, and coma.

• Blood dyscrasias have been reported rarely.

INTERACTIONS

Drugs

☒ *Cimetidine:* Increased plasma levels of quazepam

☒ *Clozapine:* Isolated cases of cardiorespiratory collapse have been reported, causal relationship to benzodiazepines has not been established

☒ *Disulfiram:* Increased serum quazepam concentrations

☒ *Ethanol:* Enhanced adverse psychomotor side effects of benzodiazepines

☒ *Levodopa:* Possible exacerbation of parkinsonism

☒ *Neuroleptics:* Increased sedation, respiratory depression

☒ *Omeprazole, macrolides, azole antifungals, isoniazid, digoxin, SSRI's, quinolones:* Possible increased benzodiazepine concentrations

☒ *Rifampin:* Reduced serum quazepam concentrations

SPECIAL CONSIDERATIONS

PATIENT/FAMILY EDUCATION

• Avoid alcohol and other CNS depressants

• Do not discontinue abruptly after prolonged therapy

• May cause daytime sedation, use caution while driving or performing other tasks requiring alertness

• Inform clinician if planning to become pregnant, or are pregnant, or if you become pregnant while taking this medicine

• May be habit forming

---

quetiapine

(kwe-tye′a-peen)

Rx: Seroquel

Chemical Class: Dibenzothiazepine derivative

Therapeutic Class: Antipsychotic

CLINICAL PHARMACOLOGY

Mechanism of Action: A dibenzepin derivative that antagonizes dopamine, serotonin, histamine, and alpha1-adrenergic receptors. *Therapeutic Effect:* Diminishes manifestations of psychotic disorders. Produces moderate sedation, few extrapyramidal effects, and no anticholinergic effects.

Pharmacokinetics

Well absorbed after PO administration. Protein binding: 83%. Widely distributed in tissues; CNS concentration exceeds plasma concentration. Undergoes extensive first-pass metabolism in the liver. Primarily excreted in urine. **Half-life:** 6 hr.

INDICATIONS AND DOSAGES

To manage manifestations of psychotic disorders, Bipolar disorder

PO

Adults, Elderly. Initially, 25 mg twice a day, then 25-50 mg 2-3 times a day on the second and third days, up to 300-400 mg/day in divided doses 2-3 times a day by the fourth day. Further adjustments of 25-50 mg twice a day may be made at intervals of 2 days or longer. Maintenance: 300-800 mg/day (adults); 50-200 mg/day (elderly).

Dosage in hepatic impairment, elderly or debilitated patients, and those predisposed to hypotensive reactions

These patients should receive a lower initial dose and lower dosage increases.

[$] **AVAILABLE FORMS/COST**

- Tab—Oral: 25 mg, 100's: **$163.57**; 100 mg, 100's: **$297.70**; 200 mg, 100's: **$561.60**

CONTRAINDICATIONS: None known.

PREGNANCY AND LACTATION: Pregnancy category C; excretion into breast milk unknown, breastfeeding is not recommended

SIDE EFFECTS

Frequent (19%-10%)

Headache, somnolence, dizziness

Occasional (9%-3%)

Constipation, orthostatic hypotension, tachycardia, dry mouth, dyspepsia, rash, asthenia, abdominal pain, rhinitis

Rare (2%)

Back pain, fever, weight gain

SERIOUS REACTIONS

- Overdose may produce heart block hypotension, hypokalemia, and tachycardia.

INTERACTIONS

Drugs

[3] *Antihypertensives:* Increased risk of hypotension

[3] *CYP3A inhibitors (Azole antifungals, macrolide antibiotics):* Increased plasma quetiapine concentrations

[3] *Lorazepam:* Increased plasma lorazepam concentrations

[3] *Phenytoin, carbamazepine, barbiturates, rifampin, glucocorticoids (enzyme inducers):* Decreased plasma quetiapine concentrations

[3] *Thioridazine:* Decreased plasma quetiapine concentrations

SPECIAL CONSIDERATIONS

- Limited clinical experience, but similar to clozapine and risperidone; may be effective for negative symptoms of schizophrenia; so far no agranulocytosis reported with quetiapine

PATIENT/FAMILY EDUCATION

- Avoid alcohol

quinapril

(kwin'na-pril)

Rx: Accupril

Chemical Class: Angiotensin-converting enzyme (ACE) inhibitor, nonsulfhydryl

Therapeutic Class: Antihypertensive

CLINICAL PHARMACOLOGY

Mechanism of Action: An ACE inhibitor that suppresses the renin-angiotensin-aldosterone system and prevents the conversion of angiotensin I to angiotensin II, a potent vasoconstrictor; may also inhibit angiotensin II at local vascular and renal sites. *Therapeutic Effect:* Reduces peripheral arterial resistance, BP, and pulmonary capillary wedge pressure; improves cardiac output.

Pharmacokinetics

Route	Onset	Peak	Duration
PO	1 hr	N/A	24 hr

Readily absorbed from the GI tract. Protein binding: 97%. Metabolized in the liver, GI tract, and extravascular tissue to active metabolite. Primarily excreted in urine. Minimal removal by hemodialysis. **Half-life:** 1-2 hr; metabolite, 3 hr (increased in those with impaired renal function).

INDICATIONS AND DOSAGES
Hypertension (monotherapy)
PO

Adults. Initially, 10-20 mg/day. May adjust dosage at intervals of at least 2 wk or longer. Maintenance: 20-80 mg/day as single dose or 2 divided doses. Maximum: 80 mg/day.

Elderly. Initially, 2.5-5 mg/day. May increase by 2.5-5 mg q1-2wk.

Hypertension (combination therapy)
PO

Adults. Initially, 5 mg/day titrated to patient's needs.

Elderly. Initially, 2.5-5 mg/day. May increase by 2.5-5 mg q1-2wk.

Adjunct to manage heart failure
PO

Adults, Elderly. Initially, 5 mg twice a day. Range: 20-40 mg/day.

Dosage in renal impairment
Dosage is titrated to the patient's needs after the following initial doses:

Creatinine Clearance	Initial Dose
more than 60 ml/min	10 mg
30-60 ml/min	5 mg
10-29 ml/min	2.5 mg

Ⓢ AVAILABLE FORMS/COST
• Tab—Oral: 5, 10, 20, 40 mg, 90's; all: **$113.25**

UNLABELED USES: Treatment of hypertension and renal crisis in scleroderma

CONTRAINDICATIONS: Bilateral renal artery stenosis

PREGNANCY AND LACTATION:
Pregnancy category D; ACE inhibitors can cause fetal and neonatal morbidity and death when administered to pregnant women; when pregnancy is detected, discontinue ACE inhibitors as soon as possible

SIDE EFFECTS
Frequent (7%-5%)
Headache, dizziness
Occasional (4%-2%)
Fatigue, vomiting, nausea, hypotension, chest pain, cough, syncope
Rare (less than 2%)
Diarrhea, cough, dyspnea, rash, palpitations, impotence, insomnia, drowsiness, malaise

SERIOUS REACTIONS
• Excessive hypotension (first-dose syncope) may occur in patients with CHF and in those who are severely salt or volume depleted.
• Angioedema and hyperkalemia occur rarely.
• Agranulocytosis and neutropenia may be noted in those with collagen vascular disease, including scleroderma and systemic lupus erythematosus, and impaired renal function.
• Nephrotic syndrome may be noted in those with history of renal disease.

INTERACTIONS
Drugs
❷ *Allopurinol:* Predisposition to hypersensitivity reactions
❸ *α-adrenergic blockers:* Exaggerated 1st dose hypotensive response
❸ *Aspirin:* Reduced hemodynamic effects; less likely with nonacetylated salicylates
❸ *Azathioprine:* Increased myelosuppression
❸ *Cyclosporine:* Renal insufficiency
❸ *Insulin:* Enhanced hypoglycemic response

[3] *Iron (parenteral):* Increased risk systemic reaction

[3] *Lithium:* Increased risk of serious lithium toxicity

[3] *Loop diuretics:* Initiation of ACE inhibitor therapy may cause hypotension and renal insufficiency

[3] *NSAIDs:* Inhibition of the antihypertensive response

[3] *Potassium, potassium-sparing diuretics:* Increased risk for hyperkalemia

[3] *Trimethoprim:* Additive risk of hyperkalemia, especially in patient predisposed to renal insufficiency

Labs

• ACE inhibition can account for approximately 0.5mEq/L rise in serum potassium

SPECIAL CONSIDERATIONS

PATIENT/FAMILY EDUCATION

• Caution with salt substitutes containing potassium chloride

• Rise slowly to sitting/standing position to minimize orthostatic hypotension

• Dizziness, fainting, lightheadedness may occur during 1st few days of therapy

• May cause altered taste perception or cough; persistent dry cough usually does not subside unless medication is stopped; notify clinician if these symptoms persist

MONITORING PARAMETERS

• BUN, creatinine, potassium within 2 wk after initiation of therapy (increased levels may indicate acute renal failure)

---

quinidine

Rx: Quinaglute Dura-Tabs, Quinalan, (gluconate); Quinidex Extentabs, Quinora (sulfate)

Chemical Class: Quinine isomer, dextrorotatory

Therapeutic Class: Antiarrhythmic, class IA; antimalarial

CLINICAL PHARMACOLOGY

Mechanism of Action: An antiarrhythmic that decreases sodium influx during depolarization, potassium efflux during repolarization, and reduces calcium transport across the myocardial cell membrane. Decreases myocardial excitability, conduction velocity, and contractility. *Therapeutic Effect:* Suppresses arrhythmias.

INDICATIONS AND DOSAGES

Maintenance of normal sinus rhythm after conversion of atrial fibrillation or flutter; prevention of premature atrial, AV, and ventricular contractions; paroxysmal atrial tachycardia; paroxysmal AV junctional rhythm; atrial fibrillation; atrial flutter; paroxysmal ventricular tachycardia not associated with complete heart block

PO

Adults, Elderly. 100–600 mg q4–6h. (Long-acting): 324–972 mg q8–12h.

Children: 30 mg/kg/day in divided doses q4–6h.

IV

Adults, Elderly. 200–400 mg.

Children. 2–10 mg/kg.

[S] AVAILABLE FORMS/COST

Quinidine Gluconate

• Sol, Inj—IM;IV: 80 mg/ml, 10 ml: **$22.46**

• Tab, Sus Action—Oral: 324 mg, 100's: **$31.20-$93.37**

Quinidine Polygalacturonate
• Tab, Uncoated—Oral: 275 mg, 100's: **$144.59**
Quinidine Sulfate
• Tab—Oral: 200 mg, 100's: **$4.25-$21.00**; 300 mg, 100's: **$18.70-$40.00**
• Tab, Coated, Sus Action—Oral: 300 mg, 100's: **$64.85-$87.84**
UNLABELED USES: Treatment of malaria (IV only)
CONTRAINDICATIONS: Complete AV block, intraventricular conduction defects (widening of QRS complex)
PREGNANCY AND LACTATION: Pregnancy category C; use during pregnancy has been classified in reviews of cardiovascular drugs as relatively safe for the fetus; high doses can produce oxytocic properties and potential for abortion; excreted in breast milk; compatible with breast-feeding
SIDE EFFECTS
Frequent
Abdominal pain and cramps, nausea, diarrhea, vomiting (can be immediate, intense)
Occasional
Mild cinchonism (ringing in ears, blurred vision, hearing loss) or severe cinchonism (headache, vertigo, diaphoresis, light-headedness, photophobia, confusion, delirium)
Rare
Hypotension (particularly with IV administration), hypersensitivity reaction (fever, anaphylaxis, photosensitivity reaction)
SERIOUS REACTIONS
• Cardiotoxic effects occur most commonly with IV administration, particularly at high concentrations, and are observed as conduction changes (50% widening of QRS complex, prolonged QT interval, flattened T waves, and disappearance of P wave), ventricular tachy-

cardia or flutter, frequent premature ventricular contractions (PVCs), or complete AV block.
• Quinidine-induced syncope may occur with the usual dosage.
• Severe hypotension may result from high dosages.
• Patients with atrial flutter and fibrillation may experience a paradoxical, exremely rapid ventricular rate that may be prevented by prior digitalization.
• Hepatotoxicity with jaundice due to drug hypersensitivity may occur.
INTERACTIONS
Drugs
▣ *Acetazolamide, antacids, sodium bicarbonate, thiazide diuretics:* Alkalinization of urine increases plasma quinidine concentrations
▣ *Amiloride:* Increased risk of arrhythmias in patients with ventricular tachycardia
▣ *Amiodarone, cimetidine, verapamil:* Increased plasma quinidine concentrations
▣ *Azole antifungals:* Inhibition of quinidine metabolism (CYP3A4), increased concentrations
▣ *Barbiturates, nifedipine, kaolin-pectin, phenytoin, rifampin, rifabutin:* Decreased plasma quinidine concentrations
▣ *β-blockers:* Increased concentrations of metoprolol, propranolol, and timolol
▣ *Cholinergic agents:* Reduced therapeutic effects of cholinergic drugs
❷ *Codeine:* Inhibition of codeine to its active metabolite, diminished analgesia
▣ *Cyclic antidepressants:* Increased imipramine, nortriptyline and desipramine concentrations
▣ *Dextromethorphan:* Increased dextromethorphan concentrations, toxicity may result

3 *Digitalis glycosides:* Increased digoxin and digitoxin concentrations, toxicity may result

3 *Encainide:* Increased encainide serum concentrations in rapid encainide metabolizers

3 *Haloperidol:* Increased haloperidol concentrations, toxicity

3 *Macrolides:* Increased quinidine concentrations with erythromycin, troleandomycin, clarithromycin due to CYP34A inhibition

3 *Mexiletine:* Increased mexiletine concentrations

3 *Neuromuscular blocking agents:* Enhanced effects of neuromuscular blocking agents

3 *Nifedipine:* Increased serum nifedipine concentrations, decreased serum quinidine concentrations

3 *Procainamide:* Marked increased procainamide concentrations

3 *Propafenone:* Increased propafenone concentrations and decreased concentrations of its active metabolite; net effect unknown

3 *Warfarin:* Enhanced anticoagulant response

Labs

• *False increase:* Urine 17-ketosteroids

SPECIAL CONSIDERATIONS

• 267 mg gluconate=275 mg polygalacturonate=200 mg sulfate

PATIENT/FAMILY EDUCATION

• Take with food to decrease GI upset

• Do not crush or chew sustained release tablets

MONITORING PARAMETERS

• Plasma quinidine concentration (therapeutic range 2-6 mcg/ml)

• ECG

• Liver function tests during the 1st 4-8 weeks

• CBC periodically during prolonged therapy

quinine

(kwye′-nine)

Rx: Quinine
Chemical Class: Cinchona alkaloid
Therapeutic Class: Antimalarial

CLINICAL PHARMACOLOGY

Mechanism of Action: A cinchona alkaloid that relaxes skeletal muscle by increasing the refractory period, decreasing excitability of motor end plates (curarelike), and affecting distribution of calcium with muscle fiber. Antimalaria: Depresses oxygen uptake, carbohydrate metabolism, elevates pH in intracellular organelles of parasites. *Therapeutic Effect:* Relaxes skeletal muscle; produces parasite death.

Pharmacokinetics

Rapidly absorbed mainly from upper small intestine. Protein binding: 70%-95%. Metabolized in liver. Excreted in feces, saliva, and urine. **Half-life:** 8-14 hrs (adults), 6-12 hrs (children).

INDICATIONS AND DOSAGES

Nocturnal leg cramps

PO

Adults, Elderly. 260-300 mg at bedtime as needed.

Treatment of malaria

PO

Adults, Elderly. 260-650 mg 3 times a day for 6-12 days.

Children. 10 mg/kg q8h for 5-7 days.

Dosage in renal impairment

Creatinine Clearance	Dosage Interval
10-50 ml/min	75% of normal dose or q12h
Less than 10 ml/min	30%-50% of normal dose or q24h

ⓢ AVAILABLE FORMS/COST
• Cap, Gel—Oral: 200 mg, 100's: **$10.66-$55.62**; 325 mg, 100's: **$5.05-$90.34**
• Tab—Oral: 260 mg, 100's: **$9.95-$79.20**

CONTRAINDICATIONS: Hypersensitivity to quinine (possible cross-sensitivity to quinidine), G-6-PD deficiency, tinnitus, optic neuritis, history of thrombocytopenia during previous quinine therapy, blackwater fever

PREGNANCY AND LACTATION: Pregnancy category X; excreted into breast milk; compatible with breast-feeding; use caution in infants at risk for G-6-PD deficiency

SIDE EFFECTS
Frequent
Nausea, headache, tinnitus, slight visual disturbances (mild cinchonism)
Occasional
Extreme flushing of skin with intense generalized pruritus is most typical hypersensitivity reaction; also rash, wheezing, dyspnea, angioedema.
Prolonged therapy: cardiac conduction disturbances, decreased hearing

SERIOUS REACTIONS
• Overdosage (severe cinchonism) may result in cardiovascular effects, severe headache, intestinal cramps w/vomiting and diarrhea, apprehension, confusion, seizures, blindness, and respiratory depression.
• Hypoprothrombinemia, thrombocytopenic purpura, hemoglobinuria, asthma, agranulocytosis, hypoglycemia, deafness, and optic atrophy occur rarely.

INTERACTIONS
Drugs
ⓔ *Digitalis glycosides:* Increased digoxin concentrations (especially at high quinine doses)

ⓔ *Smoking:* Reduced serum quinine concentrations
Labs
• *False increase:* 17-ketosteroids

SPECIAL CONSIDERATIONS
PATIENT/FAMILY EDUCATION
• Take with food
• May cause blurred vision, use caution driving
• Discontinue drug if flushing, itching, rash, fever, stomach pain, difficult breathing, ringing in ears, visual disturbances occur

---

quinupristin/ dalfopristin
(kwin-yoo′pris-tin/dal′foh-pris-tin)
Rx: Synercid
Chemical Class: Streptogramin combination
Therapeutic Class: Antibiotic

CLINICAL PHARMACOLOGY
Mechanism of Action: Two chemically distinct compounds that, when given together, bind to different sites on bacterial ribosomes, inhibiting protein synthesis. *Therapeutic Effect:* Bactericidal.
Pharmacokinetics
After IV administration, both are extensively metabolized in the liver, with dalfopristin to active metabolite. Protein binding: quinupristin, 23%-32%; dalfopristin, 50%-56%. Primarily eliminated in feces. **Half-life:** quinupristin, 0.85 hr; dalfopristin, 0.7 hr.

INDICATIONS AND DOSAGES
Infections due to vancomycin-resistant *Enterococcus faecium*
IV
Adults, Elderly. 7.5 mg/kg/dose q8h.

Skin and skin-structure infections
IV
Adults, Elderly. 7.5 mg/kg/dose q12h.

$ AVAILABLE FORMS/COST
• Powder, Inj—IV: 500 mg (150 mg/350 mg): **$127.84**; 600 mg (180 mg/420 mg): **$151.25**

CONTRAINDICATIONS: None known

PREGNANCY AND LACTATION: Pregnancy category B; breast milk excretion unknown

SIDE EFFECTS
Frequent
Mild erythema, pruritus, pain, or burning at infusion site (with doses greater than 7 mg/kg)
Occasional
Headache, diarrhea
Rare
Vomiting, arthralgia, myalgia

SERIOUS REACTIONS
• Antibiotic-associated colitis and other superinfections may result from bacterial imbalance.
• Hepatic function abnormalities and severe venous pain and inflammation may occur.

INTERACTIONS
Drugs
❷ *Antihistamines (astemizole, terfenadine):* Reduced antihistamine metabolism by CYP3A4 inhibition, possible prolonged QT interval

❸ *Antineoplastic agents (docetaxel, paclitaxel, vinca alkaloids):* Reduced antineoplastic metabolism by CYP3A4 inhibition

❸ *Benzodiazepines (diazepam, midazolam):* Reduced benzodiazepine metabolism by CYP3A4 inhibition

❸ *Calcium channel blockers (amlodipine, diltiazem, felodipine, isradipine, nicardipine, nifedipine, nimodipine, nisoldipine, verapamil):* Reduced calcium channel blocker metabolism by CYP3A4 inhibition

❸ *Carbamazepine:* Reduced carbamazepine metabolism by CYP3A4 inhibition

❷ *Cisapride:* Reduced cisapride metabolism by CYP3A4 inhibition, possible prolonged QT interval

❸ *Digoxin:* Decreased digoxin metabolism by GI bacteria may increase digoxin levels

❷ *Disopyramide:* Reduced disopyramide metabolism by CYP3A4 inhibition, possible prolonged QT interval

❸ *HMG-CoA reductase inhibitors (atorvastatin, fluvastatin, lovastatin, pravastatin, simvastatin):* Reduced statin metabolism by CYP3A4 inhibition

❷ *Immunosuppressives (cyclosporine, tacrolimus):* Reduced immunosuppressive metabolism by CYP3A4 inhibition

❸ *Non-nucleoside reverse transcriptase inhibitors (delavirdine, nevirapine):* Reduced NNRTI metabolism by CYP3A4 inhibition

❸ *Protease inhibitors (indinavir, ritonavir):* Reduced PI metabolism by CYP3A4 inhibition

❷ *Quinidine:* Reduced quinidine metabolism by CYP3A4 inhibition, possible prolonged QT interval

SPECIAL CONSIDERATIONS
• Most appropriate use is when Vancomycin-resistant *Enterococcus faecium* infection is documented or strongly suspected, or for therapy of methicillin resistant *Staphylococcus aureus* infection

PATIENT/FAMILY EDUCATION
• Due to high chance of drug interactions through inhibition of CYP 3A4, use caution with any additional drugs

MONITORING PARAMETERS
• CBC, ALT, AST, bilirubin, renal function

rabeprazole
(rah-bep′rah-zole)
Rx: Aciphex
Chemical Class: Benzimidazole derivative
Therapeutic Class: Antiulcer
agent

CLINICAL PHARMACOLOGY
Mechanism of Action: A proton
pump inhibitor that converts to active metabolites that irreversibly
binds to and inhibit hydrogen-potassium adenosine triphosphate, an enzyme on the surface of gastric parietal cells. Actively secretes hydrogen ions for potassium ions, resulting in an accumulation of hydrogen
ions in gastric lumen. *Therapeutic
Effect:* Increases gastric pH, reducing gastric acid production.

Pharmacokinetics
Rapidly absorbed from the GI tract
after passing through the stomach
relatively intact. Protein binding:
96%. Metabolized extensively in
the liver. Primarily excreted in urine.
Unknown if removed by hemodialysis. **Half-life:** 1–2 hr (increased with
hepatic impairment).

INDICATIONS AND DOSAGES
Gastroesophageal reflux disease
PO
Adults, Elderly. 20 mg/day for 4–8
wk. Maintenance: 20 mg/day.
Duodenal ulcer
PO
Adults, Elderly. 20 mg/day after
morning meal for 4 wk.
*Non-steroidal antiinflammatory
disorder (NSAID)-induced ulcer*
PO
Adults, Elderly. 20 mg/day.

*Pathologic hypersecretory condi-
tions*
PO
Adults, Elderly. Initially, 60 mg once
a day. May increase to 60 mg twice a
day.
Helibacter pylori infection
PO
Adults, Elderly. 20 mg 2 times a day
for 7 days (given with amoxicillin
1,000 mg and clarithromycin 500
mg)
$ **AVAILABLE FORMS/COST**
• Tab, Sus Action—Oral: 20 mg,
100's: **$427.53**
CONTRAINDICATIONS: None
known
PREGNANCY AND LACTATION:
Pregnancy category B; excretion
into breast milk unknown, use cau-
tion in nursing mothers
SIDE EFFECTS
Rare (less than 2%)
Headache, nausea, dizziness, rash,
diarrhea, malaise
SERIOUS REACTIONS
• Hyperglycemia, hypokalemia, hy-
ponatremia, and hyperlipemia occur
rarely.
INTERACTIONS
Drugs
◼ *Cyclosporine:* Potential for in-
creased cyclosporine concentra-
tions
◼ *Digoxin:* Increased serum con-
centrations of digoxin possible
◼ *Ketoconazole:* Decreased bio-
availability of ketoconazole
SPECIAL CONSIDERATIONS
• Symptomatic response does not
rule out gastric malignancy
PATIENT/FAMILY EDUCATION
• Sustained action tablets should be
swallowed whole, do not chew,
crush, or split the tablets
MONITORING PARAMETERS
• Symptom relief, mucosal healing

raloxifene
(ra-lox'-i-feen)
Rx: Evista
Chemical Class: Benzothiophene derivative
Therapeutic Class: Antiosteoporotic; selective estrogen receptor modulator (SERM)

CLINICAL PHARMACOLOGY
Mechanism of Action: A selective estrogen receptor modulator that affects some receptors like estrogen. *Therapeutic Effect:* Like estrogen, prevents bone loss and improves lipid profiles.

Pharmacokinetics
Rapidly absorbed after PO administration. Highly bound to plasma proteins (95%) and albumin. Undergoes extensive first-pass metabolism in liver. Excreted mainly in feces and, to a lesser extent, in urine. Unknown if removed by hemodialysis. **Half-life:** 27.7 hr.

INDICATIONS AND DOSAGES
Prevention or treatment of osteoporosis
PO
Adults, Elderly. 60 mg a day.

S **AVAILABLE FORMS/COST**
• Tab, Coated—Oral: 60 mg, 100's: **$269.54**

UNLABELED USES: Treatment of breast cancer in postmenopausal women, prevention of fractures

CONTRAINDICATIONS: Active or history of venous thromboembolic events, such as deep vein thrombosis, pulmonary embolism, and retinal vein thrombosis; women who are or may become pregnant

PREGNANCY AND LACTATION: Pregnancy category X; abortion and fetal anomalies noted in animal studies; unknown if excreted in milk

SIDE EFFECTS
Frequent (25%–10%)
Hot flashes, flu-like symptoms, arthralgia, sinusitis
Occasional (9%–5%)
Weight gain, nausea, myalgia, pharyngitis, cough, dyspepsia, leg cramps, rash, depression
Rare (4%–3%)
Vaginitis, UTI, peripheral edema, flatulence, vomiting, fever, migraine, diaphoresis

SERIOUS REACTIONS
• Pneumonia, gastroenteritis, chest pain, vaginal bleeding, and breast pain occur rarely.

INTERACTIONS
Drugs
❷ *Cholestyramine:* Decreased absorption and enterohepatic cycling of raloxifene
❸ *Clofibrate, indomethacin, naproxen, ibuprofen, diazepam, diazoxide:* Possible displacement of these highly protein-bound drugs
❸ *Warfarin:* Decreased PT

SPECIAL CONSIDERATIONS
• Shown to preserve bone mass, increase bone mineral density, and reduce fracture rate relative to calcium alone
• Ensure adequate dietary or supplemental calcium, vitamin D
• Not associated with endometrial proliferation; however, investigate uterine bleeding
• Risk of thromboembolic events greatest in first 4 mo, discontinue at least 72 hr prior to surgery involving immobilization. Resume when patient fully ambulatory

PATIENT/FAMILY EDUCATION
• May be taken without regard to meals
• Engage in weight-bearing exercises; do not smoke or use alcohol excessively

R

• Report leg pain or swelling, sudden chest pain, shortness of breath, vision changes

• Avoid restrictions of movement during travel. Discontinue if at bed rest.

MONITORING PARAMETERS

• Bone density tests (e.g., DEXA scan)

---

ramipril

(ram′i-pril)

Rx: Altace

Chemical Class: Angiotensin-converting enzyme (ACE) inhibitor, nonsulfhydryl

Therapeutic Class: Antihypertensive

CLINICAL PHARMACOLOGY

Mechanism of Action: An ACE inhibitor that suppresses the renin-angiotensin-aldosterone system. Decreases plasma angiotensin II, increases plasma renin activity, and decreases aldosterone secretion. *Therapeutic Effect:* Reduces peripheral arterial resistance and BP.

Pharmacokinetics

Route	Onset	Peak	Duration
PO	1-2 hr	3-6 hr	24 hr

Well absorbed from the GI tract. Protein binding: 73%. Metabolized in the liver to active metabolite. Primarily excreted in urine. Not removed by hemodialysis. **Half-life:** 5.1 hr.

INDICATIONS AND DOSAGES

Hypertension (monotherapy)

PO

Adults, Elderly. Initially, 2.5 mg/day. Maintenance: 2.5-20 mg/day as single dose or in 2 divided doses.

Hypertension (in combination with other antihypertensives)

PO

Adults, Elderly. Initially, 1.25 mg/day titrated to patient's needs.

CHF

PO

Adults, Elderly. Initially, 1.25-2.5 mg twice a day. Maximum: 5 mg twice a day.

Risk reduction for myocardial infarction stroke

PO

Adults, Elderly. Initially, 2.5 mg/day for 7 days, then 5 mg/day for 21 days, then 10 mg/day as a single dose or in divided doses.

Dosage in renal impairment

Creatinine clearance equal to or less than 40 ml/min. 25% of normal dose.

Hypertension. Initially, 1.25 mg/day titrated upward.

CHF. Initially, 1.25 mg/day, titrated up to 2.5 mg twice a day.

$ **AVAILABLE FORMS/COST**

• Cap, Gel—Oral: 1.25 mg, 100's: **$105.00**; 2.5 mg, 100's: **$133.83**; 5 mg, 100's: **$145.75**; 10 mg, 100's: **$178.88**

UNLABELED USES: Treatment of hypertension and renal crisis in scleroderma

CONTRAINDICATIONS: Bilateral renal artery stenosis

PREGNANCY AND LACTATION: Pregnancy category D; ACE inhibitors can cause fetal and neonatal morbidity and death when administered to pregnant women; when pregnancy is detected, discontinue ACE inhibitors as soon as possible

SIDE EFFECTS

Frequent (12%-5%)

Cough, headache

Occasional (4%-2%)

Dizziness, fatigue, nausea, asthenia (loss of strength)

Rare (less than 2%)
Palpitations, insomnia, nervousness, malaise, abdominal pain, myalgia
SERIOUS REACTIONS
• Excessive hypotension (first-dose syncope) may occur in patients with CHF and and in those who are severely salt or volume depleted.
• Angioedema and hyperkalemia occur rarely.
• Agranulocytosis and neutropenia may be noted in those with collagen vascular disease, including scleroderma and systemic lupus erythematosus, and impaired renal function.
• Nephrotic syndrome may be noted in those with history of renal disease.
INTERACTIONS
Drugs
❷ *Allopurinol:* Predisposition to hypersensitivity reactions
❸ *α-adrenergic blockers:* Exaggerated 1st dose hypotensive response
❸ *Aspirin:* Reduced hemodynamic effects; less likely with nonacetylated salicylates
❸ *Azathioprine:* Increased myelosuppression
❸ *Cyclosporine:* Renal insufficiency
❸ *Insulin:* Enhanced hypoglycemic response
❸ *Iron (parenteral):* Increased risk of systemic reaction
❸ *Lithium:* Increased risk of serious lithium toxicity
❸ *Loop diuretics:* Initiation of ACE inhibitor therapy may cause hypotension and renal insufficiency
❸ *NSAIDs:* Inhibition of the antihypertensive response to ACE inhibitors
❸ *Potassium, potassium-sparing diuretics:* Increased risk for hyperkalemia

❸ *Trimethoprim:* Additive risk of hyperkalemia, especially in patient predisposed to renal insufficiency
Labs
• ACE inhibition can account for approx 0.5mEq/L rise in serum potassium
SPECIAL CONSIDERATIONS
PATIENT/FAMILY EDUCATION
• Caution with salt substitutes containing potassium chloride
• Rise slowly to sitting/standing position to minimize orthostatic hypotension
• Dizziness, fainting, lightheadedness may occur during 1st few days of therapy
• May cause altered taste perception or cough; persistent dry cough usually does not subside unless medication is stopped; notify clinician if these symptoms persist
MONITORING PARAMETERS
• BUN, creatinine, potassium within 2 wk after initiation of therapy (increased levels may indicate acute renal failure)
• Potassium levels, although hyperkalemia rarely occurs

---

ranitidine
(ra-ni′ti-deen)
Rx: Zantac, Zantac EFFERdose, Zantac GELdose
OTC: Zantac 75
Chemical Class: Aminoalkyl furan derivative
Therapeutic Class: Antiulcer agent

CLINICAL PHARMACOLOGY
Mechanism of Action: An antiulcer agent that inhibits histamine action at histamine 2 receptors of gastric parietal cells. *Therapeutic Effect:* Inhibits gastric acid secretion when fasting, at night, or when stimulated

by food, caffeine, or insulin. Reduces volume and hydrogen ion concentration of gastric juice.

Pharmacokinetics

Rapidly absorbed from the GI tract. Protein binding: 15%. Widely distributed. Metabolized in the liver. Primarily excreted in urine. Not removed by hemodialysis. **Half-life:** PO, 2.5 hr; IV, 2–2.5 hr (increased with impaired renal function).

INDICATIONS AND DOSAGES

Duodenal ulcers, gastric ulcers, gastroesophageal reflux disease

PO

Adults, Elderly. 150 mg twice a day or 300 mg at bedtime. Maintenance: 150 mg at bedtime.

Children. 2–4 mg/kg/day in divided doses twice a day. Maximum: 300 mg/day.

Erosive esophagitis

PO

Adults, Elderly. 150 mg 4 times a day. Maintenance: 150 mg 2 times/day or 300 mg at bedtime.

Children. 4–10 mg/kg/day in 2 divided doses. Maximum: 600 mg/day.

Hypersecretory conditions

PO

Adults, Elderly. 150 mg twice a day. May increase up to 6 g/day.

Usual parenteral dosage

IV, IM

Adults, Elderly. 50 mg/dose q6-8h. Maximum: 400 mg/day.

Children. 2–4 mg/kg/day in divided doses q6-8h. Maximum: 200 mg/day.

Usual neonatal dosage

PO

Neonates. 2 mg/kg/day in divided doses q12h.

IV

Neonates. Initially, 1.5 mg/kg/dose; then 1.5–2 mg/kg/day in divided doses q12h.

Dosage in renal impairment

For patients with creatinine clearance less than 50 ml/min, give 150 mg PO q24h or 50 mg IV or IM q18-24h.

[$] **AVAILABLE FORMS/COST**

- Cap, Gel—Oral: 150 mg, 60's: **$102.00**; 300 mg, 100's: **$266.12**
- Granule, Effervescent—Oral: 150 mg, 60's: **$110.89**
- Sol, Inj—IM, IV: 25 mg/ml, 2 ml: **$3.99**
- Syr—Oral: 15 mg/ml, 480 ml: **$236.76**
- Tab, Coated—Oral: 75 mg, 30's: **$5.39-$9.23**; 150 mg, 100's: **$8.01-$312.23**; 300 mg, 100's: **$268.70-$286.70**
- Tab, Effervescent—Oral: 150 mg, 60's: **$121.29**

UNLABELED USES: Prevention of aspiration pneumonia

CONTRAINDICATIONS: History of acute porphyria

PREGNANCY AND LACTATION: Pregnancy category B; compatible with breast-feeding

SIDE EFFECTS

Occasional (2%)

Diarrhea

Rare (1%)

Constipation, headache (may be severe)

SERIOUS REACTIONS

- Reversible hepatitis and blood dyscrasias occur rarely.

INTERACTIONS

Drugs

[3] *Cefuroxine; cefpodoxime; enoxacin; ketoconazole:* Reduction in gastric acidity reduces absorption, decreased plasma levels, potential for therapeutic failure

[3] *Glipizide; glyburide; tolbutamide:* Increased absorption of these drugs, potential for hypoglycemia

[3] *Nifedipine, nitrendipine, nisoldipine:* Increased concentrations of these drugs

Labs
• *False positive:* Urine drugs of abuse screen

SPECIAL CONSIDERATIONS
• No advantage over other agents in this class, base selection on cost

PATIENT/FAMILY EDUCATION
• Stagger doses of ranitidine and antacids
• Dissolve effervescent tablets and granules in 6-8 oz water before drinking

MONITORING PARAMETERS
• Intragastric pH when used for stress ulcer prophylaxis, titrate dose to maintain pH >4

---

repaglinide
(re-pag'lih-nide)
Rx: Prandin
Chemical Class: Meglitinide
Therapeutic Class: Antidiabetic; hypoglycemic

CLINICAL PHARMACOLOGY
Mechanism of Action: An antihyperglycemic that stimulates release of insulin from beta cells of the pancreas by depolarizing beta cells, leading to an opening of calcium channels. Resulting calcium influx induces insulin secretion. *Therapeutic Effect:* Lowers blood glucose concentration.

Pharmacokinetics
Rapidly, completely absorbed from the GI tract. Protein binding: 98%. Metabolized in the liver to inactive metabolites. Excreted primarily in feces with a lesser amount in urine. Unknown if removed by hemodialysis. **Half-life:** 1 hr.

INDICATIONS AND DOSAGES
Diabetes mellitus
PO
Adults, Elderly. 0.5–4 mg 2–4 times a day. Maximum: 16 mg/day.

$ AVAILABLE FORMS/COST
• Tab, Coated—Oral: 0.5 mg, 1 mg, 2 mg, 100's; all: **$109.14**

CONTRAINDICATIONS: Diabetic ketoacidosis, type 1 diabetes mellitus

PREGNANCY AND LACTATION: Pregnancy category C; excretion into breast milk unknown; due to the potential for hypoglycemia in the infant, use with caution in nursing mothers

SIDE EFFECTS
Frequent (10%–6%)
Upper respiratory tract infection, headache, rhinitis, bronchitis, back pain
Occasional (5%–3%)
Diarrhea, dyspepsia, sinusitis, nausea, arthralgia, urinary tract infection
Rare (2%)
Constipation, vomiting, paresthesia, allergy

SERIOUS REACTIONS
• Hypoglycemia occurs in 16% of patients.
• Chest pain occurs rarely.

INTERACTIONS
Drugs
3 *Aspirin, β-blockers, sulfa drugs, chloramphenicol, warfarin, MAO inhibitors:* hypoglycemia
3 *Ketoconazole, miconazole, erythromycin, troglitazone, rifampicin, carbamazepine, phenobarbital, butalbital, secobarbital, or primidone:* potential increased repaglinide metabolism secondary to cytochrome P450 enzyme induction
3 *Thiazide diuretics, calcium channel blockers, β-blockers, cough, cold, or hay fever medicines (sympathomimetics), estrogen, oral contraceptives, corticosteroids, thyroid medicine, phenytoin, isoniazid, or nicotinic acid:* Hyperglycemia

R

SPECIAL CONSIDERATIONS
PATIENT/FAMILY EDUCATION
• Skip the dose of this medication if you skip a meal; take an extra dose with extra meal
• Recognize and treat hypoglycemia; maintain ready supply of glucose (glucose tablets or gel)
MONITORING PARAMETERS
• Blood glucose—biggest effect noted on postprandial values (50-75 mg/dL reductions expected); minimal effect on fasting blood glucose
• Glycosylated hemoglobin (1% to 2% reductions expected)
• Hyperglycemia/hypoglycemia signs and symptoms

reserpine
(reh-zer'-peen)
Rx: Eskaserp, Lemiserp, Reserpoid, Resine, Serpalan, Serpasil, Unitensin-R
Combinations
  Rx: with thiazide diuretics: i.e., bendroflumethazide (flumethazide), chlorothiazide, chlorthalidone (Regreton), hydrochlorothiazide (Hydropres, Hydroserpalan, Hydroserpine, Mallopress), hydroflumethiazide (Salutensin), polythiazide (Reneese), quinethazone (Hydromox R), trichloromethiazide (Metatensin, Naquival), hydrochlorothiazide and hydralazine (Hyserp, Lo-Ten, Marpres, Ser-A-Gen, Seralazide, Ser-Ap-Es, Unipres, Uni-Serp)
  Chemical Class: Rauwolfia alkaloid
  Therapeutic Class: Antihypertensive; antipsychotic; postganglionic adrenergic neuron inhibitor

CLINICAL PHARMACOLOGY
Mechanism of Action: An antihypertensive that depletes stores of catecholamines and 5-hydroxytryptamine in many organs, including the brain and adrenal medulla. Depression of sympathetic nerve function results in a decreased heart rate and a lowering of arterial blood pressure. Depletion of catecholamines and 5-hydroxytryptamine from the brain is thought to be the mechanism of the sedative and tranquilizing properties. *Therapeutic Effects:* Decrease blood pressure and heart rate; sedation.

Pharmacokinetics

Characterized by slow onset of action and sustained effects. Both cardiovascular and central nervous system effects may persist for a period of time following withdrawal of the drug. Mean maximum plasma levels were attained after a median of 3.5 hours. Bioavailability was approximately 50% of that of a corresponding intravenous dose. Protein binding: 96%. **Half life:** 33 hours.

INDICATIONS AND DOSAGES

Hypertension

PO

Adults: Usual initial dosage 0.5 mg daily for 1 or 2 weeks. For maintenance, reduce to 0.1 to 0.25 mg daily.

Children: Reserpine is not recommended for use in children. If it is to be used in treating a child, the usual recommended starting dose is 20 mcg/kg daily. The maximum recommended dose is 0.25 mg (total) daily.

Psychiatric Disorders

PO

Adults: Initial dosage 0.5 mg daily, may range from 0.1-1.0 mg. Adjust dosage upward or downward according to response.

S AVAILABLE FORMS/COST

• Tab—Oral: 0.1 mg, 100's: **$31.76**; 0.25 mg, 100's: **$45.11**

UNLABELED USES: Cerebral vasospasm, migraines, Raynaud's syndrome, reflex sympathetic dystrophy, refractory depression, tardive dyskinesia, thyrotoxic crisis.

CONTRAINDICATIONS: Hypersensitivity, mental depression or history of mental depression (especially with suicidal tendencies), active peptic ulcer, ulcerative colitis, patients receiving electroconvulsive therapy.

PREGNANCY AND LACTATION: Pregnancy category C; excreted into breast milk, no clinical reports of adverse effects in nursing infants have been located

SIDE EFFECTS

Occasional

Burning in the stomach, nausea, vomiting, diarrhea, dry mouth, nosebleed, stuffy nose, dizziness, headache, nervousness, nightmares, drowsiness, muscle aches, weight gain, redness of the eyes

Rare

Irregular heart beat, difficulty breathing, heart problems, feeling faint, swelling, gynecomastia, decreased libido

SERIOUS REACTIONS

• None known.

INTERACTIONS

Drugs

⊠ *Non-selective MAOIs:* Hypertensive reactions

Labs

• *False increase:* Serum bilirubin, urine creatinine

• *False positive:* Guiacols spot test

SPECIAL CONSIDERATIONS

• Only remaining rauwolfia derivative available

PATIENT/FAMILY EDUCATION

• May cause drowsiness or dizziness, use caution driving or participating in other activities requiring alertness

• Therapeutic effect may take 2-3 wk

MONITORING PARAMETERS

• Blood pressure, edema, drowsiness, despondency or self-depreciation, early morning insomnia, CNS depression, hypothermia, extrapyradimal tract effects

R

reteplase
(reh′te-place)

Rx: Retavase
Chemical Class: Tissue plasminogen activator (tPA)
Therapeutic Class: Thrombolytic

CLINICAL PHARMACOLOGY
Mechanism of Action: A tissue plasminogen activator that activates the fibrinolytic system by directly cleaving plasminogen to generate plasmin, an enzyme that degrades the fibrin of the thrombus. *Therapeutic Effect:* Exerts thrombolytic action.

Pharmacokinetics
Rapidly cleared from plasma. Eliminated primarily by the liver and kidney. **Half-life:** 13–16 min.

INDICATIONS AND DOSAGES
Acute MI, CHF
IV bolus
Adults, Elderly. 10 units over 2 min; repeat in 30 min.

S **AVAILABLE FORMS/COST**
• Powder—Inj: kit (2 × 10 U plus syringes, needles, etc.): **$2,872.50**
CONTRAINDICATIONS: Active internal bleeding, AV malformation or aneurysm, bleeding diathesis, history of cerebrovascular accident, intracranial neoplasm, recent intracranial or intraspinal surgery or trauma, severe uncontrolled hypertension
PREGNANCY AND LACTATION: Pregnancy category C
SIDE EFFECTS
Frequent
Bleeding at superficial sites, such as venous injection sites, catheter insertion sites, venous cutdowns, arterial punctures, and sites of recent surgical procedures, gingival bleeding

SERIOUS REACTIONS
• Bleeding at internal sites may occur, including intracranial, retroperitoneal, GI, GU, and respiratory sites.
• Lysis or coronary thrombi may produce atrial or ventricular arrhythmias and stroke.
INTERACTIONS
Drugs
❷ *Heparin, oral anticoagulants, drugs that alter platelet function (i.e., aspirin, dipyridamole, abciximab, eptifibitide, tirofiban):* May increase the risk of bleeding
SPECIAL CONSIDERATIONS
• No other IV medications should be administered in the same line

ribavirin
(rye-ba-vye′rin)

Rx: *Inhalation:* Virazole
Rx: *Oral:* Rebetol, Copegus
Combinations
　Rx: with interferon alfa-2b
　　(Rebetron)
Chemical Class: Nucleoside analog
Therapeutic Class: Antiviral

CLINICAL PHARMACOLOGY
Mechanism of Action: A synthetic nucleoside that inhibits influenza virus RNA polymerase activity and interferes with expression of messenger RNA. *Therapeutic Effect:* Inhibits viral protein synthesis and replication of viral RNA and DNA.

INDICATIONS AND DOSAGES
Chronic hepatitis C
PO (capsule or oral solution in combination with interferon alfa-2b)
Adults, Elderly. 1,000-1,200 mg/day in 2 divided doses.

Children weighing 60 kg or more. Use adult dosage. *(51-60 kg):* 400 mg 2 times/day. *(37-50 kg):*200 mg in morning, 400 mg in evening. *(24-36 kg):* 200 mg 2 times/day.

PO (capsules in combination with peginterferon alfa-2b)

Adults, Elderly. 800 mg/day in 2 divided doses.

PO (tablets in combination with peginterferon alfa-2b)

Adults, Elderly. 800-1200 mg/day in 2 divided doses.

Severe lower respiratory tract infection caused by respiratory syncytial virus (RSV)

Inhalation

Children, Infants. Use with Viratek small-particle aerosol generator at a concentration of 20 mg/ml (6 g reconstituted with 300 ml sterile water) over 12-18 hr/day for 3-7 days.

AVAILABLE FORMS/COST
• Powder, Reconst—INH: 6 g, 4's: **$5,499.38**
• Cap—Oral: 200 mg, 84's: **$927.18**
UNLABELED USES: Treatment of influenza A or B and west Nile virus
CONTRAINDICATIONS: Pregnancy, women of childbearing age who do not use contraception reliably
PREGNANCY AND LACTATION: Pregnancy category X; teratogenic in animals; contraindicated in lactating women
SIDE EFFECTS
Frequent (greater than 10%)
Dizziness, headache, fatigue, fever, insomnia, irritability, depression, emotional lability, impaired concentration, alopecia, rash, pruritus, nausea, anorexia, dyspepsia, vomiting, decreased hemoglobin, hemolysis, arthralgia, musculoskeletal pain, dyspnea, sinusitis, flu-like symptoms
Occasional (1%-10%)

Nervousness, altered taste, weakness
SERIOUS REACTIONS
• Cardiac arrest, apnea and ventilator dependence, bacterial pneumonia, pneumonia, and pneumothorax occur rarely.
• Anemia may occur if ribavirin therapy exceeds 7 days.
SPECIAL CONSIDERATIONS
PATIENT/FAMILY EDUCATION
• Female health care workers who are pregnant or may become pregnant should avoid exposure to ribavirin
MONITORING PARAMETERS
• Hematocrit

---

rifabutin
(rif′a-byoo-ten)
Rx: Mycobutin
Chemical Class: Rifamycin S derivative
Therapeutic Class: Antibiotic

CLINICAL PHARMACOLOGY
Mechanism of Action: An antitubercular that inhibits DNA-dependent RNA polymerase, an enzyme in susceptible strains of *Escherichia coli* and *Bacillus subtilis*. Rifabutin has a broad spectrum of antimicrobial activity, including against mycobacteria such as *Mycobacterium avium* complex (MAC). *Therapeutic Effect:* Prevents MAC disease.
Pharmacokinetics
Readily absorbed from the GI tract (high-fat meals delay absorption). Protein binding: 85%. Widely distributed. Crosses the blood-brain barrier. Extensive intracellular tissue uptake. Metabolized in the liver to active metabolite. Excreted in urine; eliminated in feces. Unknown if removed by hemodialysis. **Half-life:** 16-69 hr.

INDICATIONS AND DOSAGES
Prevention of MAC disease (first episode)
PO
Adults, Elderly. 300 mg as a single dose or in 2 divided doses if gastrointestinal (GI) upset occurs.
Prevention of recurrent MAC disease
PO
Adults, Elderly. 300 mg/day (in combination)
Dosage in renal impairment
Dosage is modified based on creatinine clearance. If creatinine clearance is less than 30 ml/min, reduce dosage by 50%.

AVAILABLE FORMS/COST
• Cap, Gel—Oral: 150 mg, 100's: **$653.98**

CONTRAINDICATIONS: Active tuberculosis; hypersensitivity to other rifamycins, including rifampin

PREGNANCY AND LACTATION: Pregnancy category B

SIDE EFFECTS
Frequent (30%)
Red-orange or red-brown discoloration of urine, feces, saliva, skin, sputum, sweat, or tears
Occasional (11%-3%)
Rash, nausea, abdominal pain, diarrhea, dyspepsia, belching, headache, altered taste, uveitis, corneal deposits
Rare (less than 2%)
Anorexia, flatulence, fever, myalgia, vomiting, insomnia

SERIOUS REACTIONS
• Hepatitis and thrombocytopenia occur rarely. Anemia and neutropenia may also occur.

INTERACTIONS
Drugs
▣ *Acetaminophen:* Enhanced hepatotoxicity (overdoses and possibly large therapeutic doses)
▣ *Cyclosporine:* Reduced concentration of cyclosporine
▣ *Delavirdine:* Reduced concentration of delavirdine
▣ *Eprosartan:* Reduced concentration of eprosartan
▣ *Nifedipine:* Reduced nifedipine concentrations
▣ *Oral contraceptives:* Menstrual irregularities, contraceptive failure
▣ *Oral hypoglycemics:* Reduced hypoglycemic activity
▣ *Propafenone:* Lowered propafenone concentrations, loss of antiarrhythmic efficacy
❷ *Protease inhibitors:* Increased clearance (CYP3A4 induction) and decreased protease inhibitor efficacy
▣ *Quinidine:* Marked reduction quinidine levels
▣ *Tacrolimus:* Reduced concentration of tacrolimus

SPECIAL CONSIDERATIONS
• Has liver enzyme-inducing properties similar to rifampin although less potent
• Unlike rifampin, does not appear to alter the acetylation of isoniazid

PATIENT/FAMILY EDUCATION
• May discolor bodily secretions brown-orange, soft contact lenses may be permanently stained

MONITORING PARAMETERS
• Periodic CBC with differential and platelets
• Liver function tests

rifampin

(rye'fam-pin)

Rx: Rifadin, Rimactane
Chemical Class: Rifamycin B
derivative
Therapeutic Class: Antituberculosis agent

CLINICAL PHARMACOLOGY

Mechanism of Action: An antitubercular that interferes with bacterial RNA synthesis by binding to
DNA-dependent RNA polymerase,
thus preventing its attachment to
DNA and blocking RNA transcription. *Therapeutic Effect:* Bactericidal in susceptible microorganisms.

Pharmacokinetics

Well absorbed from the GI tract
(food delays absorption). Protein
binding: 80%. Widely distributed.
Metabolized in the liver to active
metabolite. Primarily eliminated by
the biliary system. Not removed by
hemodialysis. **Half-life:** 3-5 hr (increased in hepatic impairment).

INDICATIONS AND DOSAGES

Tuberculosis

PO, IV

Adults, Elderly. 10 mg/kg/day.
Maximum: 600 mg/day.

Children. 10-20 mg/kg/day in divided doses q12-24h.

*Prevention of meningococcal in-
fections*

PO, IV

Adults, Elderly. 600 mg q12h for 2
days.

Children 1 month and older. 20
mg/kg/day in divided doses q12-
24h. Maximum: 600 mg/dose.

Infants younger than 1 mo. 10
mg/kg/day in divided doses q12h for
2 days.

Staphylococcal infections

PO, IV

Adults, Elderly. 600 mg once a day.

Children. 15 mg/kg/day in divided
doses q12h.

Staphylococcus aureus infections
(in combination with other anti-in-
fectives)

PO

Adults, Elderly. 300-600 mg twice a
day.

Neonates. 5-20 mg/kg/day in divided doses q12h.

*Prevention of Haemophilus influ-
enzae* infection

PO

Adults, Elderly. 600 mg/day for 4
days.

Children 1 mo and older. 20
mg/kg/day in divided doses q12h for
5-10 days.

Children younger than 1 mo. 10
mg/kg/day in divided doses q12h for
2 days.

AVAILABLE FORMS/COST

• Cap, Gel—Oral: 150 mg, 30's:
$36.95-$47.38; 300 mg, 100's:
$134.10-$223.87

• Powder, Inj—IV: 600 mg/vial, 1's:
$77.50-$90.28

UNLABELED USES: Prophylaxis of
H. *influenzae* type b infection; treatment of atypical mycobacterial infection and serious infections
caused by *Staphylococcus* species

CONTRAINDICATIONS: Concomitant therapy with amprenavir,
hypersensitivity to rifampin or any
other rifamycins

PREGNANCY AND LACTATION:
Pregnancy category C; compatible
with breast-feeding

SIDE EFFECTS

Expected

Red-orange or red-brown discoloration of urine, feces, saliva, skin, sputum, sweat, or tears

Occasional (5%-2%)
Hypersensitivity reaction (such as flushing, pruritus, or rash)
Rare (2%-1%)
Diarrhea, dyspepsia, nausea, candida as evidenced by sore mouth or tongue

SERIOUS REACTIONS

• Rare reactions include hepatotoxicity (risk is increased when rifampin is taken with isoniazid), hepatitis, blood dyscrasias, Stevens-Johnson syndrome, and antibiotic-associated colitis.

INTERACTIONS

Drugs

◼ *Acetaminophen:* Enhanced hepatotoxicity (overdoses and possibly large therapeutic doses)

◼ *Aminosalicylic acid:* Reduced serum concentrations of rifampin

◼ *Antidiabetics:* Diminished hypoglycemic activity of sulfonylureas

◼ *Azole antifungals, barbiturates, benzodiazepines,* β-*blockers (except nadolol), calcium channel blockers, chloramphenicol, clofibrate, cyclic antidepressants, dapsone, digitalis glycosides, disopyramide, lorcainide, methadone, mexiletine, nortriptyline, phenytoin, pirmenol, propafenone, quinidine, tocainide, theophylline, zidovudine:* Reduced serum concentrations of these drugs

◼ *Corticosteroids:* Reduced effect of corticosteroids

❷ *Cyclosporine, tacrolimus:* Reduced concentrations of these drugs, possible therapeutic failure

◼ *Isoniazid:* Increased hepatotoxic potential of isoniazid in slow acetylators or patients with pre-existing liver disease

❷ *Oral anticoagulants:* Reduced hypoprothrombinemic effect of oral anticoagulants

◼ *Oral contraceptives:* Menstrual irregularities, contraceptive failure

❷ *Protease inhibitors:* Increased clearance (CYP3A4 induction) and decreased protease inhibitor efficacy

◼ *Thyroid:* Increased elimination, increased thyroid requirements

Labs

• *Increase:* Liver function tests, uric acid

• *Interference:* Folate, vitamin B_{12}, BSP, gallbladder studies

• *False decrease:* Serum bilirubin, ALT, AST (by some methods), cholesterol, triglycerides

• *False increase:* Serum bilirubin (some methods, may also be true physiologic increase), glucose, iron, LDH, uric acid, metronidazole, phosphate, tetracycline, trimethoprim

• *False positive:* Clindamycin, erythromycin, polymyxin

SPECIAL CONSIDERATIONS

PATIENT/FAMILY EDUCATION

• Take on empty stomach, at least 1 hr before or 2 hr after meals

• May cause reddish-orange discoloration of bodily secretions, may permanently discolor soft contact lenses

MONITORING PARAMETERS

• Liver function tests at baseline and q2-4 wk during therapy

• CBC with differential and platelets at baseline and periodically throughout treatment

rifapentine

(rif-a-pen′-teen)

Rx: Priftin

Chemical Class: Rifamycin B derivative

Therapeutic Class: Antituberculosis agent

CLINICAL PHARMACOLOGY

Mechanism of Action: An antitubercular that inhibits bacterial RNA synthesis by binding to DNA-dependent RNA polymerase in *Mycobacterium tuberculosis*. This action prevents the enzyme from attaching to DNA, thereby blocking RNA transcription. *Therapeutic Effect:* Bactericidal.

INDICATIONS AND DOSAGES

Tuberculosis

PO

Adults, Elderly. Intensive phase: 600 mg twice weekly for 2 mo (interval between doses no less than 3 days). Continuation phase: 600 mg weekly for 4 mo.

[$] **AVAILABLE FORMS/COST**

- Tab, Coated—Oral: 150 mg, 32's: **$87.96**

CONTRAINDICATIONS: None known.

PREGNANCY AND LACTATION: Pregnancy category C (teratogenic in rats); excreted in breast milk, but compatible with breast-feeding

SIDE EFFECTS

Rare (less than 4%)

Red-orange or red-brown discoloration of urine, feces, saliva, skin, sputum, sweat, or tears; arthralgia, pain, nausea, vomiting, headache, dyspepsia, hypertension, dizziness, diarrhea

SERIOUS REACTIONS

- Hyperuricemia, neutropenia, proteinuria, hematuria, and hepatitis occur rarely.

INTERACTIONS

Drugs

[3] *Acetaminophen:* Enhanced hepatotoxicity

[3] *Aminosalicylic acid:* Reduced plasma concentrations of rifapentine

[3] *Azole antifungals, barbiturates, benzodiazepines, β-blockers, calcium channel blockers, chloramphenicol, clofibrate, cyclic antidepressants, dapsone, digitalis glycosides, disopyramide, lorcainide, methadone, mexiletine, phenytoin, pirmenol, propafenone, quinidine, tocainide, theophylline, zidovudine:* Reduced plasma concentrations of these drugs

[3] *Corticosteroids:* Reduced effect of corticosteroids

[2] *Cyclosporine:* Reduced plasma concentration of cyclosporine

[3] *Isoniazid:* Increased hepatotoxic potential of isoniazid in slow acetylators or patients with preexisting liver disease

[3] *Oral contraceptives:* Reduced plasma levels of these drugs with menstrual irregularity and contraceptive failure

[2] *Protease inhibitors:* Increased clearance and decreased protease inhibitor efficacy

[3] *Sulfonylureas:* Diminished hypoglycemic activity of sulfonylureas

[2] *Tacrolimus:* Reduced plasma concentration of tacrolimus

[3] *Thyroid:* Increased clearance of thyroid hormone with increased dose requirement

[2] *Warfarin:* Reduced hypoprothrombinemic effect of warfarin

Labs

- *Interference:* Folate and vitamin B_{12} levels by microbiologic assay

PATIENT/FAMILY EDUCATION
• Use an alternative method of contraception if taking oral contraceptives concurrently
• Avoid alcoholic beverages concurrently with this medication
• Rifapentine causes urine, stool, saliva, sputum, sweat, and tears to turn reddish-orange to reddish-brown and may also permanently discolor soft contact lenses; avoid wearing soft contact lenses

MONITORING PARAMETERS
• ALT, AST, alkaline phosphate, bilirubin, and CBC prior to treatment and monthly during treatment

---

rifaximin
(rye-faks′eh-men)
Rx: Xifaxan
Chemical Class: Semisynthetic rifamycin B derivative
Therapeutic Class: Antibiotic

CLINICAL PHARMACOLOGY
Mechanism of Action: An anti-infective that inhibits bacterial RNA synthesis by binding to a subunit of bacterial DNA-dependent RNA polymerase. *Therapeutic Effect:* Bactericidal.
Pharmacokinetics
Less than 0.4% absorbed after PO administration. **Half-life:** 5.85 hr.

INDICATIONS AND DOSAGES
Traveler's diarrhea
PO
Adults, Elderly, Children 12 yr and older. 200 mg 3 times a day for 3 days.
Hepatic encephalopathy
PO
Adults, Elderly. 1200 mg/day for 15-21 days.
UNLABELED USES: Treatment of hepatic encephalopathy

CONTRAINDICATIONS: Hypersensitivity to rifaximin or other rifamycin antibiotics
PREGNANCY AND LACTATION: Pregnancy category C; breast milk excretion unknown, but probably compatible with breast-feeding as its absorption is less than 1%, and the parent compound, rifampin, is compatible with breast-feeding
SIDE EFFECTS
Occasional (11%-5%)
Flatulence, headache, abdominal discomfort, rectal tenesmus, defecation urgency, nausea
Rare (4%-2%)
Constipation, fever, vomiting
SERIOUS REACTIONS
• Hypersensitivity reactions, including dermatitis, angioneurotic edema, pruritus, rash, and urticaria may occur.
• Superinfection occurs rarely.
SPECIAL CONSIDERATIONS
• Has been used for diverticular disease and hepatic encephalopathy, but not FDA approved. Not effective for traveler's diarrhea due to bacteria other than enterotoxigenic E. coli

---

riluzole
(rye′loo-zole)
Rx: Rilutek
Chemical Class: Benzothiazolamine derivative
Therapeutic Class: Amyotrophic lateral sclerosis (ALS) agent

CLINICAL PHARMACOLOGY
Mechanism of Action: An amyotrophic lateral sclerosis (ALS) agent that inhibits presynaptic glutamate release in the CNS and intereferes postsynaptically with the effects of

excitatory amino acids. *Therapeutic Effect:* Extends survival of ALS patients.

INDICATIONS AND DOSAGES
ALS
PO

Adults, Elderly. 50 mg q12h.

$ AVAILABLE FORMS/COST
• Tab—Oral: 50 mg, 60's: **$926.71**

CONTRAINDICATIONS: None significant.

PREGNANCY AND LACTATION: Pregnancy category C; excretion into breast milk unknown, use caution in nursing mothers

SIDE EFFECTS
Frequent (greater than 10%)
Nausea, asthenia, reduced respiratory function

Occasional (10%–1%)
Edema, tachycardia, headache, dizziness, somnolence, depression, vertigo, tremor, pruritus, alopecia, abdominal pain, diarrhea, anorexia, dyspepsia, vomiting, stomatitis, increased cough

SERIOUS REACTIONS
• None known.

INTERACTIONS
Drugs
⬛ *Caffeine, theophylline, amitriptyline, quinolones (CYP1A2 inhibitors):* Possible decreased riluzole elimination
⬛ *Cigarette smoking, rifampin, omeprazole (CYP1A2 inducers):* Possible increased riluzole elimination

SPECIAL CONSIDERATIONS
MONITORING PARAMETERS
• ALT, AST qmo for 3 mo, q3mo for 1 yr, then periodically thereafter; discontinue treatment if ALT or AST increases to >5 times upper limit of normal

---

rimantadine
(ri-man'ti-deen)
Rx: Flumadine
Chemical Class: Tricyclic amine
Therapeutic Class: Antiviral

CLINICAL PHARMACOLOGY
Mechanism of Action: An antiviral that appears to exert an inhibitory effect early in the viral replication cycle. May inhibit uncoating of the virus. *Therapeutic Effect:* Prevents replication of influenza A virus.

INDICATIONS AND DOSAGES
Influenza A virus
PO

Adults, Elderly. 100 mg twice a day for 7 days.

Elderly nursing home patients, patients with severe hepatic or renal impairment. 100 mg once a day for 7 days.

Prevention of influenza A virus
PO

Adults, Elderly, Children 10 yr and older. 100 mg twice a day for at least 10 days after known exposure (usually for 6-8 wk).

Children younger than 10 yr. 5 mg/kg once a day. Maximum: 150 mg.

Elderly nursing home patients, patients with severe hepatic or renal impairment. 100 mg once a day.

$ AVAILABLE FORMS/COST
• Syr—Oral: 50 mg/5 ml, 240 ml: **$46.78**
• Tab, Plain Coated—Oral: 100 mg, 100's: **$183.16-$220.03**

CONTRAINDICATIONS: Hypersensitivity to amantadine or rimantadine

PREGNANCY AND LACTATION: Pregnancy category C; concentrated in breast milk

R

SIDE EFFECTS

Occasional (3%-2%)

Insomnia, nausea, nervousness, impaired concentration, dizziness

Rare (less than 2%)

Vomiting, anorexia, dry mouth, abdominal pain, asthenia, fatigue

SERIOUS REACTIONS

• None known.

INTERACTIONS

Drugs

[3] *Triamterene:* Increased concentrations, toxicity of rimantadine

[3] *Trihexyphenidyl:* Increased CNS effects

SPECIAL CONSIDERATIONS

• PRECAUTIONS

• Resistant strains may develop during treatment (10%-30%)

• Less CNS toxicity in at risk populations

---

risedronate

(rye-se-droe'nate)

Rx: Actonel

Chemical Class: Pyrophosphate analog

Therapeutic Class: Antiosteoporotic; bisphosphonate; bone resorption inhibitor

---

CLINICAL PHARMACOLOGY

Mechanism of Action: A bisphosphonate that binds to bone hydroxyapatite and inhibits osteoclasts. *Therapeutic Effect:* Reduces bone turnover (the number of sites at which bone is remodeled) and bone resorption.

INDICATIONS AND DOSAGES

Paget's disease

PO

Adults, Elderly. 30 mg/day for 2 mo. Retreatment may occur after 2-mo post-treatment observation period.

Prevention and treatment of postmenopausal osteoporosis

PO

Adults, Elderly. 5 mg/day or 35 mg once weekly.

Glucocorticoid-induced osteoporosis

PO

Adults, Elderly. 5 mg/day.

[$] **AVAILABLE FORMS/COST**

• Tab, Coated—Oral: 5 mg, 30's: **$75.53**; 30 mg, 30's: **$528.65**; 35 mg, 4's: **$70.49**

CONTRAINDICATIONS: Hypersensitivity to other bisphosphonates, including etidronate, tiludronate, risedronate, and alendronate; hypocalcemia; inability to stand or sit upright for at least 20 minutes; renal impairment when serum creatinine clearance is greater than 5 mg/dl

PREGNANCY AND LACTATION: Pregnancy category C; breast milk excretion unknown

SIDE EFFECTS

Frequent (30%)

Arthralgia

Occasional (12%–8%)

Rash, flu-like symptoms, peripheral edema

Rare (5%–3%)

Bone pain, sinusitis, asthenia, dry eye, tinnitus

SERIOUS REACTIONS

• Overdose causes hypocalcemia, hypophosphatemia, and significant GI disturbances.

INTERACTIONS

Drugs

[3] *Antacids, calcium:* decreased absorption of risedronate

[3] *Food:* decreases bioavailability of risedronate by 50%

SPECIAL CONSIDERATIONS

PATIENT/FAMILY EDUCATION

• Administer 30 minutes before the first food/beverage/medication of the day, with 6-8 oz plain water

MONITORING PARAMETERS

• Albumin-adjusted serum calcium; N-telopeptide, alkaline phosphatase, phosphorus, osteocalcin, DEXA scan, bone and joint pain, fractures on x-ray (osteoporosis, Paget's disease)

---

risperidone
(ris-per'i-done)
Rx: Risperdal
Chemical Class: Benzisoxazole derivative
Therapeutic Class: Antipsychotic

CLINICAL PHARMACOLOGY

Mechanism of Action: A benzisoxazole derivative that may antagonize dopamine and serotonin receptors. *Therapeutic Effect:* Suppresses psychotic behavior.

Pharmacokinetics

Well absorbed from the GI tract; unaffected by food. Protein binding: 90%. Extensively metabolized in the liver to active metabolite. Primarily excreted in urine. **Half-life:** 3-20 hr; metabolite: 21-30 hr (increased in elderly).

INDICATIONS AND DOSAGES

Psychotic disorder

PO

Adults. 0.5-1 mg twice a day. May increase dosage slowly. Range: 2-6 mg/day.

Elderly. Initially, 0.25-2 mg/day in 2 divided doses. May increase dosage slowly. Range: 2-6 mg/day.

IM

Adults, Elderly. 25 mg q2wk. Maximum: 50 mg q2wk.

Mania

PO

Adults, Elderly. Initially, 2-3 mg as a single daily dose. May increase at 24 hour intervals of 1 mg/day. Range: 2-6 mg/day.

Dosage in renal impairment

Initial dosage for adults and elderly patients is 0.25-0.5 mg twice a day. Dosage is titrated slowly to desired effect.

AVAILABLE FORMS/COST

• Powder, Inj, Depot—IM: 25 mg/vial: **$277.60**; 37.5 mg/vial: **$416.41**; 50 mg/vial: **$555.21**
• Sol—Oral: 1 mg/ml, 30 ml: **$124.09**
• Tab, Coated—Oral: 0.25 mg, 60's: **$152.00**; 0.5 mg, 60's: **$201.13**; 1 mg, 60's: **$213.81**; 2 mg, 60's: **$334.76**; 3 mg, 60's: **$412.50**; 4 mg, 60's: **$548.68**
• Tab, Disintegrating—Oral: 0.5 mg, 28's: **$102.89**; 1 mg, 28's: **$120.21**; 2 mg, 28's: **$193.60**

UNLABELED USES: Autism in children, behavioral symptoms associated with dementia, Tourette's disorder

CONTRAINDICATIONS: None known.

PREGNANCY AND LACTATION: Pregnancy category C; excreted in breast milk

SIDE EFFECTS

Frequent (26%-13%)

Agitation, anxiety, insomnia, headache, constipation

Occasional (10%-4%)

Dyspepsia, rhinitis, somnolence, dizziness, nausea, vomiting, rash, abdominal pain, dry skin, tachycardia

Rare (3%-2%)

Visual disturbances, fever, back pain, pharyngitis, cough, arthralgia, angina, aggressive behavior, orthostatic hypotension, breast swelling

SERIOUS REACTIONS

• Rare reactions include tardive dyskinesia (characterized by tongue

R

protrusion, puffing of the cheeks, and chewing or puckering of the mouth) and neuroleptic malignant syndrome (marked by hyperpyrexia, muscle rigidity, change in mental status, irregular pulse or BP, tachycardia, diaphoresis, cardiac arrhythmias, rhabdomyolysis, and acute renal failure).

INTERACTIONS
Drugs
▣ *Levodopa, dopamine agonists:* Risperidone may antagonize effect

SPECIAL CONSIDERATIONS
PATIENT/FAMILY EDUCATION
• Risk of orthostatic hypotension, especially during the period of initial dose titration
• Do not operate machinery during dose titration period

---

ritonavir
(ri-tone′a-veer)
Rx: Norvir
Combinations
  Rx: with lopinavir (Kaletra)
Chemical Class: Protease inhibitor, HIV
Therapeutic Class: Antiretroviral

CLINICAL PHARMACOLOGY
Mechanism of Action: Inhibits HIV-1 and HIV-2 proteases, rendering these enzymes incapable of processing the polypeptide precursors; this results in the production of noninfectious, immature HIV particles. *Therapeutic Effect:* Impedes HIV replication, slowing the progression of HIV infection.
Pharmacokinetics
Well absorbed after PO administration (absorption increased with food). Protein binding: 98%-99%. Extensively metabolized in the liver to active metabolite. Primarily

eliminated in feces. Unknown if removed by hemodialysis. **Half-life:** 2.7-5 hr.

INDICATIONS AND DOSAGES
HIV infection
PO
Adults, Children 12 yr and older. 600 mg twice a day. If nausea occurs at this dosage, give 300 mg twice a day for 1 day, 400 mg twice a day for 2 days, 500 mg twice a day for 1 day, then 600 mg twice a day thereafter.
Children younger than 12 yr. Initially, 250 mg/m^2/dose twice a day. Increase by 50 mg/m^2/dose up to 400 mg/m^2/dose. Maximum: 600 mg/dose twice a day.

Ⓢ **AVAILABLE FORMS/COST**
• Cap—Oral: 100 mg, 168's: **$311.65**
• Sol—Oral: 80 mg/ml, 240 ml: **$335.14**

CONTRAINDICATIONS: Concurrent use of amiodarone, astemizole, bepridil, bupropion, cisapride, clozapine, encainide, flecainide, meperidine, piroxicam, propafenone, propoxyphene, quinidine, rifabutin, or terfenadine (increased risk of serious or life-threatening drug interactions, such as arrhythmias, hematologic abnormalities, and seizures); concurrent use of alprazolam, clorazepate, diazepam, estazolam, flurazepam, midazolam, triazolam, or zolpidem (may produce extreme sedation and respiratory depression)

PREGNANCY AND LACTATION: Pregnancy category B; breast milk excretion unknown; breast-feeding by HIV+ mothers not recommended

SIDE EFFECTS
Frequent
GI disturbances (abdominal pain, anorexia, diarrhea, nausea, vomiting), circumoral and peripheral paresthesias, altered taste, headache, dizziness, fatigue, asthenia

Occasional

Allergic reaction, flu-like symptoms, hypotension

Rare

Diabetes mellitus, hyperglycemia

SERIOUS REACTIONS

• None known.

INTERACTIONS

Drugs

⚠ *Amiodarone:* Increased plasma levels of amiodarone

② *Atorvastatin:* Increased risk of myopathy possible

⚠ *Astemizole:* Increased plasma levels of astemizole

③ *Barbiturates:* Increased clearance of ritonavir; reduced clearance of barbiturates

⚠ *Bepredil:* Increased plasma levels of bepredil

⚠ *Bupropion:* Increased plasma levels of bupropion

② *Carbamazepine:* Increased clearance of ritonavir; reduced clearance of carbamazepine

② *Cerivastatin:* Increased risk of myopathy possible

⚠ *Cisapride:* Increased plasma levels of cisapride

② *Clarithromycin:* Reduced clearance of ritonavir; ritonavir reduces clearance of clarithromycin; reduce clarithromycin dose for renal insufficiency

⚠ *Clorazepate:* Increased plasma levels of clorazepate

⚠ *Clozapine:* Increased plasma levels of clozapine

③ *Despiramine:* Ritonavir increases AUC of desipramine by 145%

⚠ *Diazepam:* Increased plasma levels of diazepam

③ *Didanosine:* Separate dosing by 2.5 hr to avoid formulation incompatibility

② *Disulfiram:* Ritonavir (gel capsules and solution) contain ethanol; disulfiram-like reaction possible

⚠ *Encainide:* Increased plasma levels of encainide

⚠ *Ergot alkaloids:* Increased plasma levels of ergot alkaloids

③ *Erythromycin:* Reduced clearance of ritonavir; ritonavir reduces clearance of erythromycin

⚠ *Estazolam:* Increases plasma levels of estazolam

⚠ *Flecainide:* Increased plasma levels of flecainide

⚠ *Flurazepam:* Increased plasma levels of flurazepam

③ *Indinavir:* Increased plasma level of indinavir; reduce dose to 400 mg bid when ritonavir dose is 400 mg bid

③ *Ketoconazole:* Ritonavir reduces clearance of ketoconazole; reduce ketoconazole dose

⚠ *Lovastatin:* Ritonavir reduces clearance of lovastatin

⚠ *Meperidine:* Increased plasma levels of of normeperidine which has analgesic and CNS stimulant activity (seizures)

③ *Methadone:* Ritonavir reduces methadone plasma concentration by 37%

② *Metronidazole:* Ritonavir (gel capsules and solution) contain ethanol; disulfiram-like reaction possible

⚠ *Midazolam:* Increased plasma levels of midazolam and prolonged effect

③ *Nelfinavir:* Increased plasma level of nelfinavir; reduce nelfinavir dose to 750 mg bid when ritonavir dose is 400 mg bid

③ *Oral contraceptives:* Ritonavir may reduce efficacy

③ *Phenytoin:* Increased clearance of ritonavir; reduced clearance of phenytoin

⚠ *Pimozide:* Increased plasma levels of pimozide

⚠ *Piroxicam:* Increased plasma levels of piroxicam

R

⚠ *Propafenone:* Increased plasma levels of propafenone

⚠ *Propoxyphene:* Increased plasma levels of propoxyphene

⚠ *Quinidine:* Increased plasma levels of quinidine

② *Rifabutin:* Increased clearance of ritonavir; reduced clearance of rifabutin; reduce rifabutin dose to 150 mg qod

③ *Rifampin:* Increased clearance of ritonavir

⚠ *St. John's wort (hypericum perforatum):* Substantial decrease in plasma ritonavir concentrations with loss of virologic response

③ *Saquinavir:* Decreased clearance of saquinavir; reduce dose of saquinavir (Fortovase or Invirase) to 400 bid with ritonavir 400 mg bid

② *Sildenafil:* Substantial increases in serum sildenafil concentrations

⚠ *Simvastatin:* Ritonavir reduces clearance of simvastatin

⚠ *Terfenadine:* Increased plasma levels of terfenadine

③ *Theophylline:* Ritonavir reduces theophylline plasma concentration

⚠ *Triazolam:* Increased plasma levels of triazolam and prolonged effect

③ *Troleandomycin:* Reduced clearance of ritonavir; ritonavir reduces clearance of troleandomycin

③ *Warfarin:* Decreased plasma warfarin concentrations

⚠ *Zolpidem:* Increased plasma levels of zolpidem

SPECIAL CONSIDERATIONS

• As with other protease inhibitors, ritonavir will predominantly be used in combination regimens; the ability of ritonavir (alone or in combinations) to modify clinical endpoints (e.g., time to 1st AIDS-defining illness or death) will be important in determining the ultimate role of this agent in HIV; potential for drug interaction is troublesome; as with other protease inhibitors, resistance has been problematic after several mo of treatment

PATIENT/FAMILY EDUCATION

• Store capsules in the refrigerator until dispensed; refrigeration of capsules by patient not required if used within 30 days and stored below 77°F; store oral solution at room temperature, do not refrigerate, shake well; avoid exposure to excessive heat

• Take with food

MONITORING PARAMETERS

• Therapeutic: serum HIV-1 RNA, and CD4+ cell counts (every 2-4 wk)

• Toxicity: complete blood counts, routine blood chemistry, liver function tests, and serum lipid and lipoprotein profiles

---

rivastigmine
(riv-a-stig'meen)
Rx: Exelon
Chemical Class: Carbamate derivative; cholinesterase inhibitor
Therapeutic Class: Acetylcholinesterase inhibitor

CLINICAL PHARMACOLOGY
Mechanism of Action: A cholinesterase inhibitor that inhibits the enzyme acetylcholinesterase, thus increasing the concentration of acetylcholine at cholinergic synapses and enhancing cholinergic function in the CNS. *Therapeutic Effect:* Slows the progression of symptoms of Alzheimer's disease.

Pharmacokinetics
Rapidly and completely absorbed. Protein binding: 60%. Widely distributed throughout the body. Rap-

idly and extensively metabolized. Primarily excreted in urine. **Half-life:** 1.5 hr.

INDICATIONS AND DOSAGES
Alzheimer's disease
PO

Adults, Elderly. Initially, 1.5 mg twice a day. May increase at intervals of at least 2 wk to 3 mg twice a day, then 4.5 mg twice a day, and finally 6 mg twice a day. Maximum: 6 mg twice a day.

$ AVAILABLE FORMS/COST
• Cap—Oral: 1.5, 3, 4.5, 6 mg, 60's; all: **$157.74**
• Liq—Oral: 2 mg/ml, 120 ml dispenser bottle: **$290.41**

CONTRAINDICATIONS: None known.

PREGNANCY AND LACTATION: Pregnancy category B; excretion into human breast milk unknown

SIDE EFFECTS
Frequent (47%-17%)

Nausea, vomiting, dizziness, diarrhea, headache, anorexia

Occasional (13%-6%)

Abdominal pain, insomnia, dyspepsia (heartburn, indigestion, epigastric pain), confusion, UTI, depression

Rare (5%-3%)

Anxiety, somnolence, constipation, malaise, hallucinations, tremor, flatulence, rhinitis, hypertension, flu-like symptoms, weight loss, syncope

SERIOUS REACTIONS
• Overdose may result in cholinergic crisis, characterized by severe nausea and vomiting, increased salivation, diaphoresis, bradycardia, hypotension, respiratory depression, and seizures.

INTERACTIONS
Drugs

🔟 *Anticholinergic drugs:* Interference with anticholinergic activity

🔟 *Cholinomimetics (cholinergics and other cholinesterase inhibitors i.e., bethanechol and succinylcholine):* Potential synergistic effects

🔟 *Clozapine:* Antagonistic effect on cholinesterase inhibitor activity

🔟 *Inhaled anesthetics:* Decreased neuromuscular blocking effects

🔟 *Local anesthetics:* Increased risk of local anesthetic toxicity (pseudo-cholinesterase competition)

🔟 *Neuromuscular blockers, non-depolarizing:* Antagonistic effects, reversal of neuromuscular blockade

SPECIAL CONSIDERATIONS
PATIENT/FAMILY EDUCATION
• Patient and caregiver should be advised of high incidence of gastrointestinal effects and directions for resource and resolution

MONITORING PARAMETERS
• Cognitive function (e.g., ADAS, Mini-Mental Status Exam (MMSE)), activities of daily living, global functioning, blood chemistry, complete blood counts, heart rate, blood pressure

---

rizatriptan
(rize-a-trip'tan)

Rx: Maxalt; Maxalt MLT
Chemical Class: Serotonin derivative
Therapeutic Class: Antimigraine agent

CLINICAL PHARMACOLOGY
Mechanism of Action: A serotonin receptor agonist that binds selectively to vascular receptors, producing a vasoconstrictive effect on cranial blood vessels. *Therapeutic Effect:* Relieves migraine headache.

Pharmacokinetics

Well absorbed after PO administration. Protein binding: 14%. Crosses the blood-brain barrier. Metabolized by the liver to inactive metabolite. Eliminated primarily in urine and, to a lesser extent, in feces. **Half-life:** 2–3 hr.

INDICATIONS AND DOSAGES
Acute migraine attack
PO
Adults older than 18 yr, Elderly. 5–10 mg. If headache improves, but then returns, dose may be repeated after 2 hr. Maximum: 30 mg/24 hr.

💲 AVAILABLE FORMS/COST
• Tab—Oral: 5 mg, 10 mg, 6's: **$112.79**
• Tab, Disintigrating—Oral: 5 mg, 10 mg, 6's: **$112.79**

CONTRAINDICATIONS: Basilar or hemiplegic migraine, coronary artery disease, ischemic heart disease (including angina pectoris, history of MI, silent ischemia, and Prinzmetal's angina), uncontrolled hypertension, use within 24 hours of ergotamine-containing preparations or another serotonin receptor agonist, use within 14 days of MAOIs.

PREGNANCY AND LACTATION: Pregnancy category C; use caution in nursing mothers

SIDE EFFECTS
Frequent (9%–7%)
Dizziness, somnolence, paraesthesia, fatigue
Occasional (6%–3%)
Nausea, chest pressure, dry mouth
Rare (2%)
Headache; neck, throat, or jaw pressure; photosensitivity

SERIOUS REACTIONS
• Cardiac reactions (such as ischemia, coronary artery vasospasm, and MI) and noncardiac vasospasm-related reactions (including hemorrhage and CVA), occur rarely, particularly in patients with hypertension, diabetes, or a strong family history of coronary artery disease;

obese patients; smokers; males older than 40 years; and postmenopausal women.

INTERACTIONS
Drugs
⚠ *Ergotamine-containing drugs:* Increased vasoconstriction
⚠ *MAO inhibitors:* Potential for decreased metabolism of rizatriptan
🔢 *Propranolol:* Propranolol has been shown to increase the plasma concentrations of rizatriptan by 70%; patients receiving propranolol should use 5 mg tablets (max 15 mg/24 hr)
➋ *Sibutramine:* Increased risk of serotonin syndrome

SPECIAL CONSIDERATIONS
• Safety of treating, on average, more than 4 headaches in a 30-day period has not been established
• MLT does not provide faster absorption or onset of effect because almost the entire dose is swallowed with saliva and absorbed in the GI tract

PATIENT/FAMILY EDUCATION
• Use only to treat migraine headache, not for prevention
• MLT, administration with liquid is not necessary; orally disintegrating tablet is packaged in a blister within an outer aluminum pouch, do not remove the blister from the outer pouch until just prior to dosing; blister pack should then be peeled open with dry hands and the orally disintegrating tablet placed on the tongue, where it will dissolve and be swallowed with the saliva

rofecoxib
(ro-fe-coks'ib)
Rx: Vioxx
Chemical Class: Cyclooxygenase-2 (COX-2) inhibitor
Therapeutic Class: COX-2 specific inhibitor; NSAID; nonnarcotic analgesic

CLINICAL PHARMACOLOGY
Mechanism of Action: A nonsteroidal anti-inflammatory that produces analgesic and anti-inflammatory effect by inhibiting prostaglandin synthesis. *Therapeutic Effect:* Reduces inflammatory response and intensity of pain stimulus reaching sensory nerve endings.
Pharmacokinetics
Rapid, complete absorption from the gastrointestinal (GI) tract. Protein binding: 87%. Primarily metabolized in liver. Primarily eliminated in urine with a lesser amount excreted in feces. Not removed by hemodialysis. **Half-life:** 17 hr.

INDICATIONS AND DOSAGE
Osteoarthritis
PO
Adults. Initially, 12.5 mg/day. May increase dosage to 25 mg/day. Maximum is 25 mg/day.
Rheumatoid arthritis
PO
Adults, Elderly. 25 mg/day.
Acute pain, dysmenorrhea
PO
Adults. Initially, 50 mg/day.

$ AVAILABLE FORMS/COST
• Susp—Oral: 12.5 mg/5 ml, 150 ml: **$134.28**; 25 mg/5 ml, 150 ml: **$134.28**
• Tab—Oral: 12.5 mg, 100's: **$301.36**; 25 mg, 100's: **$301.36**; 50 mg, 100's: **$440.11**

CONTRAINDICATIONS: Hypersensitivity to aspirin and NSAIDs

PREGNANCY AND LACTATION:
Pregnancy category C; (teratogenic and nonteratogenic effects in animals); decreases the diameter of the patent ductus arteriosus in animals; no adequate and controlled trials in humans; excreted into breast milk of animals

SIDE EFFECTS
Frequent (6%-5%)
Nausea (with or without vomiting), diarrhea, abdominal distress
Occasional (3%)
Dyspepsia, including heartburn, indigestion, epigastric pain
Rare (less than 2%)
Constipation, flatulence

SERIOUS REACTIONS
• None known

INTERACTIONS
Drugs
▣ *Angiotensin-converting enzyme inhibitors:* Diminished antihypertensive effects
▣ *Aspirin:* Increased risk of GI ulceration; negation of cardioprotective effects of aspirin
▣ *Diuretics (loop, thiazides):* Reduced naturetic effect
▣ *Lithium:* Elevation of plasma lithium levels, potential lithium toxicity
▣ *Rifampin:* 50% reduction of rofecoxib plasma concentrations
▣ *Warfarin:* Slight increases (10%) in PT/INRs expected; monitor appropriately
Labs
• *Transaminases:* Elevations of ALT or AST (approximately 3 or more times the upper limit of normal)

SPECIAL CONSIDERATIONS
• May be safer than conventional nonsteroidal antiinflammatory agents, particularly with respect to gastrointestinal tolerability, and of-

R

fer comparable efficacy; other complications may arise, including cardiovascular complications from selective inhibition of the COX isoenzyme

PATIENT/FAMILY EDUCATION

• Alertness for the signs and symptoms of adverse effects (e.g., GI ulceration and bleeding, renal dysfunction, hepatitis)

MONITORING PARAMETERS

• Decreased pain and stiffness of affected joints; decreased pain, cramps; baseline hemogram and fecal occult blood and routine monitoring every 6-12 months; serum electrolytes, BUN, serum creatinine, weight gain, edema, decreased urine output every 6-12 months; AST, ALT, nausea, vomiting, right upper abdominal pain, anorexia, jaundice

---

ropinirole
(ro-pin′i-role)

Rx: ReQuip
Chemical Class: Dipropylaminoethyl indolone derivative
Therapeutic Class: Anti-Parkinson's agent; dopaminergic

CLINICAL PHARMACOLOGY

Mechanism of Action: An antiparkinson agent that stimulates dopamine receptors in the striatum. *Therapeutic Effect:* Relieves signs and symptoms of Parkinson's disease.

Pharmacokinetics

Rapidly absorbed after PO administration. Protein binding: 40%. Extensively distributed throughout the body. Extensively metabolized. Steady-state concentrations achieved within 2 days. Eliminated in urine. Unknown if removed by hemodialysis. **Half-life:** 6 hr.

INDICATIONS AND DOSAGES

Parkinson's disease

PO

Adults, Elderly. Initially, 0.25 mg 3 times a day. May increase dosage every 7 days.

S   **AVAILABLE FORMS/COST**

• Tab—Oral: 0.25, 0.5, 1 mg, 100's; all: **$130.96**; 2 mg, 100's: **$133.72**; 3, 4, 5 mg, 100's; all: **$234.45**

CONTRAINDICATIONS: None known.

PREGNANCY AND LACTATION: Pregnancy category D; inhibits lactation

SIDE EFFECTS

Frequent (60%–40%)

Nausea, dizziness, somnolence

Occasional (12%–5%)

Syncope, vomiting, fatigue, viral infection, dyspepsia, diaphoresis, asthenia, orthostatic hypotension, abdominal discomfort, pharyngitis, abnormal vision, dry mouth, hypertension, hallucinations, confusion

Rare (less than 4%)

Anorexia, peripheral edema, memory loss, rhinitis, sinusitis, palpitations, impotence

SERIOUS REACTIONS

• None known.

INTERACTIONS

Drugs

▣ *Ciprofloxacin, enoxacin, pefloxacin:* Addition increases ropinirole concentrations

▣ *Dopamine antagonists:* Diminished anti-Parkinson's effect

▣ *Estrogens:* Reduced ropinirole clearance, may need to decrease ropinirole if estrogen stopped

SPECIAL CONSIDERATIONS

• Domperidone 20 mg 1 hr prior to ropinirole prevents drug-induced postural effects

• Discontinue slowly over 1 wk

rosiglitazone
(roz-ih-gli'ta-zone)
Rx: Avandia
Combinations
  Rx: with metformin (Avandamet)
Chemical Class: Thiazolidinedione
Therapeutic Class: Antidiabetic; hypoglycemic; insulin resistance reducer

CLINICAL PHARMACOLOGY
Mechanism of Action: An antidiabetic that improves target-cell response to insulin without increasing pancreatic insulin secretion. Decreases hepatic glucose output and increases insulin-dependent glucose utilization in skeletal muscle. *Therapeutic Effect:* Lowers blood glucose concentration.
Pharmacokinetics
Rapidly absorbed. Protein binding: 99%. Metabolized in the liver. Excreted primarily in urine, with a lesser amount in feces. Not removed by hemodialysis. **Half-life:** 3–4 hr.
INDICATIONS AND DOSAGES
Diabetes mellitus, combination therapy
PO
Adults, Elderly. Initially, 4 mg as a single daily dose or in divided doses twice a day. May increase to 8 mg/day after 12 wk of therapy if fasting glucose level is not adequately controlled.
Diabetes mellitus, monotherapy
Adults, Elderly. Initially, 4 mg as single daily dose or in divided doses twice a day. May increase to 8 mg/day after 12 wk of therapy.
§ **AVAILABLE FORMS/COST**
• Tab, Film-Coated—Oral: 2 mg, 60's: **$108.75**; 4 mg, 100's: **$288.54**; 8 mg, 100's: **$533.86**

• Tab, Film-Coated—Oral (with metformin): 1 mg-500 mg, 100's: **$112.50**; 2 mg-500 mg, 100's: **$168.75**; 4 mg-500 mg, 100's: **$275.00**; 2 mg-1000 mg, 60's: **$140.40**; 4 mg-1000 mg, 60's: **$210.60**
CONTRAINDICATIONS: Active hepatic disease, diabetic ketoacidosis, increased serum transaminase levels, including ALT(SGPT) greater than 2.5 times the normal serum level, type 1 diabetes mellitus
PREGNANCY AND LACTATION: Pregnancy category C; no adequate and well controlled studies in pregnant women available; abnormally high glucose levels during pregnancy associated with higher incidence of congenital anomolaies, morbidity, and mortality, insulin monotherapy preferred agent; drug detected in lactating rats; no information in humans
SIDE EFFECTS
Frequent (9%)
Upper respiratory tract infection
Occasional (4%–2%)
Headache, edema, back pain, fatigue, sinusitis, diarrhea
SERIOUS REACTIONS
• None known.
INTERACTIONS
Drugs
▣ *Fenugreek, ginseng, glucomannan:* Additive blood glucose lowering; increased risk of hypoglycemia
Labs
• Elevations of AST, ALT, bilirubin, LDH, LDL-cholesterol (15%); HDL-cholesterol (15%); decreases in hematocrit, hemoglobin, alkaline phosphatase
SPECIAL CONSIDERATIONS
• *Expected hypoglycemic effects:* Decreases in serum glucose: 50-75 mg/dL; decreases in HbA1c 1.2-1.5%

PATIENT/FAMILY EDUCATION
• Caloric restriction, weight loss, and exercise essential adjuvant therapy
• Blood draws for LFT monitoring along with routine diabetes mellitus labs; review symptoms of hepatitis (unexplained nausea, vomiting, abdominal pain, fatigue, anorexia or dark urine)
• Notify clinician of rapid increases in weight or edema or symptoms of heart failure (shortness of breath)
• OK to take with food
• Review hypoglycemia risks and symptoms when added to other hypoglycemic agents

MONITORING PARAMETERS
• "Poly" diabetes mellitus symptoms, periodic serum glucose and HbA1c measurements; LFT (AST, ALT) prior to initiation of therapy and periodically thereafter; hemoglobin/hematocrit, signs and symptoms of heart failure

---

rosuvastatin
Rx: Crestor
Chemical Class: Substituted heptenoic acid derivative
Therapeutic Class: HMG-CoA reductase inhibitor; antilipemic

CLINICAL PHARMACOLOGY
Mechanism of Action: An antihyperlipidemic that interferes with cholesterol biosynthesis by inhibiting the conversion of the enzyme HMG-CoA to mevalonate, a precursor to cholesterol. *Therapeutic Effect:* Decreases LDL cholesterol, VLDL, and plasma triglyceride levels, increases HDL concentration.

Pharmacokinetics
Protein binding: 88%. Minimal hepatic metabolism. Primarily eliminated in the feces. **Half-life:** 19 hr (increased in patients with severe renal dysfunction).

INDICATIONS AND DOSAGES
Hyperlipidemia, dyslipidemia
PO
Adults, Elderly. 5 to 40 mg/day. Usual starting dosage is 10 mg/day, with adjustments based on lipid levels; monitor q2-4wk until desired level is achieved.

Renal impairment (creatinine clearance less than 30 ml/min)
PO
Adults, Elderly. 5 mg/day; do not exceed 10 mg/day.

Concurrent cyclosporine use
PO
Adults, Elderly. 5 mg/day.

Concurrent lipid-lowering therapy
PO
Adults, Elderly. 10 mg/day.

$ **AVAILABLE FORMS/COST**
• Tab, Coated—Oral: 5, 10, 20 mg, 90's; all: **$236.25**; 40 mg, 30's: **$78.75**

CONTRAINDICATIONS: Active hepatic disease, breast-feeding, pregnancy, unexplained, persistent elevations of serum transaminase levels

PREGNANCY AND LACTATION: Pregnancy category X; not recommended for nursing mothers

SIDE EFFECTS
Rosuvastatin is generally well tolerated. Side effects are usually mild and transient.
Occasional (9%–3%)
Pharyngitis, headache, diarrhea, dyspepsia, including heartburn and epigastric distress, nausea
Rare (less than 3%)
Myalgia, asthenia or unusual fatigue and weakness, back pain

SERIOUS REACTIONS
• Lens opacities may occur.
• Hypersensitivity reaction and hepatitis occur rarely.

INTERACTIONS
Drugs
▪ *Cyclosporine:* Increase in rosuvastatin mean C_{max} and mean AUC
▪ *Warfarin:* Coadministration with stable warfarin therapy resulted in clinically significant hypoprothrombinemia (INR>4)
▪ *Gemfibrozil:* Increase in rosuvastatin mean C_{max} and mean AUC
▪ *Magnesium and aluminum containing antacids:* Decreased absorption; separate by 2 hr

SPECIAL CONSIDERATIONS
• Base statin selection on lipid-lowering prowess, cost, side effects, and availability of mortality reduction studies
• Rosuvastatin is the most potent statin on the market in its ability to decrease LDL with a significant reduction in total cholesterol, triglycerides, and increase in HDL; however, overall mortality rates are lacking
• Notable proteinuria (persistent) accompanies rosuvastatin use; clinical significance yet unknown; would hesitate to use as first line statin
• Note: not dependent on metabolism by cytochrome P450 3A4 to a clinically significant extent

PATIENT/FAMILY EDUCATION
• Report symptoms of myalgia, muscle tenderness, or weakness
• May be taken with or with out food and regardless of the time of day
• Adjunctive to diet and exercise

MONITORING PARAMETERS
• *Efficacy:* Fasting lipid panel at 3-6 months

• AST/ALT at baseline, 12 weeks, following any elevation of dose, and then periodically (discontinue if elevations persist at >3 times upper limit of normal)
• CPK in patients complaining of unexplained diffuse myalgia, muscle tenderness, or muscle weakness
• Routine urinalysis for proteinuria; may need to reduce dose with persistent proteinuria

---

salicylic acid
(sal-i-sill′ik)
OTC: Compound W, Dr. Scholl's Wart Remover Kit, DuoFilm, DuoPlant, Fostex, Freezone, Gets-it, Gordofilm, Keralyt, Mediplast, Mosco, Occlusal-HP, Off-Ezy, Panscol, Sal-Acid, Sal-Plant, Trans-Ver-Sal, Wart-Off Combinations
  Rx: with sodium thiosulfate (Versiclear)
Chemical Class: Salicylate derivative
Therapeutic Class: Keratolytic

CLINICAL PHARMACOLOGY
Mechanism of Action: A keratolytic agent that produces desquamation of hyperkeratotic epithelium by dissolution of intercellular cement and causes the cornified tissue to swell, soften, macerate, and desquamate. *Therapeutic Effect:* Decreases acne, psoriasis and wart removal

Pharmacokinetics
Absorption differs between formulations. Protein binding: 50%-80%. Bound to serum albumin. Metabolized to salicylate glucoronides and salicyluric acid. Excreted in urine.

S

INDICATIONS AND DOSAGES
Acne
Topical

Adults, Elderly, Children. Apply cream, foam, gel, liquid, pads, patch, or soap 1-3 times/day.

Callus, corn, wart Removal
Topical

Adults, Elderly, Children. Apply gel, liquid, plaster, or patch to wart 1-2 times/day.

Dandruff, psoriasis, seborrheic dermatitis
Topical

Adults, Elderly, Children. Apply cream, ointment, or shampoo 3-4 times/day.

$ AVAILABLE FORMS/COST
• Film—Top: 15%, 10's: **$10.04**; 17%, 18's: **$7.19**
• Foam—Top: 2%, 100 g: **$8.00**
• Gel—Top: 6%, 30 g: **$15.56**; 17%, 7.5, 15 g: **$5.26-$6.31**/7.5 g
• Liq—Top: 12%, 9 ml: **$2.87**; 17%, 10, 15 ml: **$1.95-$8.50**
• Plaster, Adhesive—Top: 40%, 14's: **$13.00**

UNLABELED USES: Tinea pedis
CONTRAINDICATIONS: Children less than 2 years old, diabetes, impaired circulation, hypersensitivity to salicylic acid of any of its components

PREGNANCY AND LACTATION: Pregnancy category C

SIDE EFFECTS
Occasional

Burning, erythema, irritation, pruritus, stinging

Rare

Dizziness, nausea, vomiting, diarrhea, hypoglycemia

SERIOUS REACTIONS
• Symptoms of salicylate toxicity include lethargy, hyperpnea, diarrhea, and psychic disturbances.

SPECIAL CONSIDERATIONS
PATIENT/FAMILY EDUCATION
• For external use only; avoid contact with face, eyes, genitals, mucous membranes, and normal skin surrounding warts
• May cause reddening or scaling of skin
• Soaking area in warm water for 5 min prior to application may enhance effect (remove any loose tissue with brush, washcloth, or emery board and dry thoroughly prior to application)

---

salmeterol
(sal-me'te-rol)
Rx: Serevent
Combinations
  Rx: with fluticasone (Advair)
Chemical Class: Sympathomimetic amine; β_2-adrenergic agonist
Therapeutic Class: Antiasthmatic; bronchodilator

CLINICAL PHARMACOLOGY
Mechanism of Action: An adrenergic agonist that stimulates beta$_2$-adrenergic receptors in the lungs, resulting in relaxation of bronchial smooth muscle. *Therapeutic Effect:* Relieves bronchospasm and reduces airway resistance.

Pharmacokinetics

Route	Onset	Peak	Duration
Inhalation	10–20 min	3 hr	12 hr

Low systemic absorption; acts primarily in the lungs. Protein binding: 95%. Metabolized by hydroxylation. Primarily eliminated in feces.
Half-life: 3–4 hr.

INDICATIONS AND DOSAGES

Prevention and maintenance treatment of asthma

Inhalation (Diskus)

Adults, Elderly, Children 4 yr and older. 1 inhalation (50 mcg) q12h.

Preventin of exercise-induced bronchospasm

Inhalation

Adults, Elderly, Children 4 yr and older. 1 inhalation at least 30 min before exercise.

COPD

Inhalation

Adults, Elderly. 1 inhalation q12h.

🆂 AVAILABLE FORMS/COST

• MDI—INH: 21 mcg/puffs, 6 g (60 puffs): **$56.96**; 21 mcg/puffs, 13 g (120 puffs): **$91.89**
• Powder, Disk—INH: 50 mcg/INH, 28's: **$47.23**; 50 mcg/INH, 60's: **$91.89**

CONTRAINDICATIONS: History of hypersensitivity to sympathomimetics

PREGNANCY AND LACTATION: Pregnancy category C

SIDE EFFECTS

Frequent (28%)

Headache

Occasional (7%–3%)

Cough, tremor, dizziness, vertigo, throat dryness or irritation, pharyngitis

Rare (3%)

Palpitations, tachycardia, tremors, nausea, heartburn, GI distress, diarrhea

SERIOUS REACTIONS

• Salmeterol may prolong the QT interval, which may precipitate ventricular arrhythmias.
• Hypokalemia and hyperglycemia may occur.

INTERACTIONS

Drugs

❷ *β-blockers:* Decreased action of salmeterol, cardioselective β-blockers preferable if concurrent use necessary

❸ *Furosemide:* Potential for additive hypokalemia

SPECIAL CONSIDERATIONS

PATIENT/FAMILY EDUCATION

• Patients receiving salmeterol for asthma should normally <u>also</u> be receiving regular and adequate doses of an effective asthma controller medication, such as inhaled corticosteroid
• Proper inhalation technique is vital
• Notify clinician if no response to usual doses, or if palpitations, rapid heartbeat, chest pain, muscle tremors, dizziness, headache occur
• **Do not use to treat acute symptoms or on an as-needed basis**

---

salsalate

(sal'sa-late)

Rx: Amigesic, Argesic-SA, Artha-G, Disalcid, Marthritic, Mono-Gesic, Salflex, Salsitab
Chemical Class: Salicylate derivative
Therapeutic Class: NSAID; nonnarcotic analgesic

CLINICAL PHARMACOLOGY

Mechanism of Action: An NSAID that inhibits prostaglandin synthesis, reducing the inflammatory response and the intensity of pain stimuli reaching the sensory nerve endings. *Therapeutic Effect:* Produces analgesic and anti-inflammatory effects.

INDICATIONS AND DOSAGES
Rheumatoid arthritis, osteoarthritis pain
PO

Adults, Elderly. Initially, 3 g/day in 2-3 divided doses. Maintenance: 2-4 g/day.

$ AVAILABLE FORMS/COST
• Tab, Coated—Oral: 500 mg, 100's: **$4.33-$42.78**; 750 mg, 100's: **$5.67-$55.36**

CONTRAINDICATIONS: Bleeding disorders, hypersensitivity to salicylates or NSAIDs

PREGNANCY AND LACTATION: Pregnancy category C; excreted into breast milk; use caution in nursing mothers due to potential adverse effects in nursing infant

SIDE EFFECTS
Occasional

Nausea, dyspepsia (including heartburn, indigestion, and epigastric pain)

SERIOUS REACTIONS
• Tinnitus may be the first indication that the serum salicylic acid concentration is reaching or exceeding the upper therapeutic range.
• Salsalate use may also produce vertigo, headache, confusion, drowsiness, diaphoresis, hyperventilation, vomiting, and diarrhea.
• Reye's syndrome may occur in children with chickenpox or the flu.
• Severe overdose may result in electrolyte imbalance, hyperthermia, dehydration, and blood pH imbalance.
• GI bleeding, peptic ulcer, and Reye's syndrome rarely occur.

INTERACTIONS
Labs

• *False increase:* Serum bicarbonate, CSF, protein, serum theophylline
• *False decrease:* Urine cocaine, urine estrogen, serum glucose, urine 17-hydroxycorticosteroids, urine opiates
• *False positive:* Urine ferric chloride test

SPECIAL CONSIDERATIONS
• Consider for patients with GI intolerance to aspirin or patients in whom interference with normal platelet function by aspirin or other NSAIDs is undesirable

MONITORING PARAMETERS
• AST, ALT, bilirubin, creatinine, CBC, hematocrit if patient is on long-term therapy

---

saquinavir
(sa-kwin'a-veer)
Rx: Fortovase, Invirase
Chemical Class: Protease inhibitor, HIV
Therapeutic Class: Antiretroviral

CLINICAL PHARMACOLOGY
Mechanism of Action: Inhibits HIV protease, rendering the enzyme incapable of processing the polyprotein precursors needed to generate functional proteins in HIV-infected cells. *Therapeutic Effect:* Intereferes with HIV replication, slowing the progression of HIV infection.
Pharmacokinetics

Poorly absorbed after PO administration (absorption increased with high-calorie and high-fat meals). Protein binding: 99%. Metabolized in the liver to inactive metabolite. Primarily eliminated in feces. Unknown if removed by hemodialysis. **Half-life:** 13 hr.

INDICATIONS AND DOSAGES
HIV infection in combination with other antiretrovirals
PO

Adults, Elderly. 1,200 mg Fortovase 3 times a day or 600 mg Invirase 3 times a day within 2 hr after a full meal.

Dosage adjustments when given in combination therapy:

Delavirdine: Fortovase 800 mg 3 times/day.

Lopinavir/ritonavir: Fortovase 800 mg 2 times/day.

Nelfinavir: Fortovase 800 mg 3 times/day or 1200 mg 2 times/day.

Ritonavir: Fortovase or Invirase 1000 mg 2 times/day.

S AVAILABLE FORMS/COST

• Cap—Oral (Fortovase): 200 mg, 180's: **$250.34**

• Cap—Oral (Invirase): 200 mg, 270's: **$673.91**

CONTRAINDICATIONS: Clinically significant hypersensitivity to saquinavir; concurrent use with ergot medications, lovastatin, midazolam, simvastatin, or triazolam

PREGNANCY AND LACTATION: Pregnancy category B

SIDE EFFECTS

Occasional

Diarrhea, abdominal discomfort and pain, nausea, photosensitivity, stomatitis

Rare

Confusion, ataxia, asthenia, headache, rash

SERIOUS REACTIONS

• Ketoacidosis occurs rarely.

INTERACTIONS

Drugs

▲ *Astemizole:* Increased plasma levels of astemizole

❸ *Barbiturates:* Increased clearance of saquinavir; reduced clearance of barbiturates

❷ *Carbamazepine:* Increased clearance of saquinavir, reduced clearance of carbamazepine

▲ *Cisapride:* Increased plasma levels of cisapride

❸ *Clarithromycin:* Reduced clearance of saquinavir; saquinavir reduces clearance of clarithromycin

❸ *Delavirdine:* Decreased clearance of saquinavir; reduce dose of Fortovase (saquinavir soft gel capsule) to 800 mg tid

❸ *Dexamethasone:* Reduced saquinavir level

▲ *Efavirenz:* Reduced saquinavir level

▲ *Ergot alkaloids:* Increased plasma levels of ergot alkaloids

❸ *Erythromycin:* Reduced clearance of saquinavir; saquinavir reduces clearance of erythromycin

❸ *Grapefruit juice:* Increased saquinavir level

▲ *Indinavir:* Decreased clearance of saquinavir

▲ *Lovastatin:* Saquinavir reduces clearance of lovastatin

▲ *Midazolam:* Increased plasma levels of midazolam and prolonged effect

❸ *Nelfinavir:* Decreased clearance of saquinavir; reduce dose of Fortovase (saquinavir soft gel capsule) to 800 mg tid

❸ *Oral contraceptives:* Saquinavir may reduce efficacy

❸ *Phenytoin:* Increased clearance of saquinavir; reduced clearance of phenytoin

▲ *Rifabutin:* Increased clearance of saquinavir

▲ *Rifampin:* Increased clearance of saquinavir

❸ *Ritonavir:* Decreased clearance of saquinavir; decrease saquinavir dose to 400 mg bid, or less, depending on ritonavir dose

▲ *Simvastatin:* Saquinavir reduces clearance of simvastatin

▲ *Terfenadine:* Increased plasma levels of terfenadine

▲ *Triazolam:* Increased plasma levels of triazolam and prolonged effect

S

SPECIAL CONSIDERATIONS
• Invirase and fortovase not considered bioequivalent; no food effect on Invirase when taken with ritonavir; take Fortovase with large meal
• Fortovase is the recommended formulation
• Invirase should only be considered if it is to be combined with antiretrovirals that significantly inhibit saquinavir's metabolism

---

scopolamine
(skoe-pol′a-meen)
Rx: *Transdermal:* Transderm-Scop
Rx: *Ophth:* Isopto Hyoscine
Rx: *Oral:* Scopace
Chemical Class: Belladonna alkaloid
Therapeutic Class: Anticholinergic; antiemetic; antivertigo agent; cycloplegic; mydriatic

---

CLINICAL PHARMACOLOGY
Mechanism of Action: An anticholinergic that reduces excitability of labyrinthine receptors, depressing conduction in the vestibular cerebellar pathway. *Therapeutic Effect:* Prevents motion-induced nausea and vomiting.

INDICATIONS AND DOSAGES
Prevention of motion sickness
Transdermal
Adults. 1 system q72h.

Post-operative nause or vomiting
Transdermal
Adults, Elderly. 1 system no sooner than 1 h before surgery and removed 24 h after surgery.

Ⓢ AVAILABLE FORMS/COST
• Film, Cont Rel—Transdermal: 1.5 mg, 0.5 mg/24 hr, 4 discs: **$24.94**
• Sol, Inj—IM, IV, SC: 0.4 mg/ml, 1 ml: **$1.76-$1.98**; 1 mg/ml, 1 ml: **$1.26-$1.76**

• Sol—Ophth: 0.25%, 5, 15 ml: **$20.88**/5 ml
• Tab—Oral: 0.4 mg, 100's: **$34.95**
CONTRAINDICATIONS: Angle-closure glaucoma, GI or GU obstruction, myasthenia gravis, paralytic ileus, tachycardia, thyrotoxicosis

PREGNANCY AND LACTATION: Pregnancy category C; no reports of adverse effects reported; compatible with breast-feeding

SIDE EFFECTS
Frequent (greater than 15%)
Dry mouth, somnolence, blurred vision
Rare (5%–1%)
Dizziness, restlessness, hallucinations, confusion, difficulty urinating, rash

SERIOUS REACTIONS
• None known.

INTERACTIONS
Drugs
③ *Antihistamines, phenothiazines, tricyclics:* Additive anticholinergic effect

SPECIAL CONSIDERATIONS
PATIENT/FAMILY EDUCATION
• Avoid abrupt discontinuation (taper off over 1 wk)
• Wash hands thoroughly after handling transdermal patches before contacting eyes

secobarbital

(see-koe-bar'bi-tal)

Rx: Seconal

Combinations

Rx: with amobarbital (Tuinal)

Chemical Class: Barbituric acid derivative

Therapeutic Class: Anesthesia adjunct; anticonvulsant; sedative/hypnotic

DEA Class: Schedule II

CLINICAL PHARMACOLOGY

Mechanism of Action: A barbiturate that depresses the central nervous system (CNS) activity by binding to barbiturate site at the GABA-receptor complex enhancing GABA activity and depressing reticular activity system. *Therapeutic Effect:* Produces hypnotic effect due to central nervous system (CNS) depression.

Pharmacokinetics

Well absorbed from the gastrointestinal (GI) tract. Protein binding: 52%-57%. Crosses blood-brain barrier. Widely distributed. Metabolized in liver by microsomal enzyme system to inactive and active metabolites. Primarily excreted in urine. Not removed by hemodialysis. **Half-life:** 15- 40 hrs.

INDICATIONS AND DOSAGES

Insomnia

PO

Adults. 100 mg at bedtime.

Preoperative sedation

PO

Adults. 100-300 mg 1-2 hrs. before procedure.

Children. 2-6 mg/kg 1-2 hrs. before procedure. Maximum: 100 mg/dose.

Sedation, daytime

PO

Adults. 30-50 mg 3-4 times/day.

Children. 2 mg/kg 3 times/day.

§ AVAILABLE FORMS/COST

• Cap, Gel—Oral: 100 mg, 100's: **$79.78**

UNLABELED USES: Chemotherapy-induced nausea and vomiting

CONTRAINDICATIONS: History of manifest or latent porphyria, marked liver dysfunction, marked respiratory disease in which dyspnea or obstruction is evident, and hypersensitivity to secobarbital or barbituates

PREGNANCY AND LACTATION: Pregnancy category D; small amounts excreted in breast milk, drowsiness in infant reported; compatible with breast-feeding

SIDE EFFECTS

Frequent

Somnolence

Occasional

Agitation, confusion, hyperkinesia, ataxia, CNS depression, nightmares, nervousness, psychiatric disturbance, hallucinations, insomnia, anxiety, dizziness, abnormality in thinking, hypoventilation, apnea, bradycardia, hypotension, syncope, nausea, vomiting, constipation, headache

Rare

Hypersensitivity reactions, fever, liver damage, megaloblastic anemia

SERIOUS REACTIONS

• Agranulocytosis, megaloblastic anemia, apnea, hypoventilation, bradycardia, hypotension, syncope, hepatic damage, and Stevens-Johnson syndrome rarely occur.

• Tolerance and physical dependence may occur with repeated use.

INTERACTIONS

Drugs

3 *Acetaminophen:* Enhanced hepatotoxic potential of acetaminophen overdoses

S

🔲 *Antidepressants:* Reduced serum concentration of cyclic antidepressants

🔲 *β-adrenergic blockers:* Reduced serum concentrations of β-blockers which are extensively metabolized

🔲 *Calcium channel blockers:* Reduced serum concentrations of verapamil and dihydropyridines

🔲 *Chloramphenicol:* Increased barbiturate concentrations; reduced serum chloramphenicol concentrations

🔲 *Corticosteroids:* Reduced serum concentrations of corticosteroids; may impair therapeutic effect

🔲 *Cyclosporine:* Reduced serum concentration of cyclosporine

🔲 *Digitoxin:* Reduced serum concentration of digitoxin

🔲 *Disopyramide:* Reduced serum concentration of disopyramide

🔲 *Doxycycline:* Reduced serum doxycycline concentrations

🔲 *Estrogen:* Reduced serum concentration of estrogen

🔲 *Ethanol:* Excessive CNS depression

🔲 *Griseofulvin:* Reduced griseofulvin absorption

🔲 *MAOIs:* Prolonged effect of barbiturates

🔲 *Methoxyflurane:* Enhanced nephrotoxic effect

🔲 *Narcotic analgesics:* Increased toxicity of meperidine; reduced effect of methadone; additive CNS depression

🔲 *Neuroleptics:* Reduced effect of either drug

❷ *Oral anticoagulants:* Decreased hypoprothrombinemic response to oral anticoagulants

🔲 *Oral contraceptives:* Reduced efficacy of oral contraceptives

🔲 *Phenytoin:* Unpredictable effect on serum phenytoin levels

🔲 *Propafenone:* Reduced serum concentration of propafenone

🔲 *Quinidine:* Reduced quinidine plasma concentration

🔲 *Tacrolimus:* Reduced serum concentration of tacrolimus

🔲 *Theophylline:* Reduced serum theophylline concentrations

🔲 *Valproic acid:* Increased serum concentrations of secobarbital

❷ *Warfarin:* See oral anticoagulants

Labs

• *Glucose:* Falsely low with Clinistix, Diastix

• *17-Ketosteroids:* Falsely increased in urine

• *Phenobarbital:* Falsely increased in serum

SPECIAL CONSIDERATIONS

• Compared to the benzodiazepine sedative hypnotics, secobarbital is more lethal in overdosage, has a higher tendency for abuse and addiction, and is more likely to cause drug interactions via induction of hepatic microsomal enzymes; few advantages if any in safety or efficacy over benzodiazepines

PATIENT/FAMILY EDUCATION

• Avoid driving and other dangerous activities

• Withdrawal insomnia may occur after short-term use; do not start using drug again, insomnia will improve in 1-3 nights

• May experience increased dreaming

selegiline

(seh-leg'ill-ene)
Rx: Carbex, Eldepryl
Chemical Class: Phenethyl-
amine derivative
Therapeutic Class: Anti-Par-
kinson's agent

CLINICAL PHARMACOLOGY

Mechanism of Action: An antiparkinson agent that irreversibly inhibits the activity of monoamine oxidase type B, the enzyme that breaks
down dopamine, thereby increasing
dopaminergic action. *Therapeutic
Effect:* Relieves signs and symptoms of Parkinson's disease.

Pharmacokinetics
Rapidly absorbed from the GI tract.
Crosses the blood-brain barrier. Metabolized in the liver to the active
metabolites. Primarily excreted in
urine. **Half-life:** 17 hr (amphetamine), 20 hr (methamphetamine).

INDICATIONS AND DOSAGES

*Adjunctive treatment for parkin-
sonism*
PO
Adults. 10 mg/day in divided doses,
such as 5 mg at breakfast and lunch,
given concomitantly with each dose
of carbidopa and levodopa.
Elderly. Initially, 5 mg in the morning. May increase up to 10 mg/day.

$ AVAILABLE FORMS/COST

• Cap—Oral: 5 mg, 60's: **$120.89-
$162.00**
• Tab—Oral: 5 mg, 60's: **$122.40-
$138.25**

CONTRAINDICATIONS: None
known.

PREGNANCY AND LACTATION:
Pregnancy category C; excretion in
breast milk unknown

SIDE EFFECTS

Frequent (10%–4%)
Nausea, dizziness, light-headed-
ness, syncope, abdominal discom-
fort
Occasional (3%–2%)
Confusion, hallucinations, dry
mouth, vivid dreams, dyskinesia
Rare (1%)
Headache, myalgia, anxiety, diar-
rhea, insomnia

SERIOUS REACTIONS

• Symptoms of overdose may vary
from CNS depression, characterized
by sedation, apnea, cardiovascular
collapse, and death, to severe paradoxical reactions, such as hallucinations, tremor, and seizures.
• Other serious effects may include
involuntary movements, impaired
motor coordination, loss of balance,
blepharospasm, facial grimaces,
feeling of heaviness in the lower extremities, depression, nightmares,
delusions, overstimulation, sleep
disturbance, and anger.

INTERACTIONS

Drugs
❷ *Antidepressants, serotonin reuptake inhibitors (fluoxetine, fluvoxamine, paroxetine, sertraline):*
Serious, sometimes fatal, reactions
including hyperthermia, autonomic
instability and mental status
changes
❷ *Dexfenfluramine, fenfluramine:*
Increased risk of serotonin syndrome
❷ *Dextroamphetamine:* Severe hypertension
❷ *Dextromethorphan:* Increased
risk of serotonin syndrome
❸ *Guanadrel, guanethidine:* May
inhibit the antihypertensive effects
of antihypertensive agents
❸ *Insulin:* Excessive hypoglycemia may occur when MAOIs are administered to patients with diabetes

S

3 *Levodopa:* May precipitate hypertensive crisis

⚠ *Methylphenidate:* Increased risk of hypertensive reactions

3 *Moclobemide:* Increased pressor effects of tyramine; increased risk of adverse drug or food interactions

② *Narcotic analgesics (meperidine):* Stupor, muscular rigidity, severe agitation, elevated temperature, hallucinations, and death

3 *Narcotic analgesics (morphine):* Stupor, muscular rigidity, severe agitation, elevated temperature, hallucinations, and death

⚠ *Reserpine:* Loss of antihypertensive effects

⚠ *Sibutramine:* Increased risk of serotonin syndrome

3 *Succinylcholine:* Prolonged muscle relaxation caused by succinylcholine

⚠ *Sympathomimetics (metaraminol, phenylpropanolamine, pseudoephedrine):* Additive pressor response to sympathomimetic

3 *Sympathomimetics (norepinephrine, phenylephrine):* Additive pressor response to sympathomimetic

⚠ *Venlafaxine:* Increased risk of serotonin syndrome

Labs

• *False positive:* Urine ketones, urine glucose

• *False negative:* Urine glucose (glucose oxidase)

• *False increase:* Uric acid, urine protein

SPECIAL CONSIDERATIONS

• At low doses, irreversible type B MAOI; at higher doses is metabolized to amphetamine, inhibiting both A and B subtypes of MAO

• Several placebo-controlled studies have demonstrated a significant delay in the need to initiate levodopa therapy in patients who receive selegiline in the early phase of the disease

• May have significant benefit in slowing the onset of the debilitating consequences of Parkinson's disease

---

senna

(sen'na)

OTC: Black Draught, Ex-Lax, Fletcher's Castoria, Gentlax, Lax-Pills, Senexon, Senna-Gen, Senokot, SenokotXTRA
Combinations
  OTC: with docusate (Senokot-S); with cascara sagrada (Herbal Laxative); with psyllium (Perdiem)
Chemical Class: Anthraquinone derivative
Therapeutic Class: Laxative, stimulant

CLINICAL PHARMACOLOGY

Mechanism of Action: A GI stimulant that has a direct effect on intestinal smooth musculature by stimulating the intramural nerve plexi. *Therapeutic Effect:* Increases peristalsis and promotes laxative effect.

Pharmacokinetics

Route	Onset	Peak	Duration
PO	6–12 hr	N/A	N/A
Rectal	0.5–2 hr	N/A	N/A

Minimal absorption after oral administration. Hydrolyzed to active form by enzymes of colonic flora. Absorbed drug metabolized in the liver. Eliminated in feces via biliary system.

INDICATIONS AND DOSAGES

Constipation

PO (tablets)

Adults, Elderly, Children 12 yr and older. 2 tablets at bedtime. Maximum: 4 tablets twice a day.

Children 6–11 yr. 1 tablet at bedtime. Maximum: 2 tablets twice a day.
Children 2–5 yr. 1/2 tablet at bedtime. Maximum: 1 tablet twice a day.
PO (Syrup)
Adults, Elderly, Children 12 yr and older. 10–15 ml at bedtime. Maximum: 15 ml twice a day.
Children 6–11 yr. 5–7.5 ml at bedtime. Maximum: 7.5 ml twice a day.
Children 2–5 yr. 2.5–3.75 ml at bedtime. Maximum: 3.75 ml twice a day.
PO (Granules)
Adults, Elderly, Children 12 yr and older. 1 tsp at bedtime. Maximum: 2 tsp twice a day.
Children 6–11 yr. one half (1/2) teaspoon at bedtime up to 1 teaspoon 2 times/day.
Children 2–5 yr. one quarter (1/4) teaspoon at bedtime up to one half (1/2) teaspoon 2 times/day.
Bowel evacuation
PO
Adults, Elderly, Children older than 1 yr. 75 ml between 2 p.m. and 4 p.m. on day prior to procedure.

[$] **AVAILABLE FORMS/COST**
- Liq—Oral: 33.3 mg/ml, 150 ml: **$6.01**
- Syr—Oral: 218 mg/5 ml, 60, 240 ml: **$23.36**/240 ml
- Tab—Oral: 8.6 mg, 100's: **$3.28-$21.04**; 15 mg, 30's: **$2.60-$5.39**; 25 mg, 24's: **$2.70-$5.39**; 217 mg, 90's: **$7.33**; 600 mg, 30's: **$1.31**
- Tab, Chewable—Oral: 15 mg, 48's: **$7.40**

CONTRAINDICATIONS: Abdominal pain, appendicitis, intestinal obstruction, nausea, vomiting

PREGNANCY AND LACTATION: Pregnancy category C; not excreted into breast milk; compatible with breast-feeding

SIDE EFFECTS
Frequent
Pink-red, red-violet, red-brown, or yellow-brown discoloration of urine
Occasional
Some degree of abdominal discomfort, nausea, mild cramps, griping, faintness

SERIOUS REACTIONS
- Long-term use may result in laxative dependence, chronic constipation, and loss of normal bowel function.
- Prolonged use or overdose may result in electrolyte and metabolic disturbances (such as hypokalemia, hypocalcemia, and metabolic acidosis or alkalosis), vomiting, muscle weakness, persistent diarrhea, malabsorption, and weight loss.

SPECIAL CONSIDERATIONS
- Proposed laxative of choice for narcotic-induced constipation

sertraline
(sir'trall-een)
Rx: Zoloft
Chemical Class: Naphthalenamine derivative
Therapeutic Class: Antidepressant, selective serotonin reuptake inhibitor (SSRI)

[S]

CLINICAL PHARMACOLOGY
Mechanism of Action: An antidepressant, anxiolytic, and obsessive-compulsive disorder adjunct that blocks the reuptake of the neurotransmitter serotonin at CNS neuronal presynaptic membranes, increasing its availability at postsynaptic receptor sites. *Therapeutic Effect:* Relieves depression, reduces obsessive-compulsive behavior, decreases anxiety.

Pharmacokinetics

Incompletely and slowly absorbed from the GI tract; food increases absorption. Protein binding: 98%. Widely distributed. Undergoes extensive first-pass metabolism in the liver to active compound. Excreted in urine and feces. Not removed by hemodialysis. **Half-life:** 26 hr.

INDICATIONS AND DOSAGES

Depression, obsessive-compulsive disorder

PO

Adults, Children 13-17 yr. Initially, 50 mg/day with morning or evening meal. May increase by 50 mg/day at 7-day intervals.

Elderly, Children 6-12 yr. Initially, 25 mg/day. May increase by 25–50 mg/day at 7-day intervals. Maximum: 200 mg/day.

Panic disorder, posttraumatic stress disorder, social anxiety disorder

PO

Adults, Elderly. Initially, 25 mg/day. May increase by 50 mg/day at 7-day intervals. Range: 50–200 mg/day. Maximum: 200 mg/day.

Premenstrual dysphoric disorder

PO

Adults. Initially, 50 mg/day. May increase up to 150 mg/day in 50-mg increments.

[$] **AVAILABLE FORMS/COST**

- Liq, Concentrate—Oral: 20 mg/ml, 60 ml: **$64.61**
- Tab—Oral: 25 mg, 100's: **$252.07**; 50 mg, 100's: **$272.61**; 100 mg, 100's: **$272.61**

CONTRAINDICATIONS: User within 14 days of MAOIs

PREGNANCY AND LACTATION: Pregnancy category C; excretion into breast milk unknown, use caution in nursing mother

SIDE EFFECTS

Frequent (26%–12%)

Headache, nausea, diarrhea, insomnia, somnolence, dizziness, fatigue, rash, dry mouth

Occasional (6%–4%)

Anxiety, nervousness, agitation, tremor, dyspepsia, diaphoresis, vomiting, constipation, abnormal ejaculation, visual disturbances, altered taste

Rare (less than 3%)

Flatulence, urinary frequency, paraesthesia, hot flashes, chills

SERIOUS REACTIONS

- None known.

INTERACTIONS

Drugs

[3] *Cimetidine:* Increased plasma sertraline concentrations

[3] *Cyproheptadine:* Serotonin antagonist may partially reverse antidepressant and other effects

[2] *Dexfenfluramine:* Duplicate effects on inhibition of serotonin reuptake; inhibition of dexfenfluramine metabolism (CYP2D6) exaggerates effect; both mechanisms increase risk of serotonin syndrome

[2] *Fenfluramine:* Duplicate effects on inhibition of serotonin reuptake; inhibition of dexfenfluramine metabolism (CYP2D6) exaggerates effect; both mechanisms increase risk of serotonin syndrome

[3] *Lithium:* Neurotoxicity (tremor, confusion, ataxia, dizziness, dysarthria, and absence seizures) reported in patients receiving fluoxetine-lithium combination; mechanism unknown

⚠ *MAOI's (isocarboxazid, phenelzine, tranylcypromine):* Increased CNS serotonergic effects has been associated with severe or fatal reactions with this combination

[2] *Selegiline:* Sporadic cases of mania and hypertension

3 *Sumatriptan:* Concomitant use of SSRI and sumatriptan may increase adverse effects

3 *Tricyclic antidepressants (clomipramine, desipramine, doxepin, imipramine, nortriptyline, trazodone):* Marked increases in tricyclic antidepressant levels due to inhibition of metabolism (CYP2D6)

2 *Tryptophan:* Additive serotonergic effects

3 *Warfarin:* Increased hypoprothrombinemic response to warfarin

SPECIAL CONSIDERATIONS

• SSRI of choice based on intermediate length $t_{1/2}$, linear pharmacokinetics, absence of appreciable age effect on clearance, substantially less effect on P450 enzymes, reducing potential for drug interactions

• Oral concentrate contains 12% alcohol; dropper contains natural rubber, caution if latex allergy

• Splitting 100 mg tablets to yield 50 mg dose cuts costs

PATIENT/FAMILY EDUCATION

• Oral concentrate must be diluted in water, ginger ale, lemon/lime soda, lemonade, or orange juice only, no other liquids should be used; do not mix in advance

• Avoid alcohol

---

sevelamer

(seh-vel′a-mer)

Rx: Renagel
Chemical Class: Allylamine
Therapeutic Class: Phosphate adsorbent

CLINICAL PHARMACOLOGY
Mechanism of Action: An antihyperphosphatemia agent that binds with dietary phosphorus in the GI tract, thus allowing phosphorus to be eliminated through the normal digestive process and decreasing the serum phosphorus level. *Therapeutic Effect:* Decreases incidence of hypercalcemic episodes in patients receiving calcium acetate treatment.

Pharmacokinetics
Not absorbed systemically. Unknown if removed by hemodialysis.

INDICATIONS AND DOSAGES
Hyperphosphatemia
PO
Adults, Elderly. 800–1,600 mg with each meal, depending on severity of hyperphosphatemia.

S **AVAILABLE FORMS/COST**
• Cap—Oral: 403 mg, 200's: **$142.13**
• Tab—Oral: 400 mg, 360's: **$246.51**; 800 mg, 180's: **$246.51**

CONTRAINDICATIONS: Bowel obstruction, hypophosphatemia

PREGNANCY AND LACTATION: Pregnancy category C; use caution in nursing mothers due to potential for reductions in serum levels of various vitamins

SIDE EFFECTS
Frequent (20%–11%)
Infection, pain, hypotension, diarrhea, dyspepsia, nausea, vomiting
Occasional (10%–1%)
Headache, constipation, hypertension, thrombosis, increased cough

SERIOUS REACTIONS
• None known.

INTERACTIONS
Drugs
3 *Antiarrhythmics, anticonvulsants:* Potential for decreased bioavailability of these drugs when concomitantly administered with sevelamer, administer >1 hr before or 3 hr after sevelamer

SPECIAL CONSIDERATIONS
• Has not been studied in ESRD patients not on hemodialysis
• Compared to calcium acetate, may reduce the risk of developing hypercalcemia

S

PATIENT/FAMILY EDUCATION
• A daily multivitamin supplement may prevent reduction in serum levels of vitamins D, E, K, and folic acid
• Do not chew or take caps apart prior to administration
• Space doses of sevelamer ≥1 hr before or 3 hours after concomitant medications

MONITORING PARAMETERS
• Serum phosphorus, calcium, bicarbonate, and chloride levels

---

sibutramine
(sih-byoo'tra-meen)
Rx: Meridia
Chemical Class: Cyclobutane-methamine derivative
Therapeutic Class: Anorexiant

CLINICAL PHARMACOLOGY
Mechanism of Action: A central nervous system (CNS) stimulant inhibits reuptake of serotonin (enhancing satiety) and norepinephrine (raises metabolic rate) centrally. *Therapeutic Effect:* Induces and maintains weight loss.

Pharmacokinetics
Rapidly absorbed from the gastrointestinal (GI) tract. Protein binding: 95%-97%. Metabolized in liver, undergoes first-pass metabolism. Primarily excreted in urine, minimal elimination in feces. **Half-life:** 1.1 hrs.

INDICATIONS AND DOSAGES
Weight loss
PO
Adults 16 years and older. Initially, 10 mg/day. May increase up to 15 mg/day. Maximum: 20 mg/day.

S AVAILABLE FORMS/COST
• Cap—Oral: 5 mg, 100's: **$313.76**; 10 mg, 100's: **$298.70**; 15 mg, 100's: **$386.25**

CONTRAINDICATIONS:
Anorexia nervosa, concomitant MAOI use, concomitant use of centrally acting appetite suppressants, hypersensitivity to sibutramine or any component of the formulation

PREGNANCY AND LACTATION:
Pregnancy category C; excretion into breast milk unknown, not recommended in nursing mothers

SIDE EFFECTS
Frequent
Headache, dry mouth, anorexia, constipation, insomnia, rhinitis, pharyngitis
Occasional
Back pain, flu syndrome, dizziness, nausea, asthenia (loss of strength, energy), arthralgia, nervousness, dyspepsia, sinusitis, abdominal pain, anxiety, dysmenorrheal
Rare
Depression, rash, cough, sweating, tachycardia, migraine, increased BP, paresthesia, altered taste

SERIOUS REACTIONS
• Seizures, thrombocytopenia, and deaths have been reported.
• Serotonin syndrome can occur with concomitant use of drugs that increase serotonin.
• Large doses may produce extreme nervousness and tachycardia.

INTERACTIONS
Drugs
❷ *MAO inhibitors:* Potential for the development of serotonin syndrome; at least 14 days should elapse between administration of MAO inhibitors and sibutramine

SPECIAL CONSIDERATIONS
• Primary pulmonary hypertension and cardiac valve disorders have been associated with other centrally acting weight loss agents that cause release of serotonin from nerve terminals; although sibutramine has not been associated with these effects in pre-marketing clinical stud-

ies, patients should be informed of the potential for these side effects and monitored closely for their occurrence

• Substantially increases blood pressure in some patients

• Maintenance of weight loss beyond 18 months has not been studied

MONITORING PARAMETERS

• Regular blood pressure monitoring

---

sildenafil

(sill-den'-a-fill)

Rx: Viagra

Chemical Class: CGMP specific phosphodiesterase inhibitor

Therapeutic Class: Anti-impotence agent

CLINICAL PHARMACOLOGY

Mechanism of Action: An erectile dysfunction agent that inhibits phosphodiesterase type 5, the enzyme responsible for degrading cyclic guanosine monophosphate in the corpus cavernosum of the penis, resulting in smooth muscle relaxation and increased blood flow. *Therapeutic Effect:* Facilitates an erection.

INDICATIONS AND DOSAGES

Erectile dysfunction

PO

Adults. 50 mg (30 min–4 hr before sexual activity). Range: 25–100 mg. Maximum dosing frequency is once daily.

Elderly (over 65 yr). Consider starting dose of 25 mg.

S AVAILABLE FORMS/COST

• Tab, Coated—Oral: 25 mg, 30's: **$303.79**; 50 mg, 100's: **$1,012.63**; 100 mg, 100's: **$1,012.63**

UNLABELED USES: Treatment of diabetic gastroparesis, sexual dysfunction associated with the use of selective serotonin reuptake inhibitors

CONTRAINDICATIONS: Concurrent use of sodium nitroprusside or nitrates in any form

PREGNANCY AND LACTATION: Pregnancy category B, use not recommended in women

SIDE EFFECTS

Frequent

Headache (16%), flushing (10%)

Occasional (7%-3%)

Dyspepsia, nasal congestion, UTI, abnormal vision, diarrhea

Rare (2%)

Dizziness, rash

SERIOUS REACTIONS

• Prolonged erections (lasting over 4 hours) and priapism (painful erections lasting over 6 hours) occur rarely.

INTERACTIONS

Drugs

▣ *Cimetidine, erythromycin, itraconazole, ketoconazole:* Increased sildenafil levels

▲ *Nitrates:* Cardiac arrest, death

▣ *Rifampin:* Decreased sildenafil levels

SPECIAL CONSIDERATIONS

• Tablets are priced the same regardless of dose, 100-mg tablets can be broken in half

---

silver nitrate

Rx: Silver nitrate

Chemical Class: Heavy metal

Therapeutic Class: Antibiotic; cauterizing agent

CLINICAL PHARMACOLOGY

Mechanism of Action: Free silver ions precipitate bacterial proteins by combining with chloride in tissue forming silver chloride; coagulates cellular protein to form an eschar or scab. The germicidal action is credited to precipitation of bacterial proteins by free silver ions. *Therapeutic Effect:* Inhibits growth of both gram-positive and gram-negative bacteria.

Pharmacokinetics

Minimal gastrointestinal (GI) tract and cutaneous absorption. Minimal excretion in urine.

INDICATIONS AND DOSAGES
Exuberant granulations

Applicator sticks

Adults, Elderly, Children. Apply to mucous membranes and other moist skin surfaces only on area to be treated 2-3 times/wk for 2-3 wks.

Topical, solution

Adults, Elderly, Children. Apply a cotton applicator dipped in solution on the affected area 2-3 times/wk for 2-3 wks.

Gonococcal ophthalmia neonatorum

Ophthalmic

Children. Instill 2 drops in each eye immediately after delivery.

S **AVAILABLE FORMS/COST**

• Applicators—Top: 100's: **$6.32-$8.64**

• Oint-Top: 10%, 30 g: **$32.50**

• Sol—Ophth: 1%, 1 ml, 100's: **$147.60**

• Sol—Top: 0.5%, 960 ml: **$19.33**; 10%, 30 ml: **$21.25**; 25%, 30 ml: **$33.75**; 50%, 30 ml: **$48.75**

UNLABELED USES: Children. Instill 2 drops in each eye immediately after delivery.

CONTRAINDICATIONS: Broken skin, cuts, or wounds, hypersensitivity to silver nitrate or any of its components

SIDE EFFECTS
Occasional

Ophthalmic: Chemical conjunctivitis

Topical: Burning, irritation, staining of the skin

Rare

Hyponatremia, methemoglobinemia

SERIOUS REACTIONS

• Symptoms of overdose include blackening of skin and mucous membranes, pain and burning of the mouth, salivation, vomiting, diarrhea, shock, convulsions, coma, and death.

• Methemoglobinemia is cause by absorbed silver nitrate but occurs rarely.

• Cauterization of the cornea and blindness occur rarely.

SPECIAL CONSIDERATIONS
PATIENT/FAMILY EDUCATION

• Stains skin and utensils (removable with iodine tincture followed by sodium thiosulfate solution)

---

silver sulfadiazine
(sul-fa-dye′a-zeen)

Rx: Silvadene, SSD, SSD AF, Thermazene

Chemical Class: Sulfonamide derivative

Therapeutic Class: Antibiotic, topical

CLINICAL PHARMACOLOGY
Mechanism of Action: An anti-infective that acts upon cell wall and cell membraine. Releases silver slowly in concentrations selectively toxic to bacteria. *Therapeutic Effect:* Produces bactericidal effect.

Pharmacokinetics

Variably absorbed. Significant systemic absorption may occur if applied to extensive burns. Absorbed medication excreted unchanged in urine. **Half-life:** 10 hrs (half-life increased with impaired renal function).

INDICATIONS AND DOSAGES
Burns
Topical
Adults, Elderly Children. Apply 1-2 times daily.

$ **AVAILABLE FORMS/COST**
• Cre—Top: 1%, 20, 25, 30, 50, 85, 400, 1000 g: **$21.88-$52.97**/400 g
UNLABELED USES: Treatment of minor bacterial skin infection, dermal ulcer
CONTRAINDICATIONS: Hypersensitivity to silver sulfadiazine or any component of the formulation
PREGNANCY AND LACTATION: Pregnancy category B; contraindicated in neonates (kernicterus)
SIDE EFFECTS
Side effects characteristic of all sulfonamides may occur when systemically absorbed such as extensive burn areas, anorexia, nausea, vomiting, headache, diarrhea, dizziness, photosensitivity, joint pain
Frequent
Burning feeling at treatment site
Occasional
Brown-gray skin discoloration, rash, itching
Rare
Increased sensitivity or skin to sunlight
SERIOUS REACTIONS
• If significant systemic absorption occurs, less often but serious are hemolytic anemia, hypoglycemia, diuresis, peripheral neuropathy, Stevens-Johnson syndrome, agranulocytosis, disseminated lupus erythematosus, anaphylaxis, hepatitis, and toxic nephrosis.
• Fungal superinfections may occur.
• Interstitial nephritis occurs rarely.

INTERACTIONS
Drugs
3 *Proteolytic enzymes:* Silver may inactivate enzymes
SPECIAL CONSIDERATIONS
• Prior to application, burn wounds should be cleansed and debrided (following control of shock and pain)
• Use sterile glove and tongue blade to apply medication; thin layer (1.5 mm) to completely cover wound; dressing as required only
• Continue until no chance of infection

---

simethicone
(si-meth'i-kone)
OTC: *Degas, Gas-X, Mylicon, Phazyme*
Combinations
  OTC: with calcium carbonate (*Titralac Plus*); with aluminum hydroxide, magnesium hydroxide (*Mylanta Gelisil, Maalox Extra Strength*); with calcium carbonate, magnesium hydroxide (*Tempo, Rolaids*); with Magaldrate, (*Riopan Plus*); with charcoal (*Charcoal Plus, Flatulex*)
Chemical Class: Siloxane polymer
Therapeutic Class: Antiflatulent

S

CLINICAL PHARMACOLOGY
Mechanism of Action: An antiflatulent that changes surface tension of gas bubbles, allowing easier elimination of gas. *Therapeutic Effect:* Drug dispersal, prevents formation of gas pockets in the GI tract.
Pharmacokinetics
Does not appear to be absorbed from GI tract. Excreted unchanged in feces.

INDICATIONS AND DOSAGES
Antiflatulent
PO

Adults, Elderly, Children 12 yr and older. 40–250 mg after meals and at bedtime. Maximum: 500 mg/day.

Children 2–11 yr. 40 mg 4 times a day.

Children younger than 2 yr. 20 mg 4 times a day.

💲 AVAILABLE FORMS/COST
• Cap—Oral: 125 mg, 50's: **$8.36-$9.78**; 166 mg, 60's: **$10.85**; 180 mg, 60's: **$10.99**
• Liq—Oral: 40 mg/0.6 ml, 15, 30 ml: **$2.29-$10.79**/30 ml; 62.5 mg/5 ml, 300 ml: **$5.00**
• Tab, Chewable—Oral: 80 mg, 100's: **$1.50-$15.85**; 125 mg, 60's: **$3.59-$5.10**; 150 mg, 36's: **$5.22**; 166 mg, 60's: **$10.85**
• Tab—Oral: 60 mg, 100's: **$13.57**; 95 mg, 100's: **$14.89**

UNLABELED USES: Adjunct to bowel radiography and gastroscopy
CONTRAINDICATIONS: None known

PREGNANCY AND LACTATION: Pregnancy category C
SIDE EFFECTS
None known.
SERIOUS REACTIONS
• None known.
SPECIAL CONSIDERATIONS
• Commonly prescribed, little evidence for any beneficial effect

---

simvastatin
(sim′va-sta-tin)
Rx: Zocor
Combinations
  Rx: with ezetimibe (Vytorin)
Chemical Class: Substituted hexahydronaphthalene
Therapeutic Class: HMG-CoA reductase inhibitor; antilipemic

CLINICAL PHARMACOLOGY
Mechanism of Action: A HMG-CoA reductase inhibitor that interferes with cholesterol biosynthesis by inhibiting the conversion of the enzyme HMG-CoA to mevalonate. *Therapeutic Effect:* Decreases serum LDL, cholesterol, VLDL, and plasma triglyceride levels; slightly increases serum HDL concentration.
Pharmacokinetics

Route	Onset	Peak	Duration
PO to reduce cholesterol	3 days	14 days	N/A

Well absorbed from the GI tract. Protein binding: 95%. Undergoes extensive first-pass metabolism. Hydrolyzed to active metabolite. Primarily eliminated in feces. Unknown if removed by hemodialysis.
INDICATIONS AND DOSAGES
To decrease elevated total and LDL cholesterol in hypercholesterolemia (types IIa and IIb), lower triglyceride levels, and increase HDL levels; to reduce risk of death and prevent MI in patients with heart disease and elevated cholesterol level; to reduce risk of revascularization procedures; to decrease risk of stroke or transient ischemic attack; to prevent cardiovascular events.

PO

Adults. Initially, 10–40 mg/day in evening. Dosage adjusted at 4-wk intervals.

Elderly. Initially, 10 mg/day. May increase by 5–10 mg/day q4wk. Range: 5–80 mg/day. Maximum: 80 mg/day.

§ **AVAILABLE FORMS/COST**

• Tab, Plain Coated—Oral: 5 mg, 90's: **$184.25**; 10 mg, 100's: **$237.50**; 20 mg, 100's: **$413.25**; 40 mg, 100's: **$413.25**; 80 mg, 90's: **$480.83**

CONTRAINDICATIONS: Active hepatic disease or unexplained, persistent elevations of liver function test results, age younger than 18 years, pregnancy

PREGNANCY AND LACTATION: Pregnancy category X; breast milk excretion unknown; other drugs in this class are excreted in small amounts; manufacturer recommends against breast-feeding

SIDE EFFECTS

Simvastatin is generally well tolerated. Side effects are usually mild and transient.

Occasional (3%–2%)

Headache, abdominal pain or cramps, constipation, upper respiratory tract infection

Rare (less than 2%)

Diarrhea, flatulence, asthenia (loss of strength and energy), nausea or vomiting

SERIOUS REACTIONS

• Lens opacities may occur.

• Hypersensitivity reaction and hepatitis occur rarely.

INTERACTIONS

Drugs

❷ *Azole antifungals (fluconazole, itraconazole, ketoconazole, miconazole):* Increased simvastatin levels via inhibition of metabolism with increased risk of rhabdomyolysis

❸ *Cholestyramine, colestipol:* Reduced bioavailability of simvastatin

❸ *Cyclosporine:* Concomitant administration increases risk of severe myopathy or rhabdomyolysis

❸ *Danazol:* Inhibition of metabolism (CYP3A4) thought to yield increased simvastatin levels with increased risk of rhabdomyolysis

❷ *Fluoxetine:* Inhibits CYP3A4 hepatic metabolism with risk of rhabdomyolysis

❷ *Gemfibrozil:* Small increased risk of myopathy with combination, especially at high doses of statin

❸ *Isradipine:* Isradipine probably decreases simvastatin (like lovastatin) plasma concentrations minimally

❸ *Macrolide antibiotics (clarithromycin, erythromycin, troleandomycin):* Increased simvastatin levels via inhibition of metabolism with increased risk of rhabdomyolysis

❸ *Nefazadone:* Inhibit CYP3A4 hepatic metabolism (like lovastatin) with risk of rhabdomyolysis

❸ *Niacin:* Concomitant administration increases risk of severe myopathy or rhabdomyolysis

❸ *Warfarin:* Addition of simvastatin may increase hypoprothrombinemic response to warfarin via inhibition of metabolism (CYP2C9)

SPECIAL CONSIDERATIONS

• Superior to fibrates, cholestyramine, and probucol in lowering total and LDL cholesterol levels

• Statin selection based on lipid-lowering prowess, cost, and availability

PATIENT/FAMILY EDUCATION

• Report symptoms of myalgia, muscle tenderness, or weakness

• Take daily doses in the evening for increased effect

MONITORING PARAMETERS

• Cholesterol (max therapeutic response 4-6 wk)

S

- LFT's (AST, ALT) at baseline and at 12 wk of therapy; if no change, no further monitoring necessary (discontinue if elevations persist at >3 × upper limit of normal)
- CPK at baseline and in patients complaining of diffuse myalgia, muscle tenderness, or weakness

---

sirolimus
(sir-oh-leem'-us)
Rx: Rapamune
Chemical Class: Macrolide derivative
Therapeutic Class: Immuno-suppressant

CLINICAL PHARMACOLOGY
Mechanism of Action: An immunosuppressant that inhibits T-lymphocyte proliferation induced by stimulation of cell surface receptors, mitogens, alloantigens, and lymphokines. Prevents activation of the enzyme target of rapamycin, a key regulatory kinase in cell cycle progression. *Therapeutic Effect:* Inhibits proliferation of T and B cells, essential components of the immune response; prevents organ transplant rejection.

INDICATIONS AND DOSAGES
Prevention of organ transplant rejection
PO
Adults. Loading dose: 6 mg. Maintenance: 2 mg/day.
Children 13 yr and older weighing less than 40 kg. Loading dose: 3 mg/m². Maintenance: 1 mg/m²/day.
Ⓢ **AVAILABLE FORMS/COST**
- Liq—Oral: 1 mg/ml, 60 ml: **$465.30**
- Tab—Oral: 1 mg, 100 ml: **$809.63**; 2 mg, 100's: **$1,619.25**
CONTRAINDICATIONS: Hypersensitivity to sirolimus, malignancy

PREGNANCY AND LACTATION: Pregnancy category C; excretion into breast milk unknown; use caution in nursing mothers
SIDE EFFECTS
Occasional
Hypercholesterolemia, hyperlipidemia, hypertension, rash; with high doses (5 mg/day): anemia, arthralgia, diarrhea, hypokalemia, and thrombocytopenia
SERIOUS REACTIONS
- None known.
INTERACTIONS
Drugs
Ⓑ *Azole antifungals, bromocriptine, calcium channel blockers, cimetidine, danazol, ethinyl estradiol, GI prokinetic agents, macrolide antibiotics, protease inhibitors:* Decreased metabolism or increased bioavailability of sirolimus

Ⓑ *Carbamazepine, phenobarbital, phenytoin, rifabutin, rifapentine:* Decreased sirolimus concentrations possible

Ⓑ *Cyclosporine:* Increased sirolimus concentrations when given concurrently. Sirolimus should be taken 4 hr after cyclosporine

Ⓑ *Diltiazem:* Increased sirolimus concentrations

⚠ *Grapefruit juice:* Increased sirolimus concentrations, grapefruit juice should not be administered with sirolimus

⚠ *Ketoconazole:* Significant increase in rate and extent of absorption of sirolimus, concurrent administration not recommended

⚠ *Live vaccines:* Avoid use of live vaccines, vaccinations may be less effective

❷ *Rifampin:* Sirolimus clearance significantly increased, decreased sirolimus concentrations; consider alternative therapeutic agents to rifampin

3 *St. John's wort (hypericum perforatum):* Potential for decreased plasma tacrolimus concentrations

SPECIAL CONSIDERATIONS

• Tablets and solution are not bioequivalent (tab has 27% > bioavailability), however 2 mg tabs clinically equivalent to 2 mg oral sol; not known if higher doses of oral sol are clinically equivalent to higher doses of tabs

• Allows cyclosporine dose reduction

• Experience limited with use as rescue therapy

• Black patients had higher rejection rates (56% vs 13%) than non-blacks given same regimen; no significant differences in trough sirolimus concentrations at equal doses between blacks and non-blacks

• IV formulation is under development

PATIENT/FAMILY EDUCATION

• Take medication the same each day with regard to timing of meals and other medications

• Limit UV/sunlight exposure, wear protective clothing and use sunsreen due to increased risk of skin cancer

• Due to potential risks to fetus, effective contraception should be used before, during and 12 wks after sirolimus therapy in women of childbearing potential

MONITORING PARAMETERS

• Whole-blood sirolimus levels (drawn 1 hr prior to next dose), 5-7 days after initiation or dose change. Maintain levels at 10-15 ng/ml for first month, then consider increasing to 15-20 ng/ml, especially in patients receiving little cyclosporine

• CBC, platelets, lipids

---

sodium bicarbonate
Combinations
OTC: with alginic acid, (AlOH, Mg Trisilicate Gastrocote); with sodium citrate (Citrocarbonate)
Chemical Class: Monosodium salt of carbonic acid
Therapeutic Class: Alkalinizing agent, systemic/urinary; antacid; electrolyte supplement

CLINICAL PHARMACOLOGY
Mechanism of Action: An alkalinizing agent that dissociates to provide bicarbonate ion. *Therapeutic Effect:* Neutralizes hydrogen ion concentration, raises blood and urinary pH.

Pharmacokinetics

Route	Onset	Peak	Duration
PO	15 min	N/A	1–3 hr
IV	Immediate	N/A	8–10 min

After administration, sodium bicarbonate dissociates to sodium and bicarbonate ions. With increased hydrogen ion concentrations bicarbonate ions combine with hydrogen ions to form carbonic acid, which then dissociates to CO_2, which is excreted by the lungs.

INDICATIONS AND DOSAGES
Cardiac arrest
IV
Adults, Elderly. Initially, 1 mEq/kg (as 7.5%–8.4% solution). May repeat with 0.5 mEq/kg q10min during continued cardiopulmonary arrest. Use in the postresuscitation phase is based on arterial blood pH, partial pressure of carbon dioxide in arterial blood ($PaCO_2$) and base deficit calculation.
Children, Infants. Initially, 1 mEq/kg.

Metabolic acidosis (not severe)
IV
Adults, Elderly, Children. 2–5 mEq/kg over 4–8 hr. May repeat based on laboratory values.
Metabolic acidosis (associated with chronic renal failure)
PO
Adults, Elderly. Initially, 20–36 mEq/day in divided doses.
Renal tubular acidosis (distal)
PO
Adults, Elderly. 0.5–2 mEq/kg/day in 4–6 divided doses.
Children. 2–3 mEq/kg/day in divided doses.
Renal tubular acidosis (proximal)
PO
Adults, Elderly, Children. 5–10 mEq/kg/day in divided doses.
Urine alkalinization
PO
Adults, Elderly. Initially, 4 g, then 1–2 g q4h. Maximum: 16 g/day.
Children. 84–840 mg/kg/day in divided doses.
Antacid
PO
Adults, Elderly. 300 mg–2 g 1–4 times a day.
Hyperkalemia
IV
Adults, Elderly. 1 mEq/kg over 5 minutes.

§ AVAILABLE FORMS/COST
• Sol, Inj-IV: 4.2%, 10 ml: **$3.14-$13.75**; 5%, 500 ml: **$14.06-$39.25**; 7.5%, 50 ml: **$4.46-$18.96**; 8.4%, 10 ml: **$2.89-$13.58**
• Tab, Coated—Oral: 325 mg, 1000's: **$11.55**; 650 mg, 100's: **$0.65-$4.50**
CONTRAINDICATIONS: Excessive chloride loss due to diarrhea, vomiting, or GI suctioning; hypocalcemia; metabolic or respiratory alkalosis

PREGNANCY AND LACTATION:
Pregnancy category C
SIDE EFFECTS
Frequent
Abdominal distention, flatulence, belching
SERIOUS REACTIONS
• Excessive or chronic use may produce metabolic alkalosis (characterized by irritability, twitching, paraesthesias, cyanosis, slow or shallow respirations, headache, thirst, and nausea).
• Fluid overload results in headache, weakness, blurred vision, behavioral changes, incoordination, muscle twitching, elevated BP, bradycardia, tachypnea, wheezing, coughing, and distended neck veins.
• Extravasation may occur at the IV site, resulting in tissue necrosis and ulceration.
INTERACTIONS
Drugs
▣ *Amphetamines:* Sodium bicarbonate inhibits the elimination and increases the effects of amphetamines
▣ *β-blockers:* Reduced absorption
▣ *Cefpodoxime:* Reduced absorption
▣ *Cefuroxime:* Reduced serum levels with reduced antibiotic efficacy
▣ *Ephedrine:* Large doses of sodium bicarbonate increase the serum concentrations of ephedrine
▣ *Flecainide:* Increased urine pH will increase flecainide serum concentration
▣ *Glipizide:* Enhanced rate of glipizide absorption
▣ *Glyburide:* Enhanced rate of glyburide absorption
▣ *Iron:* Reduced iron absorption
▣ *Ketoconazole:* Decreased ketoconazole absorption

⊡ *Lithium:* Sodium bicarbonate may lower lithium plasma concentrations

⊡ *Methenamine compound:* Sodium bicarbonate-induced urinary pH changes interfere with antibacterial activity of methenamine compounds

⊡ *Mexiletine:* Increased urine pH increases mexiletine concentrations

⊡ *Pseudoephedrine:* Sodium bicarbonate-induced urinary pH changes may markedly inhibit the elimination of pseudoephedrine

⊡ *Quinidine:* Sodium bicarbonate-induced urinary pH changes may increase quinidine concentrations

⊡ *Quinolones:* Reduced absorption

⊡ *Salicylates:* Sodium bicarbonate-induced urinary pH changes can decrease serum salicylate concentrations

⊡ *Tetracyclines:* Reduced absorption

Labs

• *Protein:* Falsely elevates urine protein

SPECIAL CONSIDERATIONS
PATIENT/FAMILY EDUCATION
• Milk-alkali syndrome (may result from excessive antacid use): confusion, headache, nausea, vomiting, anorexia, urinary stones, hypercalcemia
• To avoid drug interactions due to reduced absorption, separate intake by 2 hr

MONITORING PARAMETERS
• Electrolytes, blood pH, PO_2, HCO_3, during treatment
• ABGs frequently during emergencies

---

sodium chloride
OTC: *Nasal:* Afrin Saline Mist, Ayr, Breathe Free, Dristan Saline, HuMist, NSal, Ocean, Pretz, SalineX, SeaMist
OTC: *Ophth:* Adsorbonac, AK-NaCl, Muro-128, Muroptic-5
Chemical Class: Monovalent cation
Therapeutic Class: Electrolyte supplement; irrigant; moisturizing agent

---

CLINICAL PHARMACOLOGY
Mechanism of Action: Sodium is a major cation of extracellular fluid that controls water distribution, fluid and electrolyte balance, and osmotic pressure of body fluids; it also maintains acid-base balance.

Pharmacokinetics
Well absorbed from the GI tract. Widely distributed. Primarily excreted in urine.

INDICATIONS AND DOSAGES
Prevention and treatment of sodium and chloride deficiencies; source of hydration
IV
Adults, Elderly. 1–2 L/day 0.9% or 0.45% or 100 ml 3% or 5% over 1 hr; assess serum electrolyte levels before giving additional fluid.

Prevention of heat prostration and muscle cramps from excessive perspiration
PO
Adults, Elderly. 1–2 g 3 times a day.

Relief of dry and inflamed nasal membranes
Intranasal
Adults, Elderly. Use as needed.

Diagnostic aid in ophthalmoscopic exam, treatment of corneal edema
Ophthalmic solution
Adults, Elderly. Apply 1–2 drops q3–4h.
Ophthalmic ointment
Adults, Elderly. Apply once a day or as directed.

§ **AVAILABLE FORMS/COST**
• Oint—Ophth: 5%, 3.5 g: **$12.11-$15.28**
• Sol, Bacteriostatic Diluent: 0.9%, 30 ml: **$0.55-$2.14**
• Sol, Electrolyte—IV: 0.45%, 1000 ml: **$1.38-$16.79**; 0.9%, 1000 ml: **$1.38-$16.79**; 3%, 500 ml: **$1.69-$13.22**; 5%, 500 ml: **$9.49-$11.88**; 14.6%, 20 ml (for dilution): **$0.98-$2.26**; 23.4%, 30 ml (for dilution): **$0.62-$1.80**
• Sol, Isotonic—INH: 0.45%, 3 ml × 100: **$10.00-$14.00**; 0.9%, 3 ml × 100: **$5.27-$10.55**
• Sol—Genitourinary Irrigant: 0.45%, 2000 ml (hypotonic): **$6.65-$7.28**; 0.9% (isotonic), 2000 ml: **$7.28-$7.65**
• Sol—Nasal: 0.4%; 15 ml: **$3.87**; 0.9%; 45 ml: **$2.40-$4.37**
• Sol—Ophth: 5%, 15 ml: **$11.35-$12.44**
• Tab, Electrolyte—Oral: 1 g, 100's: **$4.50**

CONTRAINDICATIONS: Fluid retention, hypernatremia
PREGNANCY AND LACTATION: Pregnancy category C
SIDE EFFECTS
Frequent
Facial flushing
Occasional
Fever; irritation, phlebitis, or extravasation at injection site
Ophthalmic: Temporary burning or irritation
SERIOUS REACTIONS
• Too rapid administration may produce peripheral edema, CHF, and pulmonary edema.

• Excessive dosage may cause hypokalemia, hypervolemia, and hypernatremia.
INTERACTIONS
Drugs
▣ *Lithium:* High sodium intake may reduce serum lithium concentrations, while restriction of sodium tends to increase serum lithium
SPECIAL CONSIDERATIONS
• One g of sodium chloride provides 17.1 mEq sodium and 17.1 mEq chloride

---

sodium oxybate
(ox'ee-bate)
Rx: Xyrem
Chemical Class: Hydroxybutyrate
Therapeutic Class: Anticataplectic; central nervous system depressant

---

CLINICAL PHARMACOLOGY
Mechanism of Action: A naturally occurring inhibitory neurotransmitter that binds to gamma aminobutyric acid (GABA)-B receptors and sodium oxybate specific receptors with its highest concentrations in the basal ganglia, which meditates sleep cycles, temperature regulation, cerebral glucose metabolism and blood flow, memory, and emotion control. *Therapeutic Effect:* Reduces the number of sleep episodes.
Pharmacokinetics
Rapidly and incompletely absorbed. Absorption is delayed and decreased by a high fat meal. Protein binding: less than 1%. Widely distributed, including cerebrospinal fluid (CSF). Metabolized in liver. Excretion is less than 5% in the urine and negligible in feces. Unknown if removed by hemodialysis. **Half-life:** 20-53 min.

INDICATIONS AND DOSAGES
Cataplexy of narcolepsy
PO

Adults, Elderly. 4.5 g/day in 2 equal doses of 2.25 g, the first taken at bedtime while in bed and the second 2.5-4 hrs. later. Maximum: 9 g/day in two weekly increments of 1.5 g/day.

S **AVAILABLE FORMS/COST**
• Liq—Oral: 500 mg/ml, 180 ml, kit: **$246.44** (Xyrem is available only through restricted distribution, the Xyrem Success Program, by calling 1-877-679-9736)

UNLABELED USES: Alcohol withdrawal

CONTRAINDICATIONS: Metabolic/respiratory alkalosis, current treatment with sedative hypnotics, succinic semialdehyde dehydrogenase deficient, hypersensitivity to sodium oxybate or any component of the formulation

PREGNANCY AND LACTATION: Pregnancy category B; excretion into breast milk unknown; use caution in nursing mothers

SIDE EFFECTS
Frequent
Mild bradycardia
Occasional
Headache, vertigo, dizziness, restless legs, abdominal pain, muscle weakness
Rare
Dream-like state of confusion

SERIOUS REACTIONS
• Agitation, excitation, increased blood pressure (BP), and insomnia may occur upon abrupt discontinuation of sodium oxybate.

INTERACTIONS
Drugs
❷ *Barbiturates:* Additive CNS and respiratory depression
❷ *Benzodiazepines:* Additive CNS and respiratory depression
❷ *Centrally acting muscle relaxants:* Additive CNS and respiratory depression
❷ *Opioid analgesics:* Additive CNS and respiratory depression
❷ *Ethanol:* Additive CNS and respiratory depression

SPECIAL CONSIDERATIONS
• Sodium oxybate is effective and indicated for the treatment of cataplexy in patients with narcolepsy; it could also be effective for general anesthesia, narcolepsy, fibromyalgia syndrome, insomnia, alcoholism and opiate withdrawal, but its potential for abuse is unacceptable

PATIENT/FAMILY EDUCATION
• Prepare both doses prior to bedtime; each dose must be diluted with 2 oz (60 ml) of water in the child-resistant dosing cups before ingestion
• The first dose is to be taken at bedtime while in bed and the second taken 2.5-4 hr later while sitting in bed; patients will probably need to set an alarm to awaken for the second dose
• The second dose must be prepared before ingesting the first dose, and should be placed in close proximity to the patient's bed
• After ingesting each dose the patient should then lie down and remain in bed

MONITORING PARAMETERS
• History/physical exam: Review signs and symptoms for efficacy, toxicity and abuse, including tremor and coma
• Laboratory: Sodium and potassium plasma levels, hepatic functions, blood gas analysis

S

sodium polystyrene sulfonate

(pol-ee-stye'reen)

Rx: Kayexalate, Kionex, SPS

Chemical Class: Cation exchange resin

Therapeutic Class: Antihyperkalemic

CLINICAL PHARMACOLOGY

Mechanism of Action: An ion exchange resin that releases sodium ions in exchange primarily for potassium ions. *Therapeutic Effect:* Moves potassium from the blood into the intestine so it can be expelled from the body.

INDICATIONS AND DOSAGES

Hyperkalemia

PO

Adults, Elderly. 60 ml (15 g) 1–4 times a day.

Children. 1 g/kg/dose q6h.

Rectal

Adults, Elderly. 30–50 g as needed q6h.

Children. 1 g/kg/dose q2–6h.

[$] **AVAILABLE FORMS/COST**

- Susp—Oral: 15 g/60 ml, 60, 120, 480 ml: **$4.00-$6.35**/60 ml
- Susp—Rect: 15 g/60 ml, 120, 200 ml: **$29.50**/200 ml

CONTRAINDICATIONS: Hypernatremia, intestinal obstruction or perforation

PREGNANCY AND LACTATION: Pregnancy category C; excretion in breast milk not expected

SIDE EFFECTS

Frequent

High dosage: Anorexia, nausea, vomiting, constipation

High dosage in elderly: Fecal impaction characterized by severe stomach pain with nausea or vomiting

Occasional

Diarrhea, sodium retention marked by decreased urination, peripheral edema, and increased weight

SERIOUS REACTIONS

- Potassium deficiency may occur. Early signs of hypokalemia include confusion, delayed thought processes, extreme weakness, irritability, and EKG changes (including prolonged QT interval; widening, flattening, or inversion of T wave; and prominent U waves).
- Hypocalcemia, manifested by abdominal or muscle cramps, occurs occasionally.
- Arrhythmias and severe muscle weakness may be noted.

INTERACTIONS

Drugs

[3] *Antacids:* Combined use of magnesium- or calcium-containing antacids with resin may result in systemic alkalosis

SPECIAL CONSIDERATIONS

- Exchange efficacy of resin is approx 33%; 1 g of resin (4.1 mEq of sodium) exchanges approximately 1 mEq of potassium
- Rectal route is less effective than oral administration
- Powder formulations very hydrophobic, difficult to mix. Pre-prepared suspensions in sorbitol preferable

PATIENT/FAMILY EDUCATION

- Do not mix with orange juice

MONITORING PARAMETERS

- Serum K, Ca, Mg, Na, acid-base balance, bowel function, possibly ECG

somatropin/somatrem
Rx: *Somatropin:* Genotropin, Norditropin, Nutropin, Nutropin AQ, Humatrope, Saizen, Serostim, Zorbtive
Rx: *Somatrem:* Protropin
Chemical Class: Growth hormone; recombinant human peptide
Therapeutic Class: Anti-cachexic; growth hormone

CLINICAL PHARMACOLOGY
Mechanism of Action: A polypeptide hormone that stimulates cartilagenous growth areas of long bones, increases the number and size of skeletal muscle cells, influences the size of organs, and increases RBC mass by stimulating erythropoietin. Influences the metabolism of carbohydrates (decreases insulin sensitivity), fats (mobilizes fatty acids), minerals (retains phosphorus, sodium, potassium by promotion of cell growth), and proteins (increases protein synthesis). *Therapeutic Effect:* Stimulates growth.

Pharmacokinetics
Well absorbed after subcutaneous or IM administration. Localized primarily in the kidneys and liver. **Half-life:** IV, 20-30 min; subcutaneous, IM, 3-5 hr.

INDICATIONS AND DOSAGES
Growth hormone deficiency
Subcutaneous
Adults. 0.006 mg/kg Humatrope, Nutropin, or Nutropin AQ once daily; or 0.04-0.08 mg/kg Genotropin weekly divided into 6-7 equal doses/wk.
Children. 0.3 mg/kg Protropin weekly divided into daily doses; 0.16-0.24 mg/kg Genotropin weekly divided into daily doses;

0.18-0.3 mg/kg Humatrope weekly divided into alternate-day doses or 6 doses/wk; 0.024-0.036 mg/kg/dose Norditropin 6-7 times/wk; 0.3-0.7 mg/kg Nutropin weekly divided into daily doses; 0.06 mg/kg Saizen 3 times/wk; or 0.75mg/kg Nutropin Depot twice monthly or 1.5 mg/kg once monthly.

Chronic renal insufficiency
Subcutaneous
Children. 0.35 mg/kg Nutropin or Nutropin AQ weekly divided into daily doses.

Turner syndrome
Subcutaneous
Children. 0.375 mg/kg Humatrope, Nutropin, or Nutropin AQ weekly divided into equal doses 3-7 times/wk.

AIDS-related wasting
Subcutaneous
Adults weighing more than 55 kg. 6 mg once a day at bedtime.
Adults weighing 45-55 kg. 5mg once a day at bedtime.
Adults weighing 35-44kg. 4 mg once a day at bedtime.
Adults weighing less than 35 kg. 0.1 mg/kg once a day at bedtime.

Short bowel syndrome
Subcutaneous
Adults. 0.1 mg/kg/day (Zorbtive). Maximum: 8 mg/day.

Ⓢ AVAILABLE FORMS/COST
Somatropin
• Powder—Depot Inj: 13.5 mg, 18 mg, 22.5 mg, kit; all: **$647.45-$1,079.08**
• Powder—Inj: 0.2 mg, 0.4 mg, 0.6 mg, 0.8 mg/0.25 ml; all: **$10.07-$40.29**; 1 mg, 1.2 mg, 1.4 mg, 1.6 mg, 1.8 mg, 2 mg/0.25 ml; all: **$48.34-$95.92**; 1.5 mg/ml: **$75.54**; 4 mg/vial: **$184.16**; 5 mg/vial: **$218.75-$374.50**; 5.8 mg/ml: **$251.79**; 6 mg/vial: **$252.00**; 8 mg/vial: **$368.32**; 10 mg/vial:

$479.59; 12 mg, kit: $517.75; 13.8 mg/ml: $604.28; 24 mg, kit: $1,035.50

• Sol—Inj: 5 mg/ml, 2 ml: $441.00-$528.74

Somatrem

• Powder, Inj—M, SC: 5 mg/vial: $239.79; 10 mg/vial: $479.59

CONTRAINDICATIONS: None known.

PREGNANCY AND LACTATION: Pregnancy category C; excretion into breast milk unknown

SIDE EFFECTS

Frequent

Otitis media, other ear disorders (with Turner's syndrome)

Occasional

Carpal tunnel syndrome; gynecomastia; myalgia; swelling of hands, feet, or legs; fatigue; asthenia

Rare

Rash, pruritus, altered vision, headache, nausea, vomiting, injection site pain and swelling, abdominal pain, hip or knee pain

SERIOUS REACTIONS

• None known.

SPECIAL CONSIDERATIONS

MONITORING PARAMETERS

• Individualize doses for growth hormone inadequacy

• Check for hypothyroidism, malnutrition, antibodies or opportunistic infections (AIDs patients) if no response to initial dose

• TSH

• Evaluate if child limps

• Follow with fundoscopy (papilledema)

sorbitol

(sor'-bi-tole)

Rx: Sorbitol

Chemical Class: Polyalcoholic sugar

Therapeutic Class: Diuretic, osmotic; laxative, osmotic

CLINICAL PHARMACOLOGY

Mechanism of Action: An polyalcoholic sugar with osmotic cathartic actions. Specific mechanism unknown. *Therapeutic effect:* Catharsis, urinary irrigation.

Pharmacokinetics

Onset of action within 15-60 minutes. Poorly absorbed by both oral and rectal route. Metabolised in live to primary metabolite, fructose.

INDICATIONS AND DOSAGES

Hyperosmotic laxative

PO

Adults, Elderly, Children 12 years and older: 30-150mL as a 70% solution

Children 2- 11 years: 2mL/kg as a 70% solution

Rectal

Adults, Elderly, Children 12 years and older: 120mL as a 25-30% solution

Children 2- 11 years: 30-60mL as a 25-30% solution

Transurethral surgical procedure TOPICAL Adults, Elderly: 3-3.3% as transurethral surgical procedure irrigation

Topical

Adults, Elderly: 3-3.3% as transurethral surgical procedure irrigation

§ AVAILABLE FORMS/COST

• Sol—Irrigation: 3.3%, 4000 ml: $28.26

• Sol—Oral: 70%, 480 ml: $4.54-$25.00

CONTRAINDICATIONS: Anuria

SIDE EFFECTS

Acidosis, electrolyte loss, marked diuresis, urinary retention, edema, dryness of mouth and thirst, dehydration, pulmonary congestion, hypotension, tachycardia, angina-like pains, blurred vision, convulsions, nausea, vomiting, diarrhea, rhinitis, chills, vertigo, backache, urticaria.

SERIOUS REACTIONS

• Life threatening adverse reactions with IV sorbitol infusions have been reported in patients with fructose intolerance.

SPECIAL CONSIDERATIONS

• Just as effective as lactulose as a laxative at reduced expense

---

sotalol

(soe'ta-lole)

Rx: Betapace, Betapace AF
Chemical Class: β-adrenergic blocker, nonselective
Therapeutic Class: Antiarrhythmic, class III

CLINICAL PHARMACOLOGY

Mechanism of Action: A beta-adrenergic blocking agent that prolongs action potential, effective refractory period, and QT interval. Decreases heart rate and AV node conduction; increases AV node refractoriness. *Therapeutic Effect:* Produces antiarrhythmic activity.

Pharmacokinetics

Well absorbed from the GI tract. Protein binding: None. Widely distributed. Primarily excreted unchanged in urine. Removed by hemodialysis. **Half-life:** 12 hr (increased in the elderly and patients with impaired renal function).

INDICATIONS AND DOSAGES

Documented, life-threatening arrhythmias

PO

Adults, Elderly. Initially, 80 mg twice a day. May increase gradually at 2-to 3-day intervals. Range: 240–320 mg/day.

Dosage in renal impairment

Dosage interval is modified based on creatinine clearance.

Creatinine Clearance	Dosage Interval
30–60 ml/min	24 hr
10–30 ml/min	36–48 hr
less than 10 ml/min	Individualized

Ⓢ AVAILABLE FORMS/COST

• Tab, Coated—Oral: 80 mg, 100's: **$234.69-$320.00**; 120 mg, 100's: **$313.09-$426.94**; 160 mg, 100's: **$391.49-$533.75**; 240 mg, 100's: **$480.15-$693.81**

UNLABELED USES: Maintenance of normal heart rhythm in chronic or recurring atrial fibrillation or flutter; treatment of anxiety, chronic angina pectoris, hypertension, hypertrophic cardiomyopathy, MI, mitral valve prolapse syndrome, pheochromocytoma, thyrotoxicosis, tremors

CONTRAINDICATIONS: Bronchial asthma, cardiogenic shock, prolonged QT syndrome (unless functioning pacemaker is present), second- and third-degree heart block, sinus bradycardia, uncontrolled cardiac failure

PREGNANCY AND LACTATION: Pregnancy category B; similar drug, atenolol, frequently used in the third trimester for treatment of hypertension (many studies of efficacy and safety of atenolol in pregnancy-induced hypertension); long-term use has been associated with intrauterine growth retardation; concentrated in breast milk (levels 3-5 times those of plasma); symptoms of β-blockade possible in infant, but considered compatible with breast-feeding

SIDE EFFECTS

Frequent

Diminished sexual function, drowsiness, insomnia, unusual fatigue or weakness

Occasional

Depression, cold hands or feet, diarrhea, constipation, anxiety, nasal congestion, nausea, vomiting

Rare

Altered taste, dry eyes, itching, numbness of fingers, toes, or scalp

SERIOUS REACTIONS

• Bradycardia, CHF, hypotension, bronchospasm, hypoglycemia, prolonged QT interval, torsades de pointes, ventricular tachycardia, and premature ventricular complexes may occur.

INTERACTIONS

Drugs

▣ *Adenosine:* Bradycardia aggravated

▣ *α₁-adrenergic blockers:* Potential enhanced first dose response (marked initial drop in blood pressure), particularly on standing (especially prazocin)

▣ *Antacids:* Reduced sotalol absorption with aluminum and magnesium containing antacids, separate dose by 2 hr

⚠ *Antiarrhythmics, Class Ia (disopyramide, moricizine, quinidine, procainamide) and Class III (amiodarone, bretylium, dofetilide, ibutilide):* Concomitant therapy not recommended due to potential to prolong refractoriness, hold antiarrhythmics for at least 3 half-lives prior to doing with sotalol

❷ *β-2-receptor agonists (albuterol, isoproterenol, terbutaline):* β-agonists may have to be administered in increased dosages when used concomitantly with sotalol

▣ *Calcium channel blockers:* Possible additive effects on AV conduction or ventricular function, possible additive effects on BP

▣ *Catecholamine-depleting agents (guanethidine, reserpine):* Hypotension and marked bradycardia possible due to excessive reduction of resting sympathetic nervous tone with concomitant use

▣ *Cholinesterase inhibitors (neostigmine, physostigmine, tacrine):* Bradycardia aggravated

▣ *Cimetidine:* Renal clearance reduced; AUC increased with cimetidine coadministration

▣ *Cisapride:* Dual prolongation of QT interval; increased risk of ventricular tachyarrhythmias

▣ *Clonidine, guanabenz, guanfacine:* Exacerbation of rebound hypertension upon discontinuation of clonidine

▣ *Cocaine:* Cocaine-induced vasoconstriction potentiated; reduced coronary blood flow

▣ *Contrast media:* Increased risk of anaphylaxis

▣ *Digitalis:* Enhances bradycardia

▣ *Dipyridamole:* Bradycardia aggravated

▣ *Epinephrine, phenylephrine:* Potentiates pressor response; resultant hypertension and bradycardia

▣ *Flecainide:* Additive negative inotropic effects; case report of bradycardia, AV block, and cardiac arrest following switch from flecainide to sotalol

▣ *Fluoxetine:* Increased β-blockade activity

▣ *Hypoglycemic agents (insulin, oral antidiabetics):* Masked hypoglycemia, hyperglycemia may occur requiring dosage adjustment of insulin or antidiabetic agents

▣ *Lidocaine:* Increased serum lidocaine concentrations possible

⚠ *Macrolide antibiotics (clarithromycin, erythromycin):* Increased risk of QT prolongation and life-threatening arrhythmias
[3] *Neuroleptics:* Both drugs inhibit each other's metabolism; additive hypotension
[3] *NSAIDs:* Reduced hemodynamic effects of sotalol
⚠ *Phenothiazines:* Increased risk of QT prolongation and life-threatening arrhythmias
⚠ *Quinolone antibiotics (gatifloxacin, levofloxacin, moxifloxacin, sparfloxacin):* Increased risk of QT prolongation and life-threatening arrhythmias
[2] *Theophylline:* Antagonistic pharmacodynamic effects
⚠ *Tricyclic antidepressants:* Increased risk of QT prolongation and life-threatening arrhythmias
⚠ *Ziprasidone:* Increased risk of QT prolongation and life-threatening arrhythmias

Labs

- *Metanephrines total:* Falsely increases urine levels (may be double)

SPECIAL CONSIDERATIONS

PATIENT/FAMILY EDUCATION

- Do not discontinue abruptly; may require taper; rapid withdrawal may produce rebound hypertension or angina

MONITORING PARAMETERS

- Angina: Reduction in nitroglycerin usage; frequency, severity, onset, and duration of angina pain; heart rate
- Arrhythmias: Heart rate and rhythm; monitor QT intervals (discontinue or reduce dose if QT >520 msec)
- Congestive heart failure: Functional status, cough, dyspnea on exertion, paroxysmal nocturnal dyspnea, exercise tolerance, and ventricular function
- Hypertension: Blood pressure
- Toxicity: Blood glucose, bronchospasm, hypotension, bradycardia, depression, confusion, hallucination, sexual dysfunction
- Because of prodysrhythmic risk, begin and increase drug in setting with cardiac rhythm monitoring

---

sparfloxacin

(spar-floks'a-sin)

Rx: Zagam

Chemical Class: Fluoroquinolone derivative

Therapeutic Class: Antibiotic

CLINICAL PHARMACOLOGY

Mechanism of Action: A fluoroquinolone that interferes with DNA-gyrase in susceptible microorganisms. *Therapeutic Effect:* Inhibits DNA replication and repair. Bactericidal.

Pharmacokinetics

Well absorbed from the gastrointestinal (GI) tract after PO administration. Widely distributed. Metabolized in liver. Primarily excreted in urine with a lesser amount eliminated in the feces. **Half-life:** 16-30 hrs.

INDICATIONS AND DOSAGES

Bronchitis, pneumonia

PO

Adults 18 yrs and older, Elderly. Initially, two 200 mg tablets as a loading dose on first day. Then one 200 mg tablet q24h for a total of 10 days.

Dosage in renal impairment (creatinine clearance <50 ml/min)

PO

Adults 18 yrs and older, Elderly. Initially, two 200 mg tablets as a loading dose on first day. Then one 200 mg tablet q48h for a total of 9 days.

[$] AVAILABLE FORMS/COST

- Tab—Oral: 200 mg, 11's: **$73.58**

CONTRAINDICATIONS: Hypersensitivity to fluoroquinolones, cinoxacin, nalidixic acid

PREGNANCY AND LACTATION: Pregnancy category C; excretion into breast milk unknown; due to the potential for arthropathy and osteochondrosis, use extreme caution in nursing mothers

SIDE EFFECTS

Occasional

Photosensitivity, diarrhea, nausea, headache

Rare

Dyspepsia, dizziness, insomnia, abdominal pain, change in taste

SERIOUS REACTIONS

• Superinfection (particularly enterococcal or fungal overgrowth of nonsusceptible organisms) due to altered bacterial balance may occur (genital-anal pruritus, ulceration or changes in oral mucosa, moderate to severe diarrhea, new or increased fever).

• Hypersensitivity reactions have occurred in those receiving fluoroquinolone therapy.

INTERACTIONS

Drugs

▪ *Aluminum:* Reduced absorption of sparfloxacin; do not take within 4 hr of dose

▪ *Antacids:* Reduced absorption of sparfloxacin; do not take within 4 hr of dose

▪ *Antipyrine:* Inhibits metabolism of antipyrine; increased plasma antipyrine level

▪ *Calcium:* Reduced absorption of sparfloxacin; do not take within 4 hr of dose

▪ *Diazepam:* Inhibits metabolism of diazepam; increased plasma diazepam level

▪ *Didanosine:* Markedly reduced absorption of sparfloxacin; take sparfloxacin 2 hr before didanosine

▪ *Foscarnet:* Coadministration increases seizure risk

▪ *Iron:* Reduced absorption of sparfloxacin; do not take within 4 hr of dose

▪ *Magnesium:* Reduced absorption of sparfloxacin; do not take within 4 hr of dose

▪ *Metoprolol:* Inhibits metabolism of metoprolol; increased plasma metoprolol level

▪ *Phenytoin:* Inhibits metabolism of phenytoin; increased plasma phenytoin level

▪ *Propranolol:* Inhibits metabolism of propranolol; increased plasma propranolol level

▪ *Ropinirole:* Inhibits metabolism of ropinirole; increased plasma ropinirole level

▪ *Sodium bicarbonate:* Reduced absorption of sparfloxacin; do not take within 4 hr of dose

▪ *Sucralfate:* Reduced absorption of sparfloxacin; do not take within 4 hr of dose

▪ *Warfarin:* Inhibits metabolism of warfarin; increases hypoprothrombinemic response to warfarin

▪ *Zinc:* Reduced absorption of sparfloxacin; do not take within 4 hr of dose

SPECIAL CONSIDERATIONS

PATIENT/FAMILY EDUCATION

• Avoid direct or indirect sunlight during treatment and for 5 days after completion of therapy; drink fluids liberally

spectinomycin

(spek-ti-noe-mye'sin)

Rx: Trobicin
Chemical Class: Aminoglycoside derivative
Therapeutic Class: Antibiotic

CLINICAL PHARMACOLOGY
Mechanism of Action: An anti-infective that inhibits protein synthesis of bacterial cells. *Therapeutic Effect:* Produces bacterial cell death.

Pharmacokinetics
Rapid, complete absorption after intramuscular (IM) administration. Protein binding: Unknown. Widely distributed. Excreted unchanged in urine. Partially removed by hemodialysis. **Half-life:** 1.7 hrs.

INDICATIONS AND DOSAGES
Treatment of acute gonococcal urethritis, proctitis in males, acute gonococcal cervicitis and proctitis in females
IM

Adults, Elderly. 2 g once. In areas where antibiotic resistance is known to be prevalent, 4 g (10 ml) divided between 2 injection sites is preferred.

S AVAILABLE FORMS/COST
• Powder, Inj—IM: 400 mg/ml, 2 g: **$28.21**
UNLABELED USES: Treatment of disseminated gonorrhea
CONTRAINDICATIONS: Hypersensitivity to spectinomycin or any component of the formulation
PREGNANCY AND LACTATION: Pregnancy category B; excretion into breast milk unknown
SIDE EFFECTS
Frequent
Pain at IM injection site
Occasional
Dizziness, insomnia

Rare
Decreased urine output
SERIOUS REACTIONS
• Hypersensitivity reaction characterized as chills, fever, nausea, vomiting, urticaria, and anaphylaxis.
SPECIAL CONSIDERATIONS
• Follow with doxycycline 100 mg bid for 7 days (erythromycin if pregnant or allergic)
• Ineffective against syphilis and may mask symptoms
• Give in gluteal muscle; dose >2 g must be divided in 2 gluteal injections

spironolactone

(speer-on-oh-lak'tone)

Rx: Aldactone
Combinations
  Rx: with hydrochlorothiazide
  (Aldactazide)
Chemical Class: Aldosterone antagonist
Therapeutic Class: Antihypertensive; diuretic, potassium-sparing

CLINICAL PHARMACOLOGY
Mechanism of Action: An potassium-sparing diuretic that interferes with sodium reabsorption by competitively inhibiting the action of aldosterone in the distal tubule, thus promoting sodium and water excretion and increasing potassium retention. *Therapeutic Effect:* Produces diuresis; lowers BP; diagnostic aid for primary aldosteronism.

Pharmacokinetics

Route	Onset	Peak	Duration
PO	24–48 hr	48–72 hr	48–72 hr

Well absorbed from the GI tract (absorption increased with food). Protein binding: 91%–98%. Metabolized in the liver to active metabo-

S

lite. Primarily excreted in urine. Unknown if removed by hemodialysis.
Half-life: 0–24 hr (metabolite, 13–24 hr).

INDICATIONS AND DOSAGES
Edema
PO

Adults, Elderly. 25–200 mg/day as a single dose or in 2 divided doses.
Children. 1.5–3.3 mg/kg/day in divided doses.
Neonates. 1–3 mg/kg/day in 1-2 divided doses.

Hypertension
PO

Adults, Elderly. 25-50 mg/day in 1-2 doses/day.
Children. 1.5-3.3 mg/kg/day in divided doses.

Hypokalemia
PO

Adults, Elderly. 25-200 mg/day as a single dose or in 2 divided doses.

Hirsutism
PO

Adults, Elderly. 50-200 mg/day as a single dose or in 2 divided doses.

Primary aldosteronism
PO

Adults, Elderly. 100–400 mg/day as a single dose or in 2 divided doses.
Children. 100–400 mg/m^2/day as a single dose or in 2 divided doses.

Dosage in renal impairment
Dosage interval is modified based on creatinine clearance.

Creatinine Clearance	Interval
10–50 ml/min	Usual dose q12–24h
less than 10 ml/min	Avoid use.

$ AVAILABLE FORMS/COST
• Tab, Plain Coated—Oral: 25 mg, 100's: **$6.25-$68.18**; 50 mg, 100's: **$81.59-$119.74**; 100 mg, 100's: **$120.03-$200.75**

UNLABELED USES: Treatment of female hirsutism, polycystic ovary disease

CONTRAINDICATIONS: Acute renal insufficiency, anuria, BUN and serum creatinine levels more than twice normal values, hyperkalemia

PREGNANCY AND LACTATION: Pregnancy category D; feminization occurs in male rat fetuses; active metabolite excreted in breast milk; compatible with breast-feeding but alternate options preferred; therapy for existing hypertension can be continued throughout pregnancy with minimal risk; initiating for simple edema not recommended; few unequivocal indications for diuretic therapy in pregnancy except for pulmonary edema or congestive heart failure

SIDE EFFECTS
Frequent

Hyperkalemia (in patients with renal insufficiency and those taking potassium supplements), dehydration, hyponatremia, lethargy

Occasional

Nausea, vomiting, anorexia, abdominal cramps, diarrhea, headache, ataxia, somnolence, confusion, fever

Male: Gynecomastia, impotence, decreased libido

Female: Menstrual irregularities (including amenorrhea and postmenopausal bleeding), breast tenderness

Rare

Rash, urticaria, hirsutism

SERIOUS REACTIONS
• Severe hyperkalemia may produce arrhythmias, bradycardia, and EKG changes (tented T waves, widening QRS complex and ST segment depression). These may proceed to cardiac standstill or ventricular fibrillation.

• Cirrhosis patients are at risk for hepatic decompensation if dehydration or hyponatremia occurs.

• Patients with primary aldosteronism may experience rapid weight loss and severe fatigue during high-dose therapy.

INTERACTIONS
Drugs
3 *Ammonium chloride:* Combination may produce systemic acidosis

3 *Angiotensin-converting enzyme inhibitors:* Concurrent mechanisms to decrease potassium excretion; increased risk of hyperkalemia

3 *Angiotensin II receptor antagonists:* Concurrent mechanisms to decrease potassium excretion; increased risk of hyperkalemia

3 *Digitalis glycosides:* False or true increase in digoxin concentrations

3 *Disopyramide:* Increased potassium concentrations may enhance disopyramide effects on myocardial conduction

▲ *Mitotane:* Spironolactone antagonizes the activity of mitotane

❷ *Potassium:* Increased risk of hyperkalemia

3 *Salicylates:* Decreased diuretic (not antihypertensive effect) due to decreased tubular secretion of active metabolite

Labs
• *Corticosteroids:* Marked false increase in plasma corticosteroids
• *Cortisol:* Falsely increased fluorometric methods of measurement
• *Digoxin:* False increases in digoxin concentrations
• *17-Hydroxycorticosteroids:* False increases in urine measurements
• *17-Ketogenic steroids:* Falsely increases urine concentrations

SPECIAL CONSIDERATIONS
MONITORING PARAMETERS
• When used for diagnosis of primary hyperaldosteronism, positive results are: (long test) correction of hyperkalemia and hypertension; (short test) serum potassium increases during administration, but falls upon discontinuation

• Blood pressure, edema, urine output, ECG (if hyperkalemia exists), urine electrolytes, BUN, creatinine, gynecomastia, impotence

---

stanozolol
(stan-oh′zoe-lole)

Rx: Winstrol
Chemical Class: Anabolic steroid; testosterone derivative
Therapeutic Class: Androgen; antiangioedema agent
DEA Class: Schedule III

CLINICAL PHARMACOLOGY
Mechanism of Action: A synthetic testosterone derivative that increases circulating levels of C1 INH and C4 through an increase in general protein anabolism, and more specifically, through an increase in the synthesis of messenger RNA. *Therapeutic Effect:* Decreases swelling of the face, extremities, genitalia, bowel wall and upper respiratory tract

Pharmacokinetics
Metabolized in liver. Primarily excreted in urine. Unknown if removed by hemodialysis.

INDICATIONS AND DOSAGES
Hereditary angioedema prophylaxis
PO
Adults. Initially, 2 mg 2 times/day. Decrease at 1-3 month intervals. Maintenance: 2 mg/day.

$ **AVAILABLE FORMS/COST**
• Tab—Oral: 2 mg, 100's: **$99.45**
UNLABELED USES: Antithrombin III deficiency, arterial occlusions, hemophilia A, lichen sclerosus et atrophicus, liposclerosis, necrobio-

sis lipoidica, osteoporosis, protein C deficiency, rheumatoid arthritis, thrombosis, urticaria

CONTRAINDICATIONS: Cardiac impairment, hypercalcemia, pregnancy, prostatic or breast cancer in males, severe liver or renal disease, hypersensitivity to stanozolol or its components

PREGNANCY AND LACTATION: Pregnancy category X (masculinization); excretion into breast milk unknown; use extreme caution in nursing mothers

SIDE EFFECTS

Frequent

Gynecomastia, acne

Females: Amenorrhea or other menstrual irregularities, hirsutism deepening of voice, clitoral enlargement that may not be reversible when drug is discontinued

Occasional

Edema, nausea, insomnia, oligospermia, male pattern of baldness, bladder irritability, hypercalcemia in immobilized patients or those with breast cancer, hypercholesterolemia

SERIOUS REACTIONS

• Peliosis hepatitis or liver, spleen replaced with blood-filled cysts, hepatic neoplasms and hepatocellular carcinoma have been associated with prolonged high-dosage.

INTERACTIONS

Drugs

❷ *Oral anticoagulants:* Enhanced hypoprothrombinemic response

❸ *Antidiabetic agents:* Enhanced hypoglycemic response

❷ *Cyclosporine:* Increased cyclosporine concentrations

❸ *HMG-CoA reductase inhibitors (lovastatin, pravastatin):* Myositis risk increased

SPECIAL CONSIDERATIONS

• Anabolic steroids have potential for abuse, especially in the athlete

MONITORING PARAMETERS

• LFTs, lipids

• Growth rate in children (X-rays for bone age q6 mo)

---

stavudine (d4T)
(stav'yoo-deen)
Rx: Zerit, Zerit XR
Chemical Class: Nucleoside analog
Therapeutic Class: Antiretroviral

CLINICAL PHARMACOLOGY

Mechanism of Action: Inhibits HIV reverse transcriptase by terminating the viral DNA chain. Also inhibits RNA- and DNA-dependent DNA polymerase, an enzyme necessary for HIV replication. *Therapeutic Effect:* Impedes HIV replication, slowing the progression of HIV infection.

Pharmacokinetics

Rapidly, and completely absorbed after PO administration. Undergoes minimal metabolism. Excreted in urine. **Half-life:** 1.5 hr (increased in renal impairment).

INDICATIONS AND DOSAGES

HIV infection (in combination with other antiretrovirals)

PO

Adults weighing 60 kg or more. 40 mg twice a day.

Adults weighing less than 60 kg. 30 mg twice a day.

Children weighing 30 kg or more. 20 mg twice a day.

Children weighing less than 30 kg. 2 mg/kg/day.

HIV infection in patients with a recent history and complete resolution of peripheral neuropathy or elevated liver function test results

Adults weighing 60 kg or more. 20 mg twice a day.

Adults weighing less than 60 kg. 15 mg twice a day.

Dosage in renal impairment
Dosage and frequency are modified based on creatinine clearance and patient weight.

Creatinine Clearance	Weight 60 kg or more	Weight less than 60 kg
greater than 50 ml/min	40 mg q12h	30 mg q12h
26–50 ml/min	20 mg q12h	15 mg q12h
10–25 ml/min	20 mg q24h	15 mg q24h

§ AVAILABLE FORMS/COST
• Cap, Gel—Oral: 15 mg, 60's: **$318.09**; 20 mg, 60's: **$330.78**; 30 mg, 60's: **$351.35**; 40 mg, 60's: **$357.83**
• Cap, Sus Action—Oral: 37.5 mg, 50 mg, 75 mg, 100 mg, 30's: *cost not available*
• Powder, Reconst-Oral: 1 mg/ml, 200 ml: **$66.45**

CONTRAINDICATIONS: None known.

PREGNANCY AND LACTATION: Pregnancy category C; excreted in breast milk

SIDE EFFECTS
Frequent
Headache (55%), diarrhea (50%), chills and fever (38%), nausea and vomiting, myalgia (35%), rash (33%), asthenia (28%), insomnia, abdominal pain (26%), anxiety (22%), arthralgia (18%), back pain (20%), diaphoresis (19%), malaise (17%), depression (14%)
Occasional
Anorexia, weight loss, nervousness, dizziness, conjunctivitis, dyspepsia, dyspnea
Rare
Constipation, vasodilation, confusion, migraine, urticaria, abnormal vision

SERIOUS REACTIONS
• Peripheral neuropathy, (numbness, tingling, or pain in the hands and feet) occurs in 15% to 21% of patients.
• Ulcerative stomatitis (erythema or ulcers of oral mucosa, glossitis, gingivitis), pneumonia, and benign skin neoplasms occur occasionally.
• Pancreatitis and lactic acidosis occur rarely.

INTERACTIONS
Drugs
⚠ *Zidovudine:* Competitive inhibition of the intracellular phosphorylation of stavudine, concomitant use not recommended

SPECIAL CONSIDERATIONS
PATIENT/FAMILY EDUCATION
• Report neuropathic symptoms (numbness, tingling, or pain in the feet or hands)
MONITORING PARAMETERS
• CBC, SGOT, SGPT

---

streptokinase
(strep-toe-kye′nase)
Rx: Kabikinase, Streptase
Chemical Class: Betahemolytic steptococcus filtrate, purified
Therapeutic Class: Thrombolytic

S

CLINICAL PHARMACOLOGY
Mechanism of Action: An enzyme that activates the fibrinolytic system by converting plasminogen to plasmin, an enzyme that degrades fibrin clots. Acts indirectly by forming a complex with plasminogen, which converts plasminogen to plasmin. Action occurs within the thrombus, on its surface, and in circulating blood. *Therapeutic Effect:* Destroys thrombi.

Pharmacokinetics

Rapidly cleared from plasma by antibodies and the reticuloendothelial system. Route of elimination unknown. Duration of action continues for several hours after drug has been discontinued. **Half-life:** 23 min.

INDICATIONS AND DOSAGES

Acute evolving transmural MI (given as soon as possible after symptoms occur)

IV infusion

Adults, Elderly (1.5 million units diluted to 45 ml). 1.5 million units infused over 60 min.

Intracoronary infusion

Adults, Elderly (250,000 units diluted to 125 ml). Initially, 20,000-units (10-ml) bolus; then, 2,000 units/min for 60 min. Total dose: 140,000 units.

Pulmonary embolism, deep vein thrombosis (DVT), arterial thrombosis and embolism (given within 7 days of onset)

IV infusion

Adults, Elderly (1.5 million units diluted to 90 ml). Initially, 250,000 units infused over 30 min; then, 100,000 units/hr for 24–72 hr for arterial thrombosis or embolism, and pulmonary embolism, 72 hr for DVT.

Intra-aterial infusion

Adults, Elderly (1.5 million units diluted to 45 ml). Initially, 250,000 units infused over 30 min; then 100,000 units/hr for maintenance.

[$] **AVAILABLE FORMS/COST**

- Powder, Inj—Intracoronary; IV: 250,000 U/vial: **$93.75-$138.90**; 750,000 U/vial: **$306.58-$362.15**; 1,500,000 U/vial: **$562.50-$681.70**

CONTRAINDICATIONS: Carcinoma of the brain, cerebrovascular accident, internal bleeding, intracranial surgery, recent streptococcal infection, severe hypertension

PREGNANCY AND LACTATION: Pregnancy category C; no data available for breast-feeding

SIDE EFFECTS

Frequent

Fever, superficial bleeding at puncture sites, decreased BP

Occasional

Allergic reaction, including rash and wheezing; ecchymosis

SERIOUS REACTIONS

- Severe internal hemorrhage may occur.
- Lysis of coronary thrombi may produce life-threatening arrhythmias.

INTERACTIONS

Drugs

[3] *Heparin, oral anticoagulants, drugs that alter platelet function (i.e., aspirin, dipyridamole, abciximab, eptifibitide, tirofiben):* May increase the risk of bleeding

Labs

- *Fibrinogen:* False increase with certain methods
- *Lactate dehydrogenase isoenzymes:* False positive

streptomycin

(strep-toe-mye'sin)

Rx: Streptomycin

Chemical Class: Aminoglycoside

Therapeutic Class: Antibiotic; antituberculosis agent

CLINICAL PHARMACOLOGY

Mechanism of Action: An aminoglycoside that binds directly to the 30S ribosomal subunits causing a faulty peptide sequence to form in the protein chain. *Therapeutic effect:* Inhibits bacterial protein synthesis.

INDICATIONS AND DOSAGES
Tuberculosis
IM
Adults. 15 mg/kg/day. Maximum: 1 g/ay.
Elderly: 10 mg/kg/day. Maximum: 750 mg/day.
Children. 20–40 mg/kg/day. Maximum: 1 g/day.
Dosage in renal impairment:

Creatinine Clearance	Dosage Interval
10–50 ml/min	q24–72h
less than 10 ml/min	q72–96h

Ⓢ **AVAILABLE FORMS/COST**
• Sol, Inj-IM: 1 g/vial: **$10.31**
CONTRAINDICATIONS: Pregnancy
PREGNANCY AND LACTATION: Pregnancy category D; small amounts excreted into breast milk; compatible with breast-feeding (oral absorption poor)
SIDE EFFECTS
Occasional
Hypotension, drowsiness, headache, drug fever, paresthesia, rash, nausea, vomiting, anemia, arthralgia, weakness, tremor
SERIOUS REACTIONS
• Nephrotoxicity (as evidenced by increased BUN and serum creatinine levels and decreased creatinine clearance) may be reversible if the drug is stopped at the first sign of nephrotoxic symptoms.
• Irreversible ototoxicity (manifested as tinnitus, dizziness, ringing or roaring in the ears, and impaired hearing) and neurotoxicity (as evidenced by headache, dizziness, lethargy, tremor, and visual disturbances) occur occasionally. Symptoms of ototoxicity, nephrotoxicity, and neuromuscular toxicity may occur.

INTERACTIONS
Drugs
③ *Amphotericin B, cephalosporins, cyclosporine, NSAIDs:* Additive nephrotoxicity
③ *Carboplatin:* Additive ototoxicity
② *Ethacrynic Acid:* Additive ototoxicity
③ *Methoxyflurane:* Additive nephrotoxicity
② *Neuromuscular blocking agents:* Respiratory depression
③ *Oral anticoagulants:* Enhanced hypoprothrombinemic response
③ *Penicillins, extended-spectrum:* Inactivation of aminoglycoside
Labs
• *Protein:* Falsely increases CSF-protein
• *Sugar:* Falsely increased urine levels via copper reduction methods
• *Urea Nitrogen:* Decreases serum levels
SPECIAL CONSIDERATIONS
• Not usually used for long term therapy secondary to nephrotoxicity and ototoxicity
MONITORING PARAMETERS
• Serum drug levels; therapeutic peak levels 20-30 mcg/ml, toxic peak levels (1 hr after IM administration) >50 mcg/ml
• Keep patient well hydrated

---

succimer
(sux′sim-mer)
Rx: Chemet
Chemical Class: Dimercaprol derivative
Therapeutic Class: Antidote, heavy metal

CLINICAL PHARMACOLOGY
Mechanism of Action: An analog of dimercaprol that forms water soluble chelates with heavy metals

which are excreted renally. *Therapeutic Effect:* Treats lead intoxication in children.

Pharmacokinetics

Rapidly absorbed from the gastrointestinal (GI) tract. Extensively metabolized. Excreted in feces (39%), urine (9%-25%), and lungs (1%). Removed by hemodialysis. **Half-life:** 2 hrs-2 days.

INDICATIONS AND DOSAGES

Lead poisoning, in pediatric patients with blood lead levels about 45 mcg/L

PO

Children 12 months and older. 10 mg/kg q8h for 5 days, then 10 mg/kg q12h for 14 days.

$ AVAILABLE FORMS/COST

• Cap, Gel—Oral: 100 mg, 100's: **$595.35**

UNLABELED USES: Lead poisoning in adults, arsenic intoxication, mercury intoxication

CONTRAINDICATIONS: Hypersensitivity to succimer or any component of its formulation

PREGNANCY AND LACTATION: Pregnancy category C; excretion in breast milk unknown; discourage mothers from breast-feeding during therapy

SIDE EFFECTS

Occasional

Anorexia, diarrhea, nausea, vomiting, rash, odor to breath and urine, increased liver function tests

Rare

Neutropenia

SERIOUS REACTIONS

• Elevated blood lead levels and symptoms of intoxication may occur after succimer therapy due to redistribution of lead from bone to soft tissues and blood.

• Elevated liver function tests have been reported.

INTERACTIONS

Drugs

❷ *Other chelators (e.g., EDTA):* Coadministration not recommended

SPECIAL CONSIDERATIONS

PATIENT/FAMILY EDUCATION

• In children unable to swallow capsule, separate capsule and sprinkle beads on food or on spoon followed by fruit drink

MONITORING PARAMETERS

• Serum transaminases at start of therapy then qwk during therapy
• After therapy, monitor for rebound (because of redistribution of lead from bound stores to soft tissues, blood) qwk until stable

---

sucralfate

(soo-kral'fate)

Rx: Carafate

Chemical Class: Aluminum complex of sulfated sucrose
Therapeutic Class: Antiulcer agent

CLINICAL PHARMACOLOGY

Mechanism of Action: An antiulcer agent that forms an ulcer-adherent complex with proteinaceous exudate, such as albumin, at ulcer site. Also forms a viscous, adhesive barrier on the surface of intact mucosa of the stomach or duodenum. *Therapeutic Effect:* Protects damaged mucosa from further destruction by absorbing gastric acid, pepsin, and bile salts.

Pharmacokinetics

Minimally absorbed from the GI tract. Eliminated in feces, with small amount excreted in urine. Not removed by hemodialysis.

INDICATIONS AND DOSAGES
Active duodenal ulcers
PO

Adults, Elderly. 1 g 4 times a day (before meals and at bedtime) for up to 8 wk.
Maintenance therapy after healing of acute duodenal ulcers
PO

Adults, Elderly. 1 g twice a day.

AVAILABLE FORMS/COST
• Susp—Oral: 1 g/10 ml, 420 ml: **$40.82**
• Tab—Oral: 1 g, 100's: **$14.45-$100.85**

UNLABELED USES: Prevention and treatment of stress-related mucosal damage, especially in acutely or critically ill patients; treatment of gastric ulcer and rheumatoid arthritis; relief of GI symptoms associated with NSAIDs; treatment of gastroesophageal reflux disease

CONTRAINDICATIONS: None known

PREGNANCY AND LACTATION: Pregnancy category B; little systemic absorption, so minimal, if any, excretion into milk expected

SIDE EFFECTS
Frequent (2%)

Constipation

Occasional (less than 2%)

Dry mouth, backache, diarrhea, dizziness, somnolence, nausea, indigestion, rash, hives, itching, abdominal discomfort

SERIOUS REACTIONS
• None known.

INTERACTIONS
Drugs

▣ *Ketoconazole:* Reduces plasma levels of antifungal

▣ *Phenytoin:* Modest reduction in GI absorption of phenytoin

▣ *Quinolones:* Reduced antibiotic levels

▣ *Warfarin:* Isolated cases of reduced hypoprothrombinemic response to warfarin

SPECIAL CONSIDERATIONS
PATIENT/FAMILY EDUCATION
• Take antacids prn for pain relief, but not within ½ hr before or after sucralfate

---

sulfabenzamide / sulfacetamide / sulfathiazole

(sul-fa-ben'za-mide/sul-fa-see'ta-mide/sul-fa-thye'a-zole)

Rx: Gyne Sulf, Sulfabenzamide/Sulfacetamide/Sulfathiazole, Triple Sulfa, V.V.S.

Chemical Class: Sulfonamide derivative

Therapeutic Class: Antibiotic

CLINICAL PHARMACOLOGY
Mechanism of Action: Interferes with synthesis of folic acid that bacteria require for growth by inhibition of para-aminobenzoic acid metabolism. *Therapeutic Effect:* Prevents further bacterial growth.

Pharmacokinetics

Absorption from vagina is variable and unreliable. Primarily metabolized by acetylation. Excreted in urine. **Half-life:** unknown.

INDICATIONS AND DOSAGES
Treatment of Haemophilus vaginalis vaginitis
Vaginal

Adults, Elderly. Insert one applicatorful into vagina twice daily for 4-6 days. Dosage may then be decreased to 1/2 to 1/4 of an applicatorful twice daily.

AVAILABLE FORMS/COST
• Cre—Vag: 3.7%-2.86%-3.42%, 78, 82.5 g: **$3.94-$12.48**/82.5 g

S

• Tab—Vag: 3.7%-2.86%-3.42%, 100's: **$2.69**

CONTRAINDICATIONS: Renal dysfunction, pregnancy (or near term), hypersensitivity to sulfabenzamide, sulfacetamide, sulfathiazole or any component of preparation

PREGNANCY AND LACTATION: Pregnancy category B (category D if used near term; may cause jaundice, hemolytic anemia, and kernicterus in newborns); excreted into breast milk in low concentrations; compatible with breast-feeding in healthy, full-term infants

SIDE EFFECTS

Occasional

Local irritation

Rare

Pruritus urticaria, allergic reactions

SERIOUS REACTIONS

• Superinfection and Stevens-Johnson syndrome occur rarely.

SPECIAL CONSIDERATIONS

PATIENT/FAMILY EDUCATION

• Insert high into vagina

• Do not engage in vaginal intercourse during treatment

---

sulfacetamide
(sul-fa-see'ta-mide)
Rx: AK-Sulf, Bleph-10, Cetamide Sulster, Klaron, Ocu-Sul, Ocusulf-10, Sebizon, Sodium Sulamyd

Combinations

Rx: with prednisolone (Blephamide, Dioptimyd, Metamyd, Vasocidin, Isopto Cetapred); with sulfer (Sulfacet-R); with sulfabenzamide (Sulfathiazole, Sulfa-Gyn, Sulnac, Trysul); with phenylepherine (Vasosulf); with fluorometholone (FML-S)

Chemical Class: Sulfonamide derivative

Therapeutic Class: Antibiotic

CLINICAL PHARMACOLOGY

Mechanism of Action: Interferes with synthesis of folic acid that bacteria require for growth. *Therapeutic Effect:* Prevents further bacterial growth. Bacteriostatic.

Pharmacokinetics

Small amounts may be absorbed into the cornea. Excreted rapidly in urine. **Half-life:** 7-13 hrs.

INDICATIONS AND DOSAGES

Treatment of corneal ulcers, conjunctivitis and other superficial infections of the eye, prophylaxis after injuries to the eye/removal of foreign bodies, adjunctive therapy for trachoma and inclusion conjunctivitis

Ophthalmic

Adults, Elderly. Ointment: Apply small amount in lower conjunctival sac 1-4 times/day and at bedtime. Solution: 1-3 drops to lower conjunctival sac q2-3h. Seborrheic dermatitis, seborrheic sicca (dandruff), secondary bacterial skin infections

Topical

Adults, Elderly. Apply 1-4 times/day.

[$] **AVAILABLE FORMS/COST**

• Lotion—Top: 10%, 60 ml: **$52.21**

• Oint—Ophth: 10%, 3.5 g: **$1.65-$23.09**

• Sol—Ophth: 10%, 1, 2, 2.5, 5, 15 ml: **$1.80-$31.79**/15 ml; 15%, 2, 5, 15 ml: **$2.10**/15 ml; 30%, 15 ml: **$2.40-$25.01**

UNLABELED USES: Treatment of bacterial blepharitis, blepharoconjunctivitis, bacterial keratitis, keratoconjunctivitis

CONTRAINDICATIONS: Hypersensitivity to sulfonamides or any component of preparation (some products contain sulfite), use in combination with silver-containing products

PREGNANCY AND LACTATION: Pregnancy category B (category D if used near term); compatible with breast-feeding in healthy, full-term infants

SIDE EFFECTS

Frequent

Transient ophthalmic burning, stinging

Occasional

Headache

Rare

Hypersensitivity (erythema, rash, itching, swelling, photosensitivity)

SERIOUS REACTIONS

• Superinfection, drug-induced lupus erythematosus, Stevens-Johnson syndrome occur rarely; nephrotoxicity w/high dermatologic concentrations.

INTERACTIONS

Drugs

[2] *Silver preparations:* Incompatible with sulfacetamide

SPECIAL CONSIDERATIONS

PATIENT/FAMILY EDUCATION

• May cause sensitivity to bright light

• Do not touch tip of container to any surface

---

sulfasalazine

(sul-fa-sal'a-zeen)

Rx: Azulfidine, Azulfidine EN-Tabs

Chemical Class: Salicylate derivative; sulfonamide derivative

Therapeutic Class: Disease-modifying antirheumatic drug (DMARD); gastrointestinal antiinflammatory

CLINICAL PHARMACOLOGY

Mechanism of Action: A sulfonamide that inhibits prostaglandin synthesis, acting locally in the colon. *Therapeutic Effect:* Decreases inflammatory response, interferes with GI secretion.

Pharmacokinetics

Poorly absorbed from the GI tract. Cleaved in colon by intestinal bacteria, forming sulfapyridine and mesalamine (5-ASA). Absorbed in colon. Widely distributed. Metabolized in the liver. Primarily excreted in urine. **Half-life:** sulfapyridine, 6–14 hr; 5-ASA, 0.6–1.4 hr.

INDICATIONS AND DOSAGES

Ulcerative colitis

PO

Adults, Elderly. 1 g 3–4 times a day in divided doses q4–6h. Maintenance: 2 g/day in divided doses q6–12h. Maximum: 6 g/day.

Children. 40–75 mg/kg/day in divided doses q4–6h. Maintenance: 30–50 mg/kg/day in divided doses q4–8h. Maximum: 2 g/day. Maximum: 6 g/day.

Rheumatoid arthritis
PO

Adults, Elderly. Initially, 0.5–1 g/day for 1 wk. Increase by 0.5 g/wk, up to 3 g/day.

Juvenile rheumatoid arthritis
PO

Children. Initially, 10 mg/kg/day. May increase by 10 mg/kg/day at weekly intervals. Range: 30–50 mg/kg/day. Maximum: 2 g/day.

🅢 AVAILABLE FORMS/COST
• Tab—Oral: 500 mg, 100's: **$12.75-$38.90**
• Tab, Enteric Coated—Oral: 500 mg, 100's: **$38.42-$46.60**

UNLABELED USES: Treatment of ankylosing spondylitis

CONTRAINDICATIONS: Children younger than 2 years; hypersensitivity to carbonic anhydrase inhibitors, local anesthetics, salicylates, sulfonamides, sulfonylureas, sunscreens containing PABA, or thiazide or loop diuretics; intestinal or urinary tract obstruction; porphyria; pregnancy at term; severe hepatic or renal dysfunction

PREGNANCY AND LACTATION: Pregnancy category B; excreted into breast milk; should be given to nursing mothers with caution because significant adverse effects (bloody diarrhea) may occur in some nursing infants

SIDE EFFECTS
Frequent (33%)

Anorexia, nausea, vomiting, headache, oligospermia (generally reversed by withdrawal of drug)

Occasional (3%)

Hypersensitivity reaction (rash, urticaria, pruritus, fever, anemia)

Rare (less than 1%)

Tinnitus, hypoglycemia, diuresis, photosensitivity

SERIOUS REACTIONS
• Anaphylaxis, Stevens-Johnson syndrome, hematologic toxicity (leukopenia, agranulocytosis, hepatotoxicity, and nephrotoxicity) occur rarely.

INTERACTIONS
Drugs

🎲 *Digoxin:* Sulfasalazine reduces digoxin serum concentrations

🎲 *Folic acid:* Reduced absorption of folic acid

🎲 *Methenamine:* Combination of sulfadiazine and methenamine can result in crystalluria

🎲 *Phenytoin:* Some sulfonamides (sulfaphenazole, sulmethoxazole) increase phenytoin concentrations, requiring dosage adjustment

🎲 *Tolbutamide:* Several sulfonamides (sulfamethizole, sulfaphenazole, sulfisoxasole) can increase plasma sulfonylurea levels and enhance their hypoglycemic effects

🎲 *Warfarin:* Several sulfonamides (trimethoprim-sulfamethoxazole, sulfamethoxazole, sulfamethizole, sulfaphenazole) increase the hypoprothrombinemic response to warfarin via inhibition of metabolism

Labs

• *Bilirubin, conjugated:* Falsely increased in serum

• *Bilirubin, unconjugated:* Falsely decreased in serum

• *Creatinine:* Falsely increased in serum

• *Potassium:* Falsely decreased in serum

• *False positive:* Urinary glucose tests (Benedict's method)

SPECIAL CONSIDERATIONS
PATIENT/FAMILY EDUCATION
• Adequate hydration and urinary output are essential to prevent crystalluria and stone formation

• Avoid prolonged exposure to sunlight

MONITORING PARAMETERS

• Inflammatory bowel disease: Decrease in rectal bleeding or diarrhea in conjunction with mucosal healing

• Rheumatoid arthritis: Tender, swollen joints, visual analogue scale for pain; acute phase reactants (ESR, C-reactive protein), duration of early morning stiffness, preservation of function

• Baseline CBC with differential and liver function tests then every second week during the first 3 months of therapy, monthly during the second 3 months of therapy, then every 3 months thereafter; urinalysis and renal function tests periodically

---

sulfinpyrazone
(sul-fin-pyr′a-zone)
Rx: Anturane
Chemical Class: Pyrazolidine derivative
Therapeutic Class: Antigout agent

CLINICAL PHARMACOLOGY
Mechanism of Action: A uricosuric that increases urinary excretion of uric acid, thereby decreasing blood urate levels. *Therapeutic Effect:* Promotes uric acid excretion and reduces serum uric acid levels.
Pharmacokinetics
Rapidly and completely absorbed from gastrointestinal (GI) tract. Widely distributed. Metabolized in liver to two active metabolite, p-hydroxy-sulfinpyrazone and a sulfide analogue. Excreted primarily in urine. Not removed by hemodialysis. **Half-life:** 2.7- 6 hrs.

INDICATIONS AND DOSAGES
Gout
PO
Adults, Elderly. 100-200 mg 2 times/day. Maximum: 800 mg/day.

S AVAILABLE FORMS/COST
• Cap, Gel—Oral: 200 mg, 100's: **$27.80-$38.75**
• Tab—Oral: 100 mg, 100's: **$14.65-$59.68**

UNLABELED USES: Mitral valve replacement, myocardial infarction

CONTRAINDICATIONS: Active peptic ulcer, blood dyscrasias, GI inflammation, pregnancy (near term), hypersensitivity to sulfinpyrazone, phenylbutazone, other pyrazoles, or any of its components

PREGNANCY AND LACTATION: Pregnancy category C

SIDE EFFECTS
Frequent
Nausea, vomiting, stomach pain
Occasional
Flushed face, headache, dizziness, frequent urge to urinate, rash
Rare
Increased bleeding time, hepatic necrosis, nephrotic syndrome, uric acid stones

SERIOUS REACTIONS
• Hematological toxicity including anemia, leucopenia, agranulocytosis, thrombocytopenia, and aplastic anemia occur rarely.
• Overdose causes a drowsiness, dizziness, anorexia, abdominal pain, hemolytic anemia, acidosis, jaundice, fever, and agranulocytosis.

INTERACTIONS
Drugs
③ *Acetaminophen:* Increased metabolism of acetaminophen by about 20%; increased risk of acetaminophen toxicity
③ *β-blockers:* Reduced hypotensive effects of β-blockers

S

• *Heparinoids:* Risk of augmented bleeding and epidural or spinal hematomas is increased when used concurrently with another agent that affects hemostasis

❷ *Methotrexate:* Increased methotrexate levels with subsequent increased effect and potential toxicity

❷ *Oral anticoagulants:* Inhibit warfarin metabolism and possibly other oral anticoagulants, increasing prothrombin time response; concomitant antiplatelet effects further complicate combined therapy

❸ *Salicylates:* Inhibited uricosuric effect of each other

Labs

• *Cyclosporine:* Falsely decreased serum levels

SPECIAL CONSIDERATIONS

PATIENT/FAMILY EDUCATION

• Take with food, milk, or antacids to decrease stomach upset

• Avoid aspirin and other salicylate-containing products

• Drink plenty of fluids

MONITORING PARAMETERS

• Serum uric acid concentrations, renal function, CBC

---

sulfisoxazole

(sul-fi-sox'-a-zole)

Rx: Gantrisin

Combinations

Rx: with erythromycin (Pediazole, Sulfimycin)

Chemical Class: Sulfonamide derivative

Therapeutic Class: Antibiotic

CLINICAL PHARMACOLOGY

Mechanism of Action: An antibacterial sulphonamide that inhibits bacterial synthesis of dihydrofolic acid by preventing condensation of pteridine with aminobenzoic acid through competitive inhibition of the enzyme dihydropteroate synthetase. *Therapeutic effect:* Bacteriostatic.

Pharmacokinetics

Rapidly and completely absorbed. Small intestine is major site of absorption, but some absorption occurs in the stomach. Exists in the blood as unbound, protein-bound and conjugated forms. Sulfisoxazole is metabolized primarily by acetylation and oxidation in the liver. The free form is considered to be the therapeutically active form. Protein binding: 85%. **Half-life:** 5-8 hours.

INDICATIONS AND DOSAGES

Acute, recurrent or chronic urinary tract infections, meningococcal meningitis, acute otitis media due to Haemophilus influenzae

PO

Infants over 2 Months of Age, Children: One-half of the 24-hour dose initially then 150 mg/kg daily or 4 g/M2 daily for maintanence divided q4-6h. Maximum dose: 6 g daily.

Adults: 2-4 g initially then 4-8 g daily divided q4-6h.

Ⓢ AVAILABLE FORMS/COST

• Susp—Oral: 500 mg/5 ml, 480 ml: **$48.65**/480 ml

• Tab—Oral: 500 mg, 100's: **$3.35-$51.70**

CONTRAINDICATIONS: Patients with a known hypersensitivity to sulfonamides, children younger than 2 months (except in the treatment of congenital toxoplasmosis as adjunctive therapy with pyrimethamine), pregnant women at term, and mothers nursing infants less than 2 months of age.

PREGNANCY AND LACTATION: Pregnancy category C (if used near term; may cause jaundice, hemolytic anemia, and kernicterus in newborns); excreted into breast milk in low concentrations; compatible with breast-feeding in healthy, full-term infants

SIDE EFFECTS

Anaphylaxis, erythema multiforme (Stevens-Johnson syndrome), toxic epidermal necrolysis, exfoliative dermatitis, angioedema, arteritis and vasculitis, allergic myocarditis, serum sickness, rash, urticaria, pruritus, photosensitivity, conjunctival and scleral injection, generalized allergic reactions, generalized skin eruptions, Tachycardia, palpitations, syncope, cyanosis, goiter, diuresis, hypoglycaemia, arthralgia, myalgia, headache, dizziness, peripheral neuritis, paresthesia, convulsions, tinnitus, vertigo, ataxia, intracranial hypertension, cough, shortness of breath, pulmonary infiltrates

SERIOUS REACTIONS

• Fatalities associated with the administration of sulfonamides including Stevens-Johnson Syndrome toxic epidermal necrolysis, fulminant hepatic necrosis, agranulocytosis, aplastic anemia and other blood dyscrasias occur rarely.

• Clinical signs such as rash, sore throat, fever, arthralgia, pallor, purpura or jaundice may be early indications of serious reactions.

INTERACTIONS

Drugs

❷ *Para-aminobenzoic acid (PABA):* PABA may interfere with the antibacterial activity of sulfamethoxazole

❸ *Phenytoin:* Sulfamethoxazole increases phenytoin concentrations, requiring dosage adjustment

❸ *Tolbutamide:* Sulfisoxazole can increase plasma sulfonylurea levels and enhance their hypoglycemic effects

❸ *Warfarin:* Trimethoprim-sulfamethoxazole, sulfamethoxazole increase the hypoprothrombinemic response to warfarin via inhibition of metabolism

Labs

• *Folate:* Falsely decreased serum levels
• *Protein:* Falsely increased in CSF
• *Urobilinogen:* Decreased falsely in feces

SPECIAL CONSIDERATIONS

PATIENT/FAMILY EDUCATION

• Avoid prolonged exposure to sunlight
• Administer with glass of water

MONITORING PARAMETERS

• CBC, renal function tests, urinalysis

---

sulindac

(sul-in′dak)

Rx: Clinoril

Chemical Class: Acetic acid derivative

Therapeutic Class: NSAID; antipyretic; nonnarcotic analgesic

CLINICAL PHARMACOLOGY

Mechanism of Action: An NSAID that produces analgesic and anti-inflammatory effects by inhibiting prostaglandin synthesis. *Therapeutic Effect:* Reduces inflammatory response and intensity of pain.

Pharmacokinetics

Route	Onset	Peak	Duration
PO (Antirheumatic)	7 days	2–3 wk	N/A

Well absorbed from the GI tract. Metabolized in liver to active metabolite. Primarily excreted in urine. Not removed by hemodialysis. **Half-life:** 7.8 hr; metabolite: 16.4 hr.

INDICATIONS AND DOSAGES
Rheumatoid arthritis, osteoarthritis, ankylosing spondylitis
PO

Adults, Elderly. Initially, 150 mg twice a day; may increase up to 400 mg/day.

Acute shoulder pain, gouty arthritis, bursitis, tendinitis
PO

Adults, Elderly. 200 mg twice a day.

$ AVAILABLE FORMS/COST
• Tab—Oral: 150 mg, 100's: **$29.82-$122.54**; 200 mg, 100's: **$38.98-$150.59**

CONTRAINDICATIONS: Active peptic ulcer disease, chronic inflammation of GI tract, GI bleeding or ulceration, history of hypersensitivity to aspirin or NSAIDs

PREGNANCY AND LACTATION: Pregnancy category B (category D if used in 3rd trimester); could cause constriction of the ductus arteriosus *in utero,* persistent pulmonary hypertension of the newborn, or prolonged labor

SIDE EFFECTS
Frequent (9%–4%)

Diarrhea or constipation, indigestion, nausea, maculopapular rash, dermatitis, dizziness, headache

Occasional (3%–1%)

Anorexia, abdominal cramps, flatulence

SERIOUS REACTIONS
• Rare reactions with long-term use include peptic ulcer disease GI bleeding, gastritis, nephrotoxicity (glomerular nephritis, interstitial nephritis, nephrotic syndrome), severe hepatic reactions (cholestasis, jaundice), and severe hypersensitivity reactions (fever, chills, and joint pain).

INTERACTIONS
Drugs
▣ *Aminoglycosides:* Reduced clearance with elevated aminoglycoside levels and potential for toxicity (especially indomethacin in premature infants; other NSAIDs probably)

▣ *Anticoagulants:* Excessive hypoprothrombinemia, decreased platelet aggregation with increased risk of GI bleeding

▣ *Antihypertensives (α-blockers, angiotensin-converting enzyme inhibitors, angiotensin II receptor blockers, β-blockers, diuretics):* Inhibition of antihypertensive and other favorable hemodynamic effects

▣ *Corticosteroids:* Increased risk of GI ulceration

▣ *Cyclosporine:* Increased nephrotoxicity risk

▣ *Lithium:* Decreased clearance of lithium (mediated via prostaglandins) resulting in elevated serum lithium levels and risk of toxicity

▣ *Methotrexate:* Decreased renal secretion of methotrexate resulting in elevated methotrexate levels and risk of toxicity

▣ *Phenylpropanolamine:* Possible acute hypertensive reaction

▣ *Potassium-sparing diuretics:* Additive hyperkalemia potential

▣ *Triamterene:* Acute renal failure reported with addition of indomethacin; caution with other NSAIDs

SPECIAL CONSIDERATIONS
• No significant advantage over other NSAIDs; cost should govern use

PATIENT/FAMILY EDUCATION
• Avoid aspirin and alcoholic beverages
• Take with food, milk, or antacids to decrease GI upset

• Antirheumatic action may not be apparent for several weeks

MONITORING PARAMETERS

• Initial hemogram and fecal occult blood test within 3 mo of starting regular chronic therapy; repeat every 6-12 mo (more frequently in high-risk patients >65 years, peptic ulcer disease, concurrent steroids or anticoagulants); electrolytes, creatinine, and BUN within 3 mo of starting regular chronic therapy; repeat every 6-12 mo

sumatriptan

(soo-ma-trip'tan)

Rx: Imitrex

Chemical Class: Serotonin derivative

Therapeutic Class: Antimigraine agent

CLINICAL PHARMACOLOGY

Mechanism of Action: A serotonin receptor agonist that binds selectively to vascular receptors, producing a vasoconstrictive effect on cranial blood vessels. *Therapeutic Effect:* Relieves migraine headache.

Pharmacokinetics

Route	*Onset*	*Peak*	*Duration*
Nasal	15 min	N/A	24-48 h
PO	30 min	2 h	24-48 h
Subcutaneous	10 min	1 h	24-48 h

Rapidly absorbed after subcutaneous administration. Absorption after PO administration is incomplete, with significant amounts undergoing hepatic metabolism, resulting in low bioavailability (about 14%). Protein binding: 10%-21%. Widely distributed. Undergoes first-pass metabolism in the liver. Excreted in urine. **Half-life:** 2 hr.

INDICATIONS AND DOSAGES

Acute migraine attack

PO

Adults, Elderly. 25- 50 mg. Dose may be repeated after at least 2 hr. Maximum: 100 mg/single dose; 200 mg/24 hr.

Subcutaneous

Adults, Elderly. 6 mg. Maximum: Two 6-mg injections/24 hr (separated by at least 1 hr).

Intranasal

Adults, Elderly. 5-20 mg; may repeat in 2 hr. Maximum: 40 mg/24 hr.

[$] **AVAILABLE FORMS/COST**

• Sol, Inj—SC: 6 mg/0.5 ml, 2's: **$55.91-$117.88**

• Spray, Sol—Nasal: 5 mg/spray, 6's: **$155.08**; 20 mg/spray, 6's: **$155.08**

• Tab—Oral: 25 mg, 9's: **$110.92-$180.65**; 50 mg, 9's: **$151.26-$174.17**; 100 mg, 9's: **$161.44**

CONTRAINDICATIONS: CVA, ischemic heart disease (including angina pectoris, history of MI, silent ischemia, and Prinzmetal's angina), severe hepatic impairment, transient ischemic attack, uncontrolled hypertension, use within 14 days of MAOIs, use within 24 hr of ergotamine preparations or

PREGNANCY AND LACTATION: Pregnancy category C; excreted in breast milk in animals, no data in humans

SIDE EFFECTS

Frequent

Oral (10%-5%): Tingling, nasal discomfort

Subcutaneous (greater than 10%): Injection site reactions, tingling, warm or hot sensation, dizziness, vertigo

Nasal (greater than 10%): Bad or unusual taste, nausea, vomiting

Occasional

Oral (5%-1%): Flushing, asthenia, visual disturbances

S

Subcutaneous (10%-2%): Burning sensation, numbness, chest discomfort, drowsiness, asthenia

Nasal (5%-1%): Nasopharyngeal discomfort, dizziness

Rare

Oral (less than 1%): Agitation, eye irritation, dysuria

Subcutaneous (less than 2%): Anxiety, fatigue, diaphoresis, muscle cramps, myalgia

Nasal (less than 1%): Burning sensation

SERIOUS REACTIONS

• Excessive dosage may produce tremor, red extremities, reduced respirations, cyanosis, seizures, and paralysis.

• Serious arrhythmias occur rarely, especially in patients with hypertension, diabetes, or a strong family history of coronary artery disease; obese patients; and smokers.

INTERACTIONS

Drugs

🔳 *Ergot-containing drugs:* Potential for prolonged vasospastic reactions and additive vasoconstriction, theoretical precaution

② *Sibutramine:* Increased risk of serotonin syndrome

SPECIAL CONSIDERATIONS

• First inj should be administered under medical supervision

PATIENT/FAMILY EDUCATION

• Use only to treat migraine headache; not for prevention

---

tacrine

(tack'rin)

Rx: Cognex

Chemical Class: Cholinesterase inhibitor; monoamine acridine derivative

Therapeutic Class: Antidementia agent

CLINICAL PHARMACOLOGY

Mechanism of Action: A cholinesterase inhibitor that inhibits the enzyme acetylcholinesterase, thus increasing the concentration of acetylcholine at cholinergic synapses and enhancing cholinergic function in the CNS. *Therapeutic Effect:* Slows the progression of Alzheimer's disease.

INDICATIONS AND DOSAGES

Alzheimer's disease

PO

Adults, Elderly. Initially, 10 mg 4 times a day for 6 wk, followed by 20 mg 4 times a day for 6 wk, 30 mg 4 times a day for 12 wk, then 40 mg 4 times a day if needed.

Dosage in hepatic impairment

For patients with (SGPT)ALT greater than 3-5 times normal, decrease the dose by 40 mg/day and resume the normal dose when (SGPT)ALT returns to normal. For patients with (SGPT)ALT greater than 5 times normal, stop treatment and resume it when (SGPT)ALT returns to normal.

Ⓢ **AVAILABLE FORMS/COST**

• Cap, Gel—Oral: 10, 20, 30, 40 mg, 120's: **$350.05**

CONTRAINDICATIONS: Known hypersensitivity to tacrine, patients previously treated with tacrine who developed jaundice.

PREGNANCY AND LACTATION:
Pregnancy category C; excretion into breast milk unknown

SIDE EFFECTS

Frequent (28%-11%)
Headache, nausea, vomiting, diarrhea, dizziness

Occasional (9%-4%)
Fatigue, chest pain, dyspepsia, anorexia, abdominal pain, flatulence, constipation, confusion, agitation, rash, depression, ataxia, insomnia, rhinitis, myalgia

Rare (less than 3%)
Weight loss, anxiety, cough, facial flushing, urinary frequency, back pain, tremor

SERIOUS REACTIONS

• Overdose can cause cholinergic crisis, marked by increased salivation, lacrimation, bradycardia, respiratory depression, hypotension, and increased muscle weakness. Treatment usually consists of supportive measures and an anticholinergic such as atropine.

INTERACTIONS

Drugs

▣ *Anticholinergics:* Inhibits anticholinergic effect, centrally acting anticholinergics may inhibit effect of tacrine

▣ *β-blockers:* Additive bradycardia

▣ *Cholinergics:* Increased cholinergic effects

▣ *Cimetidine:* Increased tacrine levels

▣ *Levodopa:* Decreased levodopa effect

▣ *Quinolones:* Inhibition of tacrine metabolism

▣ *Serotonin reuptake inhibitors:* Increased tacrine concentrations

▣ *Smoking:* Markedly reduces tacrine levels

▣ *Theophylline:* Increased theophylline concentrations

SPECIAL CONSIDERATIONS

• Transaminase elevation is the most common reason for withdrawal of drug (8%); monitor ALT q wk for first 18 wk, then decrease to q 3 mo; when dose is increased, monitor qwk for 6 wk

• If elevations occur, modify dose as follows: ALT ≤3 times upper limit normal (ULN) continue current dose; ALT >3 to ≤5 times ULN reduce dose by 40 mg qd and resume dose titration when within normal limits; ALT >5 times ULN stop treatment; rechallenge may be tried if ALT is <10 times ULN

• Do not rechallenge if clinical jaundice develops

• Improvement in symptoms of dementia statistically, but perhaps not clinically significant; discontinue therapy if improvement not evident to family members and clinician

---

tacrolimus

(tak-roe-leem'us)

Rx: Prograf, Protopic
Chemical Class: Macrolide derivative
Therapeutic Class: Immunosuppressant

CLINICAL PHARMACOLOGY

Mechanism of Action: An immunologic agent that inhibits T-lymphocyte activation by binding to intracellular proteins, forming a complex, and inhibiting phosphatase activity. *Therapeutic Effect:* Suppresses the immunologically mediated inflammatory response; prevents organ transplant rejection.

Pharmacokinetics

Variably absorbed after PO administration (food reduces absorption). Protein binding: 75%–97%. Extensively metabolized in the liver. Excreted in urine. Not removed by hemodialysis. **Half-life:** 11.7 hr.

INDICATIONS AND DOSAGES

Prevention of liver transplant rejection

PO

Adults, Elderly. 0.1-0.15 mg/kg/day in 2 divided doses 12 hr apart.

Children. 0.15–0.2 mg/kg/day in 2 divided doses 12 hr apart.

IV

Adults, Elderly, Children. 0.03–0.05 mg/kg/day as a continuous infusion.

Prevention of kidney transplant rejection

PO

Adults, Elderly. 0.2 mg/kg/day in 2 divided doses 12 hr apart

IV

Adults, Elderly. 0.03-0.05 mg/kg/day as continuous infusion.

Atopic dermatitis

Topical

Adults, Elderly, Children 2 yr and older. Apply 0.03% ointment to affected area twice a day. 0.1% ointment may be used in adults and the elderly. Continue until 1 wk after symptoms have cleared.

$ **AVAILABLE FORMS/COST**

- Cap-Oral: 0.5 mg, 100's: **$227.03**; 1 mg, 100's: **$375.39**; 5 mg, 100's: **$1,858.83**
- Sol, Inj-IV: 5 mg/ml: **$125.05**
- Oint-Top: 0.03%, 30, 60, 100 g: **$60.43**/30 g; 0.1%, 30, 60, 100 g: **$64.60**/30 g

UNLABELED USES: Prevention of organ rejection in patients receiving allogeneic bone marrow, heart, pancreas, pancreatic island cell, or small-bowel transplant, treatment of autoimmune disease, severe recalcitrant psoriasis

CONTRAINDICATIONS: Concurrent use with cyclosporine (increases the risk of nephrotoxicity), hypersensitivity to HCO-60 polyoxyl 60 hydrogenated castor oil (used in solution for injection), hypersensitivity to tacrolimus

PREGNANCY AND LACTATION: Pregnancy category C; excreted in breast milk; avoid nursing

SIDE EFFECTS

Frequent (greater than 30%)

Headache, tremor, insomnia, paresthesia, diarrhea, nausea, constipation, vomiting, abdominal pain, hypertension

Occasional (29%–10%)

Rash, pruritus, anorexia, asthenia, peripheral edema, photosensitivity

SERIOUS REACTIONS

- Nephrotoxicity (characterized by increased serum creatinine level and decreased urine output), neurotoxicity (including tremor, headache, and mental status changes), and pleural effusion are common adverse reactions.
- Thrombocytopenia, leukocytosis, anemia, atelectasis, sepsis, and infection occur occasionally.

INTERACTIONS

Drugs

[3] *Azole antifungals, bromocriptine, calcium channel blockers, cimetidine, danazol, ethinyl estradiol, GI prokinetic agents, macrolide antibiotics, nefazodone, omeprazole, protease inhibitors:* Decreased metabolism or increased bioavailability of tacrolimus

[3] *Carbamazepine, phenobarbital, phenytoin, rifamycins:* Decreased tacrolimus blood levels

⚠ *Cyclosporine:* Additive/synergistic nephrotoxicity, do not coadminister, discontinue tacrolimus or cyclosporine for 24 hr before starting the other

⚠ *Live vaccines:* Avoid use of live vaccines, vaccinations may be less effective

❷ *Nephrotoxic agents (aminoglycosides, amphotericin B, cisplatin, ganciclovir):* Potential for additive/synergistic nephrotoxicity

❷ *Potassium-sparing diuretics:* Increased risk of hyperkalemia

❸ *St. John's wort (hypericum perforatum):* Potential for decreased plasma tacrolimus concentrations

SPECIAL CONSIDERATIONS
• Black patients may need higher doses in kidney transplant
• Also known as FK 506

MONITORING PARAMETERS
• Regularly assess serum creatinine, potassium, and fasting glucose
• Whole blood tacrolimus concentrations as measured by ELISA may be helpful in assessing rejection and toxicity, median trough concentrations measured after the second week of therapy ranged from 9.8 to 19.4 mg/ml

---

tadalafil
Rx: Cialis
Chemical Class: CGMP specific phosphodiesterase inhibitor
Therapeutic Class: Anti-impotence agent

CLINICAL PHARMACOLOGY
Mechanism of Action: An erectile dysfunction agent that inhibits phosphodiesterase type 5, the enzyme responsible for degrading cyclic guanosine monophosphate in the corpus cavernosum of the penis, resulting in smooth muscle relaxation and increased blood flow. *Therapeutic Effect:* Facilitates an erection.

Pharmacokinetics

Route	Onset	Peak	Duration
PO	16 min	2 hr	36 hr

Rapidly absorbed after PO administration. Drug has no effect on penile blood flow without sexual stimulation. **Half-life:** 17.5 hour.

INDICATIONS AND DOSAGES
Erectile dysfunction
PO

Adults, Elderly. 10 mg 30 min before sexual activity. Dose may be increased to 20 mg or decreased to 5 mg, based on patient tolerance. Maximum dosing frequency is once daily.

Dosage in renal impairment
For patients with a creatinine clearance of 31-50 ml/min, the starting dose is 5 mg before sexual activity once a day and the maximum dose is 10 mg no more frequently than once q48h.

For patients with a creatinine clearance of less than 31 ml/min, the starting dose is 5 mg before sexual activity once a day.

Dosage in mild or moderate hepatic impairment
Patients with Child-Pugh class A or B hepatic impairment should take no more than 10 mg once a day.

💲 **AVAILABLE FORMS/COST**
• Tab—Oral: 5 mg, 10 mg, 20 mg, 30's; all: **$303.75**

CONTRAINDICATIONS: Concurrent use of alpha-adrenergic blockers (other than the minimum dose tamsulosin), concurrent use of sodium nitroprusside or nitrates in any form, severe hepatic impairment

PREGNANCY AND LACTATION: Pregnancy category B; not indicated for use in women

T

SIDE EFFECTS
Occasional

Headache, dyspepsia, back pain, myalgia, nasal congestion, flushing

SERIOUS REACTIONS
• Prolonged erections (lasting over 4 hours) and priapism (painful erections lasting over 6 hours) occur rarely.

INTERACTIONS
Drugs

■ *Alcohol:* Substantial alcohol consumption can increase risk of blood pressure lowering effects

▲ *Alpha-adrenergic blockers:* Concurrent use with tadalafil contraindicated (except tamsulosin at 0.4 mg qd)

■ *CYP3A4 inducers (carbamazepine, phenobarbital, phenytoin, rifampin):* Decreased tadalafil levels likely

❷ *CYP3A4 inhibitors (erythromycin, itraconazole, ketoconazole, ritonavir):* Potent inhibitors significantly increase tadalafil levels, max tadalafil dose 10 mg, dosing interval not more frequent than q72 hr

▲ *Nitrates:* Concurrent use with tadalafil contraindicated

SPECIAL CONSIDERATIONS
PATIENT/FAMILY EDUCATION
• Sexual stimulation is required for an erection to occur after taking tadalafil
• Erectile function improved up to 36 hr following dose

---

tamoxifen
(ta-mox'i-fen)
Rx: Nolvadex
Chemical Class: Estrogen agonist-antagonist; triphenylethylene derivative
Therapeutic Class: Antineoplastic

CLINICAL PHARMACOLOGY
Mechanism of Action: A nonsteroidal antiestrogen that competes with estradiol for estrogen-receptor binding sites in the breasts, uterus, and vagina. *Therapeutic Effect:* Inhibits DNA synthesis and estrogen response.

Pharmacokinetics

Well absorbed from the GI tract. Metabolized in the liver. Primarily eliminated in feces by biliary system. **Half-life:** 7 days.

INDICATIONS AND DOSAGES
Adjunctive treatment of breast cancer

PO

Adults, Elderly. 20-40 mg/day. Give doses greater than 20 mg/day in divided doses.

Prevention of breast cancer in high-risk women

PO

Adults, Elderly. 20 mg/day.

Ⓢ **AVAILABLE FORMS/COST**
• Tab-Oral: 10 mg, 60's: **$110.63-$134.73**; 20 mg, 90's: **$377.10-$455.08**

UNLABELED USES: Induction of ovulation

CONTRAINDICATIONS: None known.

PREGNANCY AND LACTATION: Pregnancy category D; excretion into breast milk unknown

SIDE EFFECTS
Frequent

Women (greater than 10%): Hot flashes, nausea, vomiting

Occasional

Women (9%-1%): Changes in menstruation, genital itching, vaginal discharge, endometrial hyperplasia or polyps

Men: Impotence, decreased libido

Men and women: Headache, nausea, vomiting, rash, bone pain, confusion, weakness, somnolence

SERIOUS REACTIONS
• Retinopathy, corneal opacity, and decreased visual acuity have been noted in patients receiving extremely high dosages (240-320 mg/day) for longer than 17 months.

INTERACTIONS
Drugs

❷ *Aminoglutethimide:* Reduces tamoxifen concentrations

SPECIAL CONSIDERATIONS
• Treatment duration >5 yr may provide no further benefit and increase risk of endometrial cancer for some women; reevaluate the need for continued therapy

• The Gail Model Risk Assessment Tool is available to health care professionals by calling (800) 456-3669 (ext. 3838)

• Premenopausal women should use nonhormonal contraception during treatment

MONITORING PARAMETERS
• Endometrial biopsy indicated for abnormal vaginal bleeding

---

tamsulosin
(tam-sool'o-sin)
Rx: Flomax
Chemical Class: Quinazoline
Therapeutic Class: α_1-adrenergic blocker

CLINICAL PHARMACOLOGY
Mechanism of Action: An alpha$_1$ antagonist that targets receptors around bladder neck and prostate capsule. *Therapeutic Effect:* Relaxes smooth muscle and improves urinary flow and symptoms of prostatic hyperplasia.

Pharmacokinetics

Well absorbed and widely distributed. Protein binding: 94%-99%. Metabolized in the liver. Primarily excreted in urine. Unknown if removed by hemodialysis. **Half-life:** 9-13 hr.

INDICATIONS AND DOSAGES
Benign prostatic hyperplasia
PO

Adults. 0.4 mg once a day, approximately 30 min after same meal each day. May increase dosage to 0.8 mg if inadequate response in 2-4 wk.

§ **AVAILABLE FORMS/COST**
• Cap—Oral: 0.4 mg 100's: **$207.26**

CONTRAINDICATIONS: History of sensitivity to tamsulosin

PREGNANCY AND LACTATION: Pregnancy category B; not indicated for use in women

SIDE EFFECTS
Frequent (9%-7%)

Dizziness, somnolence

Occasional (5%-3%)

Headache, anxiety, insomnia, orthostatic hypotension

Rare (less than 2%)

Nasal congestion, pharyngitis, rhinitis, nausea, vertigo, impotence

SERIOUS REACTIONS

• First-dose syncope (hypotension with sudden loss of consciousness) may occur within 30 to 90 minutes after administration of initial dose and may be preceded by tachycardia (pulse rate of 120-160 beats/minute).

INTERACTIONS

Drugs

3 β-*blockers:* Enhanced "first-dose" phenomenon

SPECIAL CONSIDERATIONS

PATIENT/FAMILY EDUCATION

• Consider administration of first dose at bedtime; caution following first 12 hr after initiation or reinitiation of therapy for "first dose phenomenon"

---

tazarotene

(ta-zare´-oh-teen)

Rx: Avage, Tazorac
Chemical Class: Retinoid prodrug; vitamin A derivative
Therapeutic Class: Antiacne agent; antipsoriatic

CLINICAL PHARMACOLOGY

Mechanism of Action: Modulates differentiation and proliferation of epithelial tissue, binds, selectively to retinoic acid receptors. *Therapeutic effect:* Restores normal differentiation of the epidermis and reduction in epidermal inflammation.

Pharmacokinetics

Minimal systemic absorption occurs through the skin. Binding to plasma proteins is greater than 99%. Metabolism is in the skin and liver. Elimination occurs through the fecal and renal pathways. **Half-life:** 18 hours.

INDICATIONS AND DOSAGES

Psoriasis

Topical
Adults, adolescents, children >12 years. Thin film applied once daily in the evening; only cover the lesions, and area should be dry before application

Acne vulgaris

Topical
Adults, adolescents, children > 12 years. Thin film applied to affected areas once daily in the evening, after face is gently cleansed and dried.

Fine facial wrinkles, facial mottled hyperpigmentation (liver spots), hypopigmentation associated with photoaging

Topical
Adults. Thin film applied to affected areas once daily in the evening, after face is gently cleansed and dried.

AVAILABLE FORMS/COST

• Cre—Top: 0.05%, 15, 30, 60 g: **$80.23**/30 g; 0.1%, 15, 30, 60 g: **$78.20**/30 g
• Gel—Top: 0.05%, 30, 100 g: **$80.23**/30 g; 0.1%, 30, 100 g: **$85.24**/30 g

CONTRAINDICATIONS: Should not be used in pregnant women, patients with hypersensitivity to tazarotene, benzyl alcohol, or any one of its components.

PREGNANCY AND LACTATION: Pregnancy category X (some evidence to suggest potential increased safety margin vs other retinoids based on minimal absorption and short half life); excreted into breast milk of rats; no human data

SIDE EFFECTS

Frequent

Desquamation, burning or stinging, dry skin, itching, erythema, worsening of psoriasis, irritation, skin pain, pruritis, xerosis, photosensitivity

Occasional
Irritation, skin pain, fissuring, localized edema, skin discoloration, rash, desquamation, contact dermatitis, skin inflammation, bleeding, dry skin, hypertriglyceridema, peripheral edema, acne vulgaris, cheilitis

SPECIAL CONSIDERATIONS

- Attractive alternative to oral retinoid therapy in psoriasis (e.g., etretinate), primarily due to less toxicity. Structural changes to the basic retinoid structure (e.g., conformational rigidity) are claimed to enhance therapeutic efficacy and reduce the local toxicity associated with topical tretinoin (retinoic acid). However, place in therapy should await direct comparisons vs. standard regimens in terms of efficacy, toxicity, and cost

tegaserod

(teh-gas'er-od)

Rx: Zelnorm

Chemical Class: Pentylcarbazimidamide derivative

Therapeutic Class: Gastrointestinal prokinetic agent

CLINICAL PHARMACOLOGY

Mechanism of Action: An anti-irritable bowel syndrome (IBS) agent that binds to 5-HT_4 receptors in the GI tract. *Therapeutic Effect:* Triggers a peristaltic reflex in the gut, increasing bowel motility.

Pharmacokinetics
Rapidly absorbed. Widely distributed. Protein binding: 98%. Metabolized by hydrolysis in the stomach and by oxidation and conjugation of the primary metabolite. Primarily excreted in feces. **Half-life:** 11 hr.

INDICATIONS AND DOSAGES

IBS
PO
Adults, Elderly women. 6 mg twice a day for 4–6 wk.

Chronic constipation
PO
Adults. 6 mg 2 times/day.

[$] **AVAILABLE FORMS/COST**

- Tab—Oral: 2 mg, 6 mg, 60's; all: **$161.44**

CONTRAINDICATIONS: Abdominal adhesions, diarrhea, history of bowel obstruction, moderate to severe hepatic impairment, severe renal impairment, suspected sphincter of Oddi dysfunction, symptomatic gallbladder disease

PREGNANCY AND LACTATION: Pregnancy category B; excretion in human milk unknown, use caution in nursing mothers (excreted in milk of lactating rats with a high milk to plasma ratio)

SIDE EFFECTS

Frequency (greater than 5%)
Headache, abdominal pain, diarrhea, nausea, flatulence

Occasional (5%–2%)
Dizziness, migraine, back pain, extremity pain

SERIOUS REACTIONS

- None known.

SPECIAL CONSIDERATIONS

PATIENT/FAMILY EDUCATION

- Take before a meal
- Consult prescriber if severe diarrhea or diarrhea accompanied by cramping, abdominal pain, or dizziness occurs

T

telithromycin
(tell-ith'roe-my-sin)
Rx: Ketek
Chemical Class: Macrolide
derivative
Therapeutic Class: Antibiotic

CLINICAL PHARMACOLOGY
Mechanism of Action: A ketolide
that blocks protein synthesis by
binding to ribosomal receptor sites
on the bacterial cell wall. *Therapeutic Effect:* Bactericidal.
Pharmacokinetics
Protein binding: 60%-70%. More of
drug is concentrated in WBCs than
in plasma, and drug is eliminated
more slowly from WBCs than from
plasma. Partially metabolized by the
liver. Minimally excreted in feces
and urine. **Half-life:** 10 hr.

INDICATIONS AND DOSAGES
Chronic bronchitis, sinusitis
PO
Adults, Elderly. 800 mg once a day
for 5 days.
Community-acquired pneumonia
PO
Adults, Elderly. 800 mg once a day
for 7-10 days.

CONTRAINDICATIONS: Hypersensitivity to macrolide antibiotics,
concurrent use of cisapride or pimozide

PREGNANCY AND LACTATION:
Pregnancy category C; excreted in
breast milk of rats; unknown if excreted in human milk

SIDE EFFECTS
Occasional (11%-4%)
Diarrhea, nausea, headache, dizziness
Rare (3%-2%)
Vomiting, loose stools, altered taste,
dry mouth, flatulence, visual disturbances

SERIOUS REACTIONS
• Hepatic dysfunction, severe hypersensitivity reaction, and atrial arrhythmias occur rarely.
• Antibiotic-associated colitis and
other superinfections may result
from altered bacterial balance.

INTERACTIONS
Drugs
▣ *Intraconazole, ketoconazole
(C3A4 inhibitors):* increased
telithromycin levels
❷ *Simvastatin, lovastatin, atrovastation, midazolam , triazolam (CYP
34A substrates):* increased levels of
these drugs and risk of myopathy
▣ *Metoprolol (CYP 2D6 substrates):* increased metoprolol levels but half-life unchanged
▣ *Digoxin, theophylline:* increased
peak and trough levels
▣ *Sotalol:* decreased telithromycin
absorption
❷ *Rifampin, phenytoin, carbamazepine, phenobarbital:* decreased
(approx 80% with rifampin) levels
of telithromycin
⚠ *Cisapride, pimozide:* increased
levels of these drugs, contraindicated per manufacturer
▣ *Carbamazepine, cyclosporine,
tacrolimus, phenytoin, sirolimus,
hexobarbital (CYP 450 substrates):*
increased drug levels
❷ *Ergotatime, dihydroergotamine:*
ergot toxicity (vasospasm and dysethesia) reported
❷ *Quinidine, procainamide,
dofetilide:* possible arrythmia

SPECIAL CONSIDERATIONS
PATIENT/FAMILY EDUCATION
• May take without regard to meals,
swallow whole.
• Do not take if you or a close relative has a rare heart condition called
prolongation of the QT interval. Notify provider if you faint while on
this medication

- Do not take with diuretics or if you have low blood potassium or magnesium levels

---

telmisartan
(tel-meh-sar'-tan)
Rx: Micardis
Chemical Class: Angiotensin II receptor antagonist
Therapeutic Class: Antihypertensive

CLINICAL PHARMACOLOGY
Mechanism of Action: An angiotensin II receptor, type AT_1, antagonist that blocks vasoconstrictor and aldosterone-secreting effects of angiotensin II, inhibiting the binding of angiotensin II to the AT_1 receptors. *Therapeutic Effect:* Causes vasodilation, decreases peripheral resistance, and decreases BP.
Pharmacokinetics
Rapidly and completely absorbed after PO administration. Protein binding: 99%. Undergoes metabolism in the liver to inactive metabolite. Excreted in feces. Unknown if removed by hemodialysis. **Half-life:** 24 hr.

INDICATIONS AND DOSAGES
Hypertension
PO
Adults, Elderly. 40 mg once a day. Range: 20-80 mg/day.

S AVAILABLE FORMS/COST
- Tab—Oral: 20 mg, 40 mg, 28's: **$45.58**; 80 mg, 28's: **$49.40**

UNLABELED USES: Treatment of CHF

CONTRAINDICATIONS: None known.

PREGNANCY AND LACTATION
Pregnancy category C, first trimester—category D, second and third trimesters; drugs acting directly on the renin-angiotensin-aldosterone system are documented to cause fetal harm (hypotension, oligohydramnios, neonatal anemia, hyperkalemia, neonatal skull hypoplasia, anuria, and renal failure); neonatal limb contractures, craniofacial deformities, and hypoplastic lung development

SIDE EFFECTS
Occasional (7%-3%)
Upper respiratory tract infection, sinusitis, back or leg pain, diarrhea
Rare (1%)
Dizziness, headache, fatigue, nausea, heartburn, myalgia, cough, peripheral edema

SERIOUS REACTIONS
- Overdosage may manifest as hypotension and tachycardia. Bradycardia occurs less often.

INTERACTIONS
Drugs
▣ *Digoxin:* 49% increase in digoxin peak, 20% increase in trough digoxin concentrations

SPECIAL CONSIDERATIONS
- Potentially as or more effective than angiotensin-converting enzyme inhibitors, without cough; no evidence for reduction in morbidity and mortality as first-line agents in hypertension, yet; whether they provide the same cardiac and renal protection also still tentative; like ACE inhibitors, less effective in black patients

PATIENT/FAMILY EDUCATION
- Call your clinician immediately if note following side effects: wheezing; lip, throat, or face swelling; hives or rash

MONITORING PARAMETERS
- Baseline electrolytes, urinalysis, blood urea nitrogen and creatinine with recheck at 2-4 wk after initiation (sooner in volume-depleted patients); monitor sitting blood pres-

T

sure; watch for symptomatic hypotension, particularly in volume-depleted patients

---

temazepam
(te-maz'e-pam)
Rx: Restoril
Chemical Class: Benzodiazepine
Therapeutic Class: Hypnotic
DEA Class: Schedule IV

CLINICAL PHARMACOLOGY
Mechanism of Action: A benzodiazepine that enhances the action of the inhibitory neurotransmitter gamma-aminobutyric acid, resulting in CNS depression. *Therapeutic Effect:* Induces sleep.
Pharmacokinetics
Well absorbed from the GI tract. Protein binding: 96%. Widely distributed. Crosses the blood-brain barrier. Metabolized in the liver. Primarily excreted in urine. Not removed by hemodialysis. **Half-life:** 4-18 hr.

INDICATIONS AND DOSAGES
Insomnia
PO
Adults, Children 18 yr and older. 15-30 mg at bedtime.
Elderly, Debilitated. 7.5-15 mg at bedtime.

$ AVAILABLE FORMS/COST
• Cap, Gel—Oral: 7.5 mg, 100's: **$89.00-$237.26**; 15 mg, 100's: **$10.64-$326.33**; 30 mg, 100's: **$28.75-$364.93**

CONTRAINDICATIONS: Angle-closure glaucoma; CNS depression; pregnancy or breast-feeding; severe, uncontrolled pain; sleep apnea

PREGNANCY AND LACTATION: Pregnancy category X; may cause sedation and poor feeding in nursing infant

SIDE EFFECTS
Frequent
Somnolence, sedation, rebound insomnia (may occur for 1-2 nights after drug is discontinued), dizziness, confusion, euphoria
Occasional
Asthenia, anorexia, diarrhea
Rare
Paradoxical CNS excitement or restlessness (particularly in elderly or debilitated patients)

SERIOUS REACTIONS
• Abrupt or too-rapid withdrawal may result in pronounced restlessness, irritability, insomnia, hand tremor, abdominal or muscle cramps, vomiting, diaphoresis, and seizures.
• Overdose results in somnolence, confusion, diminished reflexes, respiratory depression, and coma.

INTERACTIONS
Drugs
▣ *Cimetidine, disulfiram:* Increased benzodiazepine levels
▣ *Clozapine:* Possible increased risk of cardiorespiratory collapse
▣ *Ethanol:* Adverse psychomotor effects
▣ *Rifampin:* Reduced benzodiazepine levels

SPECIAL CONSIDERATIONS
• Good benzodiazepine choice for elderly and patients with liver disease (phase II metabolism and lack of active metabolites)

PATIENT/FAMILY EDUCATION
• Withdrawal symptoms may occur if administered chronically and discontinued abruptly; symptoms include dysphoria, abdominal and muscle cramps, vomiting, sweating, tremor, and seizure
• May cause impairment the day following administration, exercise caution with hazardous tasks and driving

tenofovir

(ten-oh'foh-veer)
Rx: Viread
Combinations
Rx: with emtricitabine (Truvada)
Chemical Class: Nucleotide analog
Therapeutic Class: Antiviral

CLINICAL PHARMACOLOGY
Mechanism of Action: A nucleotide analogue that inhibits HIV reverse transcriptase by being incorporated into viral DNA, resulting in DNA chain termination. *Therapeutic Effect:* Slows HIV replication and reduces HIV RNA levels (viral load).
INDICATIONS AND DOSAGES
HIV infection (in combination with other antiretrovirals)
PO
Adults, Elderly, Children 18 yr and older. 300 mg once a day.
S AVAILABLE FORMS/COST
• Tab, Coated—Oral: 300 mg, 30's: **$456.00**
CONTRAINDICATIONS: None known.
PREGNANCY AND LACTATION: Pregnancy category B; breast milk excretion unknown; the CDC recommends that HIV-infected mothers not breast-feed their infants to avoid risking postnatal transmission of HIV
SIDE EFFECTS
Occasional
GI disturbances (diarrhea, flatulence, nausea, vomiting)
SERIOUS REACTIONS
• Lactic acidosis and hepatomegaly with steatosis occur rarely, but may be severe.

INTERACTIONS
Drugs
3 *Didanosine (buffered formulation):* Tenofovir decreases didanosine AUC by 44% (When co-administered with didanosine, tenofovir should be administered 2 hours before or 1 hour after administration of didanosine)
3 *Lopinavir/ritonavir:* Increases tenofovir AUC by 34%; tenofovir decreases AUC of lopinavir/ritonavir by 24% (when co-administered with lopinavir/ritonavir, tenofovir should be administered 2 hours before or 1 hour after administration of lopinavir/ritonavir)
SPECIAL CONSIDERATIONS
• For latest treatment guidelines see www.hivatis.org
PATIENT/FAMILY EDUCATION
• When co-administered with didanosine or lopinavir/ritonavir, take tenofovir 2 hours before or 1 hour after taking them
MONITORING PARAMETERS
• CBC with platelet count, renal function, liver enzymes

terazosin

(ter-a'zoe-sin)
Rx: Hytrin
Chemical Class: Quinazoline derivative
Therapeutic Class: Antihypertensive; α_1-adrenergic blocker

CLINICAL PHARMACOLOGY
Mechanism of Action: An antihypertensive and benign prostatic hyperplasia agent that blocks alpha-adrenergic receptors. Produces vasodilation, decreases peripheral resistance, and targets receptors around bladder neck and prostate. *Therapeutic Effect:* In hypertension,

decreases BP. In benign prostatic hyperplasia, relaxes smooth muscle and improves urine flow.

Pharmacokinetics

Route	Onset	Peak	Duration
PO	15 min	1-2 hr	12-24 hr

Rapidly, completely absorbed from the GI tract. Protein binding: 90%-94%. Metabolized in the liver to active metabolite. Primarily eliminated in feces via biliary system; excreted in urine. Not removed by hemodialysis. **Half-life:** 12 hr.

INDICATIONS AND DOSAGES
Mild to moderate hypertension
PO
Adults, Elderly. Initially, 1 mg at bedtime. Slowly increase dosage to desired levels. Range: 1–5 mg/day as single or 2 divided doses. Maximum: 20 mg.

Benign prostatic hyperplasia
PO
Adults, Elderly. Initially, 1 mg at bedtime. May increase up to 10 mg/day. Maximum: 20 mg/day.

$ AVAILABLE FORMS/COST
• Cap-Oral: 1 mg, 2 mg, 5 mg, 10 mg, 100's; all: **$154.34-$218.34**
• Tab-Oral: 1 mg, 2 mg, 5 mg, 10 mg, 100's; all: **$160.38**

CONTRAINDICATIONS: None known.

PREGNANCY AND LACTATION: Pregnancy category C; excretion into breast milk unknown

SIDE EFFECTS
Frequent (9%-5%)
Dizziness, headache, unusual tiredness
Rare (less than 2%)
Peripheral edema, orthostatic hypotension, myalgia, arthralgia, blurred vision, nausea, vomiting, nasal congestion, somnolence

SERIOUS REACTIONS
• First-dose syncope (hypotension with sudden loss of consciousness) may occur 30 to 90 minutes after initial dose of 2 mg or more, a too rapid increase in dosage, or addition of another antihypertensive agent to therapy. First-dose syncope may be preceded by tachycardia (pulse rate of 120-160 beats/minute).

INTERACTIONS
Drugs
◼ *Angiotensin converting enzyme inhibitors (enalapril):* Potential for exaggerated first dose hypotensive episode when α-blockers added
◼ *Nonsteroidal antiinflammatory drugs (ibuprofen, indomethacin):* NSAIDs may inhibit antihypertensive effects
◼ *β-adrenergic blockers:* Potential for exaggerated first dose hypotensive episode when α-blockers added
Labs
• False positive urinary metabolites of norepinephrine and VMA
• No effect on prostate specific antigen (PSA)

SPECIAL CONSIDERATIONS
• The doxazosin arm of the ALLHAT study was stopped early; the doxazosin group had a 25% greater risk of combined cardiovascular disease events which was primarily accounted for by a doubled risk of CHF vs the chlorthalidone group; doxazosin was also found to be less effective at controlling systolic BP an average of 3 mm Hg; may want to consider primary antihypertensives in addition to α-blockers for BPH symptoms
• Use as a single antihypertensive agent limited by tendency to cause sodium and water retention and increased plasma volume

PATIENT/FAMILY EDUCATION

• Alert patients to the possibility of syncopal and orthostatic symptoms, especially with the first dose ("1st dose syncope"); initial dose should be administered at bedtime in the smallest possible dose

terbinafine

(ter-been'a-feen)

Rx: *Tab:* Lamisil

OTC: *Cream:* Lamisil AT

OTC: Desenex Max

Chemical Class: Allylamine derivative

Therapeutic Class: Antifungal

CLINICAL PHARMACOLOGY

Mechanism of Action: A fungicidal antifungal that inhibits the enzyme squalene epoxidase, thereby interfering with fungal biosynthesis. *Therapeutic Effect:* Results in death of fungal cells.

INDICATIONS AND DOSAGES

Tinea pedis

Topical

Adults, Elderly, Children 12 yr and older. Apply twice a day until signs and symptoms significantly improve.

Tinea cruris, tinea corporis

Topical

Adults, Elderly, Children 12 yr and older. Apply 1-2 times a day until signs and symptoms significantly improve.

Onychomycosis

PO

Adults, Elderly, Children 12 yr and older. 250 mg/day for 6 wk (fingernails) or 12 wk (toenails).

Tinea versicolor

Topical Solution

Adults, Elderly. Apply to the affected area twice a day for 7 days.

Systemic mycosis

PO

Adults, Elderly. 250-500 mg/day for up to 16 mo.

[$] **AVAILABLE FORMS/COST**

• Cre—Top: 1%, 15, 30 g: **$53.23/**30 g

• Sol—Top: 1%, 30 ml: **$8.49**

• Tab—Oral: 250 mg, 100's: **$982.79**

CONTRAINDICATIONS: Oral: Children younger than 12 years, preexisting hepatic or renal impairment (creatinine clearance of 50 ml/min or less)

PREGNANCY AND LACTATION: Pregnancy category B; it is recommended that treatment of onychomycosis be delayed until after pregnancy; small amounts of terbinafine are excreted into breast milk when administered orally; not recommended in nursing mothers; avoid application to the breast when breast-feeding

SIDE EFFECTS

Frequent (13%)

Oral: Headache

Occasional (6%-3%)

Oral: Diarrhea, rash, dyspepsia, pruritus, taste disturbance, nausea

Rare

Oral: Abdominal pain, flatulence, urticaria, visual disturbance

Topical: Irritation, burning, pruritus, dryness

SERIOUS REACTIONS

• Hepatobiliary dysfunction (including cholestatic hepatitis), serious skin reactions, and severe neutropenia occur rarely.

• Ocular lens and retinal changes have been noted.

SPECIAL CONSIDERATIONS

PATIENT/FAMILY EDUCATION

• Optimal clinical effect in onychomycosis may not be apparent for several mo following completion of therapy

terbutaline

(ter-byoo'te-leen)

Rx: Brethine

Chemical Class: Sympathomimetic amine; β_2-adrenergic agonist

Therapeutic Class: Antiasthmatic; bronchodilator; tocolytic

CLINICAL PHARMACOLOGY

Mechanism of Action: An adrenergic agonist that stimulates beta$_2$-adrenergic receptors, resulting in relaxation of uterine and bronchial smooth muscle. *Therapeutic Effect:* Relieves bronchospasm and reduces airway resistance. Also inhibits uterine contractions.

INDICATIONS AND DOSAGES

Bronchospasm

PO

Adults, Elderly, Children 15 yr and older. Initially, 2.5 mg 3–4 times a day. Maintenance: 2.5–5 mg 3 times a day q6h while awake. Maximum: 15 mg/day.

Children 12–14 yr. 2.5 mg 3 times a day. Maximum: 7.5 mg/day.

Children younger than 12 yr. Initially, 0.05 mg/kg/dose q8h. May increase up to 0.15 mg/kg/dose. Maximum: 5 mg.

Subcutaneous

Adults, Children 12 yr and older. Initially, 0.25 mg. Repeat in 15–30 min if substantial improvement does not occur. Maximum: 0.5 mg/4 hr.

Children younger than 12 yr. 0.005–0.01 mg/kg/dose to a maximum of 0.4 mg/dose q15–20min for 2 doses.

Preterm labor

PO

Adults. 2.5–10 mg q4-6h.

IV

Adults. 2.5–10 mcg/min. May increase gradually q15-20 min up to 17.5–30 mcg/min.

[$] **AVAILABLE FORMS/COST**

- Sol, Inj-SC: 1 mg/ml, 1 ml: **$32.49**
- Tab-Oral: 2.5 mg, 100's: **$43.24**; 5 mg, 100's: **$62.21**

CONTRAINDICATIONS: History of hypersensitivity to sympathomimetics

PREGNANCY AND LACTATION: Pregnancy category B; compatible with breast-feeding

SIDE EFFECTS

Frequent (23%–18%)

Tremor, anxiety

Occasional (11%–10%)

Somnolence, headache, nausea, heartburn, dizziness

Rare (3%–1%)

Flushing, asthenia, mouth and throat dryness or irritation (with inhalation therapy)

SERIOUS REACTIONS

- Too-frequent or excessive use may lead to decreased drug effectiveness and severe, paradoxical bronchoconstriction.
- Excessive sympathomimetic stimulation may cause palpitations, extrasystoles, tachycardia, chest pain, a slight increase in BP followed by a substantial decrease, chills, diaphoresis, and blanching of skin.

INTERACTIONS

Drugs

[2] *β-blockers:* Decreased action of terbutaline, cardioselective β-blockers preferable if concurrent use necessary; metoprolol inhibits terbutaline metabolism

[3] *Furosemide:* Potential for additive hypokalemia

terconazole

(ter-kon'a-zole)

Rx: Terazol 3, Terazol 7

Chemical Class: Triazole derivative

Therapeutic Class: Antifungal

CLINICAL PHARMACOLOGY

Mechanism of Action: An antifungal that disrupts fungal cell membrane permeability. *Therapeutic Effect:* Produces antifungal activity.

Pharmacokinetics

Extent of systemic absorption after vaginal administration may be dependent on presence of a uterus, 5%-8% in women who had a hysterectomy versus 12%-16% in nonhysterectomy women.

INDICATIONS AND DOSAGES

Vulvovaginal candidiasis

Intravaginal

Adults, Elderly. 1 suppository vaginally at bedtime for 3 days.

Adults, Elderly. 1 applicatorful at bedtime for 7 days (0.4% cream) or for 3 days (0.8% cream).

[$] **AVAILABLE FORMS/COST**

• Cre—Vag: 0.4%, 45 g: **$33.84-$41.43**; 0.8%, 20 g: **$33.84-$41.43**

• Supp—Vag: 80 mg, 3's: **$28.94-$41.43**

CONTRAINDICATIONS: Hypersensitivity to terconazole or any component of the formulation

PREGNANCY AND LACTATION: Pregnancy category C, systemic absorption occurs; excretion into breast milk unknown

SIDE EFFECTS

Frequent

Headache, vulvovaginal burning

Occasional

Dysmenorrhea, pain in femail fenitalia, abdominal pain, fever, itching

Rare

Chills

SERIOUS REACTIONS

• Flu-like syndrome has been reported.

SPECIAL CONSIDERATIONS

• No significant advantage over less expensive OTC products

teriparatide

(ter-i-par'a-tide)

Rx: Forteo

Chemical Class: Recombinant human parathyroid hormone (rDNA origin)

Therapeutic Class: Parathyroid hormone

CLINICAL PHARMACOLOGY

Mechanism of Action: A synthetic polypeptide hormone that acts on bone to mobilize calcium; also acts on kidney to reduce calcium clearance, increase phosphate excretion. *Therapeutic effect:* Promotes an increased rate of release of calcium from bone into blood, stimulates new bone formation.

INDICATIONS AND DOSAGES

Osteoporosis

SC

Adults, Elderly. 20 mcg once daily into the thigh or abdominal wall.

[$] **AVAILABLE FORMS/COST**

• Pen device, Inj-SC: 0.75 mg/3 ml: **$624.18**

CONTRAINDICATIONS: Serum calcium above normal level, those at increased risk for osteosarcoma (Paget's disease, unexplained elevations of alkaline phosphatase, open epiphyses, prior radiation therapy that include the skeleton), hypercalcemic disorder (e.g., hyperparathyroidism), hypersensitivity to teriparatide or any of the components of the formulation

PREGNANCY AND LACTATION:
Pregnancy category C; not indicated for use in premenopausal women

SIDE EFFECTS

Occasional

Leg cramps, nausea, dizziness, headache, orthostatic hypotension, increased heart rate

SERIOUS REACTIONS

• None known.

INTERACTIONS

Drugs

▣ *Digoxin:* Transient increase in serum calcium may increase risk of digitalis toxicity

SPECIAL CONSIDERATIONS

• Treatment not recommended beyond 2 yr as safety and efficacy not established

• Postural hypotension, if it occurs, happens within 4 hr and with the first several doses; does not preclude continued treatment

• Inform patients teriparatide caused osteosarcoma in rats; clinical relevance in humans unknown

• Maximal serum calcium levels occur 4-6 hr post dose

PATIENT/FAMILY EDUCATION

• Initially administer lying down (postural hypotension)

• Inject into thigh or abdominal wall

• Refrigerate, minimize time out of refrigerator

• Recap pen to protect from light

• Discard if not used within 28 days

• Notify provider of nausea, vomiting, constipation, lethargy, muscle weakness (possible hypercalcemia)

---

testosterone

(tess-toss'ter-one)

Rx: *Testosterone aqueous:* Testamone-100, Testro AQ

Rx: *Testosterone cypionate:* Depo-Testosterone, Depotest, T-Cypionate, Virilon IM

Rx: *Testosterone enanthate:* Delatestryl, Everone, Testro-L.A.

Rx: *Testosterone propionate:* Generics only

Rx: *Transdermal:* Androderm, Testoderm, AndroGel, Testim

Rx: *Pellet:* Testopel

Chemical Class: Androgen

Therapeutic Class: Androgen; antineoplastic

DEA Class: Schedule III

CLINICAL PHARMACOLOGY

Mechanism of Action: A primary endogenous androgen that promotes growth and development of male sex organs and maintains secondary sex characteristics in androgen-deficient males. *Therapeutic Effect:* Helps relieve androgen deficiency.

Pharmacokinetics

Well absorbed after IM administration. Protein binding: 98%. Undergoes first-pass metabolism in the liver. Primarily excreted in urine. Unknown if removed by hemodialysis. **Half-life:** 10–20 min.

INDICATIONS AND DOSAGES

Male hypogonadism

IM

Adults. 50-400 mg q2-4wk.

Adolescents. Initially 40-50 mg/m^2/dose monthly until growth rate falls to prepubertal levels. 100

mg/m²/dose until growth ceases. Maintanence virilizing dose: 100 mg/m²/dose twice a month.
Sucutaneous (Pellets)
Adults, adolescents. 150-450 mg q3-6mo.
Transdermal (Patch [Testoderm])
Adults, Elderly. Start therapy with 6 mg/day patch. Apply patch to scrotal skin.
Transdermal (Patch [Testoderm TTS])
Adults, Elderly. Apply TTS patch to arm, back, or upper buttocks.
Trandermal (Patch [Androderm])
Adults, Elderly. Start therapy with 5 mg/day patch applied at night. Apply patch to abdomen, back, thighs, or upper arms.
Transdermal (Gel [AndroGel])
Adults, Elderly. Initial dose of 5 mg delivers 50 mg testosterone and is applied once daily to the abdomen, shoulders, or upper arms. May increase to 7.5 g, then to 10 g, if necessary.
Transdermal (Gel [Testim])
Adults, Elderly. Initial dose of 5 g delivers 50 mg testosterone and is applied once a day to the shoulders or upper arms. May increase to 10 g.
Buccal System (Striant)
Adults, Elderly: 30 mg q12h.
Delayed puberty
IM
Adults. 50-200 mg q2-4wk.
Adolescents. 40–50 mg/m²/dose every month for 6 mo.
Subcutaneous (Pellets)
Adults, Adolescents. 150-450 mg q3-6mo.
Breast carcinoma
IM (aqueous)
Adults. 50–100 mg 3 times a week.
IM (cypionate or ethanate)
Adults. 200–400 mg q2–4wk.
IM (propionate)
Adults. 50–100 mg 3 times a week.

[$] **AVAILABLE FORMS/COST**
Testosterone
• Film, Cont Rel—Transdermal: 2.5 mg/24 hr, 60's: **$178.64**; 4 mg/24 hr, 30's: **$131.54**; 5 mg/24 hr, 30's: **$178.64**; 6 mg/24 hr, 30's: **$131.54**
• Gel—Top: 1%, 2.5, 5 g, 30's; all: **$190.20-$199.80**
Testosterone Aqueous
• Sol, Inj-IM: 50 mg/ml, 10 ml: **$3.95-$8.95**; 100 mg/ml, 10 ml: **$6.50-$45.00**
Testosterone Cypionate
• Sol, Inj-IM: 100 mg/ml, 10 ml: **$15.05-$54.23**; 200 mg/ml, 10 ml: **$20.75-$103.46**
Testosterone Enanthate
• Sol, Inj-IM: 200 mg/ml, 10 ml: **$9.15-$18.50**
Testosterone Propionate
• Sol, Inj-IM: 100 mg/ml, 10 ml: **$5.85-$18.38**
• Cre, Oint-Top: 2%, 60 g: **$38.60**

CONTRAINDICATIONS: Cardiac impairment, hypercalcemia, pregnancy, prostate or breast cancer in males, severe hepatic or renal disease

PREGNANCY AND LACTATION: Pregnancy category X; excretion into breast milk unknown; use extreme caution in nursing mothers

SIDE EFFECTS
Frequent
Gynecomastia, acne
Females: Hirsutism, amenorrhea or other menstrual irregularities, deepening of voice, clitoral enlargement that may not be reversible when drug is discontinued
Occasional
Edema, nausea, insomnia, oligospermia, priapism, male-pattern baldness, bladder irritability, hypercalcemia (in immobilized patients or those with breast cancer), hypercholesterolemia, inflammation and pain at IM injection site

Transdermal: Pruritus, erythema, skin irritation
Rare
Polycythemia (with high dosage), hypersensitivity
SERIOUS REACTIONS
• Peliosis hepatitis (presence of blood-filled cysts in parenchyma of liver), hepatic neoplasms, and hepatocellular carcinoma have been associated with prolonged high-dose therapy.
• Anaphylactic reactions occur rarely.
INTERACTIONS
Drugs
3 *Cyclosporine:* Increased cyclosporine concentrations
2 *Oral anticoagulants:* Increased hypoprothrombinemic response
SPECIAL CONSIDERATIONS
MONITORING PARAMETERS
• LFTs, lipids, Hct
• Growth rate in children (X-rays for bone age q6 mo)

---

tetracaine
(tet′ra-cane)
Rx: Opticaine, Pontocaine
OTC: Cepacol Viractin
Chemical Class: Benzoic acid derivative
Therapeutic Class: Anesthetic, local

CLINICAL PHARMACOLOGY
Mechanism of Action: Tetracaine causes a reversible blockade of nerve conduction by decreasing nerve membrane permeability to sodium. *Therapeutic effect:* Local anesthetic.
Pharmacokinetics
Systemic absorption of tetracaine is variable. Metabolized by plasma pseudocholinesterasis. Excreted in the urine.

INDICATIONS AND DOSAGES
Anesthetize lower abdomen
Spinal
Adults. 3-4 ml (9-12 mg) of a 0.3% solution
Anesthetize perineum
Spinal
Adults. 1-2 ml (3-6 mg) of a 0.3% solution
Anesthetize upper abdomen
Spinal
Adults. 5 ml (15 mg) of a 0.3% solution
Obstetric anesthesia, low spinal (saddle block) anesthesia
Spinal
Adults. 1-2 ml (2-14 mg) of a 0.2% solution
Anesthesia of the perineum
Intrathecal
Adults. 0.5 ml (5 mg) as a 1% solution, diluted with equal amount of CSF or 10% dextrose injection.
Anesthesia of the perineum and lower extremeties
Intrathecal
Adults. 1 ml (10 mg) as a 1% solution, diluted with equal amount of CSF or 10% dextrose injection.
Anesthesia up to the costal margin
Intrathecal
Adults. 1.5-2 ml (15-20 mg) as a 1% solution, diluted with equal amount of CSF.
Topical anesthesia
Topical
Adults. Apply to the affected areas as needed. Maximum dosage is 28 g per 24 hours.
Children. Apply to the affected areas as needed. Maximum dosage is 7 g in a 24 hour period.
Topical anesthesia of nose and throat, abolish laryngeal and esophageal reflexes prior to diagnostic procedure

Topical

Adults. Direct application of a 0.25% or 0.5% topical solution or by oral inhalation of a nebulized 0.5% solution. Total dose should not exceed 20 mg.

Mild pain, burning and/or pruritis associated with herpes labialis (cold sores or fever blisters)

Topical

Adults and children 2 years and older. Apply to the affected area no more than 3-4 times a day.

Ophthalmic anesthesia

Topical

Adults. 1-2 drops of a 0.5% solution.

Ⓢ AVAILABLE FORMS/COST

• Cre—Top: 1%, 28 g: **$9.93**; 2%, 7.5 g: **$3.95**
• Gel—Top: 2%, 7.5 g: **$3.40**
• Sol, Inj-IV: 0.2%, 2 ml: **$5.53**; 0.3%, 5 ml: **$7.27**; 1%, 2 ml: **$5.85**
• Oint-Ophth: 0.5%, 3.5 g: **$16.21**
• Sol-Ophth: 0.5%, 15 ml: **$4.55-$27.02**
• Sol-Top: 2%, 30, 120 ml: **$14.73/30 ml**

CONTRAINDICATIONS: Hypersensitivity, to esther local anesthetics, sulfites, PABA, infection or inflammation at the injection site, bactermia, platelet abnormalities, thrombocytopenia, increased bleeding time, uncontrolled coagulopathy, or anticoagulant therapy, sulfonamide therapy.

PREGNANCY AND LACTATION: Pregnancy category C; excretion into breast milk unknown

SIDE EFFECTS

Frequent

Burning stinging, or tenderness, skin rash, itching, redness, or inflammation, numbness or tingling of the face or mouth, pain at the injection site, sensitivity to light, swelling of the eye or eyelid, watering or the eyes, acute ocular pain and ocular irritation (burning, stinging, or redness)

Occasional

Paresthesias, weakness and paralysis of lower extremity, hypotension, high or total spinal block, urinary retention or incontinence, fecal incontinence, headache, back pain, septic meningitis, meningismus, arachnoiditis, shivering cranial nerve palsies due to traction on nerves from loss of CSF, and loss of perineal sensation and sexual function

Rare

Anxiety, restlessness, difficulty breathing shortness of breath, dizziness, drowsiness, lightheadedness, nausea, vomiting, seizures (convulsions), slow, irregular heartbeat (palpitations), swelling of the face or mouth, skin rash, itching (hives), tremors, visual impairment.

SERIOUS REACTIONS

• Tetracaine induced CNS toxicity usually presents with symptoms of a CNS stimulation such as anxiety, apprehension, restlessness, nervousness, disorientation, confusion, dizziness, tinnitus, blurred vision, tremor, and/or seizures. Subsequently, depressive symptoms may occur including drowsiness, respiratory arrest, or coma.

• Depression or cardiac excitability and contractility may cause AV block, ventricular arrhythmias, or cardiac arrest. Symptoms of local anesthetic CNS toxicity, such as dizziness, tongue numbness, visual impairment or disturbances, and muscular twitching appear to occur before cardiotoxic effects. Cardiotoxic effects include angina, QT prolongation, PR prolongation, atrial fibrillation, sinus bradycardia, hypotension, palpitations, and cardiovascular collapse. Maternal seizures and cardiovascular collapse may oc-

T

cur following paracervical block in early pregnancy due to rapid systemic absorption.

Alert

• Tetracaine is more likely than any other topical anesthetic to cause contact reactions including, skin rash (unspecified), mucous membrane irritation, erythema, pruritis, urticaria, burning, stinging, edema, or tenderness.

Alert

• During labor and obstetric delivery, local anesthetics can cause varying degrees of maternal, fetal, and neonatal toxicities. Fetal heart rate should be monitored continuously because fetal bradycardia may occur in patients receiving tetracaine anesthesia and may be associated with fetal acidosis. Maternal hypotension can result from regional anesthesia; patient position can alleviate this problem. Spincal tetracaine may cause decreased uterine contractility or maternal expulsion efforts and alter the forces of parturition.

INTERACTIONS

Drugs

▣ *Propranolol:* Enhanced sympathomimetic side effects resulting in hypertensive reactions; acute discontinuation of β-blockers prior to local anesthesia may increase side effects of tetracaine

Labs

• *Interference:* CSF protein

SPECIAL CONSIDERATIONS

• Previously used as component of "Magic Numbing Solution" or TAC Sol (epinephrine 1:2,000, tetracaine 0.5%, cocaine 11.8%) and LET Sol (lidocaine 4%, epinephrine 0.1%, tetracaine 0.5%), which are used as topical anesthesia for repair of minor lacerations, especially in pediatric patients. Topical tetracain solutions no longer available

---

tetracycline
(tet-ra-sye′kleen)

Rx: *Systemic:* Tetralon Achromycin, Panmycin, Sumycin, Tetracap, Tetracyn

Rx: *Topical:* Topicycline

Rx: *Peridontal fiber:* Actisite

OTC: Achromycin

Chemical Class: Tetracycline

Therapeutic Class: Antibiotic

CLINICAL PHARMACOLOGY

Mechanism of Action: A tetracycline antibiotic that inhibits bacterial protein synthesis by binding to ribosomes. *Therapeutic Effect:* Bacteriostatic.

Pharmacokinetics

Readily absorbed from the GI tract. Protein binding: 30%-60%. Widely distributed. Excreted in urine; eliminated in feces through biliary system. Not removed by hemodialysis. **Half-life:** 6-11 hr (increased in impaired renal function).

INDICATIONS AND DOSAGES

Inflammatory acne vulgaris, Lyme disease, mycoplasmal disease, Legionella infections, Rocky Mountain spotted fever, chlamydial infections in patients with gonorrhea

PO

Adults, Elderly. 250-500 mg q6-12h.

Children 8 yr and older. 25-50 mg/kg/day in 4 divided doses. Maximum: 3 g/day.

Helicobacter pylori **infections**

PO

Adults, Elderly. 500 mg 2-4 times a day (in combination).

Topical

Adults, Elderly. Apply twice a day (once in the morning, once in the evening).

Dosage in renal impairment

Dosage interval is modified based on creatinine clearance.

Creatinine Clearance	Dosage Interval
50-80 ml/min	Usual dose q8-12h
10-50 ml/min	Usual dose q12-24h
less than 10 ml/min	Usual dose q24h

AVAILABLE FORMS/COST

• Cap, Gel—Oral: 100 mg, 1000's: **$31.20**; 250 mg, 100's: **$0.54-$18.96**; 500 mg, 100's: **$5.46-$14.09**

• Susp—Oral: 125 mg/5 ml, 480 ml: **$6.00-$13.98**

• Tab, Coated—Oral: 250 mg, 100's: **$8.51**; 500 mg, 100's: **$16.57**

CONTRAINDICATIONS: Children 8 years and younger, hypersensitivity to tetracyclines or sulfites

PREGNANCY AND LACTATION: Pregnancy category D (systemic), category B (topical); systemic tetracycline excreted into breast milk in low concentrations; theoretically, dental staining could occur, but serum levels in infants undetectable, so considered compatible with breast-feeding

SIDE EFFECTS

Frequent

Dizziness, light-headedness, diarrhea, nausea, vomiting, abdominal cramps, possibly severe photosensitivity

Topical: Dry, scaly skin; stinging or burning sensation

Occasional

Pigmentation of skin or mucous membranes, rectal or genital pruritus, stomatitis

Topical: Pain, redness, swelling, or other skin irritation.

SERIOUS REACTIONS

• Superinfection (especially fungal), anaphylaxis, and benign intracranial hypertension may occur.

• Bulging fontanelles occur rarely in infants.

INTERACTIONS

Drugs

③ *Antacids:* Reduced tetracycline concentrations

② *Bismuth subsalicylate:* Reduced tetracycline concentrations

③ *Calcium:* Reduced tetracycline concentrations

③ *Cholestyramine colestipol:* Reduced tetracycline concentrations

③ *Digoxin:* Decreased digoxin concentrations due to reduced GI flora

③ *Food:* Reduced tetracycline concentrations

③ *Iron:* Reduced tetracycline concentrations

③ *Magnesium:* Reduced tetracycline concentrations

② *Methoxyflurane:* Increased renal toxicity

③ *Oral contraceptives:* Possible decreased contraceptive effect

③ *Penicillin:* Impaired efficacy of penicillin

③ *Sodium bicarbonate:* Reduced tetracycline concentrations

③ *Zinc:* Reduced tetracycline concentrations

Labs

• *False negative:* Urine glucose with Clinistix or TesTape

• *False increase:* Serum glucose

• *False decrease:* Serum acetaminophen concentration, serum folate

• *Interference:* Plasma catecholamines, urinary porphyrins, CSF protein

SPECIAL CONSIDERATIONS

PATIENT/FAMILY EDUCATION

• Avoid milk products, antacids, or separate by 2 hr; take with a full glass of water

• Use in children ≤8 yr causes permanent discoloration of teeth, enamel hypoplasia, and retardation

of skeletal development; risk greatest for children <4 yr and receiving high doses
• Side effects noted for systemic administration not observed with topical formulations

---

tetrahydrozoline hydrochloride

(tet-ra-hi-droz'o-leen)

Rx: *Nasal:* Tyzine

Rx: *Ophthalmic:* Collyrium Fresh, Eyesine, Murine Plus, Optigene 3, Visine, Tetrasine
Chemical Class: Sympathomimetic amine
Therapeutic Class: Decongestant

CLINICAL PHARMACOLOGY

Mechanism of Action: A vasoconstrictor that stimulates alpha-adrenergic receptors in sympathetic nervous system. Constricts arterioles.
Therapeutic Effect: Reduces redness, irritation, and congestion.

Pharmacokinetics

May be systemically absorbed. Metabolic, elimination rates unknown.

INDICATIONS AND DOSAGES

Relief of itching, minor irritation and to control hyperemia with superficial corneal vascularity
Ophthalmic
Adults, Elderly, Children. 1-2 drops 2-4 times/day.

Relief of nasal congestion of rhinitis, the common cold, sinusitis, hay fever, or other allergies; reduces swelling and improves visualization for surgery or diagnostic procedures; opens obstructed eustachian ostia with ear inflammation

Intranasal
Adults, Elderly, Children older than 6 yrs. 2-4 drops (0.1% solution) to each nostril q4-6h (no sooner than q3h).
Children 2-6 yrs. 2-3 drops (0.05% solution) to each nostril q4-6h (no sooner than q3h).

AVAILABLE FORMS/COST
• Spray-Nasal: 0.1%, 15 ml: **$16.52**
• Sol—Nasal: 0.05%, 15 ml: **$14.93**; 0.1%, 30 ml: **$22.33**
• Sol—Ophth: 0.05%, 30 ml: **$3.15-$5.78**/30 ml

CONTRAINDICATIONS: Children less than 2 years of age, the 0.1% nasal solution is contraindicated in children less than 6 years of age, angle closure glaucoma or other serious eye diseases, hypersensitivity to tetrahydrozyline or any component of the formulation

PREGNANCY AND LACTATION: Pregnancy category C; excretion into breast milk unknown

SIDE EFFECTS
Occasional
Intranasal: Transient burning, stinging, sneezing, dryness of mucosa
Ophthalmic: Irritation, blurred vision, mydriasis
Systemic sympathomimetic effects may occur with either route: headache, hypertension, weakness, sweating, palpitations, tremors. Prolonged use may result in rebound congestion

SERIOUS REACTIONS
• Overdosage may result in CNS depression with drowsiness, decreased body temperature, bradycardia, hypotension, coma, and apnea.

SPECIAL CONSIDERATIONS
• Manage rebound congestion by stopping tetrahydrozoline: one nostril at a time, substitute systemic decongestant, substitute inhaled steroid

PATIENT/FAMILY EDUCATION
• Do not use for >3-5 days or rebound congestion may occur

---

thalidomide
(thal-e-doe-mide)
Rx: Thalomid
Chemical Class: Glutamic acid derivative
Therapeutic Class: Leprostatic

CLINICAL PHARMACOLOGY
Mechanism of Action: An immunomodulator whose exact mechanism is unknown. Has sedative, anti-inflammatory, and immunosuppressive activity, which may be due to selective inhibition of the production of tumor necrosis factor-alpha. *Therapeutic Effect:* Improves muscle wasting in HIV patients; reduces local and systemic effects of leprosy.

INDICATIONS AND DOSAGES
AIDS-related muscle wasting
PO
Adults. 100–300 mg a day.
Leprosy
PO
Adults, Elderly. Initially, 100-300 mg/day as single bedtime dose, at least 1 hr after the evening meal. Continue until active reaction subsides, then reduce dose q2-4 wk in 50 mg increments.

Ⓢ AVAILABLE FORMS/COST
• Cap—Oral: 50 mg, 28's: **$501.38**; 100 mg, 28's: **$1,496.50**; 200 mg, 28's: **$2,205.00**
NOTE: Available only under a special restricted distribution program called STEPS (System for Thalidomide Education and Prescribing Safety). (1-888-4-23546)

UNLABELED USES: Treatment of Crohn's disease, recurrent aphthous ulcers in HIV patients, wasting syndrome associated with HIV or cancer

CONTRAINDICATIONS: Neutropenia, peripheral neuropathy; pregnancy, sensitivity to thalidomide

PREGNANCY AND LACTATION: Pregnancy category X; breast milk excretion unknown

SIDE EFFECTS
Frequent
Somnolence, dizziness, mood changes, constipation, dry mouth, peripheral neuropathy
Occasional
Increased appetite, weight gain, headache, loss of libido, edema of face and limbs, nausea, alopecia, dry skin, rash, hypothyroidism

SERIOUS REACTIONS
• Neutropenia, peripheral neuropathy, and thromboembolism occur rarely.

INTERACTIONS
Drugs
Ⓔ *Barbiturates:* Additive sedative effects
Ⓔ *Chlorpromazine:* Additive sedative effects
Ⓔ *Ethanol:* Additive sedative effects
Ⓔ *Reserpine:* Additive sedative effects

SPECIAL CONSIDERATIONS
PATIENT/FAMILY EDUCATION
• Teratogenic in human whether taken by male or female
• Sedation common; usually taken at bedtime

MONITORING PARAMETERS
• Pregnancy test (weekly during first mo of use, then monthly)
• ALT, AST
• CBC

theophylline

(thee-off'-i-lin)

Rx: *Immediate release tabs:* Quibron-T, Theolair, Bronkodyl, Elixophyllin

Rx: *Liquids:* Asmalix, Aquaphyllin, Accubron, Lanophyllin, Theoclear, Theostat, Elixomin, Elixophyllin, Theolair

Rx: *Sustained release caps:* Theo-24

Rx: *Sustained release tabs:* Quibron-T/SR, Respbid, Theochron, Theo-Dur, Theolair-SR, Theo-X, Slophyllin Gyrocap, Theobid, Theoclear LA, Theospan SR, Theovent, Theosave, Uniphyl Combinations

> **Rx:** with guaifenesin (Elixophyllin-GG, Quibron, Slo-Phyllin-GG); with potassium iodide (Elixophylline KI)

Chemical Class: Xanthine derivative

Therapeutic Class: COPD agent; antiasthmatic; bronchodilator

CLINICAL PHARMACOLOGY

Mechanism of Action: An antiasthmatic medication with two distinct actions in the airways of patients with reversible obstruction; smooth muscle relaxation and suppression of the response of airways to stimuli. Mechanisms of action are not known with certainty. It is known theophylline increases force of contraction of diaphragmatic muscles by enhancing calcium uptake through adenosine-mediated channels. *Therapeutic effect:* Causes bronchodilation and decreased airway reactivity.

Pharmacokinetics

The pharmacokinetics of theophylline vary widely among similar patients and cannot be predicted by age, sex, body weight or other demographic characteristics. Rapidly and completely absorbed after oral administration in solution or immediate-release solid oral dosage form. Distributed freely into fat-free tissues. Extensively metabolized in liver. **Half-life:** 4-8 hours.

INDICATIONS AND DOSAGES

Chronic asthma/lung diseases

PO

Adults: Acute symptoms: 5 mg/kg as a loading dose, maintenance 3 mg/kg every 8 hours (non-smokers), 3 mg/kg every 6 hours (smokers), 2 mg/kg every 8 hours (older patients), 1-2 mg/kg every 12 hours (CHF); IV 5 mg/kg load over 20 minutes, maintenance 0.2 mg/kg/hour (CHF, elderly), 0.43 mg/kg/hour (non-smokers), 0.7 mg/kg/hour (young adult smokers).

Slow titration: initial dose 16 mg/kg/day or 400mg daily, whichever is less, doses divided every 6-8 hours

Dosage adjustment after serum theophylline measurement: Serum level 5-10 mcg/ml, maintain dose by 25%, recheck level in 3 days. Serum level 10-20 mcg/ml, maintain dosage if tolerated, recheck level every 6-12 months. Serum level 20-25 mcg/ml, decrease dose by 10%, recheck level in 3 days. Serum level 25-30 mcg/ml, skip next dose, decrease dose by 25%, recheck level in 3 days. Serum level > 30 mcg/ml, skip next 2 doses, decrease dose by 50%, recheck level in 3 days.

Children 9-16 years: 5 mg/kg as a loading dose, maintenance 3 mg/kg every 6 hours; IV 5 mg/kg load over 20 minutes, maintenance 0.7 mg/kg/hour.

Children 1-9 years: 5 mg/kg as a loading dose, maintenance 4 mg/kg every 6 hours; IV 5 mg/kg load over 20 minutes, maintenance 0.8 mg/kg/hour.

Infants: [(0.2 X age in weeks) +5] X kg = 24 hour dose in mg; divide into every 8 hour dosing (6 weeks to 6 months), every 6 hour dosing (6-12 months); IV 5 mg/kg load over 20 minutes, maintenance dose in mg/kg/hour [(0.0008 X age in weeks) + 0.21]

$ AVAILABLE FORMS/COST

• Cap—Oral: 100 mg, 100's: **$39.02-$49.45**; 200 mg, 100's: **$51.93-$65.72**; 300 mg, 100's: **$20.82**

• Cap, Gel, Sus Action—Oral: 50 mg, 100's: **$17.33-$25.68**; 65 mg, 100's: **$17.00**; 75 mg, 100's: **$19.75-$28.34**; 100 mg, 100's: **$19.61-$20.55**; 125 mg, 100's: **$25.75-$39.21**; 200 mg, 100's: **$30.70-$46.68**; 300 mg, 100's: **$36.55-$54.98**; 100 mg/24 hr, 100's: **$45.07**; 200 mg/24 hr, 100's: **$67.18**; 300 mg/24 hr, 100's: **$82.87**; 400 mg/24 hr, 100's: **$116.03**

• Elixir—Oral: 80 mg/15 ml, 480 ml: **$3.23-$95.05**

• Sol, Inj-IV: 0.4 mg/ml, 1000 ml: **$15.92**; 0.8 mg/ml, 1000 ml: **$7.30-$16.42**; 1.6 mg/ml, 500 ml: **$5.45-$16.21**; 2 mg/ml, 100 ml: **$5.87-$12.76**; 3.2 mg/ml, 250 ml: **$6.27-$10.95**; 4 mg/ml, 100 ml: **$6.00-$10.71**

• Sol—Oral: 80 mg/15 ml, 480 ml: **$2.50-$7.31**

• Syr—Oral: 80 mg/15 ml, 480 ml: **$14.78-$27.58**

• Tab, Coated, Sus Action—Oral: 100 mg, 100's: **$11.25-$22.75**; 200 mg, 100's: **$7.58-$61.71**; 300 mg, 100's: **$10.23-$68.13**; 450 mg, 100's: **$31.45-$57.55**; 600 mg, 100's: **$129.89-$155.97**; 400 mg/24 hr, 100's: **$110.34**; 600 mg/24 hr, 100's: **$159.79**

• Tab-Oral: 100 mg, 100's: **$29.00**; 125 mg, 100's: **$53.19**; 200 mg, 30's: **$11.19**; 250 mg, 100's: **$79.26**; 300 mg, 100's: **$54.00-$60.48**

UNLABELED USES: Apnea, bradycardia of prematurity

CONTRAINDICATIONS: Hypersensitivity to theophylline or any component of the formulation, active peptic ulcer disease, underlying seizure disorders unless receiving appropriate anti-convulsant medication.

PREGNANCY AND LACTATION: Pregnancy category C; no reports of malformations; compatible with breast-feeding with precaution that rapidly absorbed preparations may cause irritability in the infant

SIDE EFFECTS

Anxiety, dizziness, headache, insomnia, lightheadedness, muscle twitching, restlessness, seizures, dysrhythmias, fluid retention with tachycardia, hypotension, palpitations, pounding heartbeat, sinus tachycardia, anorexia, bitter taste, diarrhea, dyspepsia, gastroesophageal reflux, nausea, vomiting, urinary frequency, increased respiratory rate, flushing, urticaria

SERIOUS REACTIONS

• Severe toxicity from theophylline overdose is a relatively rare event.

INTERACTIONS

Drugs

▣ *Adenosine:* Inhibited hemodynamic effects of adenosine

▣ *Allopurinol, amiodarone, cimetidine, ciprofloxacin, disulfiram, erythromycin, interferon alfa, isoniazid, methimazole, metoprolol, norfloxacin, pefloxacin, pentoxyfylline, propafenone, propylthiouracil, radioactive iodine, tacrine, thiabendazole, ticlopidine, verapamil:* Increased theophylline concentrations

❸ *Aminoglutethamide, barbiturates, carbamazepine, moricizine, phenytoin, rifampin, ritonavir, thyroid hormone:* Reduced theophylline levels; decreased serum phenytoin concentrations

❸ *β-blockers:* Reduced bronchodilating response to theophylline

❷ *Enoxacin, fluvoxamine, mexiletine, propranolol, troleandomycin:* Markedly increased theophylline concentrations

❸ *Imipenem:* Some patients on theophylline have developed seizures following the addition of imipenem

❸ *Lithium:* Reduced lithium concentrations

❸ *Smoking:* Increased theophylline dosing requirements

Labs
• *False increase:* Serum barbiturate concentrations, urinary uric acid
• *False decrease:* Serum bilirubin
• *Interference:* Plasma somatostatin

SPECIAL CONSIDERATIONS

PATIENT/FAMILY EDUCATION
• Contents of beaded capsules may be sprinkled over food for children

MONITORING PARAMETERS
• Blood levels; therapeutic level is 10-20 mcg/ml (6-14 mcg/ml for apnea, bradycardia of prematurity); toxicity may occur with small increase above 20 mcg/ml and occasionally at levels below this; obtain serum levels 1-2 hr after administration for immediate release products and 5-9 hr after the am dose for sustained release formulations
• Recent evidence indicates that blood levels of 8-12 mcg/ml may provide adequate therapeutic effect with a lower risk of adverse events

• Signs of toxicity include nausea, vomiting, anxiety, insomnia, seizures, ventricular dysrhythmias

---

thiabendazole
(thye-a-ben′-da-zole)
Rx: Mintezol
Chemical Class: Benzimidazole derivative
Therapeutic Class: Antihelmintic

CLINICAL PHARMACOLOGY
Mechanism of Action: An anthelmintic agent that inhibits helminth-specific mitochondrial fumarate reductase. *Therapeutic Effect:* Suppresses parasite production.

Pharmacokinetics
Rapidly and well absorbed from the gastrointestinal (GI) tract. Rapidly metabolized in liver. Primarily excreted in urine; partially eliminated in feces. Removed **Half-life:** 1.2 hrs.

INDICATIONS AND DOSAGES:
Dose is based on patient's body weight

Cutaneous lava migrans (creeping eruption)
PO
Adults, Elderly, Children. 50 mg/kg/day q12h for 2 days. Maximum: 3 g/day.

Intestinal roundworms
PO
Adults, Elderly, Children. 50 mg/kg/day q12h for 2 days. Maximum: 3 g/day.

Strongloidiasis (thread worms)
PO
Adults, Elderly, Children. 50 mg/kg/day q12h for 2 days. Maximum: 3 g/day.

Trichinosis
PO

Adults, Elderly, Children. 50 mg/kg/day q12h for 2-4 days. Maximum: 3 g/day.

Visceral larva migrans
PO

Adults, Elderly, Children. 50 mg/kg/day q12h for 7 days. Maximum: 3 g/day.

🅢 AVAILABLE FORMS/COST
• Susp—Oral: 500 mg/5 ml, 120 ml: **$26.32**
• Tab, Chewable—Oral: 500 mg, 36's: **$45.35**

UNLABELED USES: Angiostrongyliasis, capillaria infestations, dracunculus infestations, pediculosis capitis, tinea infections

CONTRAINDICATIONS: Prophylactic treatment of pinworm infestation, hypersensitivity to thiabendazole or its components

PREGNANCY AND LACTATION: Pregnancy category C

SIDE EFFECTS
Occasional

Dizziness, drowsiness, nausea, vomiting, diarrhea

Rare

Erythema multiform, liver damage

SERIOUS REACTIONS
• Overdose includes symptoms of altered mental status and visual problems.
• Erythema multiform, liver damage, and Stevens-Johnsons syndrome occur rarely.

INTERACTIONS
Drugs

🅳 *Carbamazepine:* Decreased thiabendazole concentrations, therapeutic failure possible

🅳 *Theophylline:* May inhibit metabolism of xanthines, potentially elevating serum concentrations

SPECIAL CONSIDERATIONS
PATIENT/FAMILY EDUCATION
• Take after meals; chew before swallowing
• Proper hygiene after bowel movement, including handwashing technique; change bed linen

---

thiamine (vitamin B₁)
(thy'a-min)
Rx: Thiamine
OTC: Thiamilate
Chemical Class: Vitamin B complex
Therapeutic Class: Vitamin

CLINICAL PHARMACOLOGY
Mechanism of Action: A water-soluble vitamin that combines with adenosine triphosphate in the liver, kidneys, and leukocytes to form thiamine diphosphate, a coenzyme that is necessary for carbohydrate metabolism. *Therapeutic Effect:* Prevents and reverses thiamine deficiency.

Pharmacokinetics

Readily absorbed from the GI tract, primarily in duodenum, after IM administration. Widely distributed. Metabolized in the liver. Primarily excreted in urine.

INDICATIONS AND DOSAGES
Dietary supplement
PO

Adults, Elderly. 1–2 mg/day.
Children. 0.5–1 mg/day.
Infants. 0.3–0.5 mg/day.

Thiamine deficiency
PO

Adults, Elderly. 5–30 mg/day, as a single dose or in 3 divided doses, for 1 mo.
Children. 10–50 mg/day in 3 divided doses.

T

Thiamine deficiency in patients who are critically ill or have malabsorption syndrome
IV, IM
Adults, Elderly. 5–100 mg, 3 times a day.
Children. 10–25 mg/day.
Metabolic disorders
PO
Adults, Elderly, Children. 10–20 mg/day; increased up to 4 g/day in divided doses.

$ **AVAILABLE FORMS/COST**
- Sol, Inj-IM, IV: 100 mg/ml, 1 ml: **$1.00-$2.11**
- Tab—Oral: 50 mg, 100's: **$2.17-$2.30**; 100 mg, 100's: **$1.88-$4.50**; 500 mg, 100's: **$7.35**

CONTRAINDICATIONS: None known.

PREGNANCY AND LACTATION: Pregnancy category A; excreted into breast milk; U.S. recommended daily allowance for thiamine during lactation is 1.5-1.6 mg; supplement women with inadequate intake; compatible with breast-feeding

SIDE EFFECTS
Frequent
Pain, induration, and tenderness at IM injection site

SERIOUS REACTIONS
- IV administration may result in a rare, severe hypersensitivity reaction marked by a feeling of warmth, pruritus, urticaria, weakness, diaphoresis, nausea, restlessness, tightness in throat, angioedema, cyanosis, pulmonary edema, GI tract bleeding, and cardiovascular collapse.

SPECIAL CONSIDERATIONS
- Worsening of Wernicke's encephalopathy is possible following glucose administration, administer thiamine before or along with dextrose-containing fluids
- Single vitamin B_1 deficiency is rare—suspect multiple vitamin deficiencies

thiethylperazine
(thye-eth-il-per'azeen)
Rx: Torecan
Chemical Class: Piperazine phenothiazine derivative
Therapeutic Class: Antiemetic

CLINICAL PHARMACOLOGY
Mechanism of Action: A piperazine phenothiazine that acts centrally to block dopamine receptors in chemoreceptor trigger zone (CTZ) in central nervous system (CNS). *Therapeutic Effect:* Relieves nausea and vomiting.

INDICATIONS AND DOSAGES
Nausea or vomiting
PO/Rectal/IM
Adults, Elderly. 10 mg 1-3 times/day.

$ **AVAILABLE FORMS/COST**
- Sol, Inj-IV: 5 mg/ml, 2 ml: **$4.84**
- Tab-Oral: 10 mg, 100's: **$61.13**

CONTRAINDICATIONS: Comatose states, severe CNS depression, pregnancy, hypersensitivity to phenothiazines

PREGNANCY AND LACTATION: Pregnancy category C; excretion into breast milk unknown, use caution in nursing mothers

SIDE EFFECTS
Frequent
Drowsiness, dizziness
Occasional
Blurred vision, decreased color/night vision, fever, headache, orthostatic hypotension, rash, ringing in ears, constipation, dry mouth, decreased sweating.

SERIOUS REACTIONS

• Extrapyramidal symptoms manifested as torticollis (neck muscle spasm), oculogyric crisis (rolling back of eyes), and akathisia (motor restlessness, anxiety) occur rarely.

INTERACTIONS

Drugs

▣ *Anticholinergics, antiparkinson drugs, antidepressants:* Increased anticholinergic action

▣ *Barbiturates:* Induction, decreased effect of thiethylperazine

▣ *β-blockers:* Augmented pharmacologic action of both drugs

▣ *Bromocriptine:* Neuroleptic drugs inhibit bromocriptine's ability to lower prolactin concentration

▣ *Epinephrine:* Reversed pressor response to epinephrine

▣ *Levodopa:* Inhibited antiparkinsonian effect of levodopa

▣ *Lithium:* Lowered serum concentration of both drugs in combination

▣ *Narcotic analgesics:* Hypotension with meperidine, caution with other narcotic analgesics

▣ *Orphenadrine:* Lower thiethylperazine concentration and excessive anticholinergic effects

SPECIAL CONSIDERATIONS

• Effective antiemetic agent for the treatment of postoperative nausea and vomiting, nausea and vomiting secondary to mildly emetic chemotherapeutic agents, and vomiting secondary to radiation therapy and toxins

• No comparisons with prochlorperazine

• More extrapyramidal reactions than chlorpromazine and promazine; thiethylperazine would be less desirable than these agents in patients where the occurrence of a dystonic reaction would be hazardous (i.e., head and neck surgery patients, patients with severe pulmonary disease, patients with a history of dyskinetic reactions)

PATIENT/FAMILY EDUCATION

• Avoid hazardous activities, activities requiring alertness

MONITORING PARAMETERS

• Respiratory status initially

---

thioridazine
(thye-or-rid'a-zeen)
Rx: Mellaril
Chemical Class: Piperazine phenothiazine derivative
Therapeutic Class: Antipsychotic

CLINICAL PHARMACOLOGY
Mechanism of Action: A phenothiazine that blocks dopamine at postsynaptic receptor sites. Possesses strong anticholinergic and sedative effects. *Therapeutic Effect:* Suppresses behavioral response in psychosis; reduces locomotor activity and aggressiveness.

INDICATIONS AND DOSAGES
Psychosis
PO
Adults, Elderly, Children 12 yr and older. Initially, 25-100 mg 3 times a day; dosage increased gradually. Maximum: 800 mg/day.
Children 2-11 yr. Initially, 0.5 mg/kg/day in 2-3 divided doses. Maximum: 3 mg/kg/day.

▨ **AVAILABLE FORMS/COST**
• Conc—Oral: 30 mg/ml, 120 ml: **$15.28-$20.34**; 100 mg/ml, 120 ml: **$36.89-$43.20**
• Tab, Coated—Oral: 10 mg, 100's: **$6.25-$33.20**; 15 mg, 100's: **$7.75-$50.79**; 25 mg, 100's: **$9.50-$46.70**; 50 mg, 100's: **$12.50-$58.40**; 100 mg, 100's: **$19.50-**

$90.00; 150 mg, 100's: **$30.00-$96.64**; 200 mg, 100's: **$34.50-$129.48**

UNLABELED USES: Treatment of behavioral problems in children, dementia, depressive neurosis

CONTRAINDICATIONS: Angle-closure glaucoma, blood dyscrasias, cardiac arrhythmias, cardiac or hepatic impairment, concurrent use of drugs that prolong QT interval, severe CNS depression

PREGNANCY AND LACTATION: Pregnancy category C

SIDE EFFECTS

Occasional

Drowsiness during early therapy, dry mouth, blurred vision, lethargy, constipation or diarrhea, nasal congestion, peripheral edema, urine retention

Rare

Ocular changes, altered skin pigmentation (in those taking high doses for prolonged periods), photosensitivity, darkening of urine

SERIOUS REACTIONS

• Prolonged QT interval may produce torsades de pointes, a form of ventricular tachycardia, and sudden death.

INTERACTIONS

Drugs

▣ *Anticholinergics, antiparkinson drugs, antidepressants:* Increased anticholinergic action

▣ *Barbiturates:* Induction, decreased effect of thioridazine

▣ *β-blockers:* Augmented pharmacologic action of both drugs

▣ *Bromocriptine:* Neuroleptic drugs inhibit bromocriptine's ability to lower prolactin concentration; reverse not common

▣ *Epinephrine:* Reversed pressor response

▣ *Levodopa:* Inhibited antiparkinsonian effect

▣ *Lithium:* Lowered serum concentration of both drugs in combination

▣ *Narcotic analgesics:* Hypotension with meperidine, caution with other narcotic analgesics

▣ *Orphenadrine:* Lower thioridazine concentration and excessive anticholinergic effects

▣ *Phenylpropanolamine:* Patient on thioridazine died after single dose of phenylpropanolamine; a causal relationship was not established

Labs

• *False positive:* Pregnancy tests, serum tricyclic antidepressants screen

SPECIAL CONSIDERATIONS

• Phenothiazine with weak potency, low incidence of EPS, but high incidence of sedation, anticholinergic effects, and cardiovascular effects

PATIENT/FAMILY EDUCATION

• Arise slowly from reclining position

• Avoid abrupt withdrawal

• Use a sunscreen during sun exposure

• Caution with activities requiring complete mental alertness (e.g., driving), may cause sedation

• Provide full information on risks of tardive dyskinesia

---

thiothixene
(thye-oh-thix′een)
Rx: Navane
Chemical Class: Thioxanthene derivative
Therapeutic Class: Antipsychotic

CLINICAL PHARMACOLOGY
Mechanism of Action: An antipsychotic that blocks postsynaptic dopamine receptor sites in brain.

Has alpha-adrenergic blocking effects, and depresses the release of hypothalamic and hypophyseal hormones. *Therapeutic Effect:* Suppresses psychotic behavior.

Pharmacokinetics

Well absorbed from the GI tract after IM administration. Widely distributed. Metabolized in the liver. Primarily excreted in urine. Unknown if removed by hemodialysis. **Half-life:** 34 hr.

INDICATIONS AND DOSAGES

Psychosis

PO

Adults, Elderly, Children older than 12 yr. Initially, 2 mg 3 times a day. Maximum: 60 mg/day.

IM

Adults, Elderly, Children older than 12 yr. Initially, 4 mg 2-4 times a day. Maximum: 30 mg/day.

§ AVAILABLE FORMS/COST

• Cap, Gel—Oral: 1 mg, 100's: **$15.77-$45.44**; 2 mg, 100's: **$12.06-$67.34**; 5 mg, 100's: **$13.95-$102.24**; 10 mg, 100's: **$44.31-$132.08**; 20 mg, 100's: **$203.69**

• Conc—Oral: 5 mg/ml, 120 ml: **$36.00-$51.92**

CONTRAINDICATIONS: Blood dyscrasias, circulatory collapse, CNS depression, coma, history of seizures

PREGNANCY AND LACTATION: Pregnancy category C

SIDE EFFECTS

Expected

Hypotension, dizziness, syncope (occur frequently after first injection, occasionally after subsequent injections, and rarely with oral form)

Frequent

Transient drowsiness, dry mouth, constipation, blurred vision, nasal congestion

Occasional

Diarrhea, peripheral edema, urine retention, nausea

Rare

Ocular changes, altered skin pigmentation (in those taking high doses for prolonged periods), photosensitivity

SERIOUS REACTIONS

• The most common extrapyramidal reaction is akathisia, characterized by motor restlessness and anxiety. Akinesia, marked by rigidity, tremor, increased salivation, mask-like facial expression, and reduced voluntary movements, occurs less frequently. Dystonias, including torticollis, opisthotonos, and oculogyric crisis, occur rarely.

• Tardive dyskinesia, characterized by tongue protrusion, puffing of the cheeks, and chewing or puckering of the mouth, occurs rarely but may be irreversible. Elderly female patients have a greater risk of developing this reaction.

• Grand mal seizures may occur in epileptic patients, especially those receiving the drug by IM administration.

• Neuroleptic malignant syndrome occurs rarely.

INTERACTIONS

Drugs

3 *Anticholinergics, antiparkinson drugs, antidepressants:* Increased anticholinergic action

3 *Barbiturates:* Induction, decreased effect of thiothixene

3 *β-blockers:* Augmented pharmacologic action of both drugs

3 *Bromocriptine:* Thiothixene inhibits bromocriptine's ability to lower prolactin concentration, reverse not common

3 *Epinephrine:* Reversed pressor response

3 *Guanethidine:* Inhibited antihypertensive response to guanethidine

T

[3] *Levodopa:* Inhibited antiparkinsonian effect

[3] *Lithium:* Lowered serum concentration of both drugs in combination

[3] *Narcotic analgesics:* Hypotension with meperidine, caution with other narcotic analgesics

[3] *Orphenadrine:* Lower thiothixene concentration and excessive anticholinergic effects

SPECIAL CONSIDERATIONS

• High-potency antipsychotic with a relatively high incidence of EPS, but a low incidence of sedation, anticholinergic effects, and cardiovascular effects

PATIENT/FAMILY EDUCATION

• Informed consent regarding risks of tardive dyskinesia; orthostatic hypotension

thyroid

(thye'-roid)

Rx: Armour Thyroid, Bro-Throid, Nature-Throid, Westhroid

Chemical Class: Thyroid hormone in natural state

Therapeutic Class: Thyroid hormone

CLINICAL PHARMACOLOGY

Mechanism of Action: A natural hormone derived from animal sources, usually beef or pork, that is involved in normal metabolism, growth, and development, especially the central nervous system (CNS) of infants. Possesses catabolic and anabolic effects. Provides both levothyroxine and liothyronine hormones. *Therapeutic Effect:* Increases basal metabolic rate, enhances gluconeogenesis, stimulates protein synthesis.

Pharmacokinetics

Partially absorbed from the gastrointestinal (GI) tract. Protein binding: 99%. Widely distributed. Metabolized in liver to active, liothyronine (T_3), and inactive, reverse triiodothyronine (rT_3), metabolites. Eliminated by biliary excretion. **Half-life:** 2- 7 days.

INDICATIONS AND DOSAGES

Hypothyroidism

PO

Adults, Elderly. Initially, 15- 30 mg. May increase by 15 mg increments q2-4wks. Maintenance: 60-120 mcg/day. Use 15 mg in patients with cardiovascular disease or myxedema.

Children 12 yrs and older. 90 mg/day.

Children 6-12 yrs. 60- 90 mg/day.

Children older than 1-5 yrs. 45-60 mg/day.

Children older than 6- 12 mos. 30-45 mg/day.

Children 3 mos. and younger. 15- 30 mg/day.

[$] **AVAILABLE FORMS/COST**

• Cap-Oral: 8 mg, 100's: **$15.60**; 15 mg, 100's: **$7.00**; 30 mg, 100's: **$9.00**; 60 mg, 100's: **$9.60**; 90 mg, 100's: **$11.25**; 120 mg, 100's: **$14.25**; 150 mg, 100's: **$22.80**; 180 mg, 100's: **$14.25**; 240 mg, 100's: **$17.40**

• Tab-Oral: 15 mg, 100's: **$10.15-$15.75**; 30 mg, 100's: **$4.62-$18.50**; 60 mg, 100's: **$0.79-$16.10**; 65 mg, 100's: **$2.21-$3.69**; 90 mg, 100's: **$20.65-$25.43**; 120 mg, 100's: **$0.98-$29.79**; 130 mg, 100's: **$3.31-$21.57**; 180 mg, 100's: **$5.25-$53.63**; 240 mg, 100's: **$57.54-$70.84**; 300 mg, 100's: **$71.33-$87.81**

CONTRAINDICATIONS: Uncontrolled adrenal cortical insufficiency, untreated thyrotoxicosis, treatment of obesity, uncontrolled angina, uncontrolled hypertension, uncontrolled myocardial infarction, and hypersensitivity to any component of the formulations

PREGNANCY AND LACTATION: Pregnancy category A; little or no transplacental passage at physiologic serum concentrations; excreted into breast milk in low concentrations (inadequate to protect a hypothyroid infant; too low to interfere with neonatal thyroid screening programs)

SIDE EFFECTS
Rare

Dry skin, GI intolerance, skin rash, hives, severe headache

SERIOUS REACTIONS

• Excessive dosage produces signs and symptoms of hyperthyroidism including weight loss, palpitations, increased appetite, tremors, nervousness, tachycardia, hypertension, headache, insomnia, and menstrual irregularities.

• Cardiac arrhythmias occur rarely.

INTERACTIONS
Drugs

🔳 *Carbamazepine, phenytoin, rifampin:* Increases elimination of thyroid hormones; may increase dosage requirements

🔳 *Bile acid sequestrants:* Reduced serum thyroid hormone concentrations

🔳 *Oral anticoagulants:* Thyroid hormones increase catabolism of vitamin K–dependent clotting factors; an increase or decrease in clinical thyroid status will increase or decrease the hypoprothrombinemic response to oral anticoagulants

🔳 *Theophylline:* Reduced serum theophylline concentrations with initiation of thyroid therapy

SPECIAL CONSIDERATIONS

• Although used traditionally, natural hormones less clinically desirable due to varying potencies, inconsistent clinical effects, and more adverse stimulatory effects; synthetic derivatives (i.e., levothyroxine) preferred

MONITORING PARAMETERS

• TSH yearly

---

tiagabine
(ti-ah-ga'bean)
Rx: Gabitril
Chemical Class: Nipecotic acid derivative
Therapeutic Class: Anticonvulsant

CLINICAL PHARMACOLOGY
Mechanism of Action: An anticonvulsant that enhances the activity of gamma-aminobutyric acid, the major inhibitory neurotransmitter in the CNS. *Therapeutic Effect:* Inhibits seizures.

INDICATIONS AND DOSAGES
Adjunctive treatment of partial seizures
PO

Adults, Elderly. Initially, 4 mg once a day. May increase by 4-8 mg/day at weekly intervals. Maximum: 56 mg/day.

Children 12-18 yr. Initially, 4 mg once a day. May increase by 4 mg at week 2 and by 4-8 mg at weekly intervals thereafter. Maximum: 32 mg/day.

S AVAILABLE FORMS/COST

• Tab, Coated—Oral: 2 mg, 100's: **$155.00**; 4 mg, 100's: **$155.00**; 12 mg, 100's: **$200.00**; 16 mg, 100's: **$230.00**; 20 mg, 100's: **$218.75**

CONTRAINDICATIONS: None known.

PREGNANCY AND LACTATION: Pregnancy category C

T

SIDE EFFECTS
Frequent (34%-20%)
Dizziness, asthenia, somnolence, nervousness, confusion, headache, infection, tremor
Occasional
Nausea, diarrhea, abdominal pain, impaired concentration

SERIOUS REACTIONS
• Overdose is characterized by agitation, confusion, hostility, and weakness. Full recovery occurs within 24 hours.

INTERACTIONS
Drugs
3 *Anticonvulsants (hepatic enzyme inducers—i.e., barbiturates, carbamazepine, phenytoin, primidone):* Decreased tiagabine levels and effect
3 *Rifampin:* Decreased tiagabine levels and effect via hepatic enzyme induction
3 *Valproate:* Increased tiagabine free blood levels

SPECIAL CONSIDERATIONS
• Patients should exercise caution with initiation and dosage titration when driving, operating hazardous machinery, or other activities requiring mental concentration; patients should be advised to take the medication with food, to delay peak effects to avoid many CNS adverse effects

---

ticarcillin disodium/clavulanate potassium
(tyekar-sill'in klav'yoo-la-nate)
Rx: *Ticarcillin disodium:* Ticar
Rx: *Ticarcillin/clavulanic acid:* Timentin
Chemical Class: Penicillin derivative, extended-spectrum
Therapeutic Class: Antibiotic

CLINICAL PHARMACOLOGY
Mechanism of Action: Ticarcillin binds to bacterial cell walls, inhibiting cell wall synthesis. Clavulanate inhibits the action of bacterial beta-lactamase. *Therapeutic Effect:* Ticarcillin is bactericidal in susceptible organisms. Clavulanate protects ticarcillin from enzymatic degradation.

Pharmacokinetics
Widely distributed. Protein binding: ticarcillin 45%-60%, clavulanate 9%-30%. Minimally metabolized in the liver. Primarily excreted unchanged in urine. Removed by hemodialysis. **Half-life:** 1-1.2 hr (increased in impaired renal function).

INDICATIONS AND DOSAGES
Skin and skin-structure, bone, joint, and lower respiratory tract infections; septicemia; endometriosis
IV
Adults, Elderly. 3.1 g (3 g ticarcillin) q4-6h. Maximum: 18-24 g/day.
Children 3 mo and older. 200-300 mg (as ticarcillin) q4-6h.
UTIs
IV
Adults, Elderly. 3.1 g q6-8h.
Dosage in renal impairment
Dosage interval is modified based on creatinine clearance.

Creatinine Clearance	Dosage Interval
10-30 ml/min	Usual dose q8h
less than 10 ml/min	Usual dose q12h

§ AVAILABLE FORMS/COST
• Powder, Inj-IM, IV: 3 g/vial: **$11.40-$13.43**

Ticarcillin/Clavulanic Acid
• Powder, Inj-IV: 3 g-0.1 g/vial: **$15.70-$16.01**

CONTRAINDICATIONS: Hypersensitivity to any penicillin

PREGNANCY AND LACTATION: Pregnancy category B; excreted into breast milk in low concentrations; compatible with breast-feeding

SIDE EFFECTS
Frequent
Phlebitis or thrombophlebitis (with IV dose), rash, urticaria, pruritus, altered smell or taste
Occasional
Nausea, diarrhea, vomiting
Rare
Headache, fatigue, hallucinations, bleeding or ecchymosis

SERIOUS REACTIONS
• Overdosage may produce seizures and other neurologic reactions.
• Antibiotic-associated colitis and other superinfections may result from bacterial imbalance.
• Severe hypersensitivity reactions, including anaphylaxis, occur rarely.

INTERACTIONS
Drugs
🖪 *Aminoglycosides:* Inactivation of aminoglycosides *in vitro* and *in vivo,* reducing the aminoglycoside effect
Labs
• *False increase:* Urine glucose

SPECIAL CONSIDERATIONS
• Synergistic with aminoglycosides
• Sodium content, 5.2 mEq/g ticarcillin
• For reliable activity against *Pseudomonas,* must be dosed q4h

ticlopidine
(tye-klo′pa-deen)
Rx: Ticlid
Chemical Class: Thienopyridine derivative
Therapeutic Class: Antiplatelet agent

CLINICAL PHARMACOLOGY
Mechanism of Action: An aggregation inhibitor that inhibits the release of adenosine diphosphate from activated platelets, which prevents fibrinogen from binding to glycoprotein IIb/IIIa receptors on the surface of activated platelets. *Therapeutic Effect:* Inhibits platelet aggregation and thrombus formation.

INDICATIONS AND DOSAGES
Prevention of stroke
PO
Adults, Elderly. 250 mg twice a day.

§ AVAILABLE FORMS/COST
• Tab-Oral: 250 mg, 100's: **$186.00**

UNLABELED USES: Treatment of intermittent claudication, sickle cell disease, subarachnoid hemorrhage

CONTRAINDICATIONS: Active pathologic bleeding, such as bleeding peptic ulcer and intracranial bleeding, hematopoietic disorders, including neutropenia and thrombocytopeni; presence of hemostatic disorder; severe hepatic impairment

PREGNANCY AND LACTATION: Pregnancy category B; use caution in nursing mothers

SIDE EFFECTS
Frequent (13%–5%)
Diarrhea, nausea, dyspepsia, including heartburn, indigestion, GI discomfort, and bloating
Rare (2%–1%)
Vomiting, flatulence, pruritus, dizziness

T

SERIOUS REACTIONS
• Neutropenia occurs in approximately 2% of patients.
• Thrombotic thrombocytopenia purpura, agranulocytosis, hepatitis, cholestatic jaundice, and tinnitus occur rarely.

INTERACTIONS
Drugs
⬛ *Cyclosporine:* Potential for reduction in blood cyclosporine concentrations
⬛ *Phenytoin:* Inhibition of hepatic metabolism (CYP2C9) of phenytoin; potential for development of phenytoin toxicity, reduction in phenytoin dose may be necessary
⬛ *Theophylline:* Increased theophylline level via inhibition of metabolism, increased risk of toxicity

SPECIAL CONSIDERATIONS
• Due to the risk of life-threatening neutropenia or agranulocytosis and cost, ticlopidine should be reserved for patients intolerant to aspirin or who fail aspirin

MONITORING PARAMETERS
• CBC q2wk for 1st 3 mo of therapy, then periodically thereafter

---

tiludronate
(ti-loo'dro-nate)
Rx: Skelid
Chemical Class: Pyrophosphate analog
Therapeutic Class: Bisphosphonate; bone resorption inhibitor

CLINICAL PHARMACOLOGY
Mechanism of Action: A calcium regulator that inhibits functioning osteoclasts through disruption of cytoskeletal ring structure and inhibition of osteoclastic proton pump. *Therapeutic Effect:* Inhibits bone resorption.

INDICATIONS AND DOSAGES
Paget's disease
PO
Adults, Elderly. 400 mg once a day for 3 mo. Must take with 6–8 ounces plain water. Do not give within 2 hr of food intake. Avoid giving aspirin, calcium supplements, mineral supplements, or antacids within 2 hr of tiludronate administration.

🅢 **AVAILABLE FORMS/COST**
• Tab—Oral: 200 mg, 56's: **$472.74**
CONTRAINDICATIONS: GI disease, such as dysphagia and gastric ulcer, impaired renal function.
PREGNANCY AND LACTATION: Pregnancy category C; dose-related scoliosis; avoid exposure in children

SIDE EFFECTS
Frequent (9%–6%)
Nausea, diarrhea, generalized body pain, back pain, headache
Occasional
Rash, dyspepsia, vomiting, rhinitis, sinusitis, dizziness

INTERACTIONS
Drugs
❷ *Food:* Reduces bioavailability 90%
❷ *Antacids/calcium:* Reduces bioavailability 60-80%
⬛ *Aspirin:* Decreases bioavailability of tiludronate by 50%
⬛ *Indomethacin:* Bioavailability of NSAID increased 2-4 fold

SPECIAL CONSIDERATIONS
• Studies needed to assess place in therapy with other bisphosphonates
• Inhibition of bone loss in osteoporosis may persist up to 2 yr after 6 mo of treatment and discontinuation of drug

PATIENT/FAMILY EDUCATION
• Take with 6-8 oz plain water; do not take within 2 hr of food or other medications

timolol
(tim'oh-lole)
Rx: *Oral:* Blockadren
Rx: *Ophthalmic:* Betimol,
Timoptic, Timoptic-XE
Combinations
  Rx: Ophthalmic with dorzol
    amide (Cosopt)
Chemical Class: β-adrenergic
blocker, nonselective
Therapeutic Class: Antiangi-
nal; antiglaucoma agent;
antihypertensive

CLINICAL PHARMACOLOGY
Mechanism of Action: An antihypertensive, antimigraine, and antiglaucoma agent that blocks $beta_1$-
and $beta_2$-adrenergic receptors.
Therapeutic Effect: Reduces intraocular pressure (IOP) by reducing aqueous humor production, lowers BP, slows the heart rate, and decreases myocardial contractility.
Pharmacokinetics

Route	Onset	Peak	Dura-tion
PO	15-45 min	0.5-2.5 hr	4 hr
Oph-thalmic	30 min	1-2 hr	12-24 hr

Well absorbed from the GI tract.
Protein binding: 10%. Minimal absorption after ophthalmic administration. Metabolized in the liver.
Primarily excreted in urine. Not removed by hemodialysis. **Half-life:**
4 hr. Systemic absorption may occur
with ophthalmic administration.

INDICATIONS AND DOSAGES
Mild to moderate hypertension
PO
Adults, Elderly. Initially, 10 mg
twice a day, alone or in combination
with other therapy. Gradually increase at intervals of not less than 1
wk. Maintenance: 20-60 mg/day in
2 divided doses.

Reduction of cardiovascular mor-
tality in definite or suspected acute
MI
PO
Adults, Elderly. 10 mg twice a day,
beginning 1-4 wk after infarction.
Migraine prevention
PO
Adults, Elderly. Initially, 10 mg
twice a day. Range: 10-30 mg/day.
Reduction of IOP in open-angle
glaucoma, aphakic glaucoma, ocu-
lar hypertension, and secondary
glaucoma
Ophthalmic
Adults, Elderly, Children. 1 drop of
0.25% solution in affected eye(s)
twice a day. May be increased to 1
drop of 0.5% solution in affected
eye(s) twice a day. When IOP is controlled, dosage may be reduced to 1
drop once a day. If patient is
switched to timolol from another antiglaucoma agent, administer concurrently for 1 day. Discontinue
other agent on following day.
Ophthalmic
Adults, Elderly. Timoptic XE: 1
drop/day Istalol: Apply once daily.
Ⓢ **AVAILABLE FORMS/COST**
• Gel—Ophth: 0.25%, 2.5, 5 ml:
$26.50-$29.44/5 ml; 0.5%, 2.5, 5
ml: **$31.50-$35.72**/5 ml
• Sol—Ophth: 0.25%, 2.5, 5, 10, 15
ml: **$11.04-$38.29**/10 ml; 0.5%, 2.5,
5, 10, 15 ml: **$27.98-$44.58**/10 ml
• Tab-Oral: 5 mg, 100's: **$22.15-**
$53.45; 10 mg, 100's: **$31.80-**
$66.11; 20 mg, 100's: **$66.10-**
$108.26

UNLABELED USES: Systemic:
Treatment of anxiety, cardiac arrhythmias, chronic angina pectoris,
hypertrophic cardiomyopathy, migraine, pheochromocytoma, thyrotoxicosis, tremors
Ophthalmic: To decrease IOP in
acute or chronic angle-closure glaucoma, treatment of angle-closure

T

glaucoma during and after iridectomy, malignant glaucoma, secondary glaucoma

CONTRAINDICATIONS: Bronchial asthma, cardiogenic shock, CHF unless secondary to tachyarrhythmias, COPD, patients receiving MAOI therapy, second- or third-degree heart block, sinus bradycardia, uncontrolled cardiac failure

PREGNANCY AND LACTATION: Pregnancy category C; similar drug, atenolol, frequently used in the third trimester for treatment of hypertension (many studies of efficacy and safety of atenolol in pregnancy induced hypertension; long term use has been associated with intrauterine growth retardation; mean milk:plasma ratio, 0.80 in one study; quantity of drug ingested by breast-feeding infant unlikely to be therapeutically significant

SIDE EFFECTS

Frequent

Diminished sexual function, drowsiness, difficulty sleeping, unusual tiredness or weakness

Ophthalmic: Eye irritation, visual disturbances

Occasional

Depression, cold hands or feet, diarrhea, constipation, anxiety, nasal congestion, nausea, vomiting, bradycardia, bronchospasm

Rare

Altered taste, dry eyes, itching, numbness of fingers, toes, or scalp

SERIOUS REACTIONS

• Overdose may produce profound bradycardia, hypotension, and bronchospasm.

• Abrupt withdrawal may result in diaphoresis, palpitations, headache, and tremors.

• Timolol administration may precipitate CHF and MI in patients with cardiac disease; thyroid storm in those with thyrotoxicosis; and peripheral ischemia in those with existing peripheral vascular disease.

• Hypoglycemia may occur in patients with previously controlled diabetes.

• Ophthalmic overdose may produce bradycardia, hypotension, bronchospasm, and acute cardiac failure.

INTERACTIONS

Drugs

☒ *$α_1$-adrenergic blockers:* Potential enhanced first dose response (marked initial drop in blood pressure, particularly on standing (especially prazocin)

☒ *Amiodarone:* Combined therapy may lead to bradycardia, cardiac arrest, or ventricular dysrhythmia

☒ *Antidiabetics:* β-blockers increase blood glucose and impair peripheral circulation; altered response to hypoglycemia by prolonging the recovery of normoglycemia, causing hypertension, and blocking tachycardia

☒ *Clonidine:* Hypertension occurring upon withdrawal of clonidine may be exacerbated by timolol

☒ *Digoxin:* Additive prolongation of atrioventricular (AV) conduction time

☒ *Dihydropyridine calcium channel blockers:* Additive hypotension (kinetic and dynamic)

☒ *Diltiazem:* Potentiates β-adrenergic effects; hypotendion, left ventricular failure, and AV conduction disturbances problemmatic in elderly, patients with left ventricular dysfunction, aortic stenosis, or with large doses of either drug

☒ *Disopyramide:* Additive negative inotropic cardiac effects

☒ *Epinephrine:* Enhanced pressor response (hypertension and bradycardia)

③ *Hypoglycemic agents:* Masked hypoglycemia, hyperglycemia

③ *Isoproterenol:* Reduced isoproterenol efficacy in asthma

③ *Methyldopa:* Potential for development of hypertension in the presence of increased catecholamines

③ *Nonsteroidal anti-inflammatory drugs:* Reduced antihypertensive effects of timolol

③ *Phenylephrine:* Potential for hypertensive episodes when administered together

③ *Prazosin:* First-dose response to prazosin may be enhanced by β-blockade

③ *Quinidine:* Increased timolol concentrations

③ *Tacrine:* Additive bradycardia

③ *Theophylline:* Antagonistic pharmacodynamic effects

③ *Verapamil:* Potentiates β-adrenergic effects; hypotendion, left ventricular failure, and AV conduction disturbances problemmatic in elderly, patients with left ventricular dysfunction, aortic stenosis, or with large doses of either drug

SPECIAL CONSIDERATIONS

• Currently available β-blockers appear to be equally effective; cardioselective or combined α- and β-adrenergic blockade are less likely to cause undesirable effects and may be preferred

PATIENT/FAMILY EDUCATION

• Do not discontinue abruptly; may require taper; rapid withdrawal may produce rebound hypertension or angina

MONITORING PARAMETERS

• Angina: reduction in nitroglycerin usage; frequency, severity, onset, and duration of angina pain; heart rate

• Arrhythmias: heart rate

• Congestive heart failure: functional status, cough, dyspnea on exertion, paroxysmal nocturnal dyspnea, exercise tolerance, and ventricular function

• Hypertension: Blood pressure

• Migraine headache: reduction in the frequency, severity, and duration of attacks

• Post myocardial infaction: left ventricular function, lower resting heart rate

• Toxicity: blood glucose, bronchospasm, hypotension, bradycardia, depression, confusion, hallucination, sexual dysfunction

---

tinidazole

(ty-ni′da-zole)
Rx: Tindamax
Chemical Class: Nitroimidazole derivative
Therapeutic Class: Antibiotic; antiprotozoal

CLINICAL PHARMACOLOGY

Mechanism of Action: A nitroimidazole derivative that is converted to the active metabolite by reduction of cell extracts of *Trichomonas*. The active metabolite causes DNA damage in pathogens. *Therapeutic Effect:* Produces antiprotozoal effect.

Pharmacokinetics

Rapidly and completely absorbed. Protein binding: 12%. Distributed in all body tissues and fluids; crosses blood-brain barrier. Significantly metabolized. Primarily excreted in urine; partially eliminated in feces. **Half-life:** 12-14 hr.

INDICATIONS AND DOSAGES

Intestinal amebiasis

PO

Adults, Elderly. 2 g/day for 3 days.
Children 3 yr and older. 50 mg/kg/day (up to 2 g) for 3 days.

Amebic hepatic abscess
PO
Adults, Elderly. 2 g/day for 3-5 days.
Children 3 yr and older. 50 mg/kg/day (up to 2 g) for 3-5 days.
Giardiasis
PO
Adults, Elderly. 2 g as a single dose.
Children 3 yr and older. 50 mg/kg (up to 2 g) as a single dose.
Trichomoniasis
PO
Adults, Elderly. 2 g as a single dose.

CONTRAINDICATIONS: First trimester of pregnancy, hypersensitivity to nitroimidazole derivatives

PREGNANCY AND LACTATION: Pregnancy category C; contraindicated in 1st trimester; unsafe in lactating women

SIDE EFFECTS
Occasional (4%-2%)
Metallic or bitter taste, nausea, weakness, fatigue or malaise
Rare (less than 2%)
Epigastric distress, anorexia, vomiting, headache, dizziness, red-brown or darkened urine

SERIOUS REACTIONS
• Peripheral neuropathy, characterized by paresthesia, is usually reversible if tinidazole treatment is stopped as soon as neurologic symptoms appear.
• Superinfection, hypersensitivity reaction, and seizures occur rarely.

SPECIAL CONSIDERATIONS
• Also effective for bacterial vaginosis, but not FDA approved

PATIENT/FAMILY EDUCATION
• For trichimoniasis, treat sexual partner; tinidazole may induce candidiasis

MONITORING PARAMETERS
• CBC with WBC differential if retreatment is necessary

---

tinzaparin
(tin-za-pair′in)
Rx: Innohep
Chemical Class: Heparin derivative, depolymerized; low-molecular weight heparin
Therapeutic Class: Anticoagulant

CLINICAL PHARMACOLOGY
Mechanism of Action: A low-molecular-weight heparin that inhibits factor Xa. Causes less inactivation of thrombin, inhibition of platelets, and bleeding than standard heparin. Does not significantly influence bleeding time, PT, aPTT. *Therapeutic Effect:* Produces anticoagulation.
Pharmacokinetics
Well absorbed after subcutaneous administration. Primarily eliminated in urine. **Half-life:** 3–4 hr.

INDICATIONS AND DOSAGES
Deep vein thrombosis
Subcutaneous
Adults, Elderly. 175 anti-Xa international units/kg once a day. Continue for at least 6 days and until patient is sufficiently anticoagulated with warfarin (International Normalizing Ratio [INR] of 2 or more for 2 consecutive days).

§ **AVAILABLE FORMS/COST**
• Sol, Inj-SC: 20,000 anti-Xa IU/ml, 2 ml: **$168.00**

CONTRAINDICATIONS: Active major bleeding, concurrent heparin therapy, hypersensitivity to heparin or pork products, thrombocytopenia associated with positive in vitro test for antiplatelet antibody

PREGNANCY AND LACTATION: Pregnancy category B; low-molecular-weight heparins have been used to prevent and treat thromboembolic disease during pregnancy in lieu of warfarin which is a known teratogen; excretion into breast milk unknown but thought to be minimal based on pharmacokinetic parameters, use caution in nursing mothers

SIDE EFFECTS

Frequent (16%)

Injection site reaction, such as inflammation, oozing, nodules, and skin necrosis

Rare (less than 2%)

Nausea, asthenia, constipation, epistaxis

SERIOUS REACTIONS

• Overdose may lead to bleeding complications ranging from local ecchymoses to major hemorrhage. Antidote: Dose of protamine sulfate (1% solution) should be equal to dose of tinzaparin injected. One mg protamine sulfate neutralizes 100 units of tinzaparin. A second dose of 0.5 mg tinzaparin per 1 mg protamine sulfate may be given if aPTT tested 2–4 hours after the initial infusion remains prolonged.

INTERACTIONS

Drugs

◧ *Antiplatelet agents (aspirin, ticlopidine, clopidogrel, dipyridamole, NSAIDs), thrombolytics:* Increased risk of hemorrhage

◧ *Oral anticoagulants:* Additive anticoagulant effects

Labs

• *Increase:* AST, ALT

SPECIAL CONSIDERATIONS

• Cannot be used interchangeably with unfractionated heparin or other low-molecular-weight heparin products

PATIENT/FAMILY EDUCATION

• Administer by deep SC inj into abdominal wall; alternate inj sites

• Do not rub inj site after completion of the inj

• Report any unusual bruising or bleeding to clinician

MONITORING PARAMETERS

• Periodic CBC with platelets

• Monitoring aPTT is not required

• Consider anti-Factor Xa monitoring in patients with impaired renal function, during pregnancy, and in very small or obese patients

---

tioconazole

(tyo-con´a-zole)

OTC: Vagistat-1, Monistat-1

Chemical Class: Imidazole derivative

CLINICAL PHARMACOLOGY

Mechanism of Action: An imidazole derivative that inhibits synthesis of ergosterol (vital component of fungal cell formation). *Therapeutic Effect:* Damaging fungal cell membrane. Fungistatic.

Pharmacokinetics

Negliglble absorption from vaginal application.

INDICATIONS AND DOSAGES

Vulvovaginal candidiasis

Intravaginal

Adults, Elderly. 1 applicatorful just before bedtime as a single dose.

Ⓢ **AVAILABLE FORMS/COST**

• Oint—Vag: 6.5%, 4.6 g single dose: **$14.38-$24.19**

CONTRAINDICATIONS: Hypersensitivity to tioconazole or other imidazole antifungal agents

PREGNANCY AND LACTATION: Pregnancy category C; excretion into breast milk unknown

SIDE EFFECTS

Frequent (25%)

Headache

Occasional (6%-1%)

Burning, itching

Rare (less than 1%)

Irritation, vaginal pain, dysuria, dryness of vaginal secretions, vulvar edema/ swelling

T

SERIOUS REACTIONS
• None reported.

SPECIAL CONSIDERATIONS
• Similar in efficacy to miconazole, econazole, and clotrimazole for the topical management of fungal skin infections; choice determined by cost and availability; additional efficacy vs. trichomoniasis with longer course of therapy

---

tiopronin
(tye-o-pro′-nin)
Rx: Thiola
Chemical Class: Thiol derivative
Therapeutic Class: Anti-kidney stone agent

CLINICAL PHARMACOLOGY
Mechanism of Action: A sulfhydryl compound with similar properties to those of penicillamine and glutathione that undergoes thiol-disulfide exchange with cysteine to form tiopronin-cysteine, a mixed disulfide. This disulfide is water soluble, unlike cysteine, and does not crystallize in the kidneys. May break disulfide bonds present in bronchial secretions and break the mucus complexes. *Therapeutic Effect:* Decreases cysteine excretion.

Pharmacokinetics
Moderately absorbed from the gastrointestinal (GI) tract. Primarily excreted in urine. Following oral administration, up to 48% of dose appears in urine during the first 4 hours and up to 78% by 72 hours. **Half-life:** 53 hrs.

INDICATIONS AND DOSAGES
Crystinuria
PO
Adults, Elderly. Initially, 800 mg in 3 divided doses. Adjust and maintain crystine concentration below its solubility limit (usually less than 250 mg/L).

Children 9 yrs and older. 15 mg/kg/day in 3 divided doses. Adjust and maintain crystine concentration below its solubility limit (usually less than 250 mg/L).

S **AVAILABLE FORMS/COST**
• Tab-Oral: 100 mg, 100's: **$71.25**

UNLABELED USES: Cataracts, epilepsy, hepatitis, rheumatoid arthritis
CONTRAINDICATIONS: History of agranulocytosis, aplastic anemia, or thrombocytopenia while on tiopronin, pregnancy and lactation, hypersensitivity to tiopronin or its components

PREGNANCY AND LACTATION:
Pregnancy category C; excreted in breast milk and may cause adverse effects in nursing infant, mothers taking tiopronin should avoid nursing

SIDE EFFECTS
Frequent
Pain, swelling, tenderness of skin, rash, hives, itching, oral ulcers
Occasional
GI upset, taste or smell impairment, bloody or cloudy urine, chills, difficulty in breathing, high blood pressure, hoarseness, joint pain, swelling of feet or lower legs, tenderness of glands
Rare
Chest pain, cough, difficulty in chewing, talking, swallowing, double vision, general feeling of discomfort, illness, weakness, muscle weakness, spitting up blood, swelling of lymph glands

SERIOUS REACTIONS
• Hematologic abnormalities, including myelosupression, unusual bleeding, drug fever, renal complications, and lupus erythematous-

like reaction including fever, arthralgia, and lymphadenopathy rarely occur.

SPECIAL CONSIDERATIONS

• May be associated with fever and less severe adverse reactions than d-penicillamine

---

tiotropium
(ty-oh'-tro-pee-um)

Rx: Spiriva
Chemical Class: Quaternary ammonium compound
Therapeutic Class: COPD agent; bronchodilator

CLINICAL PHARMACOLOGY

Mechanism of Action: An anticholinergic that binds to recombinant human muscarinic receptors at the smooth muscle, resulting in long-acting bronchial smooth-muscle relaxation. *Therapeutic Effect:* Relieves bronchospasm.

Pharmacokinetics

Route	Onset	Peak	Duration
Inhalation	N/A	N/A	24-36 hr

Binds extensively to tissue. Protein binding: 72%. Metabolized by oxidation. Excreted in urine. **Half-life:** 5-6 days

INDICATIONS AND DOSAGES

COPD

Inhalation

Adults, Elderly. 18 mcg (1 capsule)/day via *HandiHaler* inhalation device.

CONTRAINDICATIONS: History of hypersensitivity to atropine or its derivatives, including ipratropium

PREGNANCY AND LACTATION: Pregnancy category C; based on rodent studies, tiotropium is excreted into breast milk; the excretion in human milk is unknown but due to quaternary chemical structure, low degree of systemic absorption following INH and minimal systemic absorption following oral ingestion the expected exposure in a nursing infant would not be high; carefully assess risks and benefits in nursing mothers

SIDE EFFECTS

Frequent (16%-6%)

Dry mouth, sinusitis, pharyngitis, dyspepsia, UTI, rhinitis

Occasional (5%-4%)

Abdominal pain, peripheral edema, constipation, epistaxis, vomiting, myalgia, rash, oral candidiasis

SERIOUS REACTIONS

• Angina pectoris, depression, and flulike symptoms occur rarely.

INTERACTIONS

Drugs

3 *Iptratropium:* Potential for additive anticholinergic effects

SPECIAL CONSIDERATIONS

• Compared to ipratropium is more expensive, but once daily administration will likely improve adherence with therapy

PATIENT/FAMILY EDUCATION

• Capsules should NOT be swallowed

• Refer to product information for instructions on how to administer tiotropium via the HandiHaler device

• Should NOT be used for immediate relief of breathing problems, i.e. as a rescue medication

• Do NOT store capsules in the HandiHaler

MONITORING PARAMETERS

• Improvement in symptoms; reduction in the need for rescue short-acting beta2-agonists

tirofiban
(tye-roe-fye'ban)
Rx: Aggrastat
Chemical Class: Glycoprotein
(GP) IIb/IIIa inhibitor
Therapeutic Class: Antiplatelet
agent

CLINICAL PHARMACOLOGY
Mechanism of Action: An antiplatelet and antithrombotic agent
that binds to platelet receptor glycoprotein IIb/IIIa, preventing binding
of fibrinogen. *Therapeutic Effect:*
Inhibits platelet aggregation and
thrombus formation.
Pharmacokinetics
Poorly bound to plasma proteins;
unbound fraction in plasma: 35%.
Limited metabolism. Primarily
eliminated in the urine (65%) and, to
a lesser amount, in the feces. Removed by hemodialysis. **Half-life:**
2 hr. Clearance is significantly decreased in severe renal impairment
(creatinine clearance less than 30
ml/min).

INDICATIONS AND DOSAGES
Inhibition of platelet aggregation
IV
Adults, Elderly. Initially, 0.4
mcg/kg/min for 30 min; then continue at 0.1 mcg/kg/min through
procedure and for 12–24 hrs after
procedure.
*Severe renal insufficiency (creati-
nine clearance less than 30 ml/min)*
Adults, Elderly. Half the usual rate
of infusion.

AVAILABLE FORMS/COST
• Sol, Inj-IV: 250 mcg/ml, 25 ml
(vial): **$243.24**; 50 mcg/ml, 250 ml
(premixed): **$496.20**
CONTRAINDICATIONS: Active internal bleeding or a history of bleeding diathesis within previous 30
days, arteriovenous malformation
or aneurysm, history of intracranial
hemorrhage, history of thrombocytopenia after prior exposure to
tirofiban, intracranial neoplasm,
major surgical procedure within
previous 30 days, severe hypertension, stroke
PREGNANCY AND LACTATION:
Pregnancy category B; excretion
into breast milk unknown; use caution in nursing mothers
SIDE EFFECTS
Occasional (6%–3%)
Pelvis pain, bradycardia, dizziness,
leg pain
Rare (2%–1%)
Edema and swelling, vasovagal reaction, diaphoresis, nausea, fever,
headache
SERIOUS REACTIONS
• Signs and symptoms of overdose
include generally minor mucocutaneous bleeding and bleeding at the
femoral artery access site.
• Thrombocytopenia occurs rarely.
INTERACTIONS
Drugs
▣ *Antithrombotics (aspirin, heparin, warfarin, ticlopidine, clopidogrel):* Increased risk of bleeding
SPECIAL CONSIDERATIONS
• When bleeding cannot be controlled with pressure discontinue
INF
• Most major bleeding occurs at arterial access site for cardiac catheterization; prior to pulling femoral
artery sheath, discontinue heparin
for 3-4 hr and document activated
clotting time (ACT) <180 sec or
aPTT <45 sec; achieve sheath hemostasis ≥4 hr before discharge
• In clinical studies, patients received ASA unless it was contraindicated
• Tirofiban, eptifibitide, and abciximab can all decrease the incidence
of cardiac events associated with
acute coronary syndromes; direct

comparisons are needed to establish which, if any, is superior; for angioplasty, until more data become available, abciximab appears to be the drug of choice

MONITORING PARAMETERS

• Platelet count, hemoglobin, hematocrit, PT/aPTT (baseline, within 6 hr following bolus dose, then daily thereafter)

---

tizanidine
(tye-zan'i-deen)
Rx: Zanaflex
Chemical Class: Imidazoline derivative
Therapeutic Class: Skeletal muscle relaxant

CLINICAL PHARMACOLOGY
Mechanism of Action: A skeletal muscle relaxant that increases presynaptic inhibition of spinal motor neurons mediated by alpha$_2$-adrenergic agonists, reducing facilitation to postsynaptic motor neurons. *Therapeutic Effect:* Reduces muscle spasticity.

Pharmacokinetics

Route	Onset	Peak	Duration
PO	N/A	1-2 hr	3-6 hr

Metabolized in the liver. **Half-life:** 4-8 hr.

INDICATIONS AND DOSAGES
Muscle spasticity
PO
Adults, Elderly. Initially 2-4 mg, gradually increased in 2- to 4-mg increments and repeated q6-8h. Maximum: 3 doses/day or 36 mg /24 hr.

S AVAILABLE FORMS/COST
• Tab—Oral: 2 mg, 100's: **$115.00-$149.60**; 4 mg, 100's: **$135.77-$215.37**

UNLABELED USES: Spasticity associated with multiple sclerosis or spinal cord injury

CONTRAINDICATIONS: None known.

PREGNANCY AND LACTATION: Pregnancy category C; lipid soluble, may pass into breast milk

SIDE EFFECTS
Frequent (49%-41%)
Dry mouth, somnolence, asthenia
Occasional (16%-4%)
Dizziness, UTI, constipation
Rare (3%)
Nervousness, amblyopia, pharyngitis, rhinitis, vomiting, urinary frequency

SERIOUS REACTIONS
• Hypotension (a reduction in either diastolic or systolic BP) may be associated with bradycardia, orthostatic hypotension and, rarely, syncope. The risk of hypotension increases as dosage increases; BP may decrease within 1 hour after administration.

INTERACTIONS
Drugs
❷ *Clonidine, guanabenz, guanadrel, guanethidine, guanfacine:* Potential for hypotension, avoid concurrent use
❸ *Oral contraceptives:* Decreased clearance of tizanidine

SPECIAL CONSIDERATIONS
PATIENT/FAMILY EDUCATION
• Arise slowly from a reclining position

T

tobramycin sulfate
(toe-bra-mye'-sin)
Rx: *Systemic:* Nebcin
Rx: *Ophthalmic:* AKTob, Tobralcon, Tobrex, Tomycine, Tobrasol
Rx: *Nebulizer:* Tobi
Combinations
  Rx: Ophthalmic: with dexamethasone (Tobradex)
Chemical Class: Aminoglycoside
Therapeutic Class: Antibiotic

CLINICAL PHARMACOLOGY
Mechanism of Action: An aminoglycoside antibiotic that irreversibly binds to protein on bacterial ribosomes. *Therapeutic Effect:* Interferes with protein synthesis of susceptible microorganisms.
Pharmacokinetics
Rapid, complete absorption after IM administration. Protein binding: 30%. Widely distributed (doesn't cross the blood-brain barrier; low concentrations in CSF. Excreted unchanged in urine. Removed by hemodialysis. **Half-life:** 2-4 hr (increased in impaired renal function and neonates; decreased in cystic fibrosis and febrile or burn patients).

INDICATIONS AND DOSAGES
Skin and skin-structure, bone, joint, respiratory tract, postoperative, intraabdominal, and burn wound infections; complicated UTIs; septicemia; meningitis
IV, IM
Adults, Elderly. 3-6 mg/kg/day in 3 divided doses or 4-6.6 mg/kg once a day.
Superficial eye infections, including blepharitis, conjunctivitis, keratitis, and corneal ulcers

Ophthalmic Ointment
Adults, Elderly. Usual dosage, apply a thin strip to conjunctiva q8-12h (q3-4h for severe infections).
Ophthalmic Solution
Adults, Elderly. Usual dosage, 1-2 drops in affected eye q4h (2 drops/hr for severe infections).
Bronchopulmonary infections in patients with cystic fibrosis
Inhalation Solution
Adults. Usual dosage, 60-80 mg twice a day for 28 days, then off for 28 days.
Children. 40-80 mg 2-3 times/day.
Dosage in renal impairment
Dosage and frequency are modified based on the degree of renal impairment and the serum drug concentration. After a loading dose of 1-2 mg/kg, the maintenance dose and frequency are based on serum creatinine levels and creatinine clearance.

AVAILABLE FORMS/COST
• Powder, Inj-IV: 40 mg/ml, 2 ml vial: **$3.82-$13.69**
• Oint—Ophth: 0.3%, 3.5 g: **$25.60-$51.13**
• Sol-INH: 60 mg/ml, 5 ml: **$54.01**
• Sol-Ophth: 0.3%, 5 ml: **$5.37-$47.76**

CONTRAINDICATIONS: Hypersensitivity to tobramycin, other aminoglycosides (cross-sensitivity), and their components
PREGNANCY AND LACTATION: Pregnancy category D (ophth category B); excreted into breast milk; given poor oral absorption, toxicity minimal; limited to modification of bowel flora and interference with interpretation of culture results if fever workup required

SIDE EFFECTS
Occasional
IM: Pain, induration
IV: Phlebitis, thrombophlebitis
Topical: Hypersensitivity reaction (fever, pruritus, rash, urticaria)

Ophthalmic: Tearing, itching, redness, eyelid swelling

Rare

Hypotension, nausea, vomiting

SERIOUS REACTIONS

• Nephrotoxicity (as evidenced by increased BUN and serum creatinine levels and decreased creatinine clearance) may be reversible if the drug is stopped at the first sign of nephrotoxic symptoms.

• Irreversible ototoxicity (manifested as tinnitus, dizziness, ringing or roaring in ears, and hearing loss) and neurotoxicity (manifested as headache, dizziness, lethargy, tremor, and visual disturbances) occur occasionally. The risk of these reactions increases with higher dosages or prolonged therapy and when the solution is applied directly to the mucosa.

• Superinfections, particularly fungal infections, may result from bacterial imbalance with any administration route.

• Anaphylaxis may occur.

INTERACTIONS

Drugs

3️⃣ *Amphotericin B:* Synergistic nephrotoxicity

2️⃣ *Atracurium:* Tobramycin potentiates respiratory depression by atracurium

3️⃣ *Carbenicillin:* Potential for inactivation of tobramycin in patients with renal failure

3️⃣ *Carboplatin:* Additive nephrotoxicity or ototoxicity

3️⃣ *Cephalosporins:* Increased potential for nephrotoxicity in patients with preexisting renal disease

3️⃣ *Cisplatin:* Additive nephrotoxicity or ototoxicity

3️⃣ *Cyclosporine:* Additive nephrotoxicity

2️⃣ *Ethacrynic acid:* Additive ototoxicity

3️⃣ *Indomethacin:* Reduced renal clearance of tobramycin in premature infants

3️⃣ *Methoxyflurane:* Additve nephrotoxicity

2️⃣ *Neuromuscular blocking agents:* Tobramycin potentiates respiratory depression by neuromuscular blocking agents

3️⃣ *NSAIDs:* May reduce renal clearance of tobramycin

3️⃣ *Penicillins (extended spectrum):* Potential for inactivation of tobramycin in patients with renal failure

3️⃣ *Piperacillin:* Potential for inactivation of tobramycin in patients with renal failure

2️⃣ *Succinylcholine:* Tobramycin potentiates respiratory depression by succinylcholine

3️⃣ *Ticarcillin:* Potential for inactivation of tobramycin in patients with renal failure

3️⃣ *Vancomycin:* Additive nephrotoxicity or ototoxicity

2️⃣ *Vecuronium:* Tobramycin potentiates respiratory depression by vecuronium

SPECIAL CONSIDERATIONS

• Gentamicin is 1st-line aminoglycoside of choice; differences in toxicity between gentamicin and tobramycin not likely to be clinically important in most patients with normal renal function given short courses of treatment; consider tobramycin in patients who are more likely to develop toxicity (prolonged and/or recurrent aminoglycoside therapy, those with renal failure) and in patients infected with *Pseudomonas aeruginosa* because of increased antibacterial activity

• Has been administered via nebulizer to treat resistant pneumonia in patients with cystic fibrosis

MONITORING PARAMETERS

• Serum Ca, Mg, Na; serum concentrations, peak (30 min following IV INF or 1 hr after IM inj) and trough (just prior to next dose); prolonged concentrations above 12 mcg/ml or trough levels above 2 mcg/ml may indicate tissue accumulation; such accumulation, advanced age, and cumulative dosage may contribute to ototoxicity and nephrotoxicity; perform serum concentration assays after 2 or 3 doses, so that the dosage can be adjusted if necessary, and at 3- to 4-day intervals during therapy; in the event of changing renal function, more frequent serum concentrations should be obtained and the dosage or dosage interval adjusted according to more detailed guidelines

---

tocainide

(toe-kay′nide)

Rx: Tonocard

Chemical Class: Lidocaine derivative

Therapeutic Class: Antiarrhythmic, class IB

CLINICAL PHARMACOLOGY

Mechanism of Action: An amide-type local anesthetic that shortens the action potential duration and decreases the effective refractory period and automaticity in the His-Purkinje system of the myocardium by blocking sodium transport across myocardial cell membranes. *Therapeutic Effect:* Suppresses ventricular arrhythmias.

INDICATIONS AND DOSAGES

Suppression and prevention of ventricular arrhythmias

PO

Adults, Elderly. Initially, 400 mg q8h. Maintenance: 1.2-1.8 g/day in divided doses q8h. Maximum: 2,400 mg/day.

AVAILABLE FORMS/COST

• Tab, Plain Coated—Oral: 400 mg, 100's: **$88.18**; 600 mg, 100's: **$106.40**

CONTRAINDICATIONS: Hypersensitivity to local anesthetics, second- or third-degree AV block

PREGNANCY AND LACTATION: Pregnancy category C; excreted into breast milk; not recommended in nursing mothers

SIDE EFFECTS

Tocainide is generally well tolerated.

Frequent (10%-3%)

Minor, transient light-headedness, dizziness, nausea, paraesthesia, rash, tremor

Occasional (3%-1%)

Clammy skin, night sweats, myalgia

Rare (less than 1%)

Restlessness, nervousness, disorientation, mood changes, ataxia (muscular incoordination), visual disturbances

SERIOUS REACTIONS

• High dosage may produce bradycardia or tachycardia, hypotension, palpitations, increased ventricular arrhythmias, premature ventricular contractions (PVCs), chest pain, and exacerbation of CHF.

INTERACTIONS

Drugs

▨ *Antacids:* Antacids which increase urinary pH may increase tocainide serum concentrations

▨ *Rifampin:* Reduction of serum tocainide concentrations

SPECIAL CONSIDERATIONS

• Can be considered oral lidocaine; antidysrhythmic drugs have not been shown to improve survival in patients with ventricular dysrhythmias; class I antidysrhythmic drugs (e.g., tocainide) have increased the risk of death when used in patients with non-life-threatening dysrhythmias

• Initiate therapy in facilities capable of providing continuous ECG monitoring and managing life-threatening dysrhythmias

MONITORING PARAMETERS

• Blood concentrations (therapeutic concentrations 4-10 mcg/ml)

---

tolazamide
(tole-az'-a-mide)
Rx: Tolinase
Chemical Class: Sulfonylurea (1st generation)
Therapeutic Class: Antidiabetic; hypoglycemic

CLINICAL PHARMACOLOGY
Mechanism of Action: A first-generation sulfonylurea that promotes release of insulin from beta cells of pancreas. *Therapeutic Effect:* Lowers blood glucose concentration.

Pharmacokinetics
Well absorbed from the gastrointestinal (GI) tract. Extensively metabolized in liver to five metabolites, three which are active. Primarily excreted in urine. Unknown if removed by hemodialysis. **Half-life:** 7 hrs.

INDICATIONS AND DOSAGES
Diabetes mellitus
PO
Adults, Elderly. Initially, 100- 250 mg once a day, with breakfast or first main meal. Maintenance: 100- 1000 mg once a day. May increase by increments of 100-250 mg at weekly, based on blood glucose response. May increase by 100 -250 mg/day at weekly intervals. Maximum: 1000

mg/day. Doses more than 500 mg/day should be given in 2 divided doses with meals.

Ⓢ AVAILABLE FORMS/COST
• Tab-Oral: 100 mg, 100's: **$12.50-$50.86**; 250 mg, 100's: **$16.40-$112.86**; 500 mg, 100's: **$35.00-$138.60**

UNLABELED USES: *None known.*

CONTRAINDICATIONS: Diabetic complications, such as ketosis, acidosis, and diabetic coma, sole therapy for type 1 diabetes mellitus, hypersensitivity to tolazamide or its components

PREGNANCY AND LACTATION: Pregnancy category C; inappropriate for use during pregnancy due to inadequacy for blood glucose control, potential for prolonged neonatal hypoglycemia, and risk for congenital abnormalities; insulin is the drug of choice for control of blood sugars during pregnancy; breast milk excretion data is not available—again, the potential for neonatal hypoglycemia dictates caution in nursing mothers

SIDE EFFECTS
Frequent
Altered taste sensation, dizziness, drowsiness, weight gain, constipation, diarrhea, heartburn, nausea, vomiting, stomach fullness, headache
Occasional
Increased sensitivity of skin to sunlight, peeling of skin, itching, rash

SERIOUS REACTIONS
• Severe hypoglycemia may occur due to overdosage and insufficient food intake, especially with increased glucose demands.

• GI hemorrhage, cholestatic hepatic jaundice, leukopenia, thrombocytopenia, pancytopenia, agranulocytosis and aplastic or hemolytic anemia occurs rarely.

INTERACTIONS

Drugs

[3] *Anabolic steroids, chloramphenicol, clofibrate, cyclic antidepressants, MAOIs, sulfonamides:* Enhanced hypoglycemic effects

[3] *β-blockers:* Alter response to hypoglycemia, increase blood glucose concentrations

[3] *Clonidine:* Diminished symptoms of hypoglycemia

[3] *Ethanol:* Altered glycemic control, usually hypoglycemia

[3] *Oral anticoagulants:* Dicoumarol, not warfarin, enhances hypoglycemic response

[3] *Oral contraceptives:* Impaired glucose tolerance

[3] *Rifampin:* Reduced serum levels, reduced hypoglycemic activity

SPECIAL CONSIDERATIONS

- Similar clinical effect as second generations (e.g., glyburide, glipizide); usually less expensive

PATIENT/FAMILY EDUCATION

- Home blood glucose monitoring
- Multiple drug interactions, including alcohol and salicylates
- Symptoms of hypoglycemia: tingling lips/tongue, nausea, confusion, fatigue, sweating, hunger, visual changes (spots)

MONITORING PARAMETERS

- Self-monitored blood glucoses; glycosolated hemoglobin q3-6 mo

tolbutamide

(tole-byoo'ta-mide)

Rx: Orinase

Chemical Class: Sulfonylurea (1st generation)

Therapeutic Class: Antidiabetic; hypoglycemic

CLINICAL PHARMACOLOGY

Mechanism of Action: A first-generation sulfonylurea that promotes the release of insulin from beta cells of pancreas. *Therapeutic Effect:* Lowers blood glucose concentration.

Pharmacokinetics

Route	*Onset*	*Peak*	*Duration*
PO	1 hr	5-8 hrs	12-24 hrs
IV	N/A	30-45 min	90-181 min

Well absorbed from the gastrointestinal (GI) tract. Protein binding: 80%-99%. Extensively metabolized in liver to 2 inactive metabolites, primarily via oxidation. Excreted in urine. Removed by hemodialysis. **Half-life:** 4.5- 6.5 hrs.

INDICATIONS AND DOSAGES

Diabetes mellitus

PO

Adults. Initially, 1 g daily, with breakfast or first main meal, or in divided doses. Maintenance: 0.25- 3 g once a day. After dose of 2 g is reached, dosage should be increased in increments of up to 2 mg q1-2wks, based on blood glucose response. Maximum: 3 g/day.

Endocrine tumor diagnosis

IV

Adults. 1 g infused over 2-3 minutes.

[$] **AVAILABLE FORMS/COST**

- Tab-Oral: 500 mg, 100's: **$3.65-$28.30**

CONTRAINDICATIONS: Diabetic ketoacidosis with or without coma, sole therapy for type 1 diabetes mellitus, use in children, hypersensitivity to tolbutamide or any component of its formulation

PREGNANCY AND LACTATION: Pregnancy category C; inappropriate for use during pregnancy due to inadequacy for blood glucose control, potential for prolonged neonatal hypoglycemia, and risk of congenital abnormalities; insulin is the drug of choice for control of blood sugars during pregnancy; milk-to-plasma ratio of 0.25 reported; the potential for neonatal hypoglycemia dictates caution in nursing mothers

SIDE EFFECTS

Frequent

Increased sensitivity of skin to sunlight, peeling of skin, itching, rash, dizziness, drowsiness, weight gain, constipation, diarrhea, heartburn, nausea, headache, pain at injection site

Occasional

Altered taste sensation, constipation, vomiting, stomach fullness

SERIOUS REACTIONS

• Severe hypoglycemia may occur because of overdosage or insufficient food intake, especially with increased glucose demands.

• Cardiovascular mortality has been reported higher in patients treated with tolbutamide.

• GI hemorrhage, cholestatic hepatic jaundice, leukopenia, thrombocytopenia, pancytopenia, agranulocytosis and aplastic or hemolytic anemia occurs rarely.

INTERACTIONS

Drugs

3 *Anabolic steroids, aspirin, chloramphenicol, MAOIs, sulfonamides:* Enhanced hypoglycemic effects

3 *β-blockers:* Alter response to hypoglycemia

⚠ *Ethanol:* Altered glycemic control, usually hypoglycemia; "Antabuse"-like reaction

3 *Fluconazole, halofenate, itraconazole, ketoconazole, miconazole:* Increased serum concentrations of tolbutamide and other sulfonylureas

3 *Oral anticoagulants:* Dicoumarol, not warfarin, enhances hypoglycemic response to tolbutamide

2 *Phenylbutazone:* Increased hypoglycemic action

3 *Rifabutin, rifampin:* Reduced serum levels, reduced hypoglycemic activity

Labs

• *False increase:* Serum AST, CSF protein

• *Interference:* Urinary albumin

SPECIAL CONSIDERATIONS

• Possible differences exist for tolbutamide (short duration of action, hepatic clearance), potential preferred choice in older patients with poor general physical status and renal impairment

PATIENT/FAMILY EDUCATION

• Multiple drug interactions, including alcohol and salicylates

• Symptoms of hypoglycemia: tingling lips/tongue, nausea, confusion, fatigue, sweating, hunger, visual changes (spots)

MONITORING PARAMETERS

• Self-monitored blood glucoses; glycosolated hemoglobin q 3-6 mo

tolcapone
(toll'ka-pone)
Rx: Tasmar
Chemical Class: Catechol-o-methyl-tranferase (COMT) inhibitor; nitrocatechol
Therapeutic Class: Anti-Parkinson's agent

CLINICAL PHARMACOLOGY
Mechanism of Action: An antiparkinson agent that inhibits the enzyme catechol-*O*-methyltransferase (COMT), potentiating dopamine activity and increasing the duration of action of levodopa. *Therapeutic Effect:* Relieves signs and symptoms of Parkinson's disease.

Pharmacokinetics
Rapidly absorbed after PO administration. Protein binding: 99%. Metabolized in the liver. Eliminated primarily in urine (60%) and, to a lesser extent, in feces (40%). Unknown if removed by hemodialysis. **Half-life:** 2-3 hr.

INDICATIONS AND DOSAGES
Adjunctive treatment of Parkinson's disease
PO
Adults, Elderly. Initially, 100-200 mg 3 times a day concomitantly with each dose of carbidopa and levodopa. Maximum: 600 mg/day.

§ AVAILABLE FORMS/COST
• Tab, Film Coated—Oral: 100 mg, 90's: **$227.71**; 200 mg, 90's: **$244.41**

CONTRAINDICATIONS: None known.

PREGNANCY AND LACTATION: Pregnancy category C; use caution in nursing mothers

SIDE EFFECTS
Alert
Frequency of side effects increases with dosage. The following effects are based on a 200-mg dose.

Frequent (35%-16%)
Nausea, insomnia, somnolence, anorexia, diarrhea, muscle cramps, orthostatic hypotension, excessive dreaming
Occasional (11%-4%)
Headache, vomiting, confusion, hallucinations, constipation, diaphoresis, bright yellow urine, dry eyes, abdominal pain, dizziness, flatulence
Rare (3%-2%)
Dyspepsia, neck pain, hypotension, fatigue, chest discomfort

SERIOUS REACTIONS
• Upper respiratory tract infection and UTI occur in 7%-5% of patients.
• Too-rapid withdrawal from therapy may produce withdrawal-emergent hyperpyrexia, characterized by fever, muscular rigidity, and altered LOC.
• Dyskinesia and dystonia occur frequently.

INTERACTIONS
Drugs
❷ *Nonselective MAO inhibitors (phenelzine, tranycypromine):* Inhibition of the majority of the pathways responsible for normal catecholamine metabolism
❸ *Warfarin:* Possible increased hypoprothrombinemic effect of warfarin

SPECIAL CONSIDERATIONS
• Because of the risk of liver failure, use only in patients who are experiencing symptom fluctuations and are not responding to, or are not candidates for, other adjunctive therapies
• Withdraw drug from patients who fail to show substantial clinical benefit within 3 wk of initiation
• Consider having patients sign informed consent alerting them to potential risks and benefits of this drug

PATIENT/FAMILY EDUCATION
• Monitor for signs of liver disease (clay-colored stools, jaundice, dark urine, right upper quadrant tenderness, pruritus, fatigue, appetite loss, lethargy)

MONITORING PARAMETERS
• ALT/AST at baseline then q2 wk for first yr of therapy, q4 wk for next 6 mo, then q8 wk thereafter; repeat this cycle if dose increased to 200 mg tid; **discontinue tolcapone if ALT or AST exceeds upper limit of normal or if clinical signs and symptoms suggest onset of hepatic failure**

---

tolmetin
(tole′met-in)
Rx: Tolectin
Chemical Class: Acetic acid derivative
Therapeutic Class: NSAID; antipyretic; nonnarcotic analgesic

CLINICAL PHARMACOLOGY
Mechanism of Action: A nonsteroidal anti-inflammatory that produces analgesic and anti-inflammatory effect by inhibiting prostaglandin synthesis. *Therapeutic Effect:* Reduces inflammatory response and intensity of pain stimulus reaching sensory nerve endings.

Pharmacokinetics
Rapidly absorbed from the gastrointestinal (GI) tract. Metabolized in liver. Excreted in urine. Minimally removed by hemodialysis. **Half-life:** 5 hrs.

INDICATIONS AND DOSAGES
Rheumatoid arthritis, osteoarthritis
PO
Adults, Elderly. Initially, 400 mg 3 times/day (including 1 dose upon arising, 1 dose at bedtime). Adjust dose at 1-2 wk intervals. Maintenance: 600-1,800 mg/day in 3-4 divided doses.

Juvenile rheumatoid arthritis
PO
Children more than 2 yrs. Initially, 20 mg/kg/day in 3-4 divided doses. Maintenance: 15-30 mg/kg/day in 3-4 divided doses.

AVAILABLE FORMS/COST
• Cap, Gel—Oral: 400 mg, 100's: **$74.50-$175.24**
• Tab—Oral: 200 mg, 100's: **$65.00**; 600 mg, 100's: **$89.89-$212.61**

UNLABELED USES: Treatment of ankylosing spondylitis, psoriatic arthritis

CONTRAINDICATIONS: Severely incapacitated, bedridden, wheelchair bound, hypersensitivity to aspirin or other NSAIDs

PREGNANCY AND LACTATION: Pregnancy category B (category D near term); small amounts excreted into breast milk, compatible with breast-feeding

SIDE EFFECTS
Occasional
Nausea, vomiting, diarrhea, abdominal cramping, dyspepsia (heartburn, indigestion, epigastric pain), flatulence, dizziness, headache, weight decrease or increase
Rare
Constipation, anorexia, rash, pruritus

SERIOUS REACTIONS
• Peptic ulcer, GI bleeding, gastritis, and severe hepatic reaction (cholestasis, jaundice) occur rarely.
• Nephrotoxicity (dysuria, hematuria, proteinuria, nephrotic syndrome) and severe hypersensitivity reaction (fever, chills, bronchospasm) occur rarely.

INTERACTIONS
Drugs
③ *Aminoglycosides:* Reduced clearance with elevated aminoglycoside levels and potential for toxicity (especially indomethacin in premature infants; other NSAIDs probably)

③ *Anticoagulants:* Excessive hypoprothrombinemia, decreased platelet aggregation with increased risk of GI bleeding

③ *Antihypertensives (α-blockers, angiotensin-converting enzyme inhibitors, angiotensin II receptor blockers, β-blockers, diuretics):* Inhibition of antihypertensive and other favorable hemodynamic effects

③ *Corticosteroids:* Increased risk of GI ulceration

③ *Cyclosporine:* Increased nephrotoxicity risk

③ *Lithium:* Decreased clearance of lithium (mediated via prostaglandins) resulting in elevated serum lithium levels and risk of toxicity

③ *Methotrexate:* Decreased renal secretion of methotrexate resulting in elevated methotrexate levels and risk of toxicity

③ *Phenylpropanolamine:* Possible acute hypertensive reaction

③ *Potassium-sparing diuretics:* Additive hyperkalemia potential

③ *Triamterene:* Acute renal failure reported with addition of indomethacin; caution with other NSAIDs

Labs
• *False positive:* Proteinuria (use dye-impregnated reagent strips), urinary drugs of abuse screen

SPECIAL CONSIDERATIONS
MONITORING PARAMETERS
• Initial hemogram and fecal occult blood test within 3 mo of starting regular chronic therapy; repeat every 6-12 mo (more frequently in high-risk patients [>65 years, peptic ulcer disease, concurrent steroids or anticoagulants]); electrolytes, creatinine, and BUN within 3 mo of starting regular chronic therapy; repeat every 6-12 mo

---

tolnaftate
(tole-naf'tate)
OTC: Absorbine Athelete's Foot Cream, Aftate, Quinsana Plus, Tinactin, Ting
Chemical Class: Carbamothioic acid derivative
Therapeutic Class: Antifungal

CLINICAL PHARMACOLOGY
Mechanism of Action: An antifungal that distorts hyphae and stunts mycelial growth in susceptible fungi. *Therapeutic Effect:* Results in fungal cell death.

INDICATIONS AND DOSAGES
Tinea pedis, tinea cruris, tinea corporis
Topical
Adults, Elderly, Children 2 yrs and older. Spray aerosol or apply 1-3 drops of solution or a small amount of cream, gel, or powder 2 times daily for 2-4 wks.

Ⓢ AVAILABLE FORMS/COST
• Cre-Top: 1%, 15, 30 g: **$1.32-$8.44**/15 g
• Oint-Top: 1%, 30 g: **$1.90**
• Powder-Top: 1%, 45, 90 g: **$1.92-$5.99**/45 g
• Sol-Top: 1%, 10, 15, 30, 60, 120 ml: **$1.60-$4.79**/10 ml
• Spray-Top: 1%, 90, 105, 120 ml: **$3.11**/105 ml

UNLABELED USES: Onchomycosis

CONTRAINDICATIONS: Nail and scalp infections, hypersensitivity to tolnaftate or any component of its formulation

PREGNANCY AND LACTATION: Pregnancy category C

SIDE EFFECTS

Rare

Irritation, burning, pruritus, contact dermatitis

SERIOUS REACTIONS

- None known.

SPECIAL CONSIDERATIONS

- Non-prescription topical antifungal agent not effective in the treatment of deeper fungal infections of the skin, nor is it reliable in the treatment of fungal infections involving the scalp or nail beds; *Candida* is resistant; useful for patients desiring self-medication of mild tinea infections; patients must be advised of limitations
- Powders generally used as adjunctive therapy, but may be acceptable as primary therapy in very mild cases

tolterodine

(tol-tare'-oh-deen)

Rx: Detrol, Detrol LA

Chemical Class: Tertiary amine

Therapeutic Class: Genitourinary muscle relaxant

CLINICAL PHARMACOLOGY

Mechanism of Action: An antispasmodic that exhibits potent antimuscarinic activity by interceding via cholinergic muscarinic receptors, thereby inhibiting urinary bladder contraction. *Therapeutic Effect:* Decreases urinary frequency, urgency.

Pharmacokinetics

Rapidly and well absorbed after PO administration. Protein binding: 96%. Extensively metabolized in the liver to active metabolite. Primarily excreted in urine. Unknown if removed by hemodialysis. **Half-life:** 1.9–3.7 hr.

INDICATIONS AND DOSAGES

Overactive bladder

PO

Adults, Elderly. 1–2 mg twice a day.

Dosage in severe renal or hepatic impairment

PO

Adults, Elderly. 1 mg twice a day.

PO (Extended-Release)

Adults, Elderly. 2–4 mg once a day.

$ **AVAILABLE FORMS/COST**

- Tab—Oral: 1 mg, 60's: **$108.25**; 2 mg, 60's: **$111.10**
- Cap, Sus Action—Oral: 2 mg, 90's: **$269.88**; 4 mg, 90's: **$276.98**

CONTRAINDICATIONS: Uncontrolled angle-closure glaucoma, urine retention

PREGNANCY AND LACTATION: Pregnancy category C; probably excreted in breast milk. Not recommended during lactation

SIDE EFFECTS

Frequent (40%)

Dry mouth

Occasional (11%–4%)

Headache, dizziness, fatigue, constipation, dyspepsia (heartburn, indigestion, epigastric discomfort), upper respiratory tract infection, UTI, dry eyes, abnormal vision (accommodation problems), nausea, diarrhea

Rare (3%)

Somnolence, chest or back pain, arthralgia, rash, weight gain, dry skin

SERIOUS REACTIONS

- Overdose can result in severe anticholinergic effects, including abdominal cramps, facial warmth, excessive salivation or lacrimation, diaphoresis, pallor, urinary urgency, blurred vision, and prolonged QT interval.

INTERACTIONS

Drugs

[3] *Clarithromycin:* Increased blood tolterodine concentration

T

⬛ *Cyclosporine:* Increased blood tolterodine concentration

⬛ *Erythromycin:* Increased blood tolterodine concentration

⬛ *Itraconazole:* Increased blood tolterodine concentration

⬛ *Ketoconazole:* Increased blood tolterodine concentration

⬛ *Vinblastine:* Increased blood tolterodine concentration

SPECIAL CONSIDERATIONS
PATIENT/FAMILY EDUCATION
• Dry mouth occurs in 40% of treated patients at a dose of 2 mg bid; incidence is dose-dependent

---

topiramate
(toe-peer′a-mate)
Rx: Topamax
Chemical Class: Sulfamate-substituted monosaccharide derivative
Therapeutic Class: Anticonvulsant

CLINICAL PHARMACOLOGY
Mechanism of Action: An anticonvulsant that blocks repetitive, sustained firing of neurons by enhancing the ability of gamma-aminobutyric acid to induce an influx of chloride ions into the neurons; may also block sodium channels. *Therapeutic Effect:* Decreases seizure activity.
Pharmacokinetics
Rapidly absorbed after PO administration. Protein binding: 13%-17%. Not extensively metabolized. Primarily excreted unchanged in urine. Removed by hemodialysis. **Half-life:** 21 hr.
INDICATIONS AND DOSAGES
Adjunctive treatment of partial seizures, Lennox-Gastant Syndrome
PO
Adults, Elderly, Children older than 17 yr. Initially, 25-50 mg for 1 wk. May increase by 25-50 mg/day at weekly intervals. Maximum: 1,600 mg/day.
Children 2-16 yr. Initially, 1-3 mg/kg/day to maximum of 25 mg.. May increase by 1-3 mg/kg/day at weekly intervals. Maintenance: 5-9 mg/kg/day in 2 divided doses.
Tonic-clonic seizures
PO
Adults, Elderly, Children. Dosage is individualized and titrated.
Migraine prevention
PO
Adults, Elderly. 100 mg/day in 2 divided doses.
Dosage in renal impairment
Expect to reduce drug dosage by 50% in patients with tonic-clonic seizures who have a creatinine clearance of less than 70 ml/min.
🅢 AVAILABLE FORMS/COST
• Cap, Enteric Coated (Sprinkle)— Oral: 15 mg, 60's: **$96.46**; 25 mg, 60's: **$116.60**
• Tab—Oral: 25 mg, 60's: **$173.98**; 100 mg, 60's: **$248.46**; 200 mg, 60's: **$290.89**
UNLABELED USES: Prevention of migraine headaches, treatment of alcohol dependence
CONTRAINDICATIONS: None known.
PREGNANCY AND LACTATION: Pregnancy category C
SIDE EFFECTS
Frequent (30%-10%)
Somnolence, dizziness, ataxia, nervousness, nystagmus, diplopia, paresthesia, nausea, tremor
Occasional (9%-3%)
Confusion, breast pain, dysmenorrhea, dyspepsia, depression, asthenia, pharyngitis, weight loss, anorexia, rash, musculoskeletal pain, ab-

dominal pain, difficulty with coordination, sinusitis, agitation, flu-like symptoms

Rare (3%-2%)

Mood disturbances, such as irritability and depression; dry mouth; aggressive behavior

SERIOUS REACTIONS

• Psychomotor slowing, impaired concentration, language problems (such as word-finding difficulties), and memory disturbances occur occasionally. These reactions are generally mild to moderate but may be severe enough to require discontinuation of drug therapy.

INTERACTIONS

Drugs

▣ *Phenytoin, carbamazepine, valproic acid:* Lowers topiramate concentrations

▣ *Ethinyl estradiol:* Increased clearance of estrogen

SPECIAL CONSIDERATIONS

PATIENT/FAMILY EDUCATION

• Drink plenty of fluids to prevent kidney stone formation

---

torsemide
(tor'se-mide)
Rx: Demadex
Chemical Class: Pyridine-sulfonamide derivative
Therapeutic Class: Antihypertensive; diuretic, loop

CLINICAL PHARMACOLOGY

Mechanism of Action: A loop diuretic that enhances excretion of sodium, chloride, potassium, and water at the ascending limb of the loop of Henle; also reduces plasma and extracellular fluid volume. *Therapeutic Effect:* Produces diuresis; lowers BP.

Pharmacokinetics

Route	Onset	Peak	Dura-tion
PO	1 hr	1–2 hr	6–8 hr
IV	10 min	1 hr	6–8 hr

Rapidly and well absorbed from the GI tract. Protein binding: 97%–99%. Metabolized in the liver. Primarily excreted in urine. Not removed by hemodialysis. **Half-life:** 3.3 hr.

INDICATIONS AND DOSAGES

Hypertension

PO

Adults, Elderly. Initially, 5 mg/day. May increase to 10 mg/day if no response in 4–6 wk. If no response, additional antihypertensive added.

CHF

PO, IV

Adults, Elderly. Initially, 10–20 mg/day. May increase by approximately doubling dose until desired therapeutic effect is attained. Doses greater than 200 mg have not been adequately studied.

Chronic renal failure

PO, IV

Adults, Elderly. Initially, 20 mg/day. May increase by approximately doubling dose until desired therapeutic effect is attained. Doses greater than 200 mg have not been adequately studied.

Hepatic cirrhosis

PO, IV

Adults, Elderly. Initially, 5 mg/day given with aldosterone antagonist or potassium-sparing diuretic. May increase by approximately doubling dose until desired therapeutic effect is attained. Doses greater than 40 mg have not been adequately studied.

Ⓢ **AVAILABLE FORMS/COST**

• Sol, Inj-IV: 10 mg/ml, 2 ml: **$6.65**

• Tab-Oral: 5 mg, 100's: **$63.40-$85.43**; 10 mg, 100's: **$70.25-$94.66**; 20 mg, 100's: **$82.06-$110.58**; 100 mg, 100's: **$304.10-$409.69**

CONTRAINDICATIONS: Anuria, hepatic coma, severe electrolyte depletion

PREGNANCY AND LACTATION: Pregnancy category B; cardiovascular disorders such as pulmonary edema, severe hypertension, or CHF are probably the only valid indications for loop diuretics during pregnancy

SIDE EFFECTS

Frequent (10%–4%)

Headache, dizziness, rhinitis

Occasional (3%–1%)

Asthenia, insomnia, nervousness, diarrhea, constipation, nausea, dyspepsia, edema, EKG changes, pharyngitis, cough, arthralgia, myalgia

Rare (less than 1%)

Syncope, hypotension, arrhythmias

SERIOUS REACTIONS

• Ototoxicity may occur with high doses or a too-rapid IV administration.

• Overdose produces acute, profound water loss; volume and electrolyte depletion; dehydration; decreased blood volume; and circulatory collapse.

INTERACTIONS

Drugs

❷ *Aminoglycosides (gentamicin, kanamycin, neomycin, streptomycin):* Additive ototoxicity (ethacrynic acid > furosemide, torsemide, bumetanide)

❸ *Angiotensin converting enzyme inhibitors:* Initiation of ACEI with intensive diuretic therapy may result in precipitous fall in blood pressure; ACEIs may induce renal insufficiency in the presence of diuretic-induced sodium depletion

❸ *Barbiturates (phenobarbital):* Reduced diuretic response

❸ *Bile acid-binding resins (cholestyramine, colestipol):* Resins markedly reduce the bioavailability and diuretic response of furosemide

❸ *Carbenoxolone:* Severe hypokalemia from coadministration

❸ *Cephalosporins (cephaloridine, cephalothin):* Enhanced nephrotoxicity with coadministration

❷ *Cisplatin:* Additive ototoxicity (ethacrynic acid > furosemide, torsemide, bumetanide)

❸ *Clofibrate:* Enhanced effects of both drugs, especially in hypoalbuminemic patients

❸ *Corticosteroids:* Concomitant loop diuretic and corticosteroid therapy can result in excessive potassium loss

❸ *Digitalis glycosides (digoxin, digitoxin):* Diuretic-induced hypokalemia may increase risk of digitalis toxicity

❸ *Nonsteroidal antiinflammatory drugs (flurbiprofen, ibuprofen, indomethacin, naproxen, piroxicam, aspirin, sulindac):* Reduced diuretic and antihypertensive effects

❸ *Phenytoin:* Reduced diuretic response

❸ *Serotonin-reuptake inhibitors (fluoxetine, paroxetine, sertraline):* Case reports of sudden death; enhanced hyponatremia proposed; causal relationships not established

❸ *Terbutaline:* Additive hypokalemia

❸ *Tubocurarine:* Prolonged neuromuscular blockade

SPECIAL CONSIDERATIONS

• Offers potential advantages over other loop diuretics, including a longer duration of action and fewer adverse electrolyte and metabolic effects; available data not extensive or convincing enough at present to recommend replacement of standard loop diuretic (furosemide); considered alternative in refractory patients

MONITORING PARAMETERS

• Urine volume, creatinine clearance, BUN, electrolytes, reduction in edema, increased diuresis, decrease in body weight, reduction in blood pressure, glucose, uric acid, serum calcium (tetany), tinnitus, vertigo, hearing loss (especially in those at risk for ototoxicity—IV doses >120 mg; concomitant ototoxic drugs; renal disease)

---

tramadol

Rx: Ultram
Combinations
  Rx: with acetaminophen (Ultracet)
Chemical Class: Cyclohexanol derivative
Therapeutic Class: Centrally acting synthetic analgesic

CLINICAL PHARMACOLOGY

Mechanism of Action: An analgesic that binds to mu-opioid receptors and inhibits reuptake of norepinephrine and serotonin. Reduces the intensity of pain stimuli reaching sensory nerve endings. *Therapeutic Effect:* Alters the perception of and emotional response to pain.

Pharmacokinetics

Route	Onset	Peak	Duration
PO	less than 1 hr	2-3 hr	4-6 hr

Rapidly and almost completely absorbed after PO administration. Protein binding: 20%. Extensively metabolized in the liver to active metabolite (reduced in patients with advanced cirrhosis). Primarily excreted in urine. Minimally removed by hemodialysis. **Half-life:** 6-7 hr.

INDICATIONS AND DOSAGES

Moderate to moderately severe pain

PO

Adults, Elderly. 50-100 mg q4-6h. Maximum: 400 mg/day for patients younger than 75 yr; 300 mg/day for patients older than 75 yr.

Dosage in renal impairment

For patients with creatinine clearance of less than 30 ml/min, increase dosing interval to q12h. Maximum: 200 mg/day.

Dosage in hepatic impairment

Dosage is decreased to 50 mg q12h.

🅢 AVAILABLE FORMS/COST

• Tab-Oral: 50 mg, 100's: **$30.17-$135.10**

• Tab-Oral (with acetaminophen): 325 mg-37.5 mg, 100's: **$102.50**

CONTRAINDICATIONS: Acute alcohol intoxication; concurrent use of centrally acting analgesics, hypnotics, opioids, or psychotropic drugs

PREGNANCY AND LACTATION: Pregnancy category C; small amounts excreted into breast milk

SIDE EFFECTS

Frequent (25%-15%)

Dizziness or vertigo, nausea, constipation, headache, somnolence

Occasional (10%-5%)

Vomiting, pruritus, CNS stimulation (such as nervousness, anxiety, agitation, tremor, euphoria, mood swings, and hallucinations), asthenia, diaphoresis, dyspepsia, dry mouth, diarrhea

Rare (less than 5%)

Malaise, vasodilation, anorexia, flatulence, rash, blurred vision, urine retention or urinary frequency, menopausal symptoms

SERIOUS REACTIONS

• Overdose results in respiratory depression and seizures.

T

• Tramadol may have a prolonged duration of action and cumulative effect in patients with hepatic or renal impairment.

INTERACTIONS

③ *Carbamazepine:* CNS depression; increased tramadol metabolism, may require significantly increased tramadol dosing for equianalgesic effects

③ *Ethanol, opioids, anesthetic agents, phenothiazines, tranquilizers, sedative-hypnotics:* CNS depression

③ *MAOIs:* Potential exaggerated norepinephrine and serotonin effects, as tramadol inhibits reuptake

③ *SSRIs:* Increased risk of seizures

SPECIAL CONSIDERATIONS

• Expensive, nonnarcotic, "narcotic"-tricyclic antidepressant combination analgesic; potential use in chronic pain; demonstrated efficacy in a variety of pain syndromes; minimal cardiovascular and respiratory side effects

• Does not completely bind to opioid receptors; caution in addicted patients

• Has more potential for abuse than previously thought

• Tolerance and withdrawal symptoms milder than with opiates

• Not chemically related to opiates

---

trandolapril
(tran-doe'la-pril)
Rx: Mavik
Combinations
 Rx: with verapamil (Tarka)
Chemical Class: Angiotensin-converting enzyme (ACE) inhibitor, nonsulfhydryl
Therapeutic Class: Antihypertensive

CLINICAL PHARMACOLOGY
Mechanism of Action: An ACE inhibitor that suppresses the renin-angiotensin-aldosterone system and prevents the conversion of angiotensin I to angiotensin II, a potent vasoconstrictor; may also inhibit angiotensin II at local vascular and renal sites. Decreases plasma angiotensin II, increases plasma renin activity, and decreases aldosterone secretion. *Therapeutic Effect:* Reduces peripheral arterial resistance and pulmonary capillary wedge pressure; improves cardiac output and exercise tolerance.

Pharmacokinetics
Slowly absorbed from the GI tract. Protein binding: 80%. Metabolized in the liver and GI mucosa to active metabolite. Primarily excreted in urine. Removed by hemodialysis. **Half-life:** 24 hr.

INDICATIONS AND DOSAGES
Hypertension (without diuretic)
PO
Adults, Elderly. Initially, 1 mg once a day in nonblack patients, 2 mg once a day in black patients. Adjust dosage at least at 7-day intervals. Maintenance: 2-4 mg/day. Maximum: 8 mg/day.
CHF
PO
Adults, Elderly. Initially, 0.5-1 mg, titrated to target dose of 4 mg/day.

$ AVAILABLE FORMS/COST
• Tab—Oral: 1 mg, 2 mg, 4 mg, 100's: **$96.11**
• Tab, Sus Action—Oral (with verapamil): 1 mg-240 mg, 2 mg-180 mg, 2 mg-240 mg, 4 mg-240 mg, 100's; all: **$206.23**

CONTRAINDICATIONS: History of angioedema from previous treatment with ACE inhibitors

PREGNANCY AND LACTATION: Pregnancy category C (1st trimester), category D (2nd and 3rd trimesters); ACE inhibitors can cause fetal and neonatal morbidity and death when administered to pregnant women; when pregnancy is detected, discontinue ACE inhibitors as soon as possible

SIDE EFFECTS
Frequent (35%-23%)
Dizziness, cough
Occasional (11%-3%)
Hypotension, dyspepsia (heartburn, epigastric pain, indigestion), syncope, asthenia (loss of strength), tinnitus
Rare (less than 1%)
Palpitations, insomnia, drowsiness, nausea, vomiting, constipation, flushed skin

SERIOUS REACTIONS
• Excessive hypotension (first-dose syncope) may occur in patients with CHF and in those who are severely salt or volume depleted.
• Angioedema and hyperkalemia occur rarely.
• Agranulocytosis and neutropenia may be noted in those with collagen vascular disease, including scleroderma and systemic lupus erythematosus, and impaired renal function.
• Nephrotic syndrome may be noted in those with history of renal disease.

INTERACTIONS
Drugs
▣ *Azathioprine:* Increased myelosuppression
▣ *Lithium:* Increased risk of serious lithium toxicity
▣ *Loop diuretics:* Initiation of ACE inhibitor therapy in the presence of intensive diuretic therapy results in a precipitous fall in blood pressure in some patients; ACE inhibitors may induce renal insufficiency in the presence of diuretic-induced sodium depletion
▣ *NSAIDs:* Inhibition of the antihypertensive response to ACE inhibitors
▣ *Potassium-sparing diuretics:* Increased risk for hyperkalemia
▣ *Trimethoprim:* Additive risk of hyperkalemia, especially in patient predisposed to renal insufficiency
Labs
• ACE inhibition can account for approximately 0.5 mEq/L rise in serum potassium

SPECIAL CONSIDERATIONS
PATIENT/FAMILY EDUCATION
• Caution with salt substitutes containing potassium chloride
• Rise slowly to sitting/standing position to minimize orthostatic hypotension
• Dizziness, fainting, lightheadedness may occur during 1st few days of therapy
• May cause altered taste perception or cough; persistent dry cough usually does not subside unless medication is stopped; notify clinician if these symptoms persist

MONITORING PARAMETERS
• BUN, creatinine, potassium within 2 wk after initiation of therapy (increased levels may indicate acute renal failure)

T

tranylcypromine
(tran-ill-sip'roe-meen)
Rx: Parnate
Chemical Class: Cyclopropy-
lamine, substituted;
nonhydrazine derivative
Therapeutic Class: Antidepressant, monoamine oxidase
inhibitor (MAOI)

CLINICAL PHARMACOLOGY
Mechanism of Action: An MAOI
that inhibits the activity of the enzyme monoamine oxidase at CNS
storage sites, leading to increased
levels of the neurotransmitters epinephrine, norepinephrine, serotonin, and dopamine at neuronal receptor sites. *Therapeutic Effect:* Relieves depression.

INDICATIONS AND DOSAGES
*Depression refractory to or intoler-
ant of other therapy*
PO
Adults, Elderly. Initially, 10 mg
twice a day. May increase by 10
mg/day at 1- to 3-wk intervals up to
60 mg/day in divided doses.

§   AVAILABLE FORMS/COST
• Tab, Plain Coated—Oral: 10 mg,
100's: **$72.38**

CONTRAINDICATIONS: CHF,
children younger than 16 years,
pheochromocytoma, severe hepatic
or renal impairment, uncontrolled
hypertension

PREGNANCY AND LACTATION:
Pregnancy category C; excreted into
breast milk

SIDE EFFECTS
Frequent
Orthostatic hypotension, restlessness, GI upset, insomnia, dizziness,
lethargy, weakness, dry mouth, peripheral edema

Occasional
Flushing, diaphoresis, rash, urinary
frequency, increased appetite, tran-
sient impotence
Rare
Visual disturbances

SERIOUS REACTIONS
• Hypertensive crisis occurs rarely
and is marked by severe hypertension, occipital headache radiating
frontally, neck stiffness or soreness,
nausea, vomiting, diaphoresis, fever
or chills, clammy skin, dilated pupils, palpitations, tachycardia or
bradycardia, and constricting chest
pain.

INTERACTIONS
Drugs
▲ *Amphetamines,   sympathomimetics, tyramine containing foods:*
Severe hypertensive reactions
③ *Antidiabetics:* Prolonged hypoglycemia
③ *Barbiturates:* Prolonged effect
of barbiturates
③ *Buproprion:* Enhanced toxicity
of buproprion, concomitant use contraindicated
③ *Buspirone:* Hypertension, concomitant use not recommended
▲ *Clomipramine, fluoxetine, fluvoxamine, paroxetine, sertraline:*
Severe or fatal reactions, serotonin
related
② *Dextromethorphan:* Psychosis
or bizarre behavior reported
② *Dopamine, guanethidine, methyldopa, reserpine:* Hypertension,
headache, and related symptoms
▲ *Entacapone, tolcapone:* Inhibition of catecholamine metabolism,
concomitant use contraindicated
▲ *Ethanol:* Hypertensive response
with alcoholic beverages containing
tyramine
▲ *Furazolidone,   procarbazine:*
Additive MAO inhibition

3 *Levodopa:* Hypertensive response; carbidopa minimizes the reaction

2 *Lithium:* Hyperpyrexia with phenelzine

⚠ *Meperidine:* Serotonin accumulation—agitation, blood pressure elevations, hyperpyrexia, *seizures*

3 *Norepinephrine:* Increased pressor response to norepinephrine

⚠ *Selective serotonin reuptake inhibitors (SSRIs):* Severe or fatal reactions (serotonin syndrome)

⚠ *Sumatriptan:* Increased sumatriptan concentrations, possible toxicity

⚠ *Tricyclic antidepressants:* Increased risk of hypertensive crisis, tricyclics should never be added to an existing MAOI regimen

⚠ *Tryptophan:* Severe or fatal reactions (serotonin syndrome)

SPECIAL CONSIDERATIONS
• Irreversible nonselective MAOI effective for typical and atypical depression; equal efficacy to other MAOIs with quicker onset of action, and an amphetamine-like activity with a higher potential for abuse; no anticholinergic or cardiac effects

PATIENT/FAMILY EDUCATION
• Therapeutic effects may take 1-4 wk
• Avoid alcohol ingestion, CNS depressants, OTC medications (cold, weight loss, hay fever, cough syrup)
• Prodromal signs of hypertensive crisis are increased headache, palpitations; discontinue drug immediately
• Do not discontinue medication abruptly after long-term use
• Avoid high-tyramine foods (aged cheese, sour cream, beer, wine, pickled products, liver, raisins, bananas, figs, avocados, meat tenderizers, chocolate, yogurt)

---

trazodone
(tray′zoe-done)
Rx: Desyrel
Chemical Class: Triazolopyridine derivative
Therapeutic Class: Antidepressant

CLINICAL PHARMACOLOGY
Mechanism of Action: An antidepressant that blocks the reuptake of serotonin at neuronal presynaptic membranes, increasing its availability at postsynaptic receptor sites. *Therapeutic Effect:* Relieves depression.

Pharmacokinetics
Well absorbed from the GI tract. Protein binding: 85%-95%. Metabolized in the liver. Primarily excreted in urine. Unknown if removed by hemodialysis. **Half-life:** 5-9 hr.

INDICATIONS AND DOSAGES
Depression
PO
Adults. Initially, 150 mg/day in equally divided doses. Increase by 50 mg/day at 3-to 4-day intervals until therapeutic response is achieved. Maximum: 600 mg/day.
Elderly. Initially, 25-50 mg at bedtime. May increase by 25-50 mg every 3-7 days. Range: 75-150 mg/day.
Children 6-18 yr. Initially, 1.5-2 mg/kg/day in divided doses. May increase gradually to 6 mg/kg/day in 3 divided doses.

$ **AVAILABLE FORMS/COST**
• Tab, Plain Coated—Oral: 50 mg, 100's: **$9.88-$217.28**; 100 mg, 100's: **$11.08-$379.69**; 150 mg, 100's: **$32.00-$327.09**; 300 mg, 100's: **$426.52-$582.18**
UNLABELED USES: Treatment of neurogenic pain

CONTRAINDICATIONS: None known.

PREGNANCY AND LACTATION: Pregnancy category C; excreted into human breast milk; effects on nursing infant unknown, but of possible concern

SIDE EFFECTS

Frequent (9%-3%)

Somnolence, dry mouth, light-headedness, dizziness, headache, blurred vision, nausea, vomiting

Occasional (3%-1%)

Nervousness, fatigue, constipation, generalized aches and pains, mild hypotension

Rare

Photosensitivity reaction

SERIOUS REACTIONS

• Priapism, diminished or improved libido, retrograde ejaculation, and impotence occur rarely.

• Trazodone appears to be less cardiotoxic than other antidepressants, although arrhythmias may occur in patients with pre-existing cardiac disease.

INTERACTIONS

Drugs

▨ *Clonidine:* Inhibited antihypertensive response to clonidine

▨ *Ethanol:* Additive impairment of motor skills; abstinent alcoholics may eliminate cyclic antidepressants more rapidly than non-alcoholics

▨ *Fluoxetine:* Increased plasma trazodone concentrations

⚠ *MAOIs:* Potential for fatal serotonin syndrome

▨ *Neuroleptics:* Additive hypotension

SPECIAL CONSIDERATIONS

• Very sedating antidepressant with minimal anticholinergic effects; good choice for elderly patients in whom sedating properties would be desirable

PATIENT/FAMILY EDUCATION

• Take with food

• Use caution driving or performing other tasks requiring alertness

---

treprostinil

(treh-prost'in-ill)

Rx: Remodulin

Chemical Class: Prostacyclin analog

Therapeutic Class: Vasodilator

CLINICAL PHARMACOLOGY

Mechanism of Action: An antiplatelet that directly dilates pulmonary and systemic arterial vascular beds, inhibiting platelet aggregation. *Therapeutic Effect:* Reduces symptoms of pulmonary arterial hypertension associated with exercise.

Pharmacokinetics

Rapidly, completely absorbed after subcutaneous infusion; 91% bound to plasma protein. Metabolized by the liver. Excreted mainly in the urine with a lesser amount eliminated in the feces. **Half-life:** 2–4 hr.

INDICATIONS AND DOSAGES

Pulmonary arterial hypertension

Continuous subcutaneous infusion

Adults, Elderly. Initially, 1.25 ng/kg/min. Reduce infusion rate to 0.625 ng/kg/min if initial dose cannot be tolerated. Increase infusion rate in increments of no more than 1.25 ng/kg/min per week for the first 4 wk and then no more than 2.5 ng/kg/min per week for the duration of infusion.

Hepatic impairment (mild to moderate)

Adults, Elderly. Decrease the initial dose to 0.625 ng/kg/min based on ideal body weight and increase cautiously.

AVAILABLE FORMS/COST
• Sol, Inj-SC: 1 mg/ml, 20 ml: **$1,300.00**; 2.5 mg/ml, 20 ml: **$3,250.00**; 5 mg/ml, 20 ml: **$6,500.00**; 10 mg/ml, 20 ml: **$7,800.00**

CONTRAINDICATIONS: None known

PREGNANCY AND LACTATION: Pregnancy category B; excretion into human breast milk unknown, use caution in nursing mothers

SIDE EFFECTS
Frequent
Infusion site pain, erythema, induration, rash
Occasional
Headache, diarrhea, jaw pain, vasodilation, nausea
Rare
Dizziness, hypotension, pruritus, edema

SERIOUS REACTIONS
• Abrupt withdrawal or sudden large reductions in dosage may result in worsening of pulmonary arterial hypertension symptoms.

INTERACTIONS
Drugs
③ *Diuretics, antihypertensives, vasodilators:* Exacerbated reductions in blood pressure, increased potential for hypotension
③ *Anticoagulants, antiplatelet agents:* Increased risk for bleeding

SPECIAL CONSIDERATIONS
PATIENT/FAMILY EDUCATION
• Patient must be able to administer drug via continuous sc INF and care for the infusion system
• Therapy may be required for prolonged periods of time
• Solutions should be administered without additional dilution

MONITORING PARAMETERS
• Blood pressure, clinical symptoms

---

tretinoin
(tret′i-noyn)
Rx: *Topical:* Avita, Retin-A, Renova
Rx: *Oral:* Vesanoid (Tretinoin/Retinoic Acid) Combinations
  Rx: with fluocinolone/hydroquinone (Tri-Luma)
Chemical Class: Retinoid; vitamin A derivative
Therapeutic Class: Antiacne agent

CLINICAL PHARMACOLOGY
Mechanism of Action: A retinoid that decreases cohesiveness of follicular epithelial cells. Increases turnover of follicular epithelial cells. Bacterial skin counts are not altered. Transdermal: Exerts its effects on growth and differentiation of epithelial cells. Antineoplastic: Induces maturation, decreases proliferation of acute promyelocytic leukemia (APL) cells *Therapeutic Effect:* Causes expulsion of blackheads; alleviates fine wrinkles, hyperpigmentation; causes repopulation of bone marrow and blood by normal hematopoietic cells.

Pharmacokinetics
Topical: Minimally absorbed. Oral: Well absorbed following oral administration. Protein binding: 95%. Metabolized in liver. Primarily excreted in urine, minimal excretion in feces. **Half-life:** 0.5-2 hrs.

INDICATIONS AND DOSAGES
Acne
Topical
Adults. Apply once daily at bedtime.
Transdermal
Transdermal
Adults. Apply to face once daily at bedtime.

Acute promyelocytic leukemia
PO

Adults. 45 mg/m2/day given as two evenly divided doses until complete remission is documented. Discontinue therapy 30 days after complete remission or after 90 days of treatment, whichever comes first.

Ⓢ **AVAILABLE FORMS/COST**
• Cap—Oral: 10 mg, 100's: **$1,876.80**
• Cre—Top: 0.025%, 20, 45 g: **$31.85-$57.94**/20 g; 0.05%, 20, 45, 60 g: **$30.20-$51.49**/20 g; 0.1%, 20, 45 g: **$38.17-$60.09**/20 g; 0.02%, 40 g: **$78.65**
• Gel—Top: 0.01%, 15, 45 g: **$25.73-$36.45**/15 g; 0.025%, 15, 20, 45 g: **$25.35-$36.76**/15 g
• Gel-Top (micronized): 0.04%, 20, 45 g: **$46.49**/20 g; 0.1%, 20, 45 g: **$46.49**/20 g
• Liq—Top: 0.05%, 28 ml: **$41.58-$78.66**

UNLABELED USES: Treatment of disorders of keratinization, including photo-aged skin, liver spots

CONTRAINDICATIONS: Sensitivity to parabens (used as preservative in gelatin capsule)

PREGNANCY AND LACTATION: Pregnancy category B; teratogenic risk when used topically is thought to be close to zero; minimal absorption occurring after topical application probably precludes detection of clinically significant amounts in breast milk

SIDE EFFECTS
Expected
Topical
Temporary change in peigmentation, photosensitivity, Local inflammatory reactions (peeling, dry skin, stinging, erythema, pruritus) are to be expected and are reversible with discontinuation of tretinoin

Frequent
PO
Headache, fever, dry skin/oral mucosa, bone pain, nausea, vomiting, rash
Occasional
PO
Mucositis, earache or feeling of fullness in ears, flushing, pruritus, increased sweating, visual disturbances, hypo/hypertension, dizziness, anxiety, insomnia, alopecia, skin changes
Rare
PO
Change in visual acuity, temporary hearing loss

SERIOUS REACTIONS
PO
• Retinoic acid syndrome (fever, dyspnea, weight gain, abnormal chest auscultatory findings, episodic hypotension) occurs commonly as does leukocytosis.
• Syndrome generally occurs during first month of therapy (sometimes occurs following first dose).
• Pseudo tumor cerebri may be noted, especially in children (headache, nausea, vomiting, visual disturbances).
• Possible tumorigenic potential when combined with ultraviolet radiation.
Topical
• Possible tumorigenic potential when combined with ultraviolet radiation.

INTERACTIONS
Drugs
❸ *Sulfur, resorcinol, benzoyl peroxide, salicylic acid:* Concomitant topical acne products may cause significant skin irritation

SPECIAL CONSIDERATIONS
• Oral therapy should be prescribed only by those knowledgeable in the treatment of APL

PATIENT/FAMILY EDUCATION
• Keep away from eyes, mouth, angles of nose, and mucous membranes
• Avoid exposure to ultraviolet light
• Acne may worsen transiently
• Normal use of cosmetics is permissible

---

triamcinolone
(trye-am-sin'oh-lone)
Rx: *Oral:* Aristocort, Aristopak
Rx: *Injectable:* Acetocot, Amcort, Aristocort, Aristocort Forte, Aristospan, Cinonide-40, Clinalog, TAC-3, Kenalog, Kenaject-40, Triam-A, Triam Forte, Triamcot, Tristoject
Rx: *Inhalation:* Azmacort
Rx: *Nasal:* Nasacort, Nasacort AQ
Rx: *Topical:* Aristocort, Cinalog, Cinolar, Kenalog, Kenalog in Orabase, Triacet, Triamcot
Chemical Class: Glucocorticoid, synthetic
Therapeutic Class: Corticosteroid, inhaled; corticosteroid, systemic; corticosteroid, topical

---

CLINICAL PHARMACOLOGY
Mechanism of Action: An adrenocortical steroid that inhibits accumulation of inflammatory cells at inflammation sites, phagocytosis, lysosomal enzyme release and synthesis, and release of mediators of inflammation. *Therapeutic Effect:* Prevents or suppresses cell-mediated immune reactions. Decreases or prevents tissue response to inflammatory process.

INDICATIONS AND DOSAGES
Immunosuppression, relief of acute inflammation
PO
Adults, Elderly. 4–60 mg/day.
IM
Adults, Elderly. 40 mg/wk (triamcinolone diacetate).
Intra-articular, intralesional
Adults, Elderly. 5–40 mg.
IM
Adults, Elderly. Initially, 2.5–60 mg/day (triamcinolone acetonide). Initially, 2.5–40 mg up to 100 mg; 2–20 mg (triamcinolone hexacetonide).
Control of bronchial asthma
Inhalation
Adults, Elderly. 2 inhalations 3–4 times a day.
Children 6–12 yr. 1–2 inhalations 3–4 times a day. Maximum: 12 inhalations/day.
Rhinitis
Intranasal
Adults, Children 6 yr and older. 2 sprays each nostril each day.
Relief of inflammation or pruritus associated with corticoid-responsive dermatoses
Topical
Adults, Elderly. 2–4 times a day. May give 1–2 times a day or as intermittent therapy.

Ⓢ **AVAILABLE FORMS/COST**
Triamcinolone
• Tab—Oral: 4 mg, 100's: **$5.50-$147.84**; 8 mg, 50's: **$107.57**
Triamcinolone Acetonide
• Aer—INH: 100 mcg/inh, 20 g, 100 sprays: **$72.58**
• Aer—Nasal: 55 mcg/inh, 10 g: **$59.85**
• Spray—Nasal: 55 mcg/inh, 16.5 g (AQ): **$67.50**
• Spray—Top: 0.147 mg/g, 63 g: **$32.98-$34.92**

• Cre—Top: 0.025%, 15, 30, 60, 80, 454 g: **$2.43-$12.75**/80 g; 0.1%, 15, 30, 60, 80, 240, 454, 480 g: **$3.15-$46.52**/80 g; 0.5%, 15, 20, 100, 240 g: **$4.00-$36.62**/15 g
• Susp, Inj—Intra-articular, IM: 40 mg/ml, 5 ml: **$8.40-$38.52**
• Susp, Inj—Intra-articular, Intradermal: 10 mg/ml, 5 ml: **$8.76**
• Susp, Inj—Intradermal: 3 mg/ml, 5 ml: **$10.43**
• Lotion—Top: 0.025%, 60 ml: **$37.79-$44.22**; 0.1%, 60 ml: **$8.78-$49.65**
• Oint—Top: 0.025%, 15, 30, 80, 454 g: **$3.50-$5.25**/80 g; 0.1%, 15, 30, 60, 80, 240, 454 g: **$5.10-$13.35**/80 g; 0.5%, 15 g: **$3.64-$5.80**/15 g
• Paste—Dental: 0.1%, 5 g: **$5.00-$17.70**
Triamcinolone Diacetate
• Susp, Inj—Intra-articular, IM: 40 mg/ml, 5 ml: **$11.48-$21.11**
Triamcinolone Hexacetonide
• Susp, Inj—IV: 5 mg/ml, 5 ml: **$1.37**; 20 mg/ml, 5 ml: **$2.11**
CONTRAINDICATIONS: Administration of live virus vaccines, especially smallpox vaccine; hypersensitivity to corticosteroids or tartrazine; IM injection or oral inhalation in children younger than 6 years; peptic ulcer disease (except life-threatening situations); systemic fungal infection
Topical: Marked circulation impairment
PREGNANCY AND LACTATION: Pregnancy category C; excreted in breast milk and could interfere with infant's growth and endogenous corticosteroid production
SIDE EFFECTS
Frequent
Insomnia, dry mouth, heartburn, nervousness, abdominal distention, diaphoresis, acne, mood swings, increased appetite, facial flushing, delayed wound healing, increased susceptibility to infection, diarrhea or constipation
Occasional
Headache, edema, change in skin color, frequent urination
Rare
Tachycardia, allergic reaction (including rash and hives), mental changes, hallucinations, depression
Topical: Allergic contact dermatitis
SERIOUS REACTIONS
• Long-term therapy may cause muscle wasting in the arms or legs, osteoporosis, spontaneous fractures, amenorrhea, cataracts, glaucoma, peptic ulcer disease, and CHF.
• Abruptly withdrawing the drug following long-term therapy may cause anorexia, nausea, fever, headache, arthralgia, rebound inflammation, fatigue, weakness, lethargy, dizziness, and orthostatic hypotension.
• Anaphylaxis occurs rarely with parenteral administration.
• Suddenly discontinuing triamcinolone may be fatal.
• Blindness has occurred rarely after intralesional injection around face and head.
INTERACTIONS
Drugs
▨ *Aminoglutethamide:* Increased clearance of steroid; doubling of dose may be necessary
▨ *Antidiabetics:* Increased blood glucose
▨ *Barbiturates, carbamazepine:* Reduced serum concentrations of corticosteroids
▨ *Cholestyramine, colestipol:* Possible reduced absorption of corticosteroids
▨ *Cyclosporine:* Possible increased concentration of both drugs, seizures

3 *Erythromycin, troleandomycin, clarithromycin, ketoconazole:* Possible enhanced steroid effect

3 *Estrogens, oral contraceptives:* Enhanced effects of corticosteroids

3 *Isoniazid:* Reduced plasma concentrations of isoniazid

3 *IUDs:* Inhibition of inflammation may decrease contraceptive effect

3 *NSAIDs:* Increased risk of GI ulceration

3 *Rifampin:* Reduced therapeutic effect of corticosteroids

3 *Salicylates:* Increased elimination of salicylates

Labs

• *False increase:* Urinary amino acids

SPECIAL CONSIDERATIONS
PATIENT/FAMILY EDUCATION

• May cause GI upset, take with meals or snacks (systemic)
• Do not give live virus vaccines to patients on prolonged systemic therapy
• Take PO as single daily dose in am
• Signs of adrenal insufficiency include fatigue, anorexia, nausea, vomiting, diarrhea, weight loss, weakness, dizziness, and low blood sugar
• Avoid abrupt withdrawal of therapy following high-dose or long-term therapy
• Increased dose of rapidly acting corticosteroids may be necessary in patients subjected to unusual stress
• To be used on a regular basis, not for acute symptoms (nasal and inhalation)
• Use bronchodilators before oral inhaler (for patients using both)
• Rinse mouth to prevent oral candidiasis
• Nasal sol may cause drying and irritation of nasal mucosa, clear nasal passages prior to use

MONITORING PARAMETERS
• Serum K and glucose
• Growth of children on prolonged therapy

---

triamterene
(try-am′ter-een)
Rx: Dyrenium
Combinations
   Rx: with hydrochlorothiazide (Dyazide, Maxzide)
Chemical Class: Pteridine derivative
Therapeutic Class: Antihypertensive; diuretic, potassium-sparing

CLINICAL PHARMACOLOGY
Mechanism of Action: A potassium-sparing diuretic that inhibits sodium, potassium, ATPase. Interferes with sodium and potassium exchange in distal tubule, cortical collecting tubule, and collecting duct. Increases sodium and decreases potassium excretion. Also increases magnesium, decreases calcium loss. *Therapeutic Effect:* Produces diuresis and lowers BP.

Pharmacokinetics

Route	Onset	Peak	Duration
PO	2–4 hr	N/A	7–9 hr

Incompletely absorbed from the GI tract. Widely distributed. Metabolized in the liver. Primarily eliminated in feces via biliary route. **Half-life:** 1.5–2.5 hr (increased in renal impairment).

INDICATIONS AND DOSAGES
Edema, hypertension
PO
Adults, Elderly. 25–100 mg/day as a single dose or in 2 divided doses. Maximum: 300 mg/day.

Children. 2–4 mg/kg/day as a single dose or in 2 divided doses. Maximum: 6 mg/kg/day or 300 mg/day.

$ AVAILABLE FORMS/COST

• Cap, Gel—Oral: 50 mg, 100's: **$106.34**; 100 mg, 100's: **$193.35**

UNLABELED USES: Treatment adjunct for hypertension, prevention and treatment of hypokalemia

CONTRAINDICATIONS: Drug-induced or pre-existing hyperkalemia, progressive or severe renal disease, severe hepatic disease

PREGNANCY AND LACTATION: Pregnancy category B; therapy for preexisting hypertension can be continued throughout pregnancy with minimal risk; initiating for simple edema not recommended; few unequivocal indications for diuretic therapy in pregnancy except for pulmonary edema or congestive heart failure; may decrease placental perfusion; excreted in cow's milk, no human data

SIDE EFFECTS

Occasional

Fatigue, nausea, diarrhea, abdominal pain, leg cramps, headache

Rare

Anorexia, asthenia, rash, dizziness

SERIOUS REACTIONS

• Triamterene use may result in hyponatremia (somnolence, dry mouth, increased thirst, lack of energy) or severe hyperkalemia (irritability, anxiety, heaviness of legs, paresthesia, hypotension, bradycardia, EKG changes [tented T waves, widening QRS complex, ST segment depression]).

• Agranulocytosis, nephrolithiasis, and thrombocytopenia occur rarely.

INTERACTIONS

Drugs

🔳 *ACE inhibitors:* Hyperkalemia in predisposed patients

🔳 *Amantadine:* Increased toxicity of amantadine

🔳 *Angiotensin II receptor antagonists:* Concurrent mechanisms to decrease potassium excretion; increased risk of hyperkalemia

🔳 *Cimetidine:* Increased triamterene bioavailability and decreased renal clearance

🔳 *NSAIDs:* Acute renal failure with indomethacin and possibly other NSAIDs

② *Potassium preparation:* Concurrent use increases the risk of hyperkalemia

Labs

• *False increase:* Serum digoxin concentrations

• *Interference:* Urinary catecholamines

SPECIAL CONSIDERATIONS

PATIENT/FAMILY EDUCATION

• Take with meals

• Avoid prolonged exposure to sunlight

• Take single daily doses in am

MONITORING PARAMETERS

• Blood pressure, edema, urine output, urine electrolytes, BUN, creatinine, ECG (if hyperkalemic), gynecomastia, impotence

---

triazolam

(trye-ay´zoe-lam)

Rx: Halcion

Chemical Class: Benzodiazepine

Therapeutic Class: Hypnotic

DEA Class: Schedule IV

CLINICAL PHARMACOLOGY

Mechanism of Action: A benzodiazepine that enhances the action of the inhibitory neurotransmitter gamma-aminobutyric acid, resulting in CNS depression. *Therapeutic Effect:* Induces sleep.

INDICATIONS AND DOSAGES
Insomnia
PO
Adults, Children older than 18 yr.
0.125-0.5 mg at bedtime.
Elderly. 0.0625-0.125 mg at bedtime.
$ AVAILABLE FORMS/COST
• Tab, Plain Coated—Oral: 0.125 mg, 100's: **$61.63**; 0.25 mg, 100's: **$64.73-$146.00**
CONTRAINDICATIONS: Angle-closure glaucoma; CNS depression; pregnancy or breast-feeding; severe, uncontrolled pain; sleep apnea
PREGNANCY AND LACTATION: Pregnancy category X (according to manufacturer); no congenital anomalies have been attributed to use during human pregnancies; other benzodiazepines have been suspected of producing fetal malformations after 1st-trimester exposure
SIDE EFFECTS
Frequent
Somnolence, sedation, dry mouth, headache, dizziness, nervousness, light-headedness, incoordination, nausea, rebound insomnia (may occur for 1-2 nights after drug is discontinued)
Occasional
Euphoria, tachycardia, abdominal cramps, visual disturbances
Rare
Paradoxical CNS excitement or restlessness (particularly in elderly or debilitated patients)
SERIOUS REACTIONS
• Abrupt or too-rapid withdrawal may result in pronounced restlessness, irritability, insomnia, hand tremors, abdominal or muscle cramps, vomiting, diaphoresis, and seizures.
• Overdose results in somnolence, confusion, diminished reflexes, respiratory depression, and coma.

INTERACTIONS
Drugs
3 *Carbamazepine, phenytoin:* Reduced effect of triazolam
3 *Cimetidine, clarithromycin, disulfiram, erythromycin, fluvoxamine, grapefruit juice, isoniazid, troleandomycin:* Increased plasma triazolam concentrations
2 *Ethanol:* Enhanced adverse psychomotor effects of benzodiazepines
2 *Fluconazole, itraconazole, ketoconazole:* Increased plasma triazolam concentrations
SPECIAL CONSIDERATIONS
• **Prescriptions should be written for short-term use (7-10 days); drug should not be prescribed in quantities exceeding a 1 mo supply**
PATIENT/FAMILY EDUCATION
• Avoid alcohol and other CNS depressants
• Do not discontinue abruptly after prolonged therapy
• May cause drowsiness or dizziness, use caution while driving or performing other tasks requiring alertness
• May be habit forming

---

trientine
(trye-en'teen)
Rx: Syprine
Chemical Class: Thiol derivative
Therapeutic Class: Antidote, copper

CLINICAL PHARMACOLOGY
Mechanism of Action: An oral chelating agent that foms complexes by binding metal ions particularly copper. *Therapeutic Effect:* Binds to copper and induces cupruresis.

Pharmacokinetics
None reported.
INDICATIONS AND DOSAGES
Wilson's disease
PO
Adults, Elderly. 750-1250 mg/day in 2-4 divided doses. Maximum: 2 g/day.
Children 12 years and older. 500-750 mg/day in 2-4 divided doses. Maximum: 1500 mg/day.

S **AVAILABLE FORMS/COST**
• Cap, Gel—Oral: 250 mg, 100's: **$112.84**
CONTRAINDICATIONS: Hypersensitivity to trientine or its components
PREGNANCY AND LACTATION: Pregnancy category C
SIDE EFFECTS
Occasional
Contact dermatitis, dystonia, muscular spasm, myasthenia gravis
SERIOUS REACTIONS
• Iron deficiency anemia and systemic lupus erythematosus rarely occur.

SPECIAL CONSIDERATIONS
PATIENT/FAMILY EDUCATION
• Take on empty stomach
MONITORING PARAMETERS
• Free serum copper (goal is <10 mcg/dl); increase daily dose only when clinical response is not adequate or concentration of free serum copper is persistently above 20 mcg/dl (determine optimal long-term maintenance dosage at 6-12 mo intervals)
• 24 hr urinary copper analysis at 6-12 mo intervals (adequately treated patients will have 0.5-1 mg copper/24 hr collection of urine)

---

trifluoperazine
(trye-floo-oh-per'a-zeen)
Rx: Stelazine
Chemical Class: Piperidine phenothiazine derivative
Therapeutic Class: Antipsychotic

CLINICAL PHARMACOLOGY
Mechanism of Action: A phenothiazine derivative that blocks dopamine at postsynaptic receptor sites. Possess strong extrapyramidal and antiemetic effects and weak anticholinergic and sedative effects. *Therapeutic Effect:* Suppresses behavioral response in psychosis; reduces locomotor activity and aggressiveness.
INDICATIONS AND DOSAGES
Psychotic disorders
PO
Adults, Elderly, Children 12 yr and older. Initially, 2-5 mg once or twice a day. Range: 15-20 mg/day. Maximum: 40 mg/day.
Children 6-11 yr. Initially, 1 mg once or twice a day. Maintenance: Up to 15 mg/day.
IM
Adults. 1-2 mg q4-6h. Maximum: 10 mg/24h.
Elderly. 1 mg q4-6h. Maximum: 6 mg/24h.
Children. 1 mg 2 times/day.

S **AVAILABLE FORMS/COST**
• Sol, Inj—IM: 2 mg/ml, 10 ml: **$67.79**
• Tab, Plain Coated—Oral: 1 mg, 100's: **$56.64**; 2 mg, 100's: **$40.30-$122.90**; 5 mg, 100's: **$43.73-$154.70**; 10 mg, 100's: **$54.63-$217.32**
CONTRAINDICATIONS: Angle-closure glaucoma, circulatory collapse, myelosuppression, severe cardiac or hepatic disease, severe hypertension or hypotension

PREGNANCY AND LACTATION:
Pregnancy category C; has been used as an antiemetic during normal labor without producing any observable effect on newborn; bulk of evidence indicates safety for mother and fetus

SIDE EFFECTS

Frequent

Hypotension, dizziness, and syncope (occur frequently after first injection, occasionally after subsequent injections, and rarely with oral form)

Occasional

Drowsiness during early therapy, dry mouth, blurred vision, lethargy, constipation or diarrhea, nasal congestion, peripheral edema, urine retention

Rare

Ocular changes, altered skin pigmentation (in those taking high doses for prolonged periods), photosensitivity

SERIOUS REACTIONS

• Extrapyramidal symptoms appear to be dose-related (particularly high doses) and are divided into 3 categories: akathisia (inability to sit still, tapping of feet), parkinsonian symptoms (such as masklike face, tremors, shuffling gait, and hypersalivation), and acute dystonias (such as torticollis, opisthotonos, and oculogyric crisis). Dystonic reactions may also produce diaphoresis and pallor.

• Tardive dyskinesia, marked by tongue protrusion, puffing of the cheeks, and chewing or puckering of the mouth, occurs rarely but may be irreversible.

• Abrupt withdrawal after long-term therapy may precipitate nausea, vomiting, gastritis, dizziness, and tremors.

• Blood dyscrasias, particularly agranulocytosis, and mild leukopenia may occur.

• Trifluoperazine may lower the seizure threshold.

INTERACTIONS

Drugs

🖪 *Anticholinergics:* Inhibited therapeutic response to antipsychotic; enhanced anticholinergic side effects

🖪 *Antidepressants:* Increased serum concentrations of some cyclic antidepressants

🖪 *Barbiturates:* Reduced effect of antipsychotic

🖪 *Bromocriptine, lithium:* Reduced effects of both drugs

🖪 *Guanethidine:* Inhibited antihypertensive response to guanethidine

🛈 *Levodopa:* Inhibited effect of levodopa on Parkinson's disease

🖪 *Narcotic analgesics:* Excessive CNS depression, hypotension, respiratory depression

🖪 *Orphenadrine:* Reduced serum neuroleptic concentrations; excessive anticholinergic effects

Labs

• *False increase:* Urinary protein

SPECIAL CONSIDERATIONS

PATIENT/FAMILY EDUCATION

• Arise slowly from reclining position

• Do not discontinue abruptly

• Use a sunscreen during sun exposure; take special precautions to stay cool in hot weather

MONITORING PARAMETERS

• Observe closely for signs of tardive dyskinesia

• Periodic CBC with platelets during prolonged therapy

trifluridine

(trye-flure'i-deen)

Rx: Viroptic

Chemical Class: Nucleoside analog

Therapeutic Class: Ophthalmic antiviral

CLINICAL PHARMACOLOGY

Mechanism of Action: An antiviral agent that incorporates into DNS causing increased rate of mutation and errors in protein formation. *Therapeutic Effect:* Prevents viral replication.

Pharmacokinetics

Intraocular solution is undetectable in serum. **Half-life:** 12 min.

INDICATIONS AND DOSAGES

Herpes simplex virus ocular infections

Ophthalmic

Adults, Elderly, Children older than 6 yrs. 1 drop onto cornea q2h while awake. Maximum: 9 drops/day. Continue until corneal ulcer has completely reepithelialized; then, 1 drop q4h while awake (minimum: 5 drops/day) for an additional 7 days.

$ **AVAILABLE FORMS/COST**

• Sol—Ophth: 1%, 7.5 ml: **$94.45-$104.95**

CONTRAINDICATIONS: Hypersensitivity to trifluridine or any component of the formulation

PREGNANCY AND LACTATION: Pregnancy category C

SIDE EFFECTS

Frequent

Transient stinging or burning with instillation

Occasional

Edema of eyelid

Rare

Hypersensitivity reaction

SERIOUS REACTIONS

• Ocular toxicity may occur if used longer than 21 days.

SPECIAL CONSIDERATIONS

PATIENT/FAMILY EDUCATION

• Notify clinician if no improvement after 7 days

trihexyphenidyl

(trye-hex-ee-fen'i-dill)

Rx: Artane, Trihexy

Chemical Class: Tertiary amine

Therapeutic Class: Anti-Parkinson's agent; anticholinergic

CLINICAL PHARMACOLOGY

Mechanism of Action: An anticholinergic agent that blocks central cholinergic receptors (aids in balancing cholinergic and dopaminergic activity). *Therapeutic Effect:* Decreases salivation, relaxes smooth muscle.

Pharmacokinetics

Well absorbed from gastrointestinal (GI) tract. Primarily excreted in urine. **Half-life:** 3.3-4.1 hrs.

INDICATIONS AND DOSAGES

Parkinsonism

PO

Adults, Elderly. Initially, 1 mg on first day. May increase by 2 mg/day at 3-5 day intervals up to 6-10 mg/day (12-15 mg/day in patients with postencephalitic parkinsonism).

Drug-induced extrapyramidal symptoms

PO

Adults, Elderly. Initially, 1 mg/day. Range: 5-15 mg/day.

$ **AVAILABLE FORMS/COST**

• Elixir—Oral: 2 mg/5 ml, 480 ml: **$30.60**

• Tab—Oral: 2 mg, 100's: **$9.09-$18.29**; 5 mg, 100's: **$18.30-$36.38**

CONTRAINDICATIONS: Angle closure glaucoma, GI obstruction, paralytic ileus, intestinal atony, severe ulcerative colitis, prostatic hypertrophy, myasthenia gravis, megacolon, hypersensitivity to trihexyphenidyl or any component of the formulation

PREGNANCY AND LACTATION: Pregnancy category C; nursing infants may be particularly sensitive to anticholinergic effects

SIDE EFFECTS

Elderly (more than 60 yrs) tend to develop mental confusion, disorientation, agitation, psychotic-like symptoms

Frequent

Drowsiness, dry mouth

Occasional

Blurred vision, urinary retention, constipation, dizziness, headache, muscle cramps

Rare

Seizures, depression, rash

SERIOUS REACTIONS

• Hypersensitivity reaction (eczema, pruritus, rash, cardiac disturbances, photosensitivity) may occur.

• Overdosage may vary from CNS depression (sedation, apnea, cardiovascular collapse, death) to severe paradoxical reaction (hallucinations, tremor, seizures).

INTERACTIONS

Drugs

☒ *Amantadine:* Potentiates the side effects of amantadine

☒ *Anticholinergics:* Increased anticholinergic side effects

☒ *Neuroleptics:* Inhibition of therapeutic response to neuroleptics; excessive anticholinergic effects

☒ *Tacrine:* Reduced therapeutic effects of both drugs

Labs

• *False increase:* Serum T_3 and T_4

PATIENT/FAMILY EDUCATION

• Do not discontinue abruptly

• Use caution in hot weather; drug may increase susceptibility to heat stroke

---

trimethobenzamide
(trye-meth-oh-ben'za-mide)
Rx: Tigan, Triban, Trimazide, Tebamide
Chemical Class: Ethanolamine derivative
Therapeutic Class: Antiemetic

CLINICAL PHARMACOLOGY

Mechanism of Action: An anticholinergic that acts at the chemoreceptor trigger zone in the medulla oblongata. *Therapeutic Effect:* Relieves nausea and vomiting.

Pharmacokinetics

Route	Onset	Peak	Duration
PO	10-40 min	N/A	3-4 hr
IM	15-30 min	N/A	2-3 hr

Partially absorbed from the GI tract. Distributed primarily to the liver. Metabolic fate unknown. Excreted in urine. **Half-life:** 7-9 hr.

INDICATIONS AND DOSAGES

Nausea and vomiting

PO

Adults, Elderly. 300 mg 3-4 times a day.

Children weighing 30-100 lb. 100-200 mg 3-4 times a day.

IM

Adults, Elderly. 200 mg 3-4 times a day.

Rectal

Adults, Elderly. 200 mg 3-4 times a day.

Children weighing 30-100 lb. 100-200 mg 3-4 times a day.

T

Children weighing less than 30 lb.
100 mg 3-4 times a day.

Ⓢ **AVAILABLE FORMS/COST**

• Cap, Gel—Oral: 100 mg, 100's: **$42.68**; 250 mg, 100's: **$27.00-$86.88**; 300 mg, 100's: **$101.34-$119.39**
• Sol, Inj—IM: 100 mg/ml, 2 ml vial: **$2.84-$6.16**
• Supp—Rect: 100 mg, 10's: **$5.75-$27.84**; 200 mg, 10's: **$6.00-$33.04**

CONTRAINDICATIONS: Hypersensitivity to benzocaine or similar local anesthetics; use of parenteral form in children or suppositories in premature infants or neonates

PREGNANCY AND LACTATION: Pregnancy category C; has been used to treat nausea and vomiting during pregnancy

SIDE EFFECTS

Frequent

Somnolence

Occasional

Blurred vision, diarrhea, dizziness, headache, muscle cramps

Rare

Rash, seizures, depression, opisthotonos, parkinsonian syndrome, Reye's syndrome (marked by vomiting, seizures)

SERIOUS REACTIONS

• A hypersensitivity reaction, manifested as extrapyramidal symptoms such as muscle rigidity and allergic skin reactions, occurs rarely.
• Children may experience paradoxical reactions, marked by restlessness, insomnia, euphoria, nervousness, and tremor.
• Overdose may produce CNS depression (manifested as sedation, apnea, cardiovascular collapse, and death) or severe paradoxical reactions (such as hallucinations, tremor, and seizures).

INTERACTIONS

Drugs

❸ *Alcohol:* Increased adverse reactions

Labs

• *False positive:* Urinary amphetamine

SPECIAL CONSIDERATIONS

• Less effective than phenothiazines

---

trimethoprim
(trye-meth'oh-prim)
Rx: Primsol, Proloprim, Trimpex
Combinations
   Rx: with sulfamethoxazole (see co-trimoxazole monograph); with polymyxin B sulfate (Polytrim Ophthalmic)
Chemical Class: Folate-antagonist, synthetic
Therapeutic Class: Antibiotic

CLINICAL PHARMACOLOGY

Mechanism of Action: A folate antagonist that blocks bacterial biosynthesis of nucleic acids and proteins by interfering with the metabolism of folinic acid. *Therapeutic Effect:* Bacteriostatic.

Pharmacokinetics

Rapidly and completely absorbed from the GI tract. Protein binding: 42%-46%. Widely distributed, including to CSF. Metabolized in the liver. Primarily excreted in urine. Moderately removed by hemodialysis. **Half-life:** 8-10 hr (increased in impaired renal function and newborns; decreased in children).

INDICATIONS AND DOSAGES

Acute, uncomplicated UTI

PO

Adults, Elderly, Children 12 yr and older. 100 mg q12h or 200 mg once a day for 10 days.

Children younger than 12 yr. 4-6 mg/kg/day in 2 divided doses for 10 days.

Dosage in renal impairment
Dosage and frequency are modified based on creatinine clearance.

Creatinine Clearance	Dosage Interval
greater than 30 ml/min	No change
15-29 ml/min	50 mg q12h

$ AVAILABLE FORMS/COST
• Sol—Oral: 50 mg/ml, 473 ml: **$66.51**
• Tab—Oral: 100 mg, 100's: **$19.29-$111.24**; 200 mg, 100's: **$42.70-$222.31**

UNLABELED USES: Prevention of bacterial UTIs, treatment of pneumonia caused by *Pneumocystis carinii*

CONTRAINDICATIONS: Infants younger than 2 months, megaloblastic anemia due to folic acid deficiency

PREGNANCY AND LACTATION: Pregnancy category C; because trimethoprim is a folate antagonist, caution should be used during the 1st trimester; excreted into breast milk in low concentrations; compatible with breast-feeding

SIDE EFFECTS
Occasional
Nausea, vomiting, diarrhea, decreased appetite, abdominal cramps, headache
Rare
Hypersensitivity reaction (pruritus, rash), methemoglobinemia (bluish fingernails, lips, or skin; fever; pale skin; sore throat; unusual tiredness), photosensitivity

SERIOUS REACTIONS
• Stevens-Johnson syndrome, erythema multiforme, exfoliative dermatitis, and anaphylaxis occur rarely.
• Hematologic toxicity (thrombocytopenia, neutropenia, leukopenia, megaloblastic anemia) is more likely to occur in elderly, debilitated, or alcoholic patients; in patients with impaired renal function; and in those receiving prolonged high dosage.

INTERACTIONS
Drugs
▣ *Dapsone:* Increased serum concentrations of both drugs
▣ *Phenytoin:* Increased serum phenytoin concentrations, potential for toxicity
▣ *Procainamide:* Increased serum concentrations of procainamide and N-acetylprocainamide

SPECIAL CONSIDERATIONS
• Good alternative to co-trimoxazole in patients taking warfarin

---

trimetrexate
(try-meh-trex-ate)
Rx: Neutrexin
Chemical Class: Dihydrofolate reductase inhibitor; substituted quinazoline
Therapeutic Class: Antiprotozoal

CLINICAL PHARMACOLOGY
Mechanism of Action: A folate antagonist that inhibits the enzyme dihydrofolate reductase (DHFR). *Therapeutic Effect:* Disrupts purine, DNA, RNA, protein synthesis, with consequent cell death.
Pharmacokinetics
Following IV administration, distributed readily into ascitic fluid. Metabolized in liver. Eliminated in urine. **Half-life:** 11-20 hrs.

T

INDICATIONS AND DOSAGES
Pneumocystis carinii pneumonia (PCP)
IV Infusion
Adults. Trimetrexate: 45 mg/m² once daily over 60-90 min. Leucovorin: 20 mg/m² over 5-10 min q6h for total daily dose of 80 mg/m², or orally as 4 doses of 20 mg/m² spaced equally throughout the day. Round up the oral dose to the next higher 25 mg increment. Recommended course of therapy: 21 days trimetrexate, 24 days leucovorin.

S AVAILABLE FORMS/COST
• Powder, Inj—IV: 25 mg, 10's: **$906.00**
UNLABELED USES: Treatment of non-small cell lung, prostate, and colorectal cancer
CONTRAINDICATIONS: Clinically significant hypersensitivity to trimetrexate, leucovorin, or methotrexate
PREGNANCY AND LACTATION: Pregnancy category D; breast milk excretion unknown, but women should not breastfeed while taking trimetrexate
SIDE EFFECTS
Occasional
Fever, rash, pruritus, nausea, vomiting, confusion
Rare
Fatigue
SERIOUS REACTIONS
• Trimetrexate given without concurrent leucovorin may result in serious or fatal hematologic, hepatic, and/or renal complications, including bone marrow suppression, oral and GI mucosal ulceration, and renal and hepatic dysfunction.
• In event of overdose, stop trimetrexate and give leucovorin 40 mg/m² q6h for 3 days.
• Anaphylaxis occurs rarely.

INTERACTIONS
Drugs
② *Cimetidine:* Reduced trimetrexate metabolism
② *Erythromycin:* Reduced trimetrexate metabolism
② *Ketoconazole:* Reduced trimetrexate metabolism
② *Rifabutin:* Increased trimetrexate metabolism
② *Rifampin:* Increased trimetrexate metabolism
SPECIAL CONSIDERATIONS
• Reserve for patients intolerant of or refractory to trimethoprim-sulfamethoxazole
• Randomized trials show trimetrexate is less effective than trimethoprim-sulfamethoxazole (failure rates 40% and 24%, respectively)
MONITORING PARAMETERS
• Check at least twice per week: CBC with platelets, hepatic and renal function

---

trimipramine
(trye-mih-prah-meen)
Rx: Surmontil
Chemical Class: Dibenzazepine derivative; tertiary amine
Therapeutic Class: Antidepressant, tricyclic

CLINICAL PHARMACOLOGY
Mechanism of Action: A tricyclic antibulimic, anticataplectic, antidepressant, antinarcoleptic, antineuralgic, antineuritic, and antipanic agent that blocks the reuptake of neurotransmitters, such as norepinephrine and serotonin, at presynaptic membranes, increasing their concentration at postsynaptic receptor sites. May demonstrate less autonomic toxicity than other tricyclic antidepressants. *Therapeutic Effect:*

Results in antidepressant effect. Anticholinergic effect controls nocturnal enuresis.

Pharmacokinetics

Rapidly, completely absorbed after PO administration, and not affected by food. Protein binding: 95%. Metabolized in liver (significant first-pass effect). Primarily excreted in urine. Not removed by hemodialysis. **Half-life:** 16-40 hrs.

INDICATIONS AND DOSAGES

Depression

PO

Adults. 50-150 mg/day at bedtime. Maximum: 200 mg/day for outpatients, 300 mg/day for inpatients.

Elderly. Initially, 25 mg/day at bedtime. May increase by 25 mg q3-7days. Maximum: 100 mg/day.

AVAILABLE FORMS/COST

• Cap, Gel—Oral: 25 mg, 100's: **$108.26**; 50 mg, 100's: **$177.11**; 100 mg, 100's: **$257.48**

CONTRAINDICATIONS: Acute recovery period after myocardial infarction (MI), within 14 days of MAOI ingestion, hypersensitivity to trimipramine or any component of the formulation

PREGNANCY AND LACTATION: Pregnancy category C; excreted into breast milk; effect on nursing infant unknown, but may be of concern

SIDE EFFECTS

Frequent

Drowsiness, fatigue, dry mouth, blurred vision, constipation, delayed micturition, postural hypotension, diaphoresis, disturbed concentration, increased appetite, urinary retention, photosensitivity.

Occasional

Gastrointestinal (GI) disturbances, such as nausea, and a metallic taste sensation.

Rare

Paradoxical reaction, marked by agitation, restlessness, nightmares, insomnia, extrapyramidal symptoms, particularly fine hand tremors.

SERIOUS REACTIONS

• High dosage may produce cardiovascular effects, such as severe postural hypotension, dizziness, tachycardia, palpitations, arrhythmias and seizures. High dosage may also result in altered temperature regulation, including hyperpyrexia or hypothermia.

• Abrupt withdrawal from prolonged therapy may produce headache, malaise, nausea, vomiting, and vivid dreams.

INTERACTIONS

Drugs

3 *Anticholinergics, propantheline:* Excessive anticholinergic effects

3 *Barbiturates, carbamazepine:* Reduced serum concentrations of cyclic antidepressants

3 *Cimetidine:* Increases trimipramine level

2 *Clonidine:* Reduced antihypertensive response to clonidine; enhanced hypertensive response with abrupt clonidine withdrawal

2 *Epinephrine, norepinephrine:* Markedly enhanced pressor response to IV epinephrine

3 *Ethanol:* Additive impairment of motor skills; abstinent alcoholics may eliminate cyclic antidepressants more rapidly than non-alcoholics

3 *Fluoxetine:* Marked increases in cyclic antidepressant plasma concentrations

2 *Guanadrel, guanethidine:* Inhibited antihypertensive response to guanethidine

⚠ *MAOIs:* Excessive sympathetic response; mania or hyperpyrexia possible

T

❷ *Moclobemide:* Potential association with fatal or non-fatal serotonin syndrome

❸ *Phenylephrine:* Markedly enhanced pressor response to IV epinephrine

❸ *Propoxyphene:* Enhanced effect of cyclic antidepressants

❸ *Quinidine:* Increased cyclic antidepressant serum concentrations

SPECIAL CONSIDERATIONS
PATIENT/FAMILY EDUCATION
• Therapeutic effects may take 2-3 wk
• Avoid rising quickly from sitting to standing, especially elderly
• Do not discontinue abruptly after long-term use
MONITORING PARAMETERS
• CBC, ECG

---

trioxsalen
(trye-ox′a-len)
Rx: Trisoralen
Chemical Class: Psoralen derivative
Therapeutic Class: Pigmenting agent

CLINICAL PHARMACOLOGY
Mechanism of Action: A member of the family of psoralens that induces the process of melanogensesis by a mechanism that is not known. *Therapeutic Effect:* Enhances pigmentation.

Pharmacokinetics
Rapidly absorbed from the gastrointestinal (GI) tract. **Half-life:** 2 hrs. (skin sensitivity to light remains for 8-12 hrs.)

INDICATIONS AND DOSAGES
Pigmentation
PO
Adults, Elderly, Children 12 yrs and older. 10 mg/day 2 hrs before exposure to UVA light or sun exposure.

Vitiligo
PO
Adults, Elderly, Children 12 yrs and older. 10 mg/day 2-4 hrs before exposure to UVA light.

Ⓢ **AVAILABLE FORMS/COST**
• Tab—Oral: 5 mg, 100's: **$238.31**
UNLABELED USES: Polymorphous light eruption, psoriasis, sunlight sensitivity
CONTRAINDICATIONS: Concomitant disease states associated with photosensitivity (acute lupus erythematosus, porphyria, leukoderma of infectious origin), concomitant use of preparations with any internal or external photosensitizing capacity, children under 12 years old, hypersensitivity to trioxsalen or any component of the formulation
PREGNANCY AND LACTATION: Pregnancy category C; excretion into breast milk unknown, use caution in nursing mothers
SIDE EFFECTS
Occasional
Gastric discomfort, photosensitivity, pruritus
SERIOUS REACTIONS
• Overdose or overexposure may result in serious blistering and burning.
INTERACTIONS
Drugs
❸ *Anthralin, coal tar, griseofulvin, phenothiazines, nalidixic acid, halogenated salicylanilides, sulfonamides, tetracyclines, thiazides:* Increased photosensitivity to these agents
SPECIAL CONSIDERATIONS
PATIENT/FAMILY EDUCATION
• Do not sunbathe during 24 hr prior to ingestion and UVA exposure
• Wear UVA-absorbing sunglasses for 24 hr following treatment to prevent cataract

- Avoid sun exposure for at least 8 hr after ingestion
- Avoid furocoumarin-containing foods (e.g., limes, figs, parsley, parsnips, mustard, carrots, celery)
- Repigmentation may begin after 2-3 wk but full effect may require 6-9 mo

---

trospium
(trose'pee-um)
Rx: Sanctura
Chemical Class: Antimuscarinic substituted amine
Therapeutic Class: Genitourinary muscle relaxant

CLINICAL PHARMACOLOGY
Mechanism of Action: An anticholinergic that antagonizes the effect of acetylcholine on muscarinic receptors, producing parasympatholytic action. *Therapeutic Effect:* Reduces smooth muscle tone in the bladder.
Pharmacokinetics
Minimally absorbed after PO administration. Protein binding: 50%-85%. Distributed in plasma. Excreted mainly in feces and, to a lesser extent, in urine. **Half life:** 20 hr.

INDICATIONS AND DOSAGES
Overactive bladder
PO
Adults. 20 mg 2 times/day.
Elderly (75 yr and older). Titrate dosage down to 20 mg once a day, based on tolerance.
Dosage in renal impairment
For patients with creatinine clearance less than 30 ml/min, dosage reduced to 20 mg once a day at bedtime.

CONTRAINDICATIONS: Decreased GI motility, gastric retention, uncontrolled angle-closure glaucoma, urine retention
PREGNANCY AND LACTATION: Pregnancy category C; breast milk excretion unknown
SIDE EFFECTS
Frequent (20%)
Dry mouth
Occasional (10%-4%)
Constipation, headache
Rare (less than 2%)
Fatigue, upper abdominal pain, dyspepsia, flatulence, dry eyes, urine retention
SERIOUS REACTIONS
- Overdose may result in severe anticholinergic effects, such as abdominal pain, nausea and vomiting, confusion, depression, diaphoresis, facial flushing, hypertension, hypotension, respiratory depression, irritability, lacrimation, nervousness, and restlessness.
- Supraventricular tachycardia and hallucinations occur rarely.
INTERACTIONS
Drugs
🖪 *Procainamide:* Additive antivagal effects at atrioventricular node
SPECIAL CONSIDERATIONS
- Studies have not shown that trospium is better than generically available drugs for the same purpose
PATIENT/FAMILY EDUCATION
- May precipitate urinary retention or narrow angle glaucoma

T

trovafloxacin / alatrofloxacin
(troh-va-flocks-ah-sin)
Rx: Trovan
Combinations
Rx: with azithromycin (Trovan/Zithromax compliance pak)
Chemical Class: Fluoroquinolone derivative
Therapeutic Class: Antibiotic

CLINICAL PHARMACOLOGY
Mechanism of Action: A fluoroquinolone that inhibits the DNA enzyme gyrase in susceptible microorganisms, interfering with bacterial DNA replication and repair. *Therapeutic Effect:* Produces bactericidal activity.
Pharmacokinetics
Well absorbed from the gastrointestinal (GI) tract. Protein binding: 76%. Widely distributed including cerebrospinal fluid (CSF). Metabolized in liver by conjugation. Excreted in feces. Not removed by hemodialysis. **Half-life:** 9-13 hrs.

INDICATIONS AND DOSAGES
Pneumonia
PO/IV
Adults, Elderly. 200 mg q24h for 7-14 days.
Skin and skin-structure infections
PO/IV
Adults, Elderly. 200 mg q24h for 10-14 days.
Gynecologic infections
IV
Adults, Elderly. 300 mg q24h for 7-14 days.
PO
Adults, Elderly. 100 mg q24h for 7-14 days.
Abdominal infection
Adults, Elderly. 300 mg q24h for 7-14 days.

Bronchitis
PO
Adults, Elderly. 100 q24h for 7-10 days.

⬛ AVAILABLE FORMS/COST
• Sol, Inj—IV (alatrofloxacin): 200 mg/40 ml, 1's: **$40.08**; 300 mg/60 ml, 1's: **$60.45**
• Tab—Oral (trovafloxacin): 100 mg, 30's: **$193.60**; 200 mg, 30's: **$234.35**

CONTRAINDICATIONS: History of hypersensitivity to other fluoroquinolones
PREGNANCY AND LACTATION: Pregnancy category C; excreted in breast milk
SIDE EFFECTS
Occasional
Diarrhea, dizziness, drowsiness, headache, lightheadedness, vaginal pain and discharge
Rare
Confusion, hallucinations, restlessness, seizures, tremors, rapid heartbeat, shortness of breath, abdominal pain, dark urine, fatigue, loss of appetite, nausea, vomiting, jaundice, pain at injection site, stomach cramps, diarrhea, tendon rupture, increased sensitivity of skin to sunlight

SERIOUS REACTIONS
• Pseudomembranous colitis as evidenced by severe abdominal pain and cramps, and severe watery diarrhea, and fever, may occur.
• Superinfection manifested as genital or anal pruritus, ulceration or changes in oral mucosa, and moderate to severe diarrhea, may occur.
• Hypersensitivity reactions, including photosensitivity as evidenced by rash, pruritus, blistering, swelling, and the sensation of the skin burning have occurred in patients receiving fluoroquinolone therapy.

INTERACTIONS
Drugs
▣ *Aluminum:* Reduced absorption of trovafloxacin; do not take within 4 hr of dose

▣ *Antacids:* Reduced absorption of trovafloxacin; do not take within 4 hr of dose

▣ *Antipyrine:* Inhibits metabolism of antipyrine; increased plasma antipyrine level

▣ *Calcium:* Reduced absorption of trovafloxacin; do not take within 4 hr of dose

▣ *Diazepam:* Inhibits metabolism of diazepam; increased plasma diazepam level

▣ *Didanosine:* Markedly reduced absorption of trovafloxacin; take trovafloxacin 2 hr before didanosine

▣ *Foscarnet:* Coadministration increases seizure risk

▣ *Iron:* Reduced absorption of trovafloxacin; do not take within 4 hr of dose

▣ *Magnesium:* Reduced absorption of trovafloxacin; do not take within 4 hr of dose

▣ *Metoprolol:* Inhibits metabolism of metoprolol; increased plasma metoprolol level

▣ *Morphine:* Reduced absorption of trovafloxacin; do not take within 2 hr of dose

▣ *Pentoxifylline:* Inhibits metabolism of pentoxifylline; increased plasma pentoxifylline level

▣ *Phenytoin:* Inhibits metabolism of phenytoin; increased plasma phenytoin level

▣ *Propranolol:* Inhibits metabolism of propranolol; increased plasma propranolol level

▣ *Ropinirole:* Inhibits metabolism of ropinirole; increased plasma ropinirole level

▣ *Sodium bicarbonate:* Reduced absorption of trovafloxacin; do not take within 4 hr of dose

▣ *Sucralfate:* Reduced absorption of trovafloxacin; do not take within 4 hr of dose

▣ *Warfarin:* Inhibits metabolism of warfarin; increases hypoprothrombinemic response to warfarin

▣ *Zinc:* Reduced absorption of trovafloxacin; do not take within 4 hr of dose

SPECIAL CONSIDERATIONS
PATIENT/FAMILY EDUCATION
• Do not take antacids (aluminum, calcium, or magnesium-containing) or iron within 2 hr of taking trovafloxacin. Take at bedtime or with food to minimize dizziness associated with trovafloxacin. Avoid excessive sunlight during treatment

MONITORING PARAMETERS
• Transaminases if given for more than 7 days

---

undecylenic acid
(un-de-sye-len'ik)
OTC: Caldesene, Cruex, Desenex, Fungoid AF, Phicon F
Chemical Class: Hendecenoic acid derivative
Therapeutic Class: Antifungal

CLINICAL PHARMACOLOGY
Mechanism of Action: An antifungal whose mechanism of action is not well understood. *Therapeutic Effect:* Fungistatic.

INDICATIONS AND DOSAGES
Tinea pedis, tinea corporis
Topical

Adults, Children 2 yrs and older. Apply 2 times/day to affected area for 4 wks.

Ⓢ **AVAILABLE FORMS/COST**
• Cre—Top: 20%, 15 g: **$5.34**
• Oint—Top: 25%, 15, 30, 454 g: **$1.80-$7.40**/30 g

U

• Powder—Top: 25%, 45, 60, 90, 165 g: **$5.36**/90 g
• Spray—Top: 19%, 54, 90, 105, 165 g: **$4.64**/105 g; 25%, 45 g: **$3.85**
CONTRAINDICATIONS: Hypersensitivity to undecylenic acid or any component of its formulation
PREGNANCY AND LACTATION: Problems not documented in breast-feeding
SIDE EFFECTS
Occasional
Skin irritation, rash
SERIOUS REACTIONS
• Hypersensitivity reactions characterized by rash, facial swelling, pruritus, and a sensation of warmth occur.

SPECIAL CONSIDERATIONS
• Newer topical antifungals more effective
• Powders are generally used as adjunctive therapy, but may be useful for primary therapy in very mild cases

---

urea
(yoor-ee'-a)
Rx: *Parenteral:* Ureaphil
Rx: *Topical:* Gordon's Urea 40%
OTC: *Topical:* Aqua Care, Carmol, Gormel, Lanaphilic UltraMide, Ureacin
Chemical Class: Carbonic acid diamide salt
Therapeutic Class: Antiglaucoma agent; osmotic agent

CLINICAL PHARMACOLOGY
Mechanism of Action: A diuretic which rapidly increases blood tonicity causing a greater urea concentration gradient in the blood than in the extravascular fluid resulting in movement of fluid from the tissues, including the brain and cerebrospi-

nal fluid into the blood. A keratolytic that dissolves the intercellular matrix and thereby softens hyperkeratotic areas by enhancing the shedding of scales. *Therapeutic effect:* Decreases ocular hypertension and cerebral edema.
Pharmacokinetics
None known

INDICATIONS AND DOSAGES
Reduction in intracranial/intraocular pressure
Adults, Elderly: 1 to 1.5 g/kg. Maximum 120 g daily.
Children 2 years and older: 0.5-1.5 g/kg
Children 2 years and younger: 0.1 g/kg may be adequate.
Skin/nail debridement
Topical
Adults, Elderly, Children: Apply urea cream, 40% to affected areas. If desired, cover with occlusive dressing. Keep dry and occlusive for 3-7 days.

Ⓢ **AVAILABLE FORMS/COST**
• Cre—Top: 10%, 90, 454 g: **$7.26**/90 g; 20%, 75, 90, 120, 454, 480 g: **$6.15**/75 g; 22%, 30 g: **$13.12**; 30%, 60 g: **$6.50**; 40%, 30, 90, 120 g: **$28.75-$29.40**/30 g
• Gel—Top: 40%, 15 ml: **$80.93**
• Lotion—Top: 10%, 240, 480 ml: **$2.95-$13.00**/240 ml; 15%, 120 g: **$5.90**; 25%, 105, 240 ml: **$10.54**/240 ml
• Oint—Top: 10%, 180, 454 g: **$3.85**/180 g
• Paste—Top: 50%, 60 g: **$14.79**
• Shampoo—Top: 10%, 240 ml: **$11.94**

UNLABELED USES: *None known.*
CONTRAINDICATIONS: Severely impaired renal function, active intracranial bleeding, marked dehydration, frank liver failure,
PREGNANCY AND LACTATION: Pregnancy category C; no data on breast-feeding available

SIDE EFFECTS
Common

Transient stinging, burning, itching, irritation, headaches, nausea, vomiting, infection at site of injection, venous thrombosis or phlebitis extending from site of injection, extravasation, hypervolemia.

Occasional

Syncope, disorientation

Rare

Transient agitated confusional state, chemical phlebitis and thrombosis near site of injection

SERIOUS REACTIONS

• No serious reactions have been noted when solutions have been infused slowly provided renal function is not seriously impaired or there is no evidence of active intracranial bleeding.

• Signs of overdosage include unusually elevated blood urea nitrogen (BUN) levels.

SPECIAL CONSIDERATIONS

• Do not infuse into lower extremity veins

• Monitor for extravasation, tissue necrosis may occur

---

urokinase
(you-oh-kine-ace)

Rx: Abbokinase, Abbokinase Open-Cath (not for systemic administration)
Chemical Class: Renal enzyme
Therapeutic Class: Thrombolytic

CLINICAL PHARMACOLOGY

Mechanism of Action: A thrombolytic agent that activates fibrinolytic system by converting plasminogen to plasmin (enzyme that degrades fibrin clots). Acts indirectly by forming complex with plasminogen, which converts plasminogen to plasmin. Action occurs within thrombus, on its surface, and in circulating blood. *Therapeutic Effect:* Destroys thrombi.

Pharmacokinetics

Rapidly cleared from circulation by liver. Small amounts eliminated in urine and via bile. **Half-life:** 20 min.

INDICATIONS AND DOSAGES
Pulmonary embolism

IV

Adults, Elderly. Initially, 4,400 IU/kg at rate of 90 ml/hr over 10 min; then, 4,400 IU/kg at rate of 15 ml/hr for 12 hrs. Flush tubing. Follow with anticoagulant therapy.

Coronary artery thrombi

Intracoronary

Adults, Elderly. 6,000 IU/min for up to 2 hrs.

Occluded IV catheter

Adults, Elderly. Disconnect IV tubing from catheter; attach a 1 ml TB syringe with 5,000 U urokinase to catheter; inject urokinase slowly (equal to volume of catheter). Connect empty 5 ml syringe; aspirate residual clot. When patency is restored, irrigate with 0.9% NaCl; reconnect IV tubing to catheter.

$ AVAILABLE FORMS/COST

• Powder, Inj—IV: 5000 U/ml, 1 ml: **$56.61**; 9000 U/vial: **$98.72** (not for systemic administration); 250,000 U/vial: **$539.78**

CONTRAINDICATIONS: Active internal bleeding, atrioventricular (AV) malformation or aneurysm, bleeding diathesis, intracranial neoplasm, intracranial or intraspinal surgery or trauma, recent (within the past 2 mos) cerebrovascular accident

PREGNANCY AND LACTATION: Pregnancy category B; no data available on breast-feeding

U

SIDE EFFECTS
Frequent

Superficial or surface bleeding at puncture sites (venous cutdowns, arterial punctures, surgical sites, IM sites, retroperitoneal/intracerebral sites); internal bleeding (GI/GU tract, vaginal).

Rare

Mild allergic reaction such as rash or wheezing

SERIOUS REACTIONS

• Severe internal hemorrhage may occur. Lysis of coronary thrombi may produce atrial/ventricular arrhythmias

INTERACTIONS
Drugs

▣ *Heparin, oral anticoagulants, drugs that alter platelet function (i.e., aspirin, dipyridamole, abciximab, eptifibitide, tirofiban):* May increase the risk of bleeding

---

ursodiol

(your-soo′dee-ol)

Rx: Actigall
Chemical Class: Ursodeoxycholic acid
Therapeutic Class: Cholelitholytic

CLINICAL PHARMACOLOGY
Mechanism of Action: A gallstone solubilizing agent that suppresses hepatic synthesis and secretion of cholesterol; inhibits intestinal absorption of cholesterol. *Therapeutic Effect:* Changes the bile of patients with gallstones from precipitating (capable of forming crystals) to cholesterol solubilizing (capable of being dissolved).

INDICATIONS AND DOSAGES
Dissolution of radiolucent, noncalcified gallstones when cholecystectomy is not recommended; treatment of biliary cirrhosis
PO

Adults, Elderly. 8–10 mg/kg/day in 2–3 divided doses. Treatment may require months. Obtain ultrasound image of gallbladder at 6-mo intervals for first year. If gallstones have dissolved, continue therapy and repeat ultrasound within 1–3 mo.

Prevention of gallstones
PO

Adults, Elderly. 300 mg twice a day.

§ AVAILABLE FORMS/COST
• Cap, Gel—Oral: 300 mg, 100's: **$257.70-$388.71**
• Tab—Oral: 250 mg, 100's: **$220.73**

UNLABELED USES: Treatment of alcoholic cirrhosis, biliary atresia, chronic hepatitis, gallstone formation, sclerosing cholangitis, prophylaxis of liver transplant rejection

CONTRAINDICATIONS: Allergy to bile acids, calcified cholesterol stones, chronic hepatic disease, radiolucent bile pigment stones, radiopaque stones

PREGNANCY AND LACTATION: Pregnancy category B; excretion into breast milk unknown

SIDE EFFECTS
Occasional

Diarrhea

SERIOUS REACTIONS

• None significant.

SPECIAL CONSIDERATIONS

• Complete dissolution may not occur; likelihood of success is low if partial stone dissolution not seen by 12 mo
• Stones recur within 5 yr in 50% of patients

PATIENT/FAMILY EDUCATION

• Administer with food to facilitate dissolution in the intestine

valacyclovir
(val-a-sye'kloe-ver)
Rx: Valtrex
Chemical Class: Acyclic purine
nucleoside analog; acyclovir
derivative
Therapeutic Class: Antiviral

CLINICAL PHARMACOLOGY
Mechanism of Action: A virustatic
antiviral that is converted to acyclovir triphosphate, becoming part of
the viral DNA chain. *Therapeutic
Effect:* Interferes with DNA synthesis and replication of herpes simplex
virus and varicella-zoster virus.
Pharmacokinetics
Rapidly absorbed after PO administration. Protein binding: 13%-18%.
Rapidly converted by hydrolysis to
the active compound acyclovir.
Widely distributed to tissues and
body fluids (including CSF). Primarily eliminated in urine. Removed
by hemodialysis. **Half-life:** 2.5-3.3
hr (increased in impaired renal function).

INDICATIONS AND DOSAGES
Herpes zoster (shingles)
PO
Adults, Elderly. 1 g 3 times a day for
7 days.
Herpes simplex (cold sores)
PO
Adults, Elderly. 2 g twice a day for 1
day.
Initial episode of genital herpes
PO
Adults, Elderly. 1 g twice a day for
10 days.
*Recurrent episodes of genital her-
pes*
PO
Adults, Elderly. 500 mg twice a day
for 3 days.

Prevention of genital herpes
PO
Adults, Elderly. 500-1,000 mg/day.
Dosage in renal impairment
Dosage and frequency are modified
based on creatinine clearance.

Creatinine Clearance	Herpes Zoster	Genital Herpes
50 ml/min or higher	1 g q8h	500 mg q12h
30-49 ml/min	1 g q12h	500 mg q12h
10-29 ml/min	1 g q24h	500 mg q24h
less than 10 ml/min	500 mg q24h	500 mg q24h

AVAILABLE FORMS/COST
• Cap—Oral: 500 mg, 42's: **$169.26**
• Tab—Oral: 1 g, 21's: **$163.26**
UNLABELED USES: To reduce the
risk of heterosexual transmission of
genital herpes
CONTRAINDICATIONS: Hypersensitivity to or intolerance of acy-
clovir, valacyclovir, or their compo-
nents
PREGNANCY AND LACTATION:
Pregnancy category B; acyclovir excreted into breast milk; safety not established but should be compatible
with breast-feeding
SIDE EFFECTS
Frequent
Herpes zoster (17%-10%): Nausea,
headache
Genital herpes (17%): Headache
Occasional
Herpes zoster (7%-3%): Vomiting,
diarrhea, constipation (50 yr or
older), asthenia, dizziness (50 yr and
older)
Genital herpes (8%-3%): Nausea,
diarrhea, dizziness
Rare
Herpes zoster (3%-1%): Abdominal
pain, anorexia
Genital herpes (3%-1%): Asthenia,
abdominal pain

V

SERIOUS REACTIONS

- None known.

SPECIAL CONSIDERATIONS

- Acyclovir 400 mg PO bid less expensive for chronic suppression of genital herpes

---

valdecoxib

(val-de-cocks'ib)

Rx: Bextra

Chemical Class: Cyclooxygenase-2 (COX-2) inhibitor

Therapeutic Class: COX-2 specific inhibitor; NSAID; nonnarcotic analgesic

Withdrawn from Market

CLINICAL PHARMACOLOGY

Mechanism of Action: An NSAID that inhibits cyclo-oxygenase-2, the enzyme responsible for producing prostaglandins, which cause pain and inflammation. *Therapeutic Effect:* Reduces inflammatory response and intensity of pain.

Pharmacokinetics

Rapidly and almost completely absorbed from the GI tract. Widely distributed. Extensively metabolized in the liver. Primarily eliminated in urine. **Half-life:** 8-11 hr.

INDICATIONS AND DOSAGES

Osteoarthritis, rheumatoid arthritis

PO

Adults, Elderly. 10 mg once a day.

Primary dysmenorrhea

PO

Adults, Elderly. 20 mg twice a day.

$ **AVAILABLE FORMS/COST**

- Tab—Oral: 10, 20 mg 100's; all: **$314.06**

CONTRAINDICATIONS: Hypersensitivity to aspirin or NSAIDs, severe hepatic or renal impairment

PREGNANCY AND LACTATION: Pregnancy category C; excreted into breast milk of animals

SIDE EFFECTS

Frequent (8%-4%)

Headache

Occasional (3%-2%)

Dizziness

Rare (less than 2%)

Dyspepsia, nausea, diarrhea, sinusitis, peripheral edema

SERIOUS REACTIONS

- None known.

INTERACTIONS

Drugs

[3] *Angiotensin-converting enzyme inhibitors:* Diminished antihypertensive effects

[3] *Aspirin:* Increased risk of GI ulceration; negation of cardioprotective effects of aspirin

[3] *Diuretics (loop, thiazides):* Reduced naturetic effect

[3] *Lithium:* Elevation of plasma lithium levels, potential lithium toxicity

SPECIAL CONSIDERATIONS

- May be safer that conventional nonsteroidal antiinflammatory agents, particularly with respect to gastrointestinal tolerability, and offer comparable efficacy. Other complications may arise, including cardiovascular complications from selective inhibition of the COX-2 isozyme (see rofecoxib)

PATIENT/FAMILY EDUCATION

- Alert for symptoms of adverse effects (e.g., GI ulceration and bleeding, renal dysfunction)

MONITORING PARAMETERS

- Improvement in clinical symptoms (pain, stiffness, mobility, swollen/tender joints); blood pressure in patients with cardiovascular disease, upper gastrointestinal tests are suggested in patients with persistent dyspepsia, nausea, cramps, hematemesis

valganciclovir
(val-gan-sye'kloh-veer)

Rx: Valcyte

Chemical Class: Acyclic purine nucleoside analog; ganciclovir derivative

Therapeutic Class: Antiviral

Creatinine Clearance	Induction Dosage	Maintenance Dosage
60 ml/min or more	900 mg twice/day	900 mg once/day
40–59 ml/min	450 mg twice/day	450 mg once/day
25–39 ml/min	450 mg once/day	450 mg q2 days
10–24 ml/min	450 mg q2 days	450 mg twice/week

CLINICAL PHARMACOLOGY

Mechanism of Action: A synthetic nucleoside that competes with viral DNA esterases and is incorporated directly into growing viral DNA chains. *Therapeutic Effect:* Interferes with DNA synthesis and viral replication.

Pharmacokinetics

Well absorbed and rapidly converted to ganciclovir by intestinal and hepatic enzymes. Widely distributed. Slowly metabolized intracellularly. Primarily excreted unchanged in urine. Removed by hemodialysis. **Half-life:** 18 hr (increased in impaired renal function).

INDICATIONS AND DOSAGES

Cytomegalovirus (CMV) retinitis in patients with normal renal function

PO

Adults. Initially, 900 mg (two 450-mg tablets) twice a day for 21 days. Maintenance: 900 mg once a day.

Prevention of CMV after transplant

PO

Adults, Elderly. 900 mg once a day beginning within 10 days of transplant and continuing until 100 days post-transplant.

Dosage in renal impairment

Dosage and frequency are modified based on creatinine clearance.

§ **AVAILABLE FORMS/COST**

• Tab—Oral: 450 mg, 60's: **$1,888.43**

CONTRAINDICATIONS: Hypersensitivity to acyclovir or ganciclovir

PREGNANCY AND LACTATION: Pregnancy category C (teratogenic in animals); breast milk excretion unknown but breast-feeding not recommended if taking valganciclovir; do not resume nursing for at least 72 hr after last dose of valganciclovir

SIDE EFFECTS

Frequent (16%-9%)

Diarrhea, neutropenia, headache

Occasional (8%-3%)

Nausea, anemia, thrombocytopenia

Rare (less than 3%)

Insomnia, paraesthesia, vomiting, abdominal pain, fever

SERIOUS REACTIONS

• Hematologic toxicity, including severe neutropenia (most common), anemia, and thrombocytopenia, may occur.

• Retinal detachment occurs rarely.

• An overdose may result in renal toxicity.

• Valganciclovir may decrease sperm production and fertility.

INTERACTIONS

Drugs

③ *Didanosine:* Didanosine may increase valganciclovir level; increased hematological toxicity possible

V

❷ *Mycophenolate:* Mycophenolate may increase valganciclovir level; valganciclovir may increase mycophenolate level; increased hematological toxicity possible

❷ *Probenecid:* Probenecid reduces ganciclovir clearance; increased hematological toxicity possible

▲ *Zidovudine:* Additive hematological toxicity

SPECIAL CONSIDERATIONS

PATIENT/FAMILY EDUCATION

• Take with food

• Do not take during pregnancy or lactation

• Men should use a condom during sex while using this medicine for at least 3 months after treatment ends because valganciclovir interferes with normal sperm formation

MONITORING PARAMETERS

• CBC, platelet count, creatinine

**valproic acid /
valproate sodium /
divalproex sodium**

Chemical Class: Carboxylic acid derivative
Therapeutic Class: Anticonvulsant

CLINICAL PHARMACOLOGY

Mechanism of Action: An anticonvulsant, antimanic, and antimigraine agent that directly increases concentration of the inhibitory neurotransmitter gamma-aminobutyric acid. *Therapeutic Effect:* Reduces seizure activity.

Pharmacokinetics

Well absorbed from the GI tract. Protein binding: 80%-90%. Metabolized in the liver. Primarily excreted in urine. Not removed by hemodialysis. **Half-life:** 6-16 hr (may be increased in hepatic impairment, the elderly, and children younger than 18 mo).

INDICATIONS AND DOSAGES

Seizures

PO

Adults, Elderly, Children 10 yr and older. Initially, 10-15 mg/kg/day in 1-3 divided doses. May increase by 5-10 mg/kg/day at weekly intervals up to 30-60 mg/kg/day. Usual adult dosage: 1,000-2,500 mg/day.

IV

Adults, Elderly, Children. Same as oral dose but given q6h.

Manic episodes

PO

Adults, Elderly. Initially, 750 mg/day in divided doses. Maximum: 60 mg/kg/day.

Prevention of migraine headaches

PO (Extended-Release tablets)

Adults, Elderly. Initially, 500 mg/day for 7 days. May increase up to 1000 mg/day.

PO (Delayed-Release tablets)

Adults, Elderly. Initially, 250 mg twice a day. May increase up to 1,000 mg/day.

Ⓢ AVAILABLE FORMS/COST

Valproic Acid

• Cap, Elastic—Oral: 250 mg, 100's: **$26.85-$216.03**

• Syr—Oral: 250 mg/5 ml, 480 ml: **$16.44-$72.75**

Divalproex Sodium

• Cap, Enteric Coated (Sprinkle)—Oral: 125 mg, 100's: **$57.78**

• Tab, Enteric Coated—Oral: 125 mg, 100's: **$57.46**; 250 mg, 100's: **$112.85**; 500 mg, 100's: **$208.11**

• Tab, Sus Action—Oral: 250 mg, 100's: **$112.84**; 500 mg, 100's: **$198.49**

Valproate Sodium

• Sol, Inj—IV: 100 mg/ml, 5 ml: **$8.38-$13.96**

UNLABELED USES: Treatment of myoclonic, simple partial, and tonic-clonic seizures

CONTRAINDICATIONS: Active hepatic disease

PREGNANCY AND LACTATION: Pregnancy category D; teratogenic; increased risk of neural tube defects (1%-2% when used between day 17-30 after fertilization); compatible with breast-feeding

SIDE EFFECTS

Frequent

Epilepsy: Abdominal pain, irregular menses, diarrhea, transient alopecia, indigestion, nausea, vomiting, tremors, weight gain or loss

Mania (22%-19%): Nausea, somnolence

Occasional

Epilepsy: Constipation, dizziness, drowsiness, headache, skin rash, unusual excitement, restlessness

Mania (12%–6%): Asthenia, abdominal pain, dyspepsia (heartburn, indigestion, epigastric distress), rash

Rare

Epilepsy: Mood changes, diplopia, nystagmus, spots before eyes, unusual bleeding or ecchymosis

SERIOUS REACTIONS

• Hepatotoxicity may occur, particularly in the first 6 months of valproic acid therapy. It may be preceded by loss of seizure control, malaise, weakness, lethargy, anorexia, and vomiting rather than abnormal serum liver function test results.

• Blood dyscrasias may occur.

INTERACTIONS

Drugs

☒ *Carbamazepine, phenytoin:* Increase, decrease, or no effect on carbamazepine and phenytoin concentrations

☒ *Cholestyramine, colestipol:* Reduced absorption of valproic acid

☒ *Clarithromycin, erythromycin, troleandomycin:* Increased valproic acid concentrations

☒ *Clonazepam:* Absence seizure reported with concurrent use

☒ *Clozapine:* Reduced serum clozapine concentrations

☒ *Felbamate:* Increased valproic acid concentrations

☒ *Isoniazid:* Increased valproic acid concentrations

☒ *Lamotrigine:* Increased plasma lamotrigine concentrations; decreased valproic acid concentrations

☒ *Nimodipine:* Increased nimodipine area under the plasma concentration-time curve

☒ *Phenobarbital, primidone:* Increased phenobarbital levels

☒ *Salicylates:* Increased valproate levels

☒ *Zidovudine:* Increased zidovudine levels

Labs

• *False increase:* Serum free fatty acids

• *False positive:* Urinary ketones

SPECIAL CONSIDERATIONS

PATIENT/FAMILY EDUCATION

• Administer with food to decrease GI side effects

• Do not administer with carbonated beverages or milk

MONITORING PARAMETERS

• Therapeutic levels (draw just before next dose) 50-100 mcg/ml

• ALT, AST, coagulation studies, and platelet count prior to and during therapy, especially first 6 mo

• Minor elevations in ALT, AST are frequent and dose related

valsartan
(val-sar′tan)
Rx: Diovan
Combinations
  Rx: with hydrochlorothiazide
    (Diovan HCT)
Chemical Class: Angiotensin II
receptor antagonist
Therapeutic Class: Antihypertensive

CLINICAL PHARMACOLOGY
Mechanism of Action: An angiotensin II receptor, type AT_1, antagonist that blocks vasoconstrictor and aldosterone-secreting effects of angiotensin II, inhibiting the binding of angiotensin II to the AT_1 receptors. *Therapeutic Effect:* Causes vasodilation, decreases peripheral resistance, and decreases BP.

Pharmacokinetics
Poorly absorbed after PO administration. Food decreases peak plasma concentration. Protein binding: 95%. Metabolized in the liver. Recovered primarily in feces and, to a lesser extent, in urine. Unknown if removed by hemodialysis. **Half-life:** 6 hr.

INDICATIONS AND DOSAGES
Hypertension
PO
Adults, Elderly. Initially, 80-160 mg/day in patients who are not volume depleted. May increase up to a Maximum: 320 mg/day.

CHF
PO
Adults, Elderly. Initially, 40 mg twice a day. May increase up to 160 mg twice a day. Maximum: 320 mg/day.

💲 AVAILABLE FORMS/COST
• Cap—Oral: 40 mg, 30's: **$41.73**; 80 mg, 100's: **$166.28**; 160 mg, 100's: **$178.78**; 320 mg, 100's: **$226.18**
• Tab—Oral (with hydrochlorothiazide): 12.5 mg-80 mg, 100's: **$178.83**; 12.5 mg-160 mg, 100's: **$194.58**; 25 mg-160 mg, 100's: **$220.65**

CONTRAINDICATIONS: Bilateral renal artery stenosis, biliary cirrhosis or obstruction, hypoaldosteronism, severe hepatic impairment

PREGNANCY AND LACTATION: Pregnancy category C, first trimester—category D, second and third trimesters; drugs acting directly on the renin-angiotensin-aldosterone system are documented to cause fetal harm (hypotension, oligohydramnios, neonatal anemia, hyperkalemia, neonatal skull hypoplasia, anuria, and renal failure); neonatal limb contractures, craniofacial deformities, and hypoplastic lung development

SIDE EFFECTS
Rare (2%-1%)
Insomnia, fatigue, heartburn, abdominal pain, dizziness, headache, diarrhea, nausea, vomiting, arthralgia, edema

SERIOUS REACTIONS
• Overdosage may manifest as hypotension and tachycardia. Bradycardia occurs less often.
• Viral infection and upper respiratory tract infection (cough, pharyngitis, sinusitis, rhinitis) occur rarely.

SPECIAL CONSIDERATIONS
• Potentially as or more effective than angiotensin-converting enzyme inhibitors, without cough; no evidence for reduction in morbidity and mortality as first-line agents in hypertension, yet; whether they provide the same cardiac and renal pro-

tection also still tentative; like ACE inhibitors, less effective in black patients

PATIENT/FAMILY EDUCATION

• Call your clinician immediately if note following side effects: wheezing; lip, throat, or face swelling; hives or rash

MONITORING PARAMETERS

• Baseline electrolytes, urinalysis, BUN and creatinine with recheck at 2-4 wk after initiation (sooner in volume-depleted patients); monitor sitting blood pressure; watch for symptomatic hypotension, particularly in volume-depleted patients

vancomycin

(van-koe-mye'sin)

Rx: Vancocin, Vancoled

Chemical Class: Tricyclic glycopeptide derivative

Therapeutic Class: Antibiotic

CLINICAL PHARMACOLOGY

Mechanism of Action: A tricyclic glycopeptide antibiotic that binds to bacterial cell walls, altering cell membrane permeability and inhibiting RNA synthesis. *Therapeutic Effect:* Bactericidal.

Pharmacokinetics

PO: Poorly absorbed from the GI tract. Primarily eliminated in feces. Parenteral: Widely distributed. Protein binding: 55%. Primarily excreted unchanged in urine. Not removed by hemodialysis. **Half-life:** 4-11 hr (increased in impaired renal function).

INDICATIONS AND DOSAGES

Treatment of bone, respiratory tract, skin and soft-tissue infections, endocarditis, peritonitis, and septicemia; prevention of bacterial endocarditis in those at risk (if penicillin is contraindicated) when undergoing biliary, dental, GI, GU, or respiratory surgery or invasive procedures

IV

Adults, Elderly. 500 mg q6h or 1 g q12h.

Children older than 1 mo. 40 mg/kg/day in divided doses q6-8h. Maximum: 3-4 g/day.

Neonates. Initially, 15 mg/kg, then 10 mg/kg q8-12h.

Staphylococcal enterocolitis, antibiotic-associated pseudomembranous colitis caused by *Clostridium difficile*

PO

Adults, Elderly. 0.5-2 g/day in 3-4 divided doses for 7-10 days.

Children. 40 mg/kg/day in 3-4 divided doses for 7-10 days. Maximum: 2 g/day.

Dosage in renal impairment

After a loading dose, subsequent dosages and frequency are modified based on creatinine clearance, the severity of the infection, and the serum concentration of the drug.

[$] **AVAILABLE FORMS/COST**

• Cap, Gel—Oral: 125 mg, 20's: **$153.96**; 250 mg, 20's: **$307.92**

• Powder, Inj—IV: 500 mg/vial: **$4.19-$8.68**; 1 g/vial: **$6.06-$16.25**

• Powder, Reconst—Oral: 250 mg/5 ml, 10, 20 ml: **$30.66**/10 ml; 500 mg/6 ml, 120 ml: **$326.95**

UNLABELED USES: Treatment of brain abscess, perioperative infections, staphylococcal or streptococcal meningitis

CONTRAINDICATIONS: None known.

PREGNANCY AND LACTATION: Pregnancy category C (oral), B (IV); excreted into breast milk, milk level 4 hr after steady state dose, 12.7

mcg/ml (similar to mother's trough level); poorly absorbed orally, systemic absorption not expected; problems limited to modification of bowel flora, allergic sensitization, and interference with interpretation of culture results during fever workup

SIDE EFFECTS

Frequent

PO: Bitter or unpleasant taste, nausea, vomiting, mouth irritation (with oral solution)

Rare

Parenteral: Phlebitis, thrombophlebitis, or pain at peripheral IV site; dizziness; vertigo; tinnitus; chills; fever; rash; necrosis with extravasation

PO: Rash.

SERIOUS REACTIONS

• Nephrotoxicity and ototoxicity may occur.

• "Red-neck" syndrome (redness on face, neck, arms, and back; chills; fever; tachycardia; nausea or vomiting; pruritus; rash; unpleasant taste) may result from too-rapid injection.

INTERACTIONS

Drugs

▣ *Aminoglycosides:* Enhanced nephrotoxicity

▣ *Indomethacin:* Increased vancomycin in neonates, possible vancomycin toxicity

▣ *Methotrexate:* Reduced methotrexate concentrations with oral vancomycin

Labs

• *False increase:* CSF protein

SPECIAL CONSIDERATIONS

MONITORING PARAMETERS

• Audiograms, BUN, creatinine, serum vancomycin concentrations

---

vardenafil

Rx: Levitra
Chemical Class: CGMP specific phosphodiesterase inhibitor
Therapeutic Class: Anti-impotence agent

CLINICAL PHARMACOLOGY

Mechanism of Action: An erectile dysfunction agent that inhibits phosphodiesterase type 5, the enzyme responsible for degrading cyclic guanosine monophosphate in the corpus cavernosum of the penis, resulting in smooth muscle relaxation and increased blood flow. *Therapeutic Effect:* Facilitates an erection.

Pharmacokinetics

Rapidly absorbed after PO administration. Extensive tissue distribution. Protein binding: 95%. Metabolized in the liver. Excreted primarily in feces; a lesser amount eliminated in urine. Drug has no effect on penile blood flow without sexual stimulation. **Half-life:** 4–5 hr.

INDICATIONS AND DOSAGES

Erectile dysfunction

PO

Adults. 10 mg approximately 1 hr before sexual activity. Dose may be increased to 20 mg or decreased to 5 mg, based on patient tolerance. Maximum dosing frequency is once daily.

Elderly (older than 65 yr). 5 mg.

Dosage in moderate hepatic impairment

PO

For patients with Child-Pugh class B hepatic impairment, dosage is 5 mg 60 min before sexual activity.

Dosage with concurrent ritonavir

PO

Adults. 2.5 mg in a 72-hr period.

Dosage with concurrent ketoconazole or itraconazole (at 400 mg/day), or indinavir
PO
Adults. 2.5 mg in a 24-hour period.
Dosage with concurrent ketoconazole or itraconazole (at 200 mg/day), or erythromycin
PO
Adults. 5 mg in a 24-hr period.

§ **AVAILABLE FORMS/COST**
• Tab, Film-Coated—Oral: 2.5 mg, 5 mg, 10 mg, 20 mg, 30's; all: **$288.75**

CONTRAINDICATIONS: Concurrent use of alpha-adrenergic blockers, sodium nitroprusside, or nitrates in any form

PREGNANCY AND LACTATION: Pregnancy category B, not indicated for use in women

SIDE EFFECTS
Occasional
Headache, flushing, rhinitis, indigestion
Rare (less than 2%)
Dizziness, changes in color vision, blurred vision

SERIOUS REACTIONS
• Prolonged erections (lasting over 4 hours) and priapism (painful erections lasting over 6 hours) occur rarely.

INTERACTIONS
Drugs
⚠ *Alpha-adrenergic blockers:* Concurrent use with vardenafil contraindicated
② *Erythromycin:* Erythromycin increases vardenafil C_{max} by factor of 4
② *Indinavir:* Indinavir increases vardenafil C_{max} by factor of 7, vardenafil reduces indinavir C_{max} by 40%
② *Itraconazole:* Itraconazole increases vardenafil C_{max} by factor of 4

② *Ketoconazole:* Ketoconazole increases vardenafil C_{max} by factor of 4
⚠ *Nitrates:* Concurrent use with vardenafil contraindicated
② *Ritonavir:* Ritonavir increases vardenafil C_{max} by factor of 13, vardenafil reduces ritonavir C_{max} by 20%

SPECIAL CONSIDERATIONS
PATIENT/FAMILY EDUCATION
• Sexual stimulation is required for an erection to occur after taking vardenafil
• Take vardenafil approximately 60 minutes before sexual activity, fatty meal may reduce effect
• Rates of erection sufficient for penetration were 65%, 75%, and 80% with 5 mg, 10 mg, and 20 mg doses, respectively
• For diabetics, rates of erection sufficient for penetration were 61% and 64% with 10 mg and 20 mg doses, respectively
• For men after radical prostatectomy, rates of erection sufficient for penetration were 47% and 48% with 10 mg and 20 mg doses, respectively

---

vasopressin
(vay-soe-press'in)
Rx: Pitressin
Chemical Class: Arginine vasopressin
Therapeutic Class: Antidiuretic; hemostatic

CLINICAL PHARMACOLOGY
Mechanism of Action: A posterior pituitary hormone that increases reabsorption of water by the renal tubules. Increases water permeability at the distal tubule and collecting duct. Directly stimulates smooth

V

muscle in the GI tract. *Therapeutic Effect:* Causes peristalsis and vasoconstriction.

Pharmacokinetics

Route	Onset	Peak	Duration
IV	N/A	N/A	0.5–1 hr
IM/Subcutaneous	1–2 hr	N/A	2–8 hr

Distributed throughout extracellular fluid. Metabolized in the liver and kidney. Primarily excreted in urine. **Half-life:** 10–20 min.

INDICATIONS AND DOSAGES

Cardiac arrest

IV

Adults, Elderly. 40 units as a one-time bolus.

Diabetes insipidus

IV infusion

Adults, Children. 0.5 mUnits/kg/hr. May double dose q30min. Maximum: 10 mUnits/kg/hr.

IM, Subcutaneous

Adults, Elderly. 5–10 units 2–4 times a day. Range: 5–60 unit/day.

Children. 2.5–10 units, 2–4 times a day.

Abdominal distention, Intestinal paresis

IM

Adults, Elderly. Initially, 5 units. Subsequent doses, 10 units q3–4h.

GI hemorrhage

IV infusion

Adults, Elderly. Initially, 0.2–0.4 unit/min progressively increased to 0.9 unit/min.

Children. 0.002–0.005 unit/kg/min. Titrate as needed. Maximum: 0.01 unit/kg/min.

Vasodilatory shock

IV

Adults, Elderly. Initially, 0.04 - 0.1 unit/min. Titrate to desired effect.

[$] **AVAILABLE FORMS/COST**

• Sol, Inj—IM, SC: 20 U/ml, 1 ml: **$5.40-$8.40**

UNLABELED USES: Adjunct in treatment of acute, massive hemorrhage

CONTRAINDICATIONS: None known

PREGNANCY AND LACTATION: Pregnancy category C; breastfeeding reported without complications

SIDE EFFECTS

Frequent

Pain at injection site (with vasopressin tannate)

Occasional

Abdominal cramps, nausea, vomiting, diarrhea, dizziness, diaphoresis, pale skin, circumoral pallor, tremors, headache, eructation, flatulence

Rare

Chest pain; confusion; allergic reaction, including rash or hives, pruritus, wheezing or difficulty breathing, facial and peripheral edema; sterile abscess (with vasopressin tannate)

SERIOUS REACTIONS

• Anaphylaxis, MI, and water intoxication have occurred.

• The elderly and very young are at higher risk for water intoxication.

SPECIAL CONSIDERATIONS

• For diabetes insipidus, vasopressin sol for injection may be administered intranasally on cotton pledgets, by nasal spray or by dropper; dose must be individualized

PATIENT/FAMILY EDUCATION

• Common adverse effects (skin blanching, abdominal cramps, and nausea) may be reduced by taking 1-2 glasses of water with the dose of vasopressin; self-limited in minutes

MONITORING PARAMETERS

• ECG, fluid and electrolyte status

• Extravasation may cause tissue necrosis

venlafaxine
(ven-la-fax'een)
Rx: Effexor, Effexor XR
Chemical Class: Phenethylamine derivative
Therapeutic Class: Antidepressant

CLINICAL PHARMACOLOGY
Mechanism of Action: A phenethylamine derivative that potentiates
CNS neurotransmitter activity by
inhibiting the reuptake of serotonin,
norepinephrine and, to a lesser degree, dopamine. *Therapeutic Effect:*
Relieves depression.

Pharmacokinetics
Well absorbed from the GI tract.
Protein binding: 25%-30%. Metabolized in the liver to active metabolite. Primarily excreted in urine. Not
removed by hemodialysis. **Half-
life:** 3-7 hr; metabolite, 9-13 hr (increased in hepatic or renal impairment.

INDICATIONS AND DOSAGES
Depression
PO
Adults, Elderly. Initially, 75 mg/day
in 2-3 divided doses with food. May
increase by 75 mg/day at intervals of
4 days or longer. Maximum: 375
mg/day in 3 divided doses.
PO (Extended-Release)
Adults, Elderly. 75 mg/day as a
single dose with food. May increase
by 75 mg/day at intervals of 4 days
or longer. Maximum: 225 mg/day.

Anxiety disorder
PO (Extended-Release)
Adults. 37.5-225 mg/day.

*Dosage in renal and hepatic im-
pairment*
Expect to decrease venlafaxine dosage by 50% in patients with moderate hepatic impairment, 25% in patients with mild to moderate renal

impairment, and 50% in patients on
dialysis (withhold dose until
completion of dialysis).

§ AVAILABLE FORMS/COST
• Cap, Sus Action—Oral: 37.5 mg,
100's: **$291.00**; 75 mg, 100's:
$326.00; 150 mg, 100's: **$355.06**
• Tab—Oral: 25 mg, 100's:
$175.06; 37.5 mg, 100's: **$180.31**;
50 mg, 100's: **$185.75**; 75 mg,
100's: **$196.88**; 100 mg, 100's:
$208.63

UNLABELED USES: Prevention of
relapses of depression; treatment of
attention-deficit hyperactivity disorder, autism, chronic fatigue syndrome, obsessive-compulsive disorder

CONTRAINDICATIONS: Use
within 14 days of MAOIs

PREGNANCY AND LACTATION:
Pregnancy category C; excretion
into breast milk unknown

SIDE EFFECTS
Frequent (greater than 20%)
Nausea, somnolence, headache, dry
mouth
Occasional (20%-10%)
Dizziness, insomnia, constipation,
diaphoresis, nervousness, asthenia,
ejaculatory disturbance, anorexia
Rare (less than 10%)
Anxiety, blurred vision, diarrhea,
vomiting, tremor, abnormal dreams,
impotence

SERIOUS REACTIONS
• A sustained increase in diastolic
BP of 10-15 mm Hg occurs occa-
sionally.

SPECIAL CONSIDERATIONS
• Do not stop abruptly

V

verapamil
(ver-ap'a-mill)
Rx: Calan, Calan SR, Covera HS, Isoptin, Isoptin SR, Verelan
Combinations
   Rx: with trandolapril (Tarka)
Chemical Class: Phenylalkylamine
Therapeutic Class: Antianginal; antiarrhythmic, class IV; antihypertensive; calcium channel blocker

CLINICAL PHARMACOLOGY
Mechanism of Action: A calcium channel blocker and antianginal, antiarrhythmic, and antihypertensive agent that inhibits calcium ion entry across cardiac and vascular smooth-muscle cell membranes. This action causes the dilation of coronary arteries, peripheral arteries, and arterioles. *Therapeutic Effect:* Decreases heart rate and myocardial contractility and slows SA and AV conduction. Decreases total peripheral vascular resistance by vasodilation.

Pharmacokinetics

Route	Onset	Peak	Duration
PO	30 min	1-2 hr	6-8 hr
PO (Extended-Release)	30 min	N/A	N/A
IV	1-2 min	3-5 min	10-60 min

Well absorbed from the GI tract. Protein binding: 90% (60% in neonates.) Undergoes first-pass metabolism in the liver to active metabolite. Primarily excreted in urine. Not removed by hemodialysis.
Half-life: 2-8 hr.

INDICATIONS AND DOSAGES
Supraventricular tachyarrhythmias, temporary control of rapid ventricular rate with atrial fibrillation or flutter
IV
Adults, Elderly. Initially, 5-10 mg; repeat in 30 min with 10-mg dose.
Children 1 to 15 yr. 0.1 mg/kg. May repeat in 30 min up to a maximum second dose of 10 mg. Not recommended in children younger than 1 yr.
Arrhythmias, including prevention of recurrent paroxysmal supraventricular tachycardia and control of ventricular resting rate in chronic atrial fibrillation or flutter (with digoxin)
PO
Adults, Elderly. 240-480 mg/day in 3-4 divided doses.
Vasospastic angina (Prinzmetal's variant), unstable (crescendo or preinfarction) angina, chronic stable (effort-associated) angina
PO
Adults. Initially, 80-120 mg 3 times a day. For elderly patients and those with hepatic dysfunction, 40 mg 3 times a day. Titrate to optimal dose. Maintenance: 240-480 mg/day in 3-4 divided doses.
PO (Covera-HS)
Adults, Elderly. 180-480 mg/day at bedtime.
Hypertension
PO
Adults, Elderly. Initially, 40-80 mg 3 times a day. Maintenance: 480 mg or less a day.
PO (Covera-HS)
Adults, Elderly. 180-480 mg/day at bedtime.
PO (Extended-Release)
Adults, Elderly. 120-240 mg/day. May give 480 mg or less a day in 2 divided doses.

PO (Verelan PM)
Adults, Elderly. 100-300 mg/day.

§ **AVAILABLE FORMS/COST**
• Cap, Sus Action—Oral: 100 mg, 100's: **$157.41**; 120 mg, 100's: **$129.05-$203.98**; 180 mg, 100's: **$135.16-$213.60**; 200 mg, 100's: **$202.74**; 240 mg, 100's: **$152.54-$241.08**; 300 mg, 100's: **$294.75**; 360 mg, 100's: **$209.94-$354.36**
• Sol, Inj—IV: 2.5 mg/ml, 2 ml: **$2.95-$3.29**
• Tab, Coated, Sus Action—Oral: 120 mg, 100's: **$86.79-$143.63**; 180 mg, 100's: **$22.93-$182.03**; 240 mg, 100's: **$50.32-$208.25**
• Tab, Plain Coated—Oral: 40 mg, 100's: **$26.15-$53.09**; 80 mg, 100's: **$7.00-$76.36**; 120 mg, 100's: **$9.56-$106.50**
• Tab, Sus Action—Oral (with trandolapril): 1 mg-240 mg, 2 mg-180 mg, 2 mg-240 mg, 4 mg-240 mg, 100's; all: **$206.23**

UNLABELED USES: Treatment of hypertrophic cardiomyopathy, vascular headaches

CONTRAINDICATIONS: Atrial fibrillation or flutter and an accessory bypass tract, cardiogenic shock, heart block, sinus bradycardia, ventricular tachycardia

PREGNANCY AND LACTATION: Pregnancy category C; excreted in breast milk (approx 25% of maternal serum); compatible with breast-feeding

SIDE EFFECTS
Frequent (7%)
Constipation
Occasional (4%-2%)
Dizziness, light-headedness, headache, asthenia (loss of strength, energy), nausea, peripheral edema, hypotension
Rare (less than 1%)
Bradycardia, dermatitis or rash

SERIOUS REACTIONS
• Rapid ventricular rate in atrial flutter or fibrillation, marked hypotension, extreme bradycardia, CHF, asystole, and second- and third-degree AV block occur rarely.

INTERACTIONS
Drugs
▪ *Amiodarone:* Cardiotoxicity with bradycardia and decreased cardiac output
▪ *Barbiturates:* Reduced plasma concentrations of verapamil
▪ *Benzodiazepines:* Marked increase in midazolam concentrations, increased sedation likely to result
▪ *β-blockers:* β-blocker serum concentrations increased *(atenolol, metoprolol, propranolol)*; increased risk of bradycardia, hypotension, AV conduction, and myocardial contractility
❷ *Carbamazepine:* Increased carbamazepine toxicity when verapamil added to chronic anticonvulsant regimens; reduced metabolism
▪ *Cimetidine:* Increased verapamil concentrations and effect by cimetidine
▪ *Cyclosporine, tacrolimus:* Increased concentrations of these drugs, nephrotoxicity possible
▪ *Dantrolene:* Hyperkalemia and myocardial depression may occur; consider a dihydropyridine calcium blocker
▪ *Diclofenac:* Reduced verapamil concentrations
▪ *Digitalis glycosides:* Increased digoxin concentrations by approximately 70%
▪ *Doxazosin, prazosin, terazosin:* Enhanced hypotensive effects
▪ *Doxorubicin:* Increased doxorubicin concentrations
▪ *Encainide:* Increased encainide concentrations

⬛ *Ethanol:* Increased ethanol concentrations, prolonged and increased levels of intoxication

⬛ *Fentanyl:* Severe hypotension or increased fluid volume requirements

⬛ *Histamine H_2-antagonists:* Increased blood levels of verapamil with cimetidine

⬛ *Hydantoins:* Serum verapamil levels may fall if used concurrently

⬛ *Imipramine:* Increased imipramine concentrations

⬛ *Lithium:* Potential for neurotoxicity

⬛ *Neuromuscular blocking agents:* Prolonged neuromuscular blockade

⬛ *Quinidine:* Quinidine toxicity via inhibition of metabolism

⬛ *Rifampin, rifabutin:* Induced metabolism; reduced verapamil concentrations

⬛ *Sulfinpyrazone:* Increased clearance of verapamil

⬛ *Theophylline:* Verapamil inhibits metabolism, increases theophylline levels

⬛ *Vitamin D:* Therapeutic efficacy of verapamil may be reduced

SPECIAL CONSIDERATIONS

• Dihydropyridine calcium channel blockers preferred over verapamil and diltiazem in patients with sinus bradycardia, conduction disturbances, and for combination with a β-blocker

• Differentiate PSVT from narrow complex ventricular tachycardia prior to IV administration; failure to do so has resulted in fatalities

vitamin A

Rx: Aquasol A
Chemical Class: Vitamin, fat soluble
Therapeutic Class: Vitamin

CLINICAL PHARMACOLOGY

Mechanism of Action: A fat-soluble vitamin that may act as a co-factor in biochemical reactions. *Therapeutic Effect:* Is essential for normal function of retina, visual adaptation to darkness, bone growth, testicular and ovarian function, and embryonic development; preserves integrity of epithelial cells.

Pharmacokinetics

Rapidly absorbed from the GI tract if bile salts, pancreatic lipase, protein, and dietary fat are present. Transported in blood to the liver, where it's metabolized; stored in parenchymal hepatic cells, then transported in plasma as retinol, as needed. Excreted primarily in bile and, to a lesser extent, in urine.

INDICATIONS AND DOSAGES

Severe vitamin A deficiency

PO

Adults, Elderly, Children 8 yr and older. 500,000 units/day for 3 days; then 50,000 units/day for 14 days, then 10,000–20,000 units/day for 2 mo.

Children 1–8 yr. 5,000 units/kg/day for 5 days, then 5,000-10,000 units/day for 2 mo.

Children younger than 1 yr. 5,000-10,000 units/day for 2 mo.

IM

Adults, Elderly, Children 8 yr and older. 100,000 units/day for 3 days; then 50,000 units/day for 14 days.

Children 1–8 yr. 17,500–35,000 units/day for 10 days.

Children younger than 1 yr. 7,500-15,000 units/day.

Malabsorption syndrome
PO
Adults, Elderly, Children 8 yr and older. 10,000-50,000 units/day.

Dietary supplement
PO
Adults, Elderly. 4,000–5,000 units/day.
Children 7–10 yr. 3,300–3,500 units/day.
Children 4–6 yr. 2,500 units/day.
Children 6 mo–3 yr. 1,500–2,000 units/day.
Neonates younger than 5 mos. 1,500 units/day.

Ⓢ AVAILABLE FORMS/COST
• Cap, Elastic—Oral: 8,000 U, 100's: **$2.03-$2.79**; 10,000 U, 100's: **$1.60-$3.25**; 25,000 U, 100's: **$2.25-$9.76**; 50,000 U, 100's: **$5.50**
• Sol, Inj—IM: 50,000 U/ml, 2 ml: **$27.67**

CONTRAINDICATIONS: Hypervitaminosis A
PREGNANCY AND LACTATION: Pregnancy category A; safety of exceeding 5000/6000 IU PO/IV recommended daily allowance (RDA) not established; naturally present in breast milk, deficiency rare, RDA during lactation is 6000 IU; danger of higher doses unknown
SIDE EFFECTS
None known.
SERIOUS REACTIONS
• Chronic overdose produces malaise, nausea, vomiting, drying or cracking of skin or lips, inflammation of tongue or gums, irritability, alopecia, and night sweats.
• Bulging fontanelles have occurred in infants.
INTERACTIONS
Drugs
❸ *Acitretin, etretinate:* Large doses of vitamin A should be avoided with these retinoids

SPECIAL CONSIDERATIONS
PATIENT/FAMILY EDUCATION
• Administer with food for better PO absorption
• Foods high in vitamin A: yellow and dark green vegetables, yellow and orange fruits, A-fortified foods, liver, egg yolks

---

vitamin D (cholecalciferol, vitamin D₃; ergocalciferol, vitamin D₂)
Rx: Calciferol, Drisdol
OTC: Calciferol, Drisdol
Chemical Class: Vitamin, fat soluble
Therapeutic Class: Vitamin

CLINICAL PHARMACOLOGY
Mechanism of Action: A fat-soluble vitamin that stimulates calcium and phosphate absorption from small intestine, promotes secretion of calcium from bone to blood, and promotes resorption of phosphate in renal tubules; also acts on bone cells to stimulate skeletal growth and on parathyroid gland to suppress hormone synthesis and secretion. *Therapeutic Effect:* Essential for absorption and utilization of calcium and phosphate and normal bone calcification. Reduces parathyroid hormone level. Improves phosphorus and calcium homeostasis in chronic renal failure.
Pharmacokinetics
Readily absorbed from small intestine. Concentrated primarily in liver and fat deposits. Activated in the liver and kidneys. Eliminated by biliary system; excreted in urine. **Half-life:** 19–48 hr for ergocalciferol.

V

INDICATIONS AND DOSAGES:
A;ertOral dosing is preferred. Administer the drug IM only in patients with GI, hepatic, or biliary disease associated with malabsorption of vitamin D.

Dietary supplement
PO
Adults, Elderly, Children. 10 mcg (400 units)/day.
Neonates. 10–20 mcg (400–800 units)/day.

Renal failure
PO
Adults, Elderly. 0.5 mg/day.
Children. 0.1–1 mg/day.

Hypoparathyroidism
PO
Adults, Elderly. 625 mcg–5 mg/day (with calcium supplements).
Children. 1.25–5 mg/day (with calcium supplements).

Nutritional rickets, osteomalacia
PO
Adults, Elderly, Children. 25–125 mcg/day for 8–12 wk.
Adults, Elderly (with malabsorption syndrome). 250–7,500 mcg/day.
Children (with malabsorption syndrome). 250–625 mcg/day.

Vitamin D–dependent rickets
PO
Adults, Elderly. 250 mcg–1.5 mg/day.
Children. 75–125 mcg/day. Maximum: 1,500 mcg/day.

Vitamin D–resistant rickets
PO
Adults, Elderly. 250–1,500 mcg/day (with phosphate supplements).
Children. Initially 1,000–2,000 mcg/day (with phosphate supplements). May increase in 250- to 600-mcg increments q3-4mo.

$ **AVAILABLE FORMS/COST**
• Cap, Elastic—Oral: 25,000 IU D$_2$, 100's: **$8.00**; 50,000 IU D$_2$, 100's: **$3.57-$36.00**

• Inj—IM: 500,000 IU/ml, D$_2$, 1 ml amp: **$35.10**
• Liq—Oral: 8000 IU/ml D$_2$, 60 ml (OTC): **$66.81-$102.04**
• Tab—Oral: 400 IU D$_2$, 100's: **$1.94-$2.44**; 50,000 IU D$_2$, 100's: **$52.59**; 400 IU D$_3$, 100's: **$2.15-$3.33**

CONTRAINDICATIONS: Hypercalcemia, malabsorption syndrome, vitamin D toxicity

PREGNANCY AND LACTATION: Pregnancy category A (400 IU/d); category D (doses above recommended daily allowance) associated with supravalvular aortic stenosis, elfin facies, and mental retardation; caution should be exercised when ergocalciferol is administered to nursing women; vitamin D and metabolites appear in breast milk; compatible with breast-feeding; but infant should be monitored for hypercalcemia if doses exceed recommended daily allowance

SIDE EFFECTS
None known.

SERIOUS REACTIONS
• Early signs and symptoms of overdose are weakness, headache, somnolence, nausea, vomiting, dry mouth, constipation, muscle and bone pain, and metallic taste.
• Later signs and symptoms of overdose include polyuria, polydipsia, anorexia, weight loss, nocturia, photophobia, rhinorrhea, pruritus, disorientation, hallucinations, hyperthermia, hypertension, and cardiac arrhythmias.

INTERACTIONS
Labs
• *Interference:* Serum cholesterol

SPECIAL CONSIDERATIONS
• IM therapy should be reserved for patients with GI, liver, or biliary disease associated with vitamin D malabsorption

• Ensure adequate calcium intake; maintain serum calcium levels between 9-10 mg/dL

MONITORING PARAMETERS

• Serum calcium and phosphorus levels (vitamin D levels also helpful, although less frequently)
• Height and weight in children
• X-ray bones monthly until condition is corrected and stabilized
• Periodically determine magnesium and alk phosphatase
• Serum calcium times phosphorous should not exceed 70 mg/dL to avoid ectopic calcification

---

vitamin E

OTC: Aquasol E, E-400, Gordon's Vite E
Chemical Class: Vitamin, fat soluble
Therapeutic Class: Vitamin

CLINICAL PHARMACOLOGY

Mechanism of Action: An antioxidant that prevents oxidation of vitamins A and C, protects fatty acids from attack by free radicals, and protects RBCs from hemolysis by oxidizing agents. *Therapeutic Effect:* Prevents and treats vitamin E deficiency.

Pharmacokinetics

Variably absorbed from the GI tract (requires bile salts, dietary fat, and normal pancreatic function). Primarily concentrated in adipose tissue. Metabolized in the liver. Primarily eliminated by biliary system.

INDICATIONS AND DOSAGES

Vitamin E deficiency

PO

Adults, Elderly. 60–75 units/day.
Children. 1 unit/kg/day.

AVAILABLE FORMS/COST

• Cap, Gel—Oral: 100 IU, 100's: **$2.70-$88.74**; 200 IU, 100's: **$3.55-$7.99**; 400 IU, 100's: **$3.12-$9.01**; 600 IU, 100's: **$7.15-$11.00**; 1000 IU, 100's: **$12.00-$16.35**
• Sol, Drops—Oral: 15 IU/0.3 ml, 12 ml: **$24.68**

UNLABELED USES: To decrease severity of tardive dyskinesia

CONTRAINDICATIONS: None known.

PREGNANCY AND LACTATION: Pregnancy category A (C if used above recommended daily allowance doses); recommended daily allowance in pregnancy is 15 IU; excreted into breast milk, 5 times richer in vitamin E than cow's milk; U.S. recommended daily allowance of vitamin E during lactation is 16 IU

SIDE EFFECTS

None known.

SERIOUS REACTIONS

• Chronic overdose may produce fatigue, weakness, nausea, headache, blurred vision, flatulence, and diarrhea.

INTERACTIONS

Drugs

🄳 *Iron:* Impaired hematological response to iron in children with iron-deficiency anemia

🄳 *Oral anticoagulants:* Vitamin E increases hypoprothombinemic response to oral anticoagulants, especially in doses >400 IU/day

SPECIAL CONSIDERATIONS

• Recommended daily allowance adult male 15 IU, adult female 12 IU

voriconazole
(vohr-ee-con'ah-zole)
Rx: Vfend
Chemical Class: Triazole derivative
Therapeutic Class: Antifungal

CLINICAL PHARMACOLOGY
Mechanism of Action: A triazole derivative that inhibits the synthesis of ergosterol, a vital component of fungal cell wall formation. *Therapeutic Effect:* Damages fungal cell wall membrane.

Pharmacokinetics
Rapidly and completely absorbed after PO administration. Widely distributed. Protein binding: 98%. Metabolized in the liver. Primarily excreted as a metabolite in urine. **Half-life:** 6 hr.

INDICATIONS AND DOSAGES
Invasive aspergillosis, other serious fungal infections caused by Scedosporium apiospermum and Fusarium species
PO
Adults, Elderly weighing 40 kg and more. Initially, 400 mg q12h for 2 doses on day 1. Maintenance: 200 mg q12h (may increase to 200 mg q12h).
Adults, Elderly weighing less than 40 kg. Initially, 200 mg q12h for 2 doses on day 1. Maintenance: 100 mg q12h (may increase to 150 mg q12h).
Usual parenteral dosage
IV
Adults, Elderly, Children. Initially, 6 mg/kg/dose q12h for 2 doses, then 4 mg/kg/dose q12h (may decrease to 3 mg/kg/dose if patient is unable to tolerate 4 mg/kg/dose).

Esophageal candidiasis
PO
Adults, Elderly weighing 40 kg ond more. 200 mg q12h for minimum of 14 days, then at least 7 days following resolution of symptoms.
Adults, Elderly weighing less than 40 kg. 100 mg q12h for minimum 14 days, then at least 7 days following resolution of symptoms.
PO

AVAILABLE FORMS/COST
• Powder, Inj—IV: 200 mg/vial: **$109.44**
• Tab–Oral: 50 mg, 30's: **$241.41**; 200 mg, 30's: **$965.63**

CONTRAINDICATIONS: Concurrent administration of carbamazepine; ergot alkaloids; pimozide or quinidine (may cause prolonged QT interval or torsades de pointes); rifabutin; rifampin; or sirolimus

PREGNANCY AND LACTATION: Pregnancy category C; breast milk excretion unknown

SIDE EFFECTS
Frequent (20%-5%)
Abnormal vision, fever, nausea, rash, vomiting
Occasional (5%-2%)
Headache, chills, hallucinations, photophobia, tachycardia, hypertension

SERIOUS REACTIONS
• Hepatotoxicity occurs rarely.

INTERACTIONS
Drugs
▣ *Alprazolam:* Increased alprazolam effect
⚠ *Astemizole:* Increased astemizole level
⚠ *Barbiturates:* Significantly increased voriconazole metabolism
⚠ *Carbamazepine:* Significantly increased voriconazole metabolism
⚠ *Cisapride:* Increased cisapride level

② *Cyclosporine:* Increased cyclosporine level (reduce cyclosporine dose to one-half)

② *Delavirdine:* Decreased or increased voriconazole metabolism

③ *Dihydropyridine calcium channel blockers:* Increased dihydropyridine level

② *Efavirenz:* Decreased or increased voriconazole metabolism

⚠ *Ergot alkaloids:* Increased ergot alkaloid level

③ *HMG-CoA Reductase Inhibitors (Statins):* Increased statin level

③ *Midazolam:* Increased midazolam effect

② *Omeprazole:* Increased omeprazole level (reduce omeprazole dose by one-half if taking 40 mg qd or more)

② *Phenytoin:* Increased voriconazole metabolism (adjust dose, see **DOSAGE**); increased phenytoin level

⚠ *Pimozide:* Increased pimozide level

⚠ *Quinidine:* Increased quinidine level

⚠ *Rifabutin:* Significantly increased voriconazole metabolism

⚠ *Rifampin:* Significantly increased voriconazole metabolism

③ *Ritonavir:* Decreased voriconazole metabolism

⚠ *Sirolimus:* Increased sirolimus level

③ *Sulfonylureas:* Increased sulfonylurea level

⚠ *Terfenadine:* Increased terfenadine level

② *Tacrolimus:* Increased tacrolimus level (reduce tacrolimus dose to one-third)

③ *Triazolam:* Increased triazolam effect

③ *Vinca Alkaloids:* Increased vinca alkaloid level

② *Warfarin:* Increased hypoprothrombinemic effect

SPECIAL CONSIDERATIONS
• Do not take PO within 1 hr of meals
• Do not drive at night while taking voriconazole

MONITORING PARAMETERS
• Visual acuity, field, and color perception if taken more than 28 days
• ALT, AST, alkaline phosphatase, bilirubin, electrolytes

---

warfarin

(war'far-in)

Rx: Coumadin

Chemical Class: Coumarin derivative

Therapeutic Class: Anticoagulant

CLINICAL PHARMACOLOGY

Mechanism of Action: A coumarin derivative that interferes with hepatic synthesis of vitamin K–dependent clotting factors, resulting in depletion of coagulation factors II, VII, IX, and X. *Therapeutic Effect:* Prevents further extension of formed existing clot; prevents new clot formation or secondary thromboembolic complications.

Pharmacokinetics

Route	Onset	Peak	Duration
PO	1.5–3 days	5–7 days	N/A

Well absorbed from the GI tract. Metabolized in the liver. Primarily excreted in urine. Not removed by hemodialysis. **Half-life:** 1.5–2.5 days.

INDICATIONS AND DOSAGES

Anticoagulant

PO

Adults, Elderly. Initially, 5–15 mg/day for 2–5 days; then adjust based on International Normalized Ratio (INR). Maintenance: 2–10 mg/day.

w

Children. Initially, 0.1–0.2 mg/kg (maximum 10 mg). Maintenance: 0.05–0.34 mg/kg/day.

Usual elderly dosage (maintenance)

PO, IV

• *Elderly.* 2–5 mg/day.

$ AVAILABLE FORMS/COST

• Powder, Inj—IV: 5 mg: **$22.58**

• Tab—Oral: 1 mg, 100's: **$53.35-$75.11**; 2 mg, 100's: **$55.67-$78.38**; 2.5 mg, 100's: **$57.45-$80.88**; 3 mg, 100's: **$62.23-$81.19**; 4 mg, 100's: **$57.83-$81.40**; 5 mg, 100's: **$58.21-$84.29**; 6 mg, 100's: **$89.10-$108.59**; 7.5 mg, 100's: **$85.43-$112.35**; 10 mg, 100's: **$88.61-$116.54**

UNLABELED USES: Preventiuon of recurrent cerebral embolism, myocardial reinfarction; treatment adjunct in transient ischemic attacks

CONTRAINDICATIONS: Neurosurgical procedures, open wounds, pregnancy, severe hypertension, severe hepatic or renal damage, uncontrolled bleeding, ulcers

PREGNANCY AND LACTATION: Pregnancy category X; use in 1st trimester carries significant risk to the fetus; exposure in the 6th-9th wk of gestation may produce a pattern of defects termed the fetal warfarin syndrome with an incidence up to 25% in some series; compatible with breast-feeding for normal, full-term infants

SIDE EFFECTS

Occasional

GI distress, such as nausea, anorexia, abdominal cramps, diarrhea

Rare

Hypersensitivity reaction, including dermatitis and urticaria, especially in those sensitive to aspirin

SERIOUS REACTIONS

• Bleeding complications ranging from local ecchymoses to major hemorrhage may occur. Drug should be discontinued immediately and vitamin K or phytonadione administered. Mild hemorrhage: 2.5–10 mg PO, IM, or IV. Severe hemorrhage: 10–15 mg IV and repeated q4h, as necessary.

• Hepatotoxicity, blood dyscrasias, necrosis, vasculitis, and local thrombosis occur rarely.

INTERACTIONS

Drugs

3 *Acetaminophen:* Repeated doses of acetaminophen may increase the hypoprothrombinemic response to warfarin

3 *Allopurinol, amiodarone, ciprofloxacin, clarithromycin, erythromycin, fluconazole, fluorouracil, fluvastatin, fluvoxamine, glucagon, isoniazid, itraconazole, ketoconazole, lovastatin, miconazole, nalidixic acid, neomycin (oral), norfloxacin, ofloxacin, propafenone, propoxyphene, quinidine, sertraline, sulfonamides, sulfonylureas, thyroid hormones, triclofos, troleandomycin, vitamin E, zafirlukast:* Enhanced hypoprothrombinemic response to warfarin

3 *Aminoglutethimide, carbamazepine, cyclophosphamide, ethchlorvynol, griseofulvin, mercaptopurine, methimazole, mitotane, nafcillin, propylthiouracil, vitamin K:* Reduced hypoprothrombinemic response to warfarin

2 *Aspirin:* Increased risk of bleeding complications

2 *Azathioprine, chloramphenicol, cimetidine, clofibrate, co-trimoxazole, danazol, dextrothyroxine, disulfiram, gemfibrozil, metronidazole, sulfinpyrazone, testosterone derivatives:* Enhanced hypoprothrombinemic response to warfarin

2 *Barbiturates, glutethimide, rifampin:* Reduced hypoprothrombinemic response to warfarin

3 *Bile acid-binding resins:* Variable effect on hypoprothrombinemic effect of warfarin

2 *Cephalosporins:* Enhanced hypoprothrombinemic response to warfarin with moxalactam, cefoperazone, cefamandole, cefotetan, and cefmetazole

3 *Chloral hydrate:* Transient increase in hypoprothrombinemic response to warfarin

3 *Ethanol:* Enhanced hypoprothrombinemic response to warfarin with acute ethanol intoxication

3 *Heparin:* Prolonged activated partial thromboplastin time in patients receiving heparin; prolonged prothrombin times in patients receiving warfarin

3 *Mesalamine:* Warfarin effect inhibited in one case report

2 *NSAIDs:* Increased risk of bleeding in anticoagulated patients

2 *Oral contraceptives:* Increase or decrease in anticoagulant response; increased risk of thromboembolic disorders

3 *Phenytoin:* Transient increase in hypoprothrombinemic response to warfarin with initiation of phenytoin therapy, followed within 1-2 wk by inhibition of hypoprothrombinemic response to warfarin

3 *Salicylates:* Increased risk of bleeding in anticoagulated patients; enhanced hypoprothrombinemic response to warfarin with large salicylate doses

Labs
• *Interference:* May cause orange-red discoloration of urine, which may interfere with some lab tests

SPECIAL CONSIDERATIONS
• Avoid use of initial doses >5 mg
• INR during 1st 5 days of therapy does not correlate with degree of anticoagulation

• Anticoagulant effect of warfarin may be reversed by administration of vitamin K or fresh frozen plasma; should only use in situations where INR is severely elevated >10, or when patient is actively bleeding

PATIENT/FAMILY EDUCATION
• Strict adherence to prescribed dosage schedule is necessary
• Avoid alcohol, salicylates, and drastic changes in dietary habits
• Do not change from one brand to another without consulting clinician

MONITORING PARAMETERS
• Dosage of anticoagulants must be individualized and adjusted according to INR determinations; it is recommended that INR determinations be performed prior to initiation of therapy, at 24-hr intervals while maintenance dosage is being established, then once or twice weekly for the following 3-4 wk, then at 1-4 wk intervals for the duration of treatment
• Maintain INR at 2-3 (2.5-3.5 for mechanical valves, recurrent systemic thromboembolism)

---

xylometazoline
(zye-loe-met-az′-oh-leen)
OTC: Otrivin, Natru-Vent
Chemical Class: Imidazoline derivative
Therapeutic Class: Decongestant

CLINICAL PHARMACOLOGY
Mechanism of Action: A sympathomimetic that directly acts on alpha-adrenergic receptors in arterioles of the nasal mucosa to produce vasoconstriction resulting in decreased blood flow. *Therapeutic Effect:* Decreased nasal congestion.

Pharmacokinetics
Onset of action occurs within 5-10 minutes for a duration of action of 5-6 hours. Well absorbed through nasal mucosa. May also be systemically absorbed from both nasal mucosa and gastrointestinal (GI) tract. **Half-life:** Unknown.

INDICATIONS AND DOSAGES
Rhinitis
Intranasal
Adults, Elderly, Children 12 yrs and older. 1- 3 drops (0.1%) in each nostril q8-10h or 1 to 2 sprays (0.1%) in each nostril q8-10h. Maximum: 3 doses/day.
Children 2- 12 yrs. 2 or 3 drops (0.05%) in each nostril q8-10h.

$ **AVAILABLE FORMS/COST**
• Sol, Drops—Nasal: 0.05%, 25 ml: **$5.38**; 0.1%, 25 ml: **$6.24**
• Sol, Spray—Nasal: 0.1%, 20 ml: **$4.88**

CONTRAINDICATIONS: Narrow-angle glaucoma, rhinitis sicca, children under 6 years, hypersensitivity to xylometazoline or other adrenergic agents

PREGNANCY AND LACTATION: Pregnancy category C

SIDE EFFECTS
Occasional
Nasal: Burning, stinging, drying nasal mucosa, sneezing, rebound congestion

SERIOUS REACTIONS
• Large doses may produce tachycardia, palpitations, lightheadedness, nausea, and vomiting.
• Overdosage in patients older than 60 years of age may produce hallucinations, CNS depression, and seizures.

SPECIAL CONSIDERATIONS
• Manage rebound congestion by stopping xylometazoline: one nostril at a time, substitute systemic decongestant, substitute inhaled steroid

PATIENT/FAMILY EDUCATION
• Do not use for >3-5 days or rebound congestion may occur

yohimbine
(yoe-him'been)
Rx: Actibine, Aphrodyne, Dayto-Himbin, Yocon, Yohimex
Chemical Class: Indolalkylamine derivative
Therapeutic Class: Anti-impotence agent

CLINICAL PHARMACOLOGY
Mechanism of Action: An herb that produces genital blood vessel dilation, improves nerve impulse transmission to genital area. Increases penile blood flow, central sympathetic excitation impulses to genital tissues. *Therapeutic Effect:* Improves sexual vigor, affects impotence.

Pharmacokinetics
Rapidly absorbed. Extensive metabolism in liver and kidneys. Minimal excretion in urine as unchanged drug. **Half-life:** 36 min.

INDICATIONS AND DOSAGES
Impotence
PO
Adults, Elderly. 5.4 mg 3 times/day.
Orthostatic hypotension
PO
Adults, Elderly. 12.5 mg/day.

$ **AVAILABLE FORMS/COST**
• Tab—Oral: 5 mg, 100's: **$27.50**; 5.4 mg, 100's: **$7.00-$64.39**

UNLABELED USES: Treatment of SSRI-induced sexual dysfunction, weight loss, sympathicolytic and mydriatic, aphrodisiac

CONTRAINDICATIONS: Renal disease, hypersensitivity to yohimbine or any component of the formulation

PREGNANCY AND LACTATION:
Do not use during pregnancy
SIDE EFFECTS
Excitement, tremors, insomnia, anxiety, hypertension, tachycardia, dizziness, headache, irritability, salivation, dilated pupils, nausea, vomiting, hypersensitivity reaction
SERIOUS REACTIONS
• Paralysis, severe hypotension, irregular heartbeats, and cardiac failure may occur. Overdose can be fatal.

---

zafirlukast
(za-feer'loo-kast)
Rx: Accolate
Chemical Class: Tolylsulfonyl benzamide derivative
Therapeutic Class: Antiasthmatic; leukotriene receptor antagonist

---

CLINICAL PHARMACOLOGY
Mechanism of Action: An antiasthmic that binds to leukotriene receptors, inhibiting bronchoconstriction due to sulfur dioxide, cold air, and specific antigens, such as grass, cat dander, and ragweed. *Therapeutic Effect:* Reduces airway edema and smooth muscle constriction; alters cellular activity associated with the inflammatory process.
Pharmacokinetics
Rapidly absorbed after PO administration (food reduces absorption). Protein binding: 99%. Extensively metabolized in the liver. Primarily excreted in feces. Unknown if removed by hemodialysis. **Half-life:** 10 hr.
INDICATIONS AND DOSAGES
Bronchial asthma
PO
Adults, Elderly, Children 12 yr and older. 20 mg twice a day.

Children 5–11 yr. 10 mg twice a day.
⬛ AVAILABLE FORMS/COST
• Tab—Oral: 10, 20 mg, 60's: **$76.91**
CONTRAINDICATIONS: None known.
PREGNANCY AND LACTATION:
Pregnancy category C; breast milk excretion unknown
SIDE EFFECTS
Frequent (13%)
Headache
Occasional (3%)
Nausea, diarrhea
Rare (less than 3%)
Generalized pain, asthenia, myalgia, fever, dyspepsia, vomiting, dizziness
SERIOUS REACTIONS
• Concurrent administration of inhaled corticosteroids increases the risk of upper respiratory tract infection.
INTERACTIONS
Drugs
⬛ *Astemizole, terfenadine:* Zafirlukast inhibits drug metabolism with potential for cardiac dysrhythmias
⬛ *Warfarin:* Zafirlukast increases hypoprothrombinemic effect
SPECIAL CONSIDERATIONS
PATIENT/FAMILY EDUCATION
• Take regularly, even during symptom-free periods
MONITORING PARAMETERS
• ALT, AST, CBC

zalcitabine (ddc)
(zal-site'a-been)
Rx: Hivid
Chemical Class: Nucleoside
analog
Therapeutic Class: Antiretroviral

CLINICAL PHARMACOLOGY
Mechanism of Action: A nucleoside reverse transcriptase inhibitor that inhibits viral DNA synthesis. *Therapeutic Effect:* Prevents replication of HIV-1.
Pharmacokinetics
Readily absorbed from the GI tract (absorption decreased by food). Protein binding: 4%. Undergoes phosphorylation intracellularly to the active metabolite. Primarily excreted in urine. Removed by hemodialysis. **Half-life:** 1-3 hr; metabolite, 2.6-10 hr (increased in impaired renal function).

INDICATIONS AND DOSAGES
HIV infection (in combination with other antiretrovirals)
PO
Adults, Children 13 yr and older. 0.75 mg q8h.
Children younger than 13 yr. 0.01 mg/kg q8h. Range: 0.005–0.01 mg/kg q8h.
Dosage in renal impairment
Dosage and frequency are modified based on creatinine clearance.

Creatinine Clearance	Dose
10-40 ml/min	0.75 mg q12h
less than 10 ml/min	0.75 mg q24h

S AVAILABLE FORMS/COST
• Tab—Oral: 0.375 mg, 100's: **$226.93**; 0.75 mg, 100's: **$284.43**
CONTRAINDICATIONS: Moderate or severe peripheral neuropathy
PREGNANCY AND LACTATION: Pregnancy category C

SIDE EFFECTS
Frequent (28%-11%)
Peripheral neuropathy, fever, fatigue, headache, rash
Occasional (10%-5%)
Diarrhea, abdominal pain, oral ulcers, cough, pruritus, myalgia, weight loss, nausea, vomiting
Rare (4%-1%)
Nasal discharge, dysphagia, depression, night sweats, confusion

SERIOUS REACTIONS
• Peripheral neuropathy (characterized by numbness, tingling, burning, and pain in the lower extremities) occurs in 17% to 31% of patients. These symptoms may be followed by sharp, shooting pain and progress to a severe, continuous, burning pain that may be irreversible if the drug is not discontinued in time.
• Pancreatitis, leukopenia, neutropenia, eosinophilia, and thrombocytopenia occur rarely.

SPECIAL CONSIDERATIONS
• Consult the most recent guidelines for HIV antiviral therapy prior to prescribing

MONITORING PARAMETERS
• Periodic CBC, serum chemistry tests, transaminase levels
• Serum amylase and triglyceride concentrations in patients with history of elevated amylase, pancreatitis, ethanol abuse, or receiving parenteral nutrition

zaleplon

(zal'e-plon)

Rx: Sonata

Chemical Class: Pyrazolopyrimidine derivative

Therapeutic Class: Sedative/hypnotic

CLINICAL PHARMACOLOGY

Mechanism of Action: A nonbenzodiazepine that enhances the action of the inhibitory neurotransmitter gamma-aminobutyric acid. *Therapeutic Effect:* Induces sleep.

INDICATIONS AND DOSAGES

Insomnia

PO

Adults. 10 mg at bedtime. Range: 5-20 mg.

Elderly. 5 mg at bedtime.

§   AVAILABLE FORMS/COST

• Cap—Oral: 5 mg, 100's: **$227.80**; 10 mg, 100's: **$280.19**

CONTRAINDICATIONS: Severe hepatic impairment

PREGNANCY AND LACTATION: Pregnancy category C; small amount excreted in breast milk, with highest excreted amount during a feeding 1 hr after zaleplon administration

SIDE EFFECTS

Expected

Somnolence, sedation, mild rebound insomnia (on first night after drug is discontinued)

Frequent (28%-7%)

Nausea, headache, myalgia, dizziness

Occasional (5%-3%)

Abdominal pain, asthenia, dyspepsia, eye pain, paresthesia

Rare (2%)

Tremors, amnesia, hyperacusis (acute sense of hearing), fever, dysmenorrhea

SERIOUS REACTIONS

• Zaleplon may produce altered concentration, behavior changes, and impaired memory.

• Taking the drug while up and about may result in adverse CNS effects, such as hallucinations, impaired coordination, dizziness, and light-headedness.

• Overdose results in somnolence, confusion, diminished reflexes, and coma.

INTERACTIONS

Drugs

❷ *Alcohol:* Additive CNS depression

❸ *Carbamazepine:* CYP3A4 inducer; may reduce efficacy of zaleplon by lowering AUC, C_{max}

❷ *Cimetidine:* Inhibits both CYP3A4 and aldehyde oxidase; concomitant administration increases zaleplon AUC and C_{max} 85%

❸ *Diphenhydramine:* Weak inhibitor of aldehyde oxidase; might reduce hepatic clearance of zaleplon; additive CNS depressant effects

❸ *Imipramine:* Additive effects on decreased alertness and psychomotor performance

❸ *Phenytoin:* CYP3A4 inducer; may reduce efficacy of zaleplon by lowering AUC, C_{max}

❸ *Phenobarbital:* CYP3A4 inducer; may reduce efficacy of zaleplon by lowering AUC, C_{max}

❸ *Rifampin:* Inducer of CYP3A4; reduced AUC, C_{max} of zaleplon 80% - may compromise efficacy

❸ *Thioridazine:* Additive effects on decreased alertness and psychomotor performance

Labs

• *Liver function tests:* Transaminases (ALT, AST), bilirubin increased

• *Cholesterol:* Increased

• *Uric acid:* Increased

Z

• *Glucose:* Increased or decreased

SPECIAL CONSIDERATIONS

• Because of the short $t_{\frac{1}{2}}$, agent best for problems with sleep latency, rather than duration of sleep or number of awakenings (e.g., shift workers)

• Abuse potential similar to benzodiazepines

• Advantage over triazolam, given big cost difference, difficult to justify, if used correctly

PATIENT/FAMILY EDUCATION

• *Timing of administration:* Immediately before bedtime or after the patient has gone to bed and has experienced difficulty falling asleep

• Do not take with alcohol or OTC cimetidine

MONITORING PARAMETERS

• Sleep latency, number of awakenings, daytime function (hangover effect), dizziness, confusion

---

zanamivir

(za-na′mi-veer)

Rx: Relenza
Chemical Class: Carboxylic acid ethyl ester
Therapeutic Class: Antiviral

CLINICAL PHARMACOLOGY

Mechanism of Action: An antiviral that appears to inhibit the influenza virus enzyme neuraminidase, which is essential for viral replication. *Therapeutic Effect:* Prevents viral release from infected cells.

INDICATIONS AND DOSAGES

Influenza virus

Inhalation

Adults, Elderly, Children 7 yr and older. 2 inhalations (one 5-mg blister per inhalation for a total dose of 10 mg) twice a day (approximately 12 hr apart) for 5 days.

Prevention of influenza virus

Inhalation

Adults, Elderly. 2 inhalations once a day for the duration of the exposure period.

Ⓢ AVAILABLE FORMS/COST

• Powder—INH: 5 mg, disk of 4 blisters, 5 disks: **$56.73**

CONTRAINDICATIONS: None known.

PREGNANCY AND LACTATION: Pregnancy category C; breast milk excretion unknown

SIDE EFFECTS

Occasional (3%-2%)

Diarrhea, sinusitis, nausea, bronchitis, cough, dizziness, headache

Rare (less than 1.5%)

Malaise, fatigue, fever, abdominal pain, myalgia, arthralgia, urticaria

SERIOUS REACTIONS

• Neutropenia may occur.

• Bronchospasm may occur in those with a history of COPD or bronchial asthma.

SPECIAL CONSIDERATIONS

• Off-label use to prevent influenza in family members of influenza patients (N Engl J Med 2000 Nov 2;343(18):1282-9): Attack rate reduced from 19% to 4%

PATIENT/FAMILY EDUCATION

• Expected benefit of zanamivir is one day of shortening of overall symptoms

• Patients with less severe symptoms get less benefit from therapy

• Influenza vaccine remains the best way to prevent influenza and use of zanamivir should not affect the evaluation of individuals for annual influenza vaccination

• Patients scheduled to use an inhaled bronchodilator at the same time as zanamivir should use their bronchodilator before taking zanamivir

• Two doses should be taken on the first day of treatment whenever possible provided there is at least 2 hours between doses

---

zidovudine
(zyde-o'vue-deen)
Rx: Retrovir
Combinations
Rx: with lamivudine (Combivir)
Chemical Class: Nucleoside analog
Therapeutic Class: Antiretroviral

CLINICAL PHARMACOLOGY
Mechanism of Action: A nucleoside reverse transcriptase inhibitor that interferes with viral RNA-dependent DNA polymerase, an enzyme necessary for viral HIV replication. *Therapeutic Effect:* Interferes with HIV replication, slowing the progression of HIV infection.
Pharmacokinetics
Rapidly and completely absorbed from the GI tract. Protein binding: 25%-38%. Undergoes first-pass metabolism in the liver. Crosses the blood-brain barrier and is widely distributed, including to CSF. Primarily excreted in urine. Minimal removal by hemodialysis. **Half-life:** 0.8-1.2 hr (increased in impaired renal function).

INDICATIONS AND DOSAGES
HIV infection
PO
Adults, Elderly, Children older than 12 yr. 200 mg q8h or 300 mg q12h.
Children 12 yr and younger. 160 mg/m^2/dose q8h. Range: 90-180 mg/m^2/dose q6-8h.
Neonates. 2 mg/kg/dose q6h.

IV
Adults, Elderly, Children older than 12 yr. 1-2 mg/kg/dose q4h.
Children 12 yr and younger. 120 mg/m^2/dose q6h.
Neonates. 1.5 mg/kg/dose q6h.

S **AVAILABLE FORMS/COST**
• Cap, Gel—Oral: 100 mg, 100's: **$205.15**
• Conc, Inj, w/Buffer—IV: 10 mg/ml, 20 ml: **$22.19**
• Syr—Oral: 50 mg/5 ml, 240 ml: **$49.24**
• Tab—Oral: 300 mg, 60's: **$369.27**
UNLABELED USES: Prophylaxis in health care workers at risk of acquiring HIV after occupational exposure
CONTRAINDICATIONS: Life-threatening allergic reactions to zidovudine or its components
PREGNANCY AND LACTATION: Pregnancy category C; indicated for pregnant women >14 wk gestation for prevention of maternal-fetus HIV transmission; excreted in breast milk; breast-feeding by HIV+ mothers not recommended

SIDE EFFECTS
Expected (46%-42%)
Nausea, headache
Frequent (20%-16%)
Abdominal pain, asthenia, rash, fever, acne
Occasional (12%-8%)
Diarrhea, anorexia, malaise, myalgia, somnolence
Rare (6%-5%)
Dizziness, paresthesia, vomiting, insomnia, dyspnea, altered taste
SERIOUS REACTIONS
• Serious reactions include anemia, which occurs most commonly after 4-6 weeks of therapy, and granulocytopenia; both effects are more likely to occur in patients who have a low Hgb level or granulocyte count before beginning therapy.

Z

• Neurotoxicity (as evidenced by ataxia, fatigue, lethargy, nystagmus, and seizures) may occur.

INTERACTIONS

Drugs

⚠ *Doxorubicin:* Antagonism of therapeutic effect; concomitant use should be avoided

▣ *Fluconazole:* Increased plasma concentrations of zidovudine

⚠ *Ganciclovir:* Increased hematologic toxicity

⚠ *Interferon-α:* Increased hematologic toxicity

▣ *Probenecid:* Increased plasma concentration of zidovudine

⚠ *Ribavirin:* Antagonism of therapeutic effect; concomitant use should be avoided

▣ *Rifampin:* Reduced plasma concentrations of zidovudine

⚠ *Stavudine:* Antagonism of therapeutic effect; concomitant use should be avoided

▣ *Valproic acid:* Increased plasma concentrations of zidovudine

SPECIAL CONSIDERATIONS

• Consult the most recent guidelines for HIV antiviral therapy prior to prescribing

PATIENT/FAMILY EDUCATION

• Close monitoring of blood counts is extremely important; does not reduce risk of transmitting HIV to others through sexual contact or blood contamination

MONITORING PARAMETERS

• CBC with differential and platelets q2wk initially for 2 mo, then q4-8 wk

---

zileuton

(zye-lew-ton)

Rx: Zyflo

Chemical Class: Urea derivative

Therapeutic Class: Antiasthmatic; lipoxygenase inhibitor

CLINICAL PHARMACOLOGY

Mechanism of Action: A leukotriene inhibitor that inhibits the enzyme responsible for producing inflammatory response. Prevents formation of leukotrienes (leukotrienes induce bronchoconstricton response, enhances vascular permeability, stimulates mucus secretion). *Therapeutic Effect:* Prevents airway edema, smooth muscle contraction, and the inflammatory process, relieving signs and symptoms of bronchial asthma.

Pharmacokinetics

Rapidly absorbed from gastrointestinal (GI) tract. Potein binding: 93%. Metabolized in liver. Primarily excreted in urine. Unknown if removed by hemodialysis. **Half-life:** 2.1-2.5 hrs.

INDICATIONS AND DOSAGES

Bronchial asthma

PO

Adults, Elderly, Children 12 yrs and older. 600 mg 4 times/day. Total daily dosage: 2400 mg.

$ AVAILABLE FORMS/COST

• Tab—Oral: 600 mg, 120's: **$106.40**

CONTRAINDICATIONS: Active liver disease, impaired liver function, hypersensitivity to zileuton or any component of the formulation

PREGNANCY AND LACTATION: Pregnancy category C; breast milk excretion unknown

SIDE EFFECTS
Frequent
Headache
Occasional
Dyspepsia, nausea, abdominal pain, asthenia (loss of strength), myalgia
Rare
Conjunctivitis, constipation, dizziness, flatulence, insomnia
SERIOUS REACTIONS
• Liver dysfunction occurs rarely and may be manifested as right upper quadrant pain, nausea, fatigue, lethargy, pruritus, jaundice or flulike symptoms.

SPECIAL CONSIDERATIONS
PATIENT/FAMILY EDUCATION
• Must be taken regularly, even during symptom free periods
• Not a bronchodilator, do not use to treat acute episodes of asthma
MONITORING PARAMETERS
• CBC, renal function, and transaminase levels periodically during 1st year of prolonged therapy

zinc oxide/zinc sulfate

Rx: *Injection:* Zinca-Pak
Rx: *Oral:* Galzin, Zincate
OTC: *Oral:* Orazinc 110, Orazinc 220, Verazinc, Zinc Sulfate 15, Zinc 15, Zinc 220; Ophthalmic: Eye-Sed
Chemical Class: Divalent cation
Therapeutic Class: Chelating agent; ophthalmic astringent; trace element

CLINICAL PHARMACOLOGY
Mechanism of Action: A mineral that acts as a co-factor for enzymes that are important for protein and carbohydrate metabolism. *Therapeutic Effect:* Zinc oxide acts as a mild astringent and skin protectant. Zinc sulfate helps maintain normal growth and tissue repair as well as skin hydration.
INDICATIONS AND DOSAGES
Mild skin irritations and abrasions (such as chapped skin, diaper rash)
Topical (oxide)
Adults, Elderly, Children. Apply as needed.
Treatment and prevention of zinc deficiency, wound healing.
PO (sulfate)
Adults, Elderly. 220 mg 3 times a day.
$ **AVAILABLE FORMS/COST**
Zinc Acetate
• Cap—Oral: 25 mg, 250's: **$155.00**; 50 mg, 250's: **$344.31**
Zinc Sulfate
• Cap, Gel—Oral: 220 mg, (50 mg zinc), 100's: **$5.82-$26.51**
• Sol, Inj—IV: 1 mg/ml, 10 ml: **$2.49**; 5 mg/ml, 5 ml: **$4.99**
• Sol—Ophth: 0.25%, 15 ml: **$3.24**
• Tab—Oral: 66 mg (15 mg zinc), 100's: **$1.45**
CONTRAINDICATIONS: None known.
PREGNANCY AND LACTATION: Pregnancy category A (in doses not exceeding recommended daily allowance); for zinc acetate, zinc has appeared in breast milk and zinc-induced copper deficiency may occur; nursing not recommended
SIDE EFFECTS
None known.
SERIOUS REACTIONS
• None known.
INTERACTIONS
Drugs
[3] *Ciprofloxacin, enoxacin, norfloxacin:* Reduced serum concentrations of these drugs
[3] *Tetracycline:* Reduced serum tetracycline concentrations

SPECIAL CONSIDERATIONS
• Acetate not recommended for initial therapy of symptomatic Wilson's disease (should be treated initially with chelating agents)

PATIENT/FAMILY EDUCATION
• Take acetate on an empty stomach

MONITORING PARAMETERS
• 24 hr urine copper, LFTs (acetate)

---

ziprasidone
(zye-pray'za-done)
Rx: Geodon
Chemical Class: Benzisothiazole derivative
Therapeutic Class: Antipsychotic

CLINICAL PHARMACOLOGY
Mechanism of Action: A piperazine derivative that antagonizes alpha-adrenergic, dopamine, histamine, and serotonin receptors; also inhibits reuptake of serotonin and norepinephrine. *Therapeutic Effect:* Diminishes symptoms of schizophrenia and depression.

Pharmacokinetics
Well absorbed after PO administration. Food increases bioavailability. Protein binding: 99%. Extensively metabolized in the liver. Not removed by hemodialysis. **Half-life:** 7 hr.

INDICATIONS AND DOSAGES
Schizophrenia
PO
Adults, Elderly. Initially, 20 mg twice a day with food. Titrate at intervals of no less than 2 days. Maximum: 80 mg twice a day.
IM
Adults, Elderly. 10 mg q2h or 20 mg q4h. Maximum: 40 mg/day.

Bipolar Mania
PO
Adults, Elderly. 40 mg 2 times/day.

ⓈAVAILABLE FORMS/COST
• Capsule—Oral: 20 mg, 40 mg, 60's; all: **$268.21**; 60 mg, 80 mg, 60's; all: **$292.09**
• Powder, Inj—IM: 20 mg vial: **$437.50**

CONTRAINDICATIONS: Conditions that prolong the QT interval, such as congenital long QT syndrome

PREGNANCY AND LACTATION: Pregnancy category C; animal, not human studies demonstrated developmental toxicity, including possible teratogenic effects at doses similar to human therapeutic doses; breast milk excretion - unknown

SIDE EFFECTS
Frequent (30%-16%)
Headache, somnolence, dizziness
Occasional
Rash, orthostatic hypotension, weight gain, restlessness, constipation, dyspepsia

SERIOUS REACTIONS
• Prolongation of QT interval may produce torsades de pointes, a form of ventricular tachycardia. Patients with bradycardia, hypokalemia, or hypomagnesemia are at increased risk.

INTERACTIONS
Drugs
⚠ *Antiarrhythmics (amiodarone, bretylium, disopyramide, dofetilide, encainide, flecainide, ibutilide, moricizine, procainamide, propafenone, quinidine, sotalol, tocainide):* Increased risk of QT prolongation and life-threatening arrhythmias
▣ *Carbamazepine:* Added carbamazepine (induces CYP3A4) decreased AUC 35%; other inducers predicted to produce similar effects: barbiturates, oxcarbazepine, phenytoin, rifampin
▣ *Ketoconazole:* Added ketoconazole (inhibits CYP3A4) results in increased AUC and C_{max} (35-40%);

other inhibitors predicted to produce similar effects: cisapride, clarithromycin, erythromycin, fluconazole, itraconazole (all azole antifungals), quinine

3 *Levodopa, dopamine agonists:* Ziprasidone may antagonize the therapeutic effects of these drugs

⚠ *Macrolide antibiotics (erythromycin, clarithromycin):* Increased risk of QT prolongation and life-threatening arrhythmias

⚠ *Phenothiazines:* Increased risk of QT prolongation and life-threatening arrhythmias

⚠ *Quinolone antibiotics (gatifloxacin, levofloxacin, moxifloxacin, sparfloxacin):* Increased risk of QT prolongation and life-threatening arrhythmias

⚠ *Tricyclic antidepressants:* Increased risk of QT prolongation and life-threatening arrhythmias

SPECIAL CONSIDERATIONS
• Atypical agents with less risk of movement disorders best for: Patients resistant to standard antipsychotic agents; patients with therapy-limiting extrapyramidal symptoms, other adverse effects; comparisons with other atypical agents, shorter half-life and bid dosing requirement potential disadvantage, but perhaps less weight gain

PATIENT/FAMILY EDUCATION
• Review presentation of cardiac (prolonged QT - torsades de pointes) and movement disorders; avoid electrolyte disturbance and drug interactions

MONITORING PARAMETERS
• Improvement of symptomatology (both positive and negative symptoms), complete blood counts, liver function tests, serum prolactin, routine chemistry (especially K^+, Mg^{++} during prolonged therapy); signs/symptoms of akathisia, abnormal movements, persistent constipation

---

zoledronic acid
(zole-eh-drone′ick)
Rx: Zometa
Chemical Class: Bisphosphonic acid
Therapeutic Class: Bisphosphonate; bone resorption inhibitor

CLINICAL PHARMACOLOGY
Mechanism of Action: A bisphosphonate that inhibits the resorption of mineralized bone and cartilage; inhibits increased osteoclastic activity and skeletal calcium release induced by stimulatory factors produced by tumors. *Therapeutic Effect:* Increases urinary calcium and phosphorus excretion; decreases serum calcium and phosphorus levels.

INDICATIONS AND DOSAGES
Hypercalcemia
IV infusion
Adults, Elderly. 4 mg IV infusion given over no less than 15 min. Retreatment may be considered, but at least 7 days should elapse to allow for full response to initial dose.

Multiple Myeloma
IV
Adults, Elderly. 4 mg q3-4wk.

◾ **AVAILABLE FORMS/COST**
• Sol, Inj—IV: 4 mg vial: **$999.39**

CONTRAINDICATIONS: Hypersensitivity to other bisphosphonates, including alendronate, etidronate, pamidronate, risedronate, and tiludronate

PREGNANCY AND LACTATION: Pregnancy category C (developmental and embryocidal effects noted in animals, no adequate and well controlled studies in pregnant women); information on excretion into human breast milk is not available

SIDE EFFECTS

Frequent (44%–26%)

Fever, nausea, vomiting, constipation

Occasional (15%–10%)

Hypotension, anxiety, insomnia, flu-like symptoms (fever, chills, bone pain, myalgia, and arthralgia), nausea, vomiting, constipation

Rare

Conjunctivitis

SERIOUS REACTIONS

• Renal toxicity may occur if IV infusion is administered in less than 15 minutes.

INTERACTIONS

Drugs

⬛ *Aminoglycosides:* Additive nephrotoxicity

⬛ *Diuretics (loop):* Additive hypocalcemia

SPECIAL CONSIDERATIONS

• Reconstitute with 5 ml sterile water, then further diluted in 100 ml 0.9% sodium chloride or 5% dextrose; do not mix with calcium-containing infusion solutions (i.e., lactated Ringer's)

• Most potent bisphosphonate available

MONITORING PARAMETERS

• Serum creatinine, electrolytes, phosphate, magnesium, CBC

zolmitriptan
(zohl-mih-trip′tan)
Rx: Zomig, Zomig ZMT
Chemical Class: Serotonin derivative
Therapeutic Class: Antimigraine agent

CLINICAL PHARMACOLOGY

Mechanism of Action: A serotonin receptor agonist that binds selectively to vascular receptors, producing a vasoconstrictive effect on cranial blood vessels. *Therapeutic Effect:* Relieves migraine headache.

Pharmacokinetics

Rapidly but incompletely absorbed after PO administration. Protein binding: 15%. Undergoes first-pass metabolism in the liver to active metabolite. Eliminated primarily in urine (60%) and, to a lesser extent, in feces (30%). **Half-life:** 3 hr.

INDICATIONS AND DOSAGES

Acute migraine attack

PO

Adults, Elderly, Children older than 18 yr. Initially, 2.5 mg or less. If headache returns, may repeat dose in 2 hr. Maximum: 10 mg/24 hr.

Intranasal

Adults, Elderly. 5 mg. May repeat in 2 hr. Maximum: 10 mg/24hr.

$ AVAILABLE FORMS/COST

• Spray-Nasal 1: 5 mg/spray, 6's: **$148.90**

• Tab, Film-Coated—Oral: 2.5 mg, 6's: **$97.96**; 5 mg, 3's: **$55.69**

• Tab, Disintigrating—Oral: 2.5 mg, 6's: **$97.96**; 5 mg, 3's: **$55.69**

CONTRAINDICATIONS: Arrhythmias associated with conduction disorders, basilar or hemiplegic migraine, coronary artery disease, ischemic heart disease (including angina pectoris, history of MI, silent ischemia, and Prinzmetal's angina), uncontrolled hypertension, use within 24 hr of ergotamine-containing preparations or another serotonin receptor agonist, use within 14 days of MAOIs, Wolff-Parkinson-White syndrome

PREGNANCY AND LACTATION: Pregnancy category C; excretion into breast milk unknown, use caution in nursing mothers

SIDE EFFECTS
Frequent (8%-6%)
Oral: Dizziness; tingling; neck, throat, or jaw pressure; somnolence
Nasal: Altered taste, paraesthesia
Occasional (5%-3%)
Oral: Warm or hot sensation, asthenia, chest pressure
Nasal: Nausea, somnolence, nasal discomfort, dizziness, asthenia, dry mouth
Rare (2%-1%)
Diaphoresis, myalgia, paresthesia

SERIOUS REACTIONS
• Cardiac reactions (including ischemia, coronary artery vasospasm, and MI) and noncardiac vasospasm-related reactions (such as hemorrhage and CVA) occur rarely, particularly in patients with hypertension, diabetes, or a strong family history of coronary artery disease; obese patients; smokers; males older than 40 years; and postmenopausal women.

INTERACTIONS
Drugs
🔳 *Cimetidine:* Increased zolmitriptan concentration
🔳 *Ergot-containing drugs:* Potential for prolonged vasospastic reactions and additive vasoconstrictions, theoretical precaution
❷ *MAO inhibitors:* Increased zolmitriptan concentrations, increased potential for serotonin-related toxicity
❷ *Sibutramine:* Increased risk for serotonin syndrome

SPECIAL CONSIDERATIONS
• Alternative to sumatriptan for the treatment of migraine headache; has not been compared head-to-head with sumatriptan; choice should be based on cost and availability
• First dose should be administered in medical office in case cardiac symptoms occur; take great care to exclude the possibility of silent cardiovascular disease prior to prescribing
• Doses >2.5 mg were not associated with more headache relief, but were associated with increased side effects; if no relief is obtained after first dose, a second dose is unlikely to provide any benefit

---

zolpidem
(zole-pi′dem)
Rx: Ambien
Chemical Class: Imidazopyridine derivative
Therapeutic Class: Hypnotic
DEA Class: Schedule IV

CLINICAL PHARMACOLOGY
Mechanism of Action: A nonbenzodiazepine that enhances the action of the inhibitory neurotransmitter gamma-aminobutyric acid. *Therapeutic Effect:* Induces sleep and improves sleep quality.
Pharmacokinetics

Route	Onset	Peak	Duration
PO	30 min	N/A	6-8hr

Rapidly absorbed from the GI tract. Protein binding: 92%. Metabolized in the liver; excreted in urine. Not removed by hemodialysis. **Half-life:** 1.4-4.5 hr (increased in hepatic impairment).

INDICATIONS AND DOSAGES
Insomnia
PO

Adults. 10 mg at bedtime.

Elderly, Debilitated. 5 mg at bedtime.

$ AVAILABLE FORMS/COST
• Tab—Oral: 5 mg, 100's: **$249.54**; 10 mg, 100's: **$306.94**

CONTRAINDICATIONS: None known.

PREGNANCY AND LACTATION: Pregnancy category B; excreted into breast milk in small amounts

SIDE EFFECTS
Occasional (7%)

Headache

Rare (less than 2%)

Dizziness, nausea, diarrhea, muscle pain

SERIOUS REACTIONS
• Overdose may produce severe ataxia, bradycardia, altered vision (such as diplopia), severe drowsiness, nausea and vomiting, difficulty breathing, and unconsciousness.

• Abrupt withdrawal of the drug after long-term use may produce asthenia, facial flushing, diaphoresis, vomiting, and tremor.

• Drug tolerance or dependence may occur with prolonged, high-dose therapy.

SPECIAL CONSIDERATIONS
PATIENT/FAMILY EDUCATION
• Take immediately prior to retiring
• Avoid alcohol
• Use caution driving or performing other tasks requiring alertness

zonisamide
(zoh-nis'a-mide)

Rx: Zonegran

Chemical Class: Sulfonamide derivative

Therapeutic Class: Anticonvulsant

CLINICAL PHARMACOLOGY
Mechanism of Action: A succinimide that may stabilize neuronal membranes and suppress neuronal hypersynchronization by blocking sodium and calcium channels. *Therapeutic Effect:* Reduces seizure activity.

Pharmacokinetics

Well absorbed after PO administration. Extensively bound to RBCs. Protein binding: 40%. Primarily excreted in urine. **Half-life:** 63 hr (plasma), 105 hr (RBCs).

INDICATIONS AND DOSAGES
Partial seizures
PO

Adults, Elderly, Children older than 16 yr. Initially, 100 mg/day for 2 wk. May increase by 100 mg/day at intervals of 2 wk or longer. Range: 100-600 mg/day.

$ AVAILABLE FORMS/COST
• Cap—Oral: 100 mg, 100's: **$230.03**

UNLABELED USES: Treatment of obesity, weight loss

CONTRAINDICATIONS: Allergy to sulfonamides

PREGNANCY AND LACTATION: Pregnancy category C (teratogenic, embryolethal in animals; no adequate and well-controlled studies in pregnant women; breast milk excretion in women unknown

SIDE EFFECTS

Frequent (17%-9%)

Somnolence, dizziness, anorexia, headache, agitation, irritability, nausea

Occasional (8%-5%)

Fatigue, ataxia, confusion, depression, impaired memory or concentration, insomnia, abdominal pain, diplopia, diarrhea, speech difficulty

Rare (4%-3%)

Paresthesia, nystagmus, anxiety, rash, dyspepsia, weight loss

SERIOUS REACTIONS

• Overdose is characterized by bradycardia, hypotension, respiratory depression, and coma.

• Leukopenia, anemia, and thrombocytopenia occur rarely.

INTERACTIONS

Drugs

3 *Carbamazepine:* Increased clearance of zonisamide via CYP3A4 induction ($t_{1/2}$ decreased to 38 hr); no appreciable effect on carbamazepine kinetics

3 *Phenytoin:* Increased clearance of zonisamide via CYP3A4 induction ($t_{1/2}$ decreased to 27 hr); no appreciable effect on phenytoin kinetics

3 *Phenobarbital:* Increased clearance of zonisamide via CYP3A4 induction ($t_{1/2}$ decreased to 38 hr)

3 *Valproic acid:* Increased clearance of zonisamide via CYP3A4 induction ($t_{1/2}$ decreased to 46 hr); no appreciable effect on valproate kinetics

Labs

• *Liver function tests (ALT/AST/LDH):* Increased

• *Glucose:* Decreased

• *Sodium:* Decreased

SPECIAL CONSIDERATIONS

• Due to long $t_{1/2}$, steady state achievable with stable dosing for 2 weeks

• Adjunctive therapy for wide variety of seizure disorders, especially those refractory to other drugs

PATIENT/FAMILY EDUCATION

• Low threshold for discussing signs and symptoms related to skin rash, liver problems, or blood problems with clinician

MONITORING PARAMETERS

• Frequency and severity of seizures, neurotoxicity, hypersensitivity reactions, serum creatinine, BUN

Z

Appendix A

Comparative Tables

The following comparative drug tables were developed by the authors to assist providers in choosing medications of a given therapeutic class. These tables allow clinicians to compare drugs on the basis of important pharmacologic or clinical characteristics. Whenever possible, the information is based on definitive drug data and should help the reader obtain maximal therapeutic effect with minimal adverse effects. When applicable, accepted clinical practice guidelines have been incorporated into the tables.

Tables:

Acid Secretion Inhibitors

Drug Name	Trade Name	Usual Adult Starting Oral Dose	Nonprescription Strength	Generic Formulation Available	Oral Liquid Available	Parenteral Formulation Available	Drug Interaction Potential	Dose Adjustment in Renal Dysfunction
H2 Blockers								
Cimetidine	Tagamet, Tagamet HB (OTC)	300 mg qid, 400 mg bid, or 800 mg hs	100 mg	Yes	Yes	Yes	++++	Yes (CrCl <30 ml/min)
Famotidine	Pepcid, Pepcid AC (OTC) Pepcid RPD Pepcid Complete (OTC)	20 mg bid or 40 mg hs	10 mg	Yes	Yes	Yes	+	Yes (CrCl <50 ml/min)
Nizatidine	Axid, Axid AR (OTC)	150 mg bid or 300 mg hs	75 mg	Yes	Yes	No	+	Yes (CrCl <50 ml/min)
Ranitidine	Zantac, Zantac 75 (OTC) Zantac EFFERdose Zantac GELdose	150 mg bid or 300 mg hs	75 mg	Yes	Yes	Yes	+	Yes (CrCl <50 ml/min)
Proton Pump Inhibitors								
Esomeprazole	Nexium	20 mg qday	NA	No	No	No	+++	No
Lansoprazole	Prevacid	15-30 mg qday	NA	No	Yes	Yes	+++	No
Omeprazole	Prilosec	20 mg qday	10 mg	Yes	Yes	No	+++	No
Pantoprazole	Protonix	40 mg qday	NA	No	No	Yes	++	No
Rabeprazole	Aciphex	20 mg qday	NA	No	No	No	++	No

Nonopioid Analgesics

Drug Name	Trade Name*	Usual Adult Dose	Maximum Adult Dose	Chemical Class	Comments
Acetaminophen*	Tylenol, Panadol, Tempra, Feverall	325-650 mg q4-6h, 10-15 mg/kg q4-6h (pediatric dose)	4000 mg/day, 2.6 g/day (maximum pediatric dose)	Para-aminophenol	Hepatotoxic in large doses, with alcohol or cirrhosis-limit dose to 2 g/day
Salicylates					
Acetylsalicylic acid (aspirin)*	Bayer, Empirin, Ecotrin, Bufferin, Ascriptin	325-975 mg q4h (3.6-5.4 g/day)	6000 mg/day	Salicylate	Antagonizes effect of probenecid; increases effect of sulfonylureas; reduces renal clearance of methotrexate
Choline magnesium trisalicylate*	Trilisate	See choline or magnesium salicylate		Combined salicylate	Less antiplatelet effects, fewer GI adverse effects
Choline salicylate	Arthropan	870 mg q3-4h	5.2 g/day	Salicylate	Fewer GI side effects than aspirin, less antiplatelet effects
Diflunisal*	Dolobid	1 g initially, then 500 mg bid-tid	1.5 g/day	Salicylate	Not metabolized to salicylate; increases acetaminophen level by 50% when coadministered
Magnesium salicylate*	Extra Strength Doan's, Magan, Mobidin	650 mg q4h or 1090 mg tid	3.6-4.8 g/day	Salicylate	Sodium-free salicylate derivative; fewer GI side effects than aspirin, less antiplatelet effects
Salsalate*	Disalcid, Salflex, Salsitab	1 g tid, 750 mg qid	3 g/day	Salicylate	Antagonizes effect of probenecid; increases effect of sulfonylureas; reduces renal clearance of methotrexate, less antiplatelet effects
Sodium salicylate*		325-650 mg q4h	4 g/day	Salicylate	Less effective than equal doses of aspirin; less antiplatelet effects
Sodium thiosalicylate*	Rexolate	100 mg qday-bid (intramuscular)	600 mg/day × 2 days (acute gout)	Salicylate	Intramuscular administration, less antiplatelet effects

*Generic products available.

Continued

Nonopioid Analgesics—cont'd

Drug Name	Trade Name*	Usual Adult Dose	Maximum Adult Dose	Chemical Class	Comment
Short-acting NSAIDs					
Diclofenac*[†]	Cataflam, Voltaren, Voltaren SR	25-75 mg bid-tid	200 mg/day	Acetic acid	Sustained-release formulation available as qday dose form; available combined with misoprostil
		125 mg bid			
Fenoprofen*[†]	Nalfon	300-600 mg tid-qid	3200 mg/day	Propionic acid	Highly protein bound (to albumin); greater renal toxicity
Ibuprofen*[†]	Advil, Menadol, Motrin, Motrin IB	300-800 mg tid/qid, 5-10 mg/kg (pediatric dose)	3200 mg/day	Propionic acid	Also approved for primary dysmenorrhea; available in combination with hydrocodone (Vicoprofen), with oxycodone (Combunox); standard NSAID
Indomethacin*	Indocin, Indocin SR	25-50 mg bid/tid, 75 mg bid	200 mg/day	Acetic acid	Available in suppository, suspension, and sustained-release forms; many off-label indications (e.g., ankylosing spondylitis, patent ductus arteriosis)
Ketoprofen*[†]	Orudis, Oruvail	25-75 mg tid-qid, 200 mg qday	300 mg/day	Propionic acid	
Ketorolac*[†]	Toradol	IM/IV: 30-60 mg initially, then 15-30 mg q6h	150 mg first day, then 120 mg/day	Pyrrolizine-carboxylic acid	Approved only for continuation of parenteral ketorolac, 5 days only; due to higher rates of GI toxicity
		PO: 10 mg q4-6h			30 mg equal to 6-12 mg morphine sulfate; 10 times more expensive; no respiratory depression but more GI and renal ADRs
Meclofenamate*[†]		50-100 mg tid/qid	400 mg/day	Fenamate	High rate of diarrhea (10%-33%), food delays rate and amount of absorption; lower incidence of hepatic toxicity
Mefenamic acid	Ponstel	500 mg, then 250 mg q6h ×7 days (max)	1 g/day	Fenamate	Primarily used for primary dysmenorrhea; less expensive alternatives

Drug	Brand	Dose	Max	Class	Comments
Tolmetin*	Tolectin, Tolectin DS	200-600 mg tid	1800 mg/day	Acetic acid	High rate of nausea (11%); solely renal excreted
Intermediate-acting NSAIDs					
Etodolac*†	Lodine	200 mg qid-500 mg bid	1200 mg/day	Pyranocarboxylic acid	Antacids reduce peak concentration by 20%; less GI bleeding
	Lodine XL	400-1000 mg/qday			
Flurbiprofen*	Ansaid	50-100 mg bid-tid	300 mg/day	Phenylalkanoic acid	May cause CNS stimulation; more GI irritation
Naproxen*	Naprosyn, EC-Naprosyn, Naprelan	250-500 mg q8-12h	1.25 g/day	Propionic acid	Approved for acute gout; may increase effect of protein-bound drugs such as phenytoin, sulfonylureas, and warfarin; available in qday dose form
Naproxen Sodium*†	Anaprox, Anaprox DS Aleve, EC-Naprosyn, Naprelan	275-550 mg q8-12h 750-1000 mg q12h	1.375 g/day	Propionic acid	Approved for acute gout; may increase effect of protein-bound drugs such as phenytoin, sulfonylureas, and warfarin; more rapidly absorbed than Naproxen
Sulindac*	Clinoril	150-200 mg q12h	400 mg/day	Acetic acid	Approved for acute gout; less renal toxicity; "renal sparing"
Long-acting NSAIDs					
Meloxicam	Mobic	7.5-15 mg qday	15 mg/day	Oxicam	15 mg IM effective; alternate parenteral NSAID
Nabumetone*	Relafen	500 mg-1g qday-bid	2 g/day	Naphyl-alkone	High rate of diarrhea (14%); metabolized to active agent; some COX-2 selectivity
Piroxicam*	Feldene	10-20 mg qday	20 mg/day	Oxicam	High rate of dyspepsia (20%); may increase effect of protein-bound drugs such as phenytoin, sulfonylureas, and warfarin
Oxaprozin*	Daypro, Daypro ALTA	600-1200 mg qday 678 mg 1-3 qday	1800 mg/day	Proprionic acid	High rate of dyspepsia (20%); may increase effect of protein-bound drugs such as phenytoin, sulfonylureas, and warfarin

*Generic products available.
†FDA approved for mild-moderate pain.

Nonopioid Analgesics—cont'd

Drug Name	Trade Name*	Usual Adult Dose	Maximum Adult Dose	Chemical Class	Comment
COX-2 selective NSAIDs					
Celecoxib[†]	Celebrex	100-200 mg bid	400 mg/day		Immediate duration; reduces risk of adenomatous colorectal polyps; caution in patients with cardiovascular disease risks
Valdecoxib	Bextra	10-20 mg qday-bid	20 mg/day		Immediate duration; higher dose for dysmenorrhea

*Generic products available.
[†]FDA approved for mild-moderate pain.

Opioid and Opioid-Like Analgesics

Drug Name	Trade Name*	Usual Adult Dose (mg) and Routes	Parenteral Dose (mg) Equal to 10 mg Morphine Sulfate IM	Oral Dose (mg) Equal to Listed Parenteral Dose	Comment
Opioid-like agents					
Buprenorphine*	Buprenex, Subutex, Suboxone	0.3-0.6 q6h IM/IV; 12-16 mg/day SL	0.3-0.6	0.4-0.8 (SL)	Mixed agonist-antagonist; SL preparation for use in treatment of opiate dependence Combined with naloxone
Butorphanol*	Stadol, Stadol NS	1-4 q3-4h IM, 1-2 q3-4h nasal; 0.5-2 q3-4 IV	2-3	NA	Mixed agonist-antagonist
Nalbuphine*	Nubain	10 q6h IM, IV, or SC	10-20	50-60	Mixed agonist-antagonist; not a controlled substance
Pentazocine*	Talacen, Talwin, TalwinNX, Talwin Compound	30-60 q3-4h IM; 50-100 q4h PO	60	180	Mixed narcotic agonist-antagonist T's & Blues: pentazocine, tripelennamine—drug abuse substitute for heroin; combinations available with aspirin, acetaminophen, naloxone
Tramadol*	Ultram	50-100 q4-6h PO	NA	NA	100 mg equianalgesic to 60 mg codeine; long-term use may cause dependence and withdrawal syndromes; toxicity includes seizures
Opioids					
Alfentanil	Alfenta	Total dose (IV) 8-245 mcg/kg (induction and maintenance)	0.4-0.8	NA	Primary use in anesthesia
Codeine*	Codeine	15-60 q4h PO	130	200	CSA Schedule II unless combined with acetaminophen or aspirin; used as cough suppressant in 10-15 mg doses (CSA Schedule V)
Fentanyl*	Sublimaze, Duragesic (transdermal), Actiq (transmucosal)	0.05-0.1 q1-2h IM or IV; 25-100 mcg/h transdermal (base dose on total morphine dose); 5-15 mcg/kg q6h transmucosal	0.1-0.2	Transdermal 25 mcg/hr	Primary use of IV/IM form is anesthesia or patient-controlled analgesia; transdermal and transmucosal forms available; costly; 25 mg transdermal equivalent to 45 mg/day sustained release morphine

*Generic products available.
CSA, Controlled Substances Act.

Continued

Opioid and Opioid-Like Analgesics—cont'd

Drug Name	Trade Name*	Usual Adult Dose (mg) and Routes	Parenteral Dose (mg) Equal to 10 mg Morphine Sulfate IM	Oral Dose (mg) Equal to Listed Parenteral Dose	Comment
Hydrocodone*	Vicodin, Vicoprofen Lortab	5-10 q4-6h PO	NA	30	Only available combined with acetaminophen, aspirin, ibuprofen, or decongestants
Hydromorphone*	Dilaudid	2 q4-6h PO; 1-2 q4-6h IM; 3 q6-8h PR	1.5-2	6-7.5	High abuse potential; slightly longer duration than morphine
Levomethadyl	Orlaam	20-40 q48-72h initially, then titrate	NA	NA	Proarrhythmic effects: use only for treatment of opiate-addicted patients with unacceptable response to other modalities
Levorphanol*	Levo-Dromoran	2 q6-8h PO	2-3	4	Long acting; $t_{1/2}$ 12-16 hr; accumulates on days 2-3
Meperidine*	Demerol	50-150 q3-4h IM; 50-150 q4h PO	75-100	300	May be used IV; metabolite normeperidine may accumulate with prolonged use causing excitation or seizures
Methadone*	Dolophine	5-10 q4-6h PO; 2.5-10 q3-4h IM, SC	10 (acute) 4 (chronic)	20 (acute) 4 (chronic)	Good potency; long $t_{1/2}$; different $t_{1/2}$ for analgesia and prevention of opiate withdrawal; accumulates with repeated dosing, requiring decreases in dose size and frequency on days 2-5
Morphine sulfate	Astramorph, Avinza, Duramorph, Kadian, MS Contin, MSIR, Oramorph SR, Roxanol	5-20 q4h IM; 10-30 q6h PR; 10 q4h SL; 10-30 mg q4h PO; 15-60 q12h PO-sustained release except Kadian (q24h)	10	30	Oral bioavailability poor; sublingual form useful for breakthrough pain; controlled-release forms not appropriate for PRN use

Oxycodone*	Percocet, Percodan, Tylox, OxyContin, Roxicodone	5-10 q4-6h PO; 10 q12h controlled release for opiate naive patient	NA	15-30	Often combined with aspirin (Percodan) or acetaminophen (Percocet, Tylox); available in long-acting form (OxyContin)
Oxymorphone	Numorphan	1-1.5 q4-6h IM; 5 q4-6h PR; 0.5 IV	1-1.5	10	Major use is perioperative
Propoxyphene	Darvon	32-100 q4h PO	NA	180-240	Less abuse potential than codeine at usual doses; no analgesic advantage over OTC analgesics
Remifentanil	Ultiva	0.05-2 mcg/kg/min IV infusion dose range	NA	NA	Primary use in anesthesia
Sufentanil	Sufenta	1-30 mcg/kg IV infusion (total dose)	0.01-0.04	NA	Primary use in anesthesia

*Generic products available.
CSA, Controlled Substances Act.

Cephalosporin Antibiotics

Drug Name (Generation in Parentheses)	Trade Name	Usual Adult Dose (g)	Adjust Dose for Renal Insufficiency	Comment
Oral				
Cefadroxil (1)	Duricef	0.5-1.0 q12-24h	Y	Cheapest in its therapeutic class
Cephalexin (1)	Keflex	0.25-0.5 q6h	Y	
Cephradine (1)	Velosef	0.5 q6h	Y	
Cefaclor (2)	Ceclor	0.25-0.5 q8h	N	
Cefpodoxime proxetil (2)	Vantin	0.1-0.4 q12h	Y	
Cefprozil (2)	Cefzil	0.25-0.5 q12h	Y	
Cefuroxime axetil (2)	Ceftin	0.25-0.5 q12h	Y	
Loracarbef (2)	Lorabid	0.2-0.4 q12h	Y	Carbacephem derivative rather than true cephalosporin
Ceftibuten (3)	Cedax	0.4 q24h	Y	
Cefdinir (3)	Omnicef	0.6 qday or 0.3 q12h	Y	
Cefditoren (3)	Spectracef	0.2-0.4 q12h	Y	
Parenteral (IV/IM)				
Cefazolin (1)	Ancef	1-2 q6-8h	Y	
Cefotetan (2)	Cefotan	1-2 q12h	Y	Covers GI anaerobes
Cefoxitin (2)	Mefoxin	1-2 q4-6h	Y	Covers GI anaerobes
Cefuroxime (2)	Zinacef, Ceftin	0.75-1.5 q8h	Y	Crosses blood-brain barrier

Cefepime (3)	Maxipime	0.5-2.0 q12h	Y	
Cefoperazone (3)	Cefobid	1-2 q8-12h	N	
Cefotaxime (3)	Claforan	1-2 q4-6h	Y	Crosses blood-brain barrier
Ceftazidime (3)	Fortaz	1-2 q6-8h	Y	
Ceftizoxime (3)	Cefizox	1-2 q6-8h	Y	Crosses blood-brain barrier
Ceftriaxone (3)	Rocephin	1-2 q12-24h	N	May be useful in outpatient therapy of endocarditis; single-dose (125 mg) therapy for gonococcal genital and pharyngeal infections; crosses blood-brain barrier

Macrolide Antibiotics

Drug Name	Trade Name	Usual Adult Dose (mg)	Comment
Azithromycin	Zithromax	500, followed by 250 q24h	Single dose therapy for chlamydial urethritis or cervicitis (1000 mg); antibacterial spectrum includes *Hemophilus influenzae*; indicated to prevent *Mycobacterium avium-intracellulare* infection (1200 mg qwk); available in parenteral form
Clarithromycin	Biaxin, Biaxin XL	250-500 q12h (Biaxin) or 500-1000 q24h (Biaxin XL)	Antibacterial spectrum includes *H. influenzae*; used to treat *Helicobacter pylori* and to prevent *Mycobacterium avium-intracellulare* infection; multiple drug interactions
Dirithromycin	Dynabac	500 q24h	Antibacterial spectrum same as erythromycin
Erythromycin	Erythromycin	250-500 q6-12h	Available as combination product with sulfisoxazole (extends spectrum to include Group A streptococci); coating does not decrease GI side effects; available in parenteral form; multiple drug interactions
Telithromycin	Ketek	800 q24h × 5-10 days	In community-acquired pneumonia covers multi-drug-resistant *S. pneumoniae*, *H. influenzae*, *M. catarrhalis*, *C. pneumoniae*, *M. pneumoniae*

Penicillin Antibiotics

Drug Name	Trade Name	Usual Adult Dose (g)	Comment
ORAL			
Penicillin V	Penicillin VK	0.25-0.5 q6h	
Broad Spectrum Penicillins			
Amoxicillin	Amoxil, Trimox	0.25-0.5 q8-12h	May take with meals
Amoxicillin-Potassium Clavulanate	Augmentin	One tablet (0.25 or 0.5 amoxicillin/0.125 clavulanate) q8h, or one tablet (0.875 amoxicillin/0.125 clavulanate) q12h	Spectrum extended to include beta-lactamase producers such as *Hemophilus influenza, Moraxella catarrhalis, Staphylococcus aureus* (except MRSA), and *Escherichia coli*
Ampicillin	Principen	0.5-1.0 q6h	Do not take with food
Penicillinase Resistant Penicillins			
Dicloxacillin Oxacillin Oral	Dynapen	0.25-0.5 q6h	Oral penicillin of choice for *S. aureus* (except MRSA)
PARENTERAL (IV)			
Penicillin G	Bicillin CR, Pfizerpen	1-3 million U q4-6h	Procaine and benzathine forms available for IM use
Broad Spectrum Penicillins			
Ampicillin	Principen	1-2 q4-6h	
Ampicillin-Sulbactam	Unasyn	1-2/0.5-1.0 q6h	Spectrum extended to include beta-lactamase producers such as *H. influenza, M. catarrhalis, S. aureus* (except MRSA), and *E. coli*

Continued

Penicillin Antibiotics—cont'd

Drug Name	Trade Name	Usual Adult Dose (g)	Comment
Carbenicillin	Geopen, Geocillin	4-5 q4-6h	Carbenicillin indanyl sodium available for oral use
Ticarcillin	Ticar	2-3 q4-6h	Spectrum extended to include beta-lactamase producers such as *S. aureus* (except MRSA), *E. coli, Klebsiella* spp., and *Bacteroides fragilis*
Ticarcillin-Potassium Clavulanate	Timentin	3.1 (3.0 ticarcillin, 0.1 potassium clavulanate) q4-6h	
Piperacillin	Pipracil	3-4 q4-6h	Spectrum includes enterococci, *Klebsiella, Enterobacter, Acinetobacter,* and *Serratia* spp.
Piperacillin-Tazobactam	Zosyn	3.375 (3.0 piperacillin, 0.375 tazobactam) q4-6h	Spectrum includes enterococci, *Klebsiella, Enterobacter, Acinetobacter,* and *Serratia* spp; extended to include beta-lactamase producers such as *S. aureus* (except MRSA) and *B. fragilis*
Penicillinase Resistant Penicillins			
Nafcillin	Unipen	0.5-2.0 q4-6h	Parenteral penicillin of choice for *S. aureus* (except MRSA)
Oxacillin		0.5-2.0 q4-6h	Parenteral penicillin of choice for *S. aureus* (except MRSA)

NOTE: MRSA = Methicillin resistant *S. aureus*.

Quinolone Antibiotics

Drug Name	Trade Name	Usual Adult Dose (mg)	Comment
Cinoxacin	Cinobac	PO: 250 q6h or 500 q12h	Approved only to treat UTIs; *Enterococcus*, *Staphylococcus*, and *Pseudomonas* spp. are resistant
Ciprofloxacin	Cipro	PO: 500-750 q12h (250 q12h for UTIs) IV: 200-400 q12h	Available for ophthalmic use; approved for *Campylobacter*, *Salmonella*, and *Shigella* infections; antibacterial spectrum includes *Mycobacterium avium-intracellulare*
Enoxacin	Penetrex	PO: 400 q12h	Approved only to treat UTIs
Gatifloxacin	Tequin	PO: 400 q24h IV: 400 q24h	Enhanced activity against gram-positive cocci and anaerobes including *Bacteroides fragilis*; no drug interaction with warfarin; useful in oral therapy of osteomyelitis
Gemifloxacin	Factive	PO: 320 q24h	Approved only to treat acute bacterial exacerbations of bronchitis and community-acquired pneumonia
Levofloxacin	Levaquin	PO: 250-750 q24h	Levo-form of ofloxacin; enhanced activity against gram-positive cocci and oral anaerobes; useful in oral therapy of osteomyelitis
Lomefloxacin	Maxaquin	PO: 400 q24h	Not effective for *Pseudomonas aeruginosa* infections outside of the urinary tract
Moxifloxacin	Avelox	PO: 400 q24h IV: 400 q24h	Enhanced activity against gram-positive cocci and anaerobes including *Bacteroides fragilis*; no drug interaction with warfarin
Norfloxacin	Noroxin	PO: 400 q12h	Available for ophthalmic use; approved only to treat UTIs and conjunctivitis
Ofloxacin	Floxin	PO: 200-400 q12h IV: 200-400 q12h	Available for ophthalmic and otic use
Trovafloxacin	Trovan	PO: 100-200 q24h	Restricted use; enhanced activity against gram-positive cocci and anaerobes including *Bacteroides fragilis*; no drug interaction with warfarin; rare reports of fatal hepatitis

Systemic Antifungal Antibiotics

Drug Name	Trade Name	Usual Adult Dose	Common Indications	Comment
Amphotericin B	Abelcet, AmBisome, Amphotec, Fungizone	IV: 0.4-0.6 mg/kg/d for 8-10 wk (nonlipid form only)	Histoplasmosis, blastomycosis, candidiasis, cryptococcosis, coccidioidomycosis, aspergillosis, mucormycosis	Used topically in bladder; causes multiple electrolyte abnormalities; give 1 mg test dose prior to giving full dose; three lipid-complexed forms available with different doses but lower nephrotoxicity and improved outcome in some trials
Caspofungin	Cancidas	IV: 70 mg loading dose, then 50 mg qday	Aspergillosis	Minimal nephrotoxicity; $360/50 mg dose
Fluconazole	Diflucan	PO or IV: 100-400 qday	Blastomycosis, histoplasmosis, candidiasis, coccidioidomycosis	Increases serum rifabutin levels and toxicity; increases effect of cyclosporine, terfenadine, astemizole, warfarin, sulfonylureas, and others; single dose oral treatment for vaginal infection
Flucytosine	Ancobon	PO: 12.5-37.5 mg/kg q6h	Cryptococcosis, candidiasis, chromoblastomycosis	Usually used in combination with amphotericin B
Griseofulvin	Fulvicin, Gris-PEG	PO: 500 mg qday-bid (microcrystalline) PO: 330 mg qday-bid (ultra microcrystalline)	Dermatophytes	Cytochrome P450 inducer; absorption enhanced when taken with fatty foods
Itraconazole	Sporanox	PO: 100-200 mg qday-bid	Onychomycosis, blastomycosis, histoplasmosis, candidiasis, coccidioidomycosis, sporotrichosis, cryptococcosis, aspergillosis	Cytochrome P450 3A inhibitor—affects cyclosporine, warfarin, sulfonylureas, and others; tablet and solution forms not interchangeable
Ketoconazole	Nizoral	PO: 200-400 mg qday-bid	Blastomycosis, histoplasmosis, candidiasis, coccidioidomycosis, dermatophytes	Cytochrome P450 3A inhibitor—affects cyclosporine, warfarin, sulfonylureas, and others; requires acid pH for absorption; reduces testosterone synthesis
Terbinafine	Lamisil	PO: 250 mg qday	Onychomycosis	Hepatic clearance increased by rifampin, decreased by cimetidine
Voriconazole	Viread	IV: 6 mg/kg q12h × 2 doses, then 4 mg/kg q12h PO: ≥40 kg: 400 mg q12h × 2 doses, then 200 mg q12h; <40 kg: 200 mg q12h × 2 doses, then 100 mg q12h	Aspergillosis, candidiasis (resistant)	Transient visual disturbances in 30% of patients

Selective Serotonin Reuptake Inhibitor (SSRI) Antidepressants

Drug Name	Brand Name	Usual Adult Dose (mg/d)	Drug and Active Metabolite ($t_{1/2}$ [hr])	Serotonin Reuptake Inhibiton	Anticholinergic Effect	Drowsiness	Degree of Cytochrome P450 System Inhibition	Comment
Citalopram	Celexa	20-40	33-37	4+	1+	0	0	Dose up to 60 mg/d occasionally needed
Escitalopram	Lexapro	10-20	27-32	4+	1+	0	0	Pharmacologically active S-enantiomer of citalopram; no advantage over citalopram
Fluoxetine*	Prozac Sarafem Prozac Weekly	20-60 (starting dose 10 in elderly)	24-72 (acute); 96-144 (chronic); (norfluoxetine: 96-384)	4+	0-1+	0	3+ (2D6)	Up to 60 mg/d for obsessive-compulsive disorder; generics available
Fluvoxamine*	Luvox	50-300	15-26 (no active metabolite)	4+	0	0	2+	Indicated only for obsessive-compulsive disorder; generics available
Paroxetine*	Paxil Paxil CR	20-60 (starting dose 10 in elderly) 25-62.5 (CR)	21 (no active metabolite)	4+	2	1+	2+ (2D6)	May cause weight gain; overall more side effects
Sertraline	Zoloft	75-200 (starting dose 12.5-25 in elderly)	26 (desmethylsertraline: 62-104)	4+	0-1+	0-1+	1+ (2D6)	Metabolite weakly active

*Generics available.

APPENDIX A

Tricyclic and Tetracyclic Antidepressants

Drug Name	Brand Name	Usual Adult Dose (mg) for Acute Therapy (Maintenance Dose is ½-⅔ of this; lower doses recommended for elderly persons)	Relative Sedation	Relative Anticholinergic Effect	Relative Delay of Cardiac Conduction	Relative Postural Hypotension	Comment
Tricyclic							
Amitriptyline	Elavil	75-300	3+	4+	3+	4+	Used for chronic pain
Amoxapine	Asendin	200-400	2+	1+	1+	3+	Metabolite has neuroleptic side effect
Clomipramine	Anafranil	25-250	3+	3+	2+	4+	Primary use is for obsessive-compulsive disorder; may lower seizure threshold; may increase free plasma concentration of protein bound drugs (e.g., digoxin, warfarin)
Desipramine	Norpramin	75-300	1+	2+	3+	2+	Used for chronic pain; metabolite of imipramine
Doxepin	Sinequan	75-3004	4+	3+	1+	4+	Potent antihistamine
Imipramine	Tofranil Tofronil-PM	50-300	2+	3+	3+	3+	Used for chronic pain, panic disorder, urinary incontinence, and headache
Nortriptyline	Pamelor Aventyl	50-1502	1+	2+	2+	3+	Used for chronic pain, panic disorder, and headache; metabolite of amitriptyline

Protriptyline	Vivactil	15-60	2+	4+	2+	2+	2+	
Trimipramine	Surmontil	50-300	4+	3+	3+	3+	4+	
Tetracyclic								
Maprotiline		75-300	3+	1+	1+	1+	3+	May lower seizure threshold; brand name no longer available
Mirtazapine	Remeron Remeron Soltab	15-45	3+	2+	2+	0-1+	2+	Rarely associated with agranulocytosis; do not use with MAOIs
Heterocyclic								
Nefazodone	Serzone	200-600	+/-	1+	1+	0+	2+	Divided doses on bid schedule; do not administer with astemizole, cisapride, lovastatin, or simvastatin; may increase free plasma concentration of protein bound drugs (e.g., digoxin, warfarin); cytochrome 3A4 inhibitor; rarely associated with hepatic failure
Trazodone	Desyrel	150-600	2+	0+	0+	0+	4+	Risk of priapism in males and similar phenomenon in females; may increase free plasma concentration of protein bound drugs (e.g., digoxin, warfarin); should be given in divided doses

Miscellaneous Antidepressants, Including Foods that Interact with MAOIs

Drug Name	Brand Name	Usual Adult Dose (mg/d)	Anticholinergic Effect	Drowsiness	Orthostatic Hypotension	Cardiac Dysrhythmias	Comment
Bupropion	Wellbutrin, Wellbutrin SR, Wellbutrin XL, Zyban	225-450	0	+/-	+/-	1+	Single dose of immediate release product should not exceed 150 mg; inhibits dopamine reuptake; given bid or tid; FDA-approved as an aid to smoking cessation
Duloxetine	Cymbalta	20-60	0	0	0	0	Inhibits serotonin and norepinephrine reuptake; approved for management of diabetic peripheral neuropathy; may increase blood pressure
Venlafaxine	Effexor, Effexor XR	75-375	0	0	0	4+	Inhibits serotonin and norepinephrine reuptake; given bid or tid or as long-acting form; associated with elevated blood pressure
Monoamine oxidase inhibitors (MAOIs)							Avoid foods rich in amines (see below) and selected medications while taking MAOI and for 14 days after last dose
Isocarboxazid	Marplan	10-30	1+	1+	2+	1+	May be given as single daily dose
Phenelzine	Nardil	15-90	1+	1+	2+	1+	Given in divided doses
Tranylcypromine	Parnate	30-60	1+	1+	1+	1+	Given in divided doses

Avoid the following foods if taking MAOIs (contain tyramine and other amines, often as a result of aging or fermenting): broad beans; red wines; yeast extracts; beer with yeast; chicken or beef liver; caviar, anchovies, and pickled herring; fermented sausages (bologna, pepperoni, salami, and summer sausage); and aged cheeses (Boursault, Brie, Camembert, cheddar, Emmenthaler, Gruyere, mozzarella, parmesan, romano, Roquefort, and Stilton).

Systemic Antihistamines

Drug Name	Trade Name	Usual Adult Dose	Sedative Effects	Comment
First-Generation Agents				
Brompheniramine	BröveX, BröveX CT	12-24 mg q12h	+	Also available as an oral solution and in combination with decongestants
Carbinoxamine	Histex CT, Pediatex, Histex PD	8 mg q12h	++	Available as liquid and as time-release tablets
Chlorpheniramine	Aller-Chlor, Chlo-Amine, Chlor-Trimeton, Efidac 24	4 mg q4-6h	+	Also available as syrup, extended release tablets, and in combination with decongestants
Clemastine	Tavist, Dayhist-1	1 mg q12h	++	Also available as syrup and in combination with decongestants
Cyproheptadine	None	4 mg q8h	+	Also available as syrup
Dexchlorpheniramine	None	4-6 mg q6-8h	+	Active dextro-isomer of chlorpheniramine
Diphenhydramine	AllerMax, Banophen, Benadryl, Diphen AF, Dephenhist, Genahist, Tusstat	25-50 mg q6-8h	+++	Also available as syrup, liquid, solution, elixir, injection, and in combination with decongestants
Hydroxyzine	Atarax, Vistaril	25-100 mg q4-8h	+++	Also available as syrup; often used as antipruritic, sedative, and antiemetic
Phenindamine	Nolahist	25 mg q4-6h	+/-	Less sedating OTC alternative
Triprolidine	Zymine	2.5 mg q4-6h	+	Also available in combination with decongestant (Actifed); available as liquid

CT, chewable tablet.

Continued

Systemic Antihistamines—cont'd

Drug Name	Trade Name	Usual Adult Dose	Sedative Effects	Comment
Second-Generation Agents				
Azelastine	Astelin	0.5 mg q12h	+/–	Nasal spray
Cetirizine	Zyrtec	5-10 mg qday	+/–	Also available as syrup
Desloratidine	Clarinex, Clarinex RediTabs	5 mg qdh	+/–	Active metabolite of loratidine; RediTabs may be administered without water
Fexofenadine	Allegra	60 mg q12h	+/–	Active metabolite of terfenadine
Loratadine	Alavert, Claritin, Claritin RediTabs, Tavist ND	10 mg qday	+/–	Also available as syrup and rapidly disintegrating tablet (RediTabs); OTC
Miscellaneous Agents				
Doxepin	Sinequan, Zonalon	10-50 mg q8-24h	+++	Sedating tricyclic antidepressant; antipruritic; available as topical cream (Zonalon)
Promethazine	Phenergan	12.5 mg q6-8	++	Phenothiazine derivative; well tolerated by children; available as syrup, suppositories, and injection

Systemic Corticosteroids

Drug Name	Trade Name	Oral or Parenteral Dose for Equivalent Glucocorticoid Effect (mg)*	Relative Mineralocorticoid Effect	Biologic Half-life (hrs)†
Betamethasone	Celestone	0.75	0	36-54
Cortisone	Cortone	25	1	8-12
Dexamethasone††	Decadron, Hexadrol	0.75	0	36-54
Hydrocortisone	Cortef, Solu-Cortef	20	1	8-12
Methylprednisolone	Medrol, Solu-Medrol	4	0	18-36
Prednisolone	Predalone, Prelone	5	0.5	18-36
Prednisone	Deltasone, Orasone	5	0.5	18-36
Triamcinolone	Aristocort, Kenalog	4	0	18-36

*Not all preparations are suitable for IV injection.

†Because chemical half-life of all agents is 0.5-4.0 hrs, endogenous cortisol level can be measured 24 hrs after last corticosteroid dose (*JAMA* 1999; 282:671-676).

††Dexamethasone is only corticosteroid that does not cross-react with cortisol assay.

Inhaled Antiinflammatory Drugs

Drug Name	Trade Name	Dose per Activation	Usual Adult Dose	Maximum Adult Daily Dose (# of activations)
Respiratory Corticosteroids				
Beclomethasone	QVAR	40, 80 mcg	40-80 mcg bid	640 mcg (8-16)
Budesonide	Pulmicort Turbohaler	200 mcg	200-800 mcg bid	1,600 mcg (8)
	Pulmicort Respules	0.25-0.5 mg/2 ml	0.5 mg/day qday or divided bid	1 mg
Flunisolide	AeroBid, AeroBid-M	250 mcg	500 mcg bid	2,000 mcg (8)
Fluticasone	Flovent	44, 110, 220 mcg	88-220 mcg bid	880 mcg (4-20)
	Flovent Discus (powder), Flovent Rotadisk (powder), Advair Diskus (combined with salmeterol)	50, 100, 250 mcg	100-250 mcg bid	1000 mcg
Triamcinolone	Azmacort	100 mcg	200 mcg tid-qid or 400 mcg bid	1600 mcg (16)
Intranasal Corticosteroids				
Beclomethasone	Beconase AQ (solution with metering pump)	42 mcg	42 mcg each nostril bid-qid	336 mcg (8)
Budesonide	Rhinocort Aqua (solution with metering pump)	32 mcg	64 mcg each nostril bid	256 mcg (8)

Flunisolide	Nasalide (solution); Nasarel (solution with metering pump)	25 mcg	50 mcg each nostril bid	400 mcg (16)
Fluticasone	Flonase	50 mcg	100 mcg each nostril bid	200 mcg (4)
Mometasone	Nasonex	50 mcg	100 mcg each nostril qday	200 mcg (4)
Triamcinolone	Nasacort AQ (solution with metering pump)	55 mcg	110 mcg each nostril qday	440 mcg (8)
Noncorticosteroids				
Azelastine (intranasal)	Astelin	137 mcg	274 mcg each nostril BID; 137 mcg BID age 5-11 yr	1096 mcg (8)
Cromolyn (inhaled)	Intal	800 mcg	1600 mcg qid	6400 mcg (8)
Cromolyn (intranasal)	Nasalcrom	5.2 mg	5.2 mg each nostril q3-6 hours	62.4 mg (12)
Nedocromil (inhaled)	Tilade	1.75 mg	3.5 mg bid-qid	14 mg (8)

APPENDIX A

Inhaled Bronchodilators

Drug Name	Trade Name	Dose per Activation	Usual Adult Dose
Albuterol	Proventil, Proventil HFA, Ventolin, Ventolin HFA, Combivent (with ipratropium) Accuneb, Proventil	90 mcg	1-2 inhalations q 4-6h
		0.083%-0.5%*	2.5 mg tid-qid via nebulizer
Bitolterol	Tornalate	2 mg/ml*	2.5 mg tid-qid via nebulizer
Epinephrine	OTC: Primatene Mist	220 mcg	1-2 inhalations q 3-4 h (max 12 per day)
Formoterol	Foradil	12 mcg†	12 mcg q12h
Ipratropium	Atrovent, Combivent (with albuterol) Duoneb (with albuterol)	18 mcg 0.5/3 mg/3 ml*	2 inhalations q 4-6 h (max 12 per day) 3 ml qid via nebulizer
Levalbuterol	Xopenex	0.3-1.25 mg/3 ml*	0.63-1.25 mg tid via nebulizer
Metaproterenol	Alupent	650 mcg	2-3 inhalations q 3-4 h (max 12 per day)
Pirbuterol	Maxair	200 mcg	1-2 inhalations q 4-6 h (max 12 per day)
Salmeterol	Serevent Diskus, Advair Diskus (with fluticosone)	50 mg†	50 mcg q12h

*Solution for inhalation via nebulizer.
†Inhalation powder.

Noncontraceptive Estrogens

Drug Name	Trade Name	Available Strengths	Usual Adult Dose	Comment
Systemic				
Conjugated estrogens, oral	Premarin	0.3 mg, 0.45 mg, 0.625 mg, 0.9 mg, 1.25 mg	0.3-1.25 mg qday	Available in IV form; available in combination with medroxyprogesterone acetate (Prempro: 0.3 mg/1.5 mg, 0.45 mg/1.5 mg, 0.625 mg/2.5 mg, 0.625 mg/5 mg; Premphase: 0.625 mg and 0.625 mg/5 mg)
Conjugated estrogens, oral (synthetic)	Cenestin	0.3 mg, 0.625 mg, 0.9 mg, 1.25 mg		
Conjugated estrogens, oral (synthetic)	Enjuvia	0.625 mg, 1.25 mg		
Conjugated estrogens, parenteral	Premarin IV	25 mg/vial	25 mg IM/IV	
Esterified estrogens	Menest	0.3 mg, 0.625 mg, 1.25 mg, 2.5 mg	0.625-1.25 mg qday	Contains 80% sodium estrone sulfate; available in combination with methyltestosterone (Estratest, Syntest) 0.625 mg/1.25 mg, 1.25 mg/2.5 mg
Estradiol cypionate in oil	Depo-Estradiol	5 mg/ml	1-5 mg IM q3-4 wk	Oil suspension gives long action
Estradiol oral	Estrace	0.5 mg, 1 mg, 1.5 mg, 2 mg	0.5-2 mg qday	Dose for bone loss prevention 0.5 mg/day
Estradiol transdermal systems	Vivelle, Climara, Estraderm, Alora, Esclim, Vivelle-Dot	0.014 mg/24 hr 0.025 mg/24 hr 0.0375 mg/24 hr 0.05 mg/24 hr 0.06 mg/24 hr 0.075 mg/24 hr 0.1 mg/24 hr	0.025-0.1 mg/24 hr	Estraderm and Vivelle applied twice weekly; Climara applied weekly; dose for bone loss prevention 0.05 mg qday
Estradiol valerate in oil	Delestrogen	10 mg/ml; 20 mg/ml; 40 mg/ml	10-20 mg q 4 weeks	Oil suspension gives long action

Continued

Noncontraceptive Estrogens—cont'd

Drug Name	Trade Name	Available Strengths	Usual Adult Dose	Comment
Estropipate	Ortho-Est, Ogen	0.75 mg, 1.5 mg, 3 mg, 6 mg	0.75-1.5 mg qday	0.75 mg estropipate equivalent to 0.625 mg conjugated estrogens; dose for bone loss prevention 0.75 mg qday
Topical				
Conjugated estrogens	Premarin	0.625 mg conjugated estrogens per g	0.5-2 g cream qday	
Estradiol	Estrace	0.1 mg estradiol per g	2-4 g cream qday	
Estradiol	Estring	2 mg estradiol per ring	Insert vaginal ring and leave in place for 90 days	Low systemic estradiol exposure
Estradiol	Femring	0.05 mg/day, 0.1 mg/day		Releases 0.05-0.1 mg/day for 3 months
Estradiol	Estrogel	0.06% estradiol	½ applicator (tube) or single pump qday	Available in tubes and pumps; applied to one arm
Ethinyl estradiol/norethindrone (combination)	Femhrt	5 mcg ethinyl estradiol/1 mg norethindrone	1 tablet daily	
Estradiol/norgestimate (combination)	Prefest	1 mg estradiol (pink) 1 mg estradiol/0.9 mg norgestimate (white)	1 pink tablet qday × 3, then 1 white tablet qday × 3 continuously	In cards of 30, 15 of each tablet
Estradiol/norethindrone	CombiPatch	0.5 mg estradiol/0.14 mg norethindrone 0.5 mg estradiol/0.25 mg norethindrone	Replace patch twice weekly	
Estradiol topical emulsion	Estrasorb	1.74 g/pouch	3.48 g qday	Contents of pouch applied to each leg, rubbed in for 3 minutes until absorbed; used for systemic symptoms
Estropipate	Ogen Vaginal	1.5 mg/g		

Oral Hypoglycemic Agents

Drug	Trade Name	Dosage Range	Cost	Comments
Sulfonylureas* **First Generation**				
Chlorpropamide	Diabinese	100-500 mg/day (max 750 mg/day)	$0.13-0.98/250 mg tablet	Active metabolite—caution in elderly; ↓ renal function; 24-72 hr duration of effect; disulfiram reactions, hyponatremia
Tolazamide	Tolinase	250-500 mg qday (max 500 mg bid)	$0.16-1.13/250 mg tablet	Active metabolite—caution in elderly; ↓ renal function; 12-24 hr duration of effect
Tolbutamide	Orinase	250-3000 mg/day (divide doses bid)	$0.04-0.28/500 mg tablet	Negligible metabolites; OK with ↓ renal function; 6-12 hr duration of effect
Sulfonylureas* **Second Generation**				
Glimepiride	Amaryl	1-4 mg qday (max 8 mg/day)	$1.12/4 mg tablet	Minimal added effect > 4 mg/day
Glipizide	Glucotrol	2.5-20 mg qday (max 40 mg/day); divide doses > 10 mg qday (e.g., 10 mg BID)	$0.18-0.86/10 mg tablet	Minimal added effect > 20 mg/day; inactive metabolite; 24 hr duration of effect
	Glucotrol-XL	5-10 mg qday (max 20 mg/day)	$0.81/10 mg tablet	Extended-release product of long-acting drug (?)
Glyburide, micronized	Glynase	0.75-12 mg qday (max 12 mg/day)	$0.60-0.98/3 mg tablet	
Glyburide	DiaBeta, Micronase	1.25-10 mg qday (max 20 mg/day)	$0.25-1.10/5 mg tablet	Minimal added effect > 10 mg/day; active metabolite with duration longer than parent
Meglitinides[†]				
Nateglinide	Starlix	60-120 mg tid, ac	$1.09/60 mg tablet	Multiple doses per day

*Mechanism: stimulate pancreatic insulin secretion (i.e., secretagogues).
[†]Mechanism: quick acting secretagogues.

Continued

Oral Hypoglycemic Agents—cont'd

Drug	Trade name	Dosage range	Cost	Comments
Meglitinides—cont'd				
Repaglinide	Prandin	0.5-4 mg tid ac (max 16 mg/day)	$1.09/2 mg tablet	Multiple doses per day
Biguanides‡				
Metformin	Glucophage	250-1000 mg bid; (max 2550 mg/day)	$0.58-1.67/1000 mg tablet	Excreted unchanged in urine; avoid in low clearance states (e.g., decreased renal function, CHF) because predisposed to lactic acidosis; caution in pre-radiological studies requiring contrast material; minimal added effect >2000 mg/day
	Glucophage XR		$0.74-0.83/500 mg tablet	
with Glipizide	Metaglip		$1.07/500 mg-5 mg tablet	
with Glyburide	Glucovance		$1.07/500 mg-5 mg tablet	
Thiazolidinediones¶				
Pioglitazone	Actos	15-30 mg qday (max 45 mg/day)	$5.54/30 mg tablet	Caution: weight gain, fluid retention, CHF
Rosiglitazone	Avandia	4-8 mg qday (max 8 mg/day)	$5.34/8 mg tablet	Caution: weight gain, fluid retention, CHF
with metformin	Avandamet		$2.75/4 mg-500 mg tablet	
α-Glucosidase Inhibitors§				
Acarbose	Precose	50-100 mg tid ac (max 100 mg tid)	$0.73/50 mg tablet	GI adverse effects expectedly
Miglitol	Glyset	50-100 mg tid ac (max 100 mg tid)	$0.75/50 mg tablet	GI adverse effects expectedly

‡Mechanism: decrease hepatic glucose production and increase insulin sensitivity.
¶Activate peroxisome proliferative-activated receptors, "insulin sensitizer."
§Inhibit starch breakdown, attenuate postprandial hyperglycemia.

Insulins

Preparation	Onset (hr)	Peak Effect (hr)	Duration (hr)	Mixing Compatibility	Availability
Rapid-Acting Insulins					
Regular	0.5	2-4	6-8	All	V, PF, PEN
Semilente	1-1.5	5-10	12-16	Lente	V
Lispro	0.25	0.5-1.5	3.4-4.5	Ultralente, NPH	V, PEN, DISP
Aspart	0.25	1-3	3-5	NPH (if injected immediately after mixing)	PEN
Glulisine	0.3	0.6	5	NPH	V
Intermediate-Acting Insulins					
Zinc (Lente)	1-3	6-12	18-24	Regular, semilente	V
Isophane (NPH)	1-1.5	6-12	18-24	Regular	V, PF, PEN
Long-Acting Insulins					
Glargine	1.1	5 (no pronounced peak)	24	None	V
Protamine zinc (PZI)	4-8	14-24	3	Regular	V
Zinc, extended (Ultralente)	4-8	10-30	>36	Regular, semilente	V
Premixed Insulins					
NPH/regular					
70/30	0.5	2-12	18-24		V, PF, DISP
50/50	0.5	2-12	16-24		V
NPH/Lispro					
75/25	0.25	0.5-1.5	3.4-4.5		V, PF
NPH/Aspart					
70/30	0.25 (attenuated)	1-3	3.5		PF

V, Vials; *PF,* prefilled syringes; *PEN,* pen cartridges; *DISP,* disposable pen device.

Lipid Lowering Agents

Drug	Brand Name	Usual Adult Dose	Lipid-Lowering Effect	Cost($) per Dose
Bile Acid Binding Resins				
Cholestyramine	LoCholest, Preva Lite, Questran	8-16 mg/day; max 24 g/day divided bid-tid	LDL ↓ 15%-25% HDL ↑ 3%-5% TG no change or ↑	$0.81-2.80/4 g powder
Colestipol	Colestid	5-30 g qday or divided		$1.12/5 g powder
Colesevelam	Welchol	625 mg tablets; 3-6 tablets bid or 3 tablets bid		$0.89/625 mg tablet
Niacin	Immediate-release: various, generic Extended-release: Niaspan, Niacor, Slo-Niacin	1.5-6 g/day divided bid-tid (following gradual titration)	LDL ↓ 15%-25% HDL ↑ 15%-25% TG ↓ 20%-50%	IR: $0.02-0.71/500 mg tablet ER: $0.04-1.10/500 mg tablet
Fibric Acid Derivatives			LDL ↓ 0-20% HDL ↑ 10%-20% TG ↓ 20%-50%	
Clofibrate	Atromid-S	1-2 g daily in divided doses		$0.20-0.27/500 mg capsule
Fenofibrate	Tricor	54-160 mg qday		$1.57/134 mg capsule
Gemfibrozil	Lopid	600 mg bid		$0.90-1.39/600 mg tablet

HMG CoA Reductase Inhibitors			LDL ↓ 18%-55% HDL ↑ 5%-15% TG ↓ 7%-30%	
Atorvastatin	Lipitor	10-80 mg qday		$3.64/20 mg tablet
Fluvastatin, Fluvastatin XL	Lescol	20-80 mg qpm		$1.85/40 mg tablet; $2.38/80 mg XL tablet
Lovastatin, Lovastatin ER	Mevacor, Altocor, Advicor (with niacin), generic	10-80 mg qpm		$4.27/40 mg tablet; $1.97/40 mg ER tablet
Pravastatin	Pravachol	10-80 qpm		$4.52/40 mg tablet
Rosuvastatin	Crestor	5-40 qday		
Simvastatin	Zocor Vytorin (with ezetimibe)	5-80 qpm		$4.13/20 mg tablet
Cholesterol Absorption Inhibitor				
Ezetimibe	Zetia	10 qday	LDL ↓ 19% HDL ↓ 4% TG ↓ 7%-9%	$2.55/10 mg tablet

Topical Steroids

Potency Category	Drug Name	Trade Name	Type of Preparation
I (very high)	Augmented betamethasone dipropionate (0.05%)	Diprolene	Ointment, gel, lotion
	Clobetasol propionate (0.05%)	Temovate	Cream, ointment, scalp application, gel
		Embeline	Lotion, foam
	Diflorasone diacetate (0.05%)	Psorcon	Ointment
	Halobetasol propionate (0.05%)	Ultravate	Cream, ointment
II (high)	Amcinonide (0.1%)	Cyclocort	Cream, ointment, lotion
	Augmented betamethasone dipropionate (0.05%)	Diprolene AF	Cream
	Betamethasone dipropionate (0.05%)	Diprosone, Maxivate	Cream, ointment
		Teladar	Cream
	Betamethasone valerate (0.1%)		Ointment
	Desoximetasone (0.25%)	Topicort	Cream, ointment
	Diflorasone diacetate (0.05%)	Florone, Psorcon E, Maxiflor	Cream, ointment
	Fluocinolone acetonide (0.2%)	Synalar-HP, Flurosyn	Cream, ointment
	Fluocinonide (0.05%)	Lidex, Lidex E, Fluonex	Cream, ointment, solution, gel
	Halcinonide (0.1%)	Halog, Halog-E	Cream, ointment, solution
	Triamcinolone acetonide (0.5%)	Aristocort, Flutex, Kenalog	Cream, ointment
		Aristocort A	Cream, ointment
III (intermediate)	Betamethasone benzoate (0.025%)		Lotion
	Betamethasone dipropionate (0.05%)	Diprosone, Maxivate	Cream, lotion, foam (1.2 mg/g)
	Betamethasone valerate (0.1%)	Luxiq, Beta-Val, Psorion	Cream
	Clocortolone pivalate (0.1%)	Cloderm	Cream, gel
	Desoximetasone (0.05%)	Topicort	Cream, ointment
	Fluocinolone acetonide (0.025%)	Flurosyn, Synalar	Cream, ointment, lotion (0.05%)
	Flurandrenolide (0.025%, 0.05%)	Cordran, Cordran SP	Tape (4 mcg/cm²)
	Fluticasone propionate (0.005%, 0.05%)	Cutivate	Cream (0.05%), ointment (0.005%)
	Hydrocortisone butyrate (0.1%)	Locoid	Cream, ointment, solution
	Hydrocortisone valerate (0.2%)	Westcort	Cream, ointment
	Mometasone furoate (0.1%)	Elocon	Cream, ointment, lotion

	Triamcinolone acetonide (0.025%, 0.1%)	Aristocort, Aristocort A, Delta-Tritex, Flutex, Kenalog	Cream, ointment (0.1%)
		Kenalog, Kenonel,	Cream (0.1%)
			Cream, ointment (0.025%)
		Flutex	Cream (0.025%)
		Kenalog	Lotion (0.025%, 0.1%)
IV (low)	Alclometasone dipropionate (0.05%)	Aclovate	Cream, ointment
	Desonide (0.05%)	DesOwen, Tridesilon, LoKara	Cream, ointment, lotion
	Dexamethasone (0.01%, 0.04%)	Aeroseb-Dex	Aerosol (0.01%)
		Decaspray	Aerosol (0.04%)
	Dexamethasone sodium phosphate (0.1%)	Decadron Phosphate	Cream
	Fluocinolone acetonide (0.01%)	Flurosyn, Synalar	Cream
		Synalar	Solution
		Capex	Shampoo
		Derma-Smoothe/FS	Oil
	Hydrocortisone (0.25%, 0.5%, 1%, 2.5%)	Cetacort	Lotion (0.25%)
		Cortizone-5, and others	Cream, ointment (0.5%)
		Cetacort	Lotion (0.5%)
		Hycort, Hytone, and others	Cream, ointment (1%)
		Acticort, Ala-Cort, and others	Lotion (1%)
		Scalpicin, T/Scalp	Liquid (1%)
		Extra Strength CortaGel	Gel (1%)
		Penecort, Texacort	Solution (1%)
		Maximum Strength Cortaid, Procort	Spray (1%)
		Maximum Strength Cortaid Faststick	Stick, roll-on (1%)
		Ala-Scalp	Lotion (2%)
		Hytone and others	Cream, ointment (2.5%)
		Hytone, LactiCare-HC	Lotion (2.5%)
	Hydrocortisone acetate (0.5%, 1%)	Cortaid with Aloe, Lanacort-5, and others	Cream, ointment (0.5%)
		Maximum Strength Cortaid and others	Cream, ointment (1%)

Topical Antifungal Agents

Drug Name	Trade Name	Usual Adult Dose	Spectrum/Comment
Vaginal Preparations for Candidiasis			
Butoconazole	Femstat	2% vaginal cream, 5 g qhs × 3d (6d if pregnant)	Pregnancy category C
Clotrimazole	FemCare, Gyne-Lotrimin, Mycelex	1% vaginal cream, 1 applicatorful qhs × 7d; 100 mg vaginal tablet qhs × 7d; 500 mg vaginal tablet × 1	Pregnancy category B
Miconazole	Monistat	1% vaginal cream, 1 applicatorful qhs × 7d; 100 mg vaginal tablet qhs × 7d; 200 mg vaginal tablet × 3	Pregnancy category C
Nystatin	Mycostatin	100,000 units vaginal tablet qday × 14d	Pregnancy category A
Terconazole	Terazol	0.8% vaginal cream 1 applicatorful (5g) or 80 mg vaginal suppositories qhs × 3d	Pregnancy category C
Tioconazole	Vagistat	6.5% vaginal ointment, 1 applicatorful qhs × 1	Pregnancy category C
Dermatologic Preparations			
Amphotericin	Fungizone	3% cream, lotion, ointment, suspension	Candida
Butenafine	Mentax	1% cream	Tinea
Ciclopirox	Loprox	1% cream, ointment	Tinea, Candida, Tinea versicolor

Clioquinol	Vioform	3% cream, ointment	Tinea
Clotrimazole	Lotrimin, Mycelex	1% cream, lotion, solution	OTC-Tinea; Rx-Tinea, Candida, Tinea versicolor
Econazole	Spectazole	1% cream	Tinea, Candida, Tinea versicolor
Haloprogin	Halotex	1% cream, solution	Tinea, Tinea versicolor
Iodoquinol	Vytone	1% cream	Tinea, Candida
Ketoconazole	Nizoral	2% cream, shampoo	Tinea, Candida, Tinea versicolor; scalp seborrheic dermatitis
Miconazole	Micatin, Monistat-Derm	2% cream, powder, spray	Tinea, Candida, Tinea versicolor
Naftifine	Naftin	1% cream, gel	Tinea, Candida
Nystatin	Mycostatin, Nilstat, Nystex	100,000 units per gram, cream, ointment, powder	Candida
Oxiconazole	Oxistat	1% cream, lotion	Tinea, Candida, Tinea versicolor
Selenium sulfide	Selsun Blue, Exsel	1%, 2.5% lotion, shampoo	Tinea versicolor; scalp seborrheic dermatitis
Sertaconazole	Ertaczo	2% cream	Tinea
Sulconazole	Exelderm	1% cream, solution	Tinea, Candida, Tinea versicolor
Terbinafine	Lamisil	1% cream	Tinea, Candida, Tinea versicolor
Tolnaftate	Aftate, Tinactin, Desenex	1% cream, gel, powder, solution, spray liquid, spray powder	Tinea, Tinea versicolor
Undecylenic acid	Cruex, Desenex, Pedi-Pro, Caldesene, Protectol	8-20% cream, foam, ointment, powder, soap	Tinea

Nucleoside Reverse Transcriptase Inhibitors*

Drug Name	Trade Name	Usual Adult Dose (mg)	Dose Change in Renal Insufficiency	Drug Interactions	Comment
Abacavir	Ziagen, Trizivir, Epzicom	300 q12h	No	Amprenavir	Hypersensitivity in 2-5% of recipients; rechallenge may be fatal; available as oral solution
Didanosine (ddI)	Videx, Videx EC	125-200 q12h on empty stomach (pills) or 250-400 q24h	Reduce dose if CrCl < 60 ml/min	Dapsone, ganciclovir, itraconazole, methadone, quinolones	Enteric coated form preferred; available as a powder (not bioequivalent to pills)
Entricitabine	Emtriva, Truvada	200 mg q24h	Yes	None	No advantage over lamivudine
Lamivudine (3TC)	Epivir, Combivir, Trizivir	150 q12h, 300 q24h	Reduce dose if CrCl < 50 ml/min	None	Available as oral solution; available in combination with zidovudine
Stavudine (D4T)	Zerit, Zerit XR	30-40 q12h, 75-100 q24h	Reduce dose if CrCl < 50 ml/min	Additive neuropathic effect with dapsone, isoniazid, metronidazole, phenytoin, vincristine	Antagonism with zidovudine; available as oral solution
Tenofovir	Viread, Truvada	300 q24h	Do not use if CrCl < 60 ml/min	Cidofovir, ganciclovir	Take with food; associated with renal tubular injury
Zalcitabine (ddC)	Hivid	0.75 q8h	Reduce dose if CrCl < 60 ml/min	Antacids, amphotericin, foscarnet, aminoglycosides, probenecid, cimetidine, pentamidine	
Zidovudine (AZT)	Retrovir, Combivir, Trizivir	100-200 q8h or 300 q12h	Reduce dose if CrCl < 10 ml/min	Ganciclovir, interferon, probenecid, rifampin, valproic acid	Available as syrup, injection; available in combination with lamivudine; avoid with ribavirin

*See *www.aidsinfo.nih.gov* for most current information.

Non-Nucleoside Reverse Transcriptase Inhibitors*

Drug Name	Trade Name	Usual Adult Dose (mg)	Dose Change in Renal Insufficiency	Drug Interactions	Comment
Delavirdine	Rescriptor	400 tid	No	Antacids, astemizole, barbiturates, carbamazepine, cisapride, clarithromycin, dapsone, didanosine, ergotamines, H2 blockers, indinavir, midazolam, nelfinavir, nifedipine, phenytoin, proton pump inhibitors, quinidine, rifabutin, rifampin, saquinavir, terfenadine, triazolam, warfarin, zidovudine	Do not use as monotherapy due to resistance induction; separate dosing with didanosine or antacids by 1 hour; cytochrome P-4503A4 inhibitor; coadministration with astemizole, cisapride, ergotamines, H2 blockers, lovastatin, midazolam, proton pump inhibitors, rifabutin, rifampin, simvastatin, terfenadine, triazolam not recommended
Efavirenz	Sustiva	600 qday	No	Amprenavir, astemizole, barbiturates, carbamazepine, cisapride, clarithromycin, ergotamines, ethinyl estradiol, indinavir, lopinavir, lovastatin, midazolam, nelfinavir, nifedipine, phenytoin, rifabutin, rifampin, ritonavir, saquinavir, simvastatin, terfenadine, triazolam, warfarin	Do not use as monotherapy due to resistance induction; CNS side effects very frequent; cytochrome P-450 mixed inducer and inhibitor; coadministration with astemizole, cisapride, clarithromycin, ergotamines, midazolam, saquinavir, terfenadine, triazolam not recommended
Nevirapine	Viramune	200 qday for 14d, then 200 bid	No	Clarithromycin, erythromycin, ethinyl estradiol, indinavir, ketoconazole, lopinavir, methadone, nelfinavir, rifabutin, rifampin, ritonavir, saquinavir	Do not use as monotherapy due to resistance induction; cytochrome P-4503A4 inducer; coadministration with ketoconazole, rifampin not recommended; may affect methadone dose needed; available as elixir

*See www.aidsinfo.nih.gov for most current information.

Protease Inhibitors*

Drug Name	Trade Name	Usual Adult Dose (mg)	Dose Change in Renal Insufficiency	Selected Drug Interactions (see individual monographs for complete list)	Comment
Amprenavir	Agenerase	1200 q12h	No	Astemizole, cisapride, ergot alkaloids, lovastatin, midazolam, rifampin, simvastatin, terfenadine, triazolam	Capsules of amprenavir contain 109 IU of vitamin E; liquid contains 46 IU per mL
Atazanavir	Reyataz	400 q24h	No	Astemizole, cisapride, ergot alkaloids, lovastatin, midazolam, rifampin, simvastatin, terfenadine, triazolam	First once daily protease inhibitor
Indinavir	Crixivan	800 q8h	No	Astemizole, cisapride, ergot alkaloids, lovastatin, midazolam, rifampin, saquinavir, simvastatin, terfenadine, triazolam	Do not take with large meal; associated with nephrolithiasis
Lopinavir	Kaletra	400 q12h with ritonavir 100 q12h	No	Astemizole, cisapride, ergot alkaloids, flecainide, lovastatin, midazolam, pimozide, propafenone, rifampin, simvastatin, terfenadine, triazolam	Only available in combination with ritonavir; capsules contain 133.3 mg lopinavir plus 33.3 mg ritonavir
Nelfinavir	Viracept	750 tid	No	Astemizole, cisapride, ergot alkaloids, lovastatin, midazolam, rifampin, simvastatin, terfenadine, triazolam	Diarrhea most common side effect
Ritonavir	Norvir	600 q12h	No	Amiodarone, astemizole, bepredil, bupropion, cisapride, clorazepate, clozapine, diazepam, encainide, ergot alkaloids, estazolam, flecainide, flurazepam, lovastatin, meperidine, midazolam, pimozide, piroxicam, propafenone, propoxyphene, simvastatin, terfenadine, triazolam, zolpidem	Take with food; start with 300 mg q12h, increase over 14 days in 100 mg increments to 600 mg q12h; used in low dose to boost effect of other protease inhibitors
Saquinavir	Invirase (hard capsule), Fortovase (soft capsule)	Hard capsule: 400 q12h with ritonavir; soft capsule: 1200 q8h	No	Astemizole, cisapride, efavirenz, ergot alkaloids, indinavir, lovastatin, midazolam, rifabutin, rifampin, simvastatin, terfenadine, triazolam	Take with high fat meal to enhance bioavailability; available in more bioavailable gel capsule form (Fortovase)

*See www.aidsinfo.nih.gov for most current information.

Ophthalmic Agents: Glaucoma

Drug	Brand Name	Strength	Indications	Dose	Duration of Effect (hr)	Comments
Sympathomimetics*						
Apraclonidine	Iopidine	0.5%-1%	Ocular hypertension, postoperative (1%); glaucoma, open angle (0.5%)	1 hr before laser surgery and on completion (1%); bid/tid (0.5%)	7-12	Relatively selective α_2-adrenergic agonist
Brimonidine	Alphagan Alphagen P	0.2% 0.15%	↑ IOP	tid	12	α_2-Adrenergic receptor agonist
Dipivefrin	Propine, AKPro	0.1%	Glaucoma, open angle; ↑ IOP	q12h	12	Prodrug metabolized to epinephrine in vivo
Epinepherine	Epifrin, Glaucon	0.5%-2%	Glaucoma, open angle	qday-bid	12	α- and β-adrenergic agonist
Beta Blockers*						
Betaxolol	Betoptic Betoptic S	0.5% 0.25%	↑ IOP; glaucoma, open angle	bid	12	β_1 selective; onset <30 min; max effect 2 hr
Carteolol	Ocupress	1%	↑ IOP; glaucoma, open angle	bid	12	β_1 and β_2; max effect 2 hr
Levobetaxolol	Betaxon	0.5%	↑IOP; glaucoma, open angle	bid	12	β_1 selective; onset < 30 min; max effect 2 hr
Levobunolol	AK-beta, Betagan	0.25%-0.5%	↑ IOP; glaucoma, open angle	qday (0.5%); bid (0.25%)	12-24	β_1 and β_2; onset < 60 min; max effect 2-6 hr
Metipranolol	Optipranolol	0.3%	↑ IOP; glaucoma, open angle	bid	12-24	β_1 and β_2; onset ≤ 30 min; max effect approx 2 hr

***Sympathomimetics**—mechanism of action: ↓ IOP via aqueous suppression (↓ production, ↑ outflow). These are additive effects when used with miotics.

Beta blockers—mechanism of action: ↓ IOP via aqueous suppression (↓ production). Standard drug packaging colors: blue, yellow, or both. Use alone or in combination with other agents. Beta blockers are more effective than pilocarpine or epinephrine. There is no effect on pupil size or accommodation. *Continued*

Ophthalmic Agents: Glaucoma—cont'd

Drug	Brand Name	Strength	Indications	Dose	Duration of Effect (hr)	Comments
Beta Blockers*— cont'd						
Timolol	Timoptic, Betimol, Timoptic-XE	0.25%-0.5%	↑ IOP; open angle glaucoma	bid; XE qday	12-24	β_1 and β_2; onset < 30 min; max effect 2 hr; XE preparation is "gel forming"
Miotics, Direct Acting*						
Acetylcholine	Miochol-E	1%	Miosis during surgery	prn rapid effect (sec)	10-20 min	For use during surgery when rapid miosis is required
Carbachol	Carbostat, Miostat Isopto Carbachol, Carboptic	0.01% 0.75%-3%	Miosis during surgery Glaucoma	prn—single use tid	6-8	Intraocular Topical
Pilocarpine	Akarpine, Adsorbocarpine, Isopto Carpine, Pilocar, Piloptic, Pilostat, Pilopine HS, Pilagen, Ocusert Pilo	0.25%-10%; ocular therapeutic systems	↑ IOP; open angle glaucoma; acute angle closure glaucoma; mydriasis; preoperative and postoperative	Solution: tid-qid Gel: HS Ocusert: weekly	4-8	
Miotics, Cholinester-ase Inhibitors*						
Demecarium	Humorsol	0.038%-0.25%	Open angle glaucoma; accommodative esotropia	bid-biw	Miosis: 3-10 days; ↓ IOP: 7-28 days	Reversible cholinesterase binding, long acting
Echothiophate	Phospholine Iodide	0.06%-0.25%	↑ IOP; open angle glaucoma; accommodative esotropia	bid	Miosis: 1-4 weeks; ↓ IOP: 7-28 days	Irreversible cholinesterase binding; tolerance may develop after prolonged use, rest period restores response to drug

Carbonic Anhydrase Inhibitors*					
Dorzolamide	Trusopt	2%	↑ IOP (ocular hypertension; open angle glaucoma)	tid	8
Brinzolamide	Azopt	1%	↑ IOP (ocular hypertension; open angle glaucoma)	tid	4 weeks
Prostaglandin Analogues*					
Bimatoprost	Lumigan	0.03%	↑ IOP (ocular hypertension; open angle glaucoma)	hs	24	Onset: 4 hr, peak: 8-12 hr; eye pigment changes (increasing brown pigmentation)
Latanoprost	Xalatan	0.005%	↑ IOP (ocular hypertension; open angle glaucoma)	hs	24	Onset: 3-4 hr, peak: 8-12 hr; eye pigment changes (increasing brown pigmentation)
Travoprost	Travatan	0.004%	↑ IOP (ocular hypertension; open angle glaucoma)	hs	24	Onset: 2 hrs; peak: 12 hrs eye pigment; changes (increasing brown pigmentation)
Unoprostone	Rescula	0.15%	↑ IOP (ocular hypertension; open angle glaucoma)	bid	10	Eye pigment changes (increasing brown pigmentation)

Miotics, direct acting—mechanism of action: ↓ IOP via aqueous suppression (↓ outflow). Standard drug packaging color: green. Formerly first step in glaucoma treatment but yielded to beta blockers. Dark pigmented irides may require higher doses. There is an effect on accommodation.

Miotics, cholinesterase inhibitors—mechanism of action: ↓ IOP via (indirectly) ↓ resistance to aqueous outflow. Standard drug package color: green. Contraindications include angle closure glaucoma and demecarium during pregnancy. Side effects and systemic toxicity are more common and of greater significance than those of direct-acting miotics.

Carbonic anhydrase inhibitors—mechanism of action: ↓ IOP via ↓ aqueous humor secretion. May be used concomitantly with other agents.

Prostaglandin analogues—mechanism of action: ↓ IOP via selective prostenoid receptor agonism, enhancing uveoscleral outflow. Concomitant use with other topical agents to ↓ IOP is appropriate. Reserve for patients who do not respond adequately to or are intolerant of other agents.

Ophthalmic Agents: Mydriatics

Drug	Brand Name	Preparations	Dose	Mydriasis		Cycloplegia		
				Peak (min)	Recovery (days)	Peak (min)	Recovery (days)	
Atropine	Isopto atropine, Atropine Care, Atropisol	Ointment 1%, solution 0.5%, 1%, 2%	Uveitis: qid Refraction: 1 hr before exam	30-40	7-10	60-180	6-12	
Cyclopentolate	AK-Pentolate, Cyclogyl, Pentolair	0.5%, 1%, 2%	Refraction: 5-10 min before exam; repeat in 5-10 min pm	30-60	1	25-75	0.25-1	
Homatropine	Isopto Homatropine	2%, 5%	Uveitis: q3-4h Refraction: 1 hr before exam	40-60	1-3	30-60	1-3	
Scopolamine	Isopto Hyoscine	0.25%	Uveitis: qid Refraction: 1 hr before exam	20-30	3-7	30-60	3-7	
Tropicamide	Mydriacyl, Opticyl	0.5%, 1%	Refraction: 5-15 min before exam; may repeat within 20-30 min	0.25	20-35	20-35	<0.25	
Miotic*								
Dapiprazole	Rev-Eyes	0.5%	Post-procedure; repeat 5 min later	Reversal (min): 30-120 (post phenylepherine or tropicamide)				

*Miotic—mechanism of action: α = adrenergic blockade producing miosis, no activity or ciliary muscle contraction or IOP; indications: reversal of iatrogenically induced mydriasis via adrenergic or parasympatholytic agents.

Ophthalmic Agents: Antiinflammatory

Drug	Brand Name	Strength	Indications	Dose	Comments
Nonsteroidal Antiinflammatory Agents*					
Diclofenac	Voltaren	0.1%	Postoperative inflammation—cataract extraction; corneal refractive surgery	qid 24 hr before, 2 weeks after; qid 1 hr before, 15 min after, then × 3 days or less	Standard package color: grey; unlabeled uses: cystoid macular edema, inflammation after cataract, glaucoma laser surgery, and uveitis syndromes
Flurbiprofen	Ocufen	0.03%	Intraoperative miosis	q30min × 4 starting 2 hr preoperative	Contraindications: epithelial herpes, simplex keratitis, soft contact lenses; unlabeled use: cystoid macular edema
Ketorolac	Acular	0.5%	Seasonal allergic conjunctivitis; postoperative inflammation—cataract extraction	qid prn; qid × 2 weeks	
Suprofen	Profenal	1%	Inhibition of intraoperative miosis	q1h × 3 preoperatively	On day before surgery, may instill qid while patient is awake
Corticosteroids†					
Dexamethasone	AK-Dex, Decadron, Maxidex	0.05%–0.1%	Ocular inflammatory conditions	Solution: q1–2h to response, then qid; ointment: qid to response, then bid-qday	Warnings: prolonged use may result in glaucoma, optic nerve damage, defects in visual acuity and fields of vision, posterior subcapsular cataract formation, secondary ocular infections, and delay healing after cataract surgery

Nonsteroidal antiinflammatory agents—mechanism of action: inhibition of cyclooxygenase enzyme essential for biosynthesis of prostaglandins (mediators of intraocular inflammation), no effect on IOP, inhibition of miosis independent of cholinergic mechanisms.

†*Corticosteroids*—mechanism of action: antiinflammatory actions due to potentiation of epinephrine vasoconstriction, stabilization of lysosomal membranes, retardation of macrophage movement, prevention of kinin release, inhibition of lymphocyte and neutrophil function, inhibition of prostaglandin synthesis, and decrease in antibody production regardless of source (mechanical, chemical, or immunological).

Continued

Ophthalmic Agents: Antiinflammatory—cont'd

Drug	Brand Name	Strength	Indications	Dose	Comments
Corticosteroids†—cont'd					
Fluorometholone	Fluor-Op, FML, Flarex	0.1%-0.25%	Ocular inflammatory conditions	bid-qid	Contraindications: acute epithelial herpes simplex keratitis, fungal diseases of eye, vaccinia and varicella and other viral disease of the cornea and conjunctiva, ocular tuberculosis
Loteprednol	Lotemax, Alrex	0.2%-0.5%	Ocular inflammatory conditions; postoperative inflammation	qid	
Medrysone	HMS	1%	Ocular inflammatory conditions	Up to qid	
Prednisolone	Pred Mild, Econopred, PredForte, AK-Pred, Inflamase	0.12%-1%	Ocular inflammatory conditions	q1-2h initially, then qid	
Rimexolone	Vexol	1%	Ocular inflammatory conditions; postoperative inflammation	qid	For anterior uveitis, q1h while patient is awake × 1 week then q2h while patient is awake × 1 week then prn until resolution

†**Corticosteroids**—mechanism of action: antiinflammatory actions due to potentiation of epinephrine vasoconstriction, stabilization of lysosomal membranes, retardation of macrophage movement, prevention of kinin release, inhibition of lymphocyte and neutrophil function, inhibition of prostaglandin synthesis, and decrease in antibody production regardless of source (mechanical, chemical, or immunological).

Ophthalmic Agents: Miscellaneous Indications

Drug	Brand Name	Dose	Comment
Age-Related Macular Degeneration			
Pegaptanib	Macugen	0.25-0.30 mg/eye by injection	Pegylated anti–vascular endothelial growth factor (anti-VEGF) aptamer; antiangiogenic and antipermeability properties; used with or without photodynamic therapy

Ophthalmic Agents: Allergy and Congestion

Drug	Brand Name	Strengths	Indications	Dose	Comments
Mast Cell Stabilizers*					
Cromolyn	Crolom	4%	Conjunctivitis: vernal kerato-conjunctivitis, vernal conjunctivitis, vernal keratitis	4-6 x per day	Symptomatic response evident within a few days but often longer; appropriate use requires regular, non-prn dosing
Lodoxamide	Alomide	0.1%	Conjunctivitis: vernal kerato-conjunctivitis, vernal conjunctivitis, vernal keratitis	qid	
Nedocromil	Alocril	2%	Allergic conjunctivitis	bid	Continue therapy until exposure to allergen terminated even when symptoms absent
Pemirolast	Alamast	0.1%	Allergic conjunctivitis	qid	Complete response may take up to 4 wk
Antihistamines†					
Azelastine	Optivar	0.5 mg/ml	Allergic conjunctivitis	bid	Symptomatic response evident rapidly, without rebound congestion; appropriate use includes both chronic and prm dosing

Continued

Mast cell stabilizers—mechanism of action: inhibition of type I immediate hypersensitivity reaction via mast cell stabilization.
†Antihistamines—mechanism of action: selective histamine (H₁) antagonists.

Ophthalmic Agents: Allergy and Congestion—cont'd

Drug	Brand Name	Strengths	Indications	Dose	Comments
Antihistamines†—cont'd					
Emedastine		0.05%	Allergic conjunctivitis	qid	
Epinastine		0.05%	Allergic conjunctivitis	bid	
Ketotifen		0.025%	Allergic conjunctivitis	q8-12h	Selective, noncompetitive histamine antagonist and mast cell stabilizer
Levocabastine	Livostin	0.05%	Allergic conjunctivitis	qid	
Olopatadine	Pantanol	0.1%	Allergic conjunctivitis	bid (6-8 hr interval)	
Vasoconstrictors‡					
Naphazoline	OTC: 20/20 eye drops, Allerest, Clear Eyes, Degest 2, Naphcon, Allergy Drops, VasoClear, Comfort Rx: AK-Con, Albalon, Nafazair, Naphcon Forte, Vasocon	0.012%, 0.02%, 0.03% 0.1%	Relief of eye redness due to minor irritation	q3-4h prm	Duration of action: 3-4 hr
Oxymetazoline	OTC: OcuClear, Visine LR	0.025%,	Relief of eye redness due to minor irritation	q6h prm	Duration of action: 4-6 hr

Phenylepherine	OTC (0.12%): AK-Nefrin, Prefrin, Relief	0.12%	OTC: Relief of eye redness due to minor irritation	up to qid prn	Duration of action: 0.5-1.5 hr
	Rx: AK-Dilate, Mydfrin, Neo-Synephrine, Phenoptic	2.5%, 10%	Rx: Pupil dilation in uveitis (posterior synechiae), open angle glaucoma, refraction without cycloplegia before surgery, ophthalmoscopic examination, diagnostic procedures (funduscopy)	Mydriasis produced in 15-30 min and lasts 1-3 hr	
Tetrahydrozoline	OTC: Collyrium Fresh, Eye drops, Eyesine, Geneye, Mallazine, Murine, Optigene, Tetrasine, Visine	0.05%	Relief of eye redness due to minor irritation	qid	Duration of action: 1-4 hr

†**Antihistamines**—mechanism of action: selective histamine (H$_1$) antagonists.

‡**Vasoconstrictors**—mechanism of action: sympathomimetic

α: Pupil dilation, increase in outflow of aqueous humor, vasoconstriction.

β: Relaxation of ciliary muscle, decrease in formation of aqueous humor.

Contraindications: Narrow angle or anatomically narrow (occludable) angle and no glaucoma; rebound congestion occurs with frequent or extended use.

Appendix B

Bibliography

1. Mosby's Drug Consult, St. Louis, Mosby, 2005.
2. Briggs GG, Freeman RK, Yaffe SJ. Drugs in pregnancy and lactation, 6th ed. Baltimore, Williams and Wilkins, 2002.
3. Shepard TH, Lemire RJ. Catalog of teratogenic agents, 11th ed. Baltimore, Johns Hopkins University Press, 2004.
4. Young DS. Effects of Drugs on Clinical Lab Tests, 4th ed. Washington D.C., 1995, American Association for Clinical Press. (Available electronically as Young's Effects online.)

Therapeutic Index

The therapeutic index is arranged by condition/disorder. *Italics* indicate category of drug.

Index

Entries can be identified as follows: generic name, Trade Name.

Entries can be identified as follows: generic name, Trade Name.

Entries can be identified as follows: generic name, Trade Name.

Entries can be identified as follows: generic name, Trade Name

---

Entries can be identified as follows: generic name. Trade Name.

Entries can be identified as follows: generic name, Trade Name.

Entries can be identified as follows: generic name, Trade Name.

Entries can be identified as follows: generic name. Trade Name.

Entries can be identified as follows: generic name, Trade Name.

Entries can be identified as follows: generic name, Trade Name.

Entries can be identified as follows: generic name, Trade Name

---

Entries can be identified as follows: generic name, Trade Name.

IDEAL BODY WEIGHT (IBW)

ADULTS (>18 YRS):
Male IBW (kg) = 50 + 2.3 for each inch over 60 inches
Female IBW (kg) = 45.5 + 2.3 for each inch over 60 inches

CHILDREN:
Age 1 to 18 yrs, height <60 inches: IBW (kg) = $[1.65 \times height^2 (cm)]/1000$

BODY MASS INDEX (BMI)

$$BMI = \frac{weight\ (kg)}{height^2\ (m)}$$

Normal range:
   Male: 21.9-22.4
   Female: 21.3-22.1

CREATININE CLEARANCE CALCULATION

ADULTS (AGE >18; SERUM CREAT <5 MG/DL AND NOT CHANGING RAPIDLY):

$$CrCl\ (ml/min) = \frac{(140 - age)\ (weight\ in\ kg)}{(serum\ creat\ [mg/dl])\ (72)}$$

NOTES: 1. Multiply by 0.85 for females
       2. Use the following value for weight:
         a. If actual weight <IBW, use actual weight
         b. If actual weight is 100%-130% of IBW, use IBW
         c. If actual weight >130% of IBW, easiest approximation is by
           using IBW + (actual weight – IBW)/3
       3. Accuracy reduced in muscle wasting diseases (e.g., neuromuscular disease) and amputees

CHILDREN:
CrCl ($ml/min/1.73m^2$) = $[0.48 \times height\ (cm)]/serum\ creat\ (mg/dl)$

Conversion Information

WEIGHTS AND MEASURES

PREFIXES FOR FRACTIONS

deci = 10^{-1} micro = 10^{-6}
centi = 10^{-2} nano = 10^{-9}
milli = 10^{-3} pico = 10^{-12}

TEMPERATURE MEASURES

$°C = 5/9 \times (°F - 32)$
$°F = 9/5 \times (°C) + 32$

PERCENTAGE EQUIVALENTS

0.1% solution contains: 1 mg per ml
1% solution contains: 10 mg per ml
10% solution contains: 100 mg per ml

MILLIEQUIVALENT CONVERSIONS

1 mEq Na = 23 mg Na = 58.5 mg NaCl
1 g Na = 2.54 g NaCl = 43 mEq Na
1 g NaCl = 0.39 g Na = 17 mEq Na

1 mEq K = 39 mg K = 74.5 mg KCl
1 g K = 1.91 g KCl = 26 mEq K
1 g KCl = 0.52 g K = 13 mEq K

1 mEq Ca = 20 mg Ca
1 g Ca = 50 mEq Ca

1 mEq Mg = 0.12 g $MgSO_4 \cdot 7H_2O$
1 g Mg = 10.2 g $MgSO_4 \cdot 7H_2O$ = 82 mEq Mg

10 mmol P_i = 0.31 g P_i = 0.95 g PO_4
1 g P_i = 3.06 g PO_4 = 32 mmol P_i

METRIC CONVERSIONS

VOLUME MEASUREMENTS

Teaspoonful = 5 ml
Tablespoonful = 15 ml
Fluid ounce = 30 ml
Pint = 473 ml
Quart = 946 ml